Targeted Radionuclide Therapy

Targeted Radionuclide Therapy

EDITOR

Tod W. Speer, M.D.

Department of Human Oncology
University of Wisconsin School of Medicine and Public Health
Aspirus Regional Cancer Center
Wausau, Wisconsin

Wolters Kluwer | Lippincott Williams & Wilkins
Health

Philadelphia · Baltimore · New York · London
Buenos Aires · Hong Kong · Sydney · Tokyo

Senior Executive Editor: Jonathan W. Pine, Jr.
Senior Product Manager: Emilie Moyer
Senior Manufacturing Manager: Benjamin Rivera
Senior Marketing Manager: Angela Panetta
Senior Designer: Stephen Druding
Production Service: MPS Limited, a Macmillan Company

© 2011 by LIPPINCOTT WILLIAMS & WILKINS, a WOLTERS KLUWER business
Two Commerce Square
2001 Market Street
Philadelphia, PA 19103 USA
LWW.com

Printed in China

Library of Congress Cataloging-in-Publication Data

Targeted radionuclide therapy / editor, Tod W. Speer.
      p. ; cm.
   Includes bibliographical references.
   Summary: "Radioimmunotherapy, also known as systemic targeted radiation therapy, uses antibodies, antibody fragments, or compounds as carriers to guide radiation to the targets. It is a topic rapidly increasing in importance and success in treatment of cancer patients. This book represents a comprehensive amalgamation of the radiation physics, chemistry, radiobiology, tumor models, and clinical data for targeted radionuclide therapy. It outlines the current challenges and provides a glimpse at future directions. With significant advances in cell biology and molecular engineering, many targeting constructs are now available that will safely deliver these highly cytotoxic radionuclides in a targeted fashion"—Provided by publisher.
   ISBN 978-0-7817-9693-4
   1. Cancer—Radioimmunotherapy. I. Speer, Tod W.
   [DNLM: 1. Neoplasms—radiotherapy. 2. Radioisotopes—therapeutic use. 3. Radiotherapy—methods. QZ 269]
   RC271.R26T37 2011
   616.99'40642—dc22

                                                                2010031113

To purchase additional copies of this book, call our customer service department at (800) 638-3030 or fax orders to (301) 223-2320. International customers should call (301) 223-2300.

Visit Lippincott Williams & Wilkins on the Internet: at LWW.com. Lippincott Williams & Wilkins customer service representatives are available from 8:30 am to 6 pm, EST.

10 9 8 7 6 5 4 3 2 1

RRS1009

To my wife Lori, who is the most wonderful woman in the world and who has always stood by my side.

To my children, Thomas, Alexandria, Carl, and Tod II, who have been my gifts and make this world a better place.

To my Grandfather, Andrew Marshal Beacom Speer, MD, who cared for so many people in rural Pittsburgh as a family practice physician and fought for our freedom in the Pacific during WWII.

To my father, Thomas Andrew Scott Speer, MD, who worked with Jonas E. Salk on the polio vaccine at the University of Pittsburgh Medical School and departed from this world much too soon.

To my mother, Betty Lou Speer, who showed me the beauty and love in the world through her artwork.

To my teachers, who touched my life in countless ways.

To my colleagues, who support and challenge me daily.

To my patients, who have taught me courage, perseverance, and hope.

To our students, who will live, learn, and carry the torch.

To the greatest Healer, our Lord and Savior, Jesus Christ.

—TOD W. SPEER

Hope sees the invisible,
Feels the intangible,
And achieves the impossible.
—Anonymous

CONTENTS

Frits Aarts, MD, PhD
Radboud University Nijmegen
    Medical Centre
Department of Surgery
Nijmegen, The Netherlands

Fares Al-Ejah, PhD
Signal Transduction Lab
Cancer & Cell Biology Division, QIMR
Herston, Australia

Peter Anderson, MD, PhD
Department of Pediatrics
University of Texas MD Anderson
    Cancer Center
Houston, Texas

Frank Atkins, PhD
Division of Nuclear Medicine
Washington Hospital Center
Washington, DC

Bulent Aydogan, PhD
The University of Chicago
Chicago, Illinois

Neil H. Bander, MD
Bernard and Josephine Chaus
    Professor of Urologic Oncology
Department of Urology
Weill Medical College of Cornell
    University and New York
    Presbyterian Hospital
New York, New York

Jacques Barbet, PhD
Cancer Research Center
University of Nantes
INSERM
Nantes, France

Manuel Bardiès, PhD
INSERM
Nantes, France

Darryl Barton, MD
Department of Human Oncology
University of Wisconsin School of
    Medicine and Public Health
Aspirus Regional Cancer Center
Wausau, Wisconsin

Surinder K. Batra, PhD
Department of Biochemistry and
    Molecular Biology
Department of Pathology and
    Microbiology
Eppley Institute for Research in Cancer
    and Allied Diseases
University of Nebraska Medical Center
Omaha, Nebraska

Annette G. Beck-Sickinger, PhD
Institute of Biochemistry Leipzig
    University
Leipzig, Germany

Peter Bernhardt, PhD
Department of Radiation Physics
Institution of Clinical Science
Sahlgrenska Academy
Gothenburg University
Gothenburg, Sweden

Robert P. Bleichrodt, MD, PhD
Radboud University Nijmegen
    Medical Centre
Department of Surgery
Nijmegen, The Netherlands

Otto C. Boerman, PhD
Department of Nuclear Medicine
Radboud University Nijmegen
    Medical Centre
Nijmegen, The Netherlands

Martin W. Brechbiel, PhD
The National Institutes of Health
National Cancer Institute
Canter for Cancer Research
Radioimmune & Inorganic
    Chemistry Section
Cancer Institute, The National
    Institutes of Health
Bethesda, Maryland

Michael P. Brown, MBBS, FRACP, FRCPA
Experimental Therapeutics Laboratory,
    Hanson Institute
Adelaide, South Australia, Australia
Cancer Clinical Trials Unit
Royal Adelaide Hospital Cancer Centre
School of Medicine,
    The University of Adelaide
Adelaide, South Australia

H. Bulstrode
Nuclear Medicine
Royal Free Hospital
London, United Kingdom

Michael Burdick, MD
Department of Radiation Oncology
Cleveland Clinic Taussig Cancer
    Center
Lerner College of Medicine
Cleveland, Ohio

Ingrid J. G. Burvenich, PhD
Tumour Targeting Laboratory
Ludwig Institute for Cancer Research
Austin Hospital
Heidelberg, Australia

John R. Buscombe, MD, FRCP
Nuclear Medicine
Royal Free Hospital
London, United Kingdom

Jennifer Buskerud, BS, RT(R)(T), CMD
Medical Dosimetrist
Aspirus Regional Cancer Center
Wausau, Wisconsin

Michael Campoli, MD
Department of Dermatology
University of Colorado Health Science
    Center
Denver, Colorado

Jörgen Carlsson PhD
Division of Biomedical Radiation
    Sciences
Rudbeck Laboratory
Uppsala University
Uppsala, Sweden

Arturo Casadevall, MD, PhD
Microbiology and Immunology and
    Medicine
Albert Einstein College of Medicine of
    Yeshiva University
Bronx, New York

Jean-François Chatal, MD, PhD
Arronax Cyclotron
University of Nantes
Nantes, France

Ekaterina Dadachova, PhD
Departments of Nuclear Medicine,
    Microbiology and Immunology
Albert Einstein College of Medicine of
    Yeshiva University
Bronx, New York

Daniella DiCara, PhD
Growth Factors Group, Department of
    Oncology
University of Cambridge
Cambridge, United Kingdom

Jörgen Elgqvist, PhD
Department of Oncology
The Sahlgrenska Academy
University of Gothenburg
Gothenburg, Sweden

William Erwin, MS
MD Anderson Cancer Center
Houston, Texas

Soldano Ferrone, MD, PhD
Departments of Surgery of
    Immunology and Pathology
University of Pittsburgh Cancer
    Institute
Pittsburgh, Pennsylvania

Fredrik Frejd, PhD
Division of Biomedical Radiation
    Sciences
Rudbeck Laboratory
Uppsala University, Sweden
Affibody AB
Bromma, Sweden

Mikaela Friedman, PhD
Division of Molecular Biotechnology,
    School of Biotechnology
Royal Institute of Technology (KTH)
Stockholm, Sweden

Michael Garkavij, MD, PhD
Department of Oncology
Lund University
Lund, Sweden

Katarina Sjögreen Gleisner, PhD
Department of Medical Radiation
    Physics
Lund University
Lund, Sweden

David M. Goldenberg, ScD, MD
Garden State Cancer Center
Center for Molecular Medicine and
    Immunology
Belleville, New Jersey

Stanley J. Goldsmith, MD
Department of Radiology
Weill Medical College of Cornell
    University and New York-
    Presbyterian Hospital
New York, New York

Thijs Hendriks, PhD
Radboud University Nijmegen
    Medical Centre
Department of Surgery
Nijmegen, The Netherlands

Dawn Henrich, BS, RT(R)(T), CMD
Medical Dosimetrist
Aspirus Regional Cancer Center
Wausau, Wisconsin

Ragnar Hultborn, MD, PhD
Department of Oncology
The Sahlgrenska Academy
University of Gothenburg
Gothenburg, Sweden

John L. Humm, PhD
Memorial Sloan Kettering Cancer
    Center
New York, New York

Maneesh Jain, PhD
Department of Biochemistry and
    Molecular Biology
College of Medicine
University of Nebraska Medical Center
Omaha, Nebraska

Doo-Il Jeoung, MD
School of Biological Sciences
College of Natural Sciences
Kangwon University
Chunchon, Korea

Amin I. Kassis, PhD
Department of Radiology
Harvard Medical School
Boston, Massachusetts

Sukhwinder Kaur, PhD
Department of Biochemistry and
    Molecular Biology
University of Nebraska Medical Center
Omaha, Nebraska

Andrew Kennedy, MD, FACRO
Wake Radiology Oncology
Cary, North Carolina
Adjuvant Associate Professor
Department of Mechanical and
    Aerospace Engineering; Department
    of Biomedical Engineering
North Carolina State University
Raleigh, North Carolina

Françoise Kraeber-Bodéré, MD, PhD
Nuclear Medicine Department
University Hospital
Nuclear Medicine Department
René Gauducheau Cancer Center
Cancer Research Center
University of Nantes
INSERM
Nantes, France

Laura Kulik, MD
Department of Medicine
Division of Hepatology
Robert H. Lurie Comprehensive
    Cancer Center
Northwestern University
Chicago, Illinois

Kanchan Kulkarni, MBBS
Division of Nuclear Medicine
Washington Hospital Center
Washington, DC

Robert J. Lewandowski, MD
Department of Radiology
Section of Interventional Radiology
Robert H Lurie Comprehensive Cancer
    Center
Northwestern University
Chicago, Illinois

Jeffrey P. Limmer, MS Ed, MSc, DABR
Honorary Associate-UW Madison
    Department of Human Oncology
School of Medicine and Public Health
Chief Medical Physicist
Aspirus Regional Cancer Center
Wausau, Wisconsin

Ola Linden, MD, PhD
Department of Oncology
Lund University
Lund, Sweden

Sture Lindegren, PhD
Department of Radiation Physics
The Sahlgrenska Academy
University of Gothenburg
Gothenburg, Sweden

Michael Ljungberg, PhD
Department of Medical Radiation
    Physics
Lund University
Lund, Sweden

Roger M. Macklis, MD
Department of Radiation Oncology
Cleveland Clinic Taussig Cancer
    Center
Lerner College of Medicine
Cleveland, Ohio

Christopher McNamara, MD
Department of Haematology
Royal Free Hospital
Hampstead, United Kingdom

Sotiris Missailidis, PhD
Department of Chemistry and
    Analytical Sciences
The Open University
Milton Keynes, United Kingdom

Shakeel Modak, MD
Department of Pediatrics
Memorial Sloan-Kettering Cancer
    Center
New York, New York

Giancarlo Morelli, PhD
Institute of Biostructures and
    Biomaging
CNR and Department of Biological
    Sciences
University of Naples
Naples, Italy

Firas Mourtada, MSE, PhD, DABR
MD Anderson Cancer Center
Houston, Texas

David M. Nanus, MD
Department of Urology
Division of Hematology and Medical
    Oncology, Department of Medicine
Weill Medical College of Cornell
    University and New York-
    Presbyterian Hospital
New York, New York

Marika Nestor, PhD
Unit of Otolaryngology and Head & Neck Surgery
Department of Surgical Sciences;
Unit of Biomedical Radiation Science
Department of Oncology, Radiology and Clinical Immunology
Rudbeck Laboratory;
Unit of Biomedical Radiation Sciences
Uppsala University
Uppsala, Sweden

Rune Nilsson, PhD
Department of Oncology
Lund University
Lund, Sweden

Ahuva Nissim, PhD
Bone and Joint Research Unit, William Harvey Research Institute
Barts and The London, Queen Mary's School of Medicine and Dentistry
University of London
London, United Kingdom

Larry Norton, MD
Breast Cancer Medicine Service
Department of Medicine
Memorial Sloan-Kettering Cancer Center
New York, New York

John Okosun, PhD
Department of Haematology
Royal Free Hospital
Hampstead, United Kingdom

Egbert Oosterwijk, PhD
Radboud University Nijmegen Medical Centre
Department of Urology
Experimental Urology
Nijmegen, The Netherlands

Kim Orchard, MB, BS, BSc, PhD, FRCP, FRCPath
Department of Haematology
Cancer Science Division
Southampton University Hospitals
University of Southampton
Southampton, United Kingdom

Stanley Order, MD, FACR
Director, Center for Molecular Medicine
Isotope Solutions, Inc.
Garden City, New York

Aurore Oudoux, MD
Nuclear Medicine Department
University Hospital
Nantes, France

Wim J.G. Oyen, MD, PhD
Department of Nuclear Medicine
Radboud University Nijmegen Medical Centre
Nijmegen, The Netherlands

John M. Pagel, MD, PhD
Clinical Research Division
Fred Hutchinson Cancer Research Center
Department of Medicine, Division of Medical Oncology
University of Washington
Seattle, Washington

Stig Palm, PhD
Dosimetry & Medical Radiation Physics Section
International Atomic Energy Agency
Vienna, Austria

Carlo Pedone, PhD
Institute of Biostructures and Biomaging
CNR and Department of Biological Sciences
University of Naples
Naples, Italy

Alan Perkins, BSc, MSc, PhD, SRCS, FIPEM, ARCP
Academic Medical Physics
School of Clinical Sciences
University of Nottingham
Nottingham, United Kingdom

Ahsun Riaz, MD
Department of Radiology
Section of Interventional Radiology
Robert H. Lurie Comprehensive Cancer Center
Northwestern University
Chicago, Illinois

John C. Roeske, PhD
Department of Radiation Oncology
Loyola University Medical Center
Maywood, Illinois

Pierre-Yves Salaun, MD, PhD
Nuclear Medicine Department
René Gauducheau Cancer Center
Nantes, France

Riad Salem, MD, MBA
Department of Radiology
Section of Interventional Radiology
Robert H. Lurie Comprehensive Cancer Center
Northwestern University
Chicago, Illinois

Michele Saviano, PhD
Institute of Biostructures and Biomaging
CNR and Department of Biological Sciences
University of Naples
Naples, Italy

Andrew M. Scott, MB BS, MD, FRACP, DDU
Tumour Targeting Laboratory
Ludwig Institute for Cancer Research
Austin Hospital
Heidelberg, Australia

Robert M. Sharkey, PhD
Garden State Cancer Center
Center for Molecular Medicine and Immunology
Belleville, New Jersey

Tod W. Speer, MD
Department of Human Oncology
University of Wisconsin School of Medicine and Public Health
Aspirus Regional Cancer Center
Wausau, Wisconsin

Stefan Ståhl, MD, PhD
Division of Molecular Biotechnology, School of Biotechnology
AlbaNova University Center
Royal Institute of Technology (KTH)
Stockholm, Sweden

Sven-Erik Strand, PhD
Department of Medical Radiation Physics
Lund University
Lund, Sweden

Scott T. Tagawa, MD
Division of Hematology and Medical Oncology,
Department of Medicine
Weill Medical College of Cornell University and New York-Presbyterian Hospital
New York, New York

Nidale Tarek, MD
Department of Pediatrics
Memorial Sloan-Kettering Cancer Center
New York, New York

Jan Tennvall, MD, PhD
Department of Oncology
Department of Medical Radiation Physics
Lund University
Lund, Sweden

Diego Tesauro, PhD
Institute of Biostructures and
  Biomaging
CNR and Department of Biological
  Sciences
University of Naples
Naples, Italy

Bruce Thomadsen, PhD
Department of Medical Physics
University of Wisconsin School of
  Medicine and Public Health
Madison, Wisconsin

Greg M. Thurber, PhD
Department Chemical Engineering
Massachusetts Institute of Technology
Cambridge, Massachusetts

Vladimir Tolmachev, PhD
Division of Biomedical Radiation
  Sciences
Department of Medical Sciences,
  Nuclear Medicine
Rudbeck Laboratory
Uppsala University
Uppsala, Sweden

Tiffany A. Traina, MD
Breast Cancer Medicine Service
Department of Medicine
Memorial Sloan-Kettering Cancer
  Center
New York, New York

Shankar Vallabhajosula, PhD
Department of Radiology
Weill Medical College of Cornell
  University and New York-
  Presbyterian Hospital
New York, New York

Denise VanderKooy, RT(R)(T), CMD
Medical Dosimetrist
Aspirus Regional Cancer Center
Wausau, Wisconsin

Douglas Van Nostrand, MD, FACP, FACNP
Professor of Medicine
Georgetown University Medical
  Center
Washington, DC

Betty Vogds, MS
Clinical Medical Physicist
Aspirus Regional Cancer Center
Wausau, Wisconsin

Paul E. Wallner, DO, FACR, FAOCR, FASTRO
Senior Vice President
21st Century Oncology, Inc.
Fort Myers, Florida

Roland B. Walter, MD, PhD
Clinical Research Division
Fred Hutchinson Cancer Research
  Center
Department of Medicine
Division of Hematology
University of Washington
Seattle, Washington

James Welsh, MS, MD, FACRO
Clinical Professor of Human Oncology
  and Medical Physics
University of Wisconsin Dept. of
  Human Oncology
Medical Director/Chief of Oncology
UW Cancer Center-Riverview
Madison, Wisconsin

Lawrence E. Williams, PhD
Research Professor Department of
  Cancer Immunotherapeutics and
  Tumor Immunology Beckman
  Research Institute City of Hope
  National Medical Center
Duarte, California

Aaron D. Wilson, PhD
The National Institutes of Health
National Cancer Institute
Canter for Cancer Research
Radioimmune & Inorganic Chemistry
  Section
Cancer Institute, The National
  Institutes of Health
Bethesda, Maryland

Jeffrey Y.C. Wong
Division of Radiation Oncology and
  Radiation Research
Radioimmunotherapy
Beckman Research Institute
City of Hope National Medical Center
Duarte, California

Paul J. Yazaki
Division of Cancer
Immunotherapeutics and Tumor
  Immunology
Beckman Research Institute
City of Hope National Medical Center
Duarte, California

Pat B. Zanzonico, PhD
Memorial Sloan-Kettering Cancer
  Center
New York, New York

Denise Zwanziger, PhD
Institute of Biochemistry Leipzig
  University
Leipzig, Germany

The Editor of this book is a practicing radiation oncologist expert in targeted radionuclide therapy (TRT) and a personal friend. He has assembled an eminently qualified, international list of contributors from varied disciplines to address the topic. Coverage of the subject is comprehensive. It extends from the underlying sciences, the biology of cancer, and the radiobiology and radiation safety of radionuclides, to the chemistry, development of established and novel drug conjugates and clinical data. This form of systemic radiotherapy may be categorized as "unsealed source" brachytherapy. The material in this book is timely and highly relevant to current drug development. The term "targeted" distinguishes new classes of drugs from the common anticancer chemotherapeutic agents. To increase effectiveness, radionuclides have been conjugated to the targeting vehicle to deliver radiation to the disease site. The radionuclide emissions from these drug conjugates destroy the targeted malignant cells and spare the surrounding normal tissue.

It must be understood that 80% to 90% of patients with locoregional cancer are cured by using combinations of surgery, radiotherapy, and chemotherapy. However, patients with distant metastases or multifocal disease are often not cured. This reality is brought to fruition in spite of state-of-the-art systemic, multiple-drug chemotherapy and aggressive locoregional radiotherapy and surgery. Continued failure of sequential therapies results in a progressively chemoresistant and fragile clinical state. Although chemotherapeutic drugs can be highly cytotoxic, they are typically less cytotoxic than radionuclides, and they are less effective when there is high volume metastatic disease. In this clinical setting, treatment often becomes palliative. These patients, however; often remain responsive to radiotherapy. TRT, targeted against the disease (cancer) by a vehicle, is a useful strategy for the delivery of systemic radiotherapy for the treatment of metastatic and radiosensitive cancers. TRT also appears to be an effective adjuvant therapy or an effective treatment to be used as part of a combined modality regimen.

TRT has favorably influenced outcomes in disease sites, such as colorectal cancer, ovarian cancer, and glioblastoma, when used as an adjuvant. If TRT is to be meaningful beyond radiosensitive cancers or the adjuvant setting, radiation dose-intensification is required. For dose-intensification, advantage may be gained if the dose-limiting tissue (bone marrow) is displaced to a more radioresistant tissue, for example, from the bone marrow to the liver, kidney, or lungs. These tissues are approximately 10 times more radioresistant than bone marrow. Newer strategies (i.e., pretargeted approaches) and novel drugs and radionuclides (i.e., antibody fragments and alpha-emitting radionuclides) are attractive for dose-intensification. However, it should not be forgotten that a single dose of 131I-tositumomab or 90Y-ibritumomab has proven efficacy for treating non-Hodgkin lymphoma when other drugs have failed, thereby reflecting the potency of TRT.

Cancer treatment requires selection of the preferred drug(s) and drug dose(s) for each patient. Designs for dose selection of anticancer drugs differ from designs for other drugs because of the toxicity of many anticancer drugs. These designs have serious problems. Some patients get less effective, and others, less safe drug amounts because of patient population-based designs. There are interpatient differences in drug distribution and pharmacokinetics that are unrelated to patient size. Selection of a safe and effective drug dose can be as important as selection of the right drug for a patient. When using external beam radiotherapy and brachytherapy, radiation oncologists use image guidance to increase radiation dose to the target volume. If a radionuclide is attached to the targeting vehicle for TRT, then the radiation distributions provide information for the prediction of tissue response, because the radiation effect on a tissue reflects both the absorbed radiation dose by the tissue and its innate radiosensitivity. Fixed, population-based or individualized dosing has been historically used to prescribe the administered radionuclide activity. Radiation dosimetry will then be useful to maximize the likelihood for a safe and effective treatment. A goal for TRT is to ensure that each patient receives an administered radionuclide activity sufficient to deliver a radiation dose to the cancer that is effective and without undesired effects to normal tissue. Accordingly, drug-based imaging will have an increasingly important role in TRT. With this technique, an understanding of the radiation dose distributions, radiobiology and dose-limiting toxicities will be available prior to therapy for a patient and provide the basis for selection of the drug and drug dose for that patient. Personalized drug dosing of this magnitude is attractive and most necessary.

TRT is an exciting and continually expanding anticancer therapeutic modality. It has garnered its origins from the convergence of physics, chemistry, biology, and clinical oncology. At the time of this writing, 79 TRT trials are registered with the National Institutes of Health. New technological advances hold promise for the ability of future dose escalation and intensification, as well as normal tissue protection. Concepts such as pretargeting and fractionation are in their infancy for trial development. TRT delivery based on prescribed and patient-specific radiation dose rather than on radionuclide dose or patient size should lead to continued realization of its potential to be effective, safe, and, someday soon, practice changing!

Sally J. DeNardo, MD, Professor Emeritus
Internal Medicine and Radiology
University of California at Davis
Sacramento, California

Gerald L. DeNardo, MD, Professor Emeritus
Internal Medicine, Radiology and Pathology
University of California at Davis
Sacramento, California

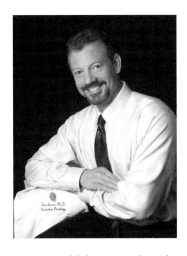

The concept of targeted therapy was first proposed in 1898 by Paul Ehrlich. As testimony to the complexity and challenges of such an endeavor, it was not until a half a century later when Pressman used the first antibody (rabbit) to target and identify a malignancy (Wagner osteogenic sarcoma). In 1952, Nungester was the first to demonstrate that melanoma patients could be treated with an I-131 labeled polyclonal antibody. With this technique, patients experienced a favorable response. Hence, the visions of Dr. Ehrlich and the basic principles of radioimmunotherapy were brought to fruition. However, antibodies were difficult to produce and isolate. As a result, the next several decades bore witness largely to the use of nontargeting radioconjugates consisting of amino acids, cholesterol compounds, and hormones. In 1975, Kohler and Milstein published their now esteemed hybridoma technique for the production of monoclonal antibodies. Physicians and researchers had the long awaited means to consistently produce a carrier molecule, for the selected radionuclide, that could accurately target tumor-associated antigens.

The modern exegesis for targeting agents does not limit the use of carrier molecules to mere antibodies. Successful targeting of tumor cells, with high affinity, can also be accomplished with antibody fragments, peptides, and affinity ligands. As the research and clinical arena ever so modestly disengage from intact antibodies as the carrier molecule for the radionuclide, the impact of the immune system has been somewhat abrogated. Typically, the in vivo antibody–receptor complex would be potentially involved with intracellular signal transduction, compliment-dependent cytotoxicity, or antibody-dependent cellular cytotoxicity. With the aforementioned "new class" delivery agents, this is no longer the case. Hence, the "immunotherapy contribution" of "radioimmunotherapy" is increasingly less effective (the exception being hematologic malignancies). Perhaps a more appropriate term for this technology would simply be "targeted radionuclide therapy." Although the goal is to deliver this form of therapy systemically, it may also be administered via intratumor or a multitude of intracompartmental routes. What has not changed is the availability of some of the most cytotoxic agents known. These are the radionuclides that produce beta, Auger, and alpha radiation. For example, Po-210, largely an alpha particle emitter, can be fatal if inhaled at a dose of 10 ng (48 µCi) or ingested (i.e., Alexander Litvinenko). It has been estimated that 1 g of Po-210 could theoretically cause radiation poisoning in 100 million humans, of which 50 million would die. Alpha particles have a very high linear energy of transfer with a path length measured in only several cell diameters. Only a capricious few alpha particles need to traverse a cancer cell nucleus in order to cause a lethal event. Considering that the basic premise of successful targeted therapy is to bring the most cytotoxic agents in close proximity to the targeted cell and spare normal tissues, it doesn't take a substantial amount of intellectual extrapolation to realize the phenomenal potential of radionuclides as targeted anticancer agents.

To date, reasonable gains have been achieved using targeted radionuclide therapy for hematologic malignancies. Still, their acceptance into the oncology community has been somewhat tenuous. At the time of this writing, there are nine FDA-approved anticancer monoclonal antibodies. Only two of these approved drugs are radioconjugates (Zevalin, Bexxar). These agents were approved in 1992 and 1993, respectively. There have been none since. Progress with solid tumor targeted radionuclide therapy has been even less sanguine. China, however, has approved Licartin for hepatoma and TNT for bronchogenic carcinoma. Still, formidable barriers remain concerning target selection, tumor penetration, dosimetry, type of radionuclide, lack of inherent radiosensitivity of tumor, heterogenic expression of tumor-associated antigens, immunogenicity of targeting vector, aberrant tumor vascularity, elevated interstitial tumor pressure, tumor necrosis, hypoxia, a recusant extracellular matrix, and toxicity of the therapeutic radioconjugate. Regardless, there is a fever pitch burgeoning of biotechnology that will soon erupt into a plethora of exciting advancements that will move targeted radionuclide therapy to the forefront of cancer therapy, not only for metastatic disease, but more importantly into the adjuvant setting (FIT trial; Chapter 33). There is a not too distant horizon when personalized cancer therapy will be standard of care. To this end, targeted radionuclide therapy will be an indispensible weapon in the armament of anticancer therapy.

This book represents a comprehensive amalgamation of the radiation physics, chemistry, radiobiology, tumor models, and clinical data for targeted radionuclide therapy. It outlines the current challenges and provides a glimpse at future directions. It is hoped that these writings will inspire the next generation of radiation oncologist, medical oncologists, radiologists, and scientist to conspire and advance this promising, exciting, and most necessary field; Godspeed to the cause.

—Tod W. Speer, MD

I would like to thank the following individuals who provided opportunity, expertise, encouragement, work ethic "above and beyond the call of duty," and an occasional "gentle prodding"; Jonathan Pine, Senior Executive Editor at Lippincott Williams & Wilkins, a Wolters Kluwer Company; Emilie Moyer, Senior Product Manager, Medical Practice, Wolters Kluwer Health: Lippincott Williams & Wilkins; Susan Rockwell and Eric Johnson of Red Act Group; Arijit Biswas, Project Manager at MPS Limited (New Delhi); and to the many other individuals who worked faithfully to help bring this project to fruition.

—Tod W. Speer

Targeted Radionuclide Therapy

FIGURE 6.5 SPECT/CT image fusion window from MIM v4.1 (MIMvista Co., Cleveland, OH). **Upper panel:** CT; **middle panel:** SPECT; **lower panel:** fused CT and SPECT with the CT as the primary image.

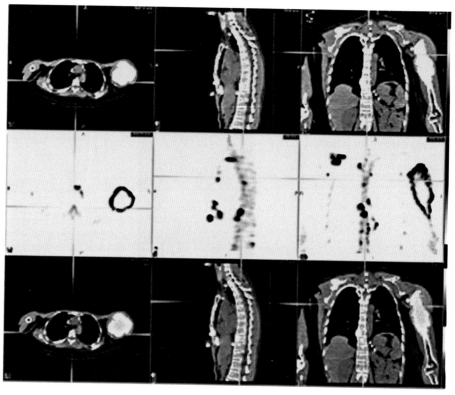

FIGURE 8.4 **(B)** Illustrative conjugate-view gamma camera whole-body scans of a thyroid cancer patient at approximately 2 hours postadministration of a 5-mCi tracer of ^{131}I-iodide. The "Posterior Mirrored" images represent the posterior image reversed about the vertical (longitudinal) axis of the patient to bring it into alignment with the anterior image prior to forming the geometric mean image (Equation 8.10).

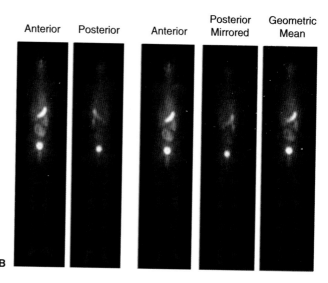

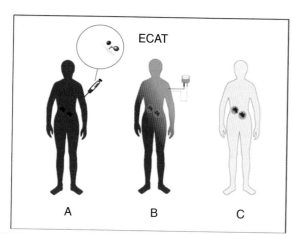

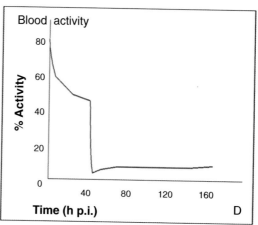

FIGURE 15.1 **The use of extracorporeal depletion in radioimmunotherapy. A:** The biotinylated radioimmunoconjugate is administered to the patient. **B:** After a suitable amount of time to allow uptake of the radioimmunoconjugate in the tumor, the radioimmunoconjugate circulating in the blood is removed by extracorporeal depletion. **C:** After depletion, a higher tumor-to-normal activity ratio is obtained, resulting in reduced side effects. **D:** Level of radioimmunoconjugate in the blood during treatment.

FIGURE 14.5 Imaging of the PC3 human prostate cancer cell line pretargeted with RS7 tri-Fab bsMAb and ^{68}Ga-labeled HP. A nude mouse bearing a subcutaneous PC3 xenograft was injected with the RS7 tri-Fab bsMAb and then 16 hours later, received an intravenous injection of the ^{68}Ga-HP. One hour later, the animal was imaged. This figure shows a posterior coronal slice in the plane of the tumor *(T)* that also captures the activity transiting through in the kidneys *(K)* into the urinary bladder *(UB).*

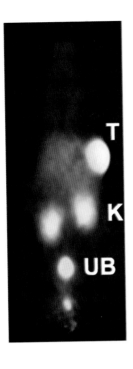

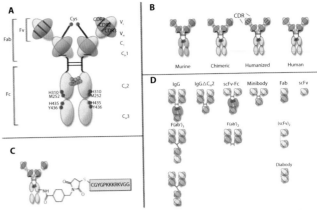

FIGURE 17.1 Antibody engineering: different strategies to improve the therapeutic index in radioimmunotherapy. **A:** Typical structure of a humanized IgG1 antibody. Following engineering strategies are presented: *Red dots,* mutations in amino acids involved in FcRn binding that influence the pharmacokinetics of the IgG; *CDR1–3,* murine CDRs grafted into a human IgG backbone to humanize the antibody; *Cys,* engineered cysteine residues for site-specific conjugation. **B:** Humanization strategies: *purple,* indicating the murine portion of the IgG and *blue,* indicating the human portion of the IgG. **C:** Introducing a nuclear localizing signal. **D:** Monospecific and bispecific fragments used in radioimmunotherapeutic strategies. Abbreviations: CDR, complementarity-determining regions; C_H, constant domain heavy chain; C_L, constant domain light chain; Fc, crystallizable fragment; Fv, variable fragment.

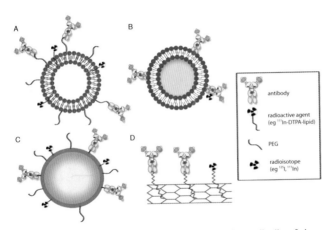

FIGURE 17.2 Targeted delivery of nanostructures using antibodies. **A:** Long-circulating immunoliposomes. **B:** Radioiodinated targeted minicells. **C:** Antibody-coated nanoparticles. **D:** Antibody-functionalized radiolabeled carbon nanotubes.

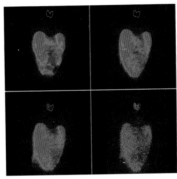

FIGURE 29.1 Consecutive anteroposterior decay-corrected scans (γ-camera) of the abdominal and thoracic area of a patient in the study by Andersson et al. (62). The thyroid uptake, which is indicated by a region of interest in each panel, was not blocked in this patient. Images were acquired at 1.5 (top left), 5 (top right), 11.5 (bottom left), and 19.5 (bottom right) hours after infusion of ^{211}At-MX35 F(ab')$_2$. The figure is reprinted by permission of the Society of Nuclear Medicine.

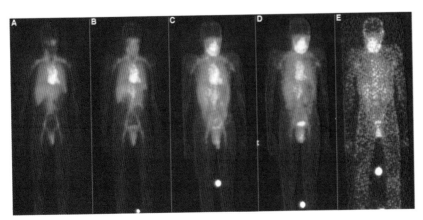

FIGURE 30.3 Whole-body scans of patient 4 acquired within 2 hours after administration of ^{186}Re-cMAb U36 and after 21, 72, and 144 hours and after 2 weeks. Immediately after injection, most prominent activity is in blood pool. This activity remains high up to 72 hours after injection. Relative uptake of radioimmunoconjugate in tumor in right oropharynx increases over time. Tumor becomes better delineated as background activity decreases. (Reprinted from Colnot DR, Quak JJ, Roos JC, et al. Phase I therapy study of ^{186}Re-labeled chimeric monoclonal antibody U36 in patients with squamous cell carcinoma of the head and neck. *J Nucl Med.* 2000;41(12):1999–2010.)

FIGURE 30.5 Frontal (*APPA*) and lateral (left and right) planar image of the head and neck region of patient after administration of ^{186}Re-BIWA-4. Accumulation of radiolabeled hMAb BIWA-4 is visible in tumor recurrence in the right nasal cavity and maxillary sinus (*red arrows*) and in two nodal metastases in the neck (*white arrows*, mid-neck; *green arrows*, low neck). It should be noted that the right neck disease is not identified on the left lateral view due to patient attenuation. (Reprinted and modified from Borjesson PK, Postema EJ, Roos JC, et al. Phase I therapy study with ^{186}Re-labeled humanized monoclonal antibody BIWA-4 (bivatuzumab) in patients with head and neck squamous cell carcinoma. *Clin Cancer Res.* 2003;9(10, pt 2):3961S–3972S.)

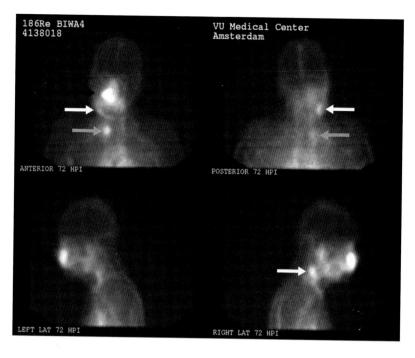

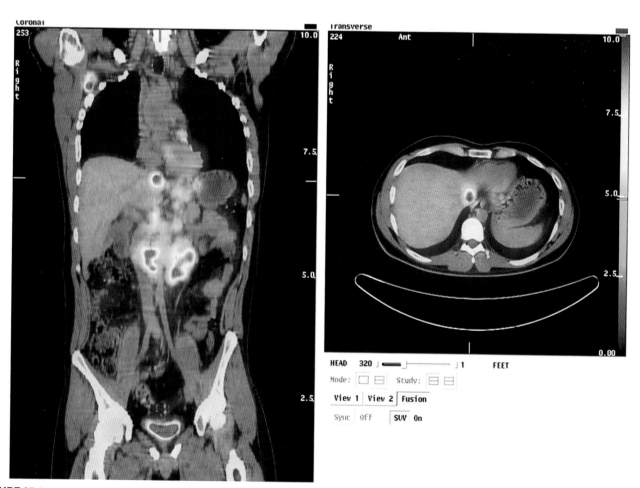

FIGURE 35.1 Fused PET imaging pre-CHT25 treatment in a Hodgkin lymphoma patient showing FDG-avid uptake above and below the diaphragm.

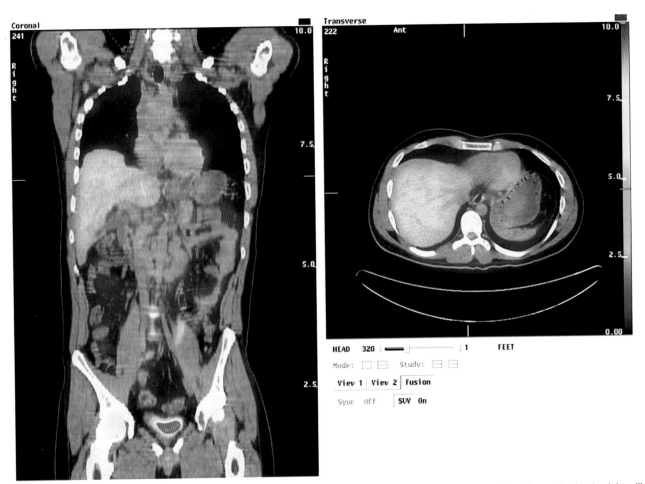

FIGURE 35.2 Same patient post-CHT25 treatment with resolution of FDG uptake in previously diseased areas. Small residual uptake remained in the right axilla.

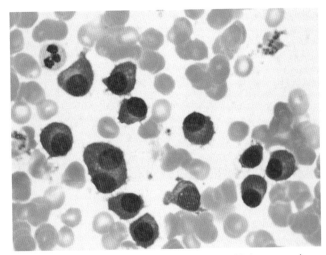

FIGURE 36.1 Malignant plasma cells from a patient with de novo myeloma.

Immunology and Targeting Constructs

Cancer Immune Surveillance and Tumor Escape Mechanisms

Michael Campoli and Soldano Ferrone

■ INTRODUCTION

More than a century ago, Paul Ehrlich proposed the idea that the host's immune system plays a critical role in preventing the growth and development of cancer (1). This concept, now known as cancer immune surveillance (Fig. 1.1), has been one of the most controversial areas in clinical oncology, given the occurrence of cancers despite a functioning immune system, and the notion of immune tolerance to normal self tissue (2). Today, although still controversial, a large body of evidence has accumulated to provide support for the concept that the host immune system interacts with developing tumors and, in some cases, plays a role in regulating tumor growth and progression (2).

Many recent studies both in animal model systems and in clinical settings have provided strong support for the existence of cancer immune surveillance. It is well established that mice lacking essential components of the innate or adaptive immune system are more susceptible to the development of spontaneous or chemically induced tumors (Table 1.1) (3–5). Moreover, polymorphisms leading to functional alterations in molecules that regulate the innate or adaptive immune system can make patients more susceptible to the development of spontaneous or chemically induced tumors (Table 1.2) (3–5). Both in animal model systems and in humans, malignant transformation of cells as a result of the accumulation of somatic mutations and deregulated onco- and/or tumor suppressor gene expression results in the expression of tumor antigens (TA), many of which are recognized by the immune system (3–7). In this regard, it is believed that TA-specific T cells play a significant role regulating tumor growth and progression in a wide range of animal tumor models (2). Similarly, TA-specific CD8(+) and CD4(+) T-cell precursors (3–5) as well as natural killer (NK) cells (8) that are capable of killing tumor cells have been identified in the peripheral blood of patients with malignant disease. In some cases, the presence of certain subsets of lymphocytes within the tumor can be a favorable prognostic sign in patients with several types of malignant disease (3–5,9). Additional evidence supporting the notion of immune surveillance in the control of human cancer is provided by the increased predisposition to the development of cancer in patients with genetically and drug-induced immune deficiencies. For example, immune-suppressed transplant patients have an increased risk of developing certain cancers such as basal cell carcinoma, squamous cell carcinoma, melanoma, lymphoma, and Kaposi sarcoma (10–13). Furthermore, patients with genetic immunodeficiency syndromes such as Wiskott-Aldrich (14) and Chediak–Higashi (15) syndrome demonstrate an increased incidence of lymphoproliferative malignancies. Lastly, the regression of occult malignant melanoma in solid organ allograft recipients after discontinuing immunosuppressive therapy suggests that the administration of immunosuppressive therapy facilitated the growth of the occult cancer through suppression of immune surveillance (16,17).

Taken together the above findings support the notion that immune surveillance plays a critical role in controlling the growth and progression of tumors. In fact it is now thought that the immune system may exert its effects on neoplastic cells through the (a) suppression of viral infection; (b) interference with the establishment of chronic inflammation-induced tumorigenesis; and (c) identification and destruction of premalignant and malignant cells (3–5). These findings, along with (a) the lack of effective treatment for advanced-stage malignancies by conventional therapies (18); (b) the identification and molecular characterization of TA (3–7); (c) the development of highly specific probes, that is, monoclonal antibodies (mAbs) (19) and cytotoxic T lymphocytes (CTLs) (20,21); and (d) the development of effective immunization strategies (20,21) have provided the justification for the development and application of immunotherapy for the treatment of malignant disease.

Despite the significant amount of evidence suggesting a role for the immune system in regulating tumor cell growth, cancer can still develop in immunocompetent hosts. Over the past 10 years, it has become apparent that, in vivo, tumor cells have evolved multiple means to escape immune surveillance either through active suppression of the immune response and/or the selection of nonimmunogenic tumor cells (immune selection) (22). Therefore, it has been suggested that tumor immune escape be added to Hanahan and Weinberg's six hallmarks of cancer, as a seventh hallmark critical to tumorigenesis (23) (Table 1.3). As a result, one of the major challenges facing tumor immunologists is the characterization of the molecular mechanisms by which

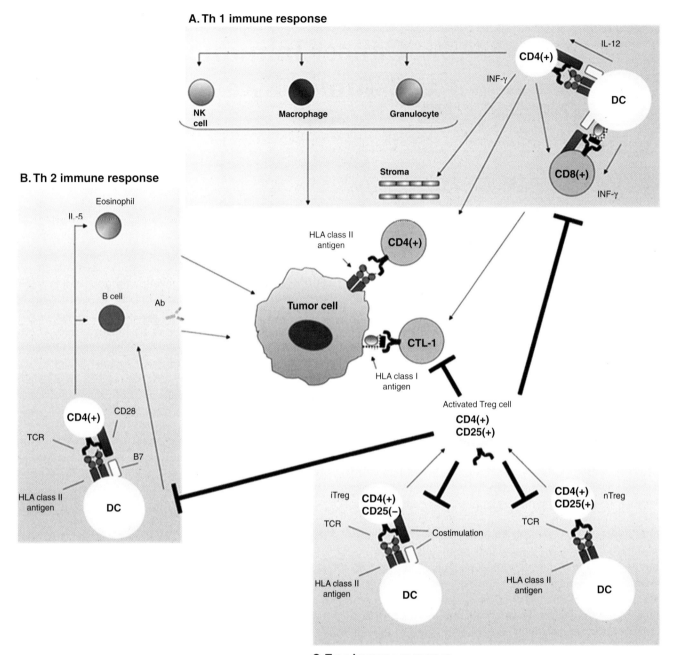

FIGURE 1.1 **Schematic representation of the generation of TA-specific T cell–based immune responses.** The immune system is believed to control tumor growth through several mechanisms. **A:** It is thought that the most effective way of mounting a TA-specific immune response is through the combined action of CD8(+) and IFN-γ–secreting CD4(+) T-helper cells (Th1). TA-specific CD8(+) T cells can be activated by antigen-presenting cells (APCs) and target tumor cells directly. The survival and persistence of CD8(+) T cells are dependent upon CD4(+) T-helper cells. Naïve CD4(+) Th1 cells recognize HLA class II antigen–peptide complexes, through their T-cell receptor (TCR), on the surface of APCs. This interaction leads to the generation of (a) Th1 cells, which promote survival and proliferation of CD8(+) T cells and (b) cytotoxic CD4(+) T cells, which can directly kill HLA class II antigen–expressing tumor cells. In addition, both CD8(+) and CD4(+) T cells secrete IFN-γ, which can further sensitize tumor cells to CD8(+) T cell–mediated killing by upregulating HLA class I antigens and APM components, promoting the recruitment of NK cells, granulocytes, and macrophages, as well as inhibiting angiogenesis within tumor stroma. **B:** Tumor cells can also be targeted by IL-5–secreting CD4(+) T-helper cells (Th2). APCs activate IL-5 Th2 cells, which induce the accumulation of eosinophils and/or provide help for the generation of a TA-specific B-cell immune response. **C:** Treg cell–mediated suppression of TA-specific CTL responses can be accomplished through the two major types of Treg cells. nTregs do not require simultaneous TCR and costimulatory signals to undergo activation and clonal expansion, while iTregs require simultaneous TCR and costimulatory signals to be activated and expanded. iTregs primarily suppress by synthesizing suppressive cytokines, while nTregs also elaborate immunosuppressive cytokines as well as through a yet undefined contact-independent mechanism.

Table **1.1**	Immunodeficient mouse strains with increased susceptibility to spontaneous and chemically induced tumors[a]
Strain	**Tumors**
SCID	T-cell lymphoma, MCA-induced sarcomas
Rag2 deficient	Adenomas, adenocarcinoma, MCA-induced sarcomas
Perforin deficient	B-cell lymphoma, MCA-induced sarcomas
IFN-γ deficient	Lymphomas, MCA-induced sarcomas
Lmp2 deficient	Uterine neoplasms, MCA-induced sarcomas
Trail deficient	Lymphomas, MCA-induced sarcomas
IL-12 deficient	Plasmocytoma and lung carcinoma, MCA-induced sarcomas

[a]A partial list of mouse strains. Adapted from Refs. 3 to 5.

Table **1.2**	Immunodeficiencies that predispose patients to the development of cancer
Gene	**Tumors**
LYST defects	Lymphomas
Perforin defects	Hodgkin and Non-Hodgkin Lyphoma
CD95 polymorphisms	Cervical cancer
HLA[a] and KIR[a] polymorphisms	Cervical cancer
NKG2D[b] polymorphisms	Increased risk of cancer at any site

[a]Human leukocyte antigen; killer-cell immunoglobulin–like receptors.
[b]Activating natural killer-cell receptor.

tumor cells evade immune recognition and destruction and the development of strategies to counteract these escape mechanisms. In this chapter, first we will review the components believed to be required for the generation and maintenance of an effective TA-specific immune response. Second, we will describe the immune escape mechanisms utilized by tumor cells to avoid a TA-specific immune response. Lastly, we will discuss potential strategies to counteract tumor immune suppression and immune escape mechanisms, since these approaches are required to improve the outcome of immunotherapy in patients with malignant disease.

Table **1.3**	Hanahan and Weinberg's six hallmarks of cancer
Self-sufficiency in growth signals	
Insensitivity to antigrowth signals	
Tissue invasion and metastasis	
Limitless replicative potential	
Sustained angiogenesis	
Evading apoptosis	

■ ESSENTIAL COMPONENTS OF AN EFFECTIVE TA-SPECIFIC IMMUNE RESPONSE

Several theories have been proposed to explain the ability of the adaptive immune system to differentiate between different stimuli, leading to immune activation or suppression. Sir F. Macfarlane Burnet (24) proposed the initial paradigm of discrimination between self and nonself. The need for a second signal or "co-stimulation" for both B- and T-cell activation was later proposed (25,26). In recent years, this paradigm was modified to incorporate phenomena found in autoimmune diseases and fetal tolerance. Specifically, Matzinger (27) formulated the "danger" model of immune activation. This model suggests that the primary role of the host's immune system is to react to cellular distress, as opposed simply to nonself (27). In this regard, "danger" signals from stressed or dying cells activate antigen-presenting cells (APCs) and provide the required costimulation or second signal to activate the adaptive immune system. The subsequent discovery of a host of endogenous "danger" signals, including but not limited to DNA, RNA, and heat shock proteins (HSPs), has provided possible molecular mechanisms underlying this hypothesis (28). Therefore, TA-specific immunity will only develop if tumors elicit "danger" signals that allow for optimal activation of APCs. It is the balance of positive and negative signals received by

APCs within the tumor microenvironment that greatly influences the activity of TA-specific immune response. To date, although the exact molecular mechanisms underlying TA-specific immunity and its role in the development and progression of malignant disease in patients have been much debated, there is ample evidence indicating that the components necessary for initiating TA-specific immune responses are present in patients with malignant disease. The role each of the components plays in the development of TA-specific T cell–based immune responses as well as the cellular interactions envisioned to take place within the tumor microenvironment are summarized in Figure 1.1. TA-specific CD8(+) CTLs and helper CD4(+) T cells and in some cases antibody-secreting B cells are essential for antitumor effector functions (3–5,20). Moreover, as in most chronic diseases, both nonspecific and specific components of the host immune response play a role in the control of tumor growth and metastasis, with some components, for example, NK cells, polymorphonuclear cells, and macrophages, thought to participate in the early phase of the response, prior to the appearance of T or B cells. As will be discussed, NK cells are likely to play a role in the elimination of tumor cells that do not express or express low levels of class I human leukocyte antigens (HLAs) (8).

Tumor antigens

Serological analysis of recombinant cDNA expression librar (SEREX) (also discussed in Part III), T cell–based, antibody-based, and reverse immunology approaches have been utilized to identify a variety of TA that are recognized by the immunocompetent host (Fig. 1.2). These TA can be broadly classified as (a) cancer–germ line antigens such as BAGE, GAGE, MAGE 1 or 3, and many others that are silent in normal tissues, with the exception of germ cells in the testes and ovaries, but are expressed in a variety of histologically distinct tumors (6,7,9); (b) differentiation-specific antigens exemplified by melanoma- and melanocyte-associated gp100, MART-1/Melan-A, and tyrosinase (6,7,9); (c) unique antigens generated by point mutations in ubiquitously expressed genes, which regulate key cellular functions, such as β-catenin, CDK4, FLICE, and MUM-1 (6,7,9); (d) overexpressed antigens, such as CEA, HMW-MAA, MDM2, and p53, which are components of normal cells, but display an increased expression in tumor cells, at least at certain stages of differentiation (6,7,9); and (e) oncogenic viral products, such as Epstein Barr virus and human papilloma virus antigens, found in lymphomas and anogenital cancers, respectively (6,7,9). Although the majority of the known TA, with the exception of mutation products, represent self-epitopes and reactive T cells undergo normal thymus selection, the presence of both TA-specific autoantibodies and T cells has been clearly documented in tumor-bearing animal models and in the circulation of normal donors and patients with cancer (6,7,29–31). In this regard, it should be stressed that changes in the expression of a number of proinflammatory cytokines, such as interleukin (IL)-1, IL-6, and tumor necrosis factor (TNF)-α, as well as proteins associated with cellular distress, such as MICA/B and ULBP, are often detected within the tumor microenvironment (8,32,33). Therefore, it is likely that both phenotypic changes in TA expression as well as cytokine secretion in the tumor microenvironment provide both antigenic abnormalities and

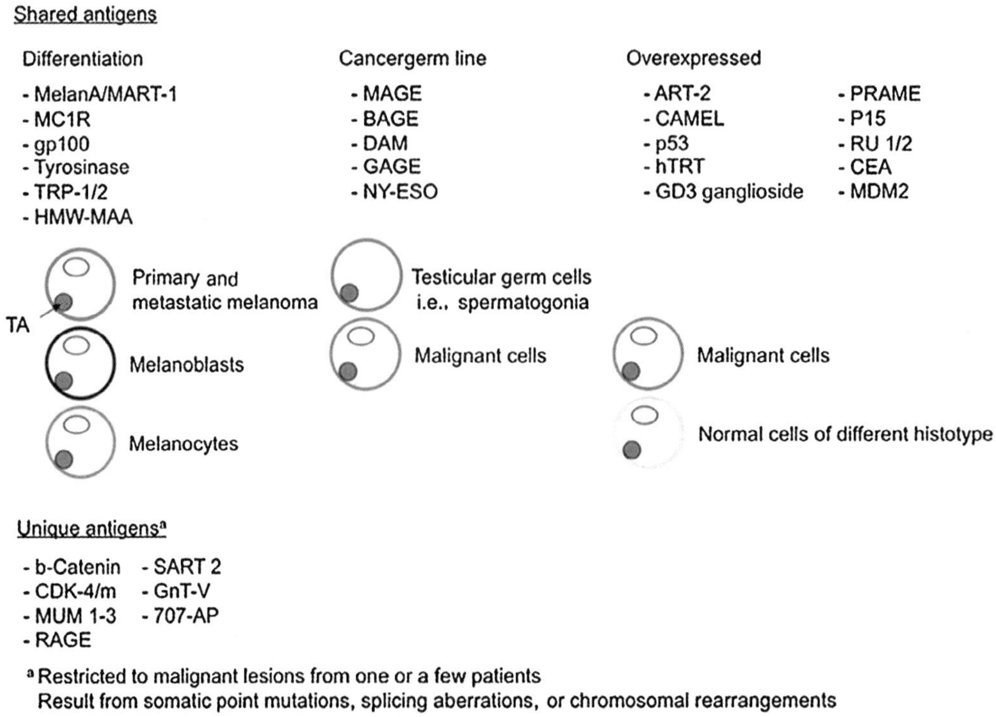

FIGURE 1.2 Classification of tumor antigens (TA). TA can be classified on the basis of their expression pattern. Distinctions can be made between shared, that is, common among different tumors, and unique, that is, expressed by a single tumor lesions. Shared TA can further be classified into three subsets: differentiation antigens, expressed by normal cells of the same histotype such as melanocytes and melanoma cells; cancer–testis antigens, expressed by tumor cells and testicular germ cells; and overexpressed antigens, expressed in normal cells and overexpressed in tumor cells.

Shared antigens

Differentiation	Cancergerm line	Overexpressed	
- MelanA/MART-1	- MAGE	- ART-2	- PRAME
- MC1R	- BAGE	- CAMEL	- P15
- gp100	- DAM	- p53	- RU 1/2
- Tyrosinase	- GAGE	- hTRT	- CEA
- TRP-1/2	- NY-ESO	- GD3 ganglioside	- MDM2
- HMW-MAA			

TA — Primary and metastatic melanoma

Melanoblasts

Melanocytes

Testicular germ cells i.e., spermatogonia

Malignant cells

Malignant cells

Normal cells of different histotype

Unique antigens[a]

- b-Catenin - SART 2
- CDK-4/m - GnT-V
- MUM 1-3 - 707-AP
- RAGE

[a] Restricted to malignant lesions from one or a few patients
Result from somatic point mutations, splicing aberrations, or chromosomal rearrangements

a "danger" signal, respectively, to activate the host's immune system and alleviate self-tolerance.

T, B, and antigen-presenting cells

The structural basis of tumor cell recognition by CTLs occurs through the interaction of T-cell receptor (TCR) with HLA class I antigens complexed to TA-derived peptides (i.e., HLA class I–TA peptide complexes) generated by the antigen-processing machinery (APM) (Fig. 1.3) (34). These complexes can be presented to T cells directly by tumor cells through a process defined as direct priming, although the tumor cell is no longer considered as the central antigen-presenting component of an ongoing TA-specific immune response. Alternatively, TA can be captured by professional APCs and processed for indirect priming of CTLs via T-helper (Th) cells. Tumor cells can also transfer TA to APCs via apoptotic or necrotic tumor cells as well as tumor-derived exosomes. TA-derived peptides are then presented to T cells through a process defined as crosspresentation (35). HSPs can also transfer TA to APCs by chaperoning TA-derived peptides, which are eventually loaded onto HLA class I and presented to naïve or activated CD8(+) T cells (36).

Dendritic cells (DCs) are the most potent APCs that initiate and regulate immune responses. Their central role in regulating immunity and tolerance is emphasized by their high

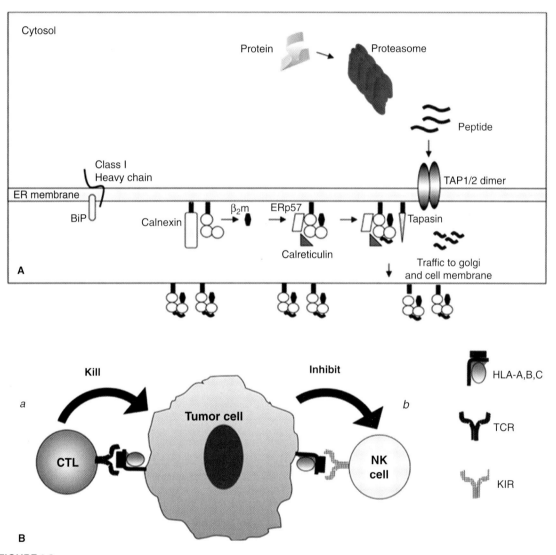

FIGURE 1.3 Generation of HLA class I antigen–TA peptide complexes. **A:** Intracellular protein antigens, which are mostly endogenous, are marked for ubiquitination within the cytosol and subsequently degraded into peptides by proteasomal cleavage. Once generated, peptides are transported into the endoplasmic reticulum (ER) through the dimeric transporter associated with antigen processing, TAP1 and TAP2. Nascent, HLA class I heavy chains are synthesized in the ER and associate with the chaperone immunoglobulin heavy chain binding protein (BiP), a universal ER chaperone involved in the translation and insertion of proteins into the ER. Following insertion into the ER, the HLA class I heavy chain associates with antigen-processing machinery components (APM), that is, calnexin, ERp57, calreticulin, and tapasin. The trimeric HLA class I–β_2m–peptide complex is then transported to the plasma membrane where it plays a major role in the interactions between target cells and T cells. **B:** Once transported to the plasma membrane, the classical HLA class I–β_2m–peptide complex plays a major role in the interactions between target cells and *(a)* activation of peptide-specific CTL through TCR; and *(b)* inhibition of T-cell subpopulations through inhibitory receptors, for example, killer-cell immunoglobulin–like receptor (KIR).

surface density of HLA antigens and costimulatory molecules as well as their ability to produce a wide array of immunostimulatory cytokines and chemokines (37). Furthermore, DCs are efficient in processing exogenous TA via the HLA class II or class I antigen pathway, directly presenting TA to CD4(+) T cells or crosspresenting TA to CD8(+) T cells, and also interact with cells of the innate immune system, that is, NK and NK T cells (38). The ability of DCs to crosspresent TA on HLA class I antigens is thought to be critical for the induction of TA-specific immunity as well as TA- and tissue-specific tolerance under steady state conditions (35).

The interaction of DCs with dying tumor cells is regulated by a balance between positive and negative signals (Fig. 1.4). The underlying premise appears to be that engagement of certain pathways may mediate tolerance or immunity. Several receptors have been shown to be important for

uptake and presentation of antigens derived from dying cells by DCs including complement, Fcγ, lectin, and toll-like receptor pathways (39–41). At least in some instances, such as the uptake of immune complexes or opsonized tumor cells, both activating and inhibitory receptors are triggered. It is noteworthy that the pathways for recognition and uptake of dying cells are not unique to DCs, since they are also utilized by macrophages. However, DCs and macrophages differ substantially in antigen processing and presentation, as well as in their capacity to prime T cells (39–42). Therefore, the immunologic consequences of antigen uptake are expected to be quite distinct for macrophages versus DCs. In particular, macrophages contain high levels of lysosomal proteases and rapidly degrade proteins, while DCs exhibit limited proteolysis, favoring antigen persistence and presentation (39–42). Furthermore, as noted earlier, DCs

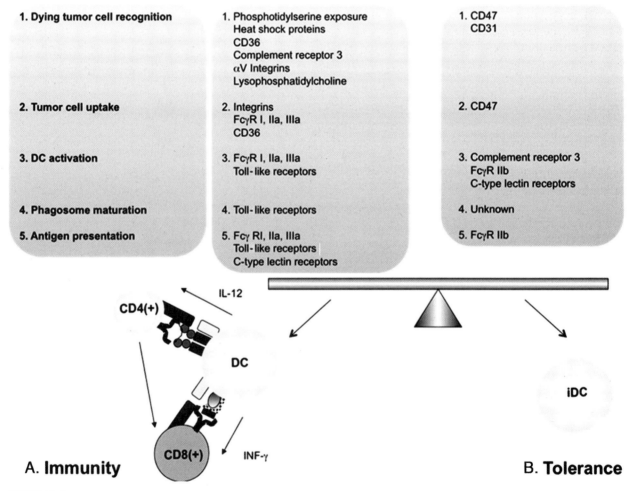

FIGURE 1.4 Factors influencing DC-based immune activation and tolerance. DCs initiate and regulate immune responses. Their central role in regulating immunity and tolerance is emphasized by their ability to influence the activity of cells from both the innate and adaptive immune system. The acquisition of genetic and epigenetic mutations activating proto-oncogenes triggers intrinsic tumor-suppressive mechanisms that induce DNA-damage responses, cellular senescence, or apoptosis. Danger signals that signal the immune system to eliminate a potentially malignant cell can come from premalignant cells in response to DNA damage. Danger signals can also be derived from apoptotic cells through the release of chemotactic factors. Opposing signals regulate the ability of DCs to induce **(A)** immunity or **(B)** tolerance to dying tumor cells in the tumor microenvironment. Positive signals often result in the production of mature DCs that are capable of increased and more effective antigen presentation. In contrast, negative signals maintain DCs in an immature state (iDCs) thereby preventing effective antigen presentation. Activation of each step requires both the presence of a positive stimulus as well as the removal of a negative one.

are also more efficient at crosspresentation of TA onto HLA class I antigens (35).

Upon encounter with pathogens or other "danger"-associated stimuli, DCs undergo a process of activation (maturation) and acquire the capacity to activate immunity (27). In contrast, immature or nonactivated DCs may only induce tolerance when they present antigen to T or B cells (27,37). The activation of immature DCs (iDCs) results in (a) increased expression of HLA antigens as well as costimulatory molecules on the cell surface and (b) increased surface area on DCs for antigen presentation (37). After internalizing TA at the tumor site, chemokine receptor 7(+) DCs traffic to tumor-draining lymph nodes, where they activate T and B cells in the paracortical cords and medullary cortex, respectively (43). It should be noted that DCs may also be present at the tumor site and are referred to as tumor-associated DCs (TADCs) (22,40). TADCs crosspresent TA to recruited CD8(+) T cells, potentially inducing their activation, proliferation, and maturation into TA-specific effector cells (22,41). In addition, TADCs, when appropriately activated, mediate the sensitization of naïve T cells that may have been recruited into the tumor site. Thus, interactions between the tumor-infiltrating T lymphocytes (TILs) and TADCs are essential for driving and maintaining the local TA-specific immune response. Optimal biologic functions and survival of T cells and DCs may be enhanced by reciprocal signaling between these two cell types via HLA class I antigen–peptide complexes and costimulatory receptor–ligand pairs (44). An additional layer of complexity is imparted by the different DC subsets that reside in or are recruited to different tissues that may carry different degrees of specialization with regard to activation of different components of the immune system (45). It is thought that these different subsets of DCs enhance the development of functionally distinct types of immune responses depending on the type of tissue. Lastly, it should be noted that DCs are also efficient at activating antigen-specific CD4(+)CD25(+) T regulatory cells (Treg) (41,46,47). The latter T cells have been shown to prevent the induction of a variety of autoimmune diseases in murine models through their ability to suppress the function and proliferation of antigen-specific CD4(+) and CD8(+) T cells (41,46,47). The immune-regulatory function of these cells has been attributed to their capacity to secrete immune-suppressive cytokines such as IL-10 and TGF-β (41,46,47). Therefore, it has been suggested that these cells play a role in the regulation of TA-specific immune responses, since tumor immunity can be thought of as an autoimmune process.

Interaction of TCRs on naïve CD8(+) T cells with HLA class I antigen–peptide complexes, together with help from activated CD4(+) T cells, leads to activation and clonal expansion of TA-specific CD8(+) CTLs. Based on our current understanding, both CD8(+) and CD4(+) T lymphocytes can be categorized into at least three functional subsets, depending on the cytokines they produce (48–50). These subsets include (a) Tc1/Th1 (type 1) cells that produce IFN-γ and IL-2; (b) Tc2/Th2 (type 2) cells that produce IL-4 and IL-5; and (c) Th3/Treg cells that produce IL-10 and/or TGF-β. As noted earlier, the latter Th3 cells dramatically suppress the function and proliferation of CD4(+) and CD8(+) T cells. Th1-biased immune responses are strongly supported by IL-12p70 (51) and are associated with the host's ability to control and eliminate intracellular pathogens and tumors. On the other hand, Th2-biased immune responses inhibit Th1 responses and do not favor the development of TA-specific cellular immunity, but rather favor humoral B-cell antibody responses. Once TA-specific CD8(+) T cells are activated, they leave the lymph node environment and make their way via the lymphatics to tumor site(s), arriving as primed, but not necessarily fully differentiated effector cells. CTLs are expected to induce programmed cell death of malignant cells that express targeted HLA class I antigen–peptide complexes, through the perforin–granzyme mechanism and/or the Fas/Fas ligand pathway (52). The latter requires the expression of Fas receptor on target cells and Fas ligand on effector CTLs.

As noted earlier, it has been hypothesized that antibody-secreting B cells also play a role in regulating tumor cell growth and progression. The latter seems likely given the clinical successes observed in patients treated with therapeutic TA-specific mAbs (Table 1.4) (19). There are many examples of TA that elicit autoantibodies in patients with a number of malignant diseases (31). These TA-specific autoantibody responses are currently being investigated as potential diagnostic tools in multiple types of cancer. It is expected that these TA-specific autoantibody responses control tumor growth through their ability to (a) induce tumor cell apoptosis; (b) trigger antibody-dependent cellular cytotoxicity (ADCC); (c) mediate complement-dependent cytotoxicity (CDC); and (d) interfere with the function of the targeted antigen and/or affect tumor cell signaling (19). More recent evidence suggests that TA-specific mAbs can induce TA-specific T-cell immune responses (19). Nevertheless, it should be stressed that the role of Th2-driven antibody responses in the control of tumor growth and progression has not yet been proven. Actually, development of TA-specific autoantibodies has been associated with poor prognosis and decreased survival in several types of malignant disease, for example, cancers of the head and neck, breast, and genitourinary tract (31). The seemingly paradoxical association between TA-specific autoantibodies and poor prognosis may be related to the formation of TA–autoantibody complexes, which skew immune responses toward Th2 cytokine profiles (31). As noted earlier, Th1- and Th2-associated cytokines act antagonistically toward one another and in general Th2 cytokines favor tumor progression. It is unclear at present whether Th2 cytokines favor tumor progression through their ability to enhance inflammation, to suppress TA-specific CTL responses, or a combination of both. The potential molecular mechanisms by which humoral immunity may influence tumor immune surveillance are summarized in Figure 1.5.

Table **1.4**   **FDA-approved TA-specific mAbs for human cancers**

mAb	Target	Isotype	FDA-Approved Disease
Rituximab	CD20	Chimeric IgG1	CD20 (+) low-grade lymphoma[a], diffuse large B-cell lymphoma[a], follicular lymphoma[a]
90Y Ibritumomab + tiuxetan	CD20	Radiolabeled murine IgG1	CD20(+) low-grade lymphoma[b]
1311 Tositumomab	CD20	Radiolabeled murine IgG1	CD20(+) low-grade lymphoma[c]
Alemtuzumab	CD52	Humanized IgG1	Chronic lymphocytic leukemia[d]
Gemtuzumab + ozogamacin	CD33	Rec. humanized IgG4-conjugated to calicheamicin	Acute myelogenous leukemia[e]
Trastuzumab	HER2/neu	Humanized IgG1	Her2/neu (+) breast cancer[f]
Cetuximab	EGFR	Chimeric IgG1	EGFR(+) colon cancer[g]
Panitumumab	EGFR	Fully human IgG2	EGFR(+) colon cancer[h]
Bevacizumab	VEGF	Humanized IgG1	Colon cancer[i], recurrent or advance non-small cell lung cancer, metastatic breast cancer

[a]Low-grade lymphoma 2nd line monotherapy; diffuse large B-cell lymphoma and follicular lymphoma: 1st line chemoimmune therapy as well as maintenance for follicular lymphoma.
[b]2nd line monotherapy and frontline adjuvant.
[c]2nd line monotherapy.
[d]1st and 2nd line monotherapy.
[e]>60 years of age, 2nd line monotherapy.
[f]2nd line monotherapy, adjuvant and 1st line chemoimmunetherapy.
[g]2nd line monotherapy or chemoimmune therapy.
[h]2nd line monotherapy.
[i]1st line chemoimmune therapy.

▨ NK cells

Unlike B and T cells, NK cells have the ability to recognize and kill target cells without prior sensitization. NK cells identify cells with reduced HLA class I antigen levels and/or increased levels of "stress"-induced ligands (2,38). In general, the balance between activating and inhibitory signals, provided by cell surface receptors, regulates NK cell activity. Typically, activation of NK cells is achieved via the triggering of NK cell–activating receptors in combination with proinflammatory cytokines. Once activated, NK cells mediate their functions through the direct killing of target cells and/or the release of cytokines (8,52–54). Even though

FIGURE 1.5 Potential role of humoral immunity in tumor immune surveillance. The tumor microenvironment is often associated with suppressed Th1-type immune responses, in combination with increased Th2-type immune responses. Th2-type immune responses lead to activation of antibody-secreting B cells that can suppress Th1-type immune responses. Furthermore, the formation of TA–antibody immune complexes leads to a proinflammatory environment that recruits neutrophils, macrophages, and mast cells, ultimately leading to a chronic inflammatory tumor-promoting state.

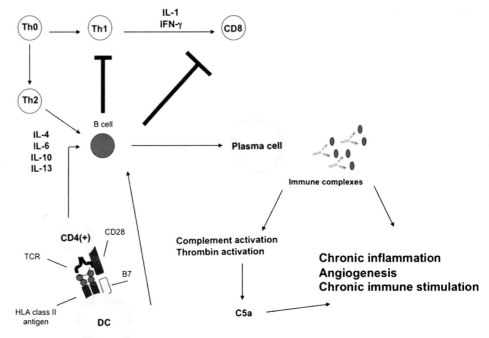

the ability to identify and destroy defective cells is the best characterized function of NK cells, there is growing evidence that NK cells may modulate the host's adaptive immune response. In this regard, NK cells have been shown to be required for the generation of antigen-specific T- and B-cell response both in vitro and in vivo (38,55,56). On the other hand, NK cells under some circumstances have also been shown to inhibit adaptive T-cell immunity. At present, little is known as to the molecular mechanism(s) through which NK cells influence adaptive immunity. In humans, both immature and mature DCs can induce resting NK-cell activation (38,55,56). Conversely, activated NK cells can also regulate the activity of DCs and this crosstalk appears to be required for the generation of an appropriate immune response (38,55,56). Whether the capacity of NK cells to modulate DC activity results from their ability to secrete Th1 cytokines or their ability to lyse iDCs is not well understood. NK cells may also modulate adaptive immunity by acting directly on effector cells. In this regard, activation of T cells is dependent on IFN-γ produced by NK cells (38,55,56). Moreover, NK cells have also been reported to stimulate autologous CD4(+) T cells, an effect that is dependent on the expression of OX40 ligand and CD86 by activated NK cells (57). A role for NK cells in the activation of B cells and the promotion of isotype class switching has also been observed (58). Conversely, NK cells have been shown to inhibit adaptive immune responses through NKG2D-dependent killing of activated T cells (38,55,56). Collectively, the available data indicate that NK cells serve a dual purpose in that they can provide help and promote the initiation of an immune response but can also curb the activity of immune effectors and thereby prevent immune-mediated damage to the host. The role NK cells play in tumor immune surveillance is less clear in humans, although a number of studies in mice provide evidence for the notion that NK cells are engaged in the eradication of tumor cells (8).

Cytokine milieu

Through secreted chemokines and cytokines, tumors can induce and amplify non-HLA–restricted, inflammatory responses in the host, leading to the accumulation of immune cells at the tumor site. Moreover, cytokines and chemokines play a key role in shaping functional attributes of both T cells and DCs in a tissue microenvironment. Like T cells, DCs are functionally heterogeneous and the polarization of DCs into distinct subsets, DC1, DC2, and DC3, appears to correspond to the functional T-cell subsets with which they interact (Th1, Th2, and Treg) (22). For example, DCs matured in the presence of Th1-type cytokines such as IFN-γ are polarized to secrete IL-12p70, a cytokine that promotes Th1-type responses (DC1); DCs matured in the presence of Th2-type cytokines such as IL-4 and IL-5 are polarized to promote Th2-type responses (DC2); and DCs matured in the presence of Treg cytokines such as IL-10 and TGF-β are believed to be polarized to downregulate

immune responses (DC3). The context of DCs' polarization and their ability to "switch" their functional potential in response to a new cytokine cocktail are being extensively studied at present, and both in vitro and in vivo experiments indicate a remarkable plasticity of this cellular population, which is clearly driven by cytokines and chemokines (59,60). Overall, it is clear that cytokines dictate the nature of the locoregional immune response, depending on the activation signals received by the T cells and DCs infiltrating the tumor microenvironment (61).

■ MECHANISMS OF TUMOR IMMUNE EVASION

The major unanswered question in human tumor immunology today is why tumors continue to progress despite the presence of TA-specific immune responses, which can be detected in patients with malignant disease whether they have been treated or not with active-specific immune therapy. In the following section, we will review the available information regarding the possible mechanisms underlying the ability of tumor cells to evade immune recognition and destruction. They include qualitative and/or quantitative defects in the generation and maintenance of TA-specific immune responses, changes in the antigenic profile of tumor cells because of their genetic instability, and/or resistance of tumor cells to immune effector cell–mediated killing.

Tumor cell–induced immune suppression

A large body of evidence has clearly demonstrated immune suppression in cancer patients and tumor-bearing animals. Table 1.5 summarizes the types of defects in immune system observed in patients with malignant disease. Many studies have demonstrated that a high percentage of T cells undergo apoptosis in patients with cancer (22,62). Furthermore, apoptosis of T cells is not limited to the tumor site, since an increased percentage of apoptotic T cells is also found in the peripheral blood of patients with head and neck squamous cell carcinoma, breast carcinoma, and melanoma (22,62). This

Table **1.5**	**Immune deviation in T cells present in the tumor microenvironment**

1. Activation of proteolytic enzymes in TILs: rapid degradation of cellular proteins.
2. Signaling defects in TIL and PBL-T
   (a) NF-κB abnormalities
   (b) ς-chain defects: either low expression or absence
   (c) Ca^{2+} flux alterations
3. Cytokine expression: absent/decreased Th1-type cytokines
4. Inhibition of lymphocyte proliferation, cytotoxic activity, or cytokine production
5. Inhibition of leukocyte migration
6. Induction of T-cell apoptosis
7. Expansion of immunosuppressive macrophages

TILs, tumor-infiltrating leukocytes.

apoptosis appears to be preferential for TA-specific CD8(+) T cells. Immune effector cells have also been found to be poorly responsive or unresponsive to traditional T cell–activating stimuli such as DC activation or TA-expressing tumor cells, in patients with malignant disease (22,62). In addition, alterations in systemic TA-specific T-cell immunity also occur in patients with malignant disease. T and NK cells from approximately half of the patients with cancer of the head and neck, breast, stomach, colon, kidney, ovary, and prostate, as well as melanoma, Hodgkin lymphoma, and acute myelocytic leukemia display a decreased in vitro response to antigens or mitogens and a decreased CD3ς chain expression (22,62). The latter is associated with the TCR–CD3 complex in T lymphocytes and Fcς RIII in NK cells and is essential for transmembrane signaling in lymphocytes (63). Circulating T cells have also been shown to be biased in their cytokine profile and function, as determined by CD3ς chain expression, proliferative index, or NF-κB activity (22,62,64). It is noteworthy that changes in signal transduction molecules are not limited to CD3ς chain, since T cells from patients with renal cell carcinoma (RCC) display a reduced level of Jak-3. The latter is a tyrosine kinase associated with the γ chain, which is common to IL-2, -4, -7, and -15 cytokine receptors (64). Moreover, T cells from RCC patients also have a diminished ability to translocate NFκBp65 (64). Regardless of the specific defect, the presence of such systemic alterations may explain, in part, the lack of correlation between immune and clinical responses in patients treated with malignant disease.

Functional impairments have also been noted in DCs. In this regard, a large body of evidence suggests that DC maturation is impaired in patients with malignant disease (65,66).

Moreover, TADCs have been shown to be functionally defective, especially in their antigen-presenting capacity in several malignant diseases (65–67). Lastly, tumor-associated macrophages (TAMs) also exhibit functional defects relative to macrophages isolated from normal tissue inflammatory sites (68). However, the functional consequences of these impairments have not yet been elucidated.

Mechanisms of tumor cell–induced immune suppression

Inflammatory and/or lytic molecules produced by tumor cells may play a role in modulating the host immune response within the tumor microenvironment. In fact, early experiments, dating back more than 30 years, provided evidence that tumor-derived factors can alter the normal functions of immune cells in vitro (64). It has been shown that serum derived from patients with malignant disease will interfere with DC differentiation and T-cell activation, as well as induce apoptosis in activated T cells (65,66). Over the years, a number of tumor-derived factors with immunosuppressive activity have been identified (Table 1.6). The unresponsiveness of the immune system in patients with cancer has been attributed to a bias toward a Th2 immune response given the paucity of Th1 cytokines (IFN-γ, IL-2, and IL-12) at the tumor site as well as the prevalence of Treg cytokines (IL-10 or TGF-β). In fact in patients with malignant disease, TILs have been shown to display a predominant Th2 or Treg phenotype associated with the local production of IL-4 or IL-10 rather than the mixed Th1/Th2 responsiveness observed in normal donors (22,64). IL-10 also inhibits differentiation and maturation of DCs as well as their ability to present antigen (65,66), thus interfering with the induction of TA-specific immune responses. It is

Table **1.6** **Tumor-associated suppressive factors**[a]		
1. The TNF family ligands: induce leukocyte apoptosis via the TNF family receptors		
FasL	Fas	
TRAIL	TRAIL-Rs	
TNF	TNFR1	
2. Small molecules		
Prostaglandin E2 (PGE2)		Inhibits leukocyte functions through increased cAMP
Histamine		Inhibits leukocyte functions through increased cAMP
Epinephrine		Inhibits leukocyte functions through increased cAMP
Inducible nitric oxide synthase		Promotes or inhibits Fas-mediated apoptosis by regulation of nitric oxide levels
H_2O_2		Has pro-oxidant activity, increases cAMP levels, causes apoptosis in NK cells, inhibits tumor-specific CTLs
3. Cytokines		
TGF-β		Inhibits perforin and granzyme mRNA expression; inhibits lymphocyte proliferation
IL-10		Inhibits production of IL-1β, IFN-γ, IL-12, and TNFα
Granulocyte–macrophage colony–stimulating factor		Promotes expansion of immunosuppressive tumor-associated macrophages
4. Tumor-associated gangliosides		Inhibit IL-2–dependent lymphocyte proliferation or induce apoptotic signals

[a]A partial list of immunosuppressive factors selected to demonstrate their diversity and a wide spectrum of effects on immune cells.

noteworthy that IL-10 may also suppress T-cell recognition of tumor cells by downregulating APM components thereby reducing HLA class I antigen–TA peptide complex expression on tumor cells (22). Tumor cell TGF-β has been shown to inhibit TA-specific T cells and reverse the immune-stimulating properties of IL-2 (69). Furthermore, TGF-β is often found at high levels in malignancies and is associated with poor prognosis and lack of response to immunotherapy (69). Prostaglandin E2 has also been implicated in tumor cell immune escape, since it can suppress Th1 immune responses while enhancing Th2 immune responses (69). In addition, IL-8 (70), soluble MIC (71), and VEGF (65,66) production has been implicated as a potential means of tumor cell escape by modulating immune effector cell function.

Different mechanisms may account for the high frequency of T-cell apoptosis observed in patients with cancer. Malignant cells have been shown to escape immune recognition by developing resistance to Fas-mediated apoptosis and acquiring expression of FasL that they may use for eliminating activated Fas$^+$ lymphocytes (22,64,72). On the other hand, chronically stimulated T cells are likely to undergo activation-induced cell death (AICD) mediated by the Fas/FasL pathway (73). In this regard, TILs, LNL, or peripheral T cells in patients with cancer experience chronic or repeated antigenic stimulation with TA and often express CD95 on the cell surface (22,64). Therefore, the chronic or acute systemic dissemination of TA may result in an excess of arginase (Ag) and "high dose" tolerance of specific T and B cells, making them particularly susceptible to AICD. More recently, the coinhibitory molecules of the B7-CD28 family, in particular B7-H1 (PD-1) that plays a role in the deletion of peripheral effector T cells, have been found to be expressed on a variety of tumor cell types (74). It has been suggested that B7-H1 expression by tumor cells may provide an additional mechanism to induce T-cell apoptosis, since administration of B7-H1–specific antagonistic mAb can enhance the therapeutic efficacy of adoptive immunotherapy with polyclonal T cells (75). Dysfunction, and ultimately, death of T cells in situ might also result from impaired TADC functions (65–67). TADCs not only process and present TA but are also important sources of IFN-α, IL-1, IL-12, IL-15, IL-18, IL-23, and IL-27, among other cytokines. They are also rich in costimulatory molecules (CD80, CD86, OX40, 4-1BBL) necessary as second signals or growth factors for T-cell differentiation, proliferation, and memory development (57,65–67). Therefore, if TADCs are dysfunctional, as suggested by data (65–67), or if they also undergo apoptosis in situ, then TADC–TIL interactions are not likely to be optimal for productive TA-specific immunity.

Elimination of DCs or DC precursors in the tumor microenvironment may, in part, contribute to an ineffective TA-specific T-cell immune response in patients with malignant disease (65–67). Analysis of gene and protein expression in DCs and DC precursors in the tumor microenvironment has demonstrated that expression of several intracellular signaling molecules is reproducibly altered in DCs coincubated with tumor cells, including IL-2Rγ, IRF2, Mcl-1, and small

Rho GTPases (65–67). The mechanisms involved in the induction of apoptosis and protection of different DC subpopulations as well as DC precursors from death signals include (a) downregulation of the antiapoptotic Bcl-2 family proteins in DCs (76); (b) accumulation of ceramides that may interfere with PI3K-mediated survival signals; or (c) production of nitric oxide (NO) species by tumor cells, which suppresses expression of cellular inhibitors of apoptosis proteins (cIAPs) or inhibitor of caspase 8—cellular FLICE inhibitory protein (cFLIP) (77).

Myeloid suppressor cells

A group of CD11b(+), Gr-1(+) cells, known as myeloid suppressor cells (MSCs), are also thought to play an important role in the suppression of TA-specific immune responses in tumor-bearing patients (78,79). MSCs represent a heterogeneous population that includes mature granulocytes, monocytes, and immature cells of the myelomonocytic lineage. There is ample evidence that tumor growth in tumor-bearing mice and in patients with all types of malignant disease is associated with an accumulation of MSCs (78,79). In vitro studies indicate that MSCs purified from tumor-bearing mice, but not from naïve mice, can suppress CD8(+) T cells. This suppression is NO independent and antigen specific and is believed to be mediated through TCR and MHC class I antigen interactions. While the molecular mechanisms underlying this phenomenon are unclear, several studies indicate that reactive oxygen species (ROS) may play a significant role. In this regard, many human tumors and cell lines are capable of secreting cytokines not limited to but including GM-CSF, IL-3, IL-6, M-CSF, and VEGF. These cytokines are capable of expanding the myeloid cell pool and may also lead to an increase in ROS production and Ag activity in MSCs (78,79). The latter enzyme indirectly increases the ROS level by decreasing L-arginine concentrations. Constant production of these factors could lead to the different levels of ROS observed in MSCs from tumor-bearing and tumor-free mice. In fact, the ROS level has been found to be threefold greater in MSCs derived from tumor-bearing mice than in tumor-free mice (78,79). The main target for ROS on T cells has been shown to be CD3ς, resulting in the suppression of CD3ς, reduced TCR signaling, and ultimately decreased Th1 cytokine secretion. ROS are short-lived substances and therefore the antigen-specific nature of their inhibition may be explained by the need for direct MSC–T cell contact (78,79). In this regard, antigen-specific interactions between T cells and APCs are much more stable and last longer than interactions in the absence of antigen. MSCs express MHC class I molecules but have low or undetectable levels of MHC class II antigens; this phenotype may explain the lack of CD4(+) T-cell suppression by MSCs (78,79).

CD4(+)CD25(+) T regulatory cells

Accumulating evidence indicates that Treg cells may also contribute to T-cell dysfunction. Treg cells prevent the induction of a variety of autoimmune diseases in murine models (41,46,47). Treg cells dramatically suppress the

FIGURE 1.6 Immune escape mechanisms utilized by tumor cells. Escape mechanisms utilized by tumor cells include loss of the HLA class I antigen–TA-derived peptide complex which can result from loss of **(A)** TA, **(B)** antigen-processing machinery components, **(C)** HLA class I antigens, **(D)** release of soluble HLA antigens and NK cell–activating ligands resulting in inhibition of DC antigen presentation, **(E)** release of immune-suppressive cytokines resulting in altered immune cell function, **(F)** overexpression of antiapoptotic proteins in tumor cells resulting in resistance to apoptosis, and **(G)** Fas ligand expression resulting in the killing of Fas+ lymphocytes.

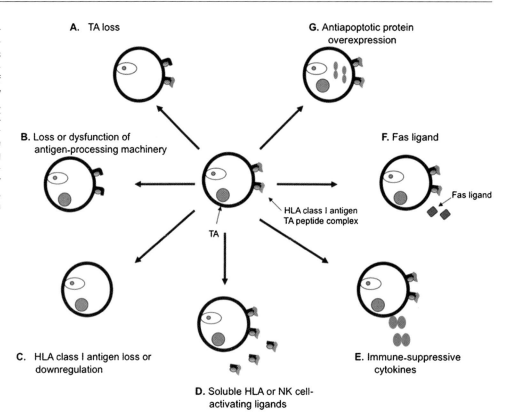

A. TA loss

G. Antiapoptotic protein overexpression

B. Loss or dysfunction of antigen-processing machinery

F. Fas ligand

Fas ligand

HLA class I antigen
TA peptide complex

TA

C. HLA class I antigen loss or downregulation

E. Immune-suppressive cytokines

D. Soluble HLA or NK cell-activating ligands

function and proliferation of CD4(+)CD25(−) and CD8(+) T cells (41,46,47). The immune-regulatory function of these cells has been attributed to their capacity to secrete immune-suppressive cytokines such as IL-10 and TGF-β, which inhibit CTL responses. As noted earlier, it has been suggested that Treg cells play a role in inhibiting TA-specific immunity, since tumor immunity can be thought of as an autoimmune process. In this regard, in vivo studies performed in murine models have shown that Treg cells, which comprise 5% to 10% of CD4(+) T cells in naïve mice, can inhibit the generation of TA-specific T-cell immune responses (41,46,47). In contrast, depletion of Treg cells has been shown to promote rejection of several tumors in mice (41,46,47). This rejection is dependent on CD8(+) and/or CD4(+) T cells depending on the mouse strain and the tumor model. In vitro studies suggest that Treg cells may suppress CD8(+) and CD4(+) T cells in an antigen nonspecific fashion through the production of TGF-β (41,46,47). In humans, Treg cells are found at a higher frequency in the peripheral blood of cancer patients and may induce peripheral ignorance of tumor cells, facilitating metastatic spread of the disease (80,81). However, their functional role in the modulation of TA-specific immune responses is yet to be elucidated.

Tumor cell escape from immune recognition and killing

Tumor cell resistance to TA-specific CTLs

Multiple immune escape mechanisms may be utilized by tumor cells to evade the host's immune response as well as recognition and destruction by host CTLs (Fig. 1.6). Because of their genetic instability (82), tumor cells may change in the expression of molecules such as TA, HLA class I antigens, and/or APM components, each of which plays a crucial role in the generation of the HLA class I antigen–TA peptide complex (83,84). The latter mediates the recognition of tumor cells by host's CTLs. Abnormalities in TA expression as well as a variable degree of inter- and intralesional heterogeneity characterize many tumors (83,84). As a result, peptides may not be generated from TA or may be formed in very low amount and the corresponding HLA class I antigen–TA peptide complexes are not formed in spite of the expression of the relevant HLA class I allospecificity. Furthermore, malignant cells may present TA-derived peptide analogs with antagonist activity resulting in suboptimal T-cell activation (83,84). These defects render malignant cells ineffective targets for TA-specific T cells.

As reviewed elsewhere (71,83,84), the frequency of HLA class I antigen loss or downregulation ranges from 16% to 80% of the various types of tumors stained with mAbs recognizing monomorphic determinants. The difference in the frequency of classical HLA class I antigen defects in various types of tumors is likely to be caused by multiple reasons. Some of them are technical in nature and include the sensitivity of the immunohistochemistry (IHC) method utilized to detect HLA antigens, the characteristics of the mAb used in the IHC reactions, and the subjective evaluation of IHC staining. Additional important variables that play a role in the different frequency of HLA class I antigen abnormalities observed in tumors of different histotype include the extent of immune selective pressure imposed on tumor cell populations, the degree of genetic instability, the time length between onset of tumor and diagnosis, the characteristics of the patient population investigated, and the histologic classification of the type of tumor analyzed.

Abnormalities in HLA class I antigen expression are caused by distinct mechanisms. They include both structural and functional defects in β_2-microglobulin, HLA class I heavy chain, and/or APM component expression (71,83,84). The APM components play a crucial role in the generation of TA-derived peptides, their loading onto HLA class I antigens, and the presentation of HLA class I antigen–peptide complexes on the surface of cells. It is noteworthy that defects in APM component expression and/or function may result in alterations in the repertoire of peptides presented by HLA class I antigens while not affecting the actual level of HLA class I antigen expression. This possibility provides a mechanism for resistance to CTL-mediated lysis of tumor cells without detectable defects in HLA class I antigen expression such as head and neck squamous cell carcinoma cells (71,83,84). The role of HLA class I antigen defects in the clinical course of the disease is highlighted by the increased frequency of HLA class I antigen abnormalities in malignant lesions in patients treated with T cell–based immunotherapy (71,83,84). Furthermore, HLA class I antigen loss has been frequently found in lesions that have recurred in patients who had experienced clinical responses following T cell–based immunotherapy (71,83,84). It is noteworthy that in some of these cases, HLA class I antigen expression can be restored by cytokines (71,83,84). Therefore, these patients, in contrast to those whose lesions possess structural defects in HLA class I antigen–encoding genes, are likely to benefit by combining T cell–based immunotherapy with administration of cytokines.

As indicated earlier, CTLs are expected to induce programmed cell death of malignant cells via the Fas/Fas ligand pathway. However, malignant cells themselves can become resistant to apoptosis through a variety of mechanisms. The mechanisms identified include loss of Fas

expression (22,64) as well as overexpression of key anti-apoptotic proteins such as two members of the IAP family (survivin and ML-IAP), bcl2, cFLIP, and NO synthetases (22,64). Alterations may appear further downstream in the death receptor signaling pathway, including functional impairment of FADD and caspase 10 by inactivation mutations (22,64). Lastly, tumor cells may escape T cell as well as NK cell granzyme-mediated killing through increased PI-9 (in mice known as SPI-6) expression (85,86). The latter is a serine protease inhibitor that inactivates granzyme B (85).

Tumor cell resistance to TA-specific antibodies

Tumor cells also utilize escape mechanisms to evade the antitumor effects of TA-specific antibodies. At present, it is difficult to precisely establish the most clinically significant means by which tumor cells avoid the antitumor effects of TA-specific antibodies given the multiple mechanisms by which endogenous and/or therapeutic TA-specific antibodies exert their antitumor effects (Table 1.7). Moreover, much of the information regarding the antitumor effects of TA-specific antibodies stems from in vitro studies, which may not accurately reflect their in vivo activity. Lastly, it should be stressed that much of the information available related to tumor cell resistance to TA-specific antibodies stems from the clinical use of therapeutic TA-specific mAb, since limited data are available about the role humoral immunity plays in tumor immune surveillance. Therefore, whether the mechanisms identified for tumor cell resistance to TA-specific therapeutic mAb can be applied to endogenous TA-specific antibodies remains to be determined.

Tumors cells may be intrinsically unresponsive to or may develop resistance to TA-specific endogenous and/or therapeutic antibodies. Resistance to TA-specific antibodies can be broadly divided into several categories. It should be noted that these mechanisms do not function independently and that they extensively interact with each other. The relative importance of each mechanism most likely varies with the type of tumor and the TA-specific antibody. First, low serum antibody levels, poor antibody tissue penetration,

Table 1.7 Molecular mechanisms underlying therapeutic efficacy of TA-specific mAb–based therapy

Immune Effector (Cell-Independent)[a]	Immune Effector (Cell-Dependent)
Induction of apoptosis	Activation of complement mediated – phagocytosis – complement-dependent cytotoxicity
Induction of alterations in intracelluar signaling Inhibition of growth factor binding to its cognate receptor Inhibition of growth factor receptor activation	Trigger antibody-dependent cellular cytotoxicity Induction of tumor cell necrosis or apoptosis leading to – Presentation of TA by APCs – Activation of CD4(+) T cell–mediated killing – Activation of B cells and eosinophils – Activation of TA-specific CTLs

[a]Ultimately results in inhibition of cancer cell proliferation, tumor-induced angiogenesis, cancer cell invasion and metastasis, as well as potentiation of antitumor activity of cytotoxic drugs and radiotherapy.

and/or TA-specific antibody affinity for the targeted TA as well as FcγR are likely to influence the ability of TA-specific antibodies to exert their antitumor effects. Second, patients' characteristics including tumor burden, functional immune status as well as FcγR polymorphisms will limit the ability of TA-specific antibodies to initiate immune effector mechanisms such as ADCC and CDC. In fact, the strongest evidence supporting ADCC as a clinically meaningful mechanism of certain therapeutic mAbs is based on studies evaluating the impact of different allelic variations of FcγR polymorphisms on clinical response (19). Third, as indicated earlier, given their genetic instability (82), tumor cells may change in the expression of TA. In this regard, poor TA surface expression and/or presence of circulating and/or altered TA limit the ability of TA-specific antibodies to bind directly to tumor cells (19). Furthermore, the epitopes recognized by TA-specific antibodies may be masked or made inaccessible through the expression of other cell surface proteins. The latter is suggested by the observation that MUC4, a membrane-associated mucin that masks membrane proteins, limits the ability of the EGFR-specific therapeutic mAb trastuzumab to bind tumor cells in vitro (19). Moreover, resistance to therapeutic EGFR-specific mAb has been suggested to reflect heterodimerization of HER2 with other receptors, which interfere with binding EGFR-specific mAb (19). Fourth, tumors may prevent TA-specific antibodies from initiating immune effector mechanisms through their ability to express molecules, which inhibit ADCC, CDC, and cell-mediated immunity (19). Fifth, alterations in signal transduction networks may render tumor cells resistant to the ability of TA-specific antibodies to modulate cell signaling as well as apoptosis. For example, elevation of the anti-apoptotic protein BCL2 has been shown to make tumor cells resistant to the CD20-specific mAb rituximab (19). Moreover, mutations and/or alterations in signaling molecules involved in key cellular signal transduction pathways allow tumor cells to bypass the blockage of one signaling pathway. This resistance is evident in non–small cell lung carcinoma (nSCLC), gastric, colorectal, pancreatic, and renal cell cancers, which demonstrate activating mutations in the *K-RAS* gene (19). The latter are believed to allow tumor cells to bypass EGFR-specific antibody-mediated inhibition of EGFR signaling through constitutive activation of *K-RAS*. Whether these findings can be applied to TA-specific antibodies in vivo remains to be determined. Lastly, it should be stressed that different cell surface receptors may share downstream signaling pathways so that despite the inhibition of one receptor by a TA-specific antibody, the downstream signaling may still be activated by other growth factors (19).

■ TOWARD IMPROVING IMMUNOTHERAPY

A significant amount of data from animal models, together with compelling data from patients with malignant disease, suggests that a functional cancer immune surveillance does exist and that it can, in some cases, suppress tumor growth.

This phenomenon along with the lack of effective treatment for advanced-stage malignant disease has provided the impetus for the development and application of immune-mediated therapies for the treatment of malignant disease. Over the past 20 years, a large number of passive immunotherapy and active-specific immunotherapy clinical trials utilizing TA-specific mAb and tumor cell (DC, HSP, cytokine, or peptide) vaccines have been conducted in patients with malignant disease. Collectively, these strategies attempt to augment protective TA-specific immunity and to disrupt the immune-regulatory circuits that are critical for maintaining tumor tolerance.

To date, significant progress has been made in the field of therapeutic TA-specific mAb. In fact, several TA-specific mAbs applicable to the treatment of several major malignant diseases have received regulatory approval and are commercially available (19). The average clinical success rate of mAb-based immune therapy is approximately 30% with a range from 0% to 80% (19). The clinical efficacy of these mAbs is manifested by the statistically significant survival prolongation and in some cases by the reduction of tumor mass in the treated patients (19). Although few in number, these mAbs have changed the face of cancer therapy, bringing us closer to more specific and more effective biologic therapy of cancer. In contrast to therapeutic TA-specific mAbs, limited progress has been made in therapies designed to augment or induce TA-specific T-cell responses in patients with malignant disease (87–89). A number of active-specific immunotherapy clinical trials have convincingly shown that vaccines (a) are able to induce and/or augment already established tumor immunity and (b) have limited or no toxicity. Despite these encouraging findings, with the exception of one trial (70), no study has demonstrated that active-specific immunotherapy can improve upon the currently available treatment modalities for malignant disease. In fact, the lack of convincing and reproducible associations between immune response and objective clinical responses to immunotherapies in patients with malignant disease has cast doubt regarding the utility of active-specific immunotherapy in general. In the remaining section, several potential strategies will be reviewed that may counteract the multiple escape mechanisms utilized by tumor cells and improve the application of immunotherapy in patients with malignant disease.

Recent progress in our understanding of the mechanisms underlying activation and proliferation of the adaptive arm of the immune response provides support for the concept that tumor cells may directly and/or indirectly lead to dysfunction and/or death of T cells as well as DCs. Therefore, it is unlikely that active-specific immunotherapy of malignant disease will be successful in the setting of tumor cell–induced immune suppression. The subsequent design of successful new therapies is likely to depend not only on reinforcement of the protective but also on inhibition of the suppressive, molecular pathways in T cells functioning within the tumor microenvironment. Unfortunately, the question of how to best protect immune effector cells from tumor cell–induced immune suppression is yet to be adequately addressed. Based on preliminary results from various laboratories, it appears that biotherapy with cytokines and/or DCs is the most effective and practical way of providing protection from apoptosis to immune effector cells (87–89). Although the mechanisms responsible for this protection are not clear, it is now recognized that DCs also play a major role in protecting T cells from apoptosis. The therapeutic implications of this finding are profound. In effect, this concept shifts the emphasis from the well-recognized role of DCs as APCs to their additional role as T-cell protectors from apoptosis-inducing signals. It should be stressed that while therapy with cytokines such as IFN-γ, IL-2, or IL-12 has been used by many investigators to treat patients with malignant disease (87–89), cytokine therapy has never been specifically directed toward preventing the death of DCs or immune effector cells. On the contrary, the rationale behind cytokine therapies has been the predicted upregulation of antitumor effector functions, especially those associated with TA–specific T cells. In retrospect, attempts to upregulate the functionality of dying cells are not likely to succeed. Enhancing both the number and function of DCs may become the primary objective of biologic therapies in cancer patients, where premature death of TA-specific CD8(+) and CD4(+) T-cell effectors occurs. To achieve adequate protection of T cells from apoptosis in the tumor microenvironment, it will be necessary to investigate mechanisms of tumor cell–induced DC immune suppression and formulate strategies for inhibition of this process, perhaps by using cytokines such as IL-7 or IL-12. New strategies for cytokine delivery as well as new cytokines themselves (IL-15 and IL-17) are also likely to be necessary to rescue dying cells or, better, to protect viable cells from death-inducing signals (90–92). Such therapeutic strategies based on creative and novel use of cytokines are both rational and practical. While the precedent exists for clinical applications of these cytokines in humans, the novelty of the suggested approach is that it targets biotherapy to the specific pathways or even affected molecules and is designed to carefully evaluate the impact of these corrective measures on immune cell function in treated patients.

More recently, attempts have been made to boost TA-specific T-cell activity and overcome immune suppression by the administration of anticytotoxic T lymphocyte–associated antigen 4 (CTLA-4) mAb (19). CTLA-4 is an immunoregulatory molecule expressed on activated T cells and a subset of Treg cells (93). This molecule is capable of downregulating T-cell activation (93). Blockade of its function has been shown to enhance TA-specific responses and potentiate the activity of cancer vaccines in animal models (93). The CTLA-4–specific ipilimumab (MDX-010) and tremelimumab (CP-675,206), which are fully human IgG1 and IgG2 mAb, respectively, are being tested in patients with nSCLC, RCC, and metastatic melanoma (19). Early studies of patients with advanced melanoma show that ipilimumab promotes antitumor activity as monotherapy and in combination with chemotherapy, cytokines, or vaccines. Adverse events observed in the clinical trials are consistent with antibody-based induction of autoimmune responses through interference with CTLA-4 engagement of its cognate ligands. Induction of these autoimmune responses in melanoma patients correlates with tumor regression (19). At present, the A3671009 phase III trial comparing tremelimumab with standard dacarbazine and temozolomide in stage IV melanoma patients has been discontinued after an interim analysis found that tremelimumab is not superior to chemotherapy (19). Since only a subgroup of patients with cancer has a clinical benefit from treatment with CTLA4-specific mAb, there is an urgent need to identify and clinically validate useful biomarkers to select patients for such treatment.

Patients' tumor cell susceptibility to immune recognition and destruction must also become a major focus of investigations in order to improve the outcome of immunotherapy. During the last few years, defects in TA, APM component, and HLA class I antigen expression have been convincingly documented in malignant lesions. Although not conclusive, the available evidence suggests that these defects may be clinically relevant. This information has been useful to focus investigators' attention on the potential role of TA, APM component, and HLA antigen defects in tumor cell escape. To date, a significant percentage of the immunotherapy clinical trials conducted have targeted only one HLA class I antigen–TA peptide complex. Clearly, abnormalities in the expression of TA, APM components, and/or HLA class I antigens will lead to alterations in HLA class I antigen–TA peptide complex expression and ultimately impair CTL recognition of tumor cells. In this regard, polyvalent vaccines, which utilize more than one TA, may be preferable to the widely used strategy to immunize patients with one TA, for several reasons. First, polyvalent vaccines have the potential to generate immune responses against the multiple TA of a particular patient's tumor. The latter provides a means to match therapeutic regimens with changing tumor antigenic profiles, which are likely to occur during the course of the disease. Second, the potential ability of polyvalent vaccines to generate immunity against multiple TA increases the probability of generating tumor immunity against unique TA that have been suggested to be more effective targets of T cell–based immunotherapy than shared TA (7). Lastly, polyvalent vaccines eliminate the requirement for patient selection based on HLA type, since they may generate immune responses restricted by each of the individual HLA types expressed in the patient to be treated. The beneficial effects on the clinical course of the disease observed in trials conducted with polyvalent vaccines support the use of this type of immunogens (87–89). The types of TA currently being utilized in clinical trials should also be re-examined. In this regard, most of the currently used TA in T cell–based immunotherapy trials represent differentiation and/or shared TA that have been identified from tumor metastases and CTLs from patients who, in the majority of cases, have failed to reject their cancer.

Moreover, many of these TA are selected on the basis of their immunogenicity and tissue distribution without paying much attention to their function in tumor cell biology. Whether any of the identified TA is a tumor rejection antigen and whether stage IV cancer patients represent the most appropriate source to identify clinically relevant TA are not known at present.

In regard to therapeutic TA-specific mAb, only little is known about why merely a limited percentage of the treated patients respond clinically to TA-specific, mAb-based immunotherapy. Except for the expression of the targeted TA in the tumor and for polymorphisms in the Fcγ receptor expressed by immune effector cells, the variables underlying the differential clinical response of the patients treated with antibody-based immunotherapy have not been identified (19). The scant information in this area has a negative impact on the optimization of the use of TA-specific mAb in immunotherapeutic strategies and represents a major obstacle to the selection of patients to be treated with mAb-based immune therapy. The customization of the variables underlying a patient's clinical response to therapy will need to be based on more precise characterization of tumor and patient factors that might predict the success of TA-specific mAb-based immune therapy. Laboratory assays are being developed to identify patients who are likely to have a response to therapy with mAb; such assays include the identification of FcγIIIR polymorphisms. Correlations between the assays that are currently available and the response to antibody therapy vary among tumor subtypes and may depend on whether antibody therapy is used alone or in combination with chemotherapy. Some studies suggest an increased benefit of rituximab therapy in patients with diffuse large B-cell lymphoma whose tumors overexpress Bcl-2 but are negative for Bcl-6 (19). Nevertheless, most analyses that have used assays that might predict responses have been retrospective, so the clinical usefulness of these assays is still uncertain. Careful and comprehensive analysis of the binding specificities of mutated mAbs to human effector cells, ideally harvested from cancer patients, would therefore be essential to predict the net effect of changing FcR interactions. An additional consideration is the expression of the FcγR variant alleles in control and disease populations, which might also influence response to therapeutic mAbs. Emphasis should also be placed on pharmacodynamic end points and surrogate markers of response in trials of novel therapies. It should be possible to check that patients have adequate levels of NK cells and monocytes before therapy and that these are responsive in ADCC assays. Once therapy has commenced, trials could be designed to assess immunologic function, for example, evidence of host cell recruitment into accessible tumor deposits and circulating cytokine levels. In addition, to examine whether other mechanisms are operating, it would be important to monitor the induction of idiotypic antibody cascades and TA-specific cell-mediated responses. Lastly, as indicated earlier, the presence of circulating and/or altered TA may negatively influence the antitumor activities of

TA-specific antibodies. Although to date, the predictive value of soluble and/or truncated TA before treatment is not clear. It is noteworthy that in one study, breast cancer patients with elevated levels of soluble HER2 have more favorable responses to the EGFR-specific therapeutic mAb trastuzumab and docetaxel, with declining levels of soluble HER2 correlating with improved disease-free survival (94,95). In addition, a meta-analysis of eight clinical trials has showed improved disease-free and overall survival in patients with at least a 20% decline in soluble HER2 levels within the first few weeks of trastuzumab-based therapy (96). Thus, monitoring circulating TA levels during treatment may be an informative serum marker for predicting response to therapeutic TA-specific mAb.

New classes of optimized TA-specific mAb will be entering clinical trials in the next decade and are likely to yield many effective new treatments for patients with malignant disease. These advances will require the identification and validation of important new functional targets, the optimization of antibody structures to promote antitumor effects, the induction and amplification of tumor–specific immune responses, the manipulation of tumor–host microenvironment interactions, and the combination of antibodies with other effective treatment modalities. Furthermore, more efficient ADCC and CDC will be achieved by overcoming the response variability caused by Fc-receptor polymorphisms. The latter may be accomplished by using mAbs with alterations in their glycosylation or Fc-domain amino acid sequences to enhance their affinity for FcR. Antibody affinity will need to be tuned and customized to inhibit binding to normal tissues, improve tumor penetration and retention, and optimize antitumor effects. The size, valence, structure, and specificity of these mAbs will also need to be modified to increase tumor specificity by accelerating systemic clearance of mAbs that have failed to bind the target of choice. Improved conjugation technologies will facilitate the development of immunoconjugates. Multifunctional mAbs will more selectively bind to tumors by targeting pairs of normal antigens that are only present together on a given tumor cell. Careful and comprehensive analysis of the binding specificities of mutated mAbs to human effector cells will be essential to predict the net effect of changing FcγR interactions. FcgRIIB expressed on follicular DCs in germinal centers has also recently been shown to be important for the regulation of B-cell recall responses (19). Whether the latter contributes to TA-specific immune responses in patients is yet to be determined (19).

It should be noted that the types of patients currently being enrolled in clinical trials as well as the criteria to evaluate clinical responses may also need to be re-evaluated. Because of ethical considerations, immunotherapy trials have been performed in patients who have failed to respond to all conventional means of treatment and usually have advanced disease. These patients are often immune suppressed and not as responsive to immunization (97). Moreover, a patient's pretreatment tumor burden has been shown to be of critical importance for the induction of a maximum TA-specific immune response (97). These findings suggest that the use of immunotherapy may only be successful when administered early during the course of the disease and/or in the adjuvant setting. In addition, the potential role of HLA type on the clinical response to active-specific immunotherapy (97) suggests that a patient's genetic makeup plays a crucial role in determining the nature of their immune response. To this end, guidelines have been established by the Cancer Vaccine Clinical Trials Working Group (21) in an attempt to improve future vaccine trials. Future studies directed at identifying genetic algorithm(s) responsible for successful tumor rejection in response to immunization may help in the selection of patients likely to benefit from specific immunization strategies. Attention must also be focused on treated patients' ability to mount effective immune responses as well as patients' tumor cell susceptibility to immune-mediated effector mechanisms. Patients should be monitored for adequate levels of DCs, monocytes, and NK cells before and during therapy. Moreover, assays should be designed to ensure that monocytes and NK cells are capable of mediating antibody-dependent cytotoxicity.

The possible role played by immune selective pressure in the generation of malignant lesions with TA or HLA class I antigen defects suggests that the use of antibody-based or T cell–based immunotherapy for the treatment of malignant disease may only be successful in a limited number of cases. Even when successful, it is likely that the immune selective pressure imposed on a tumor cell population will facilitate the emergence and expansion of resistant tumor cell subpopulations and eventually the recurrence of malignant lesions. Therefore, it will be important to combine unique types of immunologic and nonimmunologic strategies, which utilize distinct mechanisms to control tumor growth in order to counteract the selective loss of the target antigens and to activate polyclonal immune response. In addition, the concomitant targeting of normal cells, which are crucial for malignant cell survival and proliferation, may counteract the negative impact of tumor cell genetic instability on immunologic and nonimmunologic therapies.

■ CONCLUSION

Over the last decade, our understanding of how the immune system interacts with tumor cells has greatly improved. It is now clear that tumor cell–induced immune suppression and tumor immune escape both represent major obstacles in the ability of the host's immune system to control tumor growth as well as in the successful application of immunotherapy in patients with malignant disease. Furthermore, tumor cell genetic instability allows for the ability of the tumor to alter its antigenic profile and avoid immune destruction. Both of these phenomena remain important obstacles for the treatment of human malignancies through passive and active-specific immunotherapy. Understanding the molecular

mechanisms behind tumor cell–induced immune suppression and tumor cell immune escape will provide valuable insight in designing effective immunotherapeutic strategies for the treatment of malignant diseases.

■ Acknowledgments

This work was supported by an American Society for Dermatologic Surgery Cutting Edge Research Grant (M.C.) and PHS grants RO1CA110249 (SF), RO1CA113861(SF), RO1CA10494(SF), and R01CA105500(SF) awarded by the National Cancer Institute.

■ REFERENCES

1. Ehrlich P. Ueber den jetzigen. Stand der Karzinomforschung. *Ned Tijdschr Geneeskd.* 1909;5:273–290.
2. Bui JD, Schreiber RD. Cancer immunosurveillance, immunoediting and inflammation: independent or interdependent processes? *Curr Opin Immunol.* 2007;19:203–208.
3. Zitvogel L, Tesniere A, Kroemer G. Cancer despite immunosurveillance: immunoselection and immunosubversion. *Nat Rev Immunol.* 2006;6:715–727.
4. Reimana JM, Kmieciak M, Manjili MH, et al. Tumor immunoediting and immunosculpting pathways to cancer progression. *Semin Cancer Biol.* 2007;17:275–287.
5. Willimsky G, Blankenstein T. The adaptive immune response to sporadic cancer. *Immunol Rev.* 2007;220:102–112.
6. Renkvist N, Castelli C, Robbins PF, et al. A listing of human tumor antigens recognized by T cells. *Cancer Immunol Immunother.* 2001;50:51–59.
7. Parmiani G, De Filippo A, Novellino L, et al. Unique human tumor antigens: immunobiology and use in clinical trials. *J Immunol.* 2007;178:1975–1979.
8. Waldhauer I, Steinle A. NK cells and cancer immunosurveillance. *Oncogene.* 2008;27:5932–5943.
9. Prestwich RJ, Errington F, Hatfieldy P, et al. The immune system—is it relevant to cancer development, progression and treatment? *Clin Oncol.* 2008;20:101–112.
10. Vial T, Descotes J. Immunosuppressive drugs and cancer. *Toxicology.* 2003;185:229–240.
11. de Visser KE, Eichten A, Coussens LM. Paradoxical roles of the immune system during cancer development. *Nat Rev Cancer.* 2006;6:24–37.
12. Vajdic CM, McDonald SP, McCredie MR, et al. Cancer incidence before and after kidney transplantation. *JAMA.* 2006;296:2823–2831.
13. Ulrich C, Kanitakis J, Stockfleth E, et al. Skin cancer in organ transplant recipients—where do we stand today? *Am J Transplant.* 2008;8:2192–2198.
14. Bosticardo M, Marangoni F, Aiuti A, et al. Recent advances in understanding the pathophysiology of Wiskott-Aldrich syndrome. *Blood.* 2009;113:6288–6295.
15. Kaplan J, De Domenico I, Ward DM. Chediak-Higashi syndrome. *Curr Opin Hematol.* 2008;15:22–29.
16. MacKie RM, Reid R, Junor B. Fatal melanoma transferred in a donated kidney 16 years after melanoma surgery. *N Engl J Med.* 2003;348:567–568.
17. Milton CA, Barbara J, Cooper J, et al. The transmission of donor-derived malignant melanoma to a renal allograft recipient. *Clin Transplant.* 2006;20:547–550.
18. Pommier Y, Sordet O, Antony S, et al. Apoptosis defects and chemotherapy resistance: molecular interaction maps and networks. *Oncogene.* 2004;23:2934–2949.
19. Campoli M, Ferrone S. Immunotherapy of malignant disease: the coming age of therapeutic monoclonal antibodies. In: DeVita V, Hellman S, Rosenberg S, eds. *Cancer: Principles & Practice of Oncology.* Vol. 23. New York, NY: Lippincott Williams and Wilkins; 2009:1–18.
20. Mocellin S, Mandruzzato S, Bronte V, et al. Part I: Vaccines for solid tumours. *Lancet Oncol.* 2004;5:681–689.
21. Hoos A, Parmiani G, Hege K, et al. A clinical development paradigm for cancer vaccines and related biologics. Cancer Vaccine Clinical Trial Working Group. *J Immunother.* 2007;30:1–15.

22. Bronte V, Mocellin S. Suppressive influences in the immune response to cancer. *J Immunother.* 2009;32:1–11.

23. Hanahan D, Weinberg RA. The hallmarks of cancer. *Cell.* 2000;100: 57–70.

24. Burnet FM. *The Clonal Selection Theory of Acquired Immunity.* Nashville, TN: Vanderbilt University Press; 1959.

25. Bretscher P, Cohn M. A theory of self-nonself discrimination. *Science.* 1970;169:1042–1049.

26. Lafferty KJ, Cunningham AJ. A new analysis of allogeneic interactions. *Aust J Exp Biol Med Sci.* 1975;53:27–42.

27. Matzinger P. Tolerance, danger, and the extended family. *Annu Rev Immunol.* 1994;12:991–1045.

28. Gallucci S, Matzinger P. Danger signals: SOS to the immune system. *Curr Opin Immunol.* 2001;13:114–119.

29. Valmori D, Dutoit V, Lejeune F, et al. Tetramer-guided analysis of TCR beta-chain usage reveals a large repertoire of melan A-specific CD8+ T cells in melanoma patients. *J Immunol.* 2000;165:533–538.

30. Hoffmann TK, Donnenberg AD, Finkelstein SD, et al. Frequencies of tetramer+ T cells specific for the wild-type sequence p53$_{264-272}$ peptide in the circulations of patients with head and neck cancer. *Cancer Res.* 2002;62:3521–3529.

31. Tan T, Coussens LM. Humoral immunity, inflammation and cancer. *Curr Opin Immunol.* 2007;19:209–216.

32. Whiteside TL. The tumor microenvironment and its role in promoting tumor growth. *Oncogene.* 2008;27:5904–5912.

33. Kepp O, Tesniere A, Zitvogel L, et al. The immunogenicity of tumor cell death. *Curr Opin Oncol.* 2009;21:71–76.

34. Yewdell J. To DRiP or not to DRiP: generating peptide ligands for MHC class I molecules. *Mol Immunol.* 2002;39:139–146.

35. Lin ML, Zhan Y, Villadangos JA, et al. The cell biology of cross-presentation and the role of dendritic cell subsets. *Immunol Cell Biol.* 2008;86:353–362.

36. Murshid A, Gong J, Calderwood SK. Heat-shock proteins in cancer vaccines: agents of antigen cross-presentation. *Expert Rev Vaccines.* 2008;7:1019–1030.

37. Thery C, Amigorena S. The cell biology of antigen presentation in dendritic cells. *Curr Opin Immunol.* 2001;13:45–51.

38. Andoniou CE, Coudert JD, Degli-Esposti MA. Killers and beyond: NK-cell-mediated control of immune responses. *Eur J Immunol.* 2008; 38:2938–2942.

39. Dhodapkar MV, Dhodapkar KM, Palucka AK. Interactions of tumor cells with dendritic cells: balancing immunity and tolerance. *Cell Death Differ.* 2008;15:39–50.

40. Ullrich E, Bonmort M, Mignot G, et al. Tumor stress, cell death and the ensuing immune response. *Cell Death Differ.* 2008;15:21–28.

41. Pittet MJ. Behavior of immune players in the tumor microenvironment. *Curr Opin Oncol.* 2009;21:53–59.

42. Pollard J. Tumour educated macrophages promote tumour progression and metastasis. *Nat Rev Cancer.* 2004;4:71–78.

43. Liu YJ. Dendritic cell subsets and lineages and their functions in innate and adaptive immunity. *Cell.* 2001;106:259–262.

44. Curiel TJ, Wei S, Dong H, et al. Blockade of B7-H1 improves myeloid dendritic cell-mediated antitumor immunity. *Nat Med.* 2003;9:562–567.

45. Palucka AK, Ueno H, Fay J, et al. Dendritic cells: a critical player in cancer therapy? *J Immunother.* 2008;31:793–805.

46. André S, Tough DF, Lacroix-Desmazes S, et al. Surveillance of antigen-presenting cells by CD4+ CD25+ regulatory T cells in autoimmunity: immunopathogenesis and therapeutic implications. *Am J Pathol.* 2009;174:1575–1587.

47. Walker LS. Regulatory T cells overturned: the effectors fight back. *Immunology.* 2009;126:466–474.

48. Creusot RJ, Mitchison NA. How DCs control cross-regulation between lymphocytes. *Trends Immunol.* 2004;25:126–131.

49. Heath WR, Belz GT, Behrens GM, et al. Cross-presentation, dendritic cell subsets, and the generation of immunity to cellular antigens. *Immunol Rev.* 2004;199:9–26.

50. Mazzoni A, Segal DM. Controlling the Toll road to dendritic cell polarization. *J Leukoc Biol.* 2004;75:721–730.

51. Colombo MP, Trinchieri G. Interleukin-12 in anti-tumor immunity and immunotherapy. *Cytokine Growth Factor Rev.* 2002;13:155–268.

52. Barry M, Bleackley RC. Cytotoxic T lymphocytes: all roads lead to death. *Nat Rev Immunol.* 2002;2:401–409.

53. Bryceson YT, Ljunggren H. Tumor cell recognition by the NK cell activating receptor NKG2D. *Eur J Immunol.* 2008;38:2957–2961.

54. Jonjic S, Polic B, Krmpotic A. Viral inhibitors of NKG2D ligands: friends or foes of immune surveillance? *Eur J Immunol.* 2008;38:2952–2956.

55. Zimmer J, Andrès E, Hentges F. NK cells and Treg cells: a fascinating dance cheek to cheek. *Eur J Immunol.* 2008;38:2942–2945.

56. Werner H. Tolerance and reactivity of NK cells: two sides of the same coin? *Eur J Immunol.* 2008:38;2930–2933.

57. Croft M, So T, Duan W, et al. The significance of OX40 and OX40L to T-cell biology and immune disease. *Immunol Rev.* 2009;229:173–191.

58. Gao N, Jennings P, Yuan D. Requirements for the natural killer cell-mediated induction of IgG1 and IgG2a expression in B lymphocytes. *Int Immunol.* 2008;20:645–657.

59. Coffman RL, Mocci S, Ogarra A. The stability and reversibility of Th1 and Th2 populations. *Curr Top Microbiol Immunol.* 1999;238:1–12.

60. Locksley RM. Nine lives: plasticity among T helper cell subsets. *J Exp Med.* 2009;206:1643–1646.

61. Pulendran B. Modulating TH1/TH2 responses with microbes, dendritic cells, and pathogen recognition receptors. Immunol Res. 2004;29:187–196.

62. Lu B, Finn OJ. T-cell death and cancer immune tolerance. *Cell Death Differ.* 2008;15:70–79.

63. Kersh EN, Shaw AS, Allen PM. Fidelity of T cell activation through multistep T cell receptor zeta phosphorylation. *Science.* 1998;281: 572–575.

64. Whiteside TL. Tricks tumors use to escape from immune control. *Oral Oncol.* 2009;45:e119–e123.

65. Yang L, Carbone DP. Tumor-host immune interactions and dendritic cell dysfunction. *Adv Cancer Res.* 2004;92:13–27.

66. Bennaceur K, Chapman J, Brikci-Nigassa L, et al. Dendritic cells dysfunction in tumour environment. *Cancer Lett.* 2008;272:186–196.

67. Mantovani A, Allavena P, Sozzani S, et al. Chemokines in the recruitment and shaping of the leukocyte infiltrate of tumors. *Semin Cancer Biol.* 2004;14:155–160.

68. Siveen KS, Kuttan G. Role of macrophages in tumour progression. *Immunol Lett.* 2009;123:97–102.

69. Rivoltini L, Carrabba M, Huber V, et al. Immunity to cancer: attack and escape in T lymphocyte-tumor cell interaction. *Immunol Rev.* 2002;188:97–113.

70. Singh RK, Varney ML. IL-8 expression in malignant melanoma: implications in growth and metastasis. *Histol Histopathol.* 2000;15: 843–849.

71. Campoli M, Ferrone S. Tumor escape mechanisms: potential role of soluble HLA antigens and NK cells activating ligands. *Tissue Antigens.* 2008;72:321–334.

72. Ivanov VN, Bhoumik A, Ronai Z. Death receptors and melanoma resistance to apoptosis. *Oncogene.* 2003;22:3152–3161.

73. Jiang H, Chess L. How the immune system achieves self-nonself discrimination during adaptive immunity. *Adv Immunol.* 2009;102: 95–133.

74. Blank C, Mackensen A. Contribution of the PD-L1/PD-1 pathway to T-cell exhaustion: an update on implications for chronic infections and tumor evasion. *Cancer Immunol Immunother.* 2007;56:739–745.

75. Chen L. Co-inhibitory molecules of the B7-CD28 family in the control of T-cell immunity. *Nat Rev Immunol.* 2004;4:336–347.

76. Pirtskhalaishvili G, Shurin GV, Esche C, et al. Cytokine-mediated protection of human dendritic cells from prostate cancer-induced apoptosis is regulated by the Bcl-2 family of proteins. *Br J Cancer.* 2000;83:506–513.

77. Esche C, Shurin GV, Kirkwood JM, et al. Tumor necrosis factor-alpha-promoted expression of Bcl-2 and inhibition of mitochondrial cytochrome c release mediated resistance of mature dendritic cells to melanoma-induced apoptosis. *Clin Cancer Res.* 2001;7:974s–979s.

78. Mantovani A, Sica A, Allavena P, et al. Tumor-associated macrophages and the related myeloid-derived suppressor cells as a paradigm of the diversity of macrophage activation. *Hum Immunol.* 2009;70:325–330.

79. Ostrand-Rosenberg S, Sinha P. Myeloid-derived suppressor cells: linking inflammation and cancer. *J Immunol.* 2009;182:4499–4506.

80. Pentcheva-Hoang T, Corse E, Allison JP. Negative regulators of T-cell activation: potential targets for therapeutic intervention in cancer, autoimmune disease, and persistent infections. *Immunol Rev.* 2009; 229:67–87.

81. Nizar S, Copier J, Meyer B, et al. T-regulatory cell modulation: the future of cancer immunotherapy? *Br J Cancer.* 2009;100:1697–1703.

82. Onyango P. Genomics and cancer. *Curr Opin Oncol.* 2002;14:79–85.

83. Chang CC, Campoli M, Ferrone S. Classical and nonclassical HLA class I antigen and NK Cell-activating ligand changes in malignant cells: current challenges and future directions. *Adv Cancer Res.* 2005;93:189–234.

84. Campoli M, Ferrone S. HLA antigen changes in malignant cells: epigenetic mechanisms and biologic significance. *Oncogene.* 2008;27: 5869–5885.

85. Medema JP, de Jong J, Peltenburg LT, et al. Blockade of the granzyme B/perforin pathway through overexpression of the serine protease inhibitor PI-9/SPI-6 constitutes a mechanism for immune escape by tumors. *Proc Natl Acad Sci U S A.* 2001;98:11515–11520.

86. Trapani JA, Sutton VR, Smyth MJ. CTL granules: evolution of vesicles essential for combating virus infections. *Immunol Today.* 1999;20:351–356.

87. Parmiani G, Castelli C, Dalerba P, et al. Cancer immunotherapy with peptide-based vaccines: what have we achieved? Where are we going? *J Natl Cancer Inst.* 2002;94:805–818.

88. Finn OJ. Cancer immunology. *N Engl J Med.* 2008;358:2704–2715.

89. Melief CJ. Cancer immunotherapy by dendritic cells. *Immunity.* 2008;3:372–383.

90. Higano CS, Schellhammer PF, Small EJ, et al. Integrated data from 2 randomized, double-blind, placebo-controlled, phase 3 trials of active cellular immunotherapy with sipuleucel-T in advanced prostate cancer. *Cancer.* 2009;115:3670–3679.

91. Shanmugham LN, Petrarca C, Frydas S, et al. IL-15 an immunoregulatory and anti-cancer cytokine. Recent advances. *J Exp Clin Cancer Res.* 2006;25:529–536.

92. Tesmer LA, Lundy SK, Sarkar S, et al. Th17 cells in human disease. *Immunol Rev.* 2008;223:87–113.

93. Rudd CE, Taylor A, Schneider H. CD28 and CTLA-4 coreceptor expression and signal transduction. *Immunol Rev.* 2009;229:12–26.

94. Esteva FJ, Valero V, Booser D, et al. Phase II study of weekly docetaxel and trastuzumab for patients with HER-2-overexpressing metastatic breast cancer. *J Clin Oncol.* 2002;20:1800–1808.

95. Köstler WJ, Steger GG, Soleiman A, et al. Monitoring of serum Her-2/neu predicts histopathological response to neoadjuvant trastuzumab-based therapy for breast cancer. *Anticancer Res.* 2004; 24:1127–1130.

96. Anim JT, John B, Abdulsathar SSA, et al. Relationship between the expression of various markers and prognostic factors in breast cancer. *Acta Histochem.* 2005;107:87–93.

97. Campoli M, Ferrone, S. Tumor induced immune suppression and immune escape: mechanisms and impact on the outcome of immunotherapy of malignant disease. In: Disis M, ed. *Immunotherapy of Cancer.* Totowa, NJ: The Humana Press Inc.; 2005:263–284.

Methods for Development of Monoclonal Antibody Therapeutics

Danielle DiCara and Ahuva Nissim

■ INTRODUCTION

Monoclonal antibodies (mAbs) represent an almost limitless source of therapeutic and diagnostic reagents and have been significantly utilized for treatment in various diseases. Following the production of mouse mAbs by hybridoma technology, methods of antibody engineering have been developed that allow generation of antibodies against almost unlimited targets, including proteins with cross-species sequence homology and even self-antigens. The initial limitations of mouse mAb therapy, due to immunogenicity and the subsequent difficulties encountered with human hybridomas, were overcome by gradual replacement of murine with human sequences. This process began with human–mouse chimeric antibodies, followed by humanized antibodies and finally the generation of antibodies entirely from human sequences. Fully human antibodies derived both in vitro using display technologies and in vivo using transgenic mice have now been approved by the FDA, paving the way for the replacement of traditional murine antibodies with these robust technologies. In addition, antibody effector functions and pharmacokinetic properties can be tailored for a given clinical setting. Here we discuss common means of generating specific antibodies and some aspects of antibody engineering that may enhance their clinical utility.

■ GENERATION OF SPECIFIC ANTIBODIES

Monoclonal antibody development via mouse hybridoma technology

Originally, mAbs for therapy (1,2) were produced by the mouse hybridoma technology, developed by Kohler and Milstein in 1975 (3). To generate antibodies by this method, a mouse is immunized with a specific antigen, usually in the presence of an adjuvant and with several "booster" immunizations. Subsequently, B cells are removed from either the spleen or lymph nodes and fused in the laboratory with a mouse myeloma cell line such as Sp2/0, NS1, NS0, or X63Ag8, which are negative for the key nucleotide biosynthesis enzyme hypoxanthine guanine phosphoribosyltransferase (HGPRT). Unfused myeloma cells are killed by the use of selective "HAT" growth media containing

hypoxanthine–aminopterin–thymidine, which blocks de novo nucleotide biosynthesis and forces the use of the HGPRT-dependent salvage pathway, enabling only B cell–rescued myelomas to survive. Cells are then amplified, cloned by limiting dilution, and screened for antibody production (4). Early hybridomas secreted immunoglobulin chains derived from both the myeloma and the immunized B cell; however, use of immunoglobulin-negative myeloma cells soon enabled routine generation of exclusively B cell–derived antibody.

Mouse mAb administered to patients for therapy generally induced a strong anti–mouse antibody response, and this led to the development of chimeric antibodies and eventually to humanized antibodies. Chimeric antibodies consist of murine variable regions fused to human constant regions (5,6); "humanized" antibodies retain only the murine complementarity-determining regions (CDRs), grafted onto a human antibody backbone (7,8). In some cases, additional point mutations in the framework regions may be required for effective transfer of the antigen-binding properties of the CDRs (9). Similar approaches in which only parts of the CDRs are transferred to the human antibody scaffold include "resurfacing," in which only surface-exposed CDR residues are transferred (10,11), and specificity-determining residue grafting, involving only residues (both CDR and framework derived) likely to be crucial to the antibody–antigen interaction (12).

In a recent analysis of antibody trials reporting immunogenicity, the percentage of mAbs giving "marked" (observed in 15% or more of the patients) anti-antibody responses was 84%, 40%, and 9% for murine, chimeric, and humanized antibodies, respectively (13). The authors point out, however, that low immunogenicity cannot be assumed for humanized antibodies; for example, approximately 65% of patients developed an anti-antibody response on repeated administration of the humanized antibody huAb A33 (14). The human anti-human antibody (HAHA) responses in this study appeared as two distinct types of serological responses. HAHA type I (49% of patients) displayed an early onset peak of HAHA, which declined with further dosing. HAHA type II (17% of patients) was characterized by a later onset of HAHA and then by increasing levels with subsequent therapeutic dosing. The type II response correlated with infusion reactions. No patient with a type I response developed an infusion adverse event (14). To date, at least five chimeric and nine humanized antibodies have been approved by the FDA, along with three murine antibodies (15).

It is now possible to produce fully human mAbs from transgenic mice (16). Targeted disruption of endogenous heavy chain (HC) and kappa light chain (LC) loci, together with introduction of human HC and kappa LC loci, led to mice producing fully human antibodies on immunization (17,18). This technology has recently "come of age" with the regulatory approval of the fully human, mouse-derived, epidermal growth factor receptor (EGFR)-targeting mAb, panitumumab. Transgenic mouse–derived mAbs are usually high affinity due to in vivo affinity maturation and unlike fragment antibody technologies do not require reverse engineering into a complete immunoglobulin format.

Generation of human antibody fragments using display technologies

Intact antibodies are multidomain proteins consisting of target-binding variable domains and constant domains, which are responsible for effector functions. The typical antibody structure consists of four polypeptide chains: two identical HCs and two identical LCs. The domains are linked by HC–HC and HC–LC disulfide bonds (Fig. 2.1). Antibody fragments can be generated either by proteolytic digestion or by genetic engineering. Papain digestion results in cleavage of the HCs at a site N-terminal to the hinge disulfides, causing separation of the two Fab regions from each other and from the Fc. Pepsin cleaves at several locations in the Fc and generates bivalent F(ab)2 fragments. Recombinant gene technology allows generation of even smaller antigen-binding fragments, such as the single-chain fragment variable (scFv), which consists of the antigen-binding domains (VH and VL) connected by a short polypeptide linker. A variety of fragments consisting of a single antigen-binding domain have also been

developed (19,20). Antibody fragments such as scFv and domain antibodies can be expressed in *E. coli* and can readily be produced in high quantities for any application.

Antibody fragments have been used extensively in the context of display technologies. Such technologies enable generation of antigen-specific antibody fragments in vitro, which can then be reverse engineered into a full immunoglobulin if required. In vitro display technologies allow generation of antibodies against toxic or self-antigens (21,22), increased control over selection pressures, and importantly give the option of starting with human antibody sequences (23).

Phage display

The utilization of the phage display technology (24,25) for antibody selection (26) is a robust means for generation of specific antibodies. Small antibody fragments are expressed as fusion proteins on the surface of bacteriophage and physical selection ("biopanning") is used to isolate, from huge, diverse libraries, phage-bearing antibodies of the desired specificity (Fig. 2.2). In the simplest form, a protein antigen is immobilized on a plastic surface and exposed to a library of antibody–phage fusions; unbound phage are then washed away and antigen-binding phage eluted and amplified. Since each phage packages the DNA encoding the coat protein–antibody fusion, there is a physical linkage between phenotype (specific antigen binding) and genotype (antibody gene sequence), enabling phage isolated purely on their binding properties to be amplified and characterized (27). Typically a phage pool would be enriched for antigen-specific phage by several rounds of selection, with each round followed by amplification in bacteria. Biopanning on tagged antigen in solution, which is subsequently immobilized along with antigen-bound phage on tag-binding beads, enables even greater control over selection stringency and avoids adsorbing the antigen onto plastic. Phage display is highly versatile and can be used to screen against antigens not only in protein format (28), but also on cells (29,30), in tissue sections, and

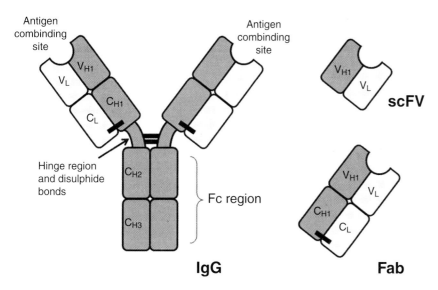

FIGURE 2.1 Representation of the subunit composition of an IgG antibody. *(Dark gray)* Heavy chain sequence; *(light gray)* light chain sequence; and *(thick black lines)* interchain disulfide bonds (intrachain disulfides are not shown).

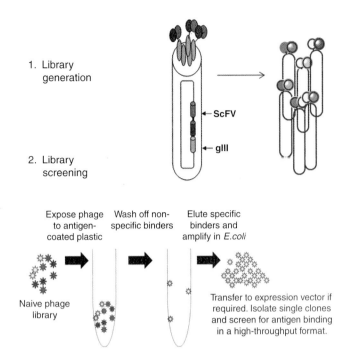

1. Library
   generation

2. Library
   screening

← ScFV

← gIII

Expose phage
to antigen-
coated plastic

Wash off non-
specific binders

Elute specific
binders and
amplify in *E.coli*

Naïve phage
library

Transfer to expression vector if
required. Isolate single clones
and screen for antigen binding
in a high-throughput format.

FIGURE 2.2 Outline of phage display library generation and screening. (1) Each phage packages the DNA sequence of the scFv–pIII fusion protein expressed on its surface. (2) In iterative selections, the phage-bearing scFv–pIII fusions are exposed to immobilized antigen. Unbound phage are removed by washing and specifically bound phage are eluted and amplified in a bacterial host.

even in vivo (31). Creative biopanning strategies can be used to select antibodies with particular properties, such as the ability to become internalized within target-expressing cells (32,33). Phage display can be used with many different antibody formats including scFv (28), Fab fragments (34), and single VH or VL domain antibodies (35).

Phage antibody libraries have been generated from immunized animals and infected humans (36). More universal nonbiased libraries were built from a pool of healthy donors producing naïve libraries, enabling further bypassing of in vivo tolerance mechanisms. Nevertheless, repertoires originating from healthy individuals are still biased due to medical histories and environmental factors. The alternative approach was to develop libraries, which are based on in vitro rearrangements of V gene segments. The concept was based on mimicking the in vivo immunoglobulin gene rearrangement artificially in vitro. The rationale was that semisynthetic repertoires are not intrinsically biased and therefore can be used for selection of antibodies against a wider range of targets (22,27), including self-antigens and antigens found difficult to target with hybridoma technology (37).

Ribosome display

Ribosome display (38,39) shares many properties with phage display, including the phenotype–genotype linkage and iterative selection on antigen in vitro. Cell-free systems are used to transcribe and translate a DNA antibody library, using conditions under which the nascent polypeptide remains noncovalently attached to the ribosome. Complex-stabilizing

conditions might include low temperature, high magnesium, and the lack of a stop codon (39,40). Selections are then performed with the antibody, mRNA, and ribosome complexes (40–42). After selection, the recovered mRNA is amplified by RT-PCR. In the related approach mRNA display, the mRNA and transcribed protein are linked covalently via a small adaptor molecule such as puromycin (39). Today ribosome display is mainly used in combination with phage display for affinity maturation of selected phage, a technique to which it is particularly suited given the intrinsic involvement of a potentially error-prone PCR step, and the ability to generate larger libraries than phage display due to the avoidance of a cell transformation step. CAT-354, a human IgG4 targeting IL-13 for the potential treatment of severe asthma (43), was developed using both phage and ribosome display and has reached phase II clinical trials.

Eukaryotic cell display

A key advantage of eukaryotic cell display systems is the availability of the eukaryotic expression system, including posttranslational modification and the presence of chaperones and foldases. Display levels of different scFv on phage can vary and have been positively correlated with their expression level in *E. coli* as soluble proteins, potentially open therefore to influences such as codon bias (44). In addition, similar to bacterial cell display (45), eukaryotic cell display exposes large numbers of antibody fragments per cell; yeast cells can display over 10^4 scFv per cell (46). This enables screening by flow cytometry. For example, yeast cells expressing myc-tagged scFv as fusions with the cell surface receptor *a*-agglutinin are incubated with fluorescently labeled antigen and cells with the highest degree of binding are then isolated by flow cytometry (46). Differences in expression are controlled by colabeling of the myc tag with a different fluorophore (46). Yeast display has been used very successfully for affinity maturation, resulting in scFv with a dissociation constant (kd) less than 50 pM and dissociation half-lives of several days (47,48).

Methods for mammalian cell display have also been reported recently (49–52). Ho and colleagues expressed myc-tagged scFv on the surface of HEK293 cells as fusions with the transmembrane domain of the PDGF receptor: similar to yeast display, cells were then exposed to a tagged antigen and screened by flow cytometry. The method was used successfully for affinity maturation of a hotspot-mutated anti-CD22 scFv (50). One limitation of this method is the potential for transfection of individual cells with multiple different antibodies, complicating selection. An alternative method starts with peripheral blood mononuclear cells isolated from immunized human volunteers, from which antigen-specific B cells are separated and a library of scFv–PDGFR transmembrane domain fusion proteins generated and expressed on the surface of BHK cells using a Sindbis virus expression system (49). A low multiplicity of infection discouraged generation of transformants expressing multiple different scFv clones. A lentivirus-mediated scFv–Fc display method has also been reported and used to demonstrate tyrosine sulfation of the displayed fusion proteins (52), illustrating the advantage of mammalian cells in providing posttranslational modification. Sulfation of tyrosine residues occurs in the trans-golgi network and has been shown to contribute substantially to the antigen-binding activity of some antibodies (53,54).

OPTIMIZING ANTIBODY UPTAKE AND PHARMACOKINETICS

Optimizing the pharmacokinetics of antibodies is an important factor in assessing their clinical potential. The nature of the desired alterations may differ between precise situations: for example, increasing antibody half-life may enhance a therapeutic effect, while decreasing the half-life may reduce off-target exposure and improve the target-to-background ratio. Pharmacokinetics depends on affinity, molecular stability, tissue penetration, and clearance as well as factors such as antigen density. Antibody effector functions, either Fc-mediated or introduced by conjugation, can also be tailored to alter pharmacokinetics and make candidate mAbs better drug candidates.

Affinity and the "binding-site barrier"

High affinity for the target antigen can improve specific delivery and reduce dosing requirements. However, increasing affinity indefinitely does not necessarily improve tumor targeting and may increase background signal or reduce tumor penetration. A seminal study on anti-HER-2/*neu* scFv demonstrated that detectable tumor retention required an affinity of at least 10^{-7} to 10^{-8} M, but that the degree of retention plateaued at an affinity of 10^{-9} M, and scFv with affinities of 10^{-10} and 10^{-11} M showed increased retention in the blood but not in the tumor (55,56). It is possible that high affinity may result in increased binding to normal tissues expressing low levels of the target antigen (compared with higher levels in the tumor): Zuckier and colleagues demonstrated this concept in vivo using beads coated with either "high-density" or "low-density" antigen that a high-affinity antibody bound to both types of bead, but a lower affinity antibody bound only to the beads coated with antigen at "high density" (57). Tumor penetration may also be affected: the "binding-site barrier" proposed after mathematical modeling studies suggested that affinity for the antigen itself may retard antibody penetration, resulting in a heterogeneous distribution throughout the tumor (58,59), and there is experimental support for this process (60). This "binding-site barrier" is distinct to any physical barrier that may be present, such as increased hydrostatic pressure due to poor local drainage, and may be partially overcome by increased antibody dose (60).

In general, however, a minimum affinity is required for specific targeting (56) and a high-affinity antibody may lead to improved overall uptake despite a more heterogeneous distribution. Affinity maturation occurs naturally in vivo but can also be performed in vitro using the display technologies (61,62). Generally some form of mutagenesis or diversification step is followed by reselection under stringent conditions. "Affinity" selections involve a limiting density of antigen, such that higher affinity antibodies outcompete lower affinity binders, while "off-rate" selections involve incubating tagged antigen–bound phage with soluble, untagged competitor antigen prior to recovery and amplification of the tagged antigen–bound phage (61). A common diversification approach is chain shuffling, in which the VL or VH domain of a selected antibody might be replaced with a large repertoire of the same type of domain (63). Barbas and colleagues described an approach termed "CDR walking," involving sequential optimization of chosen CDRs through the targeted introduction of diversity with degenerate oligonucleotides (64). Additional methods for introducing relatively random diversity include error-prone PCR (61) and the use of mutator strains of *E. coli* (65).

Size, avidity, and polymer conjugation

Antibody pharmacokinetics depends not only on the affinity, but also on the size of the antibody fragment. The term "enhanced permeability and retention" was coined to describe the phenomenon of prolonged retention within the tumor of long-circulating macromolecules, due to the enhanced permeability of tumor blood vessels combined with slow venous return and poor lymphatic drainage (66,67). Smaller proteins, however, diffuse faster and are considered to exhibit more rapid tumor penetration as well as faster clearance. Unlike scFv (~28 kD) and Fab (~55 kD), proteins approaching 70 kD are above the threshold for normal glomerular filtration (68) and clear more slowly. Antibody variable domains have been found in or engineered into a wide range of formats, from 15-kD single domains to 165-kD trivalent Fab_3 (19). Perhaps one of the simplest forms of manipulation is the shortening of the scFv VH–VL linker sequence, leading to scFv "diabodies" (69) or "triabodies" (70,71). Multiple copies of an antigen-binding fragment increase the avidity (the functional affinity) and enhance tumor targeting. A recent study by Adams and colleagues, in which a scFv, homodimeric scFv and a monovalent, heterodimeric scFv were compared for tumor targeting, suggests that the improvement in targeting with the homodimer was due to the increase in valence and independent of the increase in size (72). In a xenograft model comparing radioiodinated scFv, diabody, and IgG formats, the diabody fared favorably, with greater tumor uptake than the scFv and faster clearance from the blood than the IgG (73). Formats such as minibodies (~80 kD) and scFv–Fc (~100 kD) combine bivalency with increased size. An additional factor to be considered when Fc regions are introduced is the binding of IgG to FcRn, a pH-dependent interaction mediated by the CH2 and CH3 domains (74), which rescues the immunoglobulin from degradation and thus prolongs the serum half-life. Targeted mutation of residues key to this interaction can result in a dramatic reduction of scFv–Fc serum half-life (75).

Another means by which to prolong the half-life of antibody fragments is conjugation to polyethylene glycol (PEG), a process termed PEGylation (76). PEGylation increases molecular size, reduces renal clearance, and can improve stability to temperature, pH change, and proteolysis (77,78). Several PEGylated drugs have been approved by the FDA, including certolizumab pegol (Cimzia; UCB), a humanized TNF-specific Fab′ conjugated to PEG, which received approval in 2008 for use against Crohn disease. Certolizumab pegol has a half-life of approximately 14 days in patients, approaching that of IgG (79). In contrast to IgG, PEGylated fragments should not trigger any Fc-mediated effects, an advantage likely to be of use in the context of an anti-inflammatory therapy (80). More recently, modification with colominic acid (polysialylation) has been investigated as a more natural and biodegradable alternative to PEGylation (81). Polysialylation has been shown to increase the half-life of biologicals such as asparaginase (82) and insulin

(83) as well as single-chain Fv and Fab fragments (84,85). The method of conjugation can be important: in one example, Constantinou and colleagues found that amine-directed coupling greatly reduced the antigen-binding of an anti-CEA scFv, but were able to overcome this by site-specific thiol coupling. Similar to PEGylation, polysialylation can also reduce antigenicity, for example, prolonging the half-life of circulating asparaginase even in asparaginase-immunized mice (86). This may be an enormous benefit for applications requiring continuous or repeated dosing. Numerous factors thus impact antibody half-life in serum and uptake in tumors. For extensive further discussion on this area, the reader is directed to reviews by Beckman et al. and Thurber and colleagues (87,88).

■ ANTIBODY EFFECTOR FUNCTIONS

Antibodies can mediate biological activities via multiple mechanisms (Fig. 2.3). Even "naked," unconjugated antibodies can elicit biological responses in several ways, some

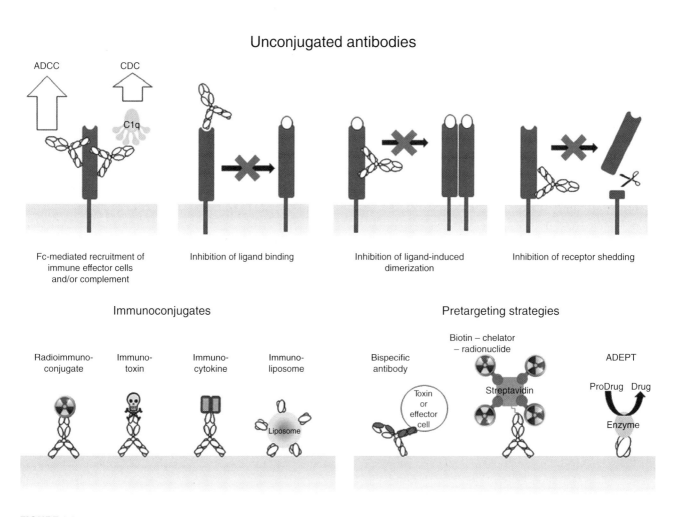

FIGURE 2.3 Potential mechanisms for antibody-mediated biological effects. Top panel: Possible mechanisms by which an unconjugated antibody specific for a cell surface receptor might affect cell signaling. **Lower panel:** Strategies for improving antibody effector functions. (Adapted from Hudis CA. Trastuzumab—mechanism of action and use in clinical practice. *N Engl J Med* 2007;357(1):39–51; Carter P. Improving the efficacy of antibody-based cancer therapies. *Nat Rev Cancer* 2001;1(2):118–129.)

mediated by the Fc region and others Fc-independent, as is illustrated by antibodies targeting growth factor receptors. It is well known that growth factor receptors and/or their activating ligands are overexpressed in cancers promoting uncontrolled cell growth and resistance to chemotherapy. Antibodies can be used for therapy by binding to the growth factor receptor and blocking the activity. Anti-EGFR cetuximab (Erbitux) is able to inhibit the tyrosine kinase activity of EGFR and block growth signals (89). In addition to inhibiting the binding of activating ligand epidermal growth factor, cetuximab binding sterically prevents EGFR from adopting the dimerization-competent conformation required for activation (90). Antibody OA-5D5 (91) antagonizes signaling from the MET receptor tyrosine kinase, a pivotal molecule in regeneration and tumor metastasis (92,93), and has been shown to inhibit growth of glioblastoma and pancreatic cancer xenografts in vivo (91,94). OA-5D5 is derived from an antibody originally identified as a MET agonist, which proved to be antagonistic only in monovalent form and was engineered into a "one-armed" format consisting of an Fc region and a single antigen-binding "arm" (91). Therefore, although a bivalent antibody format increases avidity, inappropriate receptor activation by antibody-induced dimerization may necessitate a monovalent format for certain cases. Another growth factor receptor–targeted antibody, trastuzumab (Herceptin), recognizes the HER2 protein (product of the ErbB2 oncogene, also known as ERBB2/neu). HER2 can transform cells independently of ligand when overexpressed (95); it has no known high-affinity soluble ligand but resembles the ligand-bound form of other members of the ErbB family, and is their preferred heterodimerization partner (96–98). ErbB2 amplification occurs in 30% of breast cancers and is linked to prognosis (99). The impact of trastuzumab in the clinic has been profound (100). As well as inhibiting the growth of HER2-overexpressing cell lines in vitro (101,102), experiments with mice deficient in FcγR support a considerable role for Fc-mediated functions (103). Possible activity-contributing mechanisms include prevention of receptor shedding, inhibition of HER2/EGFR heterodimerization, and increased ligand-induced EGFR downregulation (due to a trastuzumab-induced increase in EGFR homooligomerization) (104). Pertuzumab (Omnitarg, parent antibody 2C4), an anti-HER2 recognizing a different epitope to trastuzumab (96,105,106), has a greater inhibitory effect on both HER2/EGFR and HER2/ErbB3 heterodimerization (104,106,107) although, unlike trastuzumab, it does not inhibit receptor shedding. In preclinical xenograft studies pertuzumab or 2C4 demonstrated growth inhibition in models unresponsive to trastuzumab (107); in addition, growth inhibition was observed with a PEGylated Fab fragment as well as the bivalent, Fc-containing parent antibody (107). A phase III trial combining the two agents is currently underway.

In addition to epitope-dependent functions, there are now many ways to tailor antibody effector functions such as Fc-mediated tumor cell killing, using both chemical and genetic modifications (73,108). Effector functions include antibody-dependent cellular cytotoxicity (ADCC), mediated by Fc receptors (FcR), and complement-dependent cytotoxicity (CDC), mediated by binding to proteins of the complement cascade. In the case of ADCC, interaction of the Fc region (see Fig. 2.1) with FcR (particularly FcγRI and FcγRIIIA) on immune effector cells leads to lysis or phagocytosis of the antibody-bound cell (109). Alternatively, interaction of the Fc region with the series of soluble blood proteins that constitute the antibody-dependent complement activation pathway (e.g., C1q, C3, and C4) results in CDC. Choice of antibody isotype is important: human IgG1 is more efficient in supporting ADCC while IgG2 and IgG4 are less effective in mediating ADCC and CDC. While the inability of IgG4 to cross-link identical antigens makes it attractive for applications where such cross-linking is undesirable, use of this isotype is complicated by its ability to undergo Fab arm exchange in vivo, resulting in the generation of bispecific antibodies (110).

Modification of Fc-mediated functions

Modification of the Fc region now enables the tuning of many Fc-mediated functions such as ADCC and CDC (15,109). For example, it has been shown that defucosylation of Fc carbohydrates improves ADCC by enhancing binding of the antibody to FcγRIIIA (111). Many therapeutic antibodies are produced in CHO cells due to their high productivity; these cells have strong fucosylation activity (111); however, a FUT8 knockout CHO cell line was recently established to address this (112). Mutation of the Fc region has led to improvements in ADCC and CDC (113–115), as well as alterations of serum half-life (75).

Arming mAb with effector functions

The emerging display technologies resulted in many antibody fragment candidates that could potentially be suitable for therapeutic application. The selected antibody fragment can be reverse engineered into a full immunoglobulin to obtain effector function. Alternatively (or in addition), effector functions can be engineered into an antibody regardless of the characteristics, presence, or absence of an Fc region. A number of these are shown in Figure 2.3 and include the conjugation of radionuclides, drugs (73), or toxins (116,117). At least three such immunoconjugates have been approved by the FDA for cancer therapy, including two murine CD20-specific radioimmunoconjugates for non-Hodgkin lymphoma (tositumomab, a ^{131}I-labeled IgG2a (118), and ibritumomab tiuxetan, a ^{90}Y-conjugated IgG1) (119). A humanized CD33-specific IgG4 conjugated to the cytotoxic calicheamicin (gemtuzumab ozogamicin) has been approved for acute myeloid leukemia (120).

Other approaches aim to selectively stimulate the immune system. Recombinant fusion proteins termed immunocytokines combine a specific antibody with a cytokine such as TNFα (121), IL-2 (122), granulocyte/macrophage colony-stimulating factor (123–125), IL-12 (126), or IL-15 (123). As with other immunoconjugates, the aim is to achieve effective levels of the conjugated moiety in the tumor microenvironment, while avoiding systemic toxicities. Bispecific antibodies have also been generated that can, through a different epitope on each, bind both the target tissue and cytotoxic T cells, targeting the tissue for lysis (127,128). At least two bispecific antibodies of the Fc-lacking, single-chain antibody based "BiTE" (bispecific T-cell engager) format have progressed to clinical trials (129). Recently, it was reported that in a study of CD3/CD19-specific blinatumomab in relapsed non-Hodgkin lymphoma patients, complete or partial responses were observed in 11 of 38 patients, including all 7 patients in the 0.060 mg/m^2 per day group (129).

Antibody-directed enzyme prodrug therapy (ADEPT) is a pretargeting strategy involving administration of an antibody–enzyme conjugate, followed by a prodrug that is then locally converted to a cytotoxic (130). Advantages of ADEPT include amplification of the cytotoxic effect due to the involvement of a catalytic enzyme. Pretargeting systems based on the separation of the tumor targeting and radionuclide injection steps have also been used for radiotherapy (131).

■ RECENT MILESTONES IN ANTIBODY APPROVALS

▨ Human antibodies

The recent FDA approvals of adalimumab (Humira) and panitumumab (Vectibix) mark two major milestones in the development of engineered therapeutic antibodies, representing the first fully human phage-derived antibody and the first fully human transgenic mouse–derived antibody to be approved, respectively. Anti-TNFα antibody adalimumab was derived from phage display and is used to treat rheumatoid arthritis. The human mAb adalimumab appears to be less immunogenic than the chimeric infliximab (Remicade) (132), although the percentage of patients with anti-antibody responses varies widely between reports and direct comparison with infliximab is complicated by factors such as different methods of anti-antibody response detection, the type of disease being treated (e.g., Crohn disease vs. rheumatoid arthritis), and the effect of concomitant immunosuppressive treatment (132). In a cumulative report on 1062 patients from three clinical trials, approximately 5% (58/1062) of patients developed anti-adalimumab antibodies (133). Concomitant methotrexate treatment was associated with a reduction of the anti-adalimumab response rate to 1%, compared with 12% of patients on adalimumab alone (133).

More recently, the fully human EGFR-blocking antibody panitumumab was approved for EGFR-positive colorectal cancer, following a phase III multicenter, randomized trial (134,135). Panitumumab is a highly potent IgG2 derived from a transgenic "humanized" mouse, and is the first antibody derived by this method to be approved by the FDA (16). In the phase III study, panitumumab with best supportive care (BSC) resulted in a 46% decrease in the progression rate compared with BSC alone. EGFR-blocking antibody therapy has been demonstrated previously with the chimeric IgG1 cetuximab, which is approved for both colorectal cancer and head and neck squamous cell carcinoma (136). Interestingly, of the 185 patients tested for anti-panitumumab antibodies, none were found positive (135). There have also been reports of successful administration of panitumumab following adverse reactions to cetuximab (137,138). Early clinical trials reported a stronger association of skin rashes with panitumumab than cetuximab; however, skin rash in response to EGFR-directed treatment is associated with a positive response to treatment (139,140) and appears to be a class-specific effect (141).

The question of therapeutic antibody immunogenicity will surely become clearer as more human antibodies are used in the clinic. This will probably occur soon as many antibodies and antibody fragments derived from both phage display and transgenic mice are now in clinical and preclinical trials. Additional transgenic mouse–derived antibodies now in phase III development include anti-CD4, anti-CD20, two anti-CTLA-4, anti-RANKL, anti-TNFα, a neutralizing antibody against the common (p40) chain of IL-12 and IL-23 and an anti-EGFR, zalutumumab (proposed trade name: HuMax-EGFr) (16). Zalutumumab is similar to panitumumab in that both are fully human in sequence and show greater potency in mouse models than M225, the parent antibody of cetuximab (142,143); however, they differ in isotype; IgG1 zalutumumab may therefore show enhanced Fc-dependent cell killing compared with IgG2 panitumumab (16).

▨ Antibody fragments

Since 2006, two additional Fab constructs have joined abciximab (ReoPro) in the list of FDA-approved antibody fragments (4). Approved in 1994, abciximab is a chimeric IgG1 Fab that binds the platelet integrin αIIbβ3 and reduces platelet thrombus formation, and is approved by the FDA for a broad range of patients undergoing percutaneous coronary intervention and patients with unstable angina not responding to conventional medical therapy when percutaneous coronary intervention is planned within 24 hours (144). Ranibizumab (Lucentis) is a humanized VEGF-A blocker, approved for wet age-related macular degeneration, and Cimzia (certolizumab pegol) is a PEGylated, humanized anti-TNFα approved for moderate to severe Crohn disease. Single-chain Fv, miniaturized antibodies, and the V$_{HH}$-derived nanobody ALX-0081 have also entered clinical trials (4).

■ CONCLUSIONS

Initially, the range of therapeutic antibodies was very limited, but since the development of the display technologies tremendous progress has been made, mainly by the ability to directly make human mAbs of choice. Furthermore, these advances were superseded by further technologies that enabled the engineering of human-like or human antibodies to optimal affinity and effector function. Currently, there is only one human antibody approved for therapy that originated from the display technologies but many more are in clinical and preclinical trials. The recent regulatory approval of the first fully human, mouse-derived therapeutic antibody also represents a major advancement in technology. In conclusion, the development of successful mAbs for clinical application requires the integration of several characteristics including appropriate target antigen, tuned affinity, and pharmacokinetics as well as optimal isotype selection and Fc modification.

Acknowledgment

The authors would like to thank Dr Ermanno Gherardi (MRC, Cambridge) for helpful comments on the manuscript.

REFERENCES

1. Cosimi AB, Burton RC, Colvin RB, et al. Treatment of acute renal allograft rejection with OKT3 monoclonal antibody. *Transplantation.* 1981;32(6):535–539.
2. Meeker TC, Lowder J, Maloney DG, et al. A clinical trial of anti-idiotype therapy for B cell malignancy. *Blood.* 1985;65(6):1349–1363.
3. Kohler G, Milstein C. Continuous cultures of fused cells secreting antibody of predefined specificity. *Nature.* 1975;256(5517):495–497.
4. Nelson AL, Reichert JM. Development trends for therapeutic antibody fragments. *Nat Biotechnol.* 2009;27(4):331–337.
5. Boulianne GL, Hozumi N, Shulman MJ. Production of functional chimaeric mouse/human antibody. *Nature.* 1984;312(5995):643–646.
6. Morrison SL, Johnson MJ, Herzenberg LA, et al. Chimeric human antibody molecules: mouse antigen-binding domains with human constant region domains. *Proc Natl Acad Sci U S A.* 1984;81(21):6851–6855.
7. Jones PT, Dear PH, Foote J, et al. Replacing the complementarity-determining regions in a human antibody with those from a mouse. *Nature.* 1986;321(6069):522–525.
8. Verhoeyen M, Milstein C, Winter G. Reshaping human antibodies: grafting an antilysozyme activity. *Science.* 1988;239(4847):1534–1536.
9. Riechmann L, Clark M, Waldmann H, et al. Reshaping human antibodies for therapy. *Nature.* 1988;332(6162):323–327.
10. Padlan EA. A possible procedure for reducing the immunogenicity of antibody variable domains while preserving their ligand-binding properties. *Mol Immunol.* 1991;28(4–5):489–498.
11. Zhang W, Feng J, Li Y, et al. Humanization of an anti-human TNF-alpha antibody by variable region resurfacing with the aid of molecular modeling. *Mol Immunol.* 2005;42(12):1445–1451.
12. Kashmiri SV, De Pascalis R, Gonzales NR, et al. SDR grafting—a new approach to antibody humanization. *Methods.* 2005;36(1):25–34.
13. Hwang WY, Foote J. Immunogenicity of engineered antibodies. *Methods.* 2005;36(1):3–10.
14. Ritter G, Cohen LS, Williams C Jr, et al. Serological analysis of human anti-human antibody responses in colon cancer patients treated with repeated doses of humanized monoclonal antibody A33. *Cancer Res.* 2001;61(18):6851–6859.
15. Carter PJ. Potent antibody therapeutics by design. *Nat Rev Immunol.* 2006;6(5):343–357.
16. Lonberg N. Human monoclonal antibodies from transgenic mice. *Handb Exp Pharmacol.* 2008;181:69–97.
17. Green LL, Hardy MC, Maynard-Currie CE, et al. Antigen-specific human monoclonal antibodies from mice engineered with human Ig heavy and light chain YACs. *Nat Genet.* 1994;7(1):13–21.
18. Lonberg N, Taylor LD, Harding FA, et al. Antigen-specific human antibodies from mice comprising four distinct genetic modifications. *Nature.* 1994;368(6474):856–859.
19. Holliger P, Hudson PJ. Engineered antibody fragments and the rise of single domains. *Nat Biotechnol.* 2005;23(9):1126–1136.
20. Saerens D, Ghassabeh GH, Muyldermans S. Single-domain antibodies as building blocks for novel therapeutics. *Curr Opin Pharmacol.* 2008;8(5):600–608.
21. Griffiths AD, Malmqvist M, Marks JD, et al. Human anti-self antibodies with high specificity from phage display libraries. *EMBO J.* 1993;12(2):725–734.
22. Vaughan TJ, Williams AJ, Pritchard K, et al. Human antibodies with sub-nanomolar affinities isolated from a large non-immunized phage display library. *Nat Biotechnol.* 1996;14(3):309–314.
23. Marks JD, Hoogenboom HR, Bonnert TP, et al. By-passing immunization. Human antibodies from V-gene libraries displayed on phage. *J Mol Biol.* 1991;222(3):581–597.
24. Scott JK, Smith GP. Searching for peptide ligands with an epitope library. *Science.* 1990;249(4967):386–390.
25. Smith GP. Filamentous fusion phage: novel expression vectors that display cloned antigens on the virion surface. *Science.* 1985;228(4705):1315–1317.
26. Winter G, Griffiths AD, Hawkins RE, et al. Making antibodies by phage display technology. *Annu Rev Immunol.* 1994;12:433–455.
27. Hoogenboom HR. Selecting and screening recombinant antibody libraries. *Nat Biotechnol.* 2005;23(9):1105–1116.
28. McCafferty J, Griffiths AD, Winter G, et al. Phage antibodies: filamentous phage displaying antibody variable domains. *Nature.* 1990;348(6301):552–554.
29. Marks JD, Ouwehand WH, Bye JM, et al. Human antibody fragments specific for human blood group antigens from a phage display library. *Biotechnology (N Y).* 1993;11(10):1145–1149.
30. Bradbury AR, Marks JD. Antibodies from phage antibody libraries. *J Immunol Methods.* 2004;290(1–2):29–49.
31. Pasqualini R, Ruoslahti E. Organ targeting in vivo using phage display peptide libraries. *Nature.* 1996;380(6572):364–366.
32. Becerril B, Poul MA, Marks JD. Toward selection of internalizing antibodies from phage libraries. *Biochem Biophys Res Commun.* 1999;255(2):386–393.
33. Poul MA, Becerril B, Nielsen UB, et al. Selection of tumor-specific internalizing human antibodies from phage libraries. *J Mol Biol.* 2000;301(5):1149–1161.
34. Griffiths AD, Williams SC, Hartley O, et al. Isolation of high affinity human antibodies directly from large synthetic repertoires. *EMBO J.* 1994;13(14):3245–3260.
35. Holt LJ, Herring C, Jespers LS, et al. Domain antibodies: proteins for therapy. *Trends Biotechnol.* 2003;21(11):484–490.
36. Throsby M, Geuijen C, Goudsmit J, et al. Isolation and characterization of human monoclonal antibodies from individuals infected with West Nile virus. *J Virol.* 2006;80(14):6982–6992.
37. Nissim A, Hoogenboom HR, Tomlinson IM, et al. Antibody fragments from a 'single pot' phage display library as immunochemical reagents. *EMBO J.* 1994;13(3):692–698.
38. He M, Taussig MJ. Ribosome display: cell-free protein display technology. *Brief Funct Genomic Proteomic.* 2002;1(2):204–212.
39. Lipovsek D, Pluckthun A. In-vitro protein evolution by ribosome display and mRNA display. *J Immunol Methods.* 2004;290(1–2):51–67.
40. Hanes J, Pluckthun A. In vitro selection and evolution of functional proteins by using ribosome display. *Proc Natl Acad Sci U S A.* 1997;94(10):4937–4942.
41. Hanes J, Jermutus L, Weber-Bornhauser S, et al. Ribosome display efficiently selects and evolves high-affinity antibodies in vitro from immune libraries. *Proc Natl Acad Sci U S A.* 1998;95(24):14130–14135.
42. He M, Taussig MJ. Antibody–ribosome–mRNA (ARM) complexes as efficient selection particles for in vitro display and evolution of antibody combining sites. *Nucleic Acids Res.* 1997;25(24):5132–5134.
43. Blanchard C, Mishra A, Saito-Akei H, et al. Inhibition of human interleukin-13-induced respiratory and oesophageal inflammation by anti-human-interleukin-13 antibody (CAT-354). *Clin Exp Allergy.* 2005;35(8):1096–1103.
44. Scott N, Reynolds CB, Wright MJ, et al. Single-chain Fv phage display propensity exhibits strong positive correlation with overall expression levels. *BMC Biotechnol.* 2008;9:97.
45. Francisco JA, Campbell R, Iverson BL, et al. Production and fluorescence-activated cell sorting of *Escherichia coli* expressing a functional antibody fragment on the external surface. *Proc Natl Acad Sci U S A.* 1993;90(22):10444–10448.

46. Boder ET, Wittrup KD. Yeast surface display for screening combinatorial polypeptide libraries. *Nat Biotechnol*. 1997;15(6):553–557.

47. Boder ET, Midelfort KS, Wittrup KD. Directed evolution of antibody fragments with monovalent femtomolar antigen-binding affinity. *Proc Natl Acad Sci U S A*. 2000;97(20):10701–10705.

48. Graff CP, Chester K, Begent R, et al. Directed evolution of an anti-carcinoembryonic antigen scFv with a 4-day monovalent dissociation half-time at 37 degrees C. *Protein Eng Des Sel*. 2004;17(4):293–304.

49. Beerli RR, Bauer M, Buser RB, et al. Isolation of human monoclonal antibodies by mammalian cell display. *Proc Natl Acad Sci U S A*. 2008;105(38):14336–14341.

50. Ho M, Nagata S, Pastan I. Isolation of anti CD22 Fv with high affinity by Fv display on human cells. *Proc Natl Acad Sci U S A*. 2006;103(25):9637–9642.

51. Ho M, Pastan I. Mammalian cell display for antibody engineering. *Methods Mol Biol*. 2009;525:337–352, xiv.

52. Taube R, Zhu Q, Xu C, et al. Lentivirus display: stable expression of human antibodies on the surface of human cells and virus particles. *PLoS One*. 2008;3(9):e3181.

53. Baeuerle PA, Huttner WB. Tyrosine sulfation is a trans-Golgi-specific protein modification. *J Cell Biol*. 1987;105(6 pt 1):2655–2664.

54. Choe H, Li W, Wright PL, et al. Tyrosine sulfation of human antibodies contributes to recognition of the CCR5 binding region of HIV-1 gp120. *Cell*. 2003;114(2):161–170.

55. Adams GP, Schier R, Marshall K, et al. Increased affinity leads to improved selective tumor delivery of single-chain Fv antibodies. *Cancer Res*. 1998;58(3):485–490.

56. Adams GP, Schier R, McCall AM, et al. High affinity restricts the localization and tumor penetration of single-chain fv antibody molecules. *Cancer Res*. 2001;61(12):4750–4755.

57. Zuckier LS, Berkowitz EZ, Sattenberg RJ, et al. Influence of affinity and antigen density on antibody localization in a modifiable tumor targeting model. *Cancer Res*. 2000;60(24):7008–7013.

58. Baxter LT, Jain RK. Transport of fluid and macromolecules in tumors. III. Role of binding and metabolism. *Microvasc Res*. 1991;41(1):5–23.

59. Fujimori K, Covell DG, Fletcher JE, et al. Modeling analysis of the global and microscopic distribution of immunoglobulin G, F(ab')2, and Fab in tumors. *Cancer Res*. 1989;49(20):5656–5663.

60. Juweid M, Neumann R, Paik C, et al. Micropharmacology of monoclonal antibodies in solid tumors: direct experimental evidence for a binding site barrier. *Cancer Res*. 1992;52(19):5144–5153.

61. Hawkins RE, Russell SJ, Winter G. Selection of phage antibodies by binding affinity. Mimicking affinity maturation. *J Mol Biol*. 1992;226(3):889–896.

62. Levin AM, Weiss GA. Optimizing the affinity and specificity of proteins with molecular display. *Mol Biosyst*. 2006;2(1):49–57.

63. Marks JD, Griffiths AD, Malmqvist M, et al. By-passing immunization: building high affinity human antibodies by chain shuffling. *Biotechnology (N Y)*. 1992;10(7):779–783.

64. Barbas CF 3rd, Hu D, Dunlop N, et al. In vitro evolution of a neutralizing human antibody to human immunodeficiency virus type 1 to enhance affinity and broaden strain cross-reactivity. *Proc Natl Acad Sci U S A*. 1994;91(9):3809–3813.

65. Low NM, Holliger P, Winter G. Mimicking somatic hypermutation: affinity maturation of antibodies displayed on bacteriophage using a bacterial mutator strain. *J Mol Biol*. 1996;260(3):359–368.

66. Iyer AK, Khaled G, Fang J, et al. Exploiting the enhanced permeability and retention effect for tumor targeting. *Drug Discov Today*. 2006;11(17–18):812–818.

67. Matsumura Y, Maeda H. A new concept for macromolecular therapeutics in cancer chemotherapy: mechanism of tumoritropic accumulation of proteins and the antitumor agent smancs. *Cancer Res*. 1986;46(12 pt 1):6387–6392.

68. Holechek MJ. Glomerular filtration: an overview. *Nephrol Nurs J*. 2003;30(3):285–290; quiz 291–292.

69. Holliger P, Prospero T, Winter G. "Diabodies": small bivalent and bispecific antibody fragments. *Proc Natl Acad Sci U S A*. 1993;90(14):6444–6448.

70. Iliades P, Kortt AA, Hudson PJ. Triabodies: single chain Fv fragments without a linker form trivalent trimers. *FEBS Lett*. 1997;409(3):437–441.

71. Hudson PJ, Kortt AA. High avidity scFv multimers; diabodies and triabodies. *J Immunol Methods*. 1999;231(1–2):177–189.

72. Adams GP, Tai MS, McCartney JE, et al. Avidity-mediated enhancement of in vivo tumor targeting by single-chain Fv dimers. *Clin Cancer Res*. 2006;12(5):1599–1605.

73. Wu AM, Senter PD. Arming antibodies: prospects and challenges for immunoconjugates. *Nat Biotechnol*. 2005;23(9):1137–1146.

74. Burmeister WP, Huber AH, Bjorkman PJ. Crystal structure of the complex of rat neonatal Fc receptor with Fc. *Nature*. 1994;372(6504):379–383.

75. Kenanova V, Olafsen T, Crow DM, et al. Tailoring the pharmacokinetics and positron emission tomography imaging properties of anti-carcinoembryonic antigen single-chain Fv–Fc antibody fragments. *Cancer Res*. 2005;65(2):622–631.

76. Chapman AP, Antoniw P, Spitali M, et al. Therapeutic antibody fragments with prolonged in vivo half-lives. *Nat Biotechnol*. 1999;17(8):780–783.

77. Harris JM, Chess RB. Effect of pegylation on pharmaceuticals. *Nat Rev Drug Discov*. 2003;2(3):214–221.

78. Monfardini C, Schiavon O, Caliceti P, et al. A branched monomethoxypoly(ethylene glycol) for protein modification. *Bioconjug Chem*. 2002;6(1):62–69.

79. Choy EH, Hazleman B, Smith M, et al. Efficacy of a novel PEGylated humanized anti-TNF fragment (CDP870) in patients with rheumatoid arthritis: a phase II double-blinded, randomized, dose-escalating trial. *Rheumatology (Oxford)*. 2002;41(10):1133–1137.

80. Chapman AP. PEGylated antibodies and antibody fragments for improved therapy: a review. *Adv Drug Deliv Rev*. 2002;54(4):531–545.

81. Gregoriadis G, Jain S, Papaioannou I, et al. Improving the therapeutic efficacy of peptides and proteins: a role for polysialic acids. *Int J Pharm*. 2005;300(1–2):125–130.

82. Fernandes AI, Gregoriadis G. Polysialylated asparaginase: preparation, activity and pharmacokinetics. *Biochim Biophys Acta*. 1997;1341(1):26–34.

83. Jain S, Hreczuk-Hirst DH, McCormack B, et al. Polysialylated insulin: synthesis, characterization and biological activity in vivo. *Biochim Biophys Acta*. 2003;1622(1):42–49.

84. Constantinou A, Epenetos AA, Hreczuk-Hirst D, et al. Modulation of antibody pharmacokinetics by chemical polysialylation. *Bioconjug Chem*. 2008;19(3):643–650.

85. Constantinou A, Epenetos AA, Hreczuk-Hirst D, et al. Site-specific polysialylation of an antitumor single-chain Fv fragment. *Bioconjug Chem*. 2009;20:924–931.

86. Fernandes AI, Gregoriadis G. The effect of polysialylation on the immunogenicity and antigenicity of asparaginase: implication in its pharmacokinetics. *Int J Pharm*. 2001;217(1–2):215–224.

87. Beckman RA, Weiner LM, Davis HM. Antibody constructs in cancer therapy: protein engineering strategies to improve exposure in solid tumors. *Cancer*. 2007;109(2):170–179.

88. Thurber GM, Schmidt MM, Wittrup KD. Antibody tumor penetration: transport opposed by systemic and antigen-mediated clearance. *Adv Drug Deliv Rev*. 2008;60(12):1421–1434.

89. Schmitz KR, Ferguson KM. Interaction of antibodies with ErbB receptor extracellular regions. *Exp Cell Res*. 2009;315(4):659–670.

90. Li S, Schmitz KR, Jeffrey PD, et al. Structural basis for inhibition of the epidermal growth factor receptor by cetuximab. *Cancer Cell*. 2005;7(4):301–311.

91. Martens T, Schmidt NO, Eckerich C, et al. A novel one-armed anti-c-Met antibody inhibits glioblastoma growth in vivo. *Clin Cancer Res*. 2006;12(20 pt 1):6144–6152.

92. Benvenuti S, Comoglio PM. The MET receptor tyrosine kinase in invasion and metastasis. *J Cell Physiol*. 2007;213(2):316–325.

93. Birchmeier C, Birchmeier W, Gherardi E, et al. Met, metastasis, motility and more. *Nat Rev Mol Cell Biol*. 2003;4(12):915–925.

94. Jin H, Yang R, Zheng Z, et al. MetMAb, the one-armed 5D5 anti-c-Met antibody, inhibits orthotopic pancreatic tumor growth and improves survival. *Cancer Res*. 2008;68(11):4360–4368.

95. Hudziak RM, Schlessinger J, Ullrich A. Increased expression of the putative growth factor receptor p185HER2 causes transformation and tumorigenesis of NIH 3T3 cells. *Proc Natl Acad Sci U S A*. 1987;84(20):7159–7163.

96. Cho HS, Mason K, Ramyar KX, et al. Structure of the extracellular region of HER2 alone and in complex with the Herceptin Fab. *Nature*. 2003;421(6924):756–760.

97. Garrett TP, McKern NM, Lou M, et al. The crystal structure of a truncated ErbB2 ectodomain reveals an active conformation, poised to interact with other ErbB receptors. *Mol Cell*. 2003;11(2):495–505.

98. Graus-Porta D, Beerli RR, Daly JM, et al. ErbB-2, the preferred heterodimerization partner of all ErbB receptors, is a mediator of lateral signaling. *EMBO J*. 1997;16(7):1647–1655.

99. Slamon DJ, Clark GM, Wong SG, et al. Human breast cancer: correlation of relapse and survival with amplification of the HER-2/neu oncogene. *Science*. 1987;235(4785):177–182.

100. Hudis CA. Trastuzumab—mechanism of action and use in clinical practice. *N Engl J Med*. 2007;357(1):39–51.

101. Carter P, Presta L, Gorman CM, et al. Humanization of an anti-p185HER2 antibody for human cancer therapy. *Proc Natl Acad Sci U S A*. 1992;89(10):4285–4289.

102. Lewis GD, Figari I, Fendly B, et al. Differential responses of human tumor cell lines to anti-p185HER2 monoclonal antibodies. *Cancer Immunol Immunother*. 1993;37(4):255–263.

103. Clynes RA, Towers TL, Presta LG, et al. Inhibitory Fc receptors modulate in vivo cytotoxicity against tumor targets. *Nat Med*. 2000;6(4):443–446.

104. Wehrman TS, Raab WJ, Casipit CL, et al. A system for quantifying dynamic protein interactions defines a role for Herceptin in modulating ErbB2 interactions. *Proc Natl Acad Sci U S A*. 2006;103(50):19063–19068.

105. Fendly BM, Winget M, Hudziak RM, et al. Characterization of murine monoclonal antibodies reactive to either the human epidermal growth factor receptor or HER2/neu gene product. *Cancer Res*. 1990;50(5):1550–1558.

106. Franklin MC, Carey KD, Vajdos FF, et al. Insights into ErbB signaling from the structure of the ErbB2–pertuzumab complex. *Cancer Cell*. 2004;5(4):317–328.

107. Agus DB, Akita RW, Fox WD, et al. Targeting ligand-activated ErbB2 signaling inhibits breast and prostate tumor growth. *Cancer Cell*. 2002;2(2):127–137.

108. Kubota T, Niwa R, Satoh M, et al. Engineered therapeutic antibodies with improved effector functions. *Cancer Sci*. 2009;100(9):1566–1572.

109. Carter P. Improving the efficacy of antibody-based cancer therapies. *Nat Rev Cancer*. 2001;1(2):118–129.

110. van der Neut Kolfschoten M, Schuurman J, Losen M, et al. Anti-inflammatory activity of human IgG4 antibodies by dynamic Fab arm exchange. *Science*. 2007;317(5844):1554–1557.

111. Shields RL, Lai J, Keck R, et al. Lack of fucose on human IgG1 N-linked oligosaccharide improves binding to human Fcgamma RIII and antibody-dependent cellular toxicity. *J Biol Chem*. 2002;277(30):26733–26740.

112. Yamane-Ohnuki N, Kinoshita S, Inoue-Urakubo M, et al. Establishment of FUT8 knockout Chinese hamster ovary cells: an ideal host cell line for producing completely defucosylated antibodies with enhanced antibody-dependent cellular cytotoxicity. *Biotechnol Bioeng*. 2004;87(5):614–622.

113. Idusogie EE, Wong PY, Presta LG, et al. Engineered antibodies with increased activity to recruit complement. *J Immunol*. 2001;166(4):2571–2575.

114. Lazar GA, Dang W, Karki S, et al. Engineered antibody Fc variants with enhanced effector function. *Proc Natl Acad Sci U S A*. 2006;103(11):4005–4010.

115. Shields RL, Namenuk AK, Hong K, et al. High resolution mapping of the binding site on human IgG1 for Fc gamma RI, Fc gamma RII, Fc gamma RIII, and FcRn and design of IgG1 variants with improved binding to the Fc gamma R. *J Biol Chem*. 2001;276(9):6591–6604.

116. Kreitman RJ. Immunotoxins in cancer therapy. *Curr Opin Immunol*. 1999;11(5):570–578.

117. Kreitman RJ, Wilson WH, White JD, et al. Phase I trial of recombinant immunotoxin anti-Tac(Fv)-PE38 (LMB-2) in patients with hematologic malignancies. *J Clin Oncol*. 2000;18(8):1622–1636.

118. Borghaei H, Schilder RJ. Safety and efficacy of radioimmunotherapy with yttrium 90 ibritumomab tiuxetan (Zevalin). *Semin Nucl Med*. 2004;34(1 suppl 1):4–9.

119. Wahl RL. Tositumomab and (131)I therapy in non-Hodgkin's lymphoma. *J Nucl Med*. 2005;46(suppl 1):128S–140S.

120. Mylotarg. 01/23/2006 [cited 26/9/2009; FDA Label]. Available at: http://www.accessdata.fda.gov/drugsatfda_docs/label/2006/021174s020lbl.pdf.

121. Gillies SD, Young D, Lo KM, et al. Expression of genetically engineered immunoconjugates of lymphotoxin and a chimeric anti-ganglioside GD2 antibody. *Hybridoma*. 1991;10(3):347–356.

122. Gillies SD, Reilly EB, Lo KM, et al. Antibody-targeted interleukin 2 stimulates T-cell killing of autologous tumor cells. *Proc Natl Acad Sci U S A*. 1992;89(4):1428–1432.

123. Kaspar M, Trachsel E, Neri D. The antibody-mediated targeted delivery of interleukin-15 and GM-CSF to the tumor neovasculature inhibits tumor growth and metastasis. *Cancer Res*. 2007;67(10):4940–4948.

124. Tao MH, Levy R. Idiotype/granulocyte-macrophage colony-stimulating factor fusion protein as a vaccine for B-cell lymphoma. *Nature*. 1993;362(6422):755–758.

125. Zhao L, Rai SK, Grosmaire LS, et al. Construction, expression, and characterization of anticarcinoma sFv fused to IL-2 or GM-CSF. *J Hematother Stem Cell Res*. 1999;8(4):393–399.

126. Gillies SD, Lan Y, Wesolowski JS, et al. Antibody-IL-12 fusion proteins are effective in SCID mouse models of prostate and colon carcinoma metastases. *J Immunol*. 1998;160(12):6195–6203.

127. Staerz UD, Bevan MJ. Hybrid hybridoma producing a bispecific monoclonal antibody that can focus effector T-cell activity. *Proc Natl Acad Sci U S A*. 1986;83(5):1453–1457.

128. Staerz UD, Kanagawa O, Bevan MJ. Hybrid antibodies can target sites for attack by T cells. *Nature*. 1985;314(6012):628–631.

129. Bargou R, Leo E, Zugmaier G, et al. Tumor regression in cancer patients by very low doses of a T cell-engaging antibody. *Science*. 2008;321(5891):974–977.

130. Bagshawe KD, Springer CJ, Searle F, et al. A cytotoxic agent can be generated selectively at cancer sites. *Br J Cancer*. 1988;58(6):700–703.

131. Goodwin DA, Meares CF. Advances in pretargeting biotechnology. *Biotechnol Adv*. 2001;19(6):435–450.

132. Anderson PJ. Tumor necrosis factor inhibitors: clinical implications of their different immunogenicity profiles. *Semin Arthritis Rheum*. 2005;34(5 suppl 1):19–22.

133. Humira, FDA label. 21/02/2008 [cited 4/10/2009; FDA Label]. Available at: http://www.accessdata.fda.gov/drugsatfda_docs/label/2008/125057s114lbl.pdf.

134. Gibson TB, Ranganathan A, Grothey A. Randomized phase III trial results of panitumumab, a fully human anti-epidermal growth factor receptor monoclonal antibody, in metastatic colorectal cancer. *Clin Colorectal Cancer*. 2006;6(1):29–31.

135. Van Cutsem E, Peeters M, Siena S, et al. Open-label phase III trial of panitumumab plus best supportive care compared with best supportive care alone in patients with chemotherapy-refractory metastatic colorectal cancer. *J Clin Oncol*. 2007;25(13):1658–1664.

136. Rocha-Lima CM, Soares HP, Raez LE, et al. EGFR targeting of solid tumors. *Cancer Control*. 2007;14(3):295–304.

137. Helbling D, Borner M. Successful challenge with the fully human EGFR antibody panitumumab following an infusion reaction with the chimeric EGFR antibody cetuximab. *Ann Oncol*. 2007;18(5):963–964.

138. Heun J, Holen K. Treatment with panitumumab after a severe infusion reaction to cetuximab in a patient with metastatic colorectal cancer: a case report. *Clin Colorectal Cancer*. 2007;6(7):529–531.

139. Calvo E, Rowinsky EK. Clinical experience with monoclonal antibodies to epidermal growth factor receptor. *Curr Oncol Rep*. 2005;7(2):96–103.

140. Saltz L, Kies M, Abbruzzese JL, et al. The presence and intensity of the cetuximab-induced acne-like rash predicts increased survival in studies across multiple malignancies. *Proc Am Soc Clin Oncol*. 2003;22(abstr 817):204.

141. Li T, Perez-Soler R. Skin toxicities associated with epidermal growth factor receptor inhibitors. *Target Oncol*. 2009;4(2):107–119.

142. Bleeker WK, Lammerts van Bueren JJ, van Ojik HH, et al. Dual mode of action of a human anti-epidermal growth factor receptor monoclonal antibody for cancer therapy. *J Immunol*. 2004;173(7):4699–4707.

143. Yang XD, Jia XC, Corvalan JR, et al. Eradication of established tumors by a fully human monoclonal antibody to the epidermal growth factor receptor without concomitant chemotherapy. *Cancer Res*. 1999;59(6):1236–1243.

144. ReoPro. 18/06/2009 [cited 5/10/2009; FDA labeling information]. Available at: http://www.fda.gov/Drugs/DevelopmentApprovalProcess/HowDrugsareDevelopedandApproved/ApprovalApplications/TherapeuticBiologicApplications/ucm093336.htm.

Radiolabeled Peptides, Structure and Analysis

Diego Tesauro, Giancarlo Morelli, Carlo Pedone, and Michele Saviano

■ INTRODUCTION

One of the most exciting areas of research in drug design concerns the synthesis and three-dimensional (3D) structural characterization of peptides and peptidomimetic molecules that are expected to possess the same therapeutic effects as their natural peptide counterparts, with the potential added advantages of higher metabolic stability, enhanced interactions with the receptor, and improved pharmacokinetic properties (1–3). We are on the brink of a therapeutic revolution. Peptides of natural or synthetic origin are compounds involved in a variety of biologic interactions. They are hormones, protein substrates and inhibitors, opioides, sweeteners, antibiotics, releasing factors, regulators of biologic functions, cytoprotectors, and so on (4). In recent years, there has been a rapid expansion in the use of peptides as drugs or diagnostics.

A new compound best suited as a radiopharmaceutical would, after intravenous administration, travel via the blood stream to the target cells, interacting efficiently with the desired molecular pathway (5). Any radioligand that did not reach the desired target would be rapidly excreted from the body, so that the only radioactivity remaining in the body would be localized to the target site. The objective in radiopharmaceutical design is, therefore, to achieve this ideal situation. The radiopharmaceutical can be considered to have three components: (a) the targeting vector, (b) the radionuclide, and (c) a means of linking the two together that may, or may not, include a pharmacokinetic modifier (3). A major concern of conventional cancer chemotherapy is the lack of satisfactory specificity or targeting, against tumor cells, and poor antitumor activity. In order to improve these characteristics, chemotherapeutic drugs can be conjugated to targeting moieties, for example, to peptides with the ability to recognize cancer cells.

■ DESIGN, SYNTHESIS, AND STRUCTURAL CHARACTERIZATION OF BIOACTIVE POLYPEPTIDES

Three-dimensional structures in polypeptides

Peptides are formed when two or more amino acids are condensed together with the formation of a secondary amide bond, the so-called "peptide unit" (6). Several parameters

are important to consider while determining the relationship between peptide conformation, configuration, and biologic activity: (a) amino acid sequence, (b) spatial configuration of the asymmetric C^α atoms of each residue, (c) local conformation of the molecule, and (d) intramolecular and intermolecular interactions. Then, the assessment of all these parameters is the key to discovering the relationships between structure and properties of different bioactive compounds, especially for natural substances such as small molecules, protein, and biologically active compounds. The molecular conformations of a peptide chain are conveniently and precisely characterized by torsion angle (Fig. 3.1).

The backbone dihedral angles of peptides and proteins are called φ (phi, involving the backbone atoms C'–N–C^α–C'), ψ (psi, involving the backbone atoms N–C^α–C'–N), ω (omega, involving the backbone atoms C^α–C'–N–C^α), and the torsion angle χ (describing the side-chain conformation). Thus, φ controls the C'–C' distance, ψ controls the N–N distance, and ω controls the C^α–C^α distance. These three torsion angles determine the 3D shape of the peptide molecule. The ω angle in linear peptides usually presents values close to 180° corresponding to a *trans* arrangement of the peptide bond, which is energetically more favorable than the *cis* arrangement ($\omega_i = 0°$) by about 2 Kcal/mol. The *cis* arrangement is rarely found in proteins, large cyclic peptides, or in linear chains, but it is found in small cyclic peptides to reduce backbone steric hindrance. Taking into account these considerations about the peptide bond, the molecular conformation of a peptide can be described in a (φ, ψ) space by the energy of the molecule as a function of these torsion angles. The analysis of these conformational plots reported for proteins and peptides shows that all best-known secondary structures assumed by a peptide chain, such as the β-structure, the α-helix, the 3_{10}-helix, occur within the energy minima. The 3D conformation in polypeptides and proteins is classified in terms of the regions of the φ–ψ map in which they occur (Fig. 3.2) (7). These regions are classified by a letter code giving rise to a low-energy structure. The φ–ψ conformational map is divided into regions denoted by capital letters. On the left-hand portion of the map (φ ≤ 0°), six of the regions (A, C to G) comprise the distinct φ–ψ areas in which energy minima are found for numerous amino acid residues, while the region B is defined around the moderate-energy bridge region. On the right-hand portion of the map

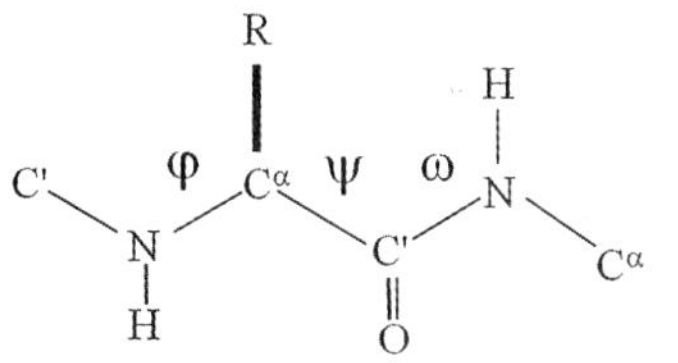

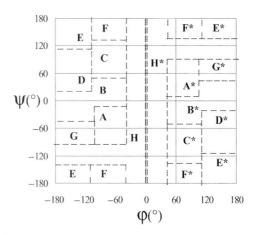

FIGURE 3.1 Schematic representation of an α-amino acid with the indentified backbone dihedral angles.

FIGURE 3.2 φ–ψ map showing the regions defining the conformational letter code.

($\phi > 0°$), regions are defined by the inversion of the left-hand half around the center of the map, and an asterisk is appended to the letters. In defining these regions, the boundaries were selected so that all related minima would fall within the same region. All amino acid computed minima fall within the allowed regions of the conformational map. These results are in general in agreement with experimental data. In fact, the statistical analysis of the conformation assumed by amino acids in x-ray protein structures reveals that almost all of the φ–ψ dihedral angles fall within the allowed regions of the conformational map.

In protein systems, α-helices and β-sheets are the major stabilizing structures. In polypeptides, the classification of secondary regular structures is more complex and is related to the specific hydrogen bond network that stabilizes the structure (8). A hydrogen bond between N–H of an amino acid sequence number "m" and C=O of a residue of the sequence number "n" is indicated as m → n (Fig. 3.3). Then, the possible folded structures in a system with four linked peptide units are 2 → 2 (or 3 → 3, or 4 → 4), 2 → 3 (or 3 → 4), 2 → 4, 3 → 1 (or 4 → 2, or 5 → 3), the 4 → 1 (or 5 → 2), and 5 → 1 intramolecular hydrogen-bonded conformations. These conformations can also be classified on the basis of the number of atoms in the ring formed by closing the hydrogen bond. Therefore, these conformations are also called C_5, C_8, C_{11}, C_7, C_{10}, and C_{13} conformations. The only

extended conformation is the C_5 conformation "i", the others are of the folded type. Another nomenclature for C_7, C_8, C_{10}, C_{11}, and C_{13} conformations is γ-, δ-, β-, ε-, and α-turn, respectively. The C_8, C_{10}, C_{11}, and C_{13} conformations can include *cis* peptide configurations. The presence of consecutive α- or β-turns gives rise to α-helical or 3_{10}-helix secondary structures, respectively.

▨ Peptide design of new drugs or diagnostics

Rational molecular design, whether it is aimed at generating novel pharmaceuticals or diagnostics, represents the basis for the development of new and selective biomolecules. The development of new, selective molecules requires knowledge at an atomic level of their conformations and how these molecules interact at the binding site (if the structure is known) or if the molecule will mimic the ligand-binding properties of existing known activities. This knowledge, combined with

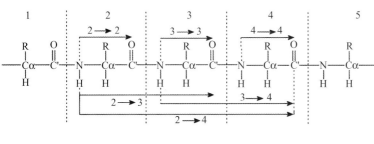

FIGURE 3.3 Schematic representation of the possible intramolecular hydrogen bonds in polypeptides (four linked peptide residues).

other chemical, physical, or biologic information, can lead to the modification and the reiteration of original proposed modeling experiments. Therefore, a thorough knowledge of 3D structure is a crucial factor in the molecular design process (9). Structure–activity relationship (SAR) studies, concerning bioactive peptides, have embraced the understanding of biologic phenomena at a molecular level with the goal of developing new selective molecules with an application in pharmacology, medicinal chemistry, and diagnostics. While developing bioactive peptides, it is necessary to fully consider various limitations and challenges that arise. In addition, the use of peptides as drugs or as diagnostic agents is limited by several factors (10):

1. Low metabolic stability toward proteolysis in the gastrointestinal tract and in the serum
2. Poor absorption after oral ingestion
3. Rapid excretion through liver and kidneys
4. Undesired effects caused by the interaction of the peptide with various receptors

Peptide probes used for imaging, unlike those used for therapy, should be cleared from the body as rapidly as possible for optimal imaging. Because the requirements for imaging and therapy are different, some considerations are necessary to determine a specific rationale for optimizing peptide probes for molecular imaging. In particular, some important questions are (2):

1. What is the range of molecular weights and the amino acid composition of the peptide backbone which enables optimal delivery to target cells, organs, and tissues and results in optimal plasma clearance?
2. What are the appropriate metrics of imaging efficacy needed to identify promising candidates of a library of peptide probes?
3. Some labels (e.g., PET or SPECT isotopes; lanthanides for MR), when free in the body, specifically accumulate in organs and pose a threat of organ toxicity or excessive radiation exposure. How can peptide probes be designed to avoid free-label toxicities?
4. What parameters, concerning peptide probe length and composition, dictate hepatic and renal clearance?
5. How do the labels (e.g., lanthanides, radioisotopes, radiometals, and fluorophores), chelators, or linkers affect imaging efficacy and renal/hepatic clearance of peptides?
6. What minimum specific activity, degree of labeling, or percentage conjugation of paramagnetic metal enables optimal imaging with peptide probes?
7. What parameters should be considered in peptide design to minimize unwanted macrophage activation, cytokine release, excessive/persistent plasma protein binding, peptide cross-linking, low solubility, and high-viscosity issues resulting from administration of peptide probes?
8. What in vitro, in silico, preclinical, or synthetic methods should be included in rational peptide design to reduce

the development time required for peptide probes to reach the market?
9. What considerations are necessary in peptide design to minimize probe degradation in vivo?
10. How can pharmacokinetic modeling of peptide probe libraries improve rational peptide design?

In recent years, in order to overcome some of these limitations, intensive efforts have been made to develop peptides or peptidomimetics with different chemical structure and possibly modified conformational preferences in solution. All biomolecular binding processes involve molecular dynamics (MD), even those apparently corresponding to the rigid lock-and-key model. Therefore, one of the goals in the design of new compounds is the introduction of constraints to reduce the conformational flexibility and to stabilize biologically active conformations of native molecules. This rational design can result in molecules endowed with high affinity and/or selectivity for one class of receptors. Structural changes and different dynamic behavior can be promoted in peptide chemistry by two basic processes: (a) modifying the sequence using specific coded or noncoded amino acids or amino acids with D configuration; (b) cyclization of the N-terminus with the C-terminus or with a side chain or with various side-chain modifications (11). Structural changes with the aim of inducing specific 3D structures in a peptide can be obtained with noncoded α- or β-amino acids. These constrained noncoded amino acids are of particular interest as "building blocks" for the preparation of analogs, since their inclusion in a peptide sequence could maintain the pharmacologic properties of the native peptide and possibly enhance resistance to biodegradation with improved bioavailability and pharmacokinetics (6,12–14). This arsenal of building blocks can be used for the rational design of new molecules with specific structure, conformation, and activity.

Many diverse approaches have been developed for the discovery of small, specific ligands that bind to the protein of interest, such as screening of natural products, development of combinatorial chemical libraries, and de novo ligand design (15). The first computational ligand design methods were developed about two decades ago. Since then, improvements have been made as a result of the increase in computational power, the availability of high-resolution protein structures, the development of combinatorial chemistry, and the advent of the genome era (16). A recent review summarizes the de novo approach in designing target specific probes for chemical genomics (17).

There are two general areas for de novo ligand design: a structure-based approach when the 3D structure of the target protein is known; a ligand-based approach when the structure of the target protein is not known, but several compounds or natural ligands for the protein are available. If the 3D structure of the ligand–receptor complex is known at atomic resolution, the ligand structure is modified, using backbone or side-chain modification including cyclization, preserving the ligand–receptor interactions. If the structure of the complex is unknown, the design will require conformational studies of the ligand and of the receptor. In this approach, before the design stage, docking programs are used to obtain a predicted ligand–receptor complex structure. These procedures use the energetics approach to determine the most favorable binding position for a specific fragment or functional group in the target site. If only the ligand structure is known, the design procedure must be preceded by an accurate conformational analysis of the molecule, using MD simulations in solution. In fact, MD simulations can give a statistical analysis of the conformational behavior and of conformational families assumed by the ligand (18). In addition, algorithms such as computational combinatorial ligand design (CCLD) have been developed to combine these approaches with database searching and virtual chemical library construction (16). Together with functional studies of the target protein, these approaches can lead to a better understanding of the structure–function relationship of the protein and lead compounds for combinatorial chemical library synthesis (19,20).

Peptide synthesis

Peptide conjugate synthesis can be performed following two alternative strategies: solution-phase synthesis and solid-phase peptide synthesis (SPPS) (21). The scope of these two methods varies largely because solution-phase synthesis is now applied only for large-scale synthesis of well-known peptides for pharmaceutical applications. In fact, the low yields and extensive purification steps (e.g., crystallization, chromatography, and distillation) make the solution-phase synthesis time-consuming for research approaches. Merrifield's SPPS (22) offers an excellent alternative approach for the synthesis of bioactive peptides. The resin is a polymer with reactive sites which chemically combine to the developing peptide chain. In recent years, the development of SPPS methodology has undergone great improvement. The most commonly used resin is a polystyrene polymer equipped with different linkers that allow cleavage under specific conditions. Two strategies are currently used that are distinguished by the N-protecting group: Boc (*tert*-butyloxycarbonyl) that can be cleaved under mild acidic conditions or Fmoc (9-fluorenylmethoxycarbonyl) that is removed under nucleophilic conditions (23). Efficient peptide bond formation is performed by the addition of activation agents. Typical reagents include carbodiimides, preformed symmetrical anhydrides, active esters, and HBTU (2-[1H-benzotriazole-1-yl]-1,1,3,3-tetramethyluronium hexafluorophosphate) like coupling reagents. By combining suitable side-chain protection groups, tailored peptides with appropriate side-chain modifications can be obtained. Both strategies follow the same cycle of stages to synthesize the peptide. The cleavage of the anchoring linkage and global deprotection of side-chain–protecting groups are achieved by incubating

peptide resin in anhydrous hydrogen fluoride in the Boc strategy and incubating in TFA (trifluoroacetic acid) following the Fmoc strategy. The peptide quality is examined routinely by analytical high-performance liquid chromatography (HPLC) to monitor the purity, in conjunction with mass spectral analysis which determines the identity. Most of the crude peptides can be purified alone by the reversed-phase HPLC to achieve the desired purity. The reversed-phase HPLC purification provides a powerful technique to purify a crude peptide with inferior quality. The peptide purity needs to be determined by analytical HPLC with two different buffer systems or even further by capillary electrophoresis. Mass spectrum by matrix-assisted laser desorption/ionization time-of-flight (MALDI-TOF) methodology is the standard analytical procedure to assess the peptide identity; moreover, data from sequence analysis and amino acid analysis can provide further detailed information on peptide homogeneity.

Methodologies for peptide modifications: production of a peptide-based radiopharmaceutical

Modified peptides can be synthesized routinely by using orthogonal protecting group strategies, resins with novel linkers and cleavage protocols. These modified peptides can be categorized as N-terminal modified, C-terminal modified, and peptides containing side-chain modifications.

Chemical modifications of radiopharmaceutical peptides are devoted to stabilize the sequence in order not to be recognized by amino peptidases and to retain binding affinity of the bioactive molecule. Peptide modification on amino acid side chains can be obtained using synthetic approaches compatible with the Fmoc strategy of SPPS. There has been a concerted effort to develop side-chain–protecting groups that utilize a different mechanism of cleavage to achieve selectivity: the protecting groups must remain chemically inert throughout the synthesis and must be removed in a facile manner to liberate the appropriate side-chain functional group. For example, within the lysine residue is a bifunctional amine, and differential protection of the amino group represents the most advantageous tool for peptide modification. Using this approach many modified peptides have been synthesized: on the lysine side chain or a peptide sequence, they typically contain branched or cyclic peptides, or a non–amino acid molecule such as a chelating agent.

To obtain peptide-based radiopharmaceuticals, the critical steps are (a) the individuation of the step where modifications may be performed without affecting binding affinity of the molecule; (b) the individuation of the method used to radiolabel the peptide molecule. As it relates to labeling of new peptide-based molecules, direct radiolabeling methods have been found to be less desirable, particularly for small peptides or peptide analogs. Such labeling schemes require rather complex chemistry and fairly sophisticated analytical methods to assess radiochemical purity and labeling efficiency.

RADIOMETALS FOR THERAPEUTIC RADIOPHARMACEUTICALS

The goal of receptor-based therapeutic radiopharmaceutical is to deliver a critical dose of radiation to the tumor cells while not causing unmanageable side effects. The selection of appropriate radionuclides is a critical factor when developing therapeutic radiopharmaceutical conjugates. Important variables include the rate of radiation delivery, half-life and specific activity of the radionuclide, tumor uptake and retention, blood clearance, and the availability of large-scale production of the radionuclide. The β-emitters have a relatively long penetration range (2 to 12 mm in tissue), which is particularly well suited for larger tumors with increased heterogeneity. The most important candidates among various radionuclides are ^{90}Y and lanthanoid radiometals. ^{90}Y is of particular interest due to its high-energy pure β-particle emission. The half-life of ^{90}Y is 2.7 days, which is short enough to achieve a critical dose rate and long enough to allow the radiopharmaceutical to be delivered. The energy of 2.3 MeV is able to penetrate tissue for a maximum depth of approximately 12.0 mm ($R_{90} = 5.2$ mm). The specific activity for ^{90}Y is high, and is well suited for receptor-based therapeutic radiopharmaceuticals. Another interesting radioisotope is ^{166}Ho. This radionuclide emits a β-particle with maximum energy of 1.85 MeV (maximum penetration range ~9 mm) and a small portion of γ-rays, which are useful for the determination of biodistribution of the therapeutic radiopharmaceutical *by using a* gamma camera. It has a half-life of 26.78 hours. A medium energy β-emitter is ^{153}Sm which emits a spectrum of β-energy (30% 0.64 MeV, 50% 0.71 MeV, and 20% 0.81 MeV). It also emits γ-rays (28% 103 keV) with a half-life of 1.95 days. The short half-life of ^{153}Sm allows for the delivery of fractionated dose regimes, while the γ-ray is useful for the determination of biodistribution of the therapeutic radiopharmaceutical via gamma camera. ^{177}Lu has three β-emissions (12% 0.176 MeV, 9% 0.384 MeV, and 79% 0.497 MeV) and two γ-emissions (6.4% 113 keV and 11% 208 keV) with a half-life of 6.75 days. Due to the low emission energy and penetration of tissues, this radionuclide is indicated for small lesions.

Within the transition metal group, Rhenium is a β-emitting radionuclide suitable for therapeutic applications. Rhenium exists as two isotopes (^{186}Re and ^{188}Re). ^{186}Re has a half-life of 3.68 days with a β-emission ($E_{max} = 1.07$ MeV, 91% abundance) and a γ-photon ($E = 137$ keV, 9% abundance) which should allow imaging during therapy. ^{188}Re has a half-life of 16.98 hours with a high-energy β-emission ($E_{max} = 2.12$ MeV, 85% abundance) and 155 keV γ-photons (15% abundance). The major advantage of using ^{188}Re in therapeutic nuclear medicine is the low cost of production of the radionuclide.

BIFUNCTIONAL CHELATING AGENTS

Coordination chemistry of radiopharmaceuticals and criteria for the selection of a BFCA

The bifunctional chelating agents (BFCAs) play a crucial role in radiolabeling of peptides. Selection of a BFCA is largely determined by the physical properties and oxidation state of the metal ion. The resulting radiopharmaceutical must have high solution stability. Since the radiopharmaceutical is manufactured, it must retain its chemical and biologic integrity. This requires that the BFCA form a metal chelate with high thermodynamic stability and kinetic inertness in vitro and in vivo to avoid the accumulation of radioactivity in normal tissue compartments and to avoid the interaction with ions involved in vital physiologic functions. Although the dissociation of the radiometal from the metal chelate could become eventually favored, the high value of the equilibrium constant has to guarantee the coordination. The most common way to achieve this aim is to use a polydentate chelator. The denticity requirement of a BFCA is largely dependent on the size and coordination geometry preference of the metal ion. Yttrium and lanthanoid metals share oxidation state +3, ionic radii, and coordination chemistry needing eight to nine donor atoms to complete the coordination sphere. Rhenium shows many oxidation states belonging to the third series of transition metals. The most popular state is +5 stabilized by a double oxo or a triple nitride bond, which favors a square pyramidal or octahedral geometry, respectively. The ion needs four or five donor atoms to obtain these stable complexes.

The preparation of a targeted radiopharmaceutical involves the covalent attachment (conjugation) of the BFCA of the radioactive isotope to the targeting vector. The BFCAs have a reactive function, which will covalently bind the bioactive molecules. This function could be an aromatic isocyanate group or an activated ester, which will react with nucleophilic sites (–NH$_2$, –SH, or –OH) of the targeting vector (24).

Another fundamental task of BFCAs is to improve blood clearance and renal excretion of the labeled conjugate, possessing high hydrophilicity. The tethering of the BFCA to a linker could enhance these properties. The linker can modulate the pharmacokinetics and the biodistribution of the probe and allow the attachment of the peptide through a metabolic resistant covalent bond.

Yttrium and lanthanoid metals in BFCA

The polyaminocarboxylate-type ligands are the BFCAs that meet the requirements to give stable Yttrium and lanthanoid complexes. They have eight or nine donor atoms able to saturate the coordination vacancy with three or four Nitrogen and four or five Oxygen atoms. Two major classes of polyaminocarboxylate were extensively studied: macrocyclic chelators such as DOTA and its derivatives (25) and the branched chelators such as DTPA and its derivatives. In

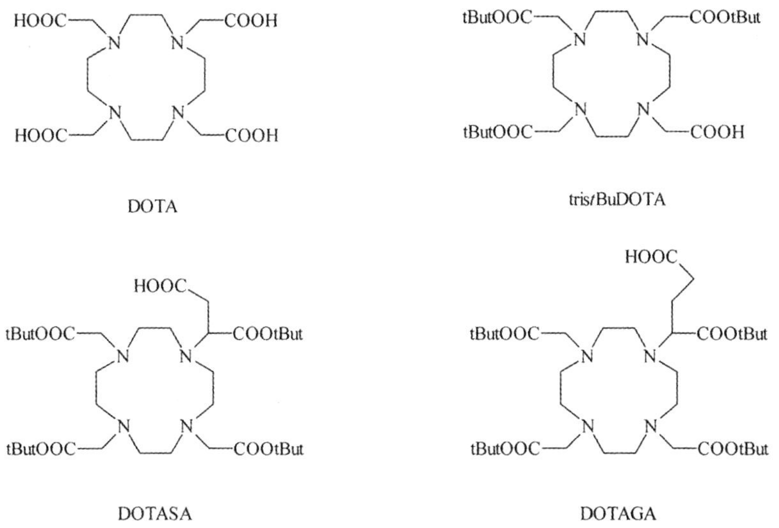

FIGURE 3.4 DOTA-like chelating agents capable of coordinating ^{90}Y and lanthanoid series elements.

DOTA

tris/BuDOTA

DOTASA

DOTAGA

both classes, the acetate groups attached to the nitrogen donor atoms have low molecular weight and respect the most favorable distance to the chelate ions.

DOTA-like chelators

DOTA (1,4,7,10-tetraazacyclododecane-1,4,7,10-tetraacetic acid) (Fig. 3.4) plays an important role in clinical applications, as it forms very stable complexes with a variety of trivalent radionuclides, such as ^{66,67,68}Ga, ^{86,90}Y, ^{111}In, ^{149}Pm, and ^{177}Lu. The macrocyclic framework forms metal complexes with high thermodynamic stability and kinetic inertness. A complete eight-coordinate structure has been reported for all DOTA complexes using four amino and four carboxy groups and often the ninth position is occupied by a water molecule. When one carboxy group is used for conjugation, the amide carbonyl oxygen occupies the eighth position around the metal. The low pK_a values result in less competition from protons, high stability of the metal complex, and minimum acid-assisted demetallation.

Two different approaches for DOTA conjugation with peptides have been developed. In the first approach, DOTA derivatives are tethered to additional side chains containing an isocyanate group or an amine for solution vector coupling. In the second approach, one of the four carboxy groups in DOTA is activated to facilitate the reaction with primary amines in the peptide and forms a stable amide bond linkage on SPPS. The tris-*tert*-butyl ester of DOTA (Fig. 3.4) has only one free carboxy group; in this way, the formation of undesired intermolecular linkages with peptides is prevented. Moreover, several DOTA derivatives have been synthesized; PA-DOTA (R-[2-(4-aminophenyl)-ethyl]-1,4,7,10-tetraazacyclododecane-1,4,7,10-tetraacetic acid) and *p*-NCS-Bz-DOTA (2-(4-isothiocyanatobenzyl)-1,4,7,10-tetraazacyclododecane-*N,N′,N″,N‴*-tetraacetic acid). Eisenwiener et al. (26) have introduced two new DOTA derivatives, DOTASA(*tBu*)$_4$, 1-(1-carboxy-2-carbo-*tert*-butoxyethyl)-4,7,10-(carbo-*tert*-butoxymethyl)-1,4,7,10-tetraazacyclododecane), and DOTAGA(*t*Bu)$_4$, 1-(1-carboxy-3-carbo-*tert*-butoxypropyl)-4,7,10-(carbo-*tert*-butoxymethyl)-1,4,7,10-tetraazacyclododecane (Fig. 3.4). The principal drawback of the use of DOTA is that high labeling efficiencies require heating the solution at 80°C during the labeling procedure that could negatively affect the peptide.

DTPA-like chelators

DTPA (*NR*-diethylenetriaminepentaacetic acid) (Fig. 3.5) is a strong chelating group able to coordinate all lanthanoid ions. The complexes in vivo are less stable than the DOTA complexes. DTPA derivatives such as cyclic DTPA (cDTPA) dianhydride and monoreactive DTPA derivative, 3,6-bis(carboxymethyl)-9-(((2-maleimidoethyl)carbamoyl)methyl)-3,6,9-triazaundecanedioic acid (mDTPA), have been used to bind bioactive molecules. For peptides containing lysine, the conjugation occurs predominantly at its ε-amino group, as this group is more basic than the αN-terminal amino group. As a result, this chelator may be inappropriate for peptides containing a lysine residue situated within the active site.

A monoreactive DTPA derivative, mDTPA, with four carboxy groups protected as *tert*-butyl esters, was introduced by Arano et al. (Fig. 3.5) (27) for both liquid- and solid-phase peptide synthesis. As with DOTA, mDTPA possesses only one free carboxy group. Another advantage is the high solubility of mDTPA in various solvents, making this BFCA appropriate for synthesis.

^{111}In-DTPA conjugates possess excellent in vivo stability (28). Much work has been dedicated to increasing the stability of complexes of Yttrium and lanthanoid ions by introducing (29) substitutions on the carbon atoms of the DTPA backbone. This modification can sterically hinder the opening of the chelate ring that occurs during radionuclide complex dissociation. The first class of modified DTPA conjugates was constructed by attaching *p*-isothiocyanatobenzyl moiety

FIGURE 3.5 DTPA-like chelating agents.

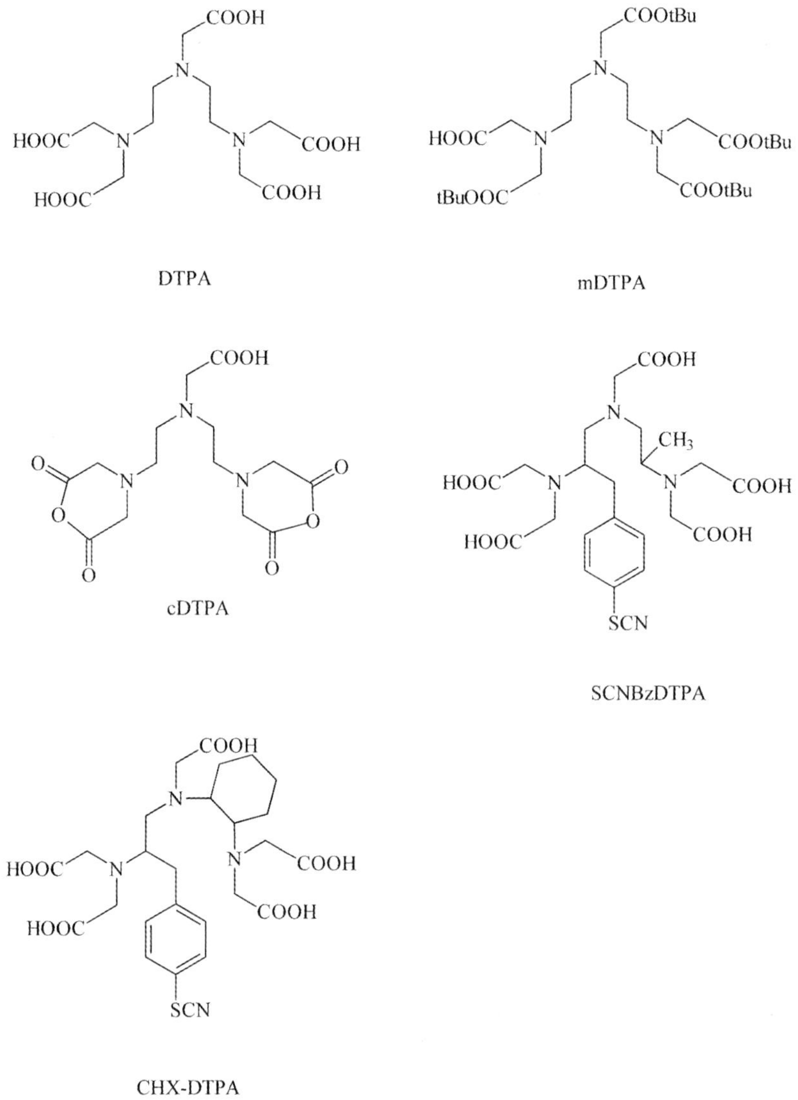

DTPA

mDTPA

cDTPA

SCNBzDTPA

CHX-DTPA

to one DTPA backbone ethylene group and appending methyl to another ethylene group in the same backbone (Fig. 3.5). The second class of modified DTPA conjugates was developed by replacing one of the ethylene groups by a cyclohexyl moiety (Fig. 3.5). These modifications increase the rigidity in the DTPA backbone and the in vivo stability of such radiopharmaceuticals (30,31).

Other polyaminocarboxylates

TETA (1,4,8,11-tetraazacyclotetradecane-1,4,8,-11-tetraacetic acid) (Fig. 3.6) forms a stable copper complex because the ion has a smaller radius than lanthanoids. In vitro studies demonstrated the serum stability of this complex. This chelating agent is used for copper radiopharmaceuticals in advanced imaging clinical trials (32).

NOTA-like chelators

NOTA (1,4,7-triazacyclononane-1,4,7-triacetic acid) (Fig. 3.6) (33), its phosphonate analog NOTP (1,4,7-triazacyclononane-N,N',N''-tris(methylenephosphonic) acid), and the

monoethyl ester of NOTP, NOTPME (1,4,7-triazacyclononane-N,N',N''-tris(methylenephosphonate monoethylester)) (34) were studied for application in radiopharmaceuticals to coordinate In and Ga ions. A monoreactive NOTA derivative, NODAGA(tBu)₃ (1-(1-carboxy-3-carbo-tert-butoxypropyl)-4,7-(carbo-tert-butoxymethyl)-1,4,7-triazacyclononane), has been synthesized (35). This BFCA is useful for the coupling to the N-terminus of peptides on solid phase and in solution. The NODAGA-peptide conjugates were labeled with ^{111}In and resulted in high yields and good specific activities. NODAGA-based derivatives carry a spacer function

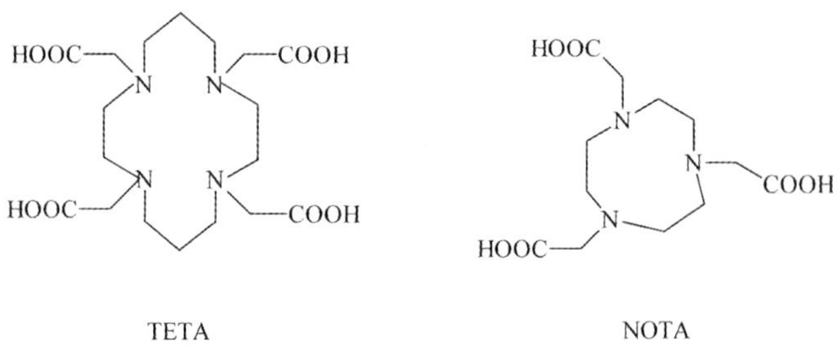

TETA

NOTA

FIGURE 3.6 Other chelating agents.

between the BFCA and the peptide which improves the receptor-binding affinity. NOTA-based octadentate ligands [2-(4,7-biscarboxymethyl[1,4,7]triazacyclononan-1-ylethyl) carbonylmethylamino]acetic acid tetrahydrochloride and [3-(4,7-biscarboxymethyl[1,4,7]triazacyclononan-1-yl-propyl) carbonylmethylamino]acetic acid tetrahydrochloride, with pendent donor groups were prepared to provide stable Y(III) complexes, for potential use in targeted radionuclide therapy. The results obtained from a preclinical biodistribution study indicate that the Yttrium complex possesses in vivo stability, comparable to the analogous DOTA complex, demonstrating an alternative to the use of DOTA derivatives for the systemic delivery of these compounds (36).

DEVELOPMENT OF RADIOLABELED PEPTIDES

The overexpression of receptors on tumor cells lead to the development of probes based on peptides to target cancer tissue. Initially, the peptides were radiolabeled with γ-emitters for SPECT or $\beta+$ for PET. The same bioactive molecules can also serve as vehicles for radiometal therapeutics, described in previous sections. It has been demonstrated that only tumors expressing a high density of receptors can be selected for peptide receptor systemic radiotherapy. Fortunately, many solid tumors meet these requirements by overexpressing the somatostatin receptor. The following sections represent a summary of the most common systems used in preclinical and clinical evaluations.

Labeled somatostatin peptide analogs

All five somatostatin-receptors (SSTRs) are found in numerous kinds of tumors (e.g., breast tumors, and small-cell lung cancer). The native peptide somatostatin (a 14-amino acid peptide) (Fig. 3.7) is rapidly degraded in vivo and has a very rapid blood clearance time ($T\frac{1}{2}$, 2 to 4 minutes). This issue resulted in the development of analogs that improved the circulating time, enhancing the stability against enzymatic cleavage. The most successful derivative is octreotide (Fig. 3.7) (37). This 8-amino acid analog, developed by Sandoz (now Novartis) is able to induce endocytosis by binding to SSTRs with high affinity, measured as a half maximal inhibitory concentration, or IC_{50}: SSTR2 ($IC_{50} = 2nM$), SSTR3 ($IC_{50} = 376$ nM), and SSTR5 ($IC_{50} = 299$ nM). Octreotide has been the subject of extensive structural studies, including NMR (38) and x-ray diffraction (39). These studies have demonstrated that octreotide adopts two conformational families in solution, differing mainly by the conformation of the C-terminal moiety. The molecule adopts an overall antiparallel β-sheet conformation, with a type II' β-turn in the D-Trp[4]-Lys[5] residues. In one conformational family, the residues after this β-turn continue the β-sheet structure, and in the second family, the residues after the β-turn adopt a 3_{10}-helical conformation. X-ray data of chelator-conjugated and metallated octapeptides are not yet available. ^{1}H- and ^{13}C-NMR data in solution are in agreement with the fast

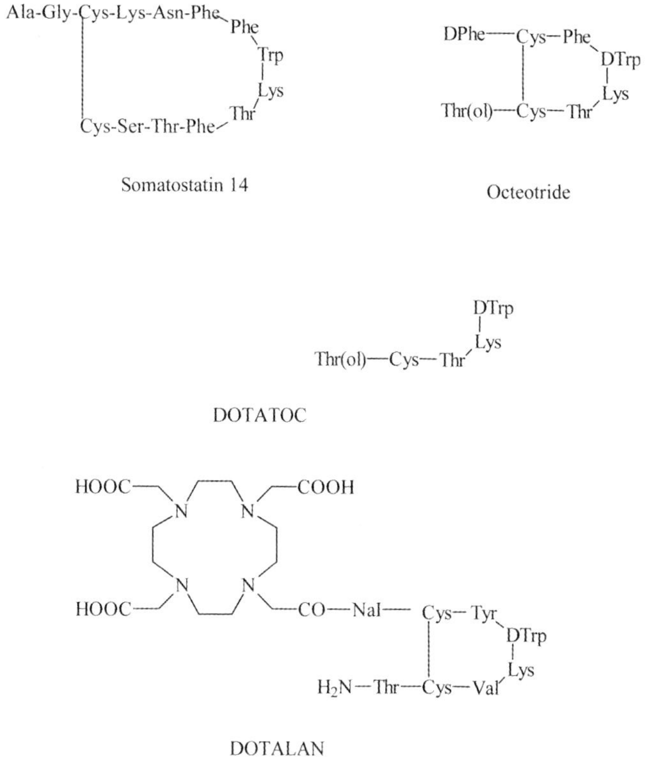

FIGURE 3.7 Somatostatin and octreotide sequences.

equilibrium of two predominant conformations, a helical and a β-sheet structure, as in octreotide (40). These residues are the biologically active portions, responsible for interacting with the receptor, while the bridging region maintains the proper orientation of the turn. Starting from the octreotide sequence, many peptide analogs were designed, all of which must conserve the critical sequence D-Trp[4]-Lys[5]. These modifications have been performed on the side-chain amino acids of this β-turn (Phe[3] and Thr[6]) (41). The peptide structure is not affected when conjugated substances are covalently bound on the N-terminus. The opportunity to modify the N-terminal position makes it possible to conjugate radiometals. The octeotride conjugate is commonly used in clinical tumor diagnosis. Many investigators have demonstrated that ^{111}In-DTPA (diethylenediaminepentaacetic acid) octreotide (Octreoscan) (Fig. 3.8) is a highly diagnostic agent for neuroendocrine tumors (NETs), which are visualized with scintigraphy (40).

Since ^{111}In emits not only γ-rays, but also therapeutic Auger and internal conversion electrons with short tissue penetration (0.02 to 10.0 and 200 to 500 μm, respectively), the first in vitro studies were performed with high doses of [^{111}In-DTPA[0]]octreotide (42). The results indicated that the high dosage of [^{111}In-DTPA[0]]octreotide can inhibit the growth cells in SSTR2-positive liver metastases, after the administration of tumor cells in the portal vein. These data indicated that [^{111}In-DTPA[0]]octreotide might be useful in the case of micrometastases, although further studies need to be performed in order to confirm this concept. Due to the low tissue penetration, further octreotide analogs labeled with β-emitting particles were

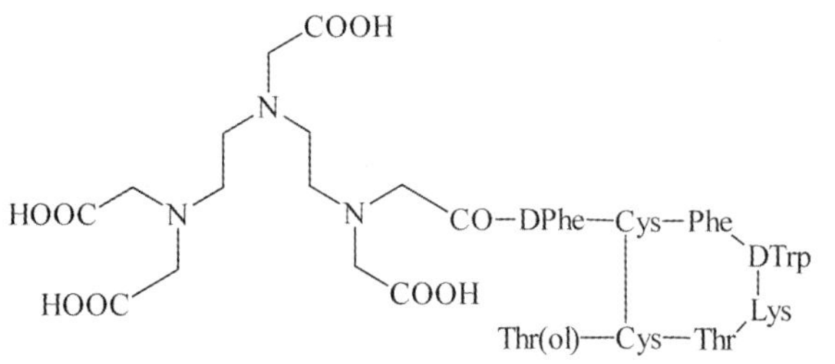

FIGURE 3.8 DTPA- and DOTA-modified somatostatin-based peptides for targeted radiotherapy.

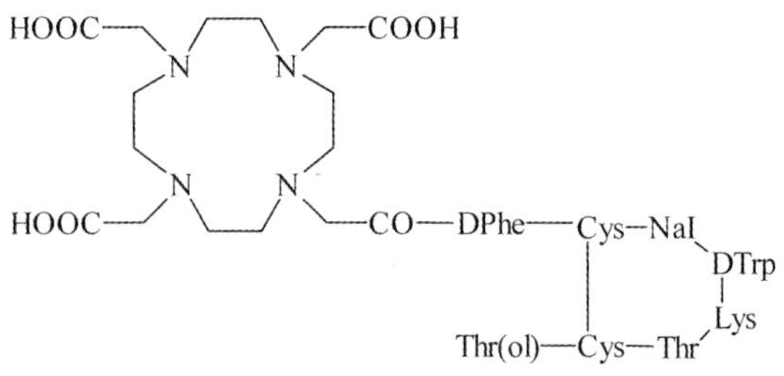

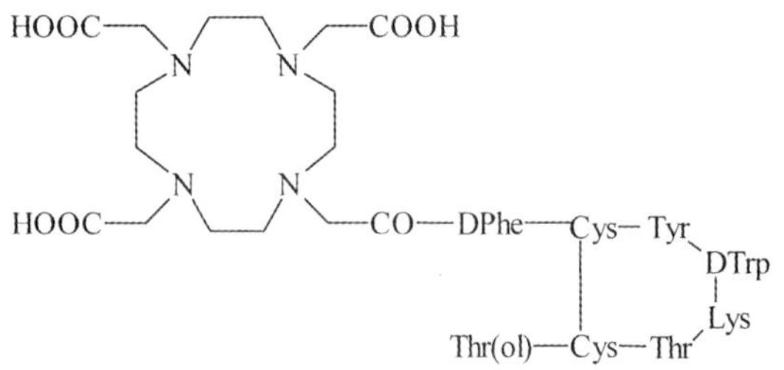

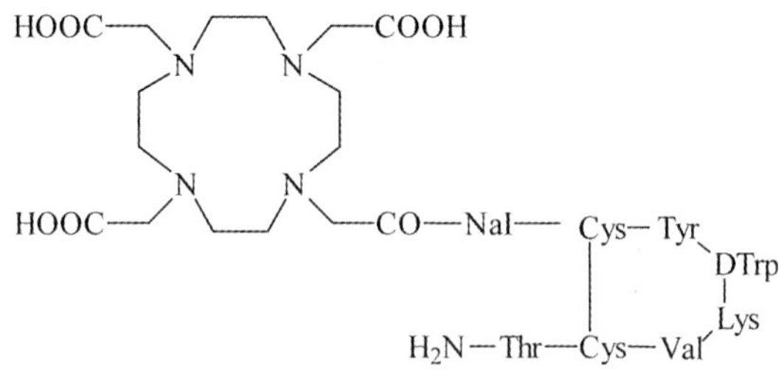

developed. The DTPA chelator was replaced by the DOTA macrocyclic chelator. DOTA shows more stability in vivo for a broad range of metallic radionuclides, some of which include ^{90}Y, ^{177}Lu, ^{188}Re, ^{67}Cu, ^{68}Ga, ^{111}In, ^{64}Cu, and ^{99m}Tc (43).

The ^{90}Y and ^{111}In DOTA analogs show more favorable biodistribution and tumor uptake in animal models compared to DPTA conjugates. Minor modifications to the peptide structure or chelate, as well as the type of radionuclide utilized, will influence the biodistribution and the binding affinity of the conjugate. Earlier studies demonstrate that the peptide in which Phe^3 is replaced by Tyr^3 (e.g., DOTA-TOC; Fig. 3.8), in order to increase hydrophilicity, exhibits improved SSTR2 affinity and a lower affinity for the SSTR3 receptor (44). For example, the IC$_{50}$ for Y-DOTA-octreotide (DOTAOC), Y-DOTA-[Tyr3]-octreotide (DOTATOC), and Y-DOTA-[Tyr3]-octreotate (DOTATATE) are 20.0, 11.0, and 1.6 nM, from lower to higher affinity, respectively (44). The ^{90}Y-DOTATOC was the first conjugate tested for peptide receptor radionuclide therapy (PRRT) in 2001–2005. Various multicenter phase 1 and 2 clinical trials have been performed (45–47). Despite the differences in protocol design, the rate of complete and partial responses (10 to 30%) consistently exceeds that obtained with [^{111}In-DTPA^0] octreotide. Very recently, a phase 2 clinical trial, reported by Iten et al., demonstrated the long-term benefit of ^{90}Y-DOTATOC when treating metastatic medullary thyroid cancer (48). In parallel, Forrer et al. performed a phase 2 study to evaluate the effectiveness and toxicity of ^{90}Y-DOTATOC and ^{177}Lu-DOTATOC in patients with surgically incurable paragangliomas. Although the therapy seems to be less effective than in gastroenteropancreatic (GEP) NETs, the usefulness of these derivatives in

incurable paragangliomas is correlated with low toxicity and long-lasting remissions (49).

DOTA-lanreotide [DOTALAN] (Fig. 3.8) labeled with ^{90}Y was the second analog used for PRRT. This analog is more lipophilic than ^{90}Y-DOTATOC. Lanreotide is an octapeptide designed from octreotide by replacing the DPhe^1 with a β-naphtyl alanine and the Thr^6 with Val. These modifications decrease the affinity of the peptide toward the SSTR2, but increase the affinity toward SSTR5. In clinical trials, two thirds of patients with NETs, treated with ^{90}Y-DOTALAN and ^{90}Y-DOTATOC, showed tumor uptake; however, the DOTALAN derivative showed a lower tumor uptake than the DOTATOC derivative. This phenomenon could be explained by the low affinity of DOTALAN for SSTR2.

The third promising analog used for PRRT is the DOTATATE conjugate. It was observed that converting the octreotide to octreotate (by replacing the C-terminal Thr(ol) of the octapeptide with a natural amino acid, Thr) results in increased receptor binding, better internalization, high tumor uptake, and improved scintigraphy (50). The same ^{177}Lu-labeled conjugate was tested in patients with metastatic NETs; moreover, Kwekkeboom et al. reported the long-term follow-up and the survival data in over 300 patients with GEP NETs (51). It was shown that this compound had few side effects and was relatively safe. In the same studies, the authors note that the residence time in tumor for this compound is higher than ^{177}Lu-DOTATOC.

Another analog has been synthesized with a more lipophilic residue, β-naphtyl alanine, in the third position [DOTA^1-Nal^3]-octreotide (DOTANOC) (Fig. 3.8) (52). This analog was selected from a 24-peptide "library" of DOTAOC derivatives (53) and it showed high affinity for SSTR2, SSTR3, and SSTR5 when complexed with [111]In. It had greater tumor uptake in comparison to ^{111}In-DOTATOC. It was concluded that this derivative (DOTANOC), when metal-complexed, exhibits the broadest affinity profile, efficiently targets SSTR2, SSTR3, SSTR5, and has improved tumor:kidney ratios in an animal model (53). Further, it has been verified by preclinical and clinical studies using ^{90}Y, ^{68}Ga, ^{111}In, and ^{177}Lu-labeled DOTANOC (53). In addition, DOTANOC and DOTATATE, labeled with ^{177}Lu, were evaluated (54). A total of 69 patients with inoperable NET were studied with 95 posttherapeutic dosimetric assessments using ^{177}Lu-DOTATATE and eight using ^{177}Lu-DOTANOC. It was concluded that the higher in vitro affinity noted with DOTANOC leads to a higher uptake in normal tissue and in a whole-body dose (54). Considering that the kidneys are the main critical organs for toxicity when PRRT is utilized, a study was undertaken to assess long-term renal function following exposure to ^{90}Y-DOTA^0,Tyr^3-octreotide (^{90}Y-DOTATOC) and ^{177}Lu-DOTA^0,Tyr^3-octreotide (^{177}Lu-DOTATATE) (55). Twenty-eight patients received a total renal dose between 18.3 and 38.7 Gy with ^{90}Y-DOTA-TOC and 37 patients received 7.3 and 26.7 Gy with ^{177}Lu-DOTATATE. Median follow-up was 2.9 and 2.4 years, respectively. All patients received renal protective amino acids during each administration of the radioligand. The median decrease in creatinine clearance per year was 7.3% and 3.8% ($p = 0.06$) with ^{90}Y-DOTATOC and ^{177}Lu-DOTATATE, respectively (55). In spite of this, therapeutic clinical studies showed that it was still necessary to use amino acid infusions to effectively decrease the kidney uptake. Also, in some cases, ^{111}In/^{177}Lu-DOTANOC exhibits higher background activity than ^{111}In-DOTATOC, probably due to the higher lipophilicity of radiolabeled DOTANOC. Recently, the use of antagonist instead of agonist receptors

was proposed as a new approach to radiolabeled peptide therapy. Ginj et al. reported promising results in a preclinical study, using an antagonist receptor that did not trigger SSTR internalization, but prevented agonist-stimulated internalization (56). If the results can be confirmed in other receptor binding studies, then the use of potent radiolabeled antagonists for in vivo tumor targeting may become a new therapeutic option for PRRT.

Other peptide receptors

In the last decade, many peptide receptors have been identified that are overexpressed in most tumors. Many of them certainly could be targeted by peptide analogs capable of delivering metal ions as contrast for SPECT and PET. In Table 3.1, a list of current eligible target related tumors is illustrated. In the following paragraphs, we will briefly summarize some of the main receptor and peptide conjugates, which may be the subject of further studies in the coming years for PRRT.

▓ Vasoactive intestinal peptide receptors

The vasoactive intestinal peptide (VIP) is a 28-amino acid peptide, neuroendocrine mediator, with a broad spectrum of functions. VIP is a vasodilator and impacts on pulmonary blood pressure. It stimulates the secretion of various hormones and regulates electrolyte and water secretion in the intestines. Patients with VIP-secreting tumors will manifest a classic "diarrhea syndrome." It has also been associated with the promotion of the growth of normal cells and cancer cells. The molecular activity of VIP is mediated by cell membrane receptors. Virgolini et al. (57) and Reubi (58) have identified the overexpression of VIP receptors on many human tumors. VIP receptors were identified on most

Table **3.1** Peptides, cancer target, and receptor candidates for peptide radiation therapy in the future		
Peptide	**Cancer Target**	**Receptor**
Somatostain analogs	Neuroendocrine, small-cell lung, breast, monocytes, and lymphocytes	Somatostatin 1–5
VIP	Non–small-cell lung, breast, colon, pancreatic, prostate, bladder, and ovarian cancer	VIP 1 and 2
Glucagon-like peptide 1	Insulinomas	Glucagon-like peptide 1 receptors
RGD analogs	Tumor-induced angiogenesis	$\alpha_v\beta_3$ Integrin
Neurotensin	Exocrine pancreatic cancer, meningioma and Ewing sarcomas, and prostate and pancreatic cancer	NT 1–3
Substance P	Glial tumors, astrocytomas, medullary thyroid, and breast cancer	NK1, NK2, and NK3
CCK/gastrin derivates	GI tumors, pancreatic adenoma, and medullary thyroid cancer	CCK1, CCK2
Neuropeptide Y	Breast, ovarian, and adrenal tumors	NPY receptors
Bombesin(7–14) Bombesin antagonist Gastrin-releasing peptide	Prostate, breast, gastric, ovarian, colon, and pancreatic cancer	GRP–bombesin

VIP, vasoactive intestinal peptide; RGD, Arg-Gly-Asp; NT, neurotensin; NK, neurokinin; CCK, cholecystokinin; NPY, neuropeptide Y; GRP, gastrin-releasing peptide.

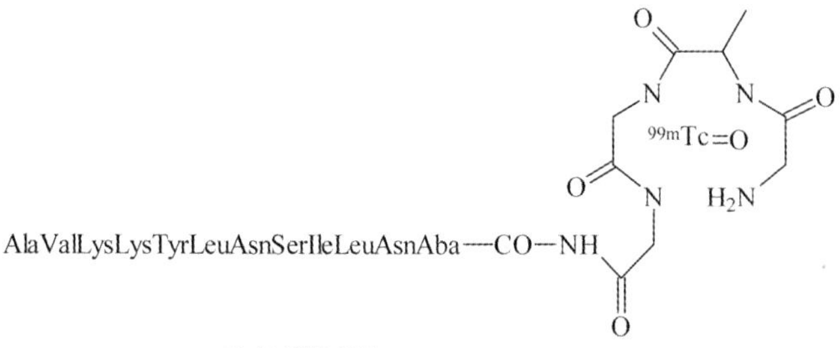

^{99m}TcTP3654

FIGURE 3.9 Structural formula of VIP conjugate to visualize VIP receptor.

adenocarcinomas and squamous cell carcinomas, using the radioligand [^{125}I-Tyr^{10}]-VIP. It was shown that VIP receptors were overexpressed to a greater degree, than SSTRs, on multiple cancer cell lines (43). Pallela et al. synthesized several compounds labeled with ^{99m}Tc (59). An initial compound failed to retain biologic activity due to manipulation of the essential bioactive N-terminus. Their most recent compound, VIP-Aba-Gly-Gly-(D)-Ala-Gly (^{99m}TcTP3654), was successfully labeled with ^{99m}Tc (Fig. 3.9) and retained biologic activity equivalent to that of native VIP (59). These results indicate a potential for SPECT imaging and radiotherapy. The low metabolic stability of VIP, however, is a potential concern for VIP receptor–based targeted therapy. Additionally, VPAC$_1$ (a subtype VIP receptor) is rather ubiquitous and expressed in most normal tissues, rendering it somewhat unsuitable for PRRT. Interestingly, VPAC$_2$, which is minimally expressed in normal tissue and overexpressed in gastrointestinal stromal tumors, may be a more reasonable model for PRRT.

Glucagon-like peptide 1 receptors

A new promising candidate for in vivo tumor targeting is the glucagon-like peptide 1 (GLP-1) receptor, a member of the glucagon receptor family (60). The GLP-1 receptor is overexpressed in human gut and lung NETs, particularly in insulinomas (61). Insulinomas have been successfully visualized scintigraphically after injection of radiolabeled GLP-1 analogs in rats and mice (62,63). Furthermore, a preclinical study has shown dramatic targeting of the GLP-1 receptor of insulinomas in the Rip1Tag2 mouse model, using the radioligand [Lys40(Ahx-DTPA-111In)NH2]exendin-4 (63). GLP-1, exendin-3, and/or exendin-4 derivatives are available and may be used for disease diagnosis and treatment. Because C-terminal conjugation does not inhibit binding of GLP-1 or exendins to their receptors, the peptides or fragments are conjugated to a lysine or an ornithine moiety. The amine group is able to bind covalently to a BFCA. Thus, the compound [(125)I]GLP-1(7-36)amide was synthesized and was synthesized and localized into RINm5F cells, a radiation-induced rat insulinoma cell line (62). In the future, more studies have to be performed so that more information becomes available about receptor concentration in tumor and in normal tissue. On the basis of their high expression in specific tumors and their low expression in normal tissues, GLP-1 receptors are very promising candidates for in vivo targeting for diagnostic and therapeutic purposes.

$\alpha_V\beta_3$ *Integrin receptors*

The integrins $\alpha_V\beta_3$ and $\alpha_V\beta_5$ play a fundamental role in angiogenesis and tumor metastasis (64,65). Integrin $\alpha_V\beta_3$ is highly expressed on the activated endothelial cells in several tumors, including melanoma, ovarian carcinoma, lung carcinoma, osteosarcoma, neuroblastoma, glioblastoma, and breast carcinoma (66,67). Integrin $\alpha_V\beta_3$, as the most abundant integrin receptor, recognizes peptide domains containing the Arg-Gly-Asp (RGD) amino acid sequence (68–70). Based on the RGD tripeptide sequence, a series of small RGD linear and cyclic peptides have been designed to antagonize the function of $\alpha_V\beta_3$ integrin, such as cyclo(RGDf-N(Me)-V), which has high activity and selectivity toward $\alpha_V\beta_3$ integrin (71). Additionally, within this compound, it should be noted that valine could be substituted for other amino acids without loss of biologic activity, enabling many different types of modifications. Systematic derivatization of the lead peptide resulted in the initial development of the above-mentioned analog, cyclo(RGDf-N(Me)-V) (EMD 121974) (72), which has entered clinical phase 2 trials as an angiogenesis inhibitor (Cilengitide) (73).

Beginning with Cilengitide, a large number of radiolabeled analogs have been developed and used as radiotracers for cancer diagnosis (SPECT and PET) and therapy. To date, a large number of reviews have summarized the potential of RGD radiolabeled peptides (74). Dijkgraaf et al. (75) reported the synthesis of four DOTA conjugated compounds. One particular compound, a cyclic RGD peptide DOTA-E-c(RGDfK), has a high affinity for $\alpha_V\beta_3$-integrin with superior tumor-targeting characteristics. With similar goals, researchers have reported the design and synthesis of a series of $\alpha_V\beta_3$ integrin–directed monomeric, dimeric, and tetrameric c[RGDfK] dendrimers. The multivalent RGD-dendrimers appeared to have enhanced affinity toward the $\alpha_V\beta_3$ integrin receptor and exhibit significantly higher tumor uptake compared to its monomeric and dimeric analogs, even though renal retention of the multimeric peptides was increased. Further studies, in athymic mice inoculated with an ovarian cancer cell line and treated with ^{177}Lu-DOTA-E-c(RGDfK), were performed. PRRT experiments in this cancer model indicated that tumor growth could be inhibited significantly by a therapeutic dose of 37 MBq of the ^{177}Lu compound. The %ID/g of tumor at 4 hours was a remarkable 38.8% (76). This level of activity far exceeds the expected %ID/g of tumor typically seen with 150-kDa monoclonal antibodies.

Recently, Del Gatto et al. reported the design, synthesis, and biologic behavior of a new and selective peptide antagonist, RGDechi (77). This peptide is a chimeric molecule consisting of a cyclic RGD sequence derived from Cilengitide to ensure receptor affinity, and two echistatin C-terminal moieties to improve the receptor selectivity, covalently linked using a Pro-Gly spacer. Studies performed on radiolabeled RGDechi derivatives showed that the peptide is suitable for selective imaging of $\alpha_V\beta_3$-expressing tumors, by SPECT and PET, and is a potential future candidate for PRRT.

Neurotensin receptors

Neurotensin (NT) is a tridecapeptide localized both in the central nervous system and in peripheral tissues (78,79). Most data confirm that NT receptors are overexpressed in different human tumors, such as pancreatic, lung, colon, prostate, and breast cancers (80,81). Overexpressed NT receptors could be targeted by radiolabeled NT analogs. The main drawback of natural NT is its rapid degradation in plasma. Structure–activity studies have already shown that the C-terminal hexapeptide NT-(8–13), Arg^8-Arg^9-Pro^{10}-Tyr^{11}-Ile^{12}-Leu^{13}, is the minimal sequence required for biologic activity. The three cleavage sites in the metabolic deactivation of NT-(8–13) are Arg^8-Arg^9, Pro^{10}-Tyr^{11}, and Tyr^{11}-Ile^{12} (82). The modification of Arg^8-Arg^9 and Tyr^{11}-Ile^{12}, of NT, results in increased plasma stability, increased affinity for the NT receptor 1 (NTR1), and good in vivo tumor uptake (83–85). One particular analog, NT-XI, allowed for the preoperative visualization of tumor in one of four patients diagnosed with pancreatic adenocarcinoma. Pathologic analysis of the tumor specimens revealed high expression of the NT receptor only in the patient with positive imaging. These data appear to confirm the potential utility of the NT analog, $[^{99m}Tc(CO)_3](N^\alpha His)Ac$-Lys-($\psi CH_2$-NH)-Arg-Pro-Tyr-Tle-Leu-), for imaging (86). However, it was shown that a rather high accumulation in the liver and kidneys occurred. The replacement of the Lys-($\psi CH_2 NH$)-Arg reduced the amide bond by an Arg-NMeArg in NT-XII and resulted in lower kidney uptake and better tumor-to-kidney ratio, while maintaining receptor affinity and in vitro plasma metabolic stability. Further improvements have been made to increase the selectivity for cancer tissue and to increase the blood clearance. Recently, a new NT analog has been designed, $(N^\alpha His)Ac$-Arg-(N-CH_3)-Arg-Pro-Dmt-Tle-Leu, NT-XIX, which shows a very slow plasma clearance when labeled with the γ-emitting radionuclide ^{99m}Tc, together with the promising results in preliminary therapeutic studies (labeled with the β-radionuclide ^{188}Re) (87).

New stable NT analogs with high receptor affinity have been synthesized by replacing arginine residues with lysine and arginine derivatives. Four ^{111}In-labeled DTPA-chelated NT analogs and one ^{111}In-labeled DOTA-chelated NT analog were evaluated in NMRI nude mice bearing NT receptor-positive HT29 tumors. It was concluded that DTPA-(Pip)Gly-Pro-(PipAm)Gly-Arg-Pro-Tyr-tBuGly-Leu-OH and the DOTA-linked counterpart had the most favorable biodistribution properties regarding tumor uptake (88).

Substance P receptors

Substance P (RPKPQQFFGLM-NH2) is an undecapeptide belonging to a family of chemically related peptides, the tachykinins which share a C-terminal amino acid sequence. This neuropeptide is involved in a variety of functions in the central and peripheral nervous systems, where it acts as a neurotransmitter and a neuromodulator, being modulated through neurokinin 1 and 2 (NK1 and NK2) receptors (89). Moreover, substance P is a potent vasodilator, modulates pain transmission, and is able to stimulate the proliferation of malignant tumor cells. The NK1 receptor is quite frequently expressed in glial tumors, but can also be detected in medullary thyroid carcinomas, small-cell lung cancers, pancreatic carcinoma as well as breast cancers (90,91). It is rarely found in gastrointestinal tumors or lymphomas.

^{111}In-DTPA-SP has been synthesized and promising results have been gained in scintigraphic visualization of thymus (92). A pilot study has been performed in advanced glioma, with local injections of ^{90}Y-DOTA–substance P, as performed previously in astrocytomas with ^{90}Y-DOTATOC (93). The high accumulation and long residence time of the tracer restricted to the tumor site has been highly encouraging and resulted in promising preliminary results (93).

A new targeting vector was developed by conjugating the chelator 1,4,7,10-tetraazacyclododecane-1-glutaric acid-4,7,10-triacetic acid (DOTAGA) to Arg^1 of substance P. This conjugate was labeling with ^{90}Y (Fig. 3.10). Following preclinical assessment, the authors conducted a pilot study in 20 patients with gliomas of WHO grades 2 to 4, primarily to assess biodistribution and short- and long-term toxicity. Secondary end points were the clinical and radiologic responses (94).

Cholecystokinin/gastrin receptors

The biologically active gastrointestinal peptides gastrin and cholecystokinin (CCK) are a family of peptides of variable length but they share five terminal amino acids at their C-terminus. CCK consists of a variety of molecular forms based upon the number of amino acids, such that CCK8 and CCK33 have 8 and 33 amino acids, respectively. CCK and gastrin hormones act as neurotransmitters in the brain and as regulators of various functions of the gastrointestinal tract, mediating several receptor subtypes. The best-characterized receptors are CCK1 (or CCK-A) and CCK2 (or CCK-B). Both receptors are overexpressed in tumors of

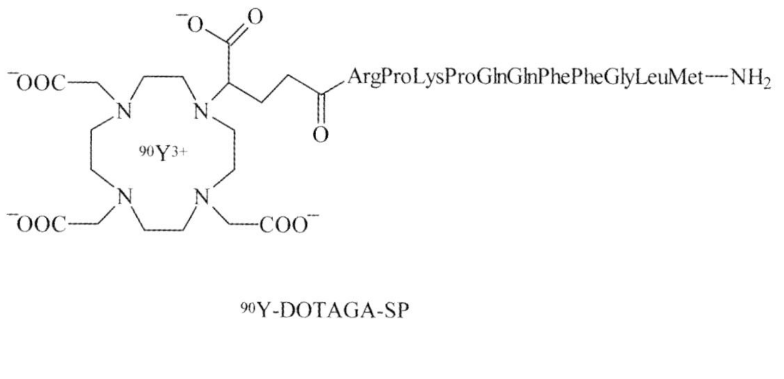

FIGURE 3.10 Substance P radiotherapeutic analog.

^{90}Y-DOTAGA-SP

neuroendocrine origin (95). In particular, the CCK2 is over-expressed in a large percentage (90%) of medullary thyroid cancers, to a lesser extent in small cell lung cancers and in GEP tumors. A wide number of conjugates have been synthesized and tested in vitro and in mice, visualizing the pathologic tissues by SPECT and PET (96).

Mutagenesis, photoaffinity, cross-linking, and NMR studies, evaluating the interaction of CCK8 with various receptors, have been performed (97–99). The results reveal that the majority of the ligand–receptor interactions in CCK2 involve the C-terminal tetrapeptide of CCK. In addition, NMR studies suggest that CCK involves the C-terminus to form specific interactions with the N-terminal arm of the CCK1 receptor (100). This knowledge base provides insight to a structure-based approach for the design of CCK analogs. A wide number of conjugates bearing the BFCA on N-terminal moiety were synthesized and tested. Most of the studies have evaluated the binding CCK octapeptide (CCK26–33 or CCK8) conjugates with DTPA, DOTA, DOTA-like, and a polydentate-chelating agent that coordinates Tc or Re isotopes. Aloj et al. evaluated the potential of ^{111}In-DTPAGlu-Gly-CCK8 (Fig. 3.11) in vitro, observing rapid internalization by cells and uptake was seen in tumor-bearing nude mice, although levels of radioactivity in the kidneys was elevated (101).

Reubi et al. tested a variety of DOTA- and DPTA-conjugated octapeptide analogs that showed specificity for the CCK-B receptors. The two lead conjugates were DTPA-[Nle28,31]-CCK(26–31) and DTPA-[d-Asp26,Nle28,31]-CCK(26–33). These radiopeptides displayed a high affinity with an IC_{50} of 1.5 nM. Animal biodistribution studies, using ^{111}In-labeled compounds, revealed that the primary clearance was renal and that the main area of uptake was in the kidneys and gastrointestinal tract. Both ligands showed high stability in human serum and underwent

biodegradation in urine. It was concluded that these two analogs show promise for imaging CCK-B–expressing tumors (96).

Behr and Behe explored the clinical utility of radiolabeled minigastrin in patients with medullary thyroid cancer on the basis of previous in vitro receptor studies. They were able to show a sensitivity of 91% imaging with ^{111}In-DTPA-dGlu(1)-minigastrin (Fig. 3.11). Eight patients with advanced metastatic disease were treated on a dose escalation study, using a ^{90}Y-labeled minigastrin conjugate. An injection was delivered every 4 to 6 weeks (30 to 50 mCi/m^2 per treatment) for a maximum of four injections. The treatment showed evidence of efficacy (two partial responses and four patients with stabilized disease), although hematologic and renal toxicity was observed (102). The main drawback for the development of PRRT using CCK2 receptors appears to be the high kidney uptake with current CCK analogs. Therefore, a new generation of CCK analogs has been designed with much less kidney uptake.

Mather et al. synthesized a small library of peptide chelators that combined relatively high tumor affinity with low renal uptake. Testing in AR42J tumor-bearing mice, they selected the peptide with the sequence DOTA-HHEAYGWMDF-NH(2), which showed the best tumor-to-kidney ratio, with saturable uptake in target organs and low uptake by nontarget tissues other than the kidney (103).

▇ Neuropeptide Y receptors

Neuropeptide Y (NPY) is a peptide, consisting of 36 amino acids, with an unusually high number of tyrosine residues (Y). NPY is widely involved in a variety of physiologic functions, mediated in humans by different receptor subtypes, the so-called Y receptors: Y_1, Y_2, Y_4, Y_5, and Y_6. Several NPY analogs, in particular Y_1 and Y_2 antagonists, are

FIGURE 3.11 Radiopeptides capable of targeting cholecystokinin/gastrin receptors.

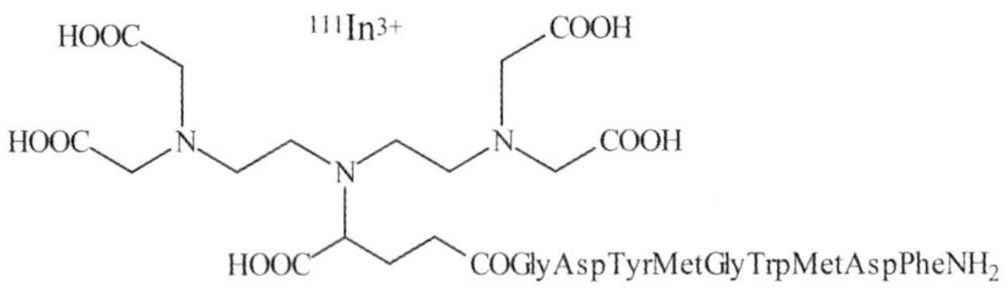

^{111}In-DTPAGlu-Gly-CCK8

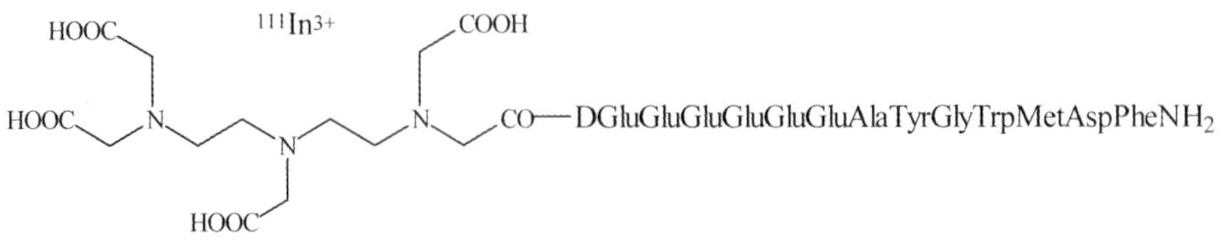

^{111}In-DTPA-DGlu-minigastrin

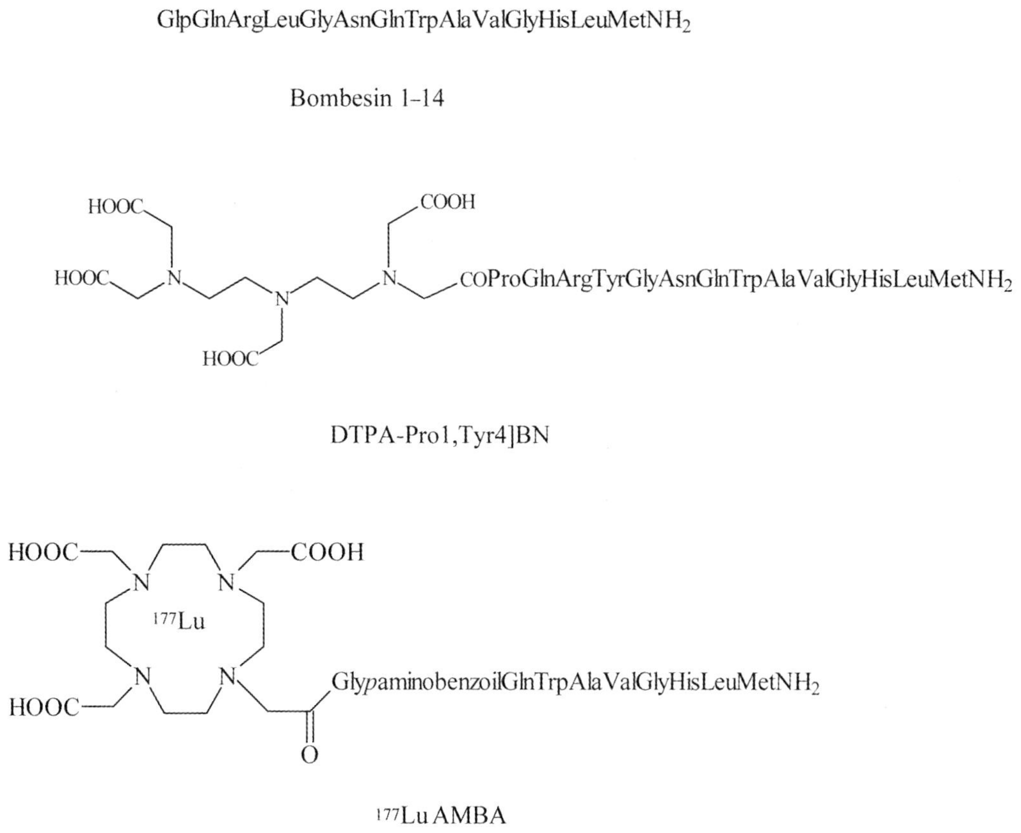
GlpGlnArgLeuGlyAsnGlnTrpAlaValGlyHisLeuMetNH2
Bombesin 1–14
HOOC
COOH
HOOC
N
N
N
COProGlnArgTyrGlyAsnGlnTrpAlaValGlyHisLeuMetNH2
HOOC
DTPA-Pro1,Tyr4]BN
HOOC
COOH
177Lu
HOOC
GlypaminobenzoilGlnTrpAlaValGlyHisLeuMetNH2
O
177Lu AMBA

FIGURE 3.12 Bombesin sequence and analogs to target GRP receptors.

being developed for potential clinical use to treat feeding disorders and anxiety (104,105). In the last decade, it has been shown that NPY might play an important role in tumors (106). The Y_1 receptor subtype is the predominant NPY receptor overexpressed in human breast tumors and metastasis. The presence of this receptor has been found in prostate cancer, in human ovarian tissue, and in renal cell carcinoma (107). The receptor selectivity is a major problem that opens a pathway to develop tools that allow the characterization of the receptors on the protein level. Selective ligands, for example fluorescent-labeled or radiolabeled, are the best approaches to address this issue. It has been shown that substitutions on C-terminal positions allow a distinction to be made between some receptor subtypes. The addition of β-aminocyclopropane carboxylic acids (β-ACCs) to the C-terminus of the NPY sequence produces a Y_1-receptor selective analog (108). Substituting a proline residue at position 34 reduces the Y_2 receptor affinity and maintains the affinity toward the Y_1 and Y_5 receptors. Introducing the turn-inducing Ala-Aib sequence in position 31 and 32, respectively, led to a Y_5-selective analog with high affinity. Currently, only iodinated radiolabeled conjugates are available for receptor Y_1 or Y_5. The covalent incorporation of radionuclides into peptides can be performed by two different chemical strategies: the direct or the indirect method (104). The introduction of a chelating agent should preferably involve the Lys^4 residue as this will not interfere with receptor binding (104).

Bombesin peptide analogs

Bombesin (BN) is a neuropeptide of 14 amino acids, originally isolated from frog skin, with a high affinity for the gastrin-releasing peptide (GRP) receptor (Fig. 3.12). The BB1, BB2, and BB3 receptors and, in particular, the GRP receptor subtype have been shown to be massively overexpressed in several human tumors (109). Interestingly, GRP overexpression is higher than SSTR2 in prostate cancer and breast cancer. Many synthetic BN peptide antagonists that bind with high affinities to GRP receptors have been synthesized to evaluate their potential to reduce or minimize the rate of growth of GRP receptor expressing cancers (110). At the same time much progress has been made in producing radiolabeled BN analogs that specifically target GRP receptor–expressing cancer cells in vitro and in vivo (111,112).

One of the analogs synthesized to target these receptors was a BN agonist [DTPA-Pro^1,Tyr^4]BN (Fig. 3.12), studied by Breeman et al. (113), which differs only from native BN by replacing $pGlu^1$ by DTPA-Pro, thus permitting labeling with ^{111}In. Additionally, the replacement of Leu^4 by Tyr potentially allowed for radioiodination. Hoffman et al. (114) demonstrated the viability of formulating radiolabeled truncated BN(8–14) as a BN agonist. The C-terminal sequence of the natural peptide retains high binding affinities for GRP receptors and they were internalized by GRP-expressing cells. A wide variety of chelating agents have been coupled to the N-terminal moiety in order to be able to coordinate ^{105}Rh, ^{99m}Tc, and ^{111}In. In a recent study, the same group evaluated DOTA through hydrocarbon spacer groups, to specifically target GRP receptor–expressing cancer cells. The length and composition of the spacer group, as well as the physicochemical properties of the radiolabeled moiety, will influence the GRP receptor–binding affinity, residualization of radioactivity in cancer cells, and pharmacokinetics of the BN conjugate. These results suggest that the ^{111}In-DOTA-X-BBN[7–14]NH$_2$ construct, where X represents a "tether" ranging between a 5- and 8-carbon spacer, is a reasonable candidate for diagnostic and therapeutic trials in patients with GRP-positive tumors (115).

Several BN analogs, replacing the unnatural or D amino acid residues, have been designed, synthesized, and characterized in vitro and in vivo. Nock et al. have reported the development of [^{99m}Tc]Demobesin 1, a potent antagonist that effectively binds to the GRP receptor with very high affinity (116). Recently, this analog was compared with BN in vitro and in vivo studies indicating that GRP receptor antagonists may be superior targeting agents in comparison to GRP receptor agonists, suggesting a paradigm shift in the field of BN radiopharmaceuticals. The same authors have also reported investigations into the design of four new agonistic BN conjugates [Demobesin 3: [N4^0,Pro^1,Tyr^4]BB; Demobesin 4: [N4^0,Pro^1,Tyr^4,Nle^{14}]BB; Demobesin 5: [(N4-Bzdig)^0]BB(7–14); and Demobesin 6: [(N4-Bzdig)^0, Nle^{14}]BB(7–14)] that can be radiolabeled with ^{99m}Tc (117). These four BN analogs, functionalized at the N-terminus with open-chain tetraamines for labeling with ^{99m}Tc, are based on agonists such as Demobesin 3 to 6. The first two analogs are based on the parent BN tetradecapeptide sequence after minor modifications (Pyr^1 has been replaced by Pro^1 to allow for N-terminal modification), while the other two are truncated peptides based on the essential residues needed for receptor interaction, the BB(7–14) motif. Demobesin 4 and 6 have undergone substitution of the oxidation-sensitive Met^{14} by Nle^{14}.

A universal ligand, [D-Tyr^6, β-Ala^{11}, Phe^{13}, Nle^{14}] bombesin (6–14), has been developed by Mantey et al. (118) and Pradhan et al. (119), which has high affinity to all of the BN receptor subtypes. From this peptide, pan-bombesin conjugates have been synthesized with high affinity to all three human BN receptor subtypes with binding affinities in the nanomolar range coordinate. DTPA and DOTA chelating agents have been covalently bonded to the N-terminus and the Phe^{13} was replaced by δ-(2-thienylcarbonyl) ornithine (Thi) because the analog shows increased metabolic stability. The DTPA and DOTA-[D-Tyr^6, β-Ala^{11}, Thi^{13}, Nle^{14}]bombesin (6–14) were able to coordinate ^{111}In and ^{90}Y, respectively.

In order to coordinate ^{177}Lu for radiotherapeutic applications, Lantry et al. (120) developed a new conjugate bearing an N-terminal moiety, dota-like chelating agent (DO3A) tethered by an organic linker (^{177}Lu AMBA) (Fig. 3.12). The organic linker seems to provide increased uptake and retention of radioactivity in tumor at 1 hour. ^{177}Lu AMBA binds with nanomolar affinity to GRP-R which has a low retention of radioactivity in kidneys, demonstrates a very favorable risk–benefit profile, and is in phase 1 clinical trials.

Further progress in developing GRP receptor–targeted radionuclides will require additional efforts in understanding the structurally sensitive mechanisms involved in the binding of these derivatives to GRP/BBN receptors, the subsequent residualization of the radiotracer in GRP receptor–expressing cancer cells, and finally, efficient clearance of nonresidualizing radiolabeled peptide from nontarget tissues. Because the number of GPR receptors in prostate and breast cancer is considerably higher than the density of SSTRs, BN receptor system may be more relevant as a clinical target than the SSTR system.

■ REFERENCES

1. Edwards CM, Cohen MA, Bloom SR. Peptides as drugs. *Q J Med.* 1999;92:1–4.
2. Agdeppa ED. Rational design for peptide drugs. *J Nucl Med.* 2006;47:22N–24N.
3. Mather SJ. Design of radiolabeled ligands for the imaging and treatment of cancer. *Mol BioSyst.* 2007;3: 30–35.
4. Hruby VJ, Matsunaga TO. Applications of synthetic peptides. In: Grant G, ed. *Synthetic Peptides.* 2nd ed. New York: Oxford University Press, 2002:292–376.
5. Han HK, Amidon GL. Targeted prodrug design to optimize drug delivery. *AAPS Pharm Sci.* 2000;2(1): DOI: 10.1208/ps020106.
6. Benedetti E. Molecular engineering in the preparation of bioactive peptides. In: Doniach S, ed. *Statistical Mechanics, Protein Structure, and Protein Substrate Interactions.* New York: Plenum Press; 1994:381–400, and references therein.
7. Zimmerman SS, Pottle MS, Némethy G, et al. Conformational analysis of the 20 naturally occurring amino acid residues using ECEPP. *Macromolecules.* 1977;10:1–7.
8. Toniolo C. Intramolecularly hydrogen-bonded peptide conformations. *CRC Crit Rev Biochem.* 1980;9:1–44.
9. Allen FH, Pitchford NA. Conformational analysis from crystallographic data. In: Codding PW, ed. *Structure-Based Drug Design.* The Netherlands: Kluwer Academic Publishers; 1998:15–26.
10. Pedone C, Morelli G, Tesauro D, et al. Peptide structure and Analysis. In: Chinol M, Paganelli G, ed. *Radionuclide Peptide Cancer Therapy.* New York: Taylor & Francis; 2006:1–30.
11. Benedetti E, Iacovino R, Saviano M. The use of uncoded α-amino acids residues in drug design. In: Codding PW, ed. *Structure-Based Drug Design.* The Netherlands: Kluwer Academic Publishers; 1998:103–112.
12. Toniolo C, Benedetti E. Old and new structures from studies of synthetic peptides rich in C$^{\alpha,\alpha}$-disbstituted glycines. *ISI Atlas Sci Biochem.* 1988;1:225–230.
13. Karle IL. Flexibility in peptide molecules and restraints imposed by hydrogen bonds, the Aib residue and core inserts. *Biopolymers.* 1996;40:157–180.
14. Saviano M, Isernia C, Rossi F, et al. Solid state structural analysis of the cyclooctapeptide cyclo-(Pro1-Pro-Phe-Phe-Ac6c-Ile-D-Ala-Val8). *Biopolymers.* 2000;53:189–199.
15. Chan TF, Zheng XFS. De novo chemical ligand design. *Drug Discov Today.* 2002;7:802–803.
16. Joseph-McCarthy D. Computational approaches to structure-based ligand design. *Pharmacol Ther.* 1999;84:179–191.
17. Zanders ED, Bailey DS, Dean PM. Probes for chemical genomics by design. *Drug Discov Today.* 2002;7:711–718.
18. Wade EC, Lüdemaann S. Computational strategies for modeling receptor flexibility in studies of receptor-ligand interactions. In: Codding PW, ed. *Structure-Based Drug Design.* The Netherlands: Kluwer Academic Publishers; 1998:41–52, and references therein.
19. Leach AR, Bryce RA, Robinson AJ. Synergy between combinatorial chemistry and de novo design. *J Mol Graph Model.* 2000;18:358–367.
20. Agrafiotis DK, Lobanov V, Salemme F. Combinatorial informatics in the post-genomic era. *Nat Rev Drug Discov.* 2002;1:337–346.
21. Bodansky M, Bodansky A. *The Practice of Peptide Synthesis.* Berlin: Springer-Verlag; 1994.
22. Marglin A, Merrifield RB. The synthesis of bovine insulin by the solid phase method. *J Am Chem Soc.* 1966;88:5051–5052.
23. Carpino LA, Han GY. 9-Fluorenylmethoxycarbonyl amino-protecting group. *J Org Chem.* 1972;37:3404–3409.

24. Liu S, Edwards DS. Bifunctional chelators for therapeutic lanthanide radiopharmaceuticals. *Bioconjug Chem.* 2001;12:7–34.

25. De León-Rodríguez LM, Kovacs Z. The synthesis and chelation chemistry of DOTA-peptide. *Bioconjug Chem.* 2008;19:392–402.

26. Eisenwiener KP, Powell P, Macke HR. A convenient synthesis of novel bifunctional prochelators for coupling to bioactive peptide for radiometal labeling. *Bioorg Med Chem Lett.* 2000;10:2133–2135.

27. Arano Y, Akizawa H, Uezono T. Conventional and high-yield synthesis of DTPA conjugated peptides: application of a monoreactive DTPA to DTPA-D-Phe[1]-octreotide synthesis. *Bioconjug Chem.* 1997; 8:442–446.

28. Breeman WAP, van Hagen PM, Kwekkeboom DJ. Somatostatin receptor scintigraphy using [^{111}In-DTPA[0]]RC-160 in humans: a comparison with [^{111}In-DTPA[0]]octreotide. *Eur J Nucl Med.* 1998;25:182–186.

29. Brechbiel MW, Gansow OA. Backbone substituted DTPA ligands for ^{90}Y radioimmunotherapy. *Bioconjug Chem.* 1991;2:187–194.

30. Kobayashi H, Wu C, Yoo TM, et al. Evaluation of the in vivo biodistribution of yttrium-labeled isomers of CHX-DTPA conjugated monoclonal antibodies. *J Nucl Med.* 1998;39:829–836.

31. Wu C, Kobayashi H, Sun B, et al. Stereochemical influence on the stability of radio-metal complexes in vivo. Synthesis and evaluation of the four stereoisomers of 2-(p-nitrobenzyl)-trans-CyDTPA. *Bioorg Med Chem.* 1997;5:1925–1934.

32. Anderson CJ, Dehdashti F, Cutler PD. ^{64}Cu-TETA-octreotide as a PET imaging agent for patients with neuroendocrine tumors. *J Nucl Med.* 2001;42:213–221.

33. McMurry TJ, Brechbiel M, Wu C, et al. Synthesis of 2-(p-thiocyanato-benzyl)-1,4,7-triazacyclononane-1,4,7-triacetic acid: application of the 4-methoxy-2,3,6-trimethylbenzenesulfonamide protecting group in the synthesis of macrocyclic polyamines. *Bioconjug Chem.* 1993;4:236–245.

34. Ramasamy R, Lazar I, Brucher E, et al. NOTPME: a phosphorus-31 NMR probe for measurement of divalent cations in biological systems. *FEBS Lett.* 1991;280:121–124.

35. Eisenwiener KP, Prata MIM, Buschmann I, et al. NODAGATOC, a new chelator-coupled somatostatin analogue labeled with [[67/68]Ga] and [^{111}In] for SPECT, PET, and targeted therapeutic applications of somatostatin receptor (hsst2) expressing tumors. *Bioconjug Chem.* 2002;13:530–541.

36. Chong H, Garmestani K, Ma D, et al. Synthesis and biological evaluation of novel macrocyclic ligands with pendent donor groups as potential yttrium chelators for radioimmunotherapy with improved complex formation kinetics. *J Med Chem.* 2002;45:3458–3468.

37. Lamberts SW, de Herder WW, Hofland LJ. Somatostatin analogs in the diagnosis and treatment of cancer. *Trends Endocrinol Metab.* 2002;13:451–457.

38. Melacini G, Zhu Q, Goodman M. Multiconformational NMR analysis of Sandostatin (octreotide): equilibrium between β-sheet and partially helical structures. *Biochemistry.* 1997;36:1233–1241.

39. Pohl E, Heine A, Sheldrick GM, et al. Structure of octreotide, a somatostatin analogue. *Acta Crystallogr D Biol Crystallogr.* 1995;51: 48–59.

40. Deshmukh MV, Voll G, Kuhlewein A, et al. NMR studies reveal structural differences between the gallium and yttrium complexes of DOTA-D-Phe[1]-Tyr[3]-octreotide. *J Med Chem.* 2005;48:1506–1514.

41. Reuter JK, Mattern R, Zhang L, et al. Syntheses and biological activities of sandostatin analogs containing stereochemical changes in positions 6 or 8. *Biopolymers.* 2000;53:497–505.

42. Capello A, Krenning EP, Bernard BF, et al. Peptide receptor radionuclide therapy in vitro using [111In-DTPA0]octreotide. *J Nucl Med.* 2003;44:98–104.

43. Heppeler A, Froidevaux S, Eberle AN, et al. Receptor targeting for tumor localization and therapy with radiopeptides. *Curr Med Chem.* 2000;7:971–994.

44. Reubi JC, Schaer JC, Waser B, et al. Affinity profiles for human somatostatin receptor subtypes SST1-SST5 of somatostatin radiotracers selected for scintigraphic and radiotherapeutic use. *Eur J Nucl Med.* 2000;27:273–282.

45. Paganelli G, Zoboli S, Bodei L, et al. Receptor-mediated radiotherapy with 90Y-DOTA-D-Phe1-Tyr3-octreotide. *Eur J Nucl Med.* 2001;28: 426–434.

46. Waldherr C, Pless M, Maecke HR, et al. The clinical value of [^{90}Y-DOTA]-D-Phe[1]-Tyr[3]-octreotide (^{90}Y-DOTATOC) in the treatment of neuroendocrine tumors: a clinical phase II study. *Ann Oncol.* 2001;12:941–945.

47. Kwekkeboom DJ, Mueller-Brand J, Paganelli G, et al. Overview of results of peptide receptor radionuclide therapy with 3 radiolabeled somatostatin analogs. *J Nucl Med.* 2005;46:62S-66S.

48. Iten F, Müller B, Schindler C, et al. Response to [[90]Yttrium-DOTA]-TOC treatment is associated with long-term survival benefit in metastasized medullary thyroid cancer: a phase II clinical trial. *Clin Cancer Res.* 2007;13:6696–6702.

49. Forrer F, Riedweg I, Maecke HR, et al. Radiolabeled DOTATOC in patients with advanced paraganglioma and pheochromocytoma. *Q J Nucl Med Mol Imaging.* 2008;52:334–340.

50. de Jong M, Breeman WAP, Bakker WH. Comparison of ^{111}In-labeled somatostatin analogues for tumor scintigraphy and radionuclide therapy. *Cancer Res.* 1998;58:437–441.

51. Kwekkeboom DJ, de Herder WW, Kam BL, et al. Treatment with the radiolabeled somatostatin analog [^{177}Lu-DOTA[0],Tyr[3]]octreotate: toxicity, efficacy, and survival. *J Clin Oncol.* 2008;26:2124–2130.

52. Wild D, Schmitt, JS, Ginj M. DOTA-NOC, a high-affinity ligand of somatostatin receptor subtypes 2, 3 and 5 for labeling with various radiometals. *Eur J Nucl Med Mol Imaging.* 2003;30:1338–1347.

53. Ginj M, Schmitt JS, Chen J, et al. Design, synthesis, and biological evaluation of somatostatin-based radiopeptides. *Chem Biol.* 2006; 13:1081–1090.

54. Wehrmann C, Senftleben S, Zachert C, et al. Results of individual patient dosimetry in peptide receptor radionuclide therapy with 177Lu DOTA-TATE and 177Lu DOTA_NOC. *Cancer Biother Radiopharm.* 2007;22:406–416.

55. Valkema R, Pauwels SA, Kvols LK, et al. Long-term follow-up of renal function after peptide receptor radiation therapy with 90Y-DOTA0,Tyr3-octreotide and 177Lu-DOTA0,Tyr3-octreotate. *J Nucl Med.* 2005;46:83S-91S.

56. Ginj M, Zhang, H, Waser B, et al. Radiolabeled somatostatin receptor antagonists are preferable to agonists for in vivo peptide receptor targeting of tumors. *Proc Natl Acad Sci U S A.* 2006;103:16436–16441.

57. Virgolini I, Yang Q, Li S, et al. Cross-competition between vasoactive intestinal peptide and somatostatin for binding to tumor cell membrane receptors. *Cancer Res.* 1994;54:690–700.

58. Reubi JC. In vitro evaluation of VIP/PACAP receptors in healthy and diseased human tissues. Clinical implications. *Ann N Y Acad Sci.* 2000;921:1–25.

59. Pallela, VR, Thakur ML, Chakder S. ^{99m}Tc-labeled vasoactive intestinal peptide receptor agonist: functional studies. *J Nucl Med.* 1999;40:352.

60. Mayo KE, Miller LJ, Bataille D, et al. International Union of Pharmacology. XXXV. The glucagon receptor family. *Pharmacol Rev.* 2003;55: 167–194.

61. Reubi JC, Waser B. Concomitant expression of several peptide receptors in neuroendocrine tumors: molecular basis for in vivo multireceptor tumor targeting. *Eur J Nucl Med Mol Imaging.* 2003;30:781–793.

62. Gotthardt M, Fischer M, Naeher I, et al. Use of the incretin hormone glucagon-like peptide-1 (GLP-1) for the detection of insulinomas: initial experimental results. *Eur J Nucl Med Mol Imaging.* 2002;29:597–606.

63. Wild D, Béhé M, Wicki A, et al. Preclinical evaluation of [Lys[40](Ahx-DTPA-^{111}In)NH[2]]exendin-4, a very promising ligand for glucagon-like peptide-1 (GLP-1) receptor targeting. *J Nucl Med.* 2006;47:2025–2033.

64. Brooks PC, Clark RA, Cheresh DA, et al. Requirement of vascular integrin alpha v beta 3 for angiogenesis. *Science.* 1994:264,569–571.

65. Felding-Habermann B, O'Toole TE, Smith JW, et al. Integrin activation controls metastasis in human breast cancer. *Proc Natl Acad Sci U S A.* 2001;98:1853–1858.

66. Albelda SM, Mette SA, Elder DE, et al. Integrin distribution in malignant melanoma: association of the β[3] subunit with tumor progression. *Cancer Res.* 1990;50:6757–6764.

67. Gasparini G, Brooks PC, Biganzoli E. Vascular integrin $\alpha_V\beta_3$: a new prognostic indicator in breast cancer. *Clin Cancer Res.* 1998;4:2625–2634.

68. Jin H, Varner J. Integrins: roles in cancer development and as treatment targets. *Br J Cancer.* 2004;90:561–565.

69. Kumar CC. Integrin $\alpha_V\beta_3$ as a therapeutic target for blocking tumor-induced angiogenesis. *Curr Drug Targets.* 2003;4:123–131.

70. Ruoslahti, E. RGD and other recognition sequences for integrins. *Annu Rev Cell Dev Biol.* 1996;12:697–715.

71. Temming K, Schiffelers RM, Molema G, et al. RGD-based strategies for selective delivery of therapeutics and imaging agents to the tumour vasculature. *Drug Resist Updat.* 2005;8:381–402.

72. Dechantsreiter MA, Planker E, Matha B, et al. N-methylated cyclic RGD peptides as highly active and selective alpha(V)beta(3) integrin antagonists. *J Med Chem.* 1999;42:3033–3040.

73. Beekman KW, Colevas AD, Cooney K, et al. Phase II evaluations of cilengitide in asymptomatic patients with androgen-independent prostate cancer: scientific rationale and study design. *Clin Genitourin Cancer.* 2006;4:299–302.

74. Okarvi SM. Peptide-based radiopharmaceuticals: future tools for diagnostic imaging of cancers and other diseases. *Med Res Rev.* 2004;24:357–397.

75. Dijkgraaf I, Rijnders AY, Soede A. Synthesis of DOTA-conjugated multivalent cyclic-RGD peptide dendrimers *via* 1,3-dipolar cycloaddition and their biological evaluation: implications for tumor targeting and tumor imaging purposes. *Org Biomol Chem.* 2007;5:935–944.

76. Dijkgraaf I, Kruijtzer JA, Frielink C, et al. $\alpha_V\beta_3$ integrin targeting of intraperitoneally growing tumors with a radiolabeled RGD peptide. *Int J Cancer.* 2007;120:605–610.

77. Del Gatto A, Zaccaro L, Grieco P, et al. Novel and selective $\alpha_V\beta_3$ receptor peptide antagonist: design, synthesis, and biological behavior. *J Med Chem.* 2006;49:3416–3420.

78. Carraway R, Leeman, SEJ. The isolation of a new hypotensive peptide, neurotensin, from bovine hypothalami. *Biol Chem.* 1973;248:6854–6861.

79. Kitabgi P, Carraway R, Leeman SE. Isolation of a tridecapeptide from bovine intestinal tissue and its partial characterization as neurotensin. *J Biol Chem.* 1976;251:7053–7058.

80. Evers BM. Neurotensin and growth in normal and neoplastic tissues. *Peptides.* 2006;27:2424–2433.

81. Carraway RE, Plona AM. Involvement of neurotensin in cancer growth: evidence, mechanisms and development of diagnostic tools. *Peptides.* 2006;27:2445–2460.

82. Kitabgi P, De Nadai F, Rovère C, et al. Biosynthesis, maturation, release and degradation of neurotensin and neuromedin. *N Ann N Y Acad Sci.* 1992;668:30–42.

83. Garcia-Garayoa E, Blaeuenstein P, Bruehlmeier M, et al. Preclinical evaluation of a new stabilized neurotensin(8–13) pseudopeptide radiolabeled with ^{99m}Tc. *J Nucl Med.* 2002;43:374–383.

84. Bruehlmeier M, Garcia Garayoa E, Blanc A, et al. Stabilization of neurotensin analogues: effect on peptide catabolism, biodistribution and tumor binding. *Nucl Med Biol.* 2002;29:321–327.

85. Maes V, Garcia-Garayoa E, Bläuenstein P, et al. Novel ^{99m}Tc-labeled neurotensin analogues with optimized biodistribution properties. *J Med Chem.* 2006;49:1833–1836.

86. Buchegger F, Bonvin F, Kosinski M, et al. Radiolabeled neurotensin analog, ^{99m}Tc-NT-XI, evaluated in ductal pancreatic adenocarcinoma patients. *J Nucl Med.* 2003;44:1649–1654.

87. Garcia-Garayoa E, Bläuenstein P, Blanc A, et al. A stable neurotensin-based radiopharmaceutical for targeted imaging and therapy of neurotensin receptor-positive tumours. *Eur J Nucl Med Mol Imaging.* 2009;36:37–47.

88. Janssen PJ, de Visser M, Verwijnen S, et al. Five stabilized ^{111}In-labeled neurotensin analogs in nude mice bearing HT29 tumors. *Cancer Biother Radiopharm.* 2007;22:374–381.

89. Hokfelt T, Pernow B, Wahren J. Substance P: a pioneer amongst neuropeptides. *J Int Med.* 2001;249:27–40.

90. Hennig IM, Laissue JA, Horisberger U. Substance P receptors in human primary neoplasms: tumoral and vascular localisation. *Int J Cancer.* 1995;61;786–792.

91. Friess H, Zhu Z, Liard V. Neurokinin-1 receptor (NK-1R) expression and its potential effects on tumor growth in human pancreatic cancer. *Lab Invest.* 2003;83;731–742.

92. van Hagen PM, Breeman WA, Reubi JC, et al. Visualization of the thymus by substance P receptor scintigraphy in man. *Eur J Nucl Med.* 1996;23:1508.

93. Schumacher T, Hofer S, Eichhorn K, et al. Local injection of the 90Y-labelled peptidic vector DOTATOC to control gliomas of WHO grades II and III: an extended pilot study. *Eur J Nucl Med.* 2002;29:486–493.

94. Kneifel S, Cordier D, Good S, et al. Local targeting of malignant gliomas by the diffusible peptidic vector 1,4,7,10-tetraazacyclododecane-1-glutaric acid-4,7,10-triacetic acid-substance P. *Clin Cancer Res.* 2006;12:3843–3850.

95. Reubi JC, Schaer JC, Waser B. Cholecystokinin(CCK)-A and CCK-B/gastrin receptors in human tumors. *Cancer Res.* 1997;57:1377–1386.

96. Reubi JC, Schaer JC, Waser B, et al. Unsulfated DTPA- and DOTA-CCK analogs as specific high-affinity ligands for CCK-B receptor-expressing human and rat tissues in vitro and in vivo. *Eur J Nucl Med.* 1998;25:481–490.

97. Ji Z, Hadac EM, Henne RM, et al. Direct identification of a distinct site of interaction between the carboxyl-terminal residue of cholecystokinin and the type A cholecystokinin receptor using photoaffinity labeling. *J Biol Chem.* 1997;272:24393–24401.

98. Kennedy K, Gigoux V, Escrieut C, et al. Identification of the two amino acids of the human cholecystokinin-A receptor that interact with the N-terminal moiety of cholecystokinin. *J Biol Chem.* 1997;272:2920–2926.

99. Giragossian C, Mierke DF. Intermolecular interactions between cholecystokinin-8 and the third extracellular loop of the cholecystokinin-2 receptor. *Biochemistry.* 2002;41:4560–4566.

100. Pellegrini M, Miercke DF. Molecular complex of cholecystokinin-8 and N-terminus of the cholecystokinin A receptor by NMR spectroscopy. *Biochemistry.* 1999;38:14775–14785.

101. Aloj L. Panico M, Caracò C, et al. In vitro and in vivo Evaluation of ^{111}In-DTPAGlu-G-CCK8 for cholecystokinin-B receptor imaging. *J Nucl Med.* 2004;45:485–494.

102. Behr TM, Behe MP. Cholecystokinin-B/gastrin receptor-targeting peptides for staging and therapy of medullary thyroid cancer and other cholecystokinin-B receptor-expressing malignancies. *Semin Nucl Med.* 2002;32:97–109.

103. Mather SJ, McKenzie AJ, Sosabowski JK, et al. Selection of radiolabeled gastrin analogs for peptide receptor-targeted radionuclide therapy. *J Nucl Med.* 2007;48:615–622.

104. Koglin N, Beck-Sickinger AG. Novel modified and radiolabeled neuropeptide Y analogues to study Y-receptor subtypes. *Neuropeptides.* 2004;38:153–161.

105. Rudolf K, Eberlein W, Engel W, et al. The first highly potent and selective non-peptide neuropeptide Y Y1 receptor antagonist: BIBP3226. *Eur J Pharmacol.* 1994;271:R11–R13.

106. Reubi JC, Gugger M, Waser B, et al. Y1-Mediated effect of neuropeptide Y in cancer: breast carcinomas as targets. *Cancer Res.* 2001;61:4636–4641.

107. Körner M, Reubi JC. NPY receptors in human cancer: a review of current knowledge. *Peptides.* 2007;28:419–425.

108. Koglin N, Zorn C, Beumer R, et al. Analogues of neuropeptide Y containing-aminocyclopropane carboxylic acids are the shortest linear peptides that are selective for the Y1 receptor. *Angew Chem Int Ed Engl.* 2003;42:202–205.

109. Markwalder R, Reubi JC. Gastrin-releasing peptide receptors in the human prostate: relation to neoplastic transformation. *Cancer Res.* 1999;59:1152–1159.

110. Qin Y, Ertl T, Cai RZ, et al. Inhibitory effect of bombesin receptor antagonist RC-3095 on the growth of human pancreatic cancer cells in vivo and in vitro. *Cancer Res.* 1994;54:1035–1041.

111. Van de Wiele C, Dumont F, Broecke RV, et al. Technetium-99m RP525, a GRP analogue for visualization of GRP receptor-expressing malignancies: a feasibility study. *Eur J Nucl Med.* 2000:27;1694–1699.

112. Scemama JL, Zahidi A, Fourmy D, et al. Interaction of $[^{125}I]$-Tyr^4-bombesin with specific receptors on normal human pancreatic membranes. *Regul Pept.* 1986;13:125–132.

113. Breeman WAP, De Jong M, Bernard BF, et al. Pre-clinical evaluation of $[^{111}$In-DTPA-Pro^1, Tyr^4 bombesin, a new radioligand for bombesin-receptor scintigraphy. *Int J Cancer.* 1999;83:657–663.

114. Hoffman TJ, Li N, Volkert WA, et al. Synthesis and characterization of ^{105}Rh labeled bombesin analogues: enhancement of GRP receptor binding affinity utilizing aliphatic carbon chain linkers. *J Label Comp Radiopharm.* 1997;40:490–493.

115. Hoffman TJ, Gali H, Smith CJ, et al. Novel series of ^{111}In-labeled bombesin analogs as potential radiopharmaceuticals for specific targeting of gastrin-releasing peptide receptors expressed on human prostate cancer cells. *J Nucl Med.* 2003;44:823–831.

116. Nock B, Nikolopoulou A, Chiotellis E, et al. $[^{99m}$Tc]Demobesin 1, a novel potent bombesin analogue for GRP receptor-targeted tumor imaging. *Eur J Nucl Med Mol Imaging.* 2003;30:247–258.

117. Nock B, Nikolopoulou A, Galanis A, et al. Potent bombesin-like peptides for GRP-receptor targeting of tumors with ^{99m}Tc: a preclinical study. *J Med Chem.* 2005;48:100–110.

118. Mantey SA, Weber HC, Sainz E, et al. Discovery of a high affinity radioligand for the human orphan receptor, bombesin receptor subtype 3, which demonstrates that it has a unique pharmacology compared with other mammalian bombesin receptors. *J Biol Chem.* 1997;272:26062–26071.

119. Pradhan TK, Katsuno T, Taylor JE, et al. Identification of a unique ligand which has high affinity for all four bombesin receptor subtypes. *Eur J Pharmacol.* 1998;343:275–287.

120. Lantry LE, Cappelletti E, Maddalena ME, et al. ^{177}Lu-AMBA: synthesis and characterization of a selective ^{177}Lu-labeled GRP-R agonist for systemic radiotherapy of prostate cancer. *J Nucl Med.* 2006;47:1144–1152.

Affibody Molecules for Targeted Radionuclide Therapy

Stefan Ståhl, Mikaela Friedman, Jörgen Carlsson, Vladimir Tolmachev, and Fredrik Frejd

■ INTRODUCTION

Targeting of tumor-associated antigens is an expanding treatment concept in clinical oncology as an alternative to or in combination with conventional treatments, such as chemotherapy, external radiation therapy, and surgery. Targeting of antigens that are uniquely or more highly expressed in tumors than in normal tissues can be used to increase the specificity and reduce the cytotoxic effect on normal tissues. Several targeting agents have been studied for clinical use, where monoclonal antibodies have been most widely used. More than 20 monoclonal antibodies are approved for therapy today, and many of them are applied in oncology. Advances in genetic engineering and in vitro selection technology have enabled high-throughput generation of monoclonal antibodies, antibody derivatives (e.g., scFvs, Fabs, diabodies, minibodies) and more recently, nonimmunoglobulin scaffold proteins. Several of these affinity proteins have been investigated for both in vivo diagnostics and therapy. Affinity proteins in tumor-targeted therapy can affect tumor progression by altering signal transduction or by delivering a payload of toxin, drug, or radionuclide. In this chapter, strategies are described for tumor targeting of solid tumors using a rather novel affinity protein, termed affibody molecules, to deliver radionuclides, for molecular imaging or radiotherapy.

For over a century, antibodies have been the dominating class of proteins used as tools for molecular recognition. Recently, however, alternative engineered proteins have emerged. There are several properties to consider in the generation of engineered binding proteins, depending on their intended use. In therapy and in vivo diagnostics, the specificity for the target protein is most essential in order not to bind to and affect normal tissues. High affinity and long tumor residence time are important parameters for a long-lasting effect in cancer therapy and to exercise good contrast for in vivo imaging. Furthermore, the size of a targeting agent is important for the pharmacokinetics and biodistribution. Large targeting agents, like antibodies (~150 kDa), have a long circulation time (biological half-life), which in general is a desirable property for therapy using nonradiolabeled antibodies. In molecular imaging, however, rapid clearance is important because it reduces background radioactivity, and thereby increases contrast of

imaging. Long residence time in the blood might also be problematic for therapy using radiolabeled antibodies, due to an increased radiation dose to the bone marrow. Smaller molecules, with a size below the threshold for kidney filtration (~60 kDa), such as certain antibody fragments, scaffold proteins, peptides, and small molecules, will be cleared much quicker from the system through excretion via the kidneys (1,2). A smaller size of the targeting agent is also favorable for the tumor penetration.

Today, a number of different targeting agents are considered for targeted imaging or therapy applications. These include (a) antibodies, (b) antibody derivatives, (c) peptides, and more recently (d) nonimmunoglobulin scaffolds (3). The latter group comprises some 50 scaffold proteins, intensely reviewed over the last years (4–8), that could be divided into four groups based on the properties of the interaction surfaces: (a) single loops on rigid framework, (b) several loop structures forming a continuous surface, (c) engineered interfaces resting on a secondary structure, and (d) oligomeric domain structures.

Candidates for suitable scaffolds should typically have a structurally rigid core that could withstand structural changes, such as amino acid substitutions or inserts in loops or side chain replacements on a contiguous surface. In order to get novel binding molecules, with specific target binding properties, the scaffold has to be suited for diversification and selection. Usually, a combinatorial protein engineering approach employs random mutagenesis of suitable amino acids to generate a synthetic library. This is followed by selection of variants with desired binding activity using different selection strategies. For the new binding molecules to compete with already established antibodies, they need to possess the same or preferably improved properties. There are several aspects to consider for a scaffold protein as described below and that is also thoroughly reviewed by Nygren and Skerra (4). The scaffold protein should preferably be relatively small and be composed of a single polypeptide chain with intrinsic stability, and the stability should also be kept in spite of the randomization of certain surface-exposed positions. The scaffold should, if possible, not be dependent on disulfide bridges for its stability, as this could limit its use under chemical labeling conditions or for use in intracellular applications. Furthermore, if the scaffold has no cysteine residues, a unique cysteine can be introduced to provide for the possibility of specific conjugation. Most of the scaffold proteins are based on naturally occurring binding proteins, which are typically engineered to improve properties such as stability. In the creation of a combinatorial library, the amino acids naturally involved in ligand interaction are the first choice for randomization. The number of positions for variation should be large enough to provide an interface for interaction with the target molecule, but not too many positions should be varied in order to avoid a decrease in the scaffold stability. An important issue to consider, when randomizing amino acid residues on a protein scaffold, is immunogenicity. This is particularly important if the binding protein is intended for in vivo applications. In addition to synthetic proteins, engineered and fully "human scaffolds" may elicit an immune response. There are, however, strategies emerging for rational reduction of protein immunogenicity, including PEGylation (9) and T-cell epitope engineering (10).

AFFIBODY MOLECULES

Affibody molecules belong to the category of scaffold proteins in which a binding interface is engineered on a secondary structure. The B-domain of protein A was chosen as starting point for a new scaffold and was engineered to increase the chemical stability (11). The resulting domain Z showed a significantly decreased Fab binding (12), but retained capability to bind IgG Fc-regions. Protein A is known to be highly soluble and stable from proteolysis and thermal degradation (13). Domain Z inherited these properties and was also shown to be a rapidly folding protein domain. The region mediating binding to the Fc part of immunoglobulins involves two of the three helices of domain Z and covers a surface area of approximately 800 Å^2, similar in size to the surfaces involved in many antigen–antibody interactions (14). The first generation affibody molecule libraries were constructed by randomization of 13 solvent accessible residues, including those involved in the Fc-binding of domain Z, thereby destroying the native Fc-interaction (15,16). Since the first isolation of affibody molecules was performed by Stahl and coworkers in 1997 (13), affibody libraries (17) have been used to select binding molecules, mostly yielding affinities in the mid-to-low nanomolar range, against many different target proteins, including human HER2 (18), transferrin (19), amyloid beta peptide (17), EGFR (20), factor VIII (21), CD25 (22), HIV gp120 (23), and CD28 (24). The affibody libraries have typically been displayed on phage, thus using phage display as selection principle. Recently, bacterial display has also been used to select high affinity affibody molecules for TNF-α (25). When necessary, the affinity has been increased by affinity maturations (21,26–28), either by helix shuffling (27) or by sequence alignment and directed combinatorial mutagenesis using a single oligonucleotide covering helix 1 and 2 (21,26,28).

The affibody molecules have a number of attractive properties useful for biotechnological applications (4), and with potential for therapy and molecular imaging (29–31). They have a small size (~7 kDa) and most of the selected affibody molecules contain no cysteine residues and have proven to be highly soluble and stable. Affibody molecules are small enough for solid-phase peptide synthesis (21,32,33), hence facilitating the introduction of desired fluorophores and also of chemical groups for direct immobilization or for radiolabeling. The absence of cysteine makes the affibody molecules suitable also for intracellular applications, as for example in targeting adenoviruses for gene therapy (34,35). It can also provide the opportunity for introduction of a unique cysteine, for example, for site-specific labeling or immobilization on a solid surface. The solvent-exposed termini of the molecule will allow for independent folding of fused proteins, and hence multimeric constructs can be created by head-to-tail genetic fusions. This can be used to increase the functional affinity (avidity) as has been seen for several affibody molecules (20,36).

In recent years the affibody molecules have been used for a wide variety of applications: as detection reagents (37–39), to inhibit receptor interaction (24), for bioseparation (19,40–42), as purification tags (43), for structure determination (44), to engineer adenovirus tropism for gene therapy applications (34,45), and as radiolabeled targeting agents for in vivo cancer diagnostics and therapy (26,28,33,46–49) (Table 4.1). Affibody molecules used in molecular imaging and radiotherapy are further discussed in Affibody Molecules in Molecular Imaging of Tumors section.

AFFIBODY MOLECULES IN MOLECULAR IMAGING OF TUMORS

The most important properties of a targeting agent for imaging may be summarized as follows:

- High specificity (i.e., absence of cross-reactivity with non-target molecules)
- High target binding affinity (low nanomolar to sub-nanomolar binding is typically desired)
- Small size (enabling fast distribution to the tumor and quick clearance from the blood and other tissue compartments)
- High structural stability for radionuclide labeling

The properties of affibody molecules thus make them highly suitable as targeting agents in molecular imaging applications. EGFR- and HER2-specific affibody molecules have been generated and their capacity as imaging agents is described below. A summary of the radioisotopes used for labeling of affibody imaging tracers is presented in Table 4.2.

Imaging of EGFR- and HER2-expressing tumors and metastases

The receptor tyrosine kinase inhibitors, epidermal growth factor receptor (EGFR) and human epidermal growth factor receptor 2 (HER2), are overexpressed in various solid

Table **4.1**	Applications of affibody molecules		
Application	**Target Protein**	**Comment**	**References**
Biotechnology			
ELISA	IgA, apolipoprotein A-1	Two-site affibody/antibody ELISA to avoid false-positive signals	(37)
Protein microarray	Taq DNA polymerase, IgA, IgE, IgG, insulin, and TNF-α	Capture ligands on protein microarrays	(38,39)
Affinity purification	Taq DNA polymerase, apolipoprotein A-1, RSV G-protein, and factor VIII	Ligands in affinity chromatography for capture of recombinant proteins from cell lysates	(21,40,42)
Depletion	IgA, transferrin, and Alzheimer Aβ peptide	Protein recovery by affinity chromatography from human plasma or serum	(17,19,41)
Ion exchange	Ion exchange chromatography media	Novel purification tag for general use as fusion partner to different target proteins	(43)
Biological research			
Structure determination	Alzheimer amyloid beta peptide	Stabilizing complex formation for structure determination	(44)
Inhibition of receptor interaction	CD28	Interference of CD28 and CD80 receptor interaction	(24)
	TNF	Blocking ligand binding to its receptor in vitro	(86)
Intracellular capture	HER2, EGFR	Reduction of cell surface level of HER2 and EGFR receptors and reduction of cell growth	(87,88)
Gene therapy (vector engineering)	HER2, HIV-1 gp120	Engineering of adenovirus tropism	(23,34,45)
	HER2	Engineering of nonviral delivery systems	(89)
Medicine			
Molecular imaging	HER2, EGFR	Radiolabeled targeting agent for cancer diagnosis Fluorescent targeting agent for superficial tumors	(26,30,47,48) (58)
Radiotherapy	HER2	Radiolabeled targeting agent for cancer therapy	(70,75,78,79,82)

ELISA, Enzyme-linked immunosorbent assay; DNA, Deoxyribonucleic acid; RSV, respiratory syncytial virus; TNF-α, tumor necrosis factor; HER2, human epidermal growth factor receptor 2; EGFR, epidermal growth factor receptor; HIV-1, human immunodeficiency virus type I.

tumors (50,51). The overexpression on primary tumors is often correlated with expression on disseminated tumor cells and metastases. Molecular imaging of these biomarkers can therefore help in receptor expression profiling, providing information for targeted therapy or assessing response to therapy.

HER2-specific affibody molecules with affinity (apparent dissociation constant) of 50 nM have been generated in phage display selection (18). Radioiodination of the affibody molecules showed retained specific binding to HER2-overexpressing cells and the ^{125}I-labeled HER2-specific affibody was found to internalize to some extent (36). When comparing monomeric and dimeric formats of the affibody molecule, the dimer demonstrated better cellular retention and was studied in mice carrying HER2-overexpressing SKOV-3 xenografts. The radioiodinated affibody molecule could be used to clearly visualize tumors by gamma-camera imaging already after 8 hours with a tumor to blood ratio of 10:1 (52). After directed molecular evolution based on the first generation affibody molecule, second

generation affibody molecules with high affinities were isolated (28). One of these variants, the $Z_{HER2:342}$, displayed several advantageous properties, including a very high affinity of 22 pM, good solubility, stability, and high tumor uptake, making it a promising candidate for further studies (28). This $Z_{HER2:342}$ binder has subsequently been extensively studied in biodistribution and molecular imaging with several different radioisotope labels. In the first study by Orlova and coworkers, the ^{125}I-labeled $Z_{HER2:342}$ demonstrated tumor uptake of approximately 9% ID/g at 4-hour pi (postinjection) and a tumor to blood ratio of 38:1 in mice carrying SKOV-3 xenografts (28). Gamma-camera imaging of these mice at 6 hours after injection of the ^{125}I-labeled $Z_{HER2:342}$ showed that the tumor could be clearly visualized with high contrast. In order to do molecular imaging using single photon emission computed tomography (SPECT), the radionuclide ^{111}In was selected because of good imaging properties, facile logistics of delivery, and well-studied labeling chemistry. The labeling was performed via isothiocyanate-benzyl-DTPA. The ^{111}In-benzyl-DTPA-$Z_{HER2:342}$

Table **4.2**　Affibody tracers for molecular imaging and therapy

Radionuclide	Mode of Labeling	Application	References
Imaging			
^{125}I (surrogate for ^{123}I)	PIB	SPECT	(28,49,52)
^{124}I	PIB	PET	(90)
^{111}In	Bz-DTPA	SPECT	(26,46,49)
	DOTA (synthetic)		(47)
	Maleimido-CHX-A″ DTPA		(56)
	Maleimido-DOTA		(57)
	CHX-A″ DTPA		(62,82)
^{99m}Tc	maGGG	SPECT	(32)
	maSSS/maGSG		(53)
	maEEE/maGEG		(54)
	maESE/maEES/maSEE		(55)
^{18}F	FBEM	PET	(59)
	FBA		(60)
^{68}Ga	DOTA (synthetic)	PET	(48,69)
^{76}Br	HPEM	PET	(77)
^{57}Co surrogate for ^{55}Co	Maleimido-DOTA	SPECT/PET	(91)
Therapy			
^{177}Lu	CHX-A″-DTPA	RIT	(70)
	DOTA		(80)
^{131}I	HPEM	RIT	(78)
^{186}Re	maGSG	RIT	(79)
^{90}Y	DOTA	RIT	(80)
^{114m}In	CHX-A″-DTPA	RIT	(75,82)

PIB, paraiodobenzoate; SPECT, single photon emission computed tomography; PET, positron emission tomography; Bz-DTPA, benzyl diethylenetriaminepentaacetic acid; maGGG, mercaptoacetyl–glycine–glycine–glycine; maGSG, mercaptoacetyl–glycyl–seryl–glycyl; HPEM, ((4-hydroxyphenyl)ethyl)maleimide.

showed retained specificity to HER2-overexpressing cells. Because of the quick blood clearance of the affibody molecule, the tumor to blood ratio was approximately 100:1 at 4-hour pi (46). Images acquired at 4-hour pi of ^{111}In-benzyl-DTPA-$Z_{HER2:342}$ in mice-bearing SKOV-3 xenografts revealed a high tumor localization of the radioactivity. Due to the residualizing properties of ^{111}In, a high uptake of radioactivity was also seen in the kidneys. The high uptake and retention of radioactivity in kidneys is a general problem for radiometal-labeled peptides and proteins with a molecular weight below approximately 60 kDa. The high uptake in the kidneys should, however, not be a problem in imaging of breast carcinoma where both primary tumor and most metastases are well separated anatomically from the kidneys.

Due to their small size, affibody molecules can be chemically synthesized. This gives the possibility to directly incorporate a chelator at a predetermined site during the synthesis process to simplify the labeling procedure. The radiometal ^{99m}Tc is one of the most commonly used radionuclides for labeling of radiopharmaceuticals in the clinic. In several studies, the affibody molecule $Z_{HER2:342}$ has

been produced by chemical synthesis incorporating a site-specifically positioned chelator, labeled with ^{99m}Tc, and then investigated in biodistribution analysis. The ^{99m}Tc-maGGG-$Z_{HER2:342}$, where the chelator is mercaptoacetyl–glycine–glycine–glycine (maGGG), showed specific targeting of HER2-expressing tumors in mice, resulting in high tumor contrast in gamma-camera imaging (33). However, this conjugate was predominantly cleared by the liver, causing high radioactivity in the intestine, which makes detection of tumors in the abdominal area difficult. By substitution of the chelating amino acids to residues with more hydrophilic character, the hepatobiliary clearance could be shifted toward renal clearance (53,54). After labeling a conjugate containing the more hydrophilic chelating sequence maEEE, ^{99m}Tc-maEEE-$Z_{HER2:342}$ displayed a 10-fold decrease in radioactivity in the intestine (54). The renal uptake was, however, increased, prompting studies of several alternative variants of synthetic affibody molecules containing a combination of serine and glutamic acid in the chelator. With maESE, the uptake in the intestinal tract could be kept low while lowering the renal retention of radioactivity with one third compared to tracers containing maEEE (55). These studies showed that peptide synthesis is an efficient way to couple chelator sequences to affibody molecules for ^{99m}Tc labeling, providing affibody molecules having alternative in vivo pharmacokinetics. Another opportunity to obtain homogenous labeling of affibody molecules is by taking advantage of the absence of cysteine in the affibody scaffold. An introduced cysteine provides a unique thiol group for site-specific labeling of a protein made either chemically or recombinantly. This was utilized in two recent studies where the affibody molecule $Z_{HER2:2395}$, a variant of the $Z_{HER2:342}$, was site-specifically conjugated with maleimido-CHX-A''-DTPA and maleimide-monamide-DOTA and labeled with ^{111}In, followed by in vitro cell binding and in vivo biodistribution studies (56,57). Affibody molecules have also been used in imaging settings other than gamma-camera, including positron emission tomography (PET) and near-infrared imaging (NIR). Recently, several groups have reported on the use of the $Z_{HER2:342}$ affibody molecule stably labeled using a site-specific cysteine and with retained specificity and affinity, for in vivo assessment of HER2 expression in NIR (labeled with Alexa Fluor) (58) and in PET (labeled with ^{18}F) (59,60).

EGFR-binding affibody molecules with moderate high affinity have been isolated with phage display selection technology. These were found to bind specifically to EGFR, both immobilized in biosensor studies and on EGFR-expressing cells (20). Further cellular assays showed that the EGFR-binding affibody molecules could be labeled with a radiohalogen or a radiometal with preserved specific binding to EGFR-expressing cells. The affibody molecule demonstrated a high uptake and good retention to EGFR-expressing A431 cells and was found to be internalized (61). All of these characteristics are important for an efficient imaging tracer. Moreover, successful targeting of EGFR-expressing tumors in tumor-bearing mice was seen in biodistribution studies and with gamma-camera imaging (62). The data suggested a potential for use of the EGFR-binding affibody tracer for molecular imaging, and in order to further improve the tumor imaging and to increase the affinity, contrast-directed evolution effort was performed. The affinity was improved approximately 30-fold and the affibody molecules showed successful targeting of A431 tumors with 4% to 6% of the injected radioactivity per gram accumulated in tumor tissue at 4-hour pi (26). Tumor targeting and biodistribution in tumor-bearing mice were studied for monomeric and dimeric constructs that were radiolabeled either with the radiohalogen ^{125}I or with the radiometal ^{111}In. The radiometal-labeled monomeric affibody construct, ^{111}In-labeled-$Z_{EGFR:1907}$, was found to provide the best tumor to organ ratio, due to high tumor localization and good tumor retention. The tumor to blood ratio was approximately 30 at 24-hour pi, and the tumor was clearly visualized by gamma-camera imaging (49). For a true comparison with other imaging agents, tracers should be studied simultaneously in the same group of mice with the xenograph. However, some comparative information

about the performance of different imaging agents can be obtained from literature. Tumor-to-blood ratio, which is often used as a measure of contrast, was below 3 at 24-hour pi for any of the anti-EGFR antibodies described, to date (63–66). Tumor-to-blood ratio was also higher for ^{111}In-labeled-$Z_{EGFR:1907}$ (T:B = 31) (49) than for EGF labeled with ^{111}In (T:B = 2.6) (64) or ^{123}I (T:B = 23) (67). Another small EGFR tracer, the EGFR-specific nanobody labeled with ^{99m}Tc showed a tumor-to-background ratio of 7.4 at 3-hour pi (68).

Affibody molecules for imaging in the clinic

Affibody molecules have also been evaluated in a clinical experimental setting (48), where a synthetic 1,4,7,10-tetraazacyclododecane-1,4,7,10-tetraacetic acid (DOTA)-chelated version of the $Z_{HER2:342}$ (ABY-002) was the first affibody molecule to be administered to humans. ^{111}In-ABY-002 was studied in a limited number of patients with recurrent breast cancer. Administration of a microdose (less than 100 µg) of ^{111}In-ABY-002 resulted in high-quality SPECT images enabling the detection even of small lesions (12 to 14 mm) as early as 2 hours pi. This approach was also successful in patients receiving Herceptin. Moreover, multiple targeting constructs and radionuclides have been reviewed as potential imaging agents for HER2 overexpressing tumors. It was concluded that smaller constructs, such as affibody molecules, had the best potential to produce high-contrast in vivo images (69).

AFFIBODY MOLECULES IN RADIONUCLIDE-BASED TARGETED THERAPY

In the case of metastatic disseminated disease, a systemic treatment is required. Chemotherapy can be efficient, but the lack of specificity often results in unwanted and dose-limiting toxicity to normal healthy organs. One way to reduce the toxicity is to accumulate the cytotoxic substance in the tumor lesion by using molecular targets that are overexpressed in cancer cells, but only expressed at low levels or not at all in normal tissues. The use of radionuclides as payloads can be advantageous because multidrug resistance to radionuclides is not readily evident. Radioimmunotherapy can be combined with many other conventional therapies and, additionally, this strategy can benefit from cross fire irradiation to kill surrounding malignant cells. There are presently two radionuclide-labeled therapeutic antibodies approved, Bexxar (^{131}I) and Zevalin (^{90}Y), both for the treatment of relapsed non-Hodgkin lymphoma. Zevalin is also approved for frontline consolidation therapy. Radionuclide-based therapy for solid tumors, however, has not yet reached a level of true success. One major issue is that it has been very difficult to deliver adequate doses of radioactivity to the tumor without delivering unacceptably high doses to critical organs. The slow blood clearance and the insufficient extravasation and tumor penetration are limiting factors of intact immunoglobulins, which have so far been the main class used as targeting agents in radionuclide therapy. Smaller targeting agents, for example, antibody derivatives and peptides have been considered in radionuclide therapy and can be advantageous in providing better tumor penetration and faster blood clearance, thereby improving tumor-to-nontumor dose ratios. However, small molecular size and fast blood clearance can lead to insufficient tumor uptake and increased renal toxicity that can limit the dose needed for efficient eradication of malignant cells. This can be overcome by modulation of size and interaction with other proteins, as discussed below.

Affibody molecules have been considered for targeted radiotherapy, but as previously noted, the small affibody molecule, labeled with residualizing radiometals, will result in high renal uptake of radioactivity. This is acceptable in molecular imaging, where gamma- or positron-emitting nuclides are used that generate low local doses, but could be a major challenge for systemic treatment using alpha- or beta-emitting nuclides. To overcome this problem, three approaches have been applied: (a) modification of blood kinetics of affibody molecules, (b) modulation of renal uptake by optimization of labeling chemistry, and (c) locoregional application of radionuclide therapy.

For systemic therapeutic applications, longer in vivo half-lives, like those observed for smaller proteins and affibody molecules are often needed for increasing the tumor load while keeping the kidney dose at a minimum. When increasing the half-life of small molecules, the bone marrow, however, often becomes the dose-limiting organ, and close attention must be paid to this issue.

Tolmachev and coworkers have shown that the fast clearance and high renal radiometal accumulation, when using affibody molecules for targeting, can be overcome by the genetic fusion of a 46 amino acid albumin-binding domain (ABD) in order to achieve a reversible interaction with human serum albumin and thereby prolonging the circulation half-life (70). The low-energy beta radionuclide ^{177}Lu was chosen for this application, since it was considered suitable in terms of both emitted radiation energy and half-life. Biodistribution in normal mice demonstrated a substantially prolonged blood clearance half-life from 0.64 ± 0.2 to 35.8 ± 0.0 hours, and the radioactivity uptake in kidney was reduced 25-fold. Biodistribution in SKOV-3 xenograft-bearing nude mice showed high tumor uptake at 24-hour pi ($19 \pm 7\%$ ID/g), and the tumor uptake was specific. In experimental radionuclide therapy of SKOV-3 microxenografts, tumor formation was completely prevented in mice administered with 17.4 or 21.6 MBq ^{177}Lu-CHX-A"-DTPA-ABD-($Z_{HER2:342}$)$_2$ (70). These results suggest that fusion with an ABD can improve the biodistribution of small tumor-targeting agents intended for radiotherapy.

Low-energy beta emitters, such as ^{177}Lu, are efficient for eradication of small tumors, while high-energy beta emitters are more optimal for the treatment of bulky lesions (71). The use of Auger emitters may also be considered for micrometastases and disseminated cells (72). Since a typical

patient would, most probably, manifest the whole range of tumor sizes, from bulky nonoperable tumors to single disseminated cells, the concept of a "radionuclide cocktail," that is, the simultaneous use of several labels with different particle energy, has been proposed (73). The use of the in vivo generator ^{114m}In/^{114}In (74) as a therapeutic label could allow for treatment of both micrometastases (due to conversion and Auger electrons of ^{114m}In) and bulky tumors (due to high-energy beta particles from the daughter nuclide ^{114}In). In addition, the low-abundance 190-keV gamma radiation from ^{114m}In would facilitate monitoring of the therapy by using SPECT. In order to select the most suitable chemistry for labeling of ABD-fused affibody molecules with ^{114m}In/^{114}In, two chelates, benzyl-DOTA (Bz-DOTA) and CHX-A"-DTPA, have been evaluated in vitro and in vivo (75). Both chelates provided stable labeling of ABD-($Z_{HER2:342}$)$_2$. The internalization rate of indium-labeled CHX-A"-DTPA-ABD-($Z_{HER2:342}$)$_2$ was somewhat higher, providing better conditions for therapy using Auger electrons. Moreover, a biodistribution study demonstrated that ^{114m}In-CHX-A"-DTPA-ABD-($Z_{HER2:342}$)$_2$ provided better tumor accumulation of radioactivity and better tumor-to-organ dose ratios than ^{114m}In-Bz-DOTA-ABD-($Z_{HER2:342}$)$_2$. The results from this study indicate that ^{114m}In-CHX-A"-DTPA-ABD-($Z_{HER2:342}$)$_2$ might be a suitable candidate for clinical applications.

The optimization of labeling chemistries has an apparent potential in the development of therapeutic conjugates. Residualizing properties of a label are important when the targeting conjugate is rapidly internalized into tumor cells as the charged chelator–radiometal complexes are retained intracellular, providing long tumor retention of radioactivity. At the same time, this mechanism causes prolonged retention of radioactivity in normal healthy organs, for example, such that it is reabsorbed by the kidneys. Previous studies demonstrated that the $Z_{HER2:342}$ affibody molecules internalize rather slowly, and the good tumor retention is due to the strong binding to membrane receptors (56,57,76). The residualizing properties are therefore not crucial for tumor targeting in this case. At the same time, labels with limited residualization would provide lower renal retention of radioactivity. These considerations were concordant with the biodistribution data concerning the $Z_{HER2:342}$-affibody molecule labeled with radioiodine using paraiodobenzoate (PIB) as a prosthetic group (28). The renal accumulation of radioactivity for radioiodinated affibody molecules was much lower than when labeled using residualizing radiometal labels, while tumor accumulation was still high. However, further reduction of renal dose was required. When using ((4-hydroxyphenyl)ethyl)maleimide (HPEM) for site-specific attachment of positron-emitting radiobromine to the affibody molecules (77), the renal accumulation of radioactivity was much lower than when using parabromobenzoate. This attracted attention to another radiohalogen, iodine-131 (^{131}I, T ½ = 8 days), which is one of the most commonly used radionuclides for targeted therapy. Since iodine is a close chemical analog of bromine, it could be expected that its biochemical behavior is also similar. In a biodistribution study comparing ^{125}I-HPEM-Z$_{HER2:342}$-C and ^{125}I-PIB-Z$_{HER2:342}$, the renal uptake was reduced nearly fourfold in the case when HPEM was used as the prosthetic group, while the tumor uptake was the same for both conjugates (78). Furthermore, the biodistribution of monomeric and dimeric forms, ^{131}I-HPEM-Z$_{HER2:342}$-C and ^{125}I-HPEM-(Z$_{HER2:342}$)$_2$-C, radiolabeled site specifically using HPEM, was compared to evaluate if dimerization provides advantages in tumor targeting. It was shown that the monomeric form provides better tumor accumulation and better tumor-to-organ dose ratios than the dimeric, presumably due to better extravasation and tumor/tissue penetration. The area under curve values for ^{131}I-HPEM-Z$_{HER2:342}$-C were 316, 122.6, 14.7, and 41.2% IA/g × h for tumor, kidney, blood, and liver, respectively. This indicates that the dose to the tumor would be much higher than the dose to healthy organs and tissues, including kidneys. These results provide good preconditions for successful radionuclide therapy using ^{131}I-HPEM-Z$_{HER2:342}$-C and suggest that the use of nonresidualizing labels for monomeric affibody molecules is a promising approach in the development of therapeutic conjugates.

A series of studies show that the biodistribution of ^{99m}Tc-labeled affibody molecules might be modified by changing the amino acid composition of mercaptoacetyl-containing peptide-based chelators (33,53,54). The biodistribution data suggested that the renal uptake of technetium-99m could partially be reduced by switching the excretion to the hepatobiliary pathway. This could be further enhanced by selection of a chelator, which provides stable attachment of the radionuclide in the blood circulation, but facilitates the catabolite excretion after intracellular catabolism in kidneys (55). Technetium isotopes are not appropriate for radionuclide therapy; however, rhenium is a chemical analog of technetium and two rhenium isotopes, ^{186}Re and ^{188}Re, hold a certain therapeutic potential. High (^{188}Re)- or medium (^{186}Re)-energy beta particles are well suited for eradication of bulky nonoperable tumors. The gamma radiation of these nuclides enables in vivo imaging of the biodistribution of rhenium-labeled conjugates, allowing for patient-specific dosimetry. In addition, ^{188}Re might be produced using a ^{188}W/^{188}Re generator, which reduces the radionuclide costs and facilitates the logistics of labeling. Thus rhenium radioisotopes are attractive for radionuclide therapy given that the labeled conjugate has a suitable biodistribution. Two synthetic affibody conjugates, mercaptoacetyl–glycyl–glycyl–glycyl (maGGG-Z$_{HER2:342}$) and mercaptoacetyl–glycyl–seryl–glycyl (maGSG-Z$_{HER2:342}$), which provided the lowest renal uptake when labeled with ^{99m}Tc, have been evaluated for targeting of ^{186}Re to HER2-overexpressing xenografts (79). Gluconate-mediated labeling of maGGG-Z$_{HER2:342}$ and maGSG-Z$_{HER2:342}$ with ^{186}Re provided a yield of more than 95% within 60 minutes. The conjugates were stable and demonstrated specific binding to HER2-expressing SKOV-3 cells. Biodistribution in normal mice demonstrated rapid blood clearance, low accumulation of

radioactivity in kidneys and in other organs, accumulating free perrhenate. Interestingly, both ^{186}Re-maGGG-Z$_{HER2:342}$ and ^{186}Re-maGSG-Z$_{HER2:342}$ demonstrated lower renal uptake than their ^{99m}Tc-labeled counterparts. ^{186}Re-maGSG-Z$_{HER2:342}$ had the lowest uptake in kidneys and was selected for further studies. Biodistribution of ^{186}Re-maGSG-Z$_{HER2:342}$ in nude mice bearing SKOV-3 xenografts showed specific targeting of tumors. Twenty-four hours after injection, the tumor uptake, 5.84 ± 0.54% IA/g, exceeded the concentration in blood more than 500-fold, and exceeded uptake in kidneys 8-fold. Dosimetric evaluation suggested that maGSG-Z$_{HER2:342}$ is a very promising therapeutic conjugate.

There is a possibility to use radiometal-labeled affibody molecules for locoregional treatment, for example, in the treatment of bladder carcinoma or for intracerebroventricular (ICV) administration in patients with brain cancer or metastases to the brain of patients with other cancers. It has been demonstrated that the DOTA-conjugated Z$_{HER2:342}$ can be stably labeled with the high-energy beta emitter ^{90}Y and the low-energy beta emitter ^{177}Lu without loosing HER2-binding specificity (80). Biodistribution of the ^{177}Lu-labeled HER2-binder in normal nude mice showed rapid clearance from the blood and low uptake in most organs (except for kidneys) indicating its potential as a targeting agent for local treatment of, for example, bladder carcinoma (80), which has been shown to have high expression of HER2 (81). To enable locoregional treatment with the ^{114m}In/^{114}In in vivo generator (see above), the isothiocyanate derivative of CHX-A″-DTPA was coupled to Z$_{HER2:342}$ (82). Labeling with both ^{111}In and ^{114m}In provided greater than 95% yield after 30 minutes at room temperature. In vitro tests demonstrated high stability of ^{114m}In-CHX-A″-DTPA-Z$_{HER2:342}$ and the radiolabeled conjugates showed high capacity for specific binding to HER2-expressing SKOV-3 ovarian carcinoma cells. ^{114m}In-CHX-A″-DTPA-Z$_{HER2:342}$ was further evaluated for specific targeting of HER2-expressing xenografts in vivo and demonstrated extremely high contrast (tumor-to-blood ratio of 200) in imaging of HER2-expressing xenografts. Breast cancer patients with HER2-expressing tumors also have a risk of developing HER2-expressing metastases in the brain, which in principle could be an interesting target for ICV administration of radiolabeled Z$_{HER2:342}$ (83).

The high expression of EGFR on some normal organs, like liver and skin, will most likely limit systemic treatment of EGFR-expressing tumors and metastases. The EGFR-targeting affibody molecule could, however, be used in locoregional treatment of glioma patients after surgery, as gliomas often exhibit significant overexpression of EGFR. Patients with glioblastoma are often treated with surgery to remove the bulky part of the tumor and the area around the tumor cavity is subsequently irradiated with external beam radiotherapy, with the goal of eradicating remaining tumor cells. Intracavitary radionuclide therapy has been proposed to be a promising modality to complement irradiation for postoperative treatment of glioblastoma, reviewed by Carlsson and coworkers (84). The small EGFR-specific affibody molecule could potentially be a good construct for reaching migrating glioma cells outside the operation cavity. Another possible local treatment modality is the intravesical treatment of urinary bladder cancer, as discussed above for HER2.

CONCLUDING REMARKS

The use of affinity proteins in tumor targeting has found applications in molecular imaging and cancer therapy. In this chapter, the potential of engineered radionuclide-conjugated affibody molecules in molecular imaging and therapy has been discussed. Despite the success of antibodies, other affinity proteins such as antibody derivatives and nonimmunoglobulin affinity proteins, including affibody molecules, are presently being considered in molecular imaging and radiotherapy.

Affibody molecules have some features that make them especially attractive as targeting agents. In addition to being able to withstand extreme chemical and temperature conditions during radiolabeling and displaying high affinity and good selectivity, they have small molecular weights. Their small size allows for more effective tissue penetration, which could be important for in vivo targeting applications. Furthermore, the small size provides the possibility of chemical synthesis. This enables incorporation of site-alternative chemical groups for specific labeling and pharmacokinetic engineering. In addition, no biologically derived materials that could contaminate the product are used. These features are unique for affibody molecules in comparison with monoclonal antibodies, antibody derivatives, and most other scaffold proteins.

Affibody molecules specific for the epidermal growth factor receptors (HER2 and EGFR), which are overexpressed on cells of solid tumors in many malignancies, have demonstrated successful tumor uptake and biodistribution in preclinical studies. Pilot clinical studies on a limited number of patients with recurrent breast cancer showed the potential for the HER2-specific affibody molecules to provide high contrast images within hours. The small size and stable scaffold are suitable for radiolabeling and provide favorable properties for imaging of tumors and metastases. For therapeutic applications, the ABD-fusion technology provides reversible binding to serum albumin and a prolonged circulation in the blood. Complete prevention of tumor formation could be seen with a radiometal-labeled affibody–ABD molecule in preclinical studies. This provides hope for the use of radiolabeled affibody molecules in future clinical trials.

After the completion of sequencing of the human genome with the recent advances in mapping of the human proteins and the understanding of their involvement in different diseases, there is now the possibility to move drug development into personalized medicine. Molecular imaging is one tool that can provide a better understanding of a single patient's disease and also help to assess the response of treatment. Among the many new affinity proteins investigated, targeting agents for molecular imaging or targeted

therapy with improved properties that will enable a more efficient and safer approach will most likely come forward. With ingenious strategies in molecular engineering, new formats are approaching that can further increase the specificity and efficacy, for example, by the use of bispecific targeting agents. A first bispecific affibody construct, binding both EGFR and HER2, was recently described (85). Many other conjugated affibody constructs have been created for evaluation (86–91). Taken together, it is evident that combinatorial protein engineering will have an impact on the generation of future targeting molecules, based on various antibody derivatives or other scaffold proteins, for the diagnosis and treatment of cancer as well as other diseases.

Acknowledgment

The authors thank Dr. Lars Abrahmsen for careful reading of the manuscript.

REFERENCES

1. Holliger P, Hudson PJ. Engineered antibody fragments and the rise of single domains. *Nat Biotechnol.* 2005;23(9):1126–1136.
2. Behr TM, Goldenberg DM, Becker W. Reducing the renal uptake of radiolabeled antibody fragments and peptides for diagnosis and therapy: present status, future prospects and limitations. *Eur J Nucl Med.* 1998;25(2):201–212.
3. Friedman M, Stahl S. Engineered affinity proteins for tumour-targeting applications. *Biotechnol Appl Biochem.* 2009;53(pt 1):1–29.
4. Nygren PÅ, Skerra A. Binding proteins from alternative scaffolds. *J Immunol Methods.* 2004;290(1–2):3–28.
5. Binz HK, Amstutz P, Pluckthun A. Engineering novel binding proteins from nonimmunoglobulin domains. *Nat Biotechnol.* 2005;23(10):1257–1268.
6. Hey T, Fiedler E, Rudolph R, et al. Artificial, non-antibody binding proteins for pharmaceutical and industrial applications. *Trends Biotechnol.* 2005;23(10):514–522.
7. Hosse RJ, Rothe A, Power BE. A new generation of protein display scaffolds for molecular recognition. *Protein Sci.* 2006;15(1):14–27.
8. Gebauer M, Skerra A. Engineered protein scaffolds as next-generation antibody therapeutics. *Curr Opin Chem Biol.* 2009;13(3):245–255.
9. Chapman AP. PEGylated antibodies and antibody fragments for improved therapy: a review. *Adv Drug Deliv Rev.* 2002;54(4):531–545.
10. Flower DR. Towards in silico prediction of immunogenic epitopes. *Trends Immunol.* 2003;24(12):667–674.
11. Nilsson B, Moks T, Jansson B, et al. A synthetic IgG-binding domain based on staphylococcal protein A. *Protein Eng.* 1987;1(2):107–113.
12. Jansson B, Uhlén M, Nygren PÅ. All individual domains of staphylococcal protein A show Fab binding. *FEMS Immunol Med Microbiol.* 1998;20(1):69–78.
13. Ståhl S, Nygren PÅ. The use of gene fusions to protein A and protein G in immunology and biotechnology. *Pathol Biol (Paris).* 1997;45(1):66–76.
14. Rees AR, Staunton D, Webster DM, et al. Antibody design: beyond the natural limits. *Trends Biotechnol.* 1994;12(5):199–206.
15. Nord K, Nilsson J, Nilsson B, et al. A combinatorial library of an alpha-helical bacterial receptor domain. *Protein Eng.* 1995;8(6):601–608.
16. Nord K, Gunneriusson E, Ringdahl J, et al. Binding proteins selected from combinatorial libraries of an alpha-helical bacterial receptor domain. *Nat Biotechnol.* 1997;15(8):772–777.
17. Grönwall C, Jonsson A, Lindström S, et al. Selection and characterization of Affibody ligands binding to Alzheimer amyloid beta peptides. *J Biotechnol.* 2007;128(1):162–183.
18. Wikman M, Steffen AC, Gunneriusson E, et al. Selection and characterization of HER2/neu-binding affibody ligands. *Protein Eng Des Sel.* 2004;17(5):455–462.
19. Grönwall C, Sjöberg A, Ramström M, et al. Affibody-mediated transferrin depletion for proteomics applications. *Biotechnol J.* 2007;2(11):1389–1398.

20. Friedman M, Nordberg E, Höidén-Guthenberg I, et al. Phage display selection of Affibody molecules with specific binding to the extracellular domain of the epidermal growth factor receptor. *Protein Eng Des Sel.* 2007;20(4):189–199.

21. Nord K, Nord O, Uhlén M, et al. Recombinant human factor VIII-specific affinity ligands selected from phage-displayed combinatorial libraries of protein A. *Eur J Biochem.* 2001;268(15):4269–4277.

22. Grönwall C, Snelders E, Palm AJ, et al. Generation of Affibody ligands binding interleukin-2 receptor alpha/CD25. *Biotechnol Appl Biochem.* 2008;50(pt 2):97–112.

23. Wikman M, Rowcliffe E, Friedman M, et al. Selection and characterization of an HIV-1 gp120-binding affibody ligand. *Biotechnol Appl Biochem.* 2006;45(pt 2):93–105.

24. Sandström K, Xu Z, Forsberg G, et al. Inhibition of the CD28-CD80 co-stimulation signal by a CD28-binding affibody ligand developed by combinatorial protein engineering. *Protein Eng.* 2003;16(9):691–697.

25. Kronqvist N, Lofblom J, Jonsson A, et al. A novel affinity protein selection system based on staphylococcal cell surface display and flow cytometry. *Protein Eng Des Sel.* 2008;21(4):247–255.

26. Friedman M, Orlova A, Johansson E, et al. Directed evolution to low nanomolar affinity of a tumor-targeting epidermal growth factor receptor-binding affibody molecule. *J Mol Biol.* 2008;376(5):1388–1402.

27. Gunneriusson E, Nord K, Uhlén M, et al. Affinity maturation of a Taq DNA polymerase specific affibody by helix shuffling. *Protein Eng.* 1999;12(10):873–878.

28. Orlova A, Magnusson M, Eriksson TL, et al. Tumor imaging using a picomolar affinity HER2 binding affibody molecule. *Cancer Res.* 2006;66(8):4339–4348.

29. Nilsson FY, Tolmachev V. Affibody molecules: new protein domains for molecular imaging and targeted tumor therapy. *Curr Opin Drug Discov Devel.* 2007;10(2):167–175.

30. Tolmachev V, Orlova A, Nilsson FY, et al. Affibody molecules: potential for in vivo imaging of molecular targets for cancer therapy. *Expert Opin Biol Ther.* 2007;7(4):555–568.

31. Orlova A, Feldwisch J, Abrahmsen L, et al. Update: affibody molecules for molecular imaging and therapy for cancer. *Cancer Biother Radiopharm.* 2007;22(5):573–584.

32. Engfeldt T, Renberg B, Brumer H, et al. Chemical synthesis of triple-labelled three-helix bundle binding proteins for specific fluorescent detection of unlabelled protein. *Chembiochem.* 2005;6(6):1043–1050.

33. Engfeldt T, Orlova A, Tran T, et al. Imaging of HER2-expressing tumours using a synthetic Affibody molecule containing the 99mTc-chelating mercaptoacetyl-glycyl-glycyl-glycyl (MAG3) sequence. *Eur J Nucl Med Mol Imaging.* 2007;34(5):722–733.

34. Magnusson MK, Henning P, Myhre S, et al. Adenovirus 5 vector genetically re-targeted by an Affibody molecule with specificity for tumor antigen HER2/neu. *Cancer Gene Ther.* 2007;14(5):468–479.

35. Myhre S, Henning P, Friedman M, et al. Re-targeted adenovirus vectors with dual specificity; binding specificities conferred by two different Affibody molecules in the fiber. *Gene Ther.* 2009;16(2):252–261.

36. Steffen AC, Wikman M, Tolmachev V, et al. In vitro characterization of a bivalent anti-HER-2 affibody with potential for radionuclide-based diagnostics. *Cancer Biother Radiopharm.* 2005;20(3):239–248.

37. Andersson M, Rönnmark J, Areström I, et al. Inclusion of a non-immunoglobulin binding protein in two-site ELISA for quantification of human serum proteins without interference by heterophilic serum antibodies. *J Immunol Methods.* 2003;283(1–2):225–234.

38. Renberg B, Shiroyama I, Engfeldt T, et al. Affibody protein capture microarrays: synthesis and evaluation of random and directed immobilization of affibody molecules. *Anal Biochem.* 2005;341(2):334–343.

39. Renberg B, Nordin J, Merca A, et al. Affibody molecules in protein capture microarrays: evaluation of multidomain ligands and different detection formats. *J Proteome Res.* 2007;6(1):171–179.

40. Nord K, Gunneriusson E, Uhlén M, et al. Ligands selected from combinatorial libraries of protein A for use in affinity capture of apolipo-protein A-1M and taq DNA polymerase. *J Biotechnol.* 2000;80(1):45–54.

41. Rönnmark J, Grönlund H, Uhlén M, et al. Human immunoglobulin A (IgA)-specific ligands from combinatorial engineering of protein A. *Eur J Biochem.* 2002;269(11):2647–2655.

42. Andersson C, Hansson M, Power U, et al. Mammalian cell production of a respiratory syncytial virus (RSV) candidate vaccine recovered using a product-specific affinity column. *Biotechnol Appl Biochem.* 2001;34(pt 1):25–32.

43. Hedhammar M, Hober S. Z(basic)—a novel purification tag for efficient protein recovery. *J Chromatogr A.* 2007;1161(1–2):22–28.

44. Hoyer W, Grönwall C, Jonsson A, et al. Stabilization of a beta-hairpin in monomeric Alzheimer's amyloid-beta peptide inhibits amyloid formation. *Proc Natl Acad Sci U S A.* 2008;105(13):5099–5104.

45. Belousova N, Mikheeva G, Gelovani J, et al. Modification of adenovirus capsid with a designed protein ligand yields a gene vector targeted to a major molecular marker of cancer. *J Virol.* 2008;82(2):630–637.

46. Tolmachev V, Nilsson FY, Widström C, et al. ^{111}In-benzyl-DTPA-Z$_{HER2:342}$, an affibody-based conjugate for in vivo imaging of HER2 expression in malignant tumors. *J Nucl Med.* 2006;47(5):846–853.

47. Orlova A, Tolmachev V, Pehrson R, et al. Synthetic affibody molecules: a novel class of affinity ligands for molecular imaging of HER2-expressing malignant tumors. *Cancer Res.* 2007;67(5):2178–2186.

48. Baum RP, Orlova A, Tolmachev V, et al. A novel molecular imaging agent for diagnosis of recurrent HER2 positive breast cancer. First time in human study using an Indium-111- or Gallium-68-labelled Affibody molecule. Abstracts of Annual Congress of the European Association of Nuclear Medicine, Athens, Greece (2006). *Eur J Nucl Med Mol Imaging.* 2006;33(suppl 14):S91.

49. Tolmachev V, Friedman M, Sandström M, et al. Affibody molecules for epidermal growth factor receptor targeting in vivo: aspects of dimerization and labeling chemistry. *J Nucl Med.* 2008;50:274–283.

50. Yarden Y, Sliwkowski MX. Untangling the ErbB signalling network. *Nat Rev Mol Cell Biol.* 2001;2(2):127–137.

51. Holbro T, Civenni G, Hynes NE. The ErbB receptors and their role in cancer progression. *Exp Cell Res.* 2003;284(1):99–110.

52. Steffen AC, Orlova A, Wikman M, et al. Affibody-mediated tumour targeting of HER-2 expressing xenografts in mice. *Eur J Nucl Med Mol Imaging.* 2006;33(6):631–638.

53. Engfeldt T, Tran T, Orlova A, et al. (99m)Tc-chelator engineering to improve tumour targeting properties of a HER2-specific Affibody molecule. *Eur J Nucl Med Mol Imaging.* 2007;34(11):1843–1853.

54. Tran T, Engfeldt T, Orlova A, et al. (99m)Tc-maEEE-Z(HER2:342), an Affibody molecule-based tracer for the detection of HER2 expression in malignant tumors. *Bioconjug Chem.* 2007;18(6):1956–1964.

55. Ekblad T, Tran T, Orlova A, et al. Development and preclinical characterization of 99mTc-labelled Affibody molecules with reduced renal uptake. *Eur J Nucl Med Mol Imaging.* 2008;35(12):2245–2255.

56. Tolmachev V, Xu H, Wallberg H, et al. Evaluation of a maleimido derivative of CHX-A''' DTPA for site-specific labeling of affibody molecules. *Bioconjug Chem.* 2008;19(8):1579–1587.

57. Ahlgren S, Orlova A, Rosik D, et al. Evaluation of maleimide derivative of DOTA for site-specific labeling of recombinant affibody molecules. *Bioconjug Chem.* 2008;19(1):235–243.

58. Lee SB, Hassan M, Fisher R, et al. Affibody molecules for in vivo characterization of HER2-positive tumors by near-infrared imaging. *Clin Cancer Res.* 2008;14(12):3840–3849.

59. Kramer-Marek G, Kiesewetter DO, Martiniova L, et al. [18F]FBEM-Z(HER2:342)-Affibody molecule-a new molecular tracer for in vivo monitoring of HER2 expression by positron emission tomography. *Eur J Nucl Med Mol Imaging.* 2008;35(5):1008–1018.

60. Namavari M, Padilla De Jesus O, Cheng Z, et al. Direct site-specific radiolabeling of an Affibody protein with 4-[18F]fluorobenzaldehyde via oxime chemistry. *Mol Imaging Biol.* 2008;10(4):177–181.

61. Nordberg E, Friedman M, Göstring L, et al. Cellular studies of binding, internalization and retention of a radiolabeled EGFR-binding affibody molecule. *Nucl Med Biol.* 2007;34(6):609–618.

62. Nordberg E, Orlova A, Friedman M, et al. In vivo and in vitro uptake of ^{111}In, delivered with the affibody molecule (ZEGFR:955)2, in EGFR expressing tumour cells. *Oncol Rep.* 2008;19(4):853–857.

63. Senekowitsch-Schmidtke R, Steiner K, Haunschild J, et al. In vivo evaluation of epidermal growth factor (EGF) receptor density on human tumor xenografts using radiolabeled EGF and anti-(EGF receptor) mAb 425. *Cancer Immunol Immunother.* 1996;42(2):108–114.

64. Reilly RM, Kiarash R, Sandhu J, et al. A comparison of EGF and MAb 528 labeled with ^{111}In for imaging human breast cancer. *J Nucl Med.* 2000;41(5):903–911.

65. Perk LR, Visser GW, Vosjan MJ, et al. (89)Zr as a PET surrogate radioisotope for scouting biodistribution of the therapeutic radio-metals (90)Y and (177)Lu in tumor-bearing nude mice after coupling to the internalizing antibody cetuximab. *J Nucl Med.* 2005;46(11):1898–1906.

66. Cai W, Chen K, He L, et al. Quantitative PET of EGFR expression in xenograft-bearing mice using 64Cu-labeled cetuximab, a chimeric anti-EGFR monoclonal antibody. *Eur J Nucl Med Mol Imaging.* 2007;34(6):850–858.

67. Wang J, Reilly RM, Chen P, et al. Fusion of the CH1 domain of IgG1 to epidermal growth factor (EGF) prolongs its retention in the blood but does not increase tumor uptake. *Cancer Biother Radiopharm.* 2002;17(6):665–671.

68. Huang L, Gainkam LO, Caveliers V, et al. SPECT imaging with 99mTc-labeled EGFR-specific nanobody for in vivo monitoring of EGFR expression. *Mol Imaging Biol.* 2008;10(3):167–175.

69. Tolmachev V. Imaging of HER-2 overexpression in tumors for guiding therapy. *Curr Pharm Des.* 2008;14:2999–3019.

70. Tolmachev V, Orlova A, Pehrson R, et al. Radionuclide therapy of HER2-positive microxenografts using a 177Lu-labeled HER2-specific Affibody molecule. *Cancer Res.* 2007;67(6):2773–2782.

71. Wheldon TE, O'Donoghue JA, Barrett A, et al. The curability of tumours of differing size by targeted radiotherapy using 131I or 90Y. *Radiother Oncol.* 1991;21(2):91–99.

72. Kassis AI. The amazing world of auger electrons. *Int J Radiat Biol.* 2004;80(11–12):789–803.

73. de Jong M, Breeman WA, Valkema R, et al. Combination radionuclide therapy using 177Lu- and 90Y-labeled somatostatin analogs. *J Nucl Med.* 2005;46 (suppl 1):13–17.

74. Tolmachev V, Bernhardt P, Forssell-Aronsson E, et al. 114mIn, a candidate for radionuclide therapy: low-energy cyclotron production and labeling of DTPA-D-phe-octreotide. *Nucl Med Biol.* 2000;27(2):183–188.

75. Tolmachev V, Wallberg H, Andersson K, et al. The influence of Bz-DOTA and CHX-A″-DTPA on the biodistribution of ABD-fused anti-HER2 Affibody molecules: implications for (114m)In-mediated targeting therapy. *Eur J Nucl Med Mol Imaging.* 2009;36(9):1460–1468.

76. Wållberg H, Orlova A. Slow internalization of anti-HER2 synthetic affibody monomer 111In-DOTA-ZHER2:342-pep2: implications for development of labeled tracers. *Cancer Biother Radiopharm.* 2008;23(4):435–442.

77. Mume E, Orlova A, Larsson B, et al. Evaluation of ((4-hydroxyphenyl) ethyl)maleimide for site-specific radiobromination of anti-HER2 affibody. *Bioconjug Chem.* 2005;16(6):1547–1555.

78. Tolmachev V, Mume E, Sjoberg S, et al. Influence of valency and labelling chemistry on in vivo targeting using radioiodinated HER2-binding Affibody molecules. *Eur J Nucl Med Mol Imaging.* 2009;36(4):692–701.

79. Orlova A, Tran TA, Ekblad T, et al. 186Re-maSGS-Z (HER2:342), a potential Affibody conjugate for systemic therapy of HER2-expressing tumours. *Eur J Nucl Med Mol Imaging.* 2010;37:260–269.

80. Fortin MA, Orlova A, Malmstrom PU, et al. Labelling chemistry and characterization of [90Y/177Lu]-DOTA-ZHER2:342-3 Affibody molecule, a candidate agent for locoregional treatment of urinary bladder carcinoma. *Int J Mol Med.* 2007;19(2):285–291.

81. Gårdmark T, Wester K, De la Torre M, et al. Analysis of HER2 expression in primary urinary bladder carcinoma and corresponding metastases. *BJU Int.* 2005;95(7):982–986.

82. Orlova A, Rosik D, Sandstrom M, et al. Evaluation of [(111/114m)In] CHX-A″-DTPA-ZHER2:342, an affibody ligand conjugate for targeting of HER2-expressing malignant tumors. *Q J Nucl Med Mol Imaging.* 2007;51(4):314–323.

83. Burstein HJ, Lieberman G, Slamon DJ, et al. Isolated central nervous system metastases in patients with HER2-overexpressing advanced breast cancer treated with first-line trastuzumab-based therapy. *Ann Oncol.* 2005;16(11):1772–1777.

84. Carlsson J, Ren ZP, Wester K, et al. Planning for intracavitary anti-EGFR radionuclide therapy of gliomas. Literature review and data on EGFR expression. *J Neurooncol.* 2006;77(1):33–45.

85. Friedman M, Lindstrom S, Ekerljung L, et al. Engineering and characterization of a bispecific HER2 x EGFR-binding affibody molecule. *Biotechnol Appl Biochem.* 2009;54(2):121–131.

86. Jonsson A, Wallberg H, Herne N, et al. Generation of tumour-necrosis-factor-alpha-specific affibody1 molecules capable of blocking receptor binding in vitro. *Biotechnol Appl Biochem.* 2009;54(2):93–103.

87. Vernet E, Konrad A, Lundberg E, et al. Affinity-based entrapment of the HER2 receptor in the endoplasmic reticulum using an affibody molecule. *J Immunol Methods.* 2008;338(1–2):1–6.

88. Vernet E, Lundberg E, Friedman M, et al. Affibody-mediated retention of the epidermal growth factor receptor in the secretory compartments leads to inhibition of phosphorylation in the kinase domain. *N Biotechnol.* 2009;25:417–423.

89. Canine BF, Wang Y, Hatefi A. Biosynthesis and characterization of a novel genetically engineered polymer for targeted gene transfer to cancer cells. *J Control Release.* 2009;138(3):188–196.

90. Orlova A, Wallberg H, Stone-Elander S, et al. On the selection of a tracer for PET imaging of HER2-expressing tumors: direct comparison of a 124I-labeled affibody molecule and trastuzumab in a murine xenograft model. *J Nucl Med.* 2009;50(3):417–425.

91. Wållberg H, Ahlgren S, Widström C, et al. Evaluation of the radiocobalt-labeled [MMA-DOTA-Cys(61)]-Z (HER2:2395)-Cys Affibody molecule for targeting of HER2-expressing tumors. *Mol Imaging Biol.* 2010;12:54–62.

Radiolabeled Aptamers for Imaging and Therapy

Sotiris Missailidis and Alan Perkins

■ INTRODUCTION

This chapter provides an overview of the field of radiolabeled aptamers for imaging and therapeutic applications, with a focus on cancer. As the number of clinically relevant radiolabeled aptamers reported so far is limited, where appropriate, other oligonucleotides equipped with radionuclides will also be presented to demonstrate further possibilities. For a more detailed discussion, the reader is encouraged to turn to the excellent reviews that have been published in the area (1–8).

Aptamers

The word "aptamer" (a chimera of the Latin "aptus" [to fit] and the Greek "meros" [part]) was coined in 1990, when three research groups simultaneously published their findings on the identification of oligonucleotides with predefined properties (9–11). As early as the 1960s, evolutionary experiments with ribonucleic acid (RNA) were described (12,13), and the development of techniques such as the polymerase chain reaction (PCR) was crucial for this breakthrough.

Aptamers are short (typically 10 to 100 bases), single- or double-stranded oligonucleotides that are selected in vitro from a random library in an evolutionary process termed SELEX (systematic evolution of ligands by exponential enrichment) (7–9) (Fig. 5.1). The key to their existence is the realization that, in addition to their two-dimensional information content (sequence), oligonucleotides also possess a three-dimensional shape (7,8,14). In fact, the seemingly simple repetitive backbone, decorated with only four base pairs, can assume a bewildering variety of shapes, more effectively populating chemical space than conventional chemical screening collections. A library of 10^{14} to 10^{15} sequences, corresponding to a 25-base fully randomized sequence, allows for sufficient diversity, which can be readily explored. However, it is possible to investigate longer structures by, for example, randomizing only some positions within the oligonucleotide sequence (8). The oligonucleotides and the target are allowed to interact and the nonbinding sequences are removed. The bound sequences are eluted, amplified by PCR, and the selection step is repeated. With each cycle of selection–amplification,

stronger binding sequences emerge. Typically, 10 to 20 rounds of selection are performed, although as little as 1 round has been described in the literature. It is common that with too few cycles, many sequences with only modest affinities are isolated, while after a sufficiently large number of rounds, the affinities of the remaining few sequences reach a plateau, as only the highest binding aptamers remain in the pool. For RNA aptamers, an additional reverse transcription step is included. It is also possible to apply the protocol to double-stranded oligonucleotides (7,8) and the selection process is amenable to automation (15,16). It is worth mentioning that aptamers can be simultaneously raised for multiple targets in complex mixtures, such as whole cells or even tissue samples. When ligands for multiple targets on human red blood cell ghosts were identified, the isolated aptamers displayed binding affinities comparable with those found against pure targets (17). In theory, it is possible to generate ligands to all targets in complex mixtures (18).

After completion of the SELEX process, the winning species are cloned, sequenced, and can be chemically synthesized. It is possible to perform the in vitro selection with modified nucleotide triphosphates that can impose enhanced stability on the aptamer, provide handles for further manipulation, or enable additional chemical reactivity, for example, photocrosslinking.

Most reported aptamers display binding constants in the low nanomolar to picomolar range. It has been argued that the exquisite selectivity observed on numerous occasions is correlated with their high specificity (19). Their ease of generation, chemical malleability, small size, high affinity and specificity, low immunogenicity, rapid blood clearance, and low production costs make them obvious alternatives to monoclonal antibodies for a number of applications (4). As they are chemically produced, their activity remains uniform from batch to batch. They have an unlimited shelf life and return to their original conformation after heat denaturation (4). Importantly, antidotes can be designed with relative ease and therefore they are easy to inhibit, should the need arise (vide infra).

A major stumbling block for the development of aptamer drugs is their low serum stability (20,21). Most unmodified RNA oligonucleotides have a serum half-life of less than 10 minutes, while deoxyribonucleic acid (DNA) is slightly

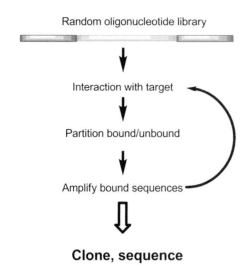

Random oligonucleotide library

↓

Interaction with target

↓

Partition bound/unbound

↓

Amplify bound sequences

⇩

Clone, sequence

FIGURE 5.1 Systematic evolution of ligands by exponential enrichment.

more stable ($t_{1/2} \sim$ several minutes to hours, depending upon the structure). The most common way to increase nuclease resistance is the incorporation of 4'-deoxy-4-thiosugars, phosphorothioate nucleosides, 2'-fluoro-, 2'-methoxy-, or 2'-aminosugars or L-sugars (vide infra).

One of the great advantages aptamers have over antibodies is their ability to recognize just about any conceivable target, from metal ions to peptides and proteins, to small organic molecules and whole cells (14,22,23). However, the actual "aptamerogenicity" of a target (i.e., whether high-affinity and high-specificity aptamers can be raised against it) has to be determined experimentally (1). There is an online database of all known aptamer sequences and targets available at http://aptamer.icmb.utexas.edu. The database is updated monthly and can be searched for target, keyword, and target type, among others (24).

Diagnostic and therapeutic relevance

Aptamers are widely used as the recognition unit of sensors (2,6) either in solution or immobilized (3). Surface immobilization is possible via physisorption, high-affinity interactions (e.g., in biotin-labeled aptamers to avidin coatings), or covalent binding through an appropriate linker. Thus, silica, gold, and polymer surfaces have been functionalized with aptamers.

A variety of aptamers have been developed to control the biological function (23,25–28). As potential antiviral agents, they could inhibit complementary DNA synthesis in human immunodeficiency virus 1 (29), avian myeloblastosis virus and Moloney murine leukemia virus (30) by binding to the respective reverse transcriptase, and the hepatitis C virus RNA-dependent RNA polymerase (31). Single-residue phosphorylation could be inhibited in the unphosphorylated C-terminal domain of GluR1 by preincubation with a phospho-Ser845 Glu1-binding aptamer (32). Intracellular expressed aptamers (intramers) are emerging as valuable tools for proteomics, genomics,

and drug discovery, in particular in the investigation of protein function (33).

Aptamers have potential in cancer therapy both as enzyme inhibitors and as target-specific carriers of drugs or imaging agents. In this context, aptamers have been produced against platelet-derived growth factor, vascular endothelial growth factor (VEGF) (34), prostate-specific membrane antigen (PSMA) (35,36), epidermal growth factor receptor (EGFR) (37), tenascin-C (38), and cancer cell lines (39,40). An anti-PSMA aptamer–toxin conjugate, consisting of 2'-F-modified RNA aptamer and gelonin (a small N-glycosidase protein) was delivered specifically to PSMA-expressing cells, which were selectively destroyed and the toxicity to nontarget cells was reduced (36). In a similar vein, conjugation of doxorubicin via an acid-labile linker to an anti–CCRF-CEM (T-cell acute lymphoblastic leukemia) aptamer resulted in the selective release of the drug in the acidic endosomal environment of those cells that internalized the conjugate (41). EGFR kinase activity could be inhibited with an anti-EGFR aptamer (37). It was found that a single-dose treatment resulted in statistically significant antitumor effect in epidermoid cancer cell–bearing nude mice. Interestingly, this aptamer was also reported to be nonspecific for EGR, also affecting insulin receptor activity (37). A 26-mer oligonucleotide, AGRO100, currently in phase II clinical trials, inhibited the proliferation in prostate, breast, and cervical cancer cells upon binding to nucleolin, and thus possibly interfering with the nuclear factor-κB pathway (42).

Modulation of aptamer activity

It may be desirable to turn on and off aptamer inhibitory activity. Light is a most convenient external stimulus for biomolecular control. It is a unique (orthogonal) signal, and as most cells do not react to a light stimulus, it enables high spatial and temporal resolution, and is noninvasive (43). It is possible to incorporate into the oligonucleotide nonnatural nucleobases bearing photolabileprotecting groups, such as the caged nucleotides shown in Figure 5.2. Upon irradiation with 366-nm light, the protecting group is cleaved and functional aptamer is obtained. The principle has been demonstrated on an antithrombin aptamer (28), which has anticoagulative activity only after the light-induced removal of a bulky protecting group from a thymidine residue that is instrumental in thrombin binding (Fig. 5.2A). In an elegant study, an antithrombin aptamer was extended with a region that contained a complementary sequence to the binding region (Fig. 5.2B). However, a mismatch was also incorporated in the form of a caged nitrophenylethyl-protected dC-residue. Upon irradiation, the mismatch was eliminated allowing the cytidine to participate in base pairing with its complementary pair in the binding site, thus inactivating the aptamer (26). The photoisomerization of azobenzene has been exploited to alternate a thrombin-binding DNA-aptamer conformation between active and inactive (25). When incorporated into the oligonucleotide, upon visible light irradiation, the azobenzene units adopted a *trans*-conformation, which rendered the aptamer

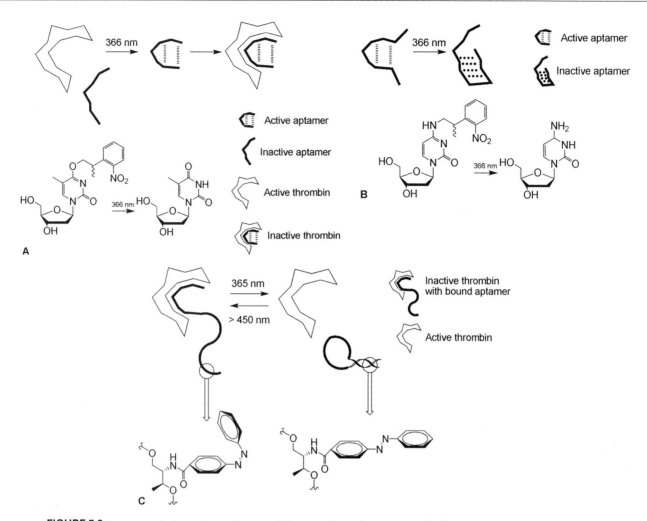

FIGURE 5.2 Aptamer activation by base pairing upon light-induced uncaging of a nucleotide (**A**). Aptamer inactivation by base pairing upon light-induced uncaging of a nucleotide (**B**). Modulation of aptamer activity *via cis–trans* isomerization of azobenzene units (**C**).

with the ability to hybridize with a complementary oligonucleotide strand attached to the recognition unit *via* a polyethylene glycol (PEG) linker. Ultraviolet (UV) irradiation resulted in *trans* → *cis* azobenzene isomerization with concomitant melting of the double strand and availability of the aptamer for thrombin binding (Fig. 5.2C). A drawback of this method is that the application of UV-visible light has poor tissue penetration. The extension of the methodology to the near infrared region should resolve this problem.

Chemical modifications

The chemical modification of aptamers is desirable for various reasons, such as imposing increased in vivo stability (21), providing attachment sites for labels (e.g., drugs, toxins, luminescent compounds, or radiometals), and for the extension of the nucleotide repertoire to access a broader range of target structures. In the context of the latter, unnatural, hydrophobic base pairs have been identified by focused screening of a library of compounds (44). Three self-pairs and a heteropair emerged that were recognized by K_f or T7 (self) and K_f, T7, and Terminator (heteropair) polymerases in vitro. Broader applications are hindered by the sluggishness of the insertion of one

of the heteropair members opposite its template. Despite the obvious need for optimization and further development, this line of research is very exciting. Polymerase tolerance for unnatural nucleoside triphosphates has been examined by several research groups (45–47). Various C5-modified dCTP or dUTP and C7-modified 7-deaza-dGTP or dATP substrates were systematically investigated with a range of polymerases (46). It was found that family A polymerases performed poorly, whereas the family B polymerases *Pwo* and Vent were much more suited to the synthesis of highly demanding templates bearing consecutive stretches of modified nucleotides. Additives, such as dimethyl sulfoxide, formamide, single-strand binding protein (SSB), betaine, and tetramethylammonium chloride (TMAC) can also have beneficial effect on the yield of the PCR (45).

Chemical modification can be carried out post-SELEX, but the product thus obtained may have altered affinity for its target. It is also possible to perform the SELEX with a nonnatural oligonucleotide pool, in which case the success of the experiment hinges on the acceptance of the modified nucleotide triphosphates by the polymerase. A range of modified nucleotide triphosphates compatible with SELEX has been reported, and is shown in Figure 5.3. The most

FIGURE 5.3 Nucleotide triphosphates compatible with enzymatic synthesis. PPP, triphosphate.

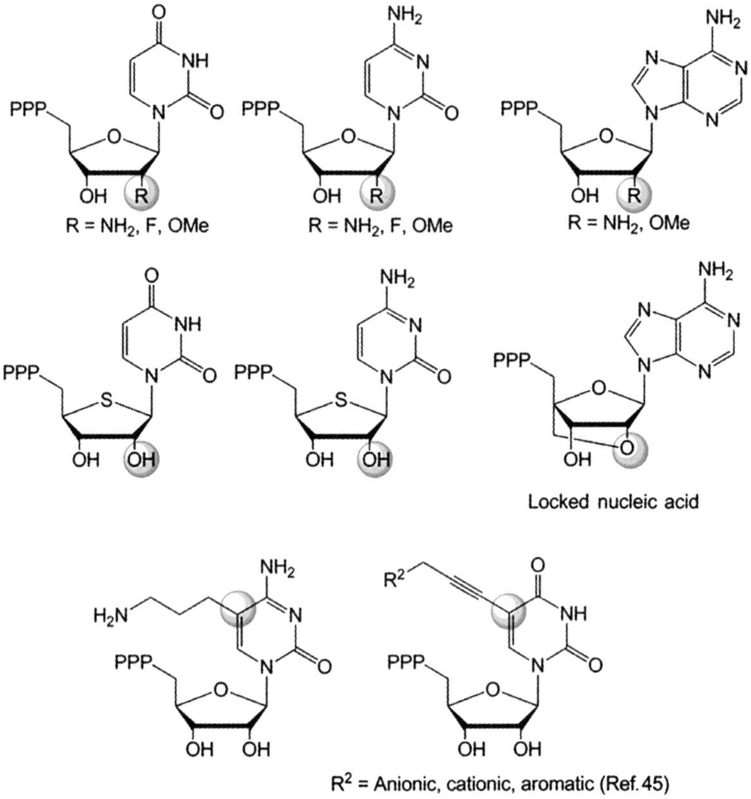

Locked nucleic acid

R^2 = Anionic, cationic, aromatic (Ref. 45)

common sites for modification are the 5-position of pyrimidines, the 2' sugar position, the 4' sugar position (replacement of the ring oxygen), and the phosphodiester linkage.

The post-SELEX labeling of DNA strands that were modified with alkyne-bearing nucleobases (48) *via* Cu(I)-catalyzed Huisgen cycloaddition was demonstrated with a range of azides, among them various fluorescent dyes (e.g., fluorescein, rhodamine, coumarin, and a cyanine dye), glucose, and a linker-equipped biotin molecule (49,50). By protecting some of the alkynes with either trimethylsilyl (TMS) or triisopropylsilyl (TIPS) groups, it was possible to introduce up to three different labels with high selectivity and efficiency (50). Although the Cu(I)-catalyzed variant of the Huisgen reaction is cytotoxic, and thus limited to fixed cells or tissues, nontoxic variants of this popular reaction have been developed, which should be possible to adapt to aptamer labeling (51–54).

Modification of the sugar moiety has yielded 2'-fluoro-, 2'-amino-, and 2'-methoxyribonucleosides (47,55,56) with better resistance to degradation and improved pharmacokinetics. All three substitutions confer significant nuclease resistance to the oligonucleotides, and in the case of amino substitution, an additional stability to alkaline hydrolysis (56). When aptamers against the same target (human keratinocyte growth factor) were raised from 2'-fluoro- or 2'-amino-deoxypyrimidine libraries, the obtained ligands displayed different thermostability, affinity, and specificity for the target, with the 2'-fluoro-aptamers having superior properties (55). Although post-SELEX modifications can have deleterious effects on ligand bioactivity, the monomer

modifications carried out pre-SELEX are rarely contributing to an increase in binding affinity, and aptamers with comparable or even improved binding properties are sometimes isolated from natural oligonucleotide pools. There are a few examples when the modification demonstrably contributed to enhanced binding, such as in the case of an ATP ligand selected from a cationic 5-(3-aminopropyl)-uridine–containing pool, where the additional positive charge under physiologic conditions presumably enables additional interactions with the α- and β-phosphates (57). For efficient enzymatic synthesis of pre-SELEX modified oligonucleotides, monomer identification by polymerases is required. A T7RNA polymerase variant that is able to incorporate multiple 2'-modified nucleotides has been selected after directed evolution (47). Additionally, oligonucleotide yields can be improved by additives (45,46) or by using a combination of polymerases (44).

Thioaptamers (*S*-oligodeoxynucleotides [*S*-ODNs]) are single- or double-stranded oligonucleotides with some (typically greater than 50%) of the phosphodiester linkages replaced by monothio- or dithiophosphate groups (20). Monothioaptamers are readily selected through standard aptamer selection methods, as α-thiotriphosphates are substrates of DNA and RNA polymerases. Monosubstitution of the phosphodiester with a sulfur potentially affords a diastereomeric mixture of compounds due to the stereogenic center established in the phosphorus. Polymerases only accept the Sp-diastereomer, giving rise to the Rp-diastereomer *via* inversion of configuration. Sp-configured thioaptamers as well as dithioate-modified aptamers have to be prepared through nonenzymatic methods, such as bead-based selections (20). Thioaptamers have significantly increased nuclease resistance in serum and urine, which is also strongly dependent on the chirality around the phosphorous atom; thus, Rp-configured thioates are cleaved by snake venom phosphodiesterase, while S1 and P1 nucleases hydrolyze Sp-configured linkages (58). As the soft sulfur atoms in the backbone are less prone to coordinate hard alkali and alkali earth metal ions (mainly Na^+ and Mg^{2+}), binding to the target requires a smaller energy investment, resulting in increased binding affinity for proteins. This also manifests itself as increased nonspecific binding, which has to be taken into consideration during aptamer selection (58,59). Thioaptamers for human recombinant basic fibroblast growth factor (bFGF) were selected from a pool of random sequences that contained at every position a phosphorothioate instead of a phosphate group. Although phosphorothioate-modified oligonucleotides bind their complementary sequences with a somewhat reduced strength, aptamer affinity for the target protein was comparable with the natural RNA aptamer. Additionally, a related protein, acid fibroblast growth factor, was recognized, but not unrelated proteins (antithrombin III, VEGF) (60). Partially or fully sulfurized phosphorothioate ODNs are synthesized analogously to their oxygenated natural counterparts *via* solid-state methods. The synthesis entails 1*H*-tetrazole-catalyzed coupling of phosphoramidates, followed by treatment of the phosphite intermediates either with elemental sulfur (S_8) in 2,6-lutidine (61) or the soluble sulfurization agent 3*H*-1,2-benzodithiole-3-one 1,1-dioxide (62). Both of these protocols afford diastereomeric mixtures of products that are separable only though tedious chromatographic steps, if at all. Furthermore, the individual diastereomers are expected to have different physicochemical properties, which, coupled with our inability to fully analyze highly complex oligonucleotide mixtures, leads to questioning the reproducibility of the syntheses. Stereoselective methods for phosphorothioates exist that exploit the stereospecific substitution of diastereomerically pure 3′-*O*-(2-thio-1,3,2-oxathiophospholanes) with the 5′-hydroxyl group of a solid-supported nucleoside (63).

The incorporation of 4′-deoxy-4′-thionucleosides into oligonucleotides imparts increased stability toward RNase compared with the natural analog. Antithrombin aptamers wherein the selection was carried out using 4′-thiouridine triphosphate (4′-thioUTP) and 4′-thiocytidine triphosphate (4′-thioCTP) furnished aptamers with 50-fold increased resistance toward RNase A, and a high binding affinity (K_d = 4.7 nM) (64). The extension of the process to 4′-thioATP and 4′-thioGTP was difficult, with the fully thioated aptamer being available only through post-SELEX synthesis, despite extensive optimization of transcription conditions. The fully thioated analog was a poorer binder of thrombin compared with the partially modified analogs (65).

The introduction of boron into the oligonucleotide can have multiple beneficial effects. Upon irradiation with thermal neutrons, the stable ^{10}B isotope undergoes nuclear fis-

sion, generating a high-energy α-particle, along with ^{7}Li. This nuclear reaction has been extensively employed in Boron Neutron Capture Therapy (66). Boron can be incorporated either in the form of a boronic acid–containing moiety that is linked to the nucleoside through a linker, or by formal substitution of one of the phosphate nonlinking oxygen atoms with a BH_3^- group, yielding boranophosphate DNA and RNA analogs. Boranophosphate ODNs and ORNs resemble their natural oxygenated counterparts electronically and sterically but have increased stabilities in water due to the low-energy P–B bond. The boranophosphate internucleotide linkage is also more stable compared with the phosphodiester bond, a highly desirable feature for the development of aptamers with increased nuclease resistance (66). It is worth noting that boron-containing compounds usually have low toxicity, and a number of boron-containing drugs have been investigated for their antineoplastic, anti-inflammatory, analgesic, and antiosteoporotic properties (66). Boronated deoxyribo- and ribonucleoside 5′-(α-P-borano) triphosphates are good substrates of DNA and RNA polymerases. However, as with monophosphothioates, monosubstitution with boron at the phosphorous affords two possible diastereomers, only one of which is usually recognized by enzymes. Boronic acid–labeled thymidine triphosphate was synthesized by linking an azido-arylboronic acid to a 5-alkyne nucleotide through a 14-atom linker in a Huisgen 1,3-dipolar cycloaddition (67). The conjugate was successfully incorporated into DNA in vitro, and the resulting DNA served as the template for PCR amplification, thus enabling the development of boronic acid–modified aptamers. SELEX carried out against ATP, using guanosine 5′-(α-P-borano) triphosphate (bG) or uridine 5′-(α-P-borano) triphosphate (bU) instead of guanosine or uridine, respectively, yielded aptamers that not only tolerated but, in some cases, required the modification for efficient binding. The dU and dG substitutions were noninterchangeable (68).

Locked nucleic acids (LNAs) are conformationally restricted nucleic acid mimics that are preorganized in an N-type conformation by virtue of a 2′-*C*,4′-oxymethylene link (69–71). The preorganization decreases the flexibility of the oligonucleotide strand, and thus the entropic penalty of binding to the target, thereby increasing binding affinity. LNA-modified oligonucleotides bind to their complementary strands with increased thermal stability and specificity compared with their natural counterpart. Furthermore, the introduction of even a single terminal LNA modification can result in a significantly enhanced nuclease resistance (69,72). LNA monomers (5′-DMT-protected 3′-phosphoramidites) are amenable to standard solid-phase oligonucleotide synthesis, extended coupling times (e.g., 10 to 15 minutes as opposed to 2 minutes for natural nucleotide phosphoramidites), and high (greater than 90%) yields (69–71). LNAs can be introduced into aptamers postselection by replacement of select bases that are not involved in the binding process (73). Alternatively, LNA triphosphates are accepted as substrates for Phusion high-fidelity DNA polymerase and 9°Nm DNA polymerase (74,75). A number of other polymerases (*Taq* DNA polymerase, Klenow enzyme, large fragment, T4 DNA polymerase, *pfu* DNA polymerase, *pfx* DNA polymerase, Speed Star HS DNA polymerase, T7 RNA polymerase, *Escherichia coli* RNA polymerase, AMV reverse transcriptase, and mutant T7 R&DNA polymerase) were also tested for their ability to incorporate LNA nucleotides but without success (74). PCR amplification using LNA triphosphates was also possible, thereby creating a potential utilization of SELEX with LNA monomers (75).

The major contributors to nucleic acid degradation in vivo are plasma exonucleases. Circularized DNA aptamers, where the 3′ and 5′ ends were connected either enzymatically (by ligases), or chemically, *via* unnatural disulfide on triethylene glycol linkers, displayed plasma half-lives up to 25 hours (76). It was possible to construct multivalent thrombin-binding aptamers by forming homo- and heterodimers and -trimers by di- and trimerizing the well-known thrombin-binding aptamers, which yielded binders with high avidity in addition to high stability (76). Mere conformational restriction of the exposed termini already improved nuclease resistance, as shown by end-paired, non-ligated aptamer dimers (76).

Probably the most elegant, but not always feasible, solution to the problem of aptamer stability is based on a selection–reflection protocol and exploits the principle that the interaction of two chiral molecules is identical in every aspect to the interaction between the corresponding enantiomers (77). Nucleases degrade specifically the naturally occurring D-sugar-containing (deoxy)nucleic acids but not the L-ribose- or L-deoxyribose-containing oligonucleotides. Thus, if a D-aptamer is raised against the unnatural (mirror image) enantiomer of a ligand, the L-aptamer (consisting of L-ribose or L-deoxyribose) recognizes the naturally occurring ligand enantiomer, while it is also resistant to nucleases (78). Such "spiegelmers" have been produced against arginine (79), adenosine (78), and vasopressin (80). An automated procedure for the SELEX of RNA speigelmers has also been reported (81). The major limitation of speigelmers is that the majority of interesting targets are available only as single isomers. Thus, while D-amino acids, peptides, L-nucleotides are readily available, the construction of, for example, mirror image cell surfaces is a major challenge.

However long the lifetimes of modified aptamers may be, some of them will eventually succumb to nucleases. An important question is the fate of the degradation products. At least in one case (2′-deoxy-2′-fluoronucleotides), it has been found that the hydrolysis products can be incorporated into cellular DNA (77).

APTAMER LABELING: GENERAL CONSIDERATIONS

There are only a handful of reports on the radiolabeling of aptamers either for imaging or therapy. The issues that need consideration are the following: (a) efficient and reliable introduction of the radiolabels, (b) stability of the conjugates in vivo, and (c) biodistribution and pharmacokinetics of the conjugates. The extensive work carried out on nonaptamer ODNs provides a firm foundation on which to address these issues. Most of the chemistry, including radiolabeling prosthetic groups, linkers, bifunctional chelators, labeling reactions, and purification procedures developed previously should translate well. For this reason, in the following examples, the work on antisense oligonucleotides will also be cited.

The stability of ODN conjugates has been discussed to some extent in the previous sections. The stability of the label (e.g., leaking of metals) is something that also needs to be investigated for every new conjugate separately (82). The same applies for the biodistribution of the labeled ODNs. It is worth noting that a number of reports have discussed the significant impact that the chelator can have on pharmacokinetics.

Aptamer labeling with ^{99m}Tc

There is a large body of work concerning the Tc labeling of oligonucleotides as antisense probes for cancer-related targets (83,84). Radiolabeled nucleic acids have been used for molecular imaging with some success; however, the method is quite new, with significant hurdles still to be overcome (84–88). Antisense oligonucleotides and aptamers have been labeled with ^{99m}Tc through complexation with N- and S-donor multidentate chelators, such as MAG_2, MAG_3, SHNH, and cyclen-based ligands (86,87), and a porphyrin (89) (Fig. 5.4).

An L-selectin-binding RNA aptamer was labeled with ^{99m}Tc. The aptamer was conjugated at the 5′ end *via* an aminohexyl linker prior to complexation to the S-protected MAG_2 chelator, which could then be deprotected under mild conditions upon treatment with dichlorodiphenyl-trichloroethane (DDT) (90).

The extracellular matrix protein tenascin-C has been one of the prime targets for aptamer development because of its abundance, its involvement in oncogenesis pathways, and its ready accessibility to circulating ligands. Its overexpression correlates well with tumor malignancy (91). An anti–tenascin-C aptamer, identified upon targeting U251 glioblastoma cells, was radiolabeled with ^{99m}Tc and ^{111}In using MAG_2, PEG-ylated MAG_2, and DTPA chelators. The radiolabeled aptamers had rapid blood clearance and high tumor-to-blood ratios. A control non-binder aptamer also cleared rapidly from the blood but was not retained in the tumor. The MAG_2-labeled aptamer cleared through renal and hepatobiliary pathways, while PEG-ylation, or DTPA-chelation (both of which increase hydrophilicity) abolished hepatobiliary clearance (92). Two LNA-stabilized anti–tenascin-C aptamers were labeled with ^{99m}Tc for biodistribution studies. Both conjugates were characterized by increased tumor uptake compared with the unmodified analog but also reduced tumor-to-kidney ratios due to their elevated kidney and liver uptake (93).

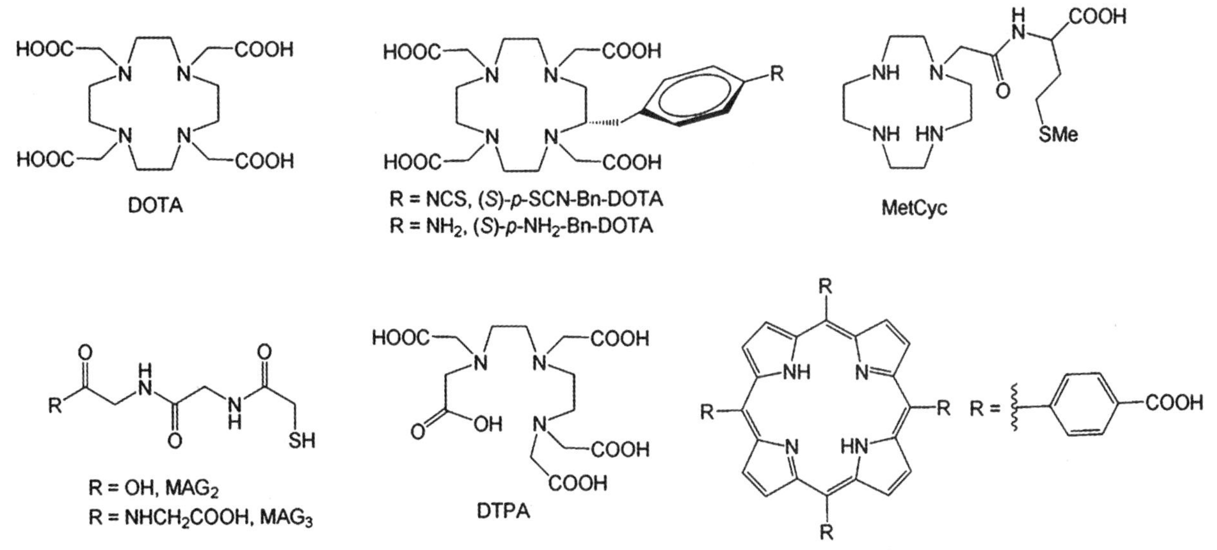

FIGURE 5.4 Bifunctional chelators used in aptamer radiometal labeling.

MUC1 is a large cell-surface glycoprotein that is overexpressed and aberrantly glycosylated in solid tumors of the breast and bladder. An aptamer against MUC1 was identified and radiolabeled with technetium and the therapeutically relevant rhenium isotope using either DOTA, a cyclen-based ligand with a methionine bioconjugatable site, or a porphyrin-tetracarboxylic acid derivative (89). DOTA and the porphyrin enable the construction of tetrameric conjugates with four binding sites and enhanced avidities. All conjugates were evaluated in a mouse breast cancer model, and it was found that the tetrameric species were retained longer in circulation than the monomeric species, while displaying similarly low immunogenicity and good tumor permeability. MUC1 was the chosen glycoprotein for two additional aptamers, one targeting the protein core, the other the tumor glycosylated glycoprotein (93). Both oligonucleotides had a 5′-aminohexyl bioconjugation site and were stabilized against nucleases *via* a 3′-inverted thymidine. Initial experiments in MCF-7 tumor-bearing mice showed that the two radiolabeled aptamers had different pharmacokinetic properties. The use of anti-MUC1 aptamers in enzyme-linked immunosorbent essays has also been described (87).

Aptamer labeling with other metals

Ethylenediaminetetraacetic acid (EDTA), DOTA, and DOTA-type chelators are the most commonly used ligands for the complexation of trivalent metal ions, for example, In^{3+}, Ga^{3+}, Y^{3+}, and the lanthanides. These ligands are available with various bioconjugatable groups (amino, carboxyl, isothiocyanate, etc.) (94–96). A phosphorothioate antisense nucleotide was coupled with SCN-Bn-EDTA through an amino group in a C-5-modified thymine. Complexation of ^{90}Y was achieved upon treatment of the EDTA-ON with ^{90}Y-acetate at room temperature, with a labeling efficiency of approximately 40%, and without loss of hybridization properties (96).

A mirror-image oligonucleotide was labeled with ^{86}Y-(S)-p-SCN-Bn-DOTA. The complex formation resulted in two isomeric compounds with slightly different hydrophilicities and biodistributions in Wistar rats. The conjugation of the two isomeric complexes to a 12-mer L-RNA *via* a 5′-aminohexyl linker afforded conjugates without significant differences (94). As with previous L-oligonucleotides, the conjugates were excreted mainly through the kidneys (94).

Two maleimide reagents were developed for the prelabeling Y-tagging of thiol-bearing oligonucleotides and peptides (95). Prelabeling, the complexation of the metal with the bifunctional chelator prior to attachment to the biomolecule, is particularly important for heat-sensitive compounds. The thiol group was introduced into the L-RNA at the 5′ end through a thiohexyl linker. In a typical labeling process, aminobenzyl-DOTA was complexed with Y^{3+}. The complex was then coupled to maleic acid. This construct could be purified by solid-phase extraction, and afterwards reacted with thiol-functionalized oligonucleotides. Postlabeling was also performed and was found to be more efficient for heat-resistant compounds.

Two high-affinity aptamers against tenascin-C have been identified using SELEX (38). Subsequently, these aptamers were labeled following the format A–B–L–C, where A represents the aptamer against tenascin-C, B is absent or represents a bridging structure, L represents a linker, and C the ligand for the metal. The bridging structure is present to allow the conjugation of further chemical structures, such as a linker (L) and is expected to be a substituted or unsubstituted lower unbranched or branched alkyl, alkene, or aldehyde, carrying an amine functionality. The linker is a chemical entity that connects the aptamer, *via* an amine group of the bridging structure or the aptamer, with the chelator C. This linker is characterized by the presence of a free mercapto (SH) functionality, which allows connection to the chelator and can be a polymeric chemical entity, including a polypeptide or a PEG molecule. The metal chelator is suitable for complexing of lanthanoid or lanthanoid-like metals (97) and includes multiple options: DO3A-maleimide, DOTA-type ligands, 1,4,7-Tris(2-mercaptoethyl)-1,4,7-triazacyclononane–type ligands, 1,4,7-triazacyclononane-1,4,7 triacetic acid–type ligands (NOTA), 1,4,7-tris(3,5-dimethyl-2-hydroxybenzyl)-1,4,7-triazacyclononane–type ligands, or tripodal ligands (97).

Aptamer labeling with halides

The radiolabeling of oligonucleotides with halides is well known and has been reported for native phosphorothioated (98), hybrid phosphodiester methylphosphonate, 2'-OMe, and spiegelmer ODNs (99). Fluorine, bromine, and iodine are generally introduced *via* prosthetic groups, typically alkylating agents such as the corresponding *N*-(4-halobenzyl)-2-bromoacetamides (100), or through a hexylamine linker with 4-([^{18}F]fluoromethyl)phenyl isothiocyanate (98). To avoid direct handling of large quantities of radioactivity and to furnish a reliable and rapid synthesis route, the automation of the radiolabel synthesis has been developed (98). The introduction of ^{18}F and ^{125}I into nonfunctional DNA and RNA spiegelmers has been demonstrated, and the pharmacokinetics of the labeled oligonucleotides has been investigated. The conjugates were metabolically stable and there was no evidence of nonspecific binding, making spiegelmers promising candidates for imaging (99). Iodination of antisense nucleotides (growth factor α and FR1 region of the Ig V_H gene) has also been carried out by capping the 5' end of the ODN with a tyramine moiety, which underwent iodination with NaI and chloramine T (101), a method that should equally be applicable to aptamer labeling.

OUTLOOK AND FUTURE PERSPECTIVES

In the two decades since aptamers entered the stage of pharmaceutical development, they have emerged as hopeful entities for imaging and therapy. Indeed, the first pharmaceutical aptamer formulation, Macugen (pegaptanib sodium injection), was approved for the treatment of age-related macular degeneration in the United States in 2004 (85). Their ease of generation, high specificity and affinity, coupled with a seemingly nonexistent immunogenicity, promises a quick solution to some of the major problems presented by antibody-based therapies. However, problems remain, for example, the limited use of modified nucleoside triphosphates as polymerase substrates. Somewhat more academic, but a very exciting question, is the extension of the four-base alphabet to enable novel binding modes and possibly the efficient recognition of thus far elusive structures.

Radiolabeling, drug delivery, and fluorescent imaging requires efficient loading of aptamers with the desired cargo. In addition to 1:1 aptamer-cargo approaches, multimeric constructs have also been described. These include multiple aptamers surrounding a single chelator (89),

several aptamers and several drug molecules arranged around a single-walled carbon nanotube (102), or a viral capsid shell (103). Additional problems that need addressing are the targeting of low-abundance or intracellular structures, the latter of which may be partially solved by conjugation to suitable internalizing receptor-specific pretargeting agents.

The dearth of radiolabeled aptamers is certainly not a sign of failure, but more that of a methodology in its infancy. With significant chemical problems already solved, it is time to use our knowledge to the targeted delivery of the vast variety of imaging and therapeutic radionuclides that are currently available. Thus, the therapeutic pair of technetium and rhenium is chemically very similar to its extensively studied counterpart. Similarly, the lessons learned from labeling experiments with indium and gallium can be applied to introduce any trivalent lanthanoid of choice, both for therapy, radioimaging, or even magnetic resonance imaging, opening new horizons on our imaging capabilities.

Another aspect crucial in the biodistribution of aptamer-based targeted radiopharmaceuticals is the choice of ligand for the metal. It has now been clearly demonstrated that different chelators can have a significant effect on the hydrophilicity and pharmacokinetic properties of an aptamer. There has been a significant amount of work looking at the pharmacokinetic properties of aptamers using tritiated bases, as a most accurate indication of the aptamer properties per se (as an example see Ref. 104). Where these have been compared with chelator-conjugated aptamers, significant differences have been obtained due to chelator labeling. Thus, the appropriate choice of a chelator and perhaps its coupling to a PEG molecule may offer the best option for the development of an aptamer as a targeted radiopharmaceutical.

Finally, consideration of other metals, such as alpha emitters, may offer the development of a new generation of labeled aptamers, with the ability to be delivered as an injection in the clinic, due to the inherent properties of alpha emitting metals. This would allow aptamers to become much more amenable to wider clinical applications and offer them flexibility of administration, opening new horizons on targeted radiopharmaceutical development.

REFERENCES

1. Mayer G. The chemical biology of aptamers. *Angew Chem Int Ed Engl.* 2009;48:2672–2689.
2. Collett JR, Cho EJ, Ellington AD. Production and processing of aptamer microarrays. *Methods.* 2005;37:4–15.
3. Balamurugan S, Obubuafo A, Soper SA, et al. Surface immobilization methods for aptamer diagnostic applications. *Anal Bioanal Chem.* 2008;390:1009–1021.
4. Nimjee SM, Rusconi CP, Sullenger BA. Aptamers: an emerging class of therapeutics. *Annu Rev Med.* 2005;56:555–583.
5. Eaton BE, Gold L, Hicke BJ, et al. Post-SELEX combinatorial optimization of aptamers. *Bioorg Med Chem.* 1997;5:1087–1096.
6. Liu J, Cao Z, Lu Y. Functional nucleic acid sensors. *Chem Rev.* 2009;109:1948–1998.
7. Famulok M, Hartig JS, Mayer G. Functional aptamers and aptazymes in biotechnology, diagnostics, and therapy. *Chem Rev.* 2007;107:3715–3743.
8. Gold L, Polisky B, Uhlenbeck O, et al. Diversity of oligonucleotide functions. *Annu Rev Biochem.* 1995;64:763–797.

9. Tuerk C, Gold L. Systematic evolution of ligands by exponential enrichment: RNA ligands to bacteriophage T4 DNA polymerase. *Science.* 1990;249:505–510.

10. Ellington AD, Szostak JW. *In vitro* selection of RNA molecules that bind specific ligands. *Nature.* 1990;346:818–822.

11. Robertson DL, Joyce GF. Selection *in vitro* of an RNA enzyme that specifically cleaves single-stranded DNA. *Nature.* 1990;344:467–468.

12. Haruna I, Nozu K, Ohtaka Y, et al. An RNA 'replicase' induced by and selective for a viral RNA: isolation and properties. *Proc Natl Acad Sci U S A.* 1963;50:905–911.

13. Millis DR, Peterson RL, Spiegelman S. An extracellular Darwinian experiment with a self-duplicating nucleic acid molecule. *Proc Natl Acad Sci U S A.* 1967;58:217–224.

14. Gold L. Oligonucleotides as research, diagnostic, and therapeutic agents. *J Biol Chem.* 1995;270:13581–13584.

15. Cox JC, Hayhurst A, Hesselberth J, et al. Automated selection of aptamers against protein targets translated *in vitro*: from gene to aptamer. *Nucleic Acids Res.* 2002;30:e108.

16. Cox JC, Rajendran M, Riedel T, et al. Automated acquisition of aptamer sequences. *Comb Chem High Throughput Screen.* 2002;5:289–299.

17. Morris KN, Jensen KB, Julin CM, et al. High affinity ligands from *in vitro* selection: Complex targets. *Proc Natl Acad Sci U S A.* 1998; 95:2902–2907.

18. Vant-Hull B, Payano-Baez A, Davis RH, et al. The mathematics of SELEX against complex targets. *J Mol Biol.* 1998;278:579–597.

19. Eaton B, Gold L, Zichi DA. Let's get specific: the relationship between specificity and affinity. *Chem Biol.* 1995;2:633–638.

20. Yang X, Gorenstein DG. Progress in thioaptamer development. *Curr Drug Targets.* 2004;5:705–715.

21. Keefe AD, Cload ST. SELEX with modified nucleotides. *Curr Opin Chem Biol.* 2008;12:448–456.

22. Morris KN, Tarasow TM, Julin CM, et al. Enrichment for RNA molecules that bind a Diels-Alder transition state analog. *Proc Natl Acad Sci U S A.* 1994;91:13028–13032.

23. Missailidis S, Hardy A. Aptamers as inhibitors of target proteins. *Expert Opin Ther Patents.* 2009;19:1–10.

24. Lee JF, Hesselberth JR, Ancel Meyers L, et al. Aptamer database. *Nucleic Acids Res.* 2004;32:D95–D100.

25. Kim Y, Phillips JA, Liu H, et al. Using photons to manipulate enzyme inhibition by an azobenzene-modified nucleic acid probe. *Proc Natl Acad Sci U S A.* 2009;106:6489–6494.

26. Heckel A, Buff MCR, Raddatz M-SL, et al. An anticoagulant with light-triggered antidote activity. *Angew Chem Int Ed Engl.* 2006;45: 6748–6750.

27. Dougan H, Weitz JI, Stafford AR, et al. Evaluation of DNA aptamers directed to thrombin as potential thrombus imaging agents. *Nucl Med Biol.* 2003;30:61–72.

28. Heckel A, Mayer G. Light regulation of aptamer activity: an anti-thrombin aptamer with caged thymidine nucleobases. *J Am Chem Soc.* 2005;127:822–823.

29. Tuerk C, MacDougal S, Gold L. RNA pseudoknots that inhibit human immunodeficiency virus type 1 reverse transcriptase. *Proc Natl Acad Sci U S A.* 1992;89:6988–6992.

30. Chen H, Gold L. Selection of high-affinity RNA ligands to reverse transcriptase: inhibition of cDNA synthesis and RNase H activity. *Biochemistry.* 1994;33:8746–8756.

31. Biroccio A, Hamm J, Incitti I, et al. Selection of RNA aptamers that are specific and high-affinity ligands of the hepatitis C virus DNA-dependent RNA polymerase. *J Virol.* 2002;76:3688–3696.

32. Liu Y, Sun Q-A, Chen Q, et al. Targeting inhibition of GluR1 Ser845 phosphorylation with an RNA aptamer that blocks AMPA receptor trafficking. *J Neurochem.* 2009;108:147–157.

33. Famulok M, Blind M, Mayer G. Intramers as promising new tools in functional proteomics. *Chem Biol.* 2001;8:931–939.

34. Cerchia L, Hamm J, Libri D, et al. Nucleic acid aptamers in cancer medicine. *FEBS Lett.* 2002;528:12–16.

35. Lupold SE, Hicke BJ, Lin Y, et al. Identification and characterization of nuclease-stabilized RNA molecules that bind human prostate cancer cells *via* the prostate-specific membrane antigen. *Cancer Res.* 2002; 62:4029–4033.

36. Chu TC, Marks JW III, Lavery LA, et al. Aptamer:toxin conjugates that specifically target prostate tumor cells. *Cancer Res.* 2006;66: 5989–5992.

37. Akhtar S, Dunnion D, Pyner D, et al. Sequence and chemistry requirements for a novel aptameric oligonucleotide inhibitor of EGF receptor tyrosine kinase activity. *Biochem Pharmacol.* 2002;63:2187–2195.

38. Hicke BJ, Marion C, Chang Y-F, et al. Tenascin-C aptamers are generated using tumor cells and purified protein. *J Biol Chem.* 2001;276: 48644–48654.

39. Shangguan D, Tang Z, Maillikaratchy P, et al. Optimization and modifications of aptamers selected from live cancer cell lines. *Chembiochem.* 2007;8:603–606.

40. Shangguan D, Cao ZC, Li Y, et al. Aptamers evolved from cultured cancer cells reveal molecular differences of cancer cells in patient samples. *Clin Chem.* 2007;53:1153–1155.

41. Huang Y-F, Shangguan D, Liu H, et al. Molecular assembly of an aptamer-drug conjugate for targeted drug delivery to tumor cells. *Chembiochem.* 2009;10:862–868.

42. Girvan AC, Teng Y, Casson LK, et al. AGRO100 inhibits activation of nuclear factor-κB NF-κB by forming a complex with NF-κB essential modulator (NEMO) and nucleolin. *Mol Cancer Ther.* 2006;5:1790–1799.

43. Mayer G, Heckel A. Biologically active molecules with a "light switch". *Angew Chem Int Ed Engl.* 2006;45:4900–4921.

44. Hwang GT, Romesberg FE. Unnatural substrate repertoire of A, B, and X family DNA polymerases. *J Am Chem Soc.* 2008;130:14872–14882.

45. Jäger S, Famulok M. Generation and enzymatic amplification of high-density functionalized DNA double strands. *Angew Chem Int Ed Engl.* 2004;43:3337–3340.

46. Jäger S, Rasched G, Kornreich-Leshem H, et al. A versatile toolbox for variable DNA functionalization at high density. *J Am Chem Soc.* 2005;127:15071–15082.

47. Chelliserrykattil J, Ellington AE. Evolution of a T7 RNA polymerase variant that transcribes 2'-O-methyl RNA. *Nat Biotechnol.* 2004;22: 1155–1160.

48. Amblard F, Cho JH, Schinazi RF. Cu(I)-catalyzed Huisgen azide-alkyne 1,3-dipolar cycloaddition reaction in nucleoside, nucleotide, and oligonucleotide chemistry. *Chem Rev.* 2009;109(9):4207–4220.

49. Gierlich J, Burley GA, Gramlich PME, et al. Click chemistry as a reliable method for the high-density postsynthetic functionalization of alkyne-modified DNA. *Org Lett.* 2006;8:3639–3642.

50. Gramlich PME, Warncke S, Gierlich J, et al. Click-click-click: single to triple modification of DNA. *Angew Chem Int Ed Engl.* 2008;47: 3442–3444.

51. Baskin JM, Prescher JA, Laughlin ST, et al. Copper-free click chemistry for dynamic *in vivo* imaging. *Proc Natl Acad Sci U S A.* 2007;104:16793–16797.

52. Sletten EM, Bertozzi CR. A hydrophilic azacyclooctyne for Cu-free click chemistry. *Org Lett.* 2008;10:3097–3099.

53. Codelli JA, Baskin JM, Agard, NJ, et al. Secon-generation difluorinated cyclooctynes for copper-free click chemistry. *J Am Chem Soc.* 2008;130:11486–11493.

54. Agard NJ, Baskin JM, Prescher JA, et al. A comparative study of bioorthogonal reactions with azides. *ACS Chem Biol.* 2006;1: 644–648.

55. Pagratis NC, Bell C, Chang Y-F, et al. Potent 2'-amino-, and 2'-fluoro-2'-deoxyribonucleotide RNA inhibitors of keratinocyte growth factor. *Nat Bitechnol.* 1997;15:68–73.

56. Pieken WA, Olsen DB, Benseler F, et al. Kinetic characterization of ribonuclease-resistant 2'-modified hammerhead ribozymes. *Science.* 1991;253:314–317.

57. Vaish NK, Larralde R, Fraley AW, et al. A novel, modification-dependent ATP-binding aptamer selected from an RNA library incorporating a cationic functionality. *Biochemistry.* 2003;42:8842–8851.

58. Stein CA, Cheng Y-C. Antisense oligonucleotides as therapeutic agents—is the bullet really magical? *Science.* 1993;261:1004–1012.

59. Stein CA. Exploiting the potential of antisense: beyond phosphoto-thioate oligodeoxynucleotides. *Chem Biol.* 1996;3:319–323.

60. Jhaveri S, Olwin B, Ellington AD. *In vitro* selection of phosphorothio-lated aptamers. *Bioorg Med Chem Lett.* 1998;8:2285–2290.

61. Stec WJ, Zon G, Uznanski B, et al. Reversed-phase high-performance liquid chromatographic separation of diastereomeric phosphoro-thioate analogues of oligodeoxyribonucleotides and other backbone-modified congeners of DNA. *J Chromatogr.* 1985;326:262–280.

62. Iyer RP, Egan W, Regan JB, et al. 3*H*-1,2-benzodithiole-3-one 1,1-dioxide as an improved sulfurizing reagent in the solid-phase synthesis of oligodeoxyribonucleoside phosphorothioates. *J Am Chem Soc.* 1990;112:1253–1254.

63. Stec WJ, Grajkowski A, Koziolkiewicz M, et al. Novel route to oligo(deoxyribonucleoside phosphorothioates). Stereocontrolled synthesis of P-chiral oligo(deoxyribonucleoside phosphorothioates). *Nucleic Acids Res.* 1991;19:5883–5888.

64. Kato Y, Minakawa N, Komatsu Y, et al. New NTP analogs: the synthesis of 4′-thioUTP and 4′-thioCTP and their utility for SELEX. *Nucleic Acids Res.* 2005;33:2942–2951.

65. Minakawa N, Sanji M, Kato Y, et al. Investigations toward the selection of fully-modified 4′-thioRNA aptamers: optimization of *in vitro* transcription steps in the presence of 4′-thioNTPs. *Bioorg Med Chem.* 2008;16:9450–9456.

66. Li P, Sergueeva ZA, Dobrikov M, et al. Nucleoside and oligonucleoside boranophosphates: chemistry and properties. *Chem Rev.* 2007; 107:4746–4796.

67. Lin N, Yan J, Huang Z, et al. Design and synthesis of boronic-acid-labeled thymidine triphosphate for incorporation into DNA. *Nucleic Acids Res.* 2007;35:1222–1229.

68. Lato SM, Ozerova NDS, He K, et al. Boron-containing aptamers to ATP. *Nucleic Acids Res.* 2002;30:1401–1407.

69. Wengel J. Synthesis of 3′-C- and 4′-C-branched oligodeoxynucleotides and the development of locked nucleic acid (LNA). *Acc Chem Res.* 1999;32:301–310.

70. Singh SK, Nielsen P, Koshkin AA, et al. LNA (locked nucleic acids): synthesis and high-affinity nucleic acid recognition. *Chem Commun.* 1998:455–456.

71. Koshkin AA, Singh SK, Nielsen P, et al. LNA (locked nucleic acids): synthesis of the adenine, cytosine, guanine, 5-methylcytosine, thymine and uracil bicyclonucleoside monomers, oligomerisation, and unprecedented nucleic acid recognition. *Tetrahedron.* 1998;54:3607–3630.

72. Vester B, Wengel J. LNA (locked nucleic acid): high-affinity targeting of complementary RNA and DNA. *Biochemistry.* 2004;43:13233–13241.

73. Schmidt KS, Borkowski S, Kurreck J, et al. Application of locked nucleic acids to improve aptamer *in vivo* stability and targeting function. *Nucleic Acids Res.* 2004;32:5757–5765.

74. Veedu RN, Vester B, Wengel J. Enzymatic incorporation of LNA nucleotides into DNA strands. *Chembiochem.* 2007;8:490–492.

75. Veedu RN, Vester B, Wengel J. Polymerase chain reaction and transcription using locked nucleic acid nucleotide triphosphates. *J Am Chem Soc.* 2008;130:8124–8125.

76. Di Giusto DA, King GC. Construction, stability, and activity of multivalent circular anticoagulant aptamers. *J Biol Chem.* 2004;279: 46483–46489.

77. Eulberg D, Klussmann S. Spiegelmers: biostable aptamers. *Chembiochem.* 2003;4,979–983.

78. Klussman S, Nolte A, Bald R, et al. Mirror-image RNA that binds D-adenosine. *Nat Biotechnol.* 1996;14:1112–1115.

79. Nolte A, Klussmann S, Bald R, et al. Mirror-design of L-oligonucleotide ligands binding to L-arginine. *Nat Biotechnol.* 1996;14:1116–1119.

80. Williams KP, Liu X-H, Schumacher TNM, et al. Bioactive and nuclease-resistant L-DNA ligand of vasopressin. *Proc Natl Acad Sci U S A.* 1997;94:11285–11290.

81. Eulberg D, Buchner K, Maasch C, et al. Development of an automated *in vitro* selection protocol to obtain RNA-based aptamers: identification of a biostable substance P antagonist. *Nucleic Acids Res.* 2005; 33:e45.

82. Winnard P Jr, Chang F, Rusckowski M, et al. Preparation and use of NHS-MAG₃ for technetium-99m labeling of DNA. *Nucl Med Biol.* 1997;24:425–432.

83. Liu M, Wang RF, Zhang CL, et al. Noninvasive imaging of human telomerase reverse transcriptase (hTERT) messenger RNA with ⁹⁹ᵐTc-radiolabeled antisense probes in malignant tumors. *J Nucl Med.* 2007; 48:2028–2036.

84. Tavitian B. *In vivo* imaging with oligonucleotides for diagnosis and drug development. *Gut.* 2003;52:iv40–iv47.

85. Perkins AC, Missailidis S. Radiolabelled aptamers for tumor imaging and therapy. *Q J Nucl Med Mol Imaging.* 2007;51:1–5.

86. Missailidis S, Perkins A. Aptamers as novel radiopharmaceuticals: their applications and future prospects in diagnosis and therapy. *Cancer Biother Radiopharm.* 2007;22:453–468.

87. Ferreira CS, Papamichael K, Guilbault G, et al. DNA aptamers against the MUC1 tumour marker: design of aptamer-antibody sandwich ELISA for the early diagnosis of epithelial tumours. *Anal Bioanal Chem.* 2008;390:1038–1050.

88. Britz-Cunningham SF, Adelstein SJ. Molecular targeting with radionuclides: state of the science. *J Nucl Med.* 2003;44:1945–1961.

89. Borbas KE, Ferreira CSM, Perkins AC, et al. Design and synthesis of mono- and multimeric targeted radiopharmaceuticals based on novel cyclen ligands coupled to anti-MUC1 aptamers for the diagnostic imaging and targeted radiotherapy of cancer. *Bioconjug Chem.* 2007; 18:1205–1212.

90. Hilger CS, Willis MC, Wolters M, et al. Synthesis of Tc-99m-labeled, modified RNA. *Tetrahedron Lett.* 1998;39:9403–9406.

91. Daniels DA, Chen H, Hicke BJ, et al. A tenascin-C aptamer identified by tumor cell SELEX: systematic evolution of ligands by exponential enrichment. *Proc Natl Acad Sci U S A.* 2003;100:15416–15421.

92. Hicke BJ, Stephens AW, Gould T, et al. Tumor targeting by an aptamer. *J Nucl Med.* 2006;47:668–678.

93. Da Pieve C, Perkins AC, Missailidis S. Anti-MUC1 aptamers: radio-labelling with ⁹⁹ᵐTc and biodistribution in MCF-7 tumour-bearing mice. *Nucl Med Biol.* 2009;36:703–710.

94. Schlesinger J, Koezle I, Bergman R, et al. An 86Y-labeled mirror-image oligonucleotide: influence of Y-DOTA isomers on the biodistribution in rats. *Bioconjug Chem.* 2008;19:928–939.

95. Schlesinger J, Fischer C, Koezle I, et al. Radiosynthesis of new [⁹⁰Y]-DOTA-based maleimide reagents suitable for the prelabeling of thiol-bearing L-oligonucleotides and peptides. *Bioconjug Chem.* 2009;20: 1340–1348.

96. Watanabe N, Sawai H, Endo K, et al. Labeling of phosphorothioate antisense oligonucleotides with yttrium-90. *Nucl Med Biol.* 1999;26: 239–243.

97. Liu S, Edwards DS. Bifunctional chelators for therapeutic lanthanide radiopharmaceuticals. *Bioconjug Chem.* 2001;12:7–34.

98. von Guggenberg E, Sader JA, Wilson JS, et al. Automated synthesis of an 18F-labelled pyridine-based alkylating agent for high yield oligonucleotide conjunction. *Appl Radiat Isot.* 2009;67:1670–1675.

99. Boisgard R, Kuhnast B, Vonhoff S, et al. In vivo biodistribution and pharmacokinetics of 18F-labelled Spiegelmers: a new class of oligonucleotidic radiopharmaceuticals. *Eur J Nucl Med Mol Imaging.* 2005;32:470–477.

100. Kühnast B, Dollé F, Terrazzino S, et al. General method to label antisense oligonucleotides with radioactive halogens for pharmacological and imaging studies. *Bioconjug Chem.* 2000;11:627–636.

101. Shen J, Wang RF, Zhang CL, et al. Study on biodistribution and imaging of radioiiodinated antisense oligonucleotides in nude mice bearing human lymphoma [in Chinese]. *Beijing Da Xue Xue Bao.* 2004; 36:655–659.

102. Villa CH, McDevitt MR, Escoria FE, et al. Synthesis and biodistribution of oligonucleotide-functionalized, tumor-targetable carbon nanotubes. *Nano Lett.* 2008;8:4221–4228.

103. Tong GJ, Hsiao SC, Carrico ZM, et al. Viral capsid DNA aptamer conjugates as multivalent cell-targeting vehicles. *J Am Chem Soc.* 2009;131: 11174–11178.

104. Boomer RM, Lewis SD, Healy JM, et al. Conjugation to polyethylene glycol polymer promotes aptamer biodistribution to healthy and inflamed tissues. *Oligonucleotides.* 2005;15:183–195.

The Science of Targeted Radionuclide Therapy

The Physics and Radiobiology of Targeted Radionuclide Therapy

Bruce Thomadsen, William Erwin, and Firas Mourtada

■ INTRODUCTION: THE PHYSICS OF RADIONUCLIDE THERAPY

Targeted radionuclide therapy integrates biology, chemistry, and physics inseparably. However, a knowledge of each of these components individually forms an essential basis for understanding of the whole. This chapter addresses the physics aspects of these treatments. A good primer for dosimetry for anyone considering radionuclide therapy is the report of Task Group 2 of the Nuclear Medicine Committee of the American Association of Physics in Medicine (1).

■ BASIC RADIATION PHYSICS

For the most part, radionuclide engines fall into three major categories: radionuclides that mostly make use of emission of alpha, electron, or gamma radiation. To complicate the classifications, many engines emit more than one type of radiation.

▨ Alpha radiation

In an atomic nucleus, the mass of all the nucleons, that is, the protons and neutrons in the nucleus, exceeds the mass of the nucleus as a whole. Some of the mass of the particles forming the nucleus converts into energy through the well-known relationship $E = mc^2$, where E stands for the energy, c is the speed of light, and m is the mass that is used. The energy thus formed serves to bind the nucleus together. The actual process is fairly complicated and involves creation, absorption, and sharing of pi mesons and need not be discussed here. Some nuclei are too large and elongated to allow the interactions between the protons and neutrons to bind all the nuclear particles (nucleons) together, and while they have a considerable amount of mass converted into binding energy, the energy per nucleon is relatively low and thus they are unstable. Individual particles in the nucleus cannot escape because they feel the nuclear attraction as they leave and fall back into the nucleus. Groups of four particles, two protons and two neutrons, continually form in the nucleus, usually to associate for a short time and then drift off into other associations. During these groupings, most of the binding for each of the particles concentrates on the other particles in the association. This grouping can escape the nucleus, taking with it some of the binding energy of the parent nucleus. Even while losing some energy to the grouping that left, the parent nucleus becomes more stable because fewer particles divide the remaining binding energy. The grouping that escaped is called an alpha particle, which is very stable, having the highest binding energy per nucleon. The alpha particle is the same as a helium nucleus. It leaves the parent nucleus with a kinetic energy equal to the difference in the binding energy of the parent nucleus before and after the particle leaves. The parent nucleus is called the daughter after the alpha particle leaves.

For a given type of nucleus, any alpha particles leaving will have one of a limited number of the kinetic energies, corresponding to the difference in the nuclear energy level of the parent's and daughter's energy states. By analyzing the energy of the alpha particles, one could potentially identify the nucleus. Often, the alpha decay will move the parent nucleus toward being more stable, but not all the way, and the daughter may undergo another alpha decay, or one of the next two processes discussed. Because alpha decay occurs in large (heavy) nuclei, they fall at the upper end of the periodic table, generally for lead and above. Alpha decay is possible for a few light nuclei, such as ^8B, but they all have very short half-lives and for the most part do not occur in nature.

▨ Isobaric decay

Nuclei have a given number of protons and neutrons. The number of positively charged protons, the atomic number, Z, determines the element. The number of neutral neutrons is the neutron number, N. The atomic mass number, $A = Z + N$, is the isobar number. Because the binding in the nucleus is mostly between the protons and the neutrons, the balance between them is very important for nuclear stability. For light nuclei, the numbers should be equal, but as the number of protons increases, stability requires more than an equal number of neutrons to offset the electric repulsion between the protons. However, an excessive number of neutrons interfere with binding, and the nucleus has to use a larger proportion of its mass converted into energy to bind the nucleons together than were it stable (balanced). To

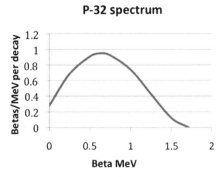

FIGURE 6.1 The beta spectrum from ^{32}P. The ordinate gives betas/MeV per decay. (Data from Cross WG, Ing H, Freedman N. A short atlas of beta-ray spectra. *Phys Med Biol.* 1983;28:1251–1260.)

adjust the balance in such a case, a neutron will turn into a proton, an electron (so charge is conserved), and an antineutrino, $\bar{\nu}$, written as

$$n \rightarrow p + e^- + \bar{\nu} + Q, \qquad \text{(Eq. 6.1)}$$

where the Q stands for the energy taken from the parent nucleus. Part of that energy is shared as kinetic energy by the electron (called a beta particle) and antineutrino as they leave the nucleus and some may be emitted as a gamma ray (see later). Because the energy is shared between the particles, either may emerge from the interaction with any combination of energy from close to zero to almost all of Q, not given to a gamma. Figure 6.1 shows a sample spectrum for the beta particles from ^{32}P. The most common energy, the mode, falls between half and a third of the greatest energy. Nuclei that undergo beta decay often come from reactors, where stable nuclei absorb neutrons to become neutron rich and unstable.

For nuclei with too many protons, one solution would be to have a proton turn into a neutron. This is not as easy as for beta decay. The mass of a neutron equals that of a proton and an electron, with just a little energy left over. To drive this conversion requires using some of the excessive energy used for binding the nucleus,

$$p + Q_{\text{excess}} = n + e^+ + \nu + Q_{\text{resultant}}. \qquad \text{(Eq. 6.2)}$$

Here, Q_{excess} denotes the amount of energy taken from the parent nucleus's binding energy. Making up for the difference in mass between the proton and the resultant neutron and positive electron (termed a positron or a beta plus) takes a little more than 1.02 MeV, and if the excess does not reach this amount, the process will not take place. The neutrino has negligible mass. As with beta decay, the $Q_{\text{resultant}}$ represents the kinetic energy of the resultant particles and energy given to a gamma. Also, as with beta decay, the energy carried by the positron will have a broad spectrum. To differentiate this process from beta decay, it is referred to as beta-plus decay or positron decay.

If a proton-rich nucleus has insufficient excessive energy to undergo beta-plus decay, a different process takes place. Sometimes when an electron ventures into the nucleus (which happens frequently, since they do not encircle the

nucleus as planets do the sun), a proton will capture the electron, as

$$p + e^- + Q_{\text{excess}} = n + \nu + Q_{\text{resultant}}. \qquad \text{(Eq. 6.3)}$$

In this process, called electron capture (or in older texts, k capture, because most often the electron captured resided in the k shell), no massive particle (i.e., one with mass greater than a neutrino) leaves the nucleus. Often, nuclei that undergo either beta-plus decay or electron capture come from particle accelerators such as cyclotrons. Most often, in a collection of nuclei that undergo beta-plus decay, some of the nuclei will decay by electron capture.

Since for beta decay the neutron turns into a proton, and for beta-plus decay or electron capture a proton turns into a neutron, the total number of nucleons remains the same, classifying the process as an isobaric decay, one where the isobar number remains constant.

Isomeric decay

Nuclei, as do atoms, have definite allowed energy levels, with a ground level that is stable. Often, following one of the transition processes described earlier, the daughter nucleus lands in an excited state. There are two methods by which they lose their extra energy and move to the ground state. The first is simply emitting the excess energy in the form of a gamma ray. A gamma ray is electromagnetic radiation similar to light, radiowaves, or microwaves, but of a much higher energy. At these high energies, the radiation appears to act more like a particle (called a photon) than waves, but a particle without mass and it always travels at the speed of light (with exceptions outside of the scope of this discussion). The energy of the photon relates to its frequency, ν, and wavelength, λ, as

$$E_\gamma = h\nu = \frac{hc}{\lambda}. \qquad \text{(Eq. 6.4)}$$

In this equation, h stands for Plank's constant, 4.136×10^{-18} keV/s, and c for the speed of light in vacuum, approximately 3×10^8 m/s. Because the nucleus shifts between discrete energy levels, the gammas emitted may have only specific energies, corresponding to the difference in the energy levels. Nuclei that differ only in their energy levels are called isomers, so these transitions are termed isomeric decay.

The alternative pathway for the excited nucleus to move to the ground state is to transfer the energy to an electron as it moves through the nucleus in a process called internal conversion. The electron, most often an inner-shell electron, takes the energy, overcomes the binding energy, and exits the atom with the remaining energy as kinetic energy. The loss of an inner-shell electron allows another electron in a higher energy orbit to drop to the more inner shell. In doing so, the dropping electron must give up energy, which it may do by emitting a photon. The energy of the photon equals the difference between the electron's higher and lower energy levels, which are discrete values characteristic of the atom, so these photons are called characteristic x-rays (x-rays originate in the atom, whereas gamma rays come from the nucleus). The dropping electron might also give its energy to another electron in its own energy level or higher. The recipient electron escapes the atom with that energy, becoming an Auger electron. Auger electrons tend to have low energies, depending on the atom. With either process, the vacancy on the higher energy level initiates another round of a dropping electron followed by elimination of the difference in energy, until there is a vacancy in an outer shell filled by an electron from outside the atom.

▨ Quantization of decay

So far, this discussion has used the term "decay" fairly loosely in its common sense as it developed historically. A better term for the processes described earlier would be "transition," since the parent nucleus changes into the daughter. That being said, decay is a good term for what happens to a collection of radioactive nuclei, called radionuclei. The radionuclei undergo transitions at random times. In the beginning, when there is a large number of radionuclei, a large number of transitions would be occurring, and many particles emitted. Over time, each of the radionuclei that transitioned reduces the number of remaining, original radionuclei. As the number of radionuclei decreases, the number of transitions happening per unit time also decreases. *Activity* is the number of transitions occurring per unit time, usually per second, in which case the unit for activity is becquerel, abbreviated as Bq. The equation relating the activity, A, and the number of radionuclei, N, is

$$A = \frac{-dN}{dt} = \lambda N, \qquad \text{(Eq. 6.5)}$$

where λ is just a proportionality constant that relates the two, and it is termed "the decay constant," which is characteristic of the particular radionuclide. The decrease, or decay, in activity follows an exponential relationship with time, t (obtained by integrating Equation 6.5):

$$A_t = A_0\, e^{-\lambda t}. \qquad \text{(Eq. 6.6)}$$

A_0 represents the activity at time $t = 0$, and A_t the activity at some time later, t. A useful characteristic of a radionuclide is the time it takes to decay to half of its original activity, or the half-life, $t_{1/2}$ given by

$$t_{1/2} = \frac{\ln(2)}{\lambda} = \frac{0.693}{\lambda}. \qquad \text{(Eq. 6.7)}$$

As noted earlier, the daughters of many radionuclides are themselves radioactive, having their characteristic half-life. Thus, looking at a source of radiation, the rate of decay may not look like it follows Equation 6.6 because of the mix of radionuclides. If the sample begins as purely the parent, each transition produces one daughter. Because the number of daughter nuclei is few, there are fewer decays per second

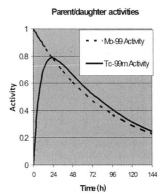

FIGURE 6.2 The relationship of the activity of a parent radionuclide (^{99}Mo) and a daughter (^{99m}Tc) **as a function of time.** The activities are relative to the initial activity of the ^{99}Mo.

compared with the parent, and the number of daughter nuclei builds. As the number of daughter nuclei increases, their rate of decay also increases. If the half-life of the daughter is short compared with that of the parent (the most common situation in medicine), the relation of the activities with respect to time looks like the curves shown in Figure 6.2. At some time, the activity of the daughter surpasses that of the parent, and then parent and daughter decay with the half-life of the parent. The ratio of the activities at this point becomes

$$\frac{A_{\text{daughter}}}{A_{\text{parent}}} = \frac{\text{parent}t_{1/2}}{\text{parent}t_{1/2} - \text{daughter}t_{1/2}}. \qquad \text{(Eq. 6.8)}$$

▨ Interactions between radiation and matter

Although this discussion only covers the necessities to understand the remaining material in this book, Attix et al., provides a more comprehensive discussion of radiologic physics for the interested reader (2). Since this text addresses radioactive materials in patients, this discussion only considers interactions between radiation and typical biologic materials.

Charged particles

At the energies of interest for radiobiology, traveling electrons and positrons (the beta and beta-plus particles) mostly interact with the outer-shell electrons of atoms they pass, with the electrons repelling the atom's electron or the positron attracting it. Either way, the passing particle may either excite the atom's electron to a higher energy level or remove the electron from the atom altogether. The process of removal of an electron from the atom is *ionization*, with the atom becoming an ion and the removed electron called a "secondary electron." The charged particle loses energy in the interaction and slows. As it slows, the radiation spends more time near the atom resulting in a higher probability of the radiation causing excitation or ionization in that atom. Thus, the farther the particle travels into matter, the slower it becomes and the higher the rate of transfer of energy from the particle to the matter. At some distance, the *range*, the particle runs out of energy and stops. If the traveling electron has a very high energy, it can remove a more inner-shell electron, producing the same cascade of events that would occur as an internal conversion. Sometimes, the traveling electron transfers a large proportion of its energy to the atomic electron, in which case the atomic electron leaves the atom with enough energy to cause some ionization and excitation by itself. These high-energy secondary electrons are termed *delta particles*.

In high Z materials, the electrons and positrons can also interact with an atomic nucleus and emit some of their energy as an x-ray, but that situation would be rare in patients. However, the positron, being antimatter, cannot exist at rest in the universe and when it has lost most of its kinetic energy, it joins with an ordinary negatively charged electron and undergoes a process called "pair annihilation." During annihilation, the two particles convert to energy, usually in the form of two photons in opposite directions, with energies equal to the rest mass of an electron (511 keV) plus half of the remaining kinetic energy.

Alpha particles, being charged particles, behave much like electrons except with a mass about 7300 times that of an electron. That large mass means that for the same energy, an alpha particle moves much more slowly than an electron and ionizes much more densely. The *linear energy transfer, LET*, specifies quantitatively the rate of energy transfer from the radiation to the matter through ionization and excitation, often in units of energy per unit length, such as electron volts per microgram. Electrons and positrons form low LET particles, whereas alpha particles are high LET. Alpha particles can activate other nuclei (make them radioactive) but that is not relevant to the present discussion.

Photons

Photons behave very differently from charged particles. Although the charged particles interact continuously with the matter through which they pass, any photon interacts only once in its existence. For the gammas and x-rays encountered in radionuclide therapy, three processes account for most of the interactions. The most common interaction is the Compton effect, where the photon interacts with a loosely bound electron (outer shell, or a valence electron) that absorbs the energy from the photon, re-emitting some of the energy as a lower-energy photon and taking the remainder of the energy as kinetic energy, thus leaving the site of the interaction. The photoelectric effect comprises another important interaction. In the photoelectric effect, the photon interacts with an inner-shell electron that uses the energy to overcome the binding to the nucleus (and gives some energy to the nucleus in recoil) and converts the rest to kinetic energy. The interaction leaves the atom with a vacancy in an inner shell, which results in a cascade of photons and/or electrons as with internal conversion. A third interaction, pair production, can occur for photons with energies greater than

1.022 MeV. In this interaction, the photon usually interacts with the nucleus and spontaneously converts into an electron and positron. The creation of the particles' rest mass takes the 1.022 MeV, and for the particle to leave the site of interaction would require more energy on the part of the incoming photon. Pair production becomes more likely with increasing photon energy and with photon interactions in material with a high atomic number. Neither of these situations are common in radionuclide therapy. The photoelectric effect, on the other hand, occurs mostly with low-energy photons (mostly below 100 keV) but again in high-atomic-number materials. The Compton effect depends little on the photon energy or atomic number of the matter. In muscle tissue, above about 20 keV, the Compton effect dominates the interactions, whereas below this energy, the photoelectric effect forms the main interaction.

The one interaction between the photon and the atom does very little to affect the medium. The effects from the photon come from the traveling electron (or positron) that the interaction produces. That traveling electron now behaves like the beta particle (discussed earlier), ionizing and exciting the matter that it passes. Thus, with respect to the effects that radiation has on matter, photons behave like the electrons they produce.

Attenuation

The intensity of radiation from a source can be specified in several ways. One of the most fundamental methods considers the particle fluence rate, $\dot{\varphi}$, which is the number of particles passing through an area per unit time. The area would be normal to the rays coming from the source and small enough so as not to worry about trying to curve the plane of the area around the source. For a very small source, the radiation follows rays in all directions, and the same number of rays spread over the surface area of a sphere surrounding the source regardless of the radius of the sphere. Since the surface area of the sphere equals $4\pi r^2$,

$$\dot{\varphi} = \frac{\text{No. of particles emitted/time}}{4\pi r^2}. \quad \text{(Eq. 6.9)}$$

Simplified,

$$\dot{\phi} \propto \frac{1}{r^2}. \quad \text{(Eq. 6.10)}$$

This relationship between the fluence rate and the distance is called the "inverse square law," which states that the intensity of radiation decreases with the square of the distance from the source. When looking at the biologic effect of radiation, rather than considering the number of particles, the energy carried by the particles forms the quantity of interest, and the corresponding measure of intensity becomes the *energy fluence rate*,

$$\dot{\varphi}_{\text{en}} = \frac{\text{Energy emitted/time}}{\text{Unit area}}. \quad \text{(Eq. 6.11)}$$

For either particles or energy, integrating the fluence rate over time results in fluence.

The intensity of radiation also varies because of the interactions with matter through which it passes as discussed in the previous section. A beam of photons of a single energy is attenuated following a simple exponential, as

$$\frac{I}{I_0} = e^{-\mu\tau}, \qquad \text{(Eq. 6.12)}$$

where I_0 stands for the original intensity of the beam and I stands for the intensity with a thickness τ of some material inserted into the beam. The attenuation coefficient, μ, is a constant equal to the fraction of the beam that the attenuating material eliminates per unit thickness, and depends on the energy of the radiation and the atomic number and density of the material. Interestingly, a beam of beta particles with a broad spectrum of energies follows a curve much like Equation 6.12. Although useful in shielding radionuclides (discussed in Chapter 10), Equation 6.12 applies only when the attenuator is relatively far from the source of the particles and the detector, and there is no other material in the near vicinity. In such a situation, the intensity of the photon beam decreases by absorption (that part of the energy of the beam that gets transmitted to the matter through ionization and excitation) and scatter (those photons that exit a Compton interaction redirected away from the original path and the characteristic x-rays following a photoelectric effect).

In a patient containing a radioactive source, as the distance from the source increases, the intensity of the radiation still varies due to the three processes in the last paragraph: distance, absorption, and scatter. The scatter may not decrease the intensity of the radiation but may increase the intensity of the beam in some situations, a phenomenon called buildup. Distance and absorption always reduce the intensity.

■ DOSE AND RELATED QUANTITIES

Intensity, as used in the previous section, while necessary for dosimetry, is seldom the quantity of interest. One of the quantities used most is *dose*, defined as the energy absorbed in the medium per unit mass. The medium absorbs the energy through the ionization produced by the interaction with the radiation. Dose often varies greatly over a volume, particularly with short-range, charged particle emitters, so the actual concept of dose becomes a differential:

$$\text{Dose} = \frac{d(\text{energy})}{d(\text{mass})}. \qquad \text{(Eq. 6.13)}$$

Although a good and clear physical quantity, dose by itself proves a poor predictor of biologic effects. The biologic results from a given dose depend on several factors, including the time course over which the delivery of the dose takes place, the LET of the radiation, and the biology (species, histology, and biologic effect under investigation).

The effects of LET and biology combine in the *relative biologic effectiveness, RBE,* which compares the effectiveness of a given type of radiation with a standard radiation, for the particular biologic end point in question. The standard radiation is actually not very standard, with the literature supporting the use of radiation from a conventional x-ray unit operating at 200 kVp or sometimes at 250 kVp, and sometimes using ^{60}Co units. Overall, the difference in RBE produced by the different "standards" remains less important than the uncertainties in the RBE values resulting from the variations due to the biologic component of the definition. In general, higher LETs produce higher RBE values (see Chapter 27 for a review of additional radiobiology principles). Because the LET varies along a charged particle track, being higher toward the end, the RBE would also change. For the most part, however, this change is not significant, since the range for alpha particles is so short and the paths for electrons continually bend around so there is no place that would be an effective end to all the paths. Thus, RBE values for radionuclides in a patient become an average along the path.

The production of biologic effects, to a great extent, requires two breaks in the deoxyribonucleic acid (DNA) in a cell's chromosomes, located in the nucleus. There are also effects resulting from damage to the cell membrane and other cellular structures, but these are less well understood and seem to be of lesser importance than the DNA. Because of the double-helix design of the DNA, if radiation breaks off a molecule from one side (by disrupting the chemical bonds through ionization), the DNA uses the remaining molecule on the other side to guide repair of the damage. This is called *repair of sublethal damage*. The repair takes place with a half time, T_{repair}, such that after the half time, half of the DNA breaks have been repaired. After two half times, only a quarter of the breaks remain, and so forth. Many types of cells appear to have two repair mechanisms active, one "short," with a half time repair on the order of 20 minutes, and one "long," with a half time repair of 1.5 to 3 hours. After repair, the DNA requires two new breaks to cause a biologic injury. Radiation with a high LET produces more biologic damage than low LET because the high density of ionization increases the probability of breaking both sides of the DNA before either has a chance for repair. Compared with a slow delivery, compressing the dose given into a short time produces a similar result—a higher effectiveness of the radiation due to the higher density of ionization. With a slow delivery, some of the one-sided DNA breaks repair before the radiation gets around to breaking the other side, which then can also repair. The *biologic effective dose (BED)* accounts, in part, for the effect of delivery duration for the dose. The somewhat simplistic basis for the BED comes from the curves relating cellular survival as a function of radiation dose. Figure 6.3 shows some example curves with typical parameters. Dose falls on the abscissa while the ordinate gives the resulting fraction of the cells surviving the dose, usually plotted as the log of the surviving fraction.

FIGURE 6.3 Survival curves for various radiation delivery approaches. Curves **A** and **B** are for acute irradiation using alpha and beta particles, respectively; **C** and **D** are for low-dose rate delivery of beta or photons, with the latter accounting for repopulation during the treatment; and **E** and **F** are for radionuclide therapy using ^{90}Y with an initial dose rate of 0.5 Gy/h, again with **F** accounting for repopulation. Notice that curve **F** begins to plateau.

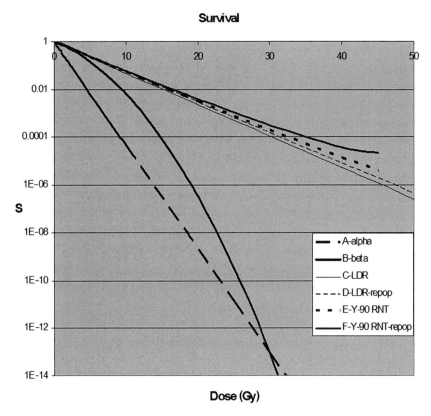

Considering curve A, which is for exposure to alpha radiation, a simple exponential describes the survival curve well. The high LET of the alpha breaks both sides of the DNA if the particle comes near enough to do any damage, and the fractional survival is given by

$$S = \frac{\text{No. of cells surviving}}{\text{Original no. of cells}} = e^{-\alpha D}. \quad \text{(Eq. 6.14)}$$

For an acute exposure to low LET radiation, shown in curve B, at low doses there is some effect, but much less than with the alpha particle because few of the interactions produce double-sided breaks. Instead, effects result when one traveling electron breaks one side and a different electron breaks the other. The killing of a cell follows the probability of two independent hits at the same place in the DNA. The low doses build a "bank of cells" with one side injured awaiting a particle to break the second side. As the dose increases, the number of these second hits increases. When the dose becomes high enough that the curve straightens, the number of first hits and second hits occur at the same rate. This low-dose-rate curve follows:

$$S = e^{-\alpha D - \beta D^2} \quad \text{(Eq. 6.15)}$$

This model for cell survival as a function of dose, referred to as the "linear-quadratic (LQ) model," performs well in many clinical situations but should not be thought of as the true description of what happens, only a pragmatic construct (3). The doses in curve B were delivered over a

time very short compared with the T_{repair} of the single-strand breaks, that is, the time it takes to repair half of the breaks. As the delivery duration for a photon or electron radiation gets longer, that is, the dose rate decreases, repair of one of the single-side breaks occurs during the exposure, reducing the effectiveness of the radiation. The equation becomes

$$S = e^{-\alpha D - \frac{2\beta D \dot{D}}{\mu} \left[1 - \frac{e^{-\mu T}}{\mu T} \right]}. \quad \text{(Eq. 6.16)}$$

In Equation 6.16, $\dot{D}$ represents the dose rate, T the total duration of the therapy, and μ the fractional rate of repair of the single-sided breaks (i.e., the fraction of the breaks repaired per unit time, usually per hour). T_{repair} and μ are related as

$$\mu = \frac{0.693}{T_{\text{repair}}}. \quad \text{(Eq. 6.17)}$$

The cell survival curve then assumes the appearance of curve C in Figure 6.3 without accounting for repopulation and D with repopulation. For alpha radiation, the survival curve would not change with a decrease in dose rate.

A useful comparison for the effect of duration and rate on the radiation delivery uses a single quantity, the *BED*, that replaces the exponents in Equations 6.15 through 6.17, so they look like Equation 6.14:

$$S = e^{-\alpha \text{BED}}. \quad \text{(Eq. 6.18)}$$

Thus, for low-dose-rate treatments with a constant dose rate, the equation for BED becomes

$$BED = D\left[1 + \frac{2\dot{D}}{\mu(\alpha/\beta)}\left(1 - \frac{e^{-\mu T}}{\mu T}\right)\right] - \frac{0.693T}{\alpha T_{dbl}}. \quad (Eq. 6.19)$$

T_{dbl} stands for the average doubling time of the tumor, that time for the number of tumor cells to double in the absence of radiation cell killing. The last term accounts for the loss of cell kill due to repopulation. This term is often ignored simply because the values for the parameters $\dot{\alpha}$ and particularly T_{dbl} are poorly known; however, the effect is important in radionuclide therapy. Cellular proliferation reduces the effectiveness of the radiation by increasing the number of surviving cells. For treatments with internal radioactivity where the dose rate decreases with time, the equation for BED becomes more complicated yet:

$$BED = D\left[1 + 2(\dot{D}_o \cdot \lambda)\left(\frac{\kappa}{(\alpha/\beta)(\mu - \lambda)}\right)\right] - \frac{0.693T}{\alpha T_{dbl}}, \quad (Eq.6.20)$$

where

$$\kappa = \left(\frac{1}{1 - e^{-\lambda T}}\right)\left\{\frac{1 - e^{-2\lambda T}}{2\lambda} - \frac{[1 - e^{-(\lambda T + \mu T)}]}{\mu + \lambda}\right\}. \quad (Eq. 6.21)$$

As the dose rate decreases, the effectiveness of the radiation at reducing the surviving fraction decreases until at some dose rate the cell killing of the radiation cannot keep up with the proliferation of the cells. At that dose rate and below, the radiation loses any curative value, although it may slow down the growth of tumor cells. Further, the situation becomes complicated at very low dose rates and the model does not work well. Figure 6.3 shows the loss in the effectiveness of radiation for cell kill as the dose rate decreases. An alternative to expressing the repopulation as the last term in Equation 6.20 is to view it as a loss in dose rate, K, so the equation becomes

$$BED = D\left[1 + 2(\dot{D}_o \cdot \lambda)\frac{\kappa}{(\alpha/\beta)(\mu - \lambda)}\right] - KT. \quad (Eq. 6.22)$$

Armpilia uses this format and suggests that K assumes a value of 0.1 Gy/day or less for prostate tumors and 0.9 Gy/day for head and neck cancers, with most other cancers existing somewhere in between (4).

For certain cases, Equation 6.19 becomes simpler. Ignoring proliferation, when the time of delivery is long compared with the half time for repair of the single-side breaks, the BED becomes

$$BED = D\left(1 + \frac{2\dot{D}}{\mu(\alpha/\beta)}\right); \quad T \gg T \quad (Eq. 6.23)$$

and when T is very short or μ is small such that $e^{-\mu T}/\mu T \underset{lim}{\Rightarrow} 1$

$$BED = D \quad (Eq. 6.24)$$

Because radiation oncologists have become so accustomed to fractionated treatments delivered at 2 Gy/day, expressing

the BED normalized to the effectiveness under this condition gives a perspective to the expected biologic results of a treatment regimen. When expressed in this manner, the BED assumes the name *normalized total dose, NTD*, which fortunately only requires division by a constant:

$$NTD = \frac{BED}{1 + (1/(\alpha/\beta))2 \, Gy}. \quad (Eq. 6.25)$$

■ THE RELATIONSHIP BETWEEN THE CHARACTERISTICS OF THE RADIONUCLIDE ENGINE AND THE BIOLOGY OF THE APPLICATION

The method of delivery greatly affects the possible choices for the radionuclide in several ways.

▨ Proximity to the target and radiation range

Much of the goal for targeted radionuclide therapy is to specifically deliver dose to the target cells and preserve as much as possible the innocent cells. The various carriers for the radionuclide engine perform this feat (sometimes more effectively than others) in different manners. Some take the radionuclide into the cell proper and may even incorporate it into the DNA. In such cases, the majority of energy should be transferred to the medium immediately around the radionuclide, suggesting the need for an alpha or low-energy electron (Auger) emitter. A typical, mid-energy alpha (~5 MeV) has a range just less than 50 μm, comparable with the 20 to 30 μm diameter of atypical cell. More precisely, the range of alpha particles is given by (5)

$$Range \, (\mu m) = \begin{cases} 7.24E_\alpha & E_\alpha < 4MeV \\ 1.60E_\alpha - 3.39 & 4MeV \le E_\alpha < 8MeV \end{cases}. \quad (Eq. 6.26)$$

Carriers that bring the radionuclide to the surface of the cell would not produce a great therapeutic effect with an alpha emitter because of the inverse square law. Since the distance from the surface to the DNA (the presumed target in this discussion) may only be about 15 μm, and because the alpha particles are emitted in all directions, it means that few would interact with the targets before running out of energy. In this case, the more penetrating beta particle would prove beneficial. A 1-MeV beta particle has a range of about 0.5 cm and typically the range varies linearly with the energy. It must be remembered, however, that beta particles from a given source have a spectrum of energies from some maximum to almost zero, with the most common between one half and a third of the maximum. The range for betas with a maximum energy, E_{max}, becomes (6)

$$Range \, (mm) = \begin{cases} 4.12E_\beta^{1.265 - 0.0954ln(E_\beta)} & 0.01 \le E_\beta < 2.5MeV \\ 5.3E_\beta - 1.06 & E_\beta \ge 2.5MeV \end{cases}. \quad (Eq. 6.27)$$

The range of the beta particle not only allows irradiation of the contents of a cell from a radionuclide on the surface, but that surface radionuclide could irradiate the DNA more than 100 cells away. The trade-off is that the alpha particle ionizes so densely that it is almost certain to disrupt the DNA that it passes through, while a sparsely ionizing beta might not cause an effect in any of the cells through which it passes. To deactivate a tumor requires getting alpha emitters into almost every cell, while the requirement for beta emitters is to get enough sources into the general vicinity to irradiate all of the cells adequately to provide a high probability for two-sided breaks in the DNA, in enough numbers, to kill the cells.

Photons, as noted earlier, do not have a range but are reduced in number through distance and absorption. Even low-energy photons, such as those from ^{125}I, still carry significant amounts of energy several centimeters from the source material, and higher energy emitters even farther. Indeed, radionuclides are seldom selected for radionuclide therapy because they emit photons. If photons are present, they come as "afterthoughts" to the emission of the charged particles of choice, as the daughter nucleus settles into the ground state. The photons potentially carry dose to neighboring structures and to the personnel who care for these patients, both undesirable consequences. On the other hand, a photon component allows imaging of the source material distribution with a gamma camera or positron emission tomography (PET) scanner, which can be helpful in many cases.

Time course

For any radioactive material in the body, the dose rate changes over time. Some materials, not usually involved in targeted radionuclide therapy, such as ^{226}Ra absorbed in the bone matrix, decay with such a long half-life, in this case approximately 1600 years, that the rate appears constant over the life of the person. The more usual situation has the radionuclide injected or infused, circulating for a while in the blood and working its way to the target or being excreted, all the time undergoing radioactive decay. In the target, the radionuclide may incorporate indefinitely or reside for a time and then move to a different compartment. The half-life of the radionuclide must fit this time course for the biologic activity of the carrier. For example, if the carrier molecule reaches the target quickly, a radionuclide with a short half-life delivers the dose over a short period, which would have the greatest effect on the cancer cells. On the other hand, some delivery carriers, particularly many antibodies, take several days for maximal integration into the tumor cells. Such applications call for a longer-lived radionuclide so that the circulating source material does not irradiate normal tissues excessively before incorporation and so a large enough quantity remains active by the time of incorporation. As discussed earlier, the delivery of the radiation must be at a dose rate that is large enough compared with the rate of proliferation of the cells to have a net

cell killing. Once the radionuclide resides in its target location, the efficacious dose begins, but at some time, the dose rate drops to the minimum dose rate for net cell kill, and the efficacious dose delivery stops. To deliver an increased dose requires a larger initial quantity injected, which will be limited by the dose to structures (typically bone marrow), other than the target, that take up the labeled carrier or are incidentally irradiated. Thus, any delivery has a window during which the treatment takes place.

The rate of clearance from the circulation also affects the choice of half-life of the radionuclide. A rapid clearance allows the use of a short half-life radionuclide. Slow clearance, coupled with a short half-life radionuclide, would result in excessive irradiation of normal tissues from the circulating radionuclide. The course for the removal of a radiolabeled carrier from the body over time often becomes complicated. Considering the decrease in radioactivity in an organ, compartment, or even the body as a whole, the general relationship is

$$\lambda_{net} = \lambda_{physical} + \sum_k \lambda_{biologic,\, k}, \quad \text{(Eq. 6.28)}$$

where λ stands for the fractional rate of increase or decrease in the activity per unit time. The term $\lambda_{physical}$ is the decay constant from Equation 6.5 and accounts for the physical decay of the radioactivity. The term, $\lambda_{biologic,k}$, represents uptake or elimination by biologic actions, of which there may be several, each denoted by the index k. Note that this term may be negative, indicating an increase in concentration (uptake) in a compartment, and this factor can change over time. Together, the physical decay and biologic uptake and/or elimination give the net fractional rate of reduction. If the biologic component could be approximated by a simple exponential elimination (many times the case, but not the rule), then each of the fractional rates would be related to their respective half time for reduction by a relationship such as Equation 6.7 giving

$$\frac{1}{t_{1/2net}} = \frac{1}{t_{1/2physical}} + \frac{1}{t_{1/2biologic}}. \quad \text{(Eq. 6.29)}$$

Because of physical decay and biologic elimination (after maximal incorporation), the dose rate decreases continually. With a dose rate that decreases following an exponential, the equation for the BED becomes

$$BED(T) = D\left[1 + \frac{2\dot{D}_o\lambda_{net}}{(\mu - \lambda_{net})(\alpha/\beta)}\frac{\dfrac{1 - e^{-2\lambda_{net}T}}{2\lambda_{net}} - \dfrac{1 - e^{-(\mu + \lambda_{net})T}}{\mu + \lambda_{net}}}{1 - e^{-\lambda_{net}T}}\right]$$

$$- \frac{0.693T}{\alpha T_{dbl}}, \quad \text{(Eq. 6.30)}$$

where T is the time since injection and $\dot{D}_o$ the initial dose rate at time $T = 0$. In Figure 6.3, curve E shows the survival curve for a radionuclide therapy using ^{90}Y, with a 64-hour half-life, ignoring the biologic component that would affect the concentration (since that would depend on the treatment site, pharmaceutical, and patient), and also ignoring repopulation; curve F includes the effect of repopulation.

The quantity more often of interest is the BED for the complete decay of the source. Ignoring proliferation, Dale gives this as (7,8)

$$\text{BED}\,(T=\infty) = D\left[1 + \frac{\dot{D}_o}{(\mu - \lambda_{\text{net}})(\alpha/\beta)}\right].\quad(\text{Eq. 6.31})$$

However, this expression does not account for the loss in cell killing due to repopulation as discussed earlier. Dale notes that the units on the last term in Equation 6.20 express the efficacious dose loss due to proliferation, and that $0.693/\alpha T_{\text{dbl}}$ equivalently becomes an efficacious dose rate below which the radiation no longer could produce a net reduction in cells (7). Approximating the decrease in activity in an organ by an exponential, the time to this critical point becomes

$$T_{\text{critical}} = -\frac{1}{\lambda_{\text{net}}}\ln\left(\frac{0.693}{\alpha\dot{D}_o T_{\text{dbl}}}\right).\quad(\text{Eq. 6.32})$$

Thus, the net treatment duration falls between $T=0$ and T_{critical}, and the effective BED would follow Equation 6.20 with $T=T_{\text{critical}}$.

For all these equations, determining the values for all the factors presents severe challenges with the current state of technology. The effects of the dynamic nature of the activity concentration and the inhomogeneous distribution of the radionuclide through the tissues and the effects on dose are discussed further later.

RADIONUCLIDE ENGINES: RADIOACTIVE SOURCES THAT PROVIDE THE PUNCH

In addition to the considerations discussed earlier, several other factors enter into the decision of which radionuclide to use in radionuclide therapy. Of the approximate 3400 possible radionuclides, most fail for very practical considerations. Most radionuclides have half-lives too short to work with or too long to provide any significant dose during the treatment. In addition, many radionuclides pose chemical problems in separation and concentration.

Consider alpha emitters. Of the approximately 400 alpha emitting radionuclides, only about 8 have appropriate combinations of half-life and energy for the emitted alpha particle. Of those, three have significant high-energy photons that make them radiation protection problems, leaving five radionuclides with clinical potential, listed in the alpha emitter section of Table 6.1. Note that two of those radionuclides have half-lives of 60 minutes or shorter, making them appropriate for mechanical delivery systems (such as labeled microspheres of nanoparticles) but not for biochemical delivery, although [213]Bi is currently in some biochemical delivery trials at the time of writing. The remaining three radionuclides, [211]At/[211]Po, [223]Ra, and [225]Ac, present the most likely candidates for targeted radionuclide therapy, although the [211]At/[211]Po presents serious production problems.

The same type of considerations applies to beta and Auger emitters, narrowing the list of potentially useful radionuclides. That being said, while Table 6.1 lists some of the properties of interest for those radionuclides most commonly considered for radionuclide therapy, it should not be considered exhaustive or even definitive. New applications of other radionuclides must be expected as the discipline grows. Emission energies are not given for Auger emitters because any dosimetry performed for these must consider very carefully the complete spectrum of emissions. Also note that many of the radionuclides listed in the Auger-emitter section are metastable nuclei and decay to other radioactive isotopes, requiring consideration of the doses and radiation hazards resulting from the daughters. Report number 37 of the American Association of Physicists in Medicine (AAPM) provides a somewhat old but still excellent reference for anyone considering therapy using Auger emitters (9).

The intention of Table 6.1 is to provide the reader with general ideas about the properties of some relevant radionuclides (9–14). Performing dosimetry requires more complete information, such as the fraction of decays that produce each energy of radiation. Such information would be too extensive for inclusion in this text.

MODELS FOR DOSE DEPOSITION

Stylized, MIRD-based dosimetry models

The conventional models, upon which internally administered radionuclide dose estimates are based, were established by the Medical Internal Radiation Dose (MIRD) Committee of the Society of Nuclear Medicine. The MIRD schema assumes a uniform distribution of activity within each source. The average absorbed dose per radioactive decay to a given target from a given source (the so-called S factor in Gy/Bq·s) is calculated by dividing the mean energy deposited per disintegration in the source by the mass of the target (which can be the volume containing the source). The S matrix has been calculated for a defined set of source and target organs and a number of standard anatomic models, for example, adult, 15-year-old, and head and brain (15–17), as well as unity density spheres simulating tumors, and voxels and cells (16–19). The product of total number of disintegrations, $\tilde{A}_s$ (cumulated activity, Bq·s), in the source material, s, and the corresponding S factor gives the dose contribution to the target, written as

$$D(t \leftarrow s) = \tilde{A}_s \times S(t \leftarrow s).\quad(\text{Eq. 6.33})$$

$\tilde{A}_s$ depends on the amount of activity administered (A_{adm}), radioactive decay (decay constant λ and time), and fractional biologic uptake and clearance in the source, s ($f_{\text{sbio}}(t)$):

$$\int_0^\infty A_s(t)\mathrm{d}t = A_{\text{adm}}\int_0^\infty f_{\text{sbio}}(t)e^{-\lambda t}\mathrm{d}t.\quad(\text{Eq. 6.34})$$

Total target dose is then the summation of all source absorbed-dose contributions. Further details and MIRD

Table **6.1**   **Some physical properties of radionuclides considered for radionuclide therapy**[a]

Beta emitters

Radionuclide	Half-Life (12) $(t_{1/2})$[b]	Most Significant Maximum (Mean) Beta Energies (Significant Auger Component, ϵ) (keV)	Range of Maximum Energy Beta (mm)	Range of Mean Energy Beta (mm)	Photon Efficacious Dose Rate Constant (13) (if Italic (14)) $((mSv \cdot m^2)/(GBq \cdot h)$
^{32}P	14.3 d	1710 (695)	5.55	3.26	
^{33}P	25.3 d	249 (76.4)	1.48	0.46	
^{47}Sc	3.35 d	441, 600 (162) ϵ	2.35	1.00	*0.0145*
^{67}Cu	2.58 d	377, 468, 561 (141) ϵ	2.08	0.87	0.0236
^{77}As	1.62 d	229 (225)	1.37	1.35	0.00170
^{89}Sr	50.5 d	1495 (585)	5.18	2.90	0.0000220
^{90}Y	2.67 d [3.19 h]	934 (934) [metastable ϵ]	3.95	3.95	*0.0783*
^{105}Rh	1.47 d	179, 79 (152) ϵ	1.10	0.94	0.0159
^{109}Pd	13.7 h	1028 (361) ϵ	4.19	2.01	*0.000405*
^{111}Ag	7.45 d	1037, 695 (350) ϵ	4.21	1.96	0.00532
^{121}Sn	1.13 d (43.9 y)	390 (116)	2.14	0.72	
^{131}I	8.03 d	606, 334, 248 (182) ϵ	2.97	1.11	0.0764
^{142}Pr	19.1 h	2162, 587 (809)	6.21	3.61	0.00810
^{143}Pr	13.6 d	934 (215)	3.95	1.30	
^{149}Pm	2.21 d	1071, 1049	4.29		0.00231
^{153}Sm	1.93 d	704, 635, 808 (224) ϵ	3.29	1.34	0.0244
^{159}Gd	18.5 h	971, 913, 607 (303) ϵ	4.05	1.74	0.0106
^{166}Ho	1.12 d	1854, 1773 (670) ϵ	5.78	3.18	0.00626
^{177}Lu	6.65 d (160 d)	149, 48, 385 (134) ϵ (for the 160 d $t_{1/2}$ 153 [40.8] ϵ)	0.92	0.83	*0.123*
^{186}Re	3.72 d	1070, 932 (347) ϵ	4.29	1.95	0.00490
^{188}Re	17.0 h	2120, 1965 (763) ϵ	6.16	3.47	0.0109
^{194}Ir	19.3 h (171 d)	2234, 1905 (800) ϵ	6.30	3.58	0.0167
^{199}Au	3.14 d	294, 244, 452 (82) ϵ	1.70	0.50	0.0186

Auger Emitters

Radionuclide	Half-Life (12) $(t_{1/2})$[b]	Photon Air Kerma Rate Constant
^{55}Fe	2.74 y	
^{67}Ga	3.26 d	0.0300
^{99m}Tc	6.01 h	0.0165
^{111}In	2.80 d	0.135
^{113m}In	1.66 h	0.0656
^{115m}In	4.49 h	0.0532
^{113}Sn	115 d	0.0484
^{123}I	13.2 h	0.0747
^{125}I	59.4 d	0.0742
^{193m}Pt	4.33 d	0.00464
^{195m}Pt	4.01 d	0.0203

Table **6.1** *(continued)*				
Alpha Emitters				
Radionuclide	**Half-Life (12) ($t_{1/2}$)^b**	**Most Significant Alpha Energies (Significant Auger Component, ε) (keV)**	**Range of Highest Energy Alpha (μm)**	**Photon Air Kerma Rate Constant**
^{211}Pb/^{211}Bi	36.1 m/2.14 m	471, 160/6623, 6278 ε	7.21	0.00983
^{213}Bi/^{213}Po	45.6 m/3.72 ms	[492, 320 (435)] 5869 (only 1.9% of decays) ε/8376	10.01	0.0314
^{211}At/^{211}Po	7.21 h/0.5 s, 25.2 s	5870/7450 ε	8.53	0.0611
^{223}Ra	11.4 d	5716, 5607, 5747, 5540 ε	5.81	0.0878
^{225}Ac	10.0 d	5830, 5793, 5791, 5732, 5637, 5724 ε	5.94	0.0517

^{a}Selection of radionuclides to include in this table mostly comes from Refs. 9–11.

^{b}Metastable state decays of dosimetric concern for radionuclides not marked with an "m" in the atomic mass number indicated in parenthesis.

mathematical formulations can be found in various MIRD publications (20–22). The MIRD-based dose calculation algorithms have been incorporated in software applications used in clinical nuclear medicine and research, such as MIRDOSE (16) and the more recent version, OLINDA (Organ Level INternal Dose Assessment)/EXM 1.0 (17). The Radiation Dose Assessment Resource (RADAR) task group Web site (www.doseinfo-radar.com) provides decay data for over 800 radionuclides; absorbed fractions for all available stylized phantoms and some voxel phantoms; kinetic data; dose factors (for all phantoms and nuclides); risk information; and other data via electronic transfer to users worldwide (23).

MIRD dose estimates based solely on generic and simplified virtual models of human anatomy lack the accuracy needed for truly patient-specific treatment planning. In particular, the dose to the skeleton, red bone marrow, stomach, and thyroid are known to be unrealistic, and the assumption of a uniform distribution is usually incorrect. Recently, investigators have improved greatly the models used for such calculations, both in the mathematical phantoms and individualized modeling (24,25). However, current dosimetric estimates come from clinical trials where the same amount of activity is usually given to most patients (perhaps with slight adjustment for total body weight), crude and systematically inaccurate planar scintigraphic estimates of radioactivity versus time are obtained, and MIRD dose calculations for the corresponding virtual model that most closely resembles the patient are attempted.

MIRD-based patient-specific dose estimation methods are based on organ mass adjustments, and sometimes tumor doses based either on the unit density sphere model or on complete self-absorption of betas or alphas only (ignoring photons). The doses from electrons and alpha particles to a region from source material, in that same region, scale linearly with mass, whereas the dose from photons scales with mass to approximately the two-thirds power (23). However, such simplistic methods are unable to account for patient-specific differences in organ or tumor shape and activity (and hence dose) heterogeneity within anatomic structures (23–25).

Dosimetry and analyses of outcome

In any form of radiotherapy, the fraction of surviving cells, healthy organ toxicity, and tumor response depend primarily on the quantity of energy deposited per unit mass, that is, radiation dose. Although dosimetry has been of some value in the preclinical phase of radiopharmaceutical development, its clinical use to optimize administered therapy to a specific patient has been limited. For instance, the lack of correlation of estimated dose with marrow toxicity for Zevalin has been attributed to large dosimetric uncertainty (26). In phase I and II clinical trials, dosimetry based on MIRD (16,17) is considered an essential component of establishing the maximum tolerated dose and dose–response relationship (27). Upon radiopharmaceutical approval, all patients are treated according to the toxicity limitations dictated by the most vulnerable of patients, leaving the majority of patients, most likely, undertreated. By the same token, it is highly probable that in successful therapies, a significant number of patients are unnecessarily overtreated. Such an approach does not tailor or optimize the therapy to the patient's own tumor profile, agent biodistribution, or normal tissue proximity. Therefore, there is a great need to improve upon the dose prediction methods to allow for meaningful patient-specific treatment planning which MIRD is lacking (28).

BED-based MIRD

Dose-rate effects are important in conventional radiotherapy because of their ability to produce differential sparing effects between normal and malignant tissue. As discussed earlier, with targeted radiotherapy, in which dose rates vary both spatially and temporally, the instantaneous dose rate is additionally relevant, since it determines whether or not any ongoing clonogenic tumor repopulation can be controlled (8). Baechler et al. applied the LQ model to targeted radionuclide therapy based on MIRD calculations (29). For internal radionuclide therapy, the dose rate to the tumor rises from an initial value of zero to a maximum value as the radioactivity is taken up by the tumor, and then decreases exponentially as the radioactivity decays and the radionuclide clears from the tumor. Similar dose-rate patterns are frequently observed for the critical normal organs as well (18). The dose rate can vary substantially among patients due to differences in kinetics (biologic half-life, metabolic rate, etc.). Dose volume histograms and BED-volume histograms can be generated for targets and critical organs such as red marrow and kidney functional components (e.g., cortex and medulla).

For late-responding tissue and continuous irradiation with exponentially decreasing dose rate, the BED is calculated using Equations 6.28 and 6.29. Average repair half times for mammalian tissues are usually on the order of 0.5 to 3 hours, with increasing evidence that tumor repair half-lives are probably shorter than those for late-responding normal tissues.

The α/β ratios provide a quantitative indication of the sensitivity of a given tumor or organ to changes in fractionation or dose rate. Because larger values of β imply an increased likelihood of potentially repairable ionizing events, it follows that tissues with smaller α/β ratios exhibit a greater dose-rate sparing effect than do those with larger values of α/β. As an example, for the kidney, the α/β value is in the range 2 to 3 Gy. Dale used a value of 2.4 Gy, as this provides results which error on the cautious side (8). A repair half time T_{μ} of 2.8 hours (corresponding to a repair rate μ of 0.25 hour^{-1}) was reported by Barone et al. (30). For the α/β ratios of red marrow cells, Fowler et al. indicate a range of 7 to 26 Gy (31). Dale assumed a value of 15 Gy for his calculations (8), and Wilder et al. used 10 Gy in their study (32). Baechler et al. assumed an α/β of 10 Gy (29). Concerning the repair half time, Dale (8) and Bolch (18) assumed 1.5 hours, while Wilder used 0.5 hour for bone marrow (32).

Image-based dosimetry using Monte Carlo, closed cone kernels, and discrete-ordinates approaches

Quantitative imaging for targeted radionuclide therapy

Targeted radionuclide therapy dosimetry has not gained wide acceptance as a clinical tool among the nuclear medical community in part because of an imbalance between the accuracy and the complexity of the procedure. Most studies have completely discarded dosimetry, instead choosing to use fixed activities for all patients or activities based on kilogram or square meter body surface area. However, there has been significant progress in recent years, especially in the fields of instrumentation, image processing, physical modeling, and radiobiology that demands a dose calculation paradigm shift. The nuclear medicine physician is at present confronted with a "dosimetric dilemma," unable to perform treatment

planning that includes advanced dosimetric calculations similar to that routinely performed in radiotherapy treatments but which are necessary to maximize the overall efficacy of the therapy.

Until the recent advent of the hybrid imaging modalities single-photon emission computed tomography (SPECT)/ computed tomography (CT) and PET/CT, more accurate quantification of the three-dimensional (3D) distribution of activity in the patient, a prerequisite for dose calculation methods such as Monte Carlo, was not possible on a routine basis. Only recently, hybrid scanners with the required compensations for attenuation, scatter, and resolution permit a much more accurate estimation of the activity within volumes of interest within the patient at different time points, as compared with the conventional and crude macroscopic, planar scintigraphic methods. For maximum accuracy, these compensations are performed as part of an iterative reconstruction method. He et al. demonstrated the need for more accurate estimation of the 3D in vivo activity distribution for targeted radionuclide therapy using reconstruction methods that include compensation for various physical effects (33). Recently, the same group reported that for practical reasons, hybrid methods consisting of a time series of planar scans plus a single time point quantitative SPECT/CT (QSPECT) are generally superior to pure planar methods and may be an acceptable alternative to the more accurate but more complicated method based on the 3D time series of QSPECT scans (34).

Another issue impacting targeted radionuclide therapy QSPECT accuracy and consistency is related to the SPECT scanner calibration traceability. Recently, the National Institute of Standards and Technology (NIST, Gaithersburg, MD) began work on establishing radioactivity standards for quantitative SPECT to reduce the uncertainty of scanner calibration to reasonable levels. Great strides are being made to use patient image data to construct individualized voxel-based models for more detailed and patient-specific dose calculations, and new findings are encouraging regarding improvement of internal dose models to provide better correlations of dose and effect (35,36). These recent advances make it likely that the relevance will soon change to be more similar to that of external beam treatment planning.

Dose point kernel dosimetry models

A dose point kernel (DPK) for a radionuclide is defined as the radial distribution of absorbed dose around an isotropic point source of radiation in an infinite homogeneous medium (typically water). The motivation behind point-kernel convolution methods is to account for nonuniform source distribution in tissue. Another alternative is the "voxel S value" approach based on MIRD schema. The DPK method is popular because of its speed in calculation (relative to Monte Carlo) and the availability of tabulated S values at the voxel level, being limited to only a few radionuclides and two voxel sizes. Several authors reported the DPK implementation in treatment planning systems for heterogeneous dose assessment of radionuclides (37–40). Although not used for the therapeutic delivery, most sources emit photons and the photons carry energy to, and deposit dose in neighboring structures. For photon sources, one should refer to MIRD pamphlet no. 2 for the DPK calculations in a water medium following Equation 6.35, where $\Phi(r)$ is the point isotropic specific absorbed fraction, defined as the fraction of the emitted photon energy absorbed per unit mass at a radial distance, r, from the source (41):

$$\Phi(r) = \left[\frac{\mu_{en}}{\rho} \frac{e^{-\mu r}}{4\pi r^2} \right] B_{en}(\mu r). \quad \text{(Eq. 6.35)}$$

In Equation 6.35, μ is the linear photon attenuation coefficient at a given energy, μ_{en} is the linear photon energy-absorption coefficient at a given energy, ρ is the mass density of the medium, and B_{en} is the energy absorption buildup factor, which accounts for the scatter contribution to dose to a point at radial distance r. Berger provided the energy deposition in water by photons isotropically emitted from point sources in spheres of various sizes (42). These evaluations were published in MIRD pamphlet no. 2, which also contains a tabulation of 75 buildup factors and related data for energy deposition in water. Nineteen monoenergetic photon sources were considered with energies ranging from 0.015 to 3 MeV. Brownell et al. evaluated the absorbed fractions for uniformly distributed and point monoenergetic photon sources in unity density and tissue equivalent materials. In this work, absorbed fractions were assessed in spheres and cylinders from 2 to 200 kg and ellipsoids from 0.3 to 6 kg, for photon energies in the 0.02 to 2.75 MeV range, published in MIRD pamphlet no. 3 (43).

All DPKs for electron point sources are derived from Monte Carlo simulations. Akabani et al. estimated beta absorbed fractions in spherical, "stylized tumors" of radii from 0.1 to 2.0 cm (44). The beta sources were uniformly distributed within the spheres and the average energy of the beta spectra was considered to be representative of the radionuclide. Monoenergetic electron sources with energies from 0.05 to 4 MeV were then considered. The calculations were performed using the Monte Carlo code EGS4 (Electron Gamma Shower, version 4) for electron and photon transport in tissue-equivalent medium by elemental composition (45). Siegel and Stabin also evaluated the absorbed fractions for electron and beta sources uniformly distributed within spheres of various sizes using the methodology developed by Berger (46). Also, Stabin and Konijnenberg re-evaluated those values using two different Monte Carlo codes: EGS4 and MCNP-4B, indicating discrepancies exceeding 10%, and recommended values averaged between the two codes. The important issue raised from this work is the considerable discrepancies that can be found using different Monte Carlo codes, demonstrating the complexity of the dose evaluation task which involves many factors, such as the values for interaction cross sections, numerical approximations, and physical models (47).

DPK accuracy was shown to be limited to homogenous tissue where there is no change in material composition or density, thus compromising accuracy in various tissue interface regions (soft tissue/bone and soft tissue/lung interface

and patient surface) (18,38,40). Furthermore, the method does not account for variations in atomic number throughout a tissue region that may influence the distribution of dose delivered by low-energy photons (18).

A compromise between MIRD and DPK was also developed. In an attempt to make real-time, patient-specific computations, a Monte Carlo–assisted voxel source kernel (MAVSK) method was developed (39). The MAVSK approach has extensive beta-dose computations performed off-line using Monte Carlo methods, so that an effective S matrix is developed initially. This matrix may then be applied to the actual patient using CT-scan data for anatomy and nuclear planar scan information for whole organ and tumor activity distributions. MAVSK scoring mesh size comparable with the CT grid size is used, assuming a voxel source with radioactivity uniformly distributed. The total energy depositions in voxels are simulated with relative errors of less than 1% at the furthest voxel. Also, voxel source kernels in lung tissue (density of 0.3 g/cm^3) are calculated. Average absorbed dose to each voxel in the 3D patient volume is then estimated by convolving the MAVSK kernel with the 3D matrix of organ uptakes as derived from the QSPECT method described earlier in section "*Quantitative Imaging for Targeted Radionuclide Therapy.*"

Monte Carlo–based models

Monte Carlo methods stochastically predict particle transport through media by tracking a statistically significant number of random particles. If enough particles are simulated, Monte Carlo will approach the true physical solution within the limits of the particle interaction data and uncertainties regarding the geometry and composition of the field being modeled. Monte Carlo is considered the current standard transport method for external radiotherapy, brachytherapy, and radionuclide therapy (48). The AAPM report 71 stated that "if the activity distribution is heterogeneous and known, a direct Monte Carlo approach is one way to estimate absorbed dose in different regions of the tumor" (49). Several authors have reported on their in-house Monte Carlo–based dose engines, in particular the most developed is 3D-ID (3D Internal Dose) from Memorial Sloan Kettering (50,51). Other codes are the SIMDOS code from the University of Lund (52), the RTDS code developed at the City of Hope Medical Center (53), MABDose (54,55), and the DOSE3D code (56). These codes rely either on standard geometrical phantoms (MABDose and DOSE3D) or on patient-specific voxel image data (3D-ID and SIMDOS). Recently, clinical results using 3D-ID have been reported for I-131 NaI treatment planning in diffuse lung metastases from thyroid carcinoma (57). The authors reported that to be able to perform the Monte Carlo calculations with practical calculation times for clinical use, activity segmentation into larger bins was needed. The rationale for segmentation was that statistical significance can be improved by pooling activity regions, especially in regions of lower activity concentration. They divided the activity into 5, 10, or 20 equally sized activity bins on the 3D lung activity map. Correspondingly, the voxels belonging to the same bin on the activity map were merged on the CT density map. The study results indicated very different dose distributions compared with a full transport simulation (50,000 tallies, 4 million histories, 4642.3 hours CPU time on 60-node Beowulf computer cluster, each computer with dual AMD Athlon processors), but choosing the 20-region activity segmentation (200,000 histories, 16.8 hours CPU time) resulted in tumor mean dose within 10% of that estimated using the full transport simulation.

Over the last decade, the use of Monte Carlo–based dose estimates have been proposed (16,51) but have still not become routine in the clinic (for a detailed description see later), due primarily to the long calculation times (e.g., several hours or more) that are needed to reduce their statistical uncertainty in low-dose regions, thereby limiting their practicality for clinical treatment planning (49). Recently, Hobbs et al. published a paper using the 3D radiobiologic dosimetry (3D-RD) system for ^{131}I treatment planning for an 11-year-old girl with differentiated papillary thyroid cancer, heavy lung involvement, and cerebral metastases (58). In this study, ^{124}I PET was used for determination of the pharmacokinetics. Dose calculation of the recommended administered activity, based on lung toxicity constraints, was available to the physician in "real time" to influence treatment decisions. In subsequent retrospective analyses, the 3D-RD calculations resulted in higher recommended administered activity than by the conventional S-value–based method (see above) with a favorable clinical outcome for this patient. The study suggested that patient-specific dosimetry permitted more aggressive treatment while adhering to patient-specific lung toxicity constraints.

Deterministic transport equation solution methods

An alternative to Monte Carlo is to solve the linear Boltzmann transport equation (LBTE) explicitly. The LBTE is the governing equation that describes the macroscopic behavior of ionizing particles (neutrons, gamma rays, electrons, etc.) as they travel through and interact with matter (59,60). As discussed earlier, the Monte Carlo method solves the LBTE via random sampling techniques that imitate propagation of radiation in the medium. One approach for solving the LBTE explicitly is via the grid-based Bolzmann solver (GBBS) (61). In GBBS, the differential form of the LBTE is then solved iteratively everywhere in the computational domain. GBBS is also known as the discrete-ordinates method (DOM). DOM has been shown to be useful for neutral particle applications such as neutron-capture therapy (62,63) and brachytherapy (64). DOM has also been used in a variety of shielding applications, where large attenuations considerably lengthen Monte Carlo computational times. Traditional DOMs have been applicable only for neutral particle transport.

Both Monte Carlo and the GBBS are convergent. That is, with sufficient input, both approaches will converge and solve the LBTE. The achievable accuracy of both approaches is equivalent and is limited only by uncertainties in the particle interaction cross section data and uncertainties in the

problem at hand. However, in reality, both methods are not perfect. In Monte Carlo, errors are stochastic and result from simulating a finite number of particles. In explicit LBTE solution methods such as the GBBS, errors are primarily systematic due to discretization of the solution variables in space, angle, and energy. In both Monte Carlo and GBBS, a trade-off exists between speed and accuracy.

Recently, the GBBS method has been evaluated for internally administered radionuclide therapy dose calculations, coupled with quantitative estimates of radioactivity and radiation transport media from a hybrid SPECT/CT scanner (65,66). The prototype for this technology is the Attila solver (67,68), the original prototype of which was developed at Los Alamos National Laboratory. The impetus for Attila was to create an efficient, generalized geometry alternative to Monte Carlo for neutral and charged particle simulations. Attila has been validated against Monte Carlo for radiotherapy applications (69,70). More recently, the accuracy of Attila's methods has been verified on arbitrary heterogeneous patient data derived from CT (71).

▓ Example of SPECT/CT voxel-based patient simulations: ^{153}Sm-EDTMP

^{153}Sm-labeled ethylenediaminetetramethylenephosphonate, EDTMP (Quadramet, EUSA Pharma (USA), Inc.), is a bone-targeted therapeutic radiopharmaceutical approved for the palliation of pain caused by metastatic bone lesions that enhance on a diagnostic radionuclide bone scan. The compound consists of ^{153}Sm, a beta emitter of medium energy (Fig. 6.4) with a physical half-life of 46.3 hours, and EDTMP, a tetraphosphonate compound that when complexed to ^{153}Sm avidly concentrates in bone. It is chemically and biologically stable and is rapidly cleared from nonosseous tissues biexponentially (fast-phase $t_{1/2}$ 14 minutes; slow-phase $t_{1/2}$ 65 minutes). ^{153}Sm-EDTMP has a beta emission with an average range of 0.5 mm and a maximum range of 3 mm. It also emits a 103-keV gamma ray photon 28.3% of the time, allowing for gamma camera planar and SPECT imaging studies of the distribution of the radionuclide. The use of 37 MBq/kg (1 mCi/kg) of ^{153}Sm-EDTMP has demonstrated

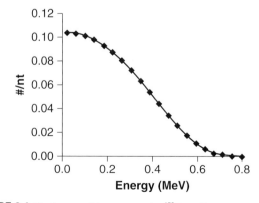

FIGURE 6.4 The beta particle spectrum for ^{153}Sm, with an average energy of 223 keV and a maximum energy of 810 keV (74).

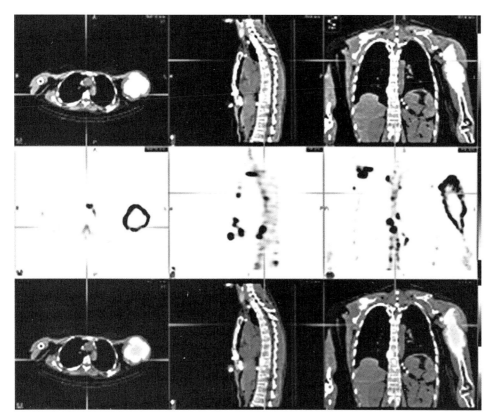

FIGURE 6.5 SPECT/CT image fusion window from MIM v4.1 (MIMvista Co., Cleveland, OH). **Upper panel:** CT; **middle panel:** SPECT; **lower panel:** fused CT and SPECT with the CT as the primary image. (Please see Color Insert).

an excellent therapeutic ratio in carcinoma metastatic to bone with myelosuppression as the major dose-limiting toxicity (72,73).

In this example, a SPECT/CT scan over the patient's chest (Fig. 6.5), including the left humerus tumor of interest, was obtained at 24 hours after a tracer injection of ^{153}Sm EDTMP with a dual-detector SPECT/6-slice CT scanner (Symbia T6, Siemens Medical Solutions USA, Inc.). An identical scan of a reference source of activity was performed, for calibration in order to convert the reconstructed SPECT voxel counts to activity (75). Ordered subset expectation maximization iterative reconstruction (16 subsets, 8 iterations) was performed, with compensations for system resolution, attenuation and scatter, 5-mm Gaussian, 3D postreconstruction filtering, and the reconstructed volume resampled to the CT field of view and slice increment dimensions.

Monte Carlo and GBBS dose calculations were performed using the DOSXYZnrc program (76) and the GBBS Attila codes, respectively. The photon dose rate was calculated using the collisional KERMA approximation rather than explicitly transporting the generated electrons. The photon, beta particle, and total absorbed dose rates calculated were compared and excellent agreement was found (66). However, for Attila, the beta particle and photon transport required about 10 minutes CPU time. DOSXYZnrc took approximately 15,000 times longer. GBBS has the potential to provide accuracy similar to MC in a much shorter time; this could be useful for voxel-based radionuclide absorbed dose estimates in a clinical setting.

Acknowledgments

The authors appreciate the contributions of James Harvey, Chief Science Officer, NorthStar Medical Radionuclides, Madison, WI.

REFERENCES

1. Wessels BW, Brill AB, Buchsbaum DJ, et al. Radiobiology of radiolabeled antibody therapy as applied to tumor dosimetry. *Med Phys.* 1993;20:601.
2. Attix F. *Introduction to Radiological Physics and Radiation Dosimetry.* New York, NY: John Wiley and Sons; 1986.
3. Barendsen GW. Dose fractionation, dose–rate and isoeffect relationships for normal-tissue responses. *Int J Radiat Oncol Biol Phys.* 1982;8:1981–1997.
4. Armpilia CI, Dale RG, Coles IP, et al. The determination of radiobiologically optimized half-lives for radionuclides used in permanent brachytherapy implants. *Int J Radiat Oncol Biol Phys.* 2003;55(2):378–385.
5. Cember H. *Introduction to Health Physics.* 3rd ed. New York, NY: McGraw-Hill; 1996.
6. Katz L, Penfold AS. Range-energy relations for electrons and the determination of beta-ray end-point energies by absorption. *Rev Mod Phys.* 1952;24:28–44.
7. Dale RG. Dose-rate effects in targeted radiotherapy. *Phys Med Biol.* 1996;41(10):1871–1884.
8. Dale R, Carabe-Fernandez A. The radiobiology of conventional radiotherapy and its application to radionuclide therapy. *Cancer Biother Radiopharm.* 2005;20(1):47–51.
9. Kereiakes JG, Rao Dandamudi V, Sastry KS, et al. Auger electron dosimetry: report no. 1 of the American Association of Physicists in Medicine Nuclear Medicine Task Group No. 6. *Med Phys.* 1992; 19(6):1361–1383.
10. O'Donoghue JA. Dosimetris principles of targeted radiotherapy. In: Abrams PG, Fritzberg, Alan R, eds. *Radioimmunotherapy of Cancer.* New York, NY: Marcel Dekker; 2000:1–20.

11. Harvey J. *Radio Immunotherapy (RIT)*. Madison, WI: University of Wisconsin; 2008.

12. National Nuclear Data Center. Interactive Chart of the Nuclides. 2010. Available at: http://www.nndc.bnl.gov/chart/. Accessed February 8, 2010.

13. Integrated Environmental Management I. Gamma Ray Dose Constants. Available at: http://www.iem-inc.com/toolgam.html. Accessed February 9, 2010.

14. Lauridsen B. Table of Exposure Rate Constants and Dose Equivalent Rate Constants. Roskilde, Denmark: Riso National Laboratory; 1982 December. Report no. R1SØ-M-2322.

15. Bouchet LG, Bolch WE, Weber DA, et al. MIRD pamphlet no. 15: radionuclide S values in a revised dosimetric model of the adult head and brain. Medical Internal Radiation Dose. *J Nucl Med.* 1999;40(3): 62S–101S.

16. Stabin MG. MIRDOSE: personal computer software for internal dose assessment in nuclear medicine. *J Nucl Med.* 1996;37(3):538–546.

17. Stabin MG, Sparkes RB, Crowe E. OLINDA/EXM: the second-generation personal computer software for internal dose assessment in nuclear medicine. *J Nucl Med.* 2005;46:1023–1027.

18. Bolch WE, Bouchet LG, Robertson JS, et al. MIRD pamphlet no. 17: the dosimetry of nonuniform activity distributions—radionuclide S values at the voxel level. Medical Internal Radiation Dose Committee. *J Nucl Med.* 1999;40(1):11S–36S.

19. Goddu S, Howell R, Bouchet L, et al. *MIRD Cellular S Values*. Reston, VA: Society of Nuclear Medicine; 1997.

20. Howell RW, Wessels BW, Loevinger R, et al. The MIRD perspective 1999. Medical Internal Radiation Dose Committee. *J Nucl Med.* 1999;40(1):3S–10S.

21. Loevinger R, Berman M. *MIRD Pamphlet No. 1: A Revised Schema for Calculating the Absorbed Dose from Biologically Distributed Radionuclides*. New York, NY: Society of Nuclear Medicine; 1976.

22. Loevinger R, Budinger T, Watson E. *MIRD Primer for Absorbed-Dose Calculations*. Revised ed. New York, NY: Society of Nuclear Medicine; 1991.

23. Stabin M, Brill AB. Physics applications in nuclear medicine: 2007. *J Nucl Med.* 2008;49(2):20N–25N.

24. Guo B, Xu XG, Shi C. Specific absorbed fractions for internal electron emitters derived for a set of anatomically realistic reference pregnant female models. *Radiat Prot Dosimetry.* 2010;138:20–28.

25. Kim S, Yoshizumi T, Toncheva G, et al. A Monte Carlo dose estimation method using a voxelized phantom for pediatric CBCT. Presented at the 54th Annual Meeting of the Health Physics Society. Minneapolis, MN, 2009.

26. Silverman DH, Delpassand ES, Torabi F, et al. Radiolabeled antibody therapy in non-Hodgkins lymphoma: radiation protection, isotope comparisons and quality of life issues. *Cancer Treat Rev.* 2004;30(2):165–172.

27. Siegel JA, Sparks RB, Sharkey RM, et al. Blood-based red marrow dosimetry: where's the beef? *J Nucl Med.* 2005;46(8):1404–1406; author reply 5–6.

28. Brill AB, Stabin M, Bouville A, et al. Normal organ radiation dosimetry and associated uncertainties in nuclear medicine, with emphasis on iodine-131. *Radiat Res.* 2006;166(1 pt 2):128–140.

29. Baechler S, Hobbs RF, Prideaux AR, et al. Extension of the biological effective dose to the MIRD schema and possible implications in radionuclide therapy dosimetry. *Med Phys.* 2008;35(3):1123–1134.

30. Barone R, Borson-Chazot F, Valkema R, et al. Patient-specific dosimetry in predicting renal toxicity with (90)Y-DOTATOC: relevance of kidney volume and dose rate in finding a dose-effect relationship. *J Nucl Med.* 2005;46(suppl 1):99S–106S.

31. Fowler J. The linear-quadratic formula and progress in fractionated radiotherapy. *Br J Radiol.* 1989;62:679–694.

32. Wilder RB, DeNardo GL, Sheri S, et al. Application of the linear-quadratic model to myelotoxicity associated with radioimmunotherapy. *Eur J Nucl Med.* 1996;23(8):953–957.

33. He B, Du Y, Song X, et al. A Monte Carlo and physical phantom evaluation of quantitative In-111 SPECT. *Phys Med Biol.* 2005;50(17): 4169–4185.

34. He B, Wahl RL, Du Y, et al. Comparison of residence time estimation methods for radioimmunotherapy dosimetry and treatment planning—Monte Carlo simulation studies. *IEEE Trans Med Imaging.* 2008;27(4):521–530.

35. Siegel JA, Yeldell D, Goldenberg DM, et al. Red marrow radiation dose adjustment using plasma FLT3-L cytokine levels: improved correlations between hematologic toxicity and bone marrow dose for radioimmunotherapy patients. *J Nucl Med.* 2003;44(1):67–76.

36. Shen S, Meredith RF, Duan J, et al. Improved prediction of myelotoxicity using a patient-specific imaging dose estimate for non-marrow-targeting (90)Y-antibody therapy. *J Nucl Med.* 2002;43(9):1245–1253.

37. Sgouros G, Barest G, Thekkumthala J, et al. Treatment planning for internal radionuclide therapy: three-dimensional dosimetry for nonuniformly distributed radionuclides. *J Nucl Med.* 1990;31(11): 1884–1891.

38. Furhang EE, Sgouros G, Chui CS. Radionuclide photon dose kernels for internal emitter dosimetry. *Med Phys.* 1996;23(5):759–764.

39. Liu A, Williams LE, Wong JY, et al. Monte Carlo-assisted voxel source kernel method (MAVSK) for internal beta dosimetry. *Nucl Med Biol.* 1998;25(4):423–433.

40. Williams LE, Liu A, Raubitschek AA, et al. A method for patient-specific absorbed dose estimation for internal beta emitters. *Clin Cancer Res.* 1999;5(10 suppl):3015s–3019s.

41. Berger M. MIRD pamphlet no. 2: energy deposition in water by photons from point isotropic sources. *J Nucl Med.* 1968;15(suppl 1):17–25.

42. Berger M. Energy deposition in water by photons from point isotropic sources. *J Nucl Med.* 1968;9(suppl 1):15–25.

43. Brownell G, Ellett W, Reddy A. MIRD pamphlet no. 3—absorbed fractions for photon dosimetry. *J Nucl Med.* 1968;15(suppl 1):29–39.

44. Akabani G, Poston JW Sr, Bolch WE. Estimates of beta absorbed fractions in small tissue volumes for selected radionuclides. *J Nucl Med.* 1991;32(5):835–839.

45. Snyder W, Ford M, Warner G. *MIRD Pamphlet No. 1, Revised—Estimates of Specific Absorbed Fractions for Photon Sources Uniformly Distributed in Various Organs of a Heterogeneous Phantom*. New York, NY: Society of Nuclear Medicine; 1978.

46. Siegel JA, Stabin MG. Absorbed fractions for electrons and beta particles in spheres of various sizes. *J Nucl Med.* 1994;35(1):152–156.

47. Stabin MG, Konijnenberg MW. Re-evaluation of absorbed fractions for photons and electrons in spheres of various sizes. *J Nucl Med.* 2000;41(1):149–160.

48. Rogers DW. Fifty years of Monte Carlo simulations for medical physics. *Phys Med Biol.* 2006;51(13):R287–R301.

49. Macey D, Williams L, Hazel B, et al. A primer for radioimmunotherapy and radionuclide therapy. AAPM Report #71. Madison, WI; 2001.

50. Furhang EE, Chui CS, Sgouros G. A Monte Carlo approach to patient-specific dosimetry. *Med Phys.* 1996;23(9):1523–1529.

51. Furhang EE, Chui CS, Kolbert KS, et al. Implementation of a Monte Carlo dosimetry method for patient-specific internal emitter therapy. *Med Phys.* 1997;24(7):1163–1172.

52. Tagesson M, Ljungberg M, Strand SE. A Monte-Carlo program converting activity distributions to absorbed dose distributions in a radionuclide treatment planning system. *Acta Oncol.* 1996;35(3):367–372.

53. Liu A, Williams LE, Lopatin G, et al. A radionuclide therapy treatment planning and dose estimation system. *J Nucl Med.* 1999;40(7):1151–1153.

54. Johnson TK, McClure D, McCourt S. MABDOSE. II: validation of a general purpose dose estimation code. *Med Phys.* 1999;26(7):1396–1403.

55. Johnson TK, McClure D, McCourt S. MABDOSE. I: characterization of a general purpose dose estimation code. *Med Phys.* 1999;26(7):1389–1395.

56. Clairand I, Ricard M, Gouriou J, et al. DOSE3D: EGS4 Monte Carlo code-based software for internal radionuclide dosimetry. *J Nucl Med.* 1999;40(9):1517–1523.

57. Song H, He B, Prideaux A, et al. Lung dosimetry for radioiodine treatment planning in the case of diffuse lung metastases. *J Nucl Med.* 2006;47(12):1985–1994.

58. Hobbs RF, Wahl RL, Lodge MA, et al. ^{124}I PET-based 3D-RD dosimetry for a pediatric thyroid cancer patient: real-time treatment planning and methodologic comparison. *J Nucl Med.* 2009;50:1844–1847.

59. Kase KR, Nelson WR. *Concepts of Radiation Dosimetry*. New York, NY: Pergamon; 1978.

60. Roesch WC. Mathematical theory of radiation fields. In: Attix FH, Roesch WC, eds. *Radiation Dosimetry*. 2nd ed. New York, NY: Academic Press; 1968.

61. Lewis EE, Miller WF. *Computational Methods of Neutron Transport*. New York, NY: Wiley; 1984.

62. Moran JM, Nigg DW, Wheeler FJ, et al. Macroscopic geometric heterogeneity effects in radiation dose distribution analysis for boron neutron capture therapy. *Med Phys.* 1992;19(3):723–732.

63. Nigg DW, Randolph PD, Wheeler FJ. Demonstration of three-dimensional deterministic radiation transport theory dose distribution analysis for boron neutron capture therapy. *Med Phys.* 1991;18(1):43–53.

64. Shapiro A, Schwartz B, Windham JP, et al. Calculated neutron dose rates and flux densities from implantable Californium-252 point and line sources. *Med Phys.* 1976;3(4):241–247.

65. Mikell J, Vassiliev O, Erwin W, et al. A novel SPECT/CT voxel-based dose calculation method for targeted radionuclide therapy. *J Nucl Med.* 2009;50(suppl 2):71P.

66. Mikell J, Vassiliev O, Erwin W, et al. Comparing a grid-based Boltzmann solver with Monte Carlo simulation for voxel-based therapeutic radionuclide dose calculations. *Med Phys.* 2009;36:2772.

67. Wareing TA, Morel JE, McGhee JM. Coupled electron-photon transport methods on 3-D unstructured grids. *Trans Am Nucl Soc.* Washington, DC; 2000.

68. Wareing TA, McGhee JM, Morel JE, et al. Discontinuous finite element SN methods on three-dimensional unstructured grids. *Nucl Sci Eng.* 2001;138(3):256–268.

69. Gifford KA, Horton JL, Wareing TA, et al. Comparison of a finite-element multigroup discrete-ordinates code with Monte Carlo for radiotherapy calculations. *Phys Med Biol.* 2006;51(9):2253–2265.

70. Gifford KA, Price MJ, Horton JL Jr, et al. Optimization of deterministic transport parameters for the calculation of the dose distribution around a high dose-rate 192Ir brachytherapy source. *Med Phys.* 2008;35(6):2279–2285.

71. Vassiliev ON, Wareing TA, Davis IM, et al. Feasibility of a multigroup deterministic solution method for three-dimensional radiotherapy dose calculations. *Int J Radiat Oncol Biol Phys.* 2008;72(1):220–227.

72. Anderson P, Nunez R. Samarium lexidronam (153Sm-EDTMP): skeletal radiation for osteoblastic bone metastases and osteosarcoma. *Expert Rev Anticancer Ther.* 2007;7(11):1517–1527.

73. Anderson PM, Wiseman GA, Dispenzieri A, et al. High-dose samarium-153 ethylene diamine tetramethylene phosphonate: low toxicity of skeletal irradiation in patients with osteosarcoma and bone metastases. *J Clin Oncol.* 2002;20(1):189–196.

74. Eckerman KF, Westfall RJ, Ryman JC, et al. Availability of nuclear decay data in electronic form, including beta spectra not previously published. *Health Phys.* 1994;67:338–345.

75. Kappadath S, Erwin W. Comparison of three sensitivity calibration methods to quantify SPECT/CT-based tumor uptake of Sm-153 EDTMP. *J Nucl Med.* 2008;49(suppl 1):398P.

76. Walters BRB, Rogers DWO. *DOSXYZnrc Users Manual.* Ottawa, Canada: National Research Council of Canada; 2002.

7

Chelation Chemistry

Aaron D. Wilson and Martin W. Brechbiel

■ INTRODUCTION

A chelate is traditionally two or more Lewis acids combined through a carbon framework. The structure of the carbon framework determines the size, relative geometry, and level of preorganization of the chelation cavity. For the purposes of radionuclide therapy, the cavity is ideally shaped when it is best suited for the incorporation and containment of a viable metallic radionuclide (RN). For targeted delivery of an RN, the chelate can be covalently bonded to a directing biomolecule (BM). A molecule that incorporates the capacity to combine an RN and a BM into a single structure is thus termed a "bifunctional chelating agent (BCA)."

The language and terms used in this chapter were selected for their practical application. For example, BM is used to refer to any sort of molecule that selectively migrates to specific tissue or site; this would include monoclonal antibodies (mAbs), antibody fragments, peptides, segments of amino acids, small molecules, dendrimers, nanoparticles, and any other potential targeting molecule or material.

A BCA is just one of a number of common names and acronym combinations used to refer to a molecule that links a metallic RN to a BM, and equivalent terms such as "bifunctional coupling agent," "bifunctional ligand," or some other reasonable derivation, with associated acronyms such as BFA or BFCA exist; the differences in language are trivial. The only substantial complication with the language is the term "chelate." "Chelate," from the Greek "chelos" meaning claw, is a biologic term used to refer to a molecule that can act as a Lewis base in multiple locations. In chemical terminology, the same molecule would usually be referred to as a "multidentate ligand" or just "ligand." However, the term "ligand" in biologic language refers to molecules that bind to proteins. Mixing of the language is also common; BCAs and metal ions are routinely termed "ligands," whereas those chelating metal ions are termed "chelates." Luckily, this is the limit of the semantic difficulties and the meaning of language can usually be inferred from context. To assist in avoiding ambiguity, we will refer to functional groups which can donate electron pairs as Lewis bases and for the sake of symmetry, electron acceptors such as protons and metallic cations (RN) will be referred to as "Lewis acids."

■ HISTORY

There are three historic fields of study that were combined to create BCAs: directed biologic targeting, coordination chemistry, and the medical application of radioisotopes. Each of these fields developed along their own course prior to convergence. The ability to target different parts of the body has been known throughout recorded history. The term "antibody" or at least the German term "antikörper" is attributed to being coined in 1891 and promoted by Ehrlich (1–3). The biologic targeting system of mAbs was characterized in the early 1970s (4–6).

Coordination chemistry draws its roots from many places, but Alfred Werner provided the principle basic science in 1893. Shortly thereafter, Alfred Werner and Paul Ehrlich made the first attempt at chelation therapy (7). In this attempt, they tried to minimize the toxic side effects of arsenic used in syphilis treatment while retaining the therapeutic value. The next major embodiments of chelation therapy focused purely on removing toxic metal from patients. In 1941, Kety and Letonoft experimented by using citrate to counter acute lead toxicity. The first widely used chelation agent was 2,3-dimercaptopropanol referred to as "British Anti-Lewisite" (BAL). BAL's common name was derived form its intended use as a counteragent to the chemical weapon dichlorovinyl arsine (Lewisite). The use of Lewisite was anticipated during World War II (WWII) but never realized. BAL remained on the sidelines through WWII and actually saw its first therapeutic use in the removal of arsenic from patients being treated for syphilis. The prototypical chelating agent, ethylenediaminetetraacetic acid (EDTA), was documented (1951) for its efficacy in removing plutonium from animals, but saw greater use in the removal of lead from human patients who had been overexposed to lead through the use of common paints (7–11). Comparative studies of various chelates were conducted as early as 1957 (12).

Henri Becquerel discovered radioactivity in 1896. Radium was isolated and characterized by the Curies in 1898 and used in therapy by 1901. This use of radioactive material would evolve into brachytherapy using radioactive "seeds" physically deposited near the treatment site such as a tumor (13). Radiotherapy and nuclear medicine have always been limited by the small number of readily available and appropriate RNs. Since the Manhattan project, there has been a significant increase in the number of easily obtained isotopes and associated advances in radiotherapy.

These three lines of inquiry were tied together in 1968 by Benisek and Richards when they converted protein amino groups into picolinamidine functional groups to act as bidentate metal chelators (14). Then in 1974, Meares and coworkers (15–17) modified EDTA to covalently attach to a BM. Since the 1970s, there has been a proliferation of complexes explored for use as BCAs for radiotherapy and imaging as well as targeted delivery of magnetic resonance imaging contrast agents. As an active field of research, the development of BCAs has been directly or indirectly reviewed several times over the last few years (18–31).

THE GOALS OF CHELATION CHEMISTRY WITHIN TARGETED RADIONUCLIDE THERAPY

The goal of chelation chemistry is to develop RN–BCA complexes that then satisfy four criteria. First, RN–BCA complexes must form rapidly under mild biologic conditions and dilute conditions. In lieu of that, there must be a viable method of preparing the RN–BCA in a therapeutic setting still constrained by constantly decaying radioactivity. Second, the RN–BCA must be kinetically stable under in vivo conditions over the course of the treatment. Third, the RN–BCA must not obstruct the BM ability to target specific tissues or sites. Fourth, the untargeted RN must ultimately clear rapidly and preferably through the renal system. The RN and BCA pairings that meet each of these requirements and successfully deliver radiation to malignant cells is a success. To achieve success, a number of features of BCA are manipulated and supplementary actions employed. These manipulations and actions, as well as the considerations behind them are the subject of this review.

BASIC FEATURES OF A BIFUNCTIONAL CHELATING AGENT

As noted, the carbon framework of a BCA determines the geometry, size, and preorganization of the cavity, which can accept a Lewis acid. However, there is more to the chelation of an RN than these criteria. The electronic characteristic of the BCA's Lewis bases is comparably important (32). The charge, pK_a (of its conjugate acid form), hard soft acid base (HSAB) character (33–36), coordination motif (κ and η), and π bonding character all influence how well a specific Lewis base bonds to a specific Lewis acid under given conditions. These are the elements that are important, for example, in differentiating the chemical reactivity of a porphyrin from that of cyclam (1,4,8, 11-tetraazacyclotetradecane).

Perhaps the most obvious electronic feature is charge and while balancing the charge of a chelate and Lewis base is not required, doing so usually improves stability. The

remaining electronic features are more sublet. The pK_a of a Lewis base suggests its strength as a σ donor and a ligand's position in the spectral chemical series. Generally, the more basic the lone pair, the stronger the donor; however, a more powerful donor is not always for the best, since biologically native Lewis acids will compete for the Lewis base. There is often no mechanism to return a Lewis base to the RN once protonated. As a result, Lewis base conjugates of weak acids, such as acetates, which readily protonate and deprotonate under biologic conditions are common in chelate chemistry.

The HSAB system deals with the polarizability and diffusivity of the orbitals involved in bonding between Lewis acids and Lewis bases (33–36). The majority of important RNs are used in high oxidation states and are located on the hard side of the scale, but there are number of metal centers such as Pb(II), Cu(II), In(III), and Bi(III) that would be considered borderline to soft. Metal centers are best stabilized when paired with Lewis bases of the proper hardness.

Lewis acid–base bonding ranges from ionic to covalent bonding as well as to various forms of weaker electrostatic interactions. Like other covalent bonds, Lewis acid–base pairs can involve more than one set of orbitals and more than one set of electron pairs. To understand such phenomenon, the π character of Lewis acids and orbital symmetries of the Lewis acid need to be considered. Commonly, the primary interaction is σ donation with the direct donation of a lone pair by the Lewis base to a vacant orbital on the Lewis acid. With available orbitals of the proper symmetry, energy, and density, additional electron density can be shared. The bonding situation can be stabilized by the ligand acting either as a π donor, delivering greater electron density to the Lewis acid, or as a π acceptor, withdrawing electron density from the nominal Lewis acid (commonly referred to as "back bonding"). Similarly, the functional group denticity (κ) and hapticity (η) are fundamental to understanding how Lewis bases and Lewis acids interact structurally. Each of these characteristics allows for better understanding of a chelate complex's stability.

Despite the importance of these subtleties, a Lewis base must meet some minimum requirements determined by the biologic environment before consideration for use in a BCA system. Many Lewis bases widely used in inorganic chemistry require inert anhydrous atmospheres. Although a number of these systems become "air-stable" once coordinated to a Lewis acid, such complexes are often unstable under in vivo conditions. Obviously, such a shortcoming would render a Lewis base useless for therapeutic use. Fortunately, many Lewis bases are stable under biologically relevant conditions and are well suited for complexing many useful RN. The major Lewis basic functional groups are listed in Table 7.1; however, there are many other more "exotic" Lewis bases that can be reached by modifying the molecular environments of oxygen, nitrogen, sulfur, phosphorous, and even carbon. Imidazole is just one example of the many Lewis bases that could also be listed here but is omitted for the sake of brevity. Table 7.1 also includes a few Lewis bases

Table **7.1**   **Major Lewis basic functional groups and coligands**

Lewis Base	Charge	Representative pK_a	HSAB	Denticity or Hapticity (Bond Order)	π Character
Carbocyclic acid	1−	~5	Hard	κ 1	π Donor
Amine	0	~11	Hard	κ 1	No significant interactions
Thiol	1−	~11	Soft	κ 1	π Donor
Hydroxamate	1−	~10	Hard	κ 1	π Donor
Amide	1−	~38	Hard	κ 1 (BO ≥ 1)	π Donor
Diazenido	2−	N/A	Hard	κ 1 (BO > 1)	π Donor
Phosphonic acid	1−, 2−	~3, ~9	Hard	κ 1	π Donor
Phosphine	0	~8	Hard	κ 1	Various π interactions
Cyclopentadien	1−	N/A	Hard	η 5 (BO > 1)	Various π interactions
Coligands					
Carbon monoxide	0	N/A	Soft	κ 1	π Acceptor
Aqua/hydroxy	0, 1−	~14	Hard	κ 1	π Donor

HSAB, hard soft acid base.

denoted as coligands that may supplement a Lewis acid's coordination sphere that is not completely filled by a BCA.

These coligands, while not part of the primary chelating ligand, can influence the rate of formation of an RN–BCA complex and the ultimate stability of the resulting RN–BCA complex under biologic conditions.

Structure and preorganization

Many chelate structures can be split into categories such as linear or macrocyclic. The macrocycles generally have a high degree of preorganization. The backbone structures of most macrocyclic molecules are constrained such that one of their most stable conformations is very similar to the conformation adopted upon coordination to a metal center. This sort of preorganization is intended to facilitate the formation as well as the biologic stability of an RN–BCA complex.

Linear chelates vary in their degree of preorganization. EDTA and DTPA have a wide range of available conformers under ambient conditions and a low degree of preorganization. The preorganization can be increased by adding steric bulk that reduces the stability of undesirable conformations, thereby increasing the relative thermodynamic stability of favorable conformations. Efforts to preorganize a chelate can be taken a step further by locking the molecule into a favorable geometry, for example, incorporation of a *trans*-cyclohexane ring into the chelate backbone (12,37). The Lewis base donors are positioned so that they become equatorial groups in the chair conformation of a cyclohexyl group, restricted to a *gauche* conformation favorable to *cis*-bidentate chelation.

Isomers

Many BCAs contain multiple stereocenters even before coordinating to an RN. Other BCAs are prochiral and form racemic

mixtures once coordinated to an RN. The synthetic methods to produce BCAs can even yield mixtures of conformational isomers (38). When there is no way to specifically control stereochemistry, the presence of a mixture can be acknowledged and research continued. Ignoring stereochemistry can be reasonable as in the case of 2-(4-isobutylphenyl)propanoic acid (ibuprofen), which racemizes under biologic conditions or a completely unreasonable assumption as in the case of thalidomide. The testing for thalidomide as a morning sickness drug was done with stereochemically pure material, but the drug was ultimately produced as a racemate, thereby including the enantiomer that was a serious teratogen.

In some cases, in vitro stability studies have failed to discern differences in bioactivity of different conformers of an RN–BCA–BM agent. These bioactivity differences only became apparent during in vivo studies (39). Although stereoscopic purity may be glossed over in early studies, once explored in detail, the stereochemistry of a BCA may prove to have a significant role in the activity of RN–BCA–BM on multiple levels.

Significant portions of BM molecules are specific stereoisomers of molecules containing many stereocenters and many native nucleophiles (Lewis acids) through which BCA can be linked. A BCA's stereochemistry may significantly influence how a BCA and a BM link. In the first place, linking a BCA to the BM usually produces distributions of BCA–BM molecules with the BCA linked to the BM in different quantities and at different positions. Differences in stereochemistry of the BCA are likely to influence this process and the resulting distribution of products. Each of the possible linkages likely differs in its biologic activity, but without practical methods to resolve the mixture on a synthetic scale, there is no way to know the magnitude of the difference in activity. Conversely, one might assume that the BCA and BM are all linked at the same position, while there is a difference in the relative stereochemistries of the connected RN–BCA complexes that could result in significant differences in the in vivo stability of the resulting RN–BCA–BM complex conformers. All of these factors remain to be explored in greater detail. With the push toward greater stereochemical control in synthetic organic chemistry and industrial drug production, improved isomer selectivity remains an obvious frontier for BCA research.

ELECTRONIC FEATURES OF RN RELEVANT TO BCA

Although metallic cations' "nuclear" characteristics such as half-life, decay pattern, and emission energies are very important selection criteria for RN, they are also comparably unimportant when selecting an appropriate chelate for the RN. A metallic cation's "electronic" characteristics actually determine the characteristics a chelate must have to form a stable complex (40). These "electronic" characteristics include oxidation state, charge, ionic radius (41), valence electron structure, orbital diffusion, and polarization as described by Pearson's HSAB model (33–36) and the ideal coordination number and geometry. Some of these characteristics are interrelated, but not in a way that makes them redundant. Although an ion's charge relates to the ion's HSAB character, they are not the same thing. Each distinct characteristic is important for understanding a Lewis acid's chelation chemistry.

An RN's electronic characteristics can be important in deciding what approximations can be applied to the ion. The RN with the proper radiologic characteristics for use in targeted radiation therapy can be from categories of the periodic table such as "main group," "f-block" ions, or "transition" metals that have either high or low D-electron counts. The coordination motifs of Lewis acids can be approximated as "ionic" spheres when the Lewis acid has a poorly defined electronic orbital structure. Thus, the "ionic" approximation works for "main group" and "f-block" ions, representing much of radiotherapy chelation chemistry, but does not reflect ions with well-defined orbital structures including many of the rhenium oxidation states and certainly ^{195m}Pt. There is a dominant geometry for each of platinum's oxidation states: Pt(II) is four-coordinate square planar, Pt(0) is four-coordinate tetrahedral, and Pt(IV) is six-coordinate octahedral. Being conscious of the valence electron structure of a Lewis acid can allow researchers to anticipate the reactivity and coordination geometry of an RN.

Our formal models of electronic structures tend to be ambiguous or deceptively "defined." For example, the "ionic radius" of a metal center is defined as half the distance between the Lewis acid and Lewis base in a crystal lattice measured from diffractometry or extrapolated from spectral features. The bond lengths between a metal center and the Lewis bases in its own coordination sphere can vary significantly; there is only more variation when different complexes are considered. For this reason, all "ionic radii" are statistical averages based on finite data sets. The "ionic radii" also varies significantly with the metal ions coordination number. In Table 7.2, the variation in ionic radius corresponds to variation in coordination number. The concepts of a fixed ionic radius or an ideal coordination number are appealing but flawed. The importance of the flaws can be demonstrated with the series represented in Table 7.2; increasing coordination numbers correlate with an increase in ionic radius which means longer bond lengths which correlate with weaker bonds. In general, the goal is to have a chelating agent fill an RN's coordination sphere with as many bonds as possible, but this goal is achieved at the expense of weakening individual bonds. Chelate stabilization effects resulting from

Table 7.2	Ionic radius and coordination number				
Core	**Charge**	**Ionic Radius (pm)[a]**	**Valence Description**	**HSAB**	**Coordination Number[a]**
Cu(II)	2+	71–87	d^9	Borderline	4–6
Ga(III)	3+	61–76	d^{10}	Soft	4–6
Y(III)	3+	90–108	Lanthanide like	Ionic	6–9
Zr(IV)	4+	59–89	d^0	Hard	4–9
Tc(V)	5+	60	d^2	Hard	6
Sm(III)	3+	96–124	Lanthanide	Ionic	6–12
Lu(III)	3+	86–103	Lanthanide	Ionic	6–9
Re(V)	5+	58	d^2	Hard	6
Pb(II)	2+	119–149	Main group	Soft	6–12
Bi(III)	3+	96–117	Main group	Soft to borderline	5–8
Ac(III)	3+	112	Actinide	Ionic	6

[a]Ref. 41

HSAB, hard soft acid base.

Adapted from Shannon RD. Revised effective ionic radii and systematic studies of interatomic distances in halides and chalcogenides. *Acta Crystallogr Sect A.* 1976; 32:751–767.

preorganization of the chelate become increasingly important the greater the coordination number of a metallic RN. This is especially true if the RN falls under the ionic approximation and lacks orbital structure to guide organization.

Even the concept of oxidation state is formalism (42). The limits of charge separation means an RN cannot be ionized more than a few times. In oxidation states of M(III) and greater, the electron density localized on the metal center is greater than that represented by its formal oxidation state; the electron density localized on the chelate is lower than that represented by their formal oxidation states. Although the large charges of most RN might only be formalisms to achieve stable complexes, they require chelates that "formally" balance their charge.

Despite the ambiguities of a metallic RN's ionic radius, valence electron configuration, ideal coordination number, HSAB character, and even charge, each of these properties is important in effectively designing an appropriate BCA. These properties determine an RN–BCA complex's thermodynamic and kinetic stability. Furthermore, since every oxidation state of every metal has unique characteristics, each must be considered independently when selecting or designing a chelate, as there is no universal chelate that will work for all metallic RNs (Table 7.2).

List of "naked" ions according to their formal oxidation states is a model that works much of the time, but in a few situations, it is better to treat an RN as a core structure that includes not only a metal center but one or more biologically inert coligands. Such considerations are useful in understanding many rhenium and technetium complexes and will be discussed in that context.

CHEMICAL CONSTRUCTION OF BCA CONTAINING RADIOTHERAPEUTICS

Prelabeling versus postlabeling

Labeling is the process through which an RN is complexed with a BCA. There are two common methods for labeling, prelabeling and postlabeling, in which the "prefix" refers to when the BCA is labeled with an RN relative to when the BCA is covalently linked to a BM. The RN is added *pre* BCA–BM linking or *post* BCA–BM linking.

Postlabeling is the vastly preferred method to prepare a radiotherapeutic. In postlabeling, a BCA is first covalently linked to a BM to create a molecule that has an extended indefinite shelf life, mostly dependant upon the stability of the BM. The BM–BCA can be complexed with the RN, albeit under conditions governed by compatibility with the BM. Ideally, this step involves nothing more than mixing the BM–BCA molecule with the RN, then isolating and purifying the desired RN–BCA–BM just prior to therapeutic application. This represents an ideal scenario.

When an RN and BCA–BM cannot be linked at ambient conditions, then another route must be employed. This other route is prelabeling in which the BCA and RN are initially combined (43). This allows for the use of synthetic conditions that would damage or destroy many BMs. The BM, often an antibody or peptide, has a limited tolerance to organic solvents, salt concentrations, redox environments, pH, and temperature. Prelabeling even allows better analytical characterization of the RN–BCA complex, allowing the demonstration of the full and desired coordination that is not feasible once linked to a BM. Characterizing an RN–BCA–BM complex is both limited and difficult due to time constraints, potential radiolysis of the components, and obvious issues of dealing with and handling radioactive products. A longer linear synthesis involving radioactive material means producing more radioactive waste, working with radioactive material for a longer period of time, resulting in higher exposure to personnel, and usually requiring more synthetic steps to be conducted at the point of application. This is especially challenging when the RN has a short half-life. The end result is that prelabeling is often unreasonable for a clinical application.

Conjugation functional groups

BCAs are covalently conjugated to BMs through activated organic functional groups, usually electrophilic centers, on the BCA (Fig. 7.1) (24,54–58). These electrophiles can react with native nucleophiles common to many large BM such as amines, sulfhydryl, imidazoles, or thioether groups. Despite an excess of open nucleophiles in many large molecules, small molecules often lack viable nucleophiles. These systems require alternative coupling methods. Nucleophiles can be synthetically added to the BM or other chemically reactive sites can be employed. Special linking segments, which will be discussed in the next section, can often assist in coupling BCA and BM.

Obviously, working with a BM with many available nucleophiles is a common situation, that is, proteins commonly express many different nucleophiles. When such BMs are reacted with BCAs, a distribution of products is formed. Populations of the BM link with multiple BCAs while others receive none in accordance to a Poisson distribution (59). Even the BM labeled only once will actually exist as a collection of BMs labeled in different positions. The resulting mixture is generally treated as a single entity with the behavior of specific forms averaged across the total population. A variety of efforts have been made to increase labeling selectivity (60,61). Yet, in most situations, how specific structural isomers contribute to the overall bioactivity is still not well understood.

Linkers

Linkers (L) can be synthetically necessary to join the BM to the BCA; pharmacokinetic modifiers (PKMs) within linkers can also impart desirable distribution characteristics. The structural and electronic characteristics of a linker such as

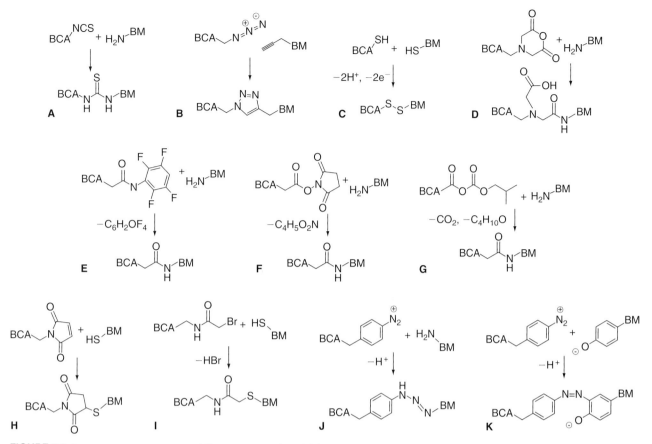

FIGURE 7.1 Conjugation functional groups: **(A)** isothiocyanate (44,45), **(B)** click chemistry (46–48), **(C)** disulfide bond, **(D)** aminodiacetic acid anhydrides such as DTPA anhydride (49–52). Activated esters: **(E)** tetrafluorophenyl ester (53), **(F)** NHS-ester maleimide/succinimide ester (54,55), **(G)** isobutylcarbonic anhydride (24), **(H)** maleimide (55,56), **(I)** haloacetamide (57), diazonium salts reacting with a **(J)** primary amine and **(K)** phenol (58).

charge, polarity, mass, reactivity, and how these properties relate to the entire RN–BCA–L–BM (or the more descriptive acronym RN–BCA–PKM–BM) structure influence the complex's biologic activity.

The PKM linker is often employed to influence renal and hepatic clearance rates. If an unmodified therapeutic agent undergoes renal clearance too quickly, it will lack time to accumulate in the desired location(s) to deliver the desired effect and/or result in unacceptable kidney damage from high radiation doses. However, it is also desirable to have a radiotherapeutic ultimately and efficiently cleared through a renal pathway. Hepatic clearance can lead to unacceptable radiation doses to the liver.

Renal clearance can often be slowed simply by increasing the therapeutic molar mass. Neutral linkers, such as hydrocarbon chains, increase lipophilicity and thus renal clearance. Polar linkers, such as a peptide sequence or inclusion of polyethylene glycol units, increase hydrophilicity and slow extraction by the liver (62–64). The rate of renal and hepatic clearance can be manipulated by adjusting the polarity and charge of the whole molecule as well as segments such as the linker between the BCA and BM.

A few chemically reactive linkers have been reported. These linkers are intended to be stable enough for the com-

plex to accumulate in the desired location and then cleave under regular metabolic conditions leading to the sequestration of the RN–BCA in the desired location or the clearance of the small molecule by renal excretion (65–69).

Scavenging

A primary goal of developing a quality radiotherapeutic is to develop an RN–BCA complex with the highest possible in vivo kinetic inertness; in lieu of a completely inert complex, it would at least be desirable to have the RN to quickly clear the renal system within the context of the RN half-life. It is common practice to use a scavenging agent, just after the incubation of an RN with BCA–BM followed by chromatography as a standard method to isolate pure RN–BCA–BM. As an added precaution, it has been proposed that the patient should be injected with a second chelating agent at a higher concentration along with the RN–BCA–BM complex. The second chelating agent is intended to scavenge any RN that is free or becomes free during the treatment and facilitating renal clearance and preventing the RN from distributing as free RN. Model in vivo studies with ^{90}Y have provided a proof of concept (70).

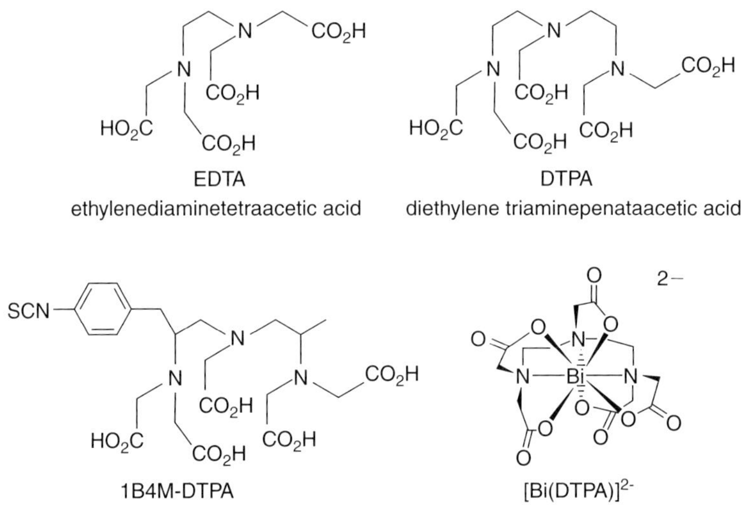

FIGURE 7.2 Structures of EDTA, DTAP, 1B4M-DPTA (31,45), and Bi(DTPA) (75).

EDTA
ethylenediaminetetraacetic acid

DTPA
diethylene triaminepenataacetic acid

1B4M-DTPA

[Bi(DTPA)]$^{2-}$

BIFUNCTIONAL CHELATE AGENTS

Polyaminopolycarboxylates

Many polyaminopolycarboxylate ligands have been used with therapeutic RNs such as ^{67}Cu, ^{90}Y, ^{111}In, ^{166}Ho, ^{177}Lu, ^{212}Pb, ^{212}Bi, and ^{213}Bi (19,24,28,71–74). Polyaminocarboxylate BCAs can be divided into two basic types, linear or straight chain backbone analogs and macrocyclic backbone analogs.

EDTA and DTPA

The straight chain backbone analogs are generally built on EDTA or DTPA backbones (31,45,75). A procedure to produce EDTA (Fig. 7.1) was first patented in Germany in 1934 and in the United States in 1936 and 1938 (76–78). The patent for the preparation of diethylenetriamine pentaacetic acid (pentetic acid, DPTA) (Fig. 7.2) was filed in 1941 and granted in 1945 (79).

Because of the well-known ability of these two ligands to chelate a wide variety of metal ions, it is not surprising that they were the early candidate chelating agents of choice for the development of BCAs. In 1974, EDTA was one of the first synthetic chelate platforms to be modified to act as a BCA (15,16). The first DPTA modified to act as a BCA was reported in 1977 (51).

The early EDTA and DTPA analogs tended to utilize a carboxylic acid for activation in coupling to BMs. These included mixed and cyclic anhydrides. Most notable of the BCA that bonds through a carboxylic acid is DTPA dianhydride (*N,N*-bis[2-(2,6-dioxo-4-morpholinyl)ethyl] glycine) first introduced as a BCA for labeling proteins in 1977 by Krejcarek and Tucker (51,52,80–85). DTPA dianhydride contains a pair of cyclic anhydride functionalities each being capable of reacting to form a covalent bond with a nucleophile. Reaction conditions can and are generally adjusted to favor the production of species where each DTPA dianhydride links to a single BM, yet it is possible for DTPA dianhydride to also serve as a crosslinker. This creates the potential to crosslink multiple BMs together, a transformation which usually results in

deleterious effects on targeting. This lack of synthetic control is partially offset by the synthetic ease with which DTPA dianhydride is obtained and applied. Yet the ease of use should not distract researchers from the inherent drawbacks (51).

The in vivo stability of these simple DTPA derivatives is handicapped as compared with chelates with more preorganization such as MX-DTPA and CHX-DTPA that also retain all five carboxylates. Tying up one of the DTPA's carboxylic arms reduces the ability of the chelate to stabilize cations under in vivo conditions. Loss of the full DTPA coordination sphere to saturate the RN using an amide as the eighth donor group has been shown to result in a complex of lesser stability in both in vivo and in vitro studies (86). This creates a situation where the RN can leak from the incomplete DTPA producing therapeutic and imaging efficacies lower than what are produced by systems using a preorganized DTPA while also contributing to toxicity with the RN, then trafficking to its inherent biologic site(s) of deposition (87).

Backbone functionalized EDTA and DTPA analogs have been developed. Functionalization to BCA has been achieved through the azo-phenyl (58), *p*-bromoacetamido-phenyl (57), carboxymethoxybenzyl (88), and the benzyl-isothiocyanate groups (44,45). It has been reported that DTPA can be functionalized through the modification of amino acids of its carbon "backbone" (89). Further development of DTPA BCAs has involved efforts to further stabilize chelate conformations, usually by providing a measure of preorganization along the chelates backbone. Toward this end, a number of additional DTPA BCA derivatives were reported (86). These derivatives include molecules in which the DTPA carbon backbone has been methylated or utilized a "built in" cyclohexyl group. The initial synthetic methodologies to prepare these methylated DPTA chelates lead to a mixture of stereo and constitutional isomers that have been referred to as "MX-DTPA," a collection of isomers of which 1B4M-DTPA is a specific example (Fig. 7.2) (31,45). Some syntheses of MX-DTPA are attributed to produce higher purities of specific conformers, such as the methods used to produce the chelate, tiuxetan. Tiuxetan is attributed to be primarily 1B4M-DTPA, named according to

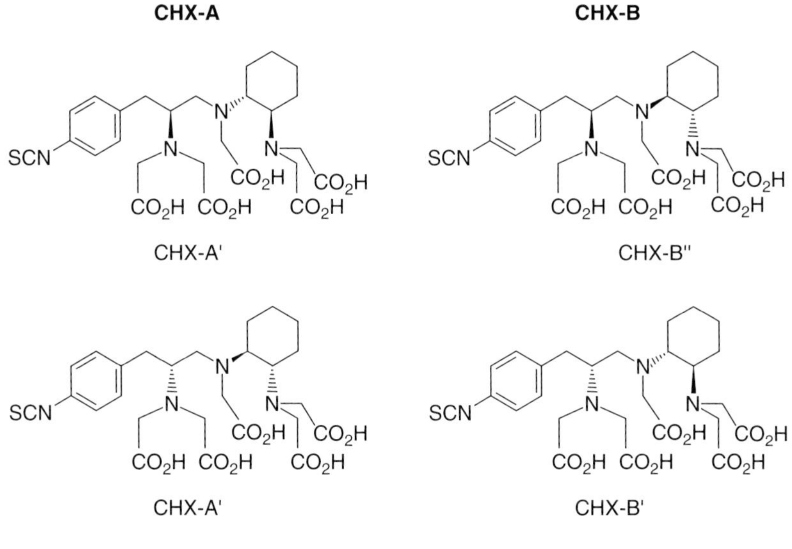

CHX-A

CHX-B

FIGURE 7.3 Stereoisomers of the CHX-DTPA, a BCA derivative of cyDTPA (39).

CHX-A'

CHX-B''

CHX-A'

CHX-B'

the convention where numbers refer to the carbons in the chelate's backbone, M refers to a methyl group, and B refers to isothiocyanatobenzyl, the functional group used to link the BCA to a BM. Even with a large amount of regiochemical purity (~90% to 95%), the molecule is still a racemic mixture of those same regioisomers. Regardless of the specific conformer, the methyl of MX-DTPA is presumed to stabilize desirable chelate conformations, increasing the level of pre-organization and stabilizing the labeled chelate structure. The observed effect is improved in vivo stability over the unmethylated DPTA derivative (38,89,90). Zevalin, the ^{90}Y Ibritumomab Tiuxetan therapeutic targeting CD20, is the first and only metallic RN–BCA–BM complex that has thus far been approved by the Food and Drug Administration (2002) for radioimmunotherapy, specifically for the treatment of non-Hodgkin lymphoma.

Presently, the ultimate DTPA backbone preorganization is probably the cyclohexyl analog. The date of the first report of *trans*-cyclohexyldiethylenetriamine pentaacetic acid (CyDPTA) is unclear, but this agent was mentioned in the patent literature as early as 1961 (91). Use of a modified CyDPTA molecule to act as a BCA was developed independently by two groups and reported between 1988 and 1991 (CHX-DPTA) (92–94). A subsequent study dealt explicitly with the stereochemistry intrinsic to the molecules based on the CyDPTA structure (39). Many BCAs avoid producing multiple stereoisomers by using chelates which do not produce stereoisomers. This is not possible for chelates such as CHX-DTPA, which contain three carbon stereocenters even before an RN is coordinated. All of this stereochemical complexity is further complicated by the coordination of an RN to CHX-DTPA. The complexation reduces the molecule's overall symmetry, producing a greater number of stable or semi-stable conformations as demonstrated in studies of lanthanides(III) with DTPA (95–98) and DTPA-monoamide (99). The study found that the single enantiomers CHX-A', CHX-A'', CHX-B', and CHX-B'' (Fig. 7.3) have significantly different abilities to stabilize radio-yttrium in vivo (39).

Regardless of the complexity of the stereochemistry, CHX-A'' DTPA is an effective chelator for ^{111}In, ^{90}Y, and ^{177}Lu, and to date is the only reported DTPA derivative to form suitably stable complexes with the above bismuth RNs, ^{212}Bi, and ^{213}Bi conjugated to mAbs or peptides in vivo (39,87,94), resulting in radioimmunoconjugates that have been used effectively in clinical trials (100). Kennel et al. investigated targeting blood vessels in lung tumors as a therapeutic approach with ^{213}Bi chelated to CHX-B to label mAb's 201B and 34A in a murine model with lung tumors of EMT-6 mammary carcinoma and IC-12 tracheal carcinoma (101).

Many conjugating functional groups have been incorporated into DTPA through the carbon backbone as well as the carboxylic acids. Many macrocyclic polyaminocarboxylate ligands and derivatives thereof have been described. These include DOTA, TETA, NOTA, DEPA, PEPA, HEHA, and others (vide infra).

DOTA

1,4,7,10-tetraazacyclododecane-1,4,7,10-tetraacetic acid (DOTA) (Fig. 7.4) is a 12-membered tetraaza macrocycle with 4 carboxylate arms providing an octadentate coordination sphere first reported in 1976 (102–104). At the time of its discovery,

DOTA

1,4,7,10-Tetraazacyclododecane-*N*,*N*',*N*'',*N*'''-tetraacetic acid

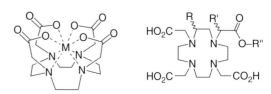

FIGURE 7.4 DOTA, DOTA coordinated at eight positions to metal M, common points (R,R' (102), and R'') at which DOTA can be functionalized to act as a BCA.

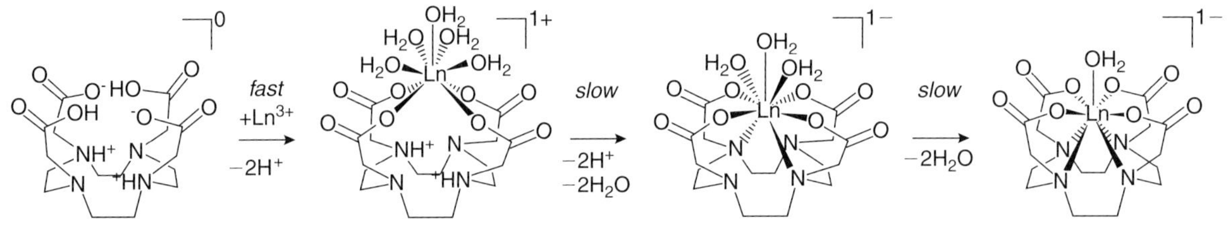

FIGURE 7.5 The intermediate involved in the full coordination of a lanthanide to DOTA (106).

DOTA was demonstrated to have the largest known formation constant for the complexation Ca^{2+} and Gd^{3+} ions. The most significant drawback to the use of DOTA has been its slow rate of complexation when compared with acyclic chelates such as DTPA and polyazamacrocycles, which do not feature ionizable chelating side arms. The slow complexation of metal centers has been attributed to various conformational intermediates (105). Moreau has presented potentiometric and EXAFS data supporting a process with three distinct steps for the coordination of a lanthanide cation to DOTA (106). The first stage of these steps is the rapid and loose electrostatic coordination of a lanthanide to DOTA's carboxylates and the loss of two protons (Fig. 7.5). The second step is slow and consists of the removal of the final two protons from DOTA and the loss of two aqua ligands from the lanthanide in exchange for two amines from DOTA. The third and final step is also slow, consisting of the lanthanides loss of two aqua ligands in exchange for two of DOTA's amines. Although the intermediates may form in hours, it may be necessary to "wait 4 to 6 weeks and even longer for their formation equilibrium to stabilize" Ln^{3+} DOTA complexes (106). Studies in which modified version of DOTA are used as the BCA, a large portion of the RN may not be fully coordinated to the BCA when the complex RN–BCA–BM is injected. It is expected that these intermediate coordination states would leak more than the fully coordinated RN–BCA yield variable and less than ideal results.

A modified version of C-functionalized DOTA, acting as a BCA, was first reported in 1988 (107). Since then there have been a handful of synthetic pathway reports to produce several different BCA DOTA derivatives. These synthetic pathways were recently reviewed in detail by Liu and Edwards (27).

Bifunctional analogs of DOTA have been used to label antibodies with ^{90}Y, ^{111}In, ^{166}Ho, ^{177}Lu, ^{212}Pb, and ^{212}Bi (19,24,28,71–74). DOTA and DTPA will complex with ^{90}Y quantitatively at low concentrations of ligand. Though both ^{90}Y-DTPA and ^{90}Y-DOTA complexes appear suitable for use in radiotherapy, ^{90}Y-DOTA complex is marginally better with higher initial clearance (108,109). A bifunctional DOTA has also been used to sequester ^{212}Pb with a mAb AE1 targeting HER2 on ovarian tumors in nude mice (110). Yet, DOTA ^{212}Bi complexes suffer from slow formation rates given that the $t_{1/2}$ of ^{212}Bi is 60 minutes (111).

TETA

1,4,8,11-tetraazacyclododecane-1,4,8,11-tetraacetic acid (TETA) (103) is similar to DOTA, but is built on the larger 14-membered 1,4,8,11-tetraazacyclododecane macrocyclic platform commonly referred to as "Cyclam" (Fig. 7.6) (112,113). The first report of TETA being functionalized to create a BCA was published in 1985 (56,114).

Crossbridging polyazamacrocyles produces bicyclic complexes that are more rigid with altered chelate cavity shapes and sizes when compared with their parent structures (115). 1,4,8,11-Tetraaza-bicyclo[6.6.2]hexadecane (CB-Cyclam) is an example of crossbridged polyazamacrocycle which has a cavity correctly sized to bind copper (116–118). The chelate 1,4,8,11-tetraaza-bicyclo[6.6.2]hexadecane-4, 11-diacetic acid (CB-TE2A) (118) is another example of a bicyclic polyaminopolycarboxylate containing two anionic ligands under biologic conditions. Crossbridged chelates have been demonstrated to have better in vivo clearance than other chelates without a crossbridge. This improved clearance is attributed to a reduction in transchelation to biologically

FIGURE 7.6 TETA, common points (R, R', R", R‴) at which TETA can be functionalized to act as a BCA, Cyclam, cross-linked TETA derivative CB-TE2A.

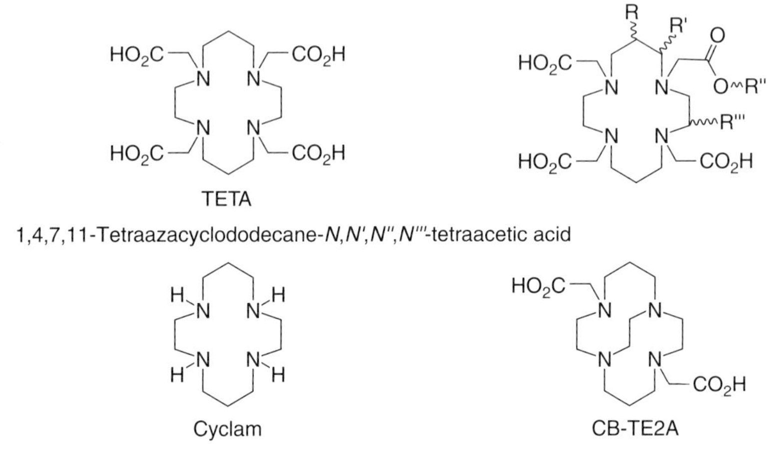

TETA

1,4,7,11-Tetraazacyclododecane-*N*,*N'*,*N"*,*N‴*-tetraacetic acid

Cyclam

CB-TE2A

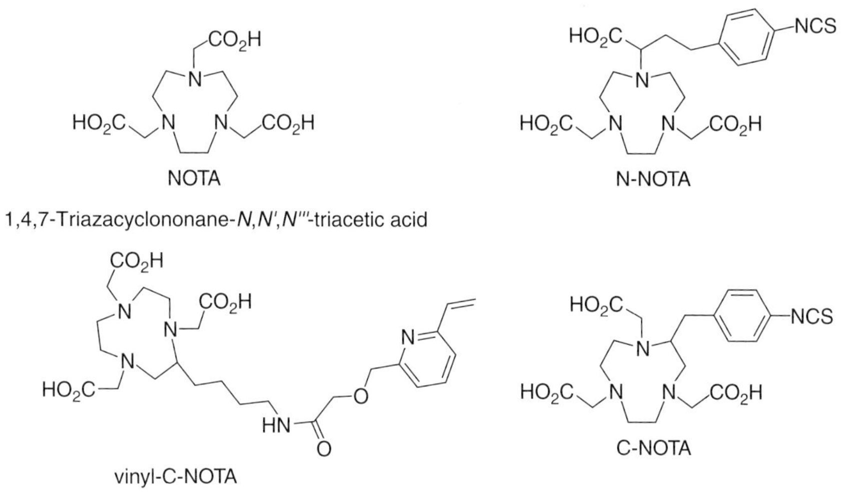

FIGURE 7.7 NOTA, vinyl-C-NOTA (122), N-NOTA (123), and C-NOTA (123,124).

NOTA

1,4,7-Triazacyclononane-*N*,*N*',*N*'''-triacetic acid

vinyl-C-NOTA

C-NOTA

native chelates (119,120). A BCA derivative of CB-TE2A was recently reported for the chelation of copper RNs (121).

NOTA

1,4,7-Triazacyclononane-1,4,7-triacetic acid (NOTA or TCTA) is assembled on a nine-membered triazacyclononane macrocycle (Fig. 7.7) (122–124). The unmodified NOTA was first reported in 1982 and a C-functionalized BCA variation was described in 1989 (122,125). The initial BCA report included triazamacrocycles consisting of 9-, 10-, 11-, and 12-membered rings in which the ethyl segments were sequentially changed to propyl groups. The relative rate of indium uptake by these triazamacrocycles was reported as 9 > 10 >> 12 > 11 member rings (122). Most subsequent work with triazamacrocycles has focused on NOTA often as a chelate for Cu(II) (126) and Ga(III) (127,128).

Other polyaminopolycarboxylate ligands

This is just a brief survey of what is a rather large array of polyaminopolycarboxylate ligands that have been investigated for use as BCAs (Fig. 7.8) (129–137). Many others chelates have been explored (138,139). Larger bifunctional macrocycles such as PCBA, PEPA, and HEHA have been

reported in the literature for use with various RNs such as ^{225}Ac(III), ^{203}Pb(II), $^{203/205}$Bi(III) (134–136,140), and ^{67}Cu(II) (29). The amines are not always fully saturated with acetates as is the case with DO2A. There are also bicyclic variations such as Et-Cyclam and polyamino polycyclic cage systems such as SarAr that have also been evaluated for use in BFC systems with ^{64}Cu(II) (130–133).

■ ALTERNATIVE SIDE CHAINS

There are many synthetic options that could be applied during the BCA synthesis to alter the chemical identity of the acetate side chains. The carboxylic acid can be substituted with an endless array of Lewis base functionalities such as amides, alcohols, pyridines, benzimidazoles, and alkanes to name just a few (141,142). Each of these modifications fundamentally alters chelation behavior. The side chain can also be extended with the addition of methylene groups or other spacers to increase the distance between the amine and side chain Lewis acid, which has a major impact on chelate stability since many metallic ions prefer a five-membered chelation ring, although some specifically do prefer a six-membered chelation ring (Fig. 7.9) (40,143–145).

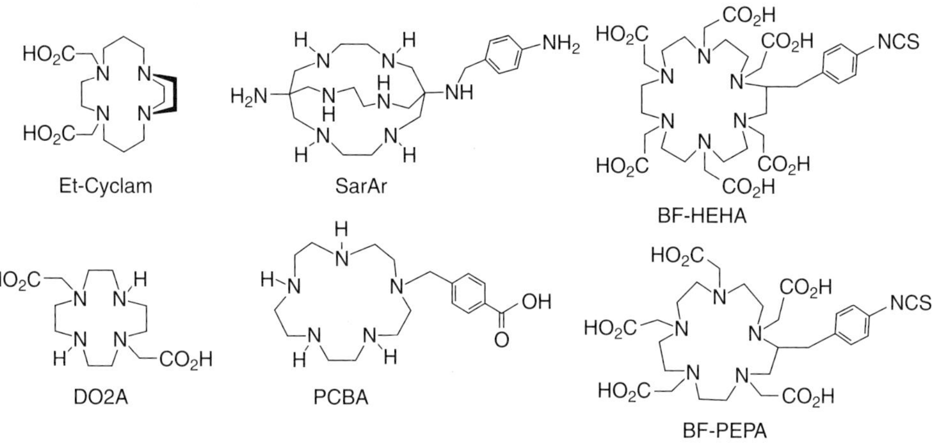

FIGURE 7.8 Et-Cyclam (129), SarAr (130–133), DO2A (129), PCBA (134,135), PEPA (136), and HEHA (137).

Et-Cyclam

SarAr

BF-HEHA

DO2A

PCBA

BF-PEPA

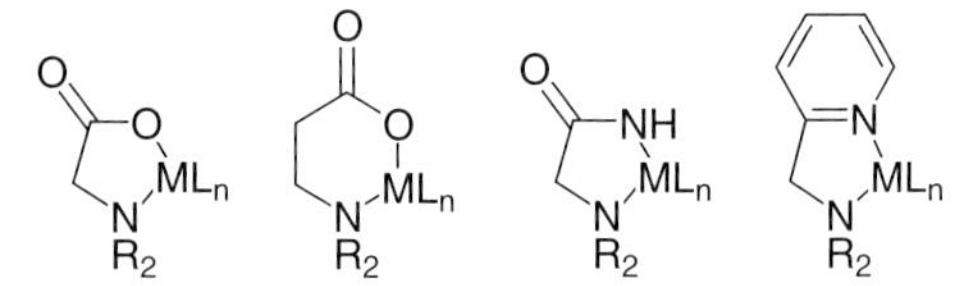

FIGURE 7.9 Examples of a five-membered and six-membered chelation rings as well as examples of amidate and pyridine side chains.

Hydroxymates

The hydroxymate functional group goes by a variety of names including hydroxamic acid. Hydroxymate-containing molecules represent a considerable fraction of documented siderophores, the molecules that organisms naturally employ to sequester iron (146,147). One example of such siderophores is deferoxamine commonly referred to as "Desferal." In addition to its use to treat iron overload (148–152) and also as a cancer therapeutic in its own right (153,154), deferoxamine also has been modified with a useful functional group to be a BCA for ^{89}Zr (155,156) and ^{67}Ga (157–159).

Trisuccin, N-[tris[2-[(N-hydroxy-amino)carbonyl]ethyl] methyl]succinamic acid is a BCA with three hydroxymate groups (Fig. 7.10). The trisuccin chelate has been used with ^{99m}Technetium and ^{188}Rhenium although the actual structures of the complexes are unknown (160–165).

One of the challenges of working with hydroxymates as chelates is developing structures that accommodate the hydroxymate's electronic preference to bond to a Lewis acid through both of its oxygen atoms (166). In the case of trisuccin, even though there are three hydroxymate groups, it seems unlikely that all three hydroxymates are coordinated to the metal center at the same time due to steric strain (167,168).

Gallium exclusive ligands

Gallium is both included and excluded from lists of therapeutic RNs but does have many gallium exclusive ligands (Fig. 7.11) (169–175). Gallium has isotopes that provide useful β^- decay for radioimmunotherapy or β^+ for positron emission tomography imaging; however, ^{67}Ga also possesses a significant Auger emission at 7.4 keV electrons

with a range of 1.63 μm (176,177). Auger emitters have a high level of cytotoxicity to cells while in the immediate vicinity of their DNA; however, this emission lacks the range of even α particles, which are limited to 50 to 100 μm depending on the α particle's initial energy. There have been several examples of Auger emitters that may have a role as a therapeutic, even if their clinical use is limited to eradication of microscopic residual disease (178,179).

The ligands explored for gallium include polyaminopolycarboxylate ligands, in particular NOTA (180). There has also been work with a modified versions of NOTA in which the carboxylate groups have been exchanged for phosphonate groups (127). Gallium(III) complexes strongly with a variety of Lewis bases which has resulted in some unique research with unique chelates. Examples of the usual chelates for a BCA include Schiff bases of [(4,6-MeO$_2$sal)$_2$BAPEN (169,170). As a soft ion, Ga(III) complexes strongly with soft thiolate ligands such as those in BAT-TECH (171,172) and tris(2-mercaptobenzyl)amine (S$_3$N) (Fig. 7.11) (173).

N$_3$S and N$_2$S$_2$

Polyamide or polyamine polythiolate ligands of the N$_3$S and N$_2$S$_2$ configuration are tetradentate basal plane chelates that were developed with the intent of stabilizing Re and Tc RNs in vivo (181,182). Similar N$_2$S$_2$ ligands, bis(thiosemicarbazone) ligands, which chelate Cu^{2+} RNs have been modified to act as BCA that can be attached to amino acids and peptides such as octreotide (183).

Bifunctional N$_3$S ligands were reported with ^{99m}Tc in 1988 (184) and soon reported for use with rhenium via a prelabeling pathway (185,186). Bifunctional N$_2$S$_2$ ligands were also first reported in 1988 for ^{99m}Tc (53,187); the vast majority of work still continues with ^{99m}Tc with a much smaller body of work concerned with Re RNs (188–191). The N$_3$S and N$_2$S$_2$ chelates have been covalently linked to BM through functional groups on their carbon backbone as well as internal and terminal amine/amides (Fig. 7.12) (23,30,53,183,192–201). The structural and functional group variations on these ligands are highly diverse, which is directly related to the large body of research into the use of ^{99m}Tc. The ligands form stable oxo-Re(V) complexes.

FIGURE 7.10 Functionalized hydroxymate-based BCAs.

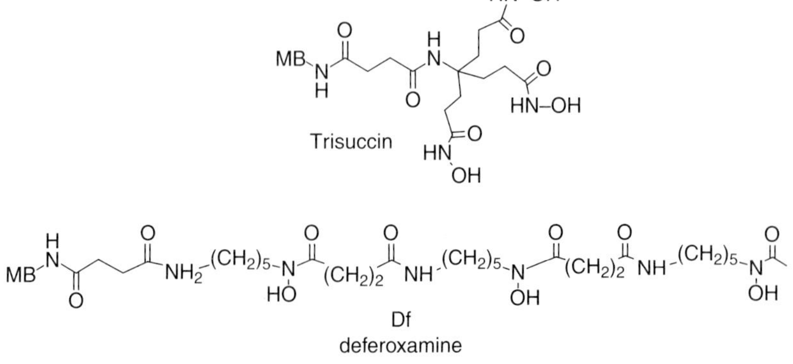

Trisuccin

Df
deferoxamine

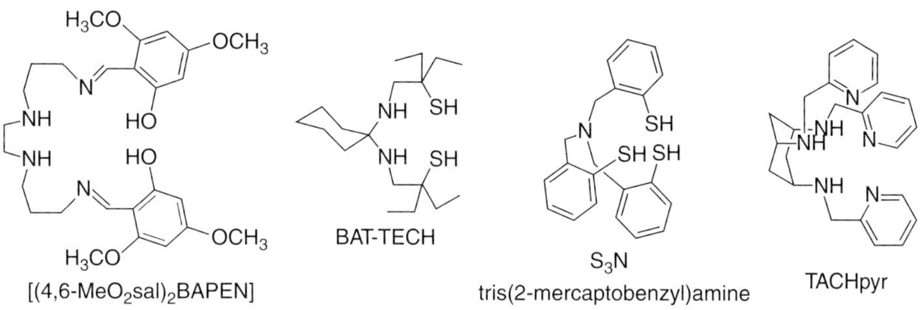

FIGURE 7.11 [(4,6-MeO$_2$sal)$_2$BAPEN] (169,170), BAT-TECH (171,172), tris(2-mercaptobenzyl)amine (S$_3$N) (173), and *N,N,N*-tris(2-pyridylmethyl)-*cis,cis*-1,3,5-triaminocyclohexane (TACHpyr) (174,175).

RHENIUM AND TECHNETIUM AND RN CORES

The chemistry of rhenium and technetium has recently been reviewed (23). Rhenium and technetium have more possible coordination environments than any other commonly used medical RN. Although it is reasonable to treat most RNs as if they are simple monatomic ions, this assumption does not necessarily make sense for all rhenium and technetium species. A number of the rhenium and technetium systems are better treated as polyatomic cores structure. The core structure includes inert coligands that are unreactive under biologic conditions as listed in Table 7.3.

Although the logic is somewhat circular, the oxo and nitrido ligands, common to several "cores," are said to help stabilize the metal center in its high oxidation. Oxidation through hydrolysis to a metal oxide is a common degradation pathway for high valent metal. Incorporating one or two oxo (or nitrido) donors into the core structure theoretically reduces the driving force to initiate an uncontrolled reaction cascade to the fully oxidized metal center.

Technetium's radio properties, specifically ^{99m}Tc ($t_{1/2} = 6$ hours; 141 keV γ-ray emission) is appropriate for imaging. Rhenium provides a complementary therapeutic RN, ^{188}Re ($t_{1/2} = 16.98$ hours) with a high-energy β^--emission ($E_{max} = 2.12$ MeV, 85% abundance) along with 155 keV γ photons (15% abundance) and ^{186}Re ($t_{1/2} = 87$ hours) with a β^--emission ($E_{max} = 1.07$ MeV) along with 137 keV γ photons (9% abundance). Rhenium and technetium belong to the same column of the periodic table and thus share similar reactivities, oxidation states, and coordination geometries. However,

labeling with ^{188}Re often requires a low pH, high temperatures, and long reaction times when compared with the facile conditions that can be used with ^{99m}Tc. Lower kinetic liability and harsher reaction conditions are expected for third-row transition metals, such as rhenium, when compared with the corresponding second row transition metal, technetium. One method to overcome these challenges is to resort to prelabeling strategies rather than postlabeling.

Diazenido

The pyridyl azide ligand, 6-hydrazinopridine-3-carboxylic acid (Hynic), forms monodentate diazenido (of organohydrazide) (Fig. 7.13) complexes with Re(V) and Tc(V). Diazenido single point of contact forms an extremely chemical inert linkage with a formal bond order greater than one. Diazenido ligands such as Hynic are limited to early transition metal centers, whereas late transition metal, main group metal, and f-block metal centers are not known or expected to support biologically stable metal-diazenido bonds (202,203). Work with aromatic hydrazides was pioneered on cold rhenium (204–206), which inspired the creation of the Hynic BCA for use with ^{99m}Tc in 1990 (207,208).

The diazenido ligands, such as Hynic, take up only one coordination site on Re(V) and Tc(V) complexes leaving five coordination sites to be filled by coligand(s). The coligand(s) play a significant role in the chemistry and biologic activity of Hynic complexes. Weak field coligands such as glucoheptonate and tricine facilitate labeling efficiency. However,

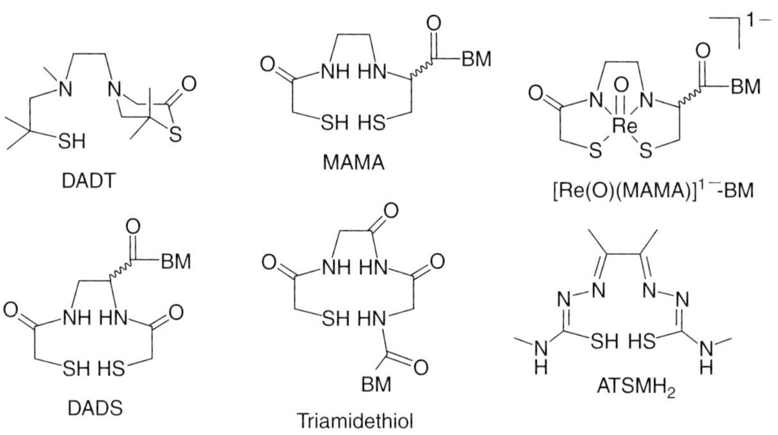

DADT

MAMA

[Re(O)(MAMA)]$^{1-}$-BM

DADS

Triamidethiol

ATSMH$_2$

FIGURE 7.12 N$_3$S and N$_2$S$_2$ are tetradentate basal plane chelates (23,30,192). Diaminedithiol (DADT) (193–196), diamidedisulfide (DADS) (53,193,197,198), monoaminemonoamide (MAMA) (119), triamidethiol (200,201), and bis(thiosemicarbazone) (ATSMH$_2$) (183).

Table **7.3**   **Polyatomic core structures of rhenium and technetium**

Core (M = Tc, Re)	Charge	Valence Description	HSAB	Ideal Coordination Number, Geometry (Preferred Chelate)
M(V) = O	3+	d^2	Hard	5, Square pyramidal (basal plain chelate)
M(V) = N	2+	d^2	Hard	5–6, (basal plain chelate)
M(V) = (O)$_2$	1+	d^2	Soft	6, Octahedral (basal plain chelate)
M(I)(CO)$_3$	1+	d^6	Soft	6, Octahedral (facial chelate)

HSAB, hard soft acid base.

these weak ligands have also been attributed to complex instability (209,210).

The in vivo stability advantage afforded by conjugating stronger field coligands and the synthetic advantages noted during coordination to Hynic, afforded by weak field coligands, have influenced synthetic methodologies. A metal center (RN) decorated with weak field coligands can be coordinated to the Hynic after which the RN's weak field ligands are exchanged for higher field ligands. Examples of higher field coligands and coligand mixtures include ethylenediamine-N,N'-diacetate (EDDA) (209–211), tricine/phosphine (212–214), tricine/pyridine (209,211,215), and tricine/acetonitrile (216).

Tricarbonyl core supporters

The tricarbonyl core is a coordination environment that is limited to Re(I) and Tc(I) as medically relevant RN. Both Re(I) and Tc(I) are transition metals with a d^6 electron configuration that favors an octahedral coordination sphere. In the wider world of inorganic chemistry, this structural format is a very common core that has been well explored. The versatility of the tricarbonyl core is only partially demonstrated in Figure 7.14. The Re(I) and Tc(I) tricarbonyl cores have three open, facially oriented, coordination sites. This geometry allows for the use of many BCA chelates, examples include tri-, bi-, and even monodentate BCAs. Notably among the BCA used with the tricarbonyl are the cyclopentadienyl (Cp) derivatives in which the Cp acts as a η 5 facial ligand filling three of the RN coordination cites (217–219). Cp tricarbonyl

FIGURE 7.13 The uncoordinated 6-hydrazinopridine-3-carboxylic acid (Hynic) and BCA variation attached to a BM and coordinating Re(V). The overall charge of the complex is dependant on the coligands and protonation state of the Hynic ligand.

complexes are common enough in organometallic chemistry to be referred to as "piano stool" complexes. The Cp ligand has a low molecular weight, lower than even the monodentate Hynic. Minimizing the size, but more importantly the chemical profile of an RN–BCA complex, minimizes how the BCA might impact bioactivity of the BM once incorporated into an RN–BCA–BM. This makes it ideal for use with small BMs such as estradiol (217).

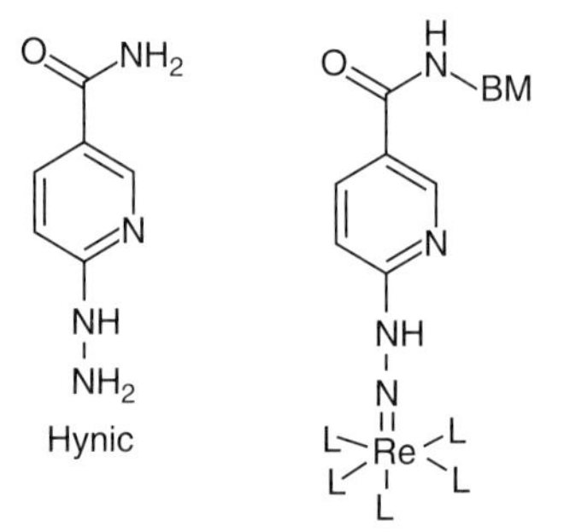

Phosphines

Phosphines are not well known as biologic Lewis bases, predominantly because of the ease with which most phosphines oxidize; simple exposure to air is enough in many cases which would severely limit their use for this application. Still, a number of systems containing phosphine chelates are used in medical imaging such as [Tc(V)(O)$_2$-(bis(di-2-ethoxyethyl)phosphino]ethane]$^+$ known as Myoview (220). Although they have not yet been functionalized as BCAs, diphospines have been explored as chelate supports for copper RNs (221). Other phosphines have been explored for use within BCA systems (222).

Phosphines featuring electron withdrawing hydroxymethyl substituents have the combined benefits of being water soluble and resistant to oxidation (222). In addition, a hydroxymethyl group coordinated to a phosphine will readily react with amines potentially allowing for coordination to BM. When P(CH$_2$OH)$_3$ is used as a coligand with bidentate ligands on tricarbonyl Tc(I) cores, reduced kidney uptake has been reported (223).

The use of protonated phosphine has been applied to preparation of synthetic organic catalysts under ambient conditions avoiding the time and resources necessary to conduct rigorous air-free techniques (224). Phosphines are protonated at pHs that are often too low for BM which may or may not require the use of a prelabeling technique if the use of protonated phosphines was imported to the synthesis of radiotherapeutics.

CONCLUSIONS

Evaluation

This chapter details a snapshot of the total BCA systems that have been reported in the literature. Suffice it to say, there are a plethora of reported BCAs. However, there is limited data actually directly comparing these systems with each other.

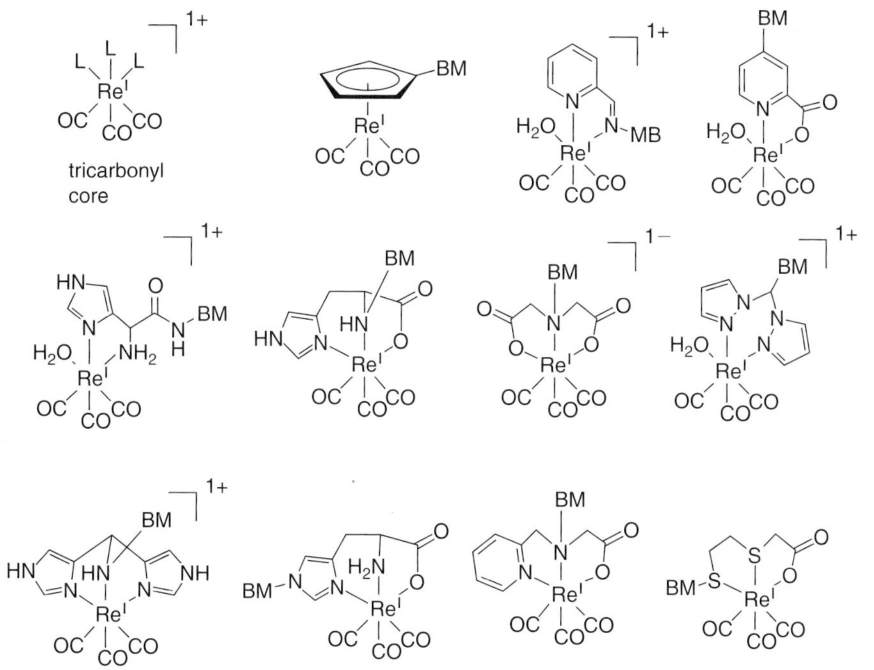

FIGURE 7.14 Collection of ligand supports for the $Re^I(CO)_3$ core.

There is a need for a "standard" method by which these systems can be compared quantitatively relative to each other.

The quality of a chelate for containing a specific ion is often discussed in terms of its stability constant ($\log(\beta)$), formation constant (K_f), binding constant (K_f), and dissociation constant (K_d). Here again the language can be a challenge. Formally, β is intended to represent a sum of formation constants, K_f. Although formation constants are often expressed in the negative log "p" scale (pK_f), the sum is β expressed in a positive log scale. Although this ensures that the relevant $\log(\beta)$ is positive, it also means these values are equivalent to negative log of dissociation constants, pK_d. Equations 7.1 through 7.3 illustrate how this relates to a BCA, chelating an RN. In this situation, β and K_f are equivalent as are $\log(\beta)$ and pK_d. Context usually indicates the specific convention, but nonetheless the use of multiple conventions is less than ideal.

$$RN + BCA \rightleftharpoons [RN - BCA]. \qquad \text{(Eq. 7.1)}$$

$$\beta = K_f = (K_d)^{-1} = [RN - BCA]/([RN][BCA]). \qquad \text{(Eq. 7.2)}$$

$$\log(\beta) = -pK_f = pK_d. \qquad \text{(Eq. 7.3)}$$

In terms of obtaining equilibrium constants, it is advantageous because multiple ways are available to measure equilibrium constants (225–228). Stability constants can clearly demonstrate the advantage of increasing the level of preorganization in derivatives of EDTA and the significant advantage DTPA has over EDTA in chelating Y^{3+}, In^{3+}, and Bi^{3+} (Table 7.4).

Yet, these noncompetitive stability constants are also oversimplifications that set a maximum possible stability when it comes to estimating RN–BCA stability under biologic conditions. The BCA must compete with protons, Ca^{2+}, Cu^{2+}, Zn^{2+}, Fe^{3+}, and other biologically abundant cations to retain the RN. The RN is also attracted to hydroxide, phosphates, amino acids, and other biologically abundant Lewis bases (229,230). Even with a perfectly complete competitive biologic stability constant, this physical measurement would still only be an indirect gauge by which to predict in vivo stability. In addition, thermodynamic *stability constants cannot accurately represent the "kinetic inertness" of an RN–BCA complex under relevant biologic conditions.*

Although in vitro and in vivo studies are components of most research projects, it is also true that every group tailors these studies to present their system in the best possible light. Although this practice is more than understandable as every group struggles to continue to publish and gain funding, it also obfuscates relevant direct comparisons

Table **7.4**	Selected stability constants ($\log(\beta)$) for acyclic polyaminocarboxylate chelates (37)			
	EDTA	**Me-EDTA**	**CDTA**	**DTPA**
Y^{3+}	18.09	18.78	19.85	22.13
In^{3+}	24.9		28.8	29.0
Bi^{3+}	27.8		32.4	35.6

between systems. A "standard" study would focus solely on the stability of the RN–BCA complex that controls for biodistribution and clearance effects which could ultimately be altered by BM and any PKM linkers.

The incorporation of functional groups to attach the chelate to a BM adds another dimension. Two different BCAs will likely link to the same BM differently at some undefined level. Labeling the BCA–BM molecule with an RN will likely have variable success. Different research projects use different BM to explore different biologic models of disease. A standard protocol to study the value of BCA would require a standard biologic model; it does not even need to be a disease model, but just a model that exposes the RN–BCA to relevant biologic conditions with an appropriate time component. The assay would need a BM which is representative of relevant BM in terms of size and ability to link to BCA. The BM would need to be stable and clear via the renal system with a reasonable half-life so that any instability in the BM would not interfere in exploring the stability of the RN–BCA component. Such a protocol would not capture the value of all systems, but it would be preferable to have a literature filled with standard comparisons with arguments for the specific values of a given system than a collection of systems, each studied on their own terms, making direct comparisons nearly impossible.

SUMMARY

Many of the well-established "stock" BCAs were first introduced in the late 1980s and early 1990s. Ultimately, research will involve tailoring BCAs for specific oxidation states of specific RNs. A "one size fits all conditions" approach does not match with the reality of the coordination chemistry of the relevant RNs. These RN–BCAs by necessity will be easy to form and extremely stable under in vivo conditions.

Perhaps the more substantial work needs to be done in developing simple methods to selectively produce conformers of RN–BCA–BM complexes. This will involve developing stereochemical and conformational selective synthesis of BCAs that also provides for selective couplings of BCA with BM in terms of stoichiometry and site-specificity. Still, refining such systems eventually reaches a point of diminishing returns. Often, biologic agents have no need to reach chemical purity expected by researcher in small molecule synthesis; a distribution of products can be good enough. The efforts to modify RN–BCA–BM complexes with PKA linkers have been very successful. PKM will surely be an important component in developing and maximizing the efficacy of any RN–BCA–BM complex for use as a therapeutic (33).

Acknowledgment

This work was supported by the Intramural Research Program of the NIH, National Cancer Institute, Center for Cancer Research.

REFERENCES

1. Lindenmann J. Origin of the terms antibody and antigen. *Scand J Immunol.* 1984;19(4):281–285.
2. Ehrlich P. Ueber Immunitat durch Vererbung und Saugung. *Z Gesamte Hyg.* 1892;12:183–203.
3. Winau F, Westphal O, Winau R. Paul Ehrlich—in search of the magic bullet. *Microbes Infect.* 2004;6(8):786–789.
4. Schwaber J, Cohen EP. Human×mouse somatic cell hybrid clone secreting immunoglobulins of both parental types. *Nature.* 1973;244(5416):444–447.
5. Kohler G, Milstein C. Continuous cultures of fused cells secreting antibody of predefined specificity. *Nature.* 1975;256(5517):495–497.
6. Cambrosio A, Keating P. Between fact and technique—the beginnings of hybridoma technology. *J Hist Biol.* 1992;25(2):175–230.
7. Andersen O. Principles and recent developments in chelation treatment of metal intoxication. *Chem Rev.* 1999;99(9):2683–2710.
8. Foreman H, Hamilton JG. The Use of Chelating Agents for Accelerating Excretion of Radioelements; 1951. Report No. AECD-3247.
9. Foreman H. Toxicology of radioactive materials. *Ann Rev Med.* 1958;9:369–386.
10. Leckie WJ, Tompsett SL. The diagnostic and therapeutic use of edathamil calcium disodium (EDTA, versene) in excessive inorganic lead absorption. *Q J Med.* 1958;27(105):65–82.
11. Rubin M, Gignac S, Bessman SP, et al. Enhancement of lead excretion in humans by disodium calcium ethylenediamine tetraacetate. *Science.* 1953;117(3050):659–660.
12. Kroll H, Korman S, Siegel E, et al. Excretion of yttrium and lanthanum chelates of cyclohexane 1,2-trans diamine tetraacetic acid and diethylenetriamine pentaacetic acid in man. *Nature.* 1957;180(4592):919–920.
13. Dutreix J, Tubiana M, Pierquin B. The hazy dawn of brachytherapy. *Radiother Oncol.* 1998;49(3):223–232.
14. Benisek WF, Richards FM. Attachment of metal-chelating functional groups to hen egg white lysozyme—an approach to introducing heavy atoms into protein crystals. *J Biol Chem.* 1968;243(16):4267–4271.
15. Sundberg MW, Meares CF, Goodwin DA, et al. Chelating agents for the binding of metal ions to macromolecules. *Nature.* 1974;250(5467):587–588.
16. Sundberg MW, Meares CF, Goodwin DA, et al. Selective binding of metal ions to macromolecules using bifunctional analogs of EDTA. *J Med Chem.* 1974;17(12):1304–1307.
17. Sundberg MW, Meares CF, Werthemann L, inventors; The Board of Trustees of the Leland Stanford Junior University, assignee. Chelating agents patent 3994966. 1976.
18. Anderson CJ, Welch MJ. Radiometal-labeled agents (non-technetium) for diagnostic imaging. *Chem Rev.* 1999;99(9):2219–2234.
19. Milenic DE, Brady ED, Brechbiel MW. Antibody-targeted radiation cancer therapy. *Nat Rev Drug Discov.* 2004;3(6):488–499.
20. Brechbiel MW. Bifunctional chelates for metal nuclides. *Q J Nucl Med Mol Imaging.* 2008;52(2):166–173.
21. Okarvi SM. Peptide-based radiopharmaceuticals and cytotoxic conjugates: potential tools against cancer. *Cancer Treat Rev.* 2008;34(1):13–26.
22. Liu S. Bifunctional coupling agents for radiolabeling of biomolecules and target-specific delivery of metallic radionuclides. *Adv Drug Deliv Rev.* 2008;60(12):1347–1370.
23. Liu G, Hnatowich DJ. Labeling biomolecules with radiorhenium: a review of the bifunctional chelators. *Anticancer Agents Med Chem.* 2007;7(3):367–377.
24. Hassfjell S, Brechbiel MW. The development of the alpha-particle emitting radionuclides Bi-212 and Bi-213, and their decay chain related radionuclides, for therapeutic applications. *Chem Rev.* 2001;101(7):2019–2036.
25. Volkert WA, Hoffman TJ. Therapeutic radiopharmaceuticals. *Chem Rev.* 1999;99(9):2269–2292.
26. Heeg MJ, Jurisson SS. The role of inorganic chemistry in the development of radiometal agents for cancer therapy. *Acc Chem Res.* 1999;32:1053–1060.
27. Liu S, Edwards DS. Bifunctional chelators for therapeutic lanthanide radiopharmaceuticals. *Bioconjug Chem.* 2001;12(1):7–34.
28. Parker D. Tumor targeting with radiolabeled macrocycle antibody conjugates. *Chem Soc Rev.* 1990;19:271–291.
29. Wadas TJ, Wong EH, Weisman GR, et al. Copper chelation chemistry and its role in copper radiopharmaceuticals. *Curr Pharm Des.* 2007;13(1):3–16.

30. Bartholoma M, Valliant J, Maresca KP, et al. Single amino acid chelates (SAAC): a strategy for the design of technetium and rhenium radiopharmaceuticals. *Chem Commun (Camb)*. 2009(5):493–512.

31. Gansow OA. Newer approaches to the radiolabeling of monoclonalantibodies by use of metal chelates. *Nucl Med Biol*. 1991;18:369–381.

32. Williams DR. Metals, ligands, and cancer. *Chem Rev*. 1972;72(3):203–213.

33. Pearson RG, Songstad J. Application of principle of hard and soft acids and bases to organic chemistry. *J Am Chem Soc*. 1967;89:1827–1836.

34. Pearson RG. Hard and soft acids and bases HSAB. 2. Underlying theories. *J Chem Educ*. 1968;45:643–648.

35. Pearson RG. Hard and soft acids and bases HSAB. 1. Fundamental principles. *J Chem Educ*. 1968;45:581–587.

36. Pearson RG. Hard and soft acids and bases—the evolution of a chemical concept. *Coord Chem Rev*. 1990;100:403–404.

37. Martell AE, Smith RM. *Critical Stability Constants*. New York, NY: Plenum Press; 1974.

38. Roselli M, Schlom J, Gansow OA, et al. Comparative biodistribution studies of DTPA-derivative bifunctional chelates for radiometal labeled monoclonal antibodies. *Nucl Med Biol*. 1991;18(4):389–394.

39. Wu C, Kobayashi H, Sun B, et al. Stereochemical influence on the stability of radio-metal complexes in vivo. Synthesis and evaluation of the four stereoisomers of 2-(p-nitrobenzyl)-trans-CyDTPA. *Bioorg Med Chem*. 1997;5(10):1925–1934.

40. Martell AE, Hancock RD, Motekaitis RJ. Factors affecting stabilities of chelate, macrocyclic and macrobicyclic complexes in solution. *Coord Chem Rev*. 1994;133:39–65.

41. Shannon RD. Revised effective ionic radii and systematic studies of interatomic distances in halides and chalcogenides. *Acta Crystallogr Sect A*. 1976;32:751–767.

42. Green MLH. A new approach to the formal classification of covalent compounds of the elements. *J Organomet Chem*. 1995;500:127–148.

43. Norenberg JP, Krenning BJ, Konings IR, et al. Bi-213-[DOTA(0),Tyr(3)] octreotide peptide receptor radionuclide therapy of pancreatic tumors in a preclinical animal model. *Clin Cancer Res*. 2006;12:897–903.

44. Meares CF, McCall MJ, Reardan DT, et al. Conjugation of antibodies with bifunctional chelating agents: isothiocyanate and bromoacetamide reagents, methods of analysis, and subsequent addition of metal ions. *Anal Biochem*. 1984;142:68–78.

45. Brechbiel MW, Gansow OA, Atcher RW, et al. Synthesis of 1-(p-isothiocyanatobenzyl) derivatives of DTPA and EDTA-antibody labeling and tumor-imaging studies. *Inorg Chem*. 1986;25:2772–2781.

46. Knor S, Modlinger A, Poethko T, et al. Synthesis of novel 1,4,7,10-tetraazacyclododecane-1,4,7,10-tetraacetic acid (DOTA) derivatives for chemoselective attachment to unprotected polyfunctionalized compounds. *Chemistry*. 2007;13:6082–6090.

47. Prasuhn DE, Yeh RM, Obenaus A, et al. Viral MRI contrast agents: coordination of Gd by native virions and attachment of Gd complexes by azide-alkyne cycloaddition. *Chem Commun*. 2007;12:1269–1271.

48. Mindt TL, Struthers H, Brans L, et al. "Click to chelate": synthesis and installation of metal chelates into biomolecules in a single step. *J Am Chem Soc*. 2006;128:15096–15097.

49. Hoare DG, Koshland DE Jr. A method for quantitative modification and estimation of carboxylic acid groups in proteins. *J Biol Chem*. 1967;242:2447–2453.

50. Paik CH, Ebbert MA, Murphy PR, et al. Factors influencing DTPA conjugation with antibodies by cyclic DTPA anhydride. *J Nucl Med*. 1983;24:1158–1163.

51. Krejcarek GE, Tucker KL. Covalent attachment of chelating groups to macromolecules. *Biochem Biophys Res Commun*. 1977;77:581–585.

52. Hnatowich DJ, Layne WW, Childs RL. The preparation and labeling of DTPA-coupled albumin. *Int J Appl Radiat Isot*. 1982;33:327–332.

53. Rao TN, Adhikesavalu D, Camerman A, et al. Technetium(V) and rhenium(V) complexes of 2,3-bis(mercaptoacetamido)propanoate. Chelate ring stereochemistry and influence on chemical and biological properties. *J Am Chem Soc*. 1990;112:5798–5804.

54. Lewis MR, Raubitschek A, Shively JE. A facile, water-soluble method for modification of proteins with DOTA. Use of elevated temperature and optimized pH to achieve high specific activity and high chelate stability in radiolabeled immunoconjugates. *Bioconjug Chem*. 1994;5:565–576.

55. Lewis MR, Shively JE. Maleimidocysteineamido-DOTA derivatives: new reagents for radiometal chelate conjugation to antibody sulfhydryl groups undergo pH-dependent cleavage reactions. *Bioconjug Chem*. 1998;9:72–86.

56. McCall MJ, Diril H, Meares CF. Simplified method for conjugating macrocyclic bifunctional chelating agents to antibodies via 2-iminothiolane. *Bioconjug Chem*. 1990;1(3):222–226.

57. Kramer SP, Goodman LE, Dorfman H, et al. Enzyme alterable alkylating agents. 6. Synthesis, chemical properties, toxicities, and clinical trial of haloacetates and haloacetamides containing enzyme-susceptible bonds. *J Natl Cancer Inst*. 1963;31:297–327.

58. Cohen LA. Group-specific reagents in protein chemistry. *Ann Rev Biochem*. 1968;37:695–726.

59. Meares CF, Goodwin DA. Linking radiometals to proteins with bifunctional chelating agents. *J Protein Chem*. 1984;3:215–228.

60. Rodwell JD, Alvarez VL, Lee C, et al. Site-specific covalent modification of monoclonal antibodies: in vitro and in vivo evaluations. *Proc Natl Acad Sci U S A*. 1986;83:2632–2636.

61. Fritzberg AR, Wilbur DS, Srinivasan A, et al., inventors; Neorx Corporation, assignee. Minimal derivatization of proteins patent 5059541. 1991.

62. Li WP, Lewis JS, Kim J, et al. DOTA-D-Tyr(1)-octreotate: a somatostatin analogue for labeling with metal and halogen radionuclides for cancer imaging and therapy. *Bioconjug Chem*. 2002;13:721–728.

63. Bailon P, Palleroni A, Schaffer CA, et al. Rational design of a potent, long-lasting form of interferon: a 40 kDa branched polyethylene glycol-conjugated interferon alpha-2a for the treatment of hepatitis C. *Bioconjug Chem*. 2001;12:195–202.

64. Yang K, Basu A, Wang M, et al. Tailoring structure-function and pharmacokinetic properties of single-chain Fv proteins by site-specific PEGylation. *Protein Eng*. 2003;16:761–770.

65. Gestin JF, Faivre-Chauvet A, Mease RC, et al. Introduction of five potentially metabolizable linking groups between 111In-cyclohexyl EDTA derivatives and F(ab')2 fragments of anti-carcinoembryonic antigen antibody—1. A new reproducible synthetic method. *Nucl Med Biol*. 1993;20:755–762.

66. Faivrechauvet A, Gestin JF, Mease RC, et al. Introduction of five potentially metabolizable linking groups between 111In-cyclohexyl EDTA derivatives and F(Ab')2 fragments of anticarcinoembryonic antigen-antibody—2. Comparative pharmacokinetics and biodistribution in human colorectal carcinoma-bearing nude mice. *Nucl Med Biol*. 1993;20:763–771.

67. Studer M, Meares CF. A convenient and flexible approach for introducing linkers on bifunctional chelating agents. *Bioconjug Chem*. 1992;3(5):420–423.

68. Li M, Meares CF. Synthesis, metal chelate stability studies, and enzyme digestion of a peptide-linked DOTA derivative and its corresponding radiolabeled immunoconjugates. *Bioconjug Chem*. 1993;4:275–283.

69. Peterson JJ, Meares CF. Enzymatic cleavage of peptide-linked radiolabels from immunoconjugates. *Bioconjug Chem*. 1999;10(4):553–557.

70. Breeman WAP, De Jong MTM, De Blois E, et al. Reduction of skeletal accumulation of radioactivity by co-injection of DTPA in [Y-90-DOTA(0),Tyr(3)]octreotide solutions containing free Y-90(3+). *Nucl Med Biol*. 2004;31(6):821–824.

71. McMurry TJ, Brechbiel M, Kumar K, et al. Convenient synthesis of bifunctional tetraaza macrocycles. *Bioconjug Chem*. 1992;3:108–117.

72. Chappell LL, Rogers BE, Khazaeli MB, et al. Improved synthesis of the bifunctional chelating agent 1,4,7,10-tetraaza-N-(1-carboxy-3-(4-nitrophenyl)propyl)-N',N'',N'''-tris(acetic acid)cyclododecane (PA-DOTA). *Bioorg Med Chem*. 1999;7:2313–2320.

73. Chappell LL, Ma D, Milenic DE, et al. Synthesis and evaluation of novel bifunctional chelating agents based on 1,4,7,10-tetraazacyclododecane-N,N',N'',N'''-tetraacetic acid for radiolabeling proteins. *Nucl Med Biol*. 2003;30:581–595.

74. Das T, Chakraborty S, Banerjee S, et al. Preparation and animal biodistribution of 166Ho labeled DOTA for possible use in intravascular radiation therapy (IVRT). *J Labelled Compd Radiopharm*. 2003;46:197–209.

75. Summers SP, Abboud KA, Farrah SR, et al. Syntheses and structures of bismuth(III) complexes with nitrilotriacetic acid, ethylenediaminetetraacetic acid, and diethylenetriaminepentaacetic acid. *Inorg Chem*. 1994;33:88–92.

76. Munz F, inventor; IG Farbenindustrie AG, assignee. [DE] Verfahren zum Unschaedlichmachen der Haertebildner des Wassers Germany patent DE000000718981A 1936 26.03. 1942.

77. Fick R, Ulrich H, inventors; IG Farbenindustrie AG, assignee. Amino nitriles and amino acids. DE patent 638071. 1936.

78. Munz F, inventor; General Aniline Works, assignee. Polyamino carboxylic acids. US patent 2130505. 1938.

79. Curme GO Jr, Chitwood HC, Clark JW, inventors; Carbide and Carbon Chemicals Corp., assignee. Amino carboxylic acids and their salts. US patent 2384816. 1945.

80. Khaw BA, Fallon JT, Strauss HW, et al. Myocardial infarct imaging of antibodies to canine cardiac myosin with indium-111-diethylenetriamine pentaacetic acid. *Science.* 1980;209(4453):295–297.

81. Kozak RW, Atcher RW, Gansow OA, et al. Bismuth-212-labeled anti-Tac monoclonal antibody: alpha-particle-emitting radionuclides as modalities for radioimmunotherapy. *Proc Natl Acad Sci U S A.* 1986; 83:474–478.

82. Macklis RM, Kinsey BM, Kassis AI, et al. Radioimmunotherapy with alpha-particle emitting immunoconjugates. *Science.* 1988;240:1024–1026.

83. Hnatowich DJ, Layne WW, Childs RL, et al. Radioactive labeling of antibody: a simple and efficient method. *Science.* 1983;220:613–615.

84. Hnatowich DJ, Lanteigne D, Childs RL, et al. Re: concerning the labeling of DTPA-coupled proteins with Tc-99m. *J Nucl Med.* 1983;24(6): 544–555.

85. Layne WW, Hnatowich DJ, Doherty PW, et al. Evaluation of the viability of In-111-labeled DTPA coupled to fibrinogen. *J Nucl Med.* 1982;23(7):627–630.

86. Sharkey RM, Mottahennessy C, Gansow OA, et al. Selection of a DTPA chelate conjugate for monoclonal-antibody targeting to a human colonic tumor in nude-mice. *Int J Cancer.* 1990;46(1):79–85.

87. Milenic DE, Garmestani K, Chappell LL, et al. In vivo comparison of macrocyclic and acyclic ligands for radiolabeling of monoclonal antibodies with 177Lu for radioimmunotherapeutic applications. *Nucl Med Biol.* 2002;29(4):431–442.

88. Sun YZ, Martell AE, Motekaitis RJ, et al. Synthesis and stabilities of the Ga(III) and In(III) chelates of a new diaminodithiol bifunctional ligand. *Tetrahedron.* 1998;54:4203–4210.

89. Yeh SM, Meares CF, Goodwin DA. Decomposition rates of radiopharmaceutical indium chelates in serum. *J Radioanal Chem.* 1979;53:327–336.

90. Camera L, Kinuya S, Garmestani K, et al. Comparative biodistribution of indium- and yttrium-labeled B3 monoclonal antibody conjugated to either 2-(p-SCN-Bz)-6-methyl-DTPA (1B4M-DTPA) or 2-(p-SCN-Bz)-1,4,7,10-tetraazacyclododecane tetraacetic acid (2B-DOTA). *Eur J Nucl Med.* 1994;2:640–646.

91. Dexter M, inventor; Geigy AG JR, assignee. [DE] Verfahren zur Herstellung von neuen alicyclischen Polyaminopolyessigsaeuren bzw. deren komplexen Metallverbindungen. 1963.

92. Mease RC, Srivastava SC. The synthesis of semi-rigid polyaminocarboxylates as new bifunctional chelating-agents. *J Nucl Med.* 1988;29: 1324–1325.

93. Brechbiel MW, Pippin CG, McMurry TJ, et al. An effective chelating agent for labeling of monoclonal antibody with Bi-212 for alpha-particle mediated radioimmunotherapy. *J Chem Soc Chem Commun.* 1991;1(17):1169–1170.

94. Brechbiel MW, Gansow OA. Synthesis of C-functionalized trans-cyclohexyldiethylenetriaminepenta-acetic acids for labeling of monoclonal antibodies with the bismuth-212 alpha-particle emitter. *J Chem Soc Perkin Trans 1.* 1992;7(9):1173–1178.

95. Konings MS, Dow WC, Love DB, et al. Gadolinium complexation by a new DTPA amide ligand-amide oxygen coordination. *Inorg Chem.* 1990;29:1488–1491.

96. Bligh SWA, Chowdhury AHMS, Mcpartlin M, et al. Neutral gadolinium(III) complexes of bulky octadentate DTPA derivatives as potential contrast agents for magnetic resonance imaging. *Polyhedron.* 1995;14:567–569.

97. Jenkins BG, Lauffer RB. Solution structure and dynamics of lanthanide(III) complexes of diethylenetriaminepentaacetate—a two-dimensional NMR analysis. *Inorg Chem.* 1988;27:4730–4738.

98. Liu S, Cheung E, Rajopadhye M, et al. Isomerism and solution dynamics of (90)Y-labeled DTPA–biomolecule conjugates. *Bioconjug Chem.* 2001;12:84–91.

99. Lammers H, Maton F, Pubanz D, et al. Structures and dynamics of lanthanide(III) complexes of sugar-based DTPA-bis(amides) in aqueous solution: a multinuclear NMR study. *Inorg Chem.* 1997;36:2527–2538.

100. Ma DH, McDevitt MR, Finn RD, et al. Rapid preparation of short-lived alpha particle emitting radioimmunopharmaceuticals. *Appl Radiat Isot.* 2001;55:463–470.

101. Kennel SJ, Stabin M, Roeske JC, et al. Radiotoxicity of bismuth-213 bound to membranes of monolayer and spheroid cultures of tumor cells. *Radiat Res.* 1999;151(3):244–256.

102. Johnson DK, Kline SJ, inventors; Abbott Laboratories, assignee. Bifunctional chelating agents patent 5057302. 1991.

103. Stetter H, Frank W. Complex-formation with tetraazacycloalkane-*N,N',N'',N'''*-tetraacetic acids as a function of ring size. *Angew Chem Int Edit Engl.* 1976;15:686.

104. Viola-Villegas N, Doyle RP. The coordination chemistry of 1,4,7,10-tetraazacyclododecane-*N,N',N'',N'''*-tetraacetic acid (H(4)DOTA): structural overview and analyses on structure-stability relationships. *Coord Chem Rev.* 2009;253:1906–1925.

105. Desreux JF. Nuclear magnetic resonance spectroscopy of lanthanide complexes with a tetraacetic tetraaza macrocycle—unusual conformation properties. *Inorg Chem.* 1980;19:1319–1324.

106. Moreau J, Guillon E, Pierrard JC, et al. Complexing mechanism of the lanthanide cations Eu^{3+}, Gd^{3+}, and Tb^{3+} with 1,4,7,10-tetrakis(carboxymethyl)-1,4,7,10-tetraazacyclododecane (dota)—characterization of three successive complexing phases: study of the thermodynamic and structural properties of the complexes by potentiometry, luminescence spectroscopy, and EXAFS. *Chemistry.* 2004;10:5218–5232.

107. Moi MK, Meares CF, DeNardo SJ. The peptide way to macrocyclic bifunctional chelating agents: synthesis of 2-(p-nitrobenzyl)-1,4,7,10-tetraazacyclododecane-*N,N',N'',N'''*-tetraacetic acid and study of its yttrium(III) complex. *J Am Chem Soc.* 1988;110(18):6266–6267.

108. Venkatesh M, Pandey U, Dhami PS, et al. Complexation studies with Y-90 from a novel Sr-90-Y-90 generator. *Radiochim Acta.* 2001;89:413–417.

109. Pandey U, Mukherjee A, Sarma HD, et al. Evaluation of 90Y-DTPA and 90Y-DOTA for potential application in intra-vascular radionuclide therapy. *Appl Radiat Isot.* 2002;57(3):313–318.

110. Horak E, Hartmann F, Garmestani K, et al. Radioimmunotherapy targeting of HER2/neu oncoprotein on ovarian tumor using lead-212-DOTA-AE1. *J Nucl Med.* 1997;38(12):1944–1950.

111. Ruegg CL, Andersonberg WT, Brechbiel MW, et al. Improved in vivo stability and tumor targeting of bismuth-labeled antibody. *Cancer Res.* 1990;50(14):4221–4226.

112. Delgado R, Felix V, Lima LM, et al. Metal complexes of cyclen and cyclam derivatives useful for medical applications: a discussion based on thermodynamic stability constants and structural data. *Dalton Trans.* 2007;26:2734–2745.

113. Barefield EK, Wagner F, Hodges KD. Synthesis of macrocyclic tetramines by metal-ion assisted cyclization reactions. *Inorg Chem.* 1976;15:1370–1377.

114. Moi MK, Meares CF, McCall MJ, et al. Copper chelates as probes of biological systems: stable copper complexes with a macrocyclic bifunctional chelating agent. *Anal Biochem.* 1985;148(1):249–253.

115. Springborg J. Adamanzanes—bi- and tricyclic tetraamines and their coordination compounds. *Dalton Trans.* 2003;9:1653–1665.

116. Weisman GR, Rogers ME, Wong EH, et al. Cross-bridged cyclam—protonation and Li+ complexation in a diamond-lattice cleft. *J Am Chem Soc.* 1990;112:8604–8605.

117. Weisman GR, Wong EH, Hill DC, et al. Synthesis and transition-metal complexes of new cross-bridged tetraamine ligands. *J Chem Soc Chem Commun.* 1996:947–948.

118. Wong EH, Weisman GR, Hill DC, et al. Synthesis and characterization of cross-bridged cyclams and pendant-armed derivatives and structural studies of their copper(II) complexes. *J Am Chem Soc.* 2000;122:10561–10572.

119. Boswell CA, Sun X, Niu W, et al. Comparative in vivo stability of copper-64-labeled cross-bridged and conventional tetraazamacrocyclic complexes. *J Med Chem.* 2004;47(6):1465–1474.

120. Sprague JE, Peng YJ, Sun XK, et al. Preparation and biological evaluation of copper-64-labeled Tyr(3)—octreotate using a cross-bridged macrocyclic chelator. *Clin Cancer Res.* 2004;10(24):8674–8682.

121. Boswell CA, Regino CA, Baidoo KE, et al. Synthesis of a cross-bridged cyclam derivative for peptide conjugation and Cu-64 radiolabeling. *Bioconjug Chem.* 2008;19(7):1476–1484.

122. Craig AS, Helps IM, Jankowski KJ, et al. Towards tumor imaging with In-111 labeled macrocycle antibody conjugates. *J Chem Soc Chem Commun.* 1989;12:794–796.

123. McMurry TJ, Brechbiel M, Wu CC, et al. Synthesis of 2-(p-thiocyanatobenzyl)-1,4,7-triazacyclononane-1,4,7-triacetic acid—application of the 4-methoxy-2,3,6-trimethylbenzenesulfonamide protecting group in the synthesis of macrocyclic polyamines. *Bioconjug Chem.* 1993;4:236–245.

124. Studer M, Meares CF. Synthesis of novel 1,4,7-triazacyclononane-*N,N',N''*-triacetic acid derivatives suitable for protein labeling. *Bioconjug Chem.* 1992;3(4):337–341.

125. Wieghardt K, Bossek U, Chaudhuri P, et al. 1,4,7-Triazacyclononane-*N,N',N"*-triacetate (TCTA), a new hexadentate ligand for divalent and trivalent metal ions crystal structures of [CrIII(TCTA)], [FeIII(TCTA)], and Na[CuII(TCTA)]. 2NaBr·8H₂O. *Inorg Chem.* 1982;21:4308–4314.

126. Prasanphanich AF, Retzloff L, Lane SR, et al. In vitro and in vivo analysis of [64Cu-NO2A-8-Aoc-BBN(7-14)NH₂]: a site-directed radiopharmaceutical for positron-emission tomography imaging of T-47D human breast cancer tumors. *Nucl Med Biol.* 2009;36(2):171–181.

127. Prata MIM, Santos AC, Geraldes CFGC, et al. Characterisation of Ga-67(3+) complexes of triaza macrocyclic ligands: biodistribution and clearance studies. *Nucl Med Biol.* 1999;26:707–710.

128. Broan CJ, Cox JPL, Craig AS, et al. Structure and solution stability of indium and gallium complexes of 1,4,7-triazacyclononanetriacetate and of yttrium complexes of 1,4,7,10-tetraazacyclododecanetetraacetate and related ligands-kinetically stable complexes for use in imaging and radioimmunotherapy-X-ray molecular structure of the indium and gallium complexes of 1,4,7-triazacyclononane-1,4,7-triacetic acid. *J Chem Soc Perkin Trans 2.* 1991;1:87–99.

129. Jones-Wilson TM, Deal KA, Anderson CJ, et al. The in vivo behavior of copper-64-labeled azamacrocyclic complexes. *Nucl Med Biol.* 1998;25:523–530.

130. Di Bartolo NM, Sargeson AM, Donlevy TM, et al. Synthesis of a new cage ligand, SarAr, and its complexation with selected transition metal ions for potential use in radioimaging. *J Chem Soc Dalton Trans.* 2001;15:2303–2309.

131. Di Bartolo N, Sargeson AM, Smith SV. New 64Cu PET imaging agents for personalised medicine and drug development using the hexa-aza cage, SarAr. *Org Biomol Chem.* 2006;4:3350–3357.

132. Voss SD, Smith SV, DiBartolo N, et al. Positron emission tomography (PET) imaging of neuroblastoma and melanoma with 64Cu-SarAr immunoconjugates. *Proc Natl Acad Sci U S A.* 2007;104(44):17489–17493.

133. Smith SV. Molecular imaging with copper-64. *J Inorg Biochem.* 2004;98(11):1874–1901.

134. Deal KA, Davis IA, Mirzadeh S, et al. Improved in vivo stability of actinium-225 macrocyclic complexes. *J Med Chem.* 1999;42(15):2988–2992.

135. Kennel SJ, Chappell LL, Dadachova K, et al. Evaluation of Ac-225 for vascular targeted radioimmunotherapy of lung tumors. *Cancer Biotherapy Radiopharm.* 2000;15(3):235–244.

136. Dadachova E, Chappell LL, Brechbiel MW. Spectrophotometric method for determination of bifunctional macrocyclic ligands in macrocyclic ligand-protein conjugates. *Nucl Med Biol.* 1999;26(8):977–982.

137. Brechbiel MW, Deal KA, Chappell LL, et al. Development of a bifunctional chelating agent suitable for radioimmunotherapy using actinium-225. *Abstr Pap Am Chem Soc.* 1999;218:U970.

138. Chong HS, Milenic DE, Garmestani K, et al. In vitro and in vivo evaluation of novel ligands for radioimmunotherapy. *Nucl Med Biol.* 2006;33(4):459–467.

139. Chong HS, Lim S, Baidoo KE, et al. Synthesis and biological evaluation of a novel decadentate ligand DEPA. *Bioorg Med Chem Lett.* 2008;18(21):5792–5795.

140. Garmestani K, Yao Z, Zhang M, et al. Synthesis and evaluation of a macrocyclic bifunctional chelating agent for use with bismuth radionuclides. *Nucl Med Biol.* 2001;28(4):409–418.

141. Keire DA, Kobayashi M. NMR studies of the metal-loading kinetics and acid-base chemistry of DOTA and butylamide-DOTA. *Bioconjug Chem.* 1999;10(3):454–463.

142. Szilagyi E, Toth E, Kovacs Z, et al. Equilibria and formation kinetics of some cyclen derivative complexes of lanthanides. *Inorg Chim Acta.* 2000;298:226–234.

143. Hancock RD, Martell AE. Ligand design for selective complexation of metal ions in aqueous solution. *Chem Rev.* 1989;89:1875–1914.

144. Redin K, Wilson AD, Newell R, et al. Studies of structural effects on the half-wave potentials of mononuclear and dinuclear nickel(II) diphosphine/dithiolate complexes. *Inorg Chem.* 2007;46(4):1268–1276.

145. Cukrowski I, Cukrowska E, Hancock RD, et al. The effect of chelate ring size on metal-ion size-based selectivity in polyamine ligands containing pyridyl and saturated nitrogen donor groups. *Anal Chim Acta.* 1995;312:307–321.

146. Miller MJ. Syntheses and therapeutic potential of hydroxamic acid based siderophores and analogs. *Chem Rev.* 1989;89:1563–1579.

147. Codd R. Traversing the coordination chemistry and chemical biology of hydroxamic acids. *Coord Chem Rev.* 2008;252:1387–1408.

148. Kontoghiorghes GJ, Pattichi K, Hadjigavriel M, et al. Transfusional iron overload and chelation therapy with deferoxamine and deferiprone (L1). *Transfus Sci.* 2000;23(3):211–223.

149. Medini I, McDonough EA, Nelson SC. A novel approach to iron chelation therapy: twice-daily subcutaneous injections of deferoxamine in the treatment of transfusional iron overload in pediatric patients. *Blood.* 1998;92:31b–31b.

150. Schafer AI, Rabinowe S, Leboff MS, et al. Long-term efficacy of deferoxamine iron chelation therapy in adults with acquired transfusional iron overload. *Arch Inter Med.* 1985;145(7):1217–1221.

151. Cooper B, Bunn HF, Propper RD, et al. Treatment of iron overload in adults with continuous parenteral desferrioxamine. *Am J Med.* 1977;63(6):958–966.

152. Propper RD, Cooper B, Rufo RR, et al. Continuous subcutaneous administration of deferoxamine in patients with iron overload. *N Engl J Med.* 1977;297:418–423.

153. Becton DL, Roberts B. Antileukemic effects of deferoxamine on human myeloid leukemia cell lines. *Cancer Res.* 1989;49(17):4809–4812.

154. Hoffbrand AV, Ganeshaguru K, Hooton JW, et al. Effect of iron deficiency and desferrioxamine on DNA synthesis in human cells. *Br J Haematol.* 1976;33(4):517–526.

155. Meijs WE, Herscheid JDM, Haisma HJ, et al. Evaluation of desferal as a bifunctional chelating agent for labeling antibodies with Zr-89. *Int J Rad Appl Instrum A.* 1992;43(12):1443–1447.

156. Govindan SV, Michel RB, Griffiths GL, et al. Deferoxamine as a chelator for Ga-67 in the preparation of antibody conjugates. *Nucl Med Biol.* 2005;32:513–519.

157. Ryser JE, Jones RML, Egeli R, et al. Colon carcinoma immunoscintigraphy by monoclonal anti-CEA antibody labeled with gallium-67-aminooxyacetyldeferoxamine. *J Nucl Med.* 1992;33(10):1766–1773.

158. Yokoyama A, Ohmomo Y, Horiuchi K, et al. Deferoxamine, a promising bifunctional chelating agent for labeling proteins with gallium: Ga-67 Df-HSA—concise communication. *J Nucl Med.* 1982;23(10):909–914.

159. Ward MC, Roberts KR, Westwood JH, et al. The effect of chelating agents on the distribution of monoclonal antibodies in mice. *J Nucl Med.* 1986;27(11):1746–1750.

160. Safavy A, Buchsbaum DJ, Khazaeli MB. Synthesis of *N*-[tris[2-[[N-(benzyloxy)amino]carbonyl]ethyl]methyl]succinamic acid, trisuccin. Hydroxamic acid derivatives as a new class of bifunctional chelating agents. *Bioconjug Chem.* 1993;4(3):194–198.

161. Safavy A, Sanders A, Qin H, et al. Conjugation of unprotected trisuccin, *N*-[tris[2-[(N-hydroxyamino)carbonyl]ethyl]methyl]succinamic acid, to monoclonal antibody CC49 by an improved active ester protocol. *Bioconjug Chem.* 1997;8(5):766–771.

162. Safavy A, Khazaeli MB, Mayo MS, et al. Synthesis, rhenium-188 labeling and biodistribution studies of a phenolic ester derivative of trisuccin. *Cancer Biother Radiopharm.* 1997;12(6):375–384.

163. Safavy A, Khazaeli MB, Kirk M, et al. Further studies on the protein conjugation of hydroxamic acid bifunctional chelating agents: group-specific conjugation at two different loci. *Bioconjug Chem.* 1999;10(1):18–23.

164. Safavy A, Khazaeli MB, Qin H, et al. Synthesis of bombesin analogs for radiolabeling with rhenium-188. *Cancer.* 1997;80(12 suppl):2354–2359.

165. Safavy A, Khazaeli MB, Safavy K, et al. Biodistribution study of 188Re-labeled trisuccin-HuCC49 and trisuccin-HuCC49ΔCH2 conjugates in athymic nude mice bearing intraperitoneal colon cancer xenografts. *Clin Cancer Res.* 1999;5(10 suppl):2994s–3000s.

166. Koshti N, Huber V, Smith P, et al. Design and synthesis of actinide specific chelators—synthesis of new cyclam tetrahydroxamate (cytrox) and cyclam tetraacetonylacetone (cytac) chelators. *Tetrahedron.* 1994;50:2657–2664.

167. King TJ, Harrison PG. Crystal and molecular structure of triphenyltin *N*-benzoyl-*N*-phenylhydroxamate. *J Chem Soc Chem Commun.* 1972;13:815–816.

168. Kongprakaiwoot N, Noll BC, Brown SN. Tetradentate bis(hydroxamate) and hydroxamate-diketonate ligands and their titanium(IV) complexes. *Inorg Chem.* 2008;47(24):11902–11909.

169. Tsang BW, Mathias CJ, Green MA. A gallium-68 radiopharmaceutical that is retained in myocardium: 68Ga[(4,6-MeO2sal)2BAPEN]+. *J Nucl Med.* 1993;34(7):1127–1131.

170. Tsang BW, Mathias CJ, Fanwick PE, et al. Structure-distribution relationships for metal-labeled myocardial imaging agents: comparison of a series of cationic gallium(III) complexes with hexadentate bis(salicylaldimine) ligands. *J Med Chem.* 1994;37(25):4400–4406.

171. Kung HF, Liu BL, Mankoff D, et al. A new myocardial imaging agent—synthesis, characterization, and biodistribution of gallium-68-bat-tech. *J Nucl Med.* 1990;31(10):1635–1640.

172. Francesconi LC, Liu BL, Billings JJ, et al. Synthesis, characterization and solid-state structure of a neutral gallium(III) amino thiolate complex—a potential radiopharmaceutical for pet imaging. *J Chem Soc Chem Commun.* 1991;2:94–95.

173. Cutler CS, Giron MC, Reichert DE, et al. Evaluation of gallium-68 tris(2-mercaptobenzyl)amine: a complex with brain and myocardial uptake. *Nucl Med Biol.* 1999;26(3):305–316.

174. Park G, Przyborowska AM, Ye N, et al. Steric effects caused by *N*-alkylation of the tripodal chelator *N*,*N′*,*N″*-tris(2-pyridylmethyl)-*cis*,*cis*-1,3,5-triaminocyclohexane (tachpyr): structural and electronic properties of the Mn(II), Co(II), Ni(II), Cu(II) and Zn(II) complexes. *Dalton Trans.* 2003;3:318–324.

175. Samuni AM, Krishna MC, DeGraff W, et al. Mechanisms underlying the cytotoxic effects of Tachpyr—a novel metal chelator. *Biochim Biophys Acta.* 2002;1571(3):211–218.

176. O'Donoghue JA, Wheldon TE. Targeted radiotherapy using Auger electron emitters. *Phys Med Biol.* 1996;41:1973–1992.

177. Howell RW. Radiation spectra for auger-electron emitting radionuclides: Report No. 2 of AAPM Nuclear Medicine Task Group No. 6. *Med Phys.* 1992;19(6):1371–1383.

178. Makrigiorgos G, Adelstein SJ, Kassis AI. Auger-electron emitters—insights gained from in vitro experiments. *Radiat Environ Biophys.* 1990;29(2):75–91.

179. Michel RB, Brechbiel MW, Mattes MJ. A comparison of 4 radionuclides conjugated to antibodies for single-cell kill. *J Nucl Med.* 2003; 44(4):632–640.

180. Griffiths GL, McBride WJ, inventors; Immunomedics, Inc., assignee. Labeling targeting agents with gallium-68 and gallium-67 patent 7011816. 2006 December 13, 2002.

181. Davison A, Jones AG, Orvig C, et al. A new class of oxotechnetium(5+) chelate complexes containing a TcON2S2 core. *Inorg Chem.* 1981;20:1629–1632.

182. Davison A, Jones AG, Orvig C, et al. A series of oxotechnetium(+5) chelate complexes containing a TcOS2N2 core. *J Nucl Med.* 1981;22: P57–P58.

183. Cowley AR, Dilworth JR, Donnelly PS, et al. Bifunctional chelators for copper radiopharmaceuticals: the synthesis of [Cu(ATSM)-amino acid] and [Cu(ATSM)-octreotide] conjugates. *Dalton Trans.* 2007;14(2): 209–217.

184. Fritzberg AR, Kasina S, Vanderheyden JL, et al., inventors; Metal-radionuclide-labeled proteins and glycoproteins and their preparation for diagnosis and therapy patent EP 284071. 1988.

185. Breitz HB, Weiden PL, Vanderheyden JL, et al. Clinical experience with rhenium-186-labeled monoclonal antibodies for radioimmunotherapy: results of phase-I trials. *J Nucl Med.* 1989;33:1099–1112.

186. Goldrosen MH, Biddle WC, Pancook J, et al. Biodistribution, pharmacokinetic, and imaging studies with rhenium-186-NR-LU-10 whole antibody in LS1741T colonic tumor-bearing mice. *Cancer Res.* 1990;50(24):7973–7978.

187. Fritzberg AR, Abrams PG, Beaumier PL, et al. Specific and stable labeling of antibodies with technetium-99m with a diamide dithiolate chelating agent. *Proc Natl Acad Sci U S A.* 1988;85(11):4025–4029.

188. Najafi A, Alauddin MM, Siegel ME, et al. Synthesis and preliminary evaluation of a new chelate N2S4 for use in labeling proteins with metallic radionuclides. *Nucl Med Biol.* 1991;18(2):179–185.

189. Najafi A, Alauddin MM, Sosa A, et al. The evaluation of rhenium-186-labeled antibodies using N2S4 chelate in vitro and in vivo using tumor-bearing nude mice. *Nucl Med Biol.* 1992;19:205–212.

190. Jeong JM, Kim YJ, Lee YS, et al. Lipiodol solution of a lipophilic agent, 188Re-TDD, for the treatment of liver cancer. *Nucl Med Biol.* 2001; 28(2):197–204.

191. Lee YS, Jeong JM, Kim YJ, et al. Synthesis of 188Re-labeled long chain alkyl diaminedithiol for therapy of liver cancer. *Nucl Med Commun.* 2002;23(3):237–242.

192. Stalteri MA, Bansal S, Hider R, et al. Comparison of the stability of technetium-labeled peptides to challenge with cysteine. *Bioconjug Chem.* 1999;10(1):130–136.

193. Baidoo KE, Lever SZ. Synthesis of a diaminedithiol bifunctional chelating agent for incorporation of technetium-99m into biomolecules. *Bioconjug Chem.* 1990;1:132–137.

194. Kung HF, Molnar M, Billings J, et al. Synthesis and biodistribution of neutral lipid-soluble Tc-99m complexes that cross the blood-brain barrier. *J Nucl Med.* 1984;25(3):326–332.

195. Lever SZ, Burns HD, Kervitsky TM, et al. Design, preparation, and biodistribution of a technetium-99m triaminedithiol complex to assess regional cerebral blood flow. *J Nucl Med.* 1985;26(11):1287–1294.

196. Oneil JP, Wilson SR, Katzenellenbogen JA. Preparation and structural characterization of monoamine-monoamide bis(thiol) oxo complexes of technetium(V) and rhenium(V). *Inorg Chem.* 1994;33:319–323.

197. Jones AG, Davison A, Lategola MR, et al. Chemical and in vivo studies of the anion oxo[*N*,*N′*-ethylenebis(2-mercaptoacetimido)]technetate(V). *J Nucl Med.* 1982;23(9):801–809.

198. Brenner D, Davison A, Listerjames J, et al. Synthesis and characterization of a series of isomeric oxotechnetium(V) diamido dithiolates. *Inorg Chem.* 1984;23:3793–3797.

199. Meegalla SK, Plossl K, Kung MP, et al. Synthesis and characterization of technetium-99m-labeled tropanes as dopamine transporter-imaging agents. *J Med Chem.* 1997;40(1):9–17.

200. Vanbilloen HP, De Roo MJ, Verbruggen AM. Complexes of technetium-99m with tetrapeptides containing one alanyl and three glycyl moieties. *Eur J Nucl Med.* 1996;23(1):40–48.

201. Vanbilloen HP, Bormans GM, Deroo MJ, et al. Complexes of Tc-99m with tetrapeptides, a new class of Tc-99m-labeled agents. *Nucl Med Biol.* 1995;22(3):325–338.

202. Sutton D. Organometallic diazo compounds. *Chem Rev.* 1993;93:995–1022.

203. Sutton D. Coordination chemistry of aryldiazonium cations—aryldiazenato (arylazo) complexes of transition metals, and aryldiazenato-nitrosyl analogy. *Chem Soc Rev.* 1975;4:443–470.

204. Duckworth VF, Douglas PG, Mason R, et al. A phenylazo-complex of rhenium(III)-structure of Re(N2C6H5)Cl2P)CH3)2C6H5!3. *J Chem Soc D Chem Commun.* 1970;17:1083.

205. Nicholson T, Zubieta J. Complexes of rhenium with benzoylazo and related ligands—crystal and molecular structures of the green chelate benzoylazo complex [ReCl2(PPH3)2(NNCOC6H4-para-Cl)],(N-alpha,o), of the analogous 1-azophthalazine chelate complex [ReCl2(PPh3)2(NNC8H5N2)](N-alpha,N1), and of the *cis*-dichloro organodiazenido complexes of the type [ReCl2(PPh3)2(NNR)NCCH3], [ReCl2(PPH3)2(NNR)NH3], [ReCl2(PPh3)2(NNR)C5H5N]—a comparison to the structure of the trans-dichlorodimethylformamide derivative[ReCl2(PPh3)2(NNCO2CH3)(Me2NCHO)]—the structural characterization of the mixed hydrazido(1-) hydrazido(2-)complexes [ReCl2(PPH3)2(NNHR)(NHNHR')], (R = R′ = −COC6H5, R = −COC6H5, R′ = −CO2CH3). *Polyhedron.* 1988;7:171–185.

206. Chatt J, Dilworth JR, Gunz HP, et al. Interaction of dinitrogen complexes of rhenium and osmium with metal salts. *J Chem Soc D Chem Commun.* 1997;2:90.

207. Abrams MJ, Juweid M, TenKate CI, et al. Technetium-99m-human polyclonal IgG radiolabeled via the hydrazino nicotinamide derivative for imaging focal sites of infection in rats. *J Nucl Med.* 1990;31(12):2022–2028.

208. Schwartz DA, Abrams MJ, Hauser MM, et al. Preparation of hydrazino-modified proteins and their use for the synthesis of technetium-99m-protein conjugates. *Bioconjug Chem.* 1991;2(5):333–336.

209. Decristoforo C, Mather SJ. Preparation, 99mTc-labeling, and in vitro characterization of HYNIC and N3S modified RC-160 and [Tyr3]octreotide. *Bioconjug Chem.* 1999;10(3):431–438.

210. Liu S, Edwards DS, Looby RJ, et al. Labeling a hydrazino nicotinamide-modified cyclic IIb/IIIa receptor antagonist with 99mTc using aminocarboxylates as coligands. *Bioconjug Chem.* 1996;7(1):63–71.

211. Decristoforo C, Mather SJ. Technetium-99m somatostatin analogues: effect of labelling methods and peptide sequence. *Eur J Nucl Med.* 1999;26(8):869–876.

212. Edwards DS, Liu S, Barrett JA, et al. New and versatile ternary ligand system for technetium radiopharmaceuticals: water soluble phosphines and tricine as coligands in labeling a hydrazinonicotinamide-modified cyclic glycoprotein IIb/IIIa receptor antagonist with 99mTc. *Bioconjug Chem.* 1997;8(2):146–154.

213. Guo WJ, Hinkle GH, Lee RJ. Tc-99m-HYNIC-folate: a novel receptor-based targeted radiopharmaceutical for tumor imaging. *J Nucl Med.* 1999;40:1563–1569.

214. Ono M, Arano Y, Uehara T, et al. Intracellular metabolic fate of radioactivity after injection of technetium-99m-labeled hydrazino nicotinamide derivatized proteins. *Bioconjug Chem.* 1999;10(3):386–394.

215. Liu S, Edwards DS, Harris AR. A novel ternary ligand system for 99mTc-labeling of hydrazino nicotinamide-modified biologically active molecules using imine-*N*-containing heterocycles as coligands. *Bioconjug Chem.* 1998;9(5):583–595.

216. Liu G, Wescott C, Sato A, et al. Nitriles form mixed-coligand complexes with 99mTc-HYNIC-Peptide. *Nucl Med Biol.* 2002;29(1):107–113.

217. Top S, Elhafa H, Vessieres A, et al. Rhenium carbonyl complexes of beta-estradiol derivatives with high affinity for the estradiol

receptor—an approach to selective organometallic radiopharmaceuticals. *J Am Chem Soc.* 1995;117:8372–8380.

218. Lavastre I, Besancon J, Brossier P, et al. The synthesis of metallocene-labeled drugs for biological assays. *Appl Organomet Chem.* 1990;4:9–17.

219. Wenzel M. Tc-99m labeling of cymantrene-analogs with different substituents—a new approach to Tc-99m radiodiagnostics. *J Labelled Compd Radiopharm.* 1992;31:641–650.

220. Kelly JD, Forster AM, Higley B, et al. Technetium-99m-tetrofosmin as a new radiopharmaceutical for myocardial perfusion imaging. *J Nucl Med.* 1993;34(2):222–227.

221. Lewis JS, Dearling JLJ, Sosabowski JK, et al. Copper bis(diphosphine) complexes: radiopharmaceuticals for the detection of multidrug resistance in tumours by PET. *Eur J Nucl Med.* 2000;27(6):638–646.

222. Katti KV, Gali H, Smith CJ, et al. Design and development of functionalized water-soluble phosphines: catalytic and biomedical implications. *Acc Chem Res.* 1999;32:9–17.

223. Smith CJ, Sieckman GL, Owen NK, et al. Radiochemical investigations of gastrin-releasing peptide receptor-specific [99mTc(X)(CO)$_3$-Dpr-Ser-Ser-Ser-Gln-Trp-Ala-Val-Gly-His-Leu-Met-(NH$_2$)] in PC-3, tumor-bearing, rodent models: syntheses, radiolabeling, and in vitro/in vivo studies where Dpr = 2,3-diaminopropionic acid and X = H$_2$O or P(CH$_2$OH)$_3$. *Cancer Res.* 2003;63(14):4082–4088.

224. Netherton MR, Fu GC. Air-stable trialkylphosphonium salts: simple, practical, and versatile replacements for air-sensitive trialkylphosphines. Applications in stoichiometric and catalytic processes. *Org Lett.* 2001;3(26):4295–4298.

225. Martell AE, Welch MJ, Motekaitis RJ. A new radiochemical method to determine the stability constants of metal chelates attached to a protein. *J Nucl Med.* 1990;31(10):1744–1745.

226. Subramanian KM, Wolf W. A new radiochemical method to determine the stability constants of metal chelates attached to a protein. *J Nucl Med.* 1990;31(4):480–488.

227. Wu SL, Horrocks WD. General method for the determination of stability constants of lanthanide ion chelates by ligand–ligand competition: laser-excited Eu^{3+} luminescence excitation spectroscopy. *Anal Chem.* 1996;68:394–401.

228. Martell AE, Motekaitis RJ. *Determination and Use of Stability Constants.* 2nd ed. New York, NY: VCH Publishers; 1992.

229. Jackson GE, Wynchank S, Woudenberg M. Gadolinium(III) complex equilibria: the implications for Gd(III) MRI contrast agents. *Magn Reson Med.* 1990;16(1):57–66.

230. Sherry AD, Cacheris WP, Kuan KT. Stability constants for gadolinium(3+) binding to model DTPA-conjugates and DTPA-proteins: implications for their use as magnetic resonance contrast agents. *Magn Reson Med.* 1988;8(2):180–190.

Radiation Dosimetry for Targeted Radionuclide Therapy

Pat B. Zanzonico

■ INTRODUCTION

Historically, nuclear medicine has been largely a diagnostic specialty, with relatively low administered activities yielding important clinical information, the benefit of which far outweighs the small potential risk associated with the attendant low normal tissue radiation doses. Average normal tissue doses received by the "standard" patient, described in package inserts for approved radiopharmaceuticals and in reports issued by authoritative bodies such as the International Commission on Radiation Units and Measurements (ICRU), may deviate from population averages. By incorporation of appropriately large quantities of therapeutic radionuclides into target and tissue-avid radiopharmaceuticals, a sufficiently high radiation dose may be delivered to produce a therapeutic response in tumor or other tissue. With such large administered activities and resulting higher normal tissue doses, serious radiation injury can occur. Radiation dosimetry for radionuclide therapy entails patient-specific determination of radiation doses to "at risk" (therapy-limiting) normal tissues as well as the target tissue(s) in order to prescribe the optimum therapeutic administered activity. In practice, however, such therapy is often administered without performing individualized dosimetry; that is, by administering the same activity to all patients. This chapter reviews the technical aspects of internal radionuclide therapy and the basic approaches to treatment planning (dose prescription) for such therapy, including patient-specific dosimetry, and the advantages and disadvantages of these various approaches.

■ RADIATION QUANTITIES AND UNITS

Definitions of various quantities used to specify radiation "dose" and of selected related quantities are presented below. This represents a comprehensive compilation of System Internationale (SI) and Report Nos. 33 and 60 (1,2) of the ICRU and Report No. 82 (3) of the National Council on Radiation Protection and Measurements (NCRP).

▨ Administered activity

Administered activity is specified by the SI unit becquerel (Bq) (one disintegration per second; dps) or some multiple

thereof. The conventional unit of activity, the curie (Ci), corresponds to 3×10^{10} dps. Note that 37 MBq equals 1 mCi and 37 kBq equals 1 μCi. It is important to distinguish the amount of radioactivity administered from the radiation dose delivered; the radiation dose takes into account the masses of tissues, the kinetics of uptake and clearance of activity in different tissues, the energy deposited in tissues, *the heterogeneity of deposition of radionuclide in the tumor, and the emission properties of the radionuclide.* The term "dose" is often used when referring to the administered activity (mCi or MBq). Strictly speaking, this is incorrect. "Dose," or more specifically "absorbed dose," is a rigorously defined physical quantity (see section "Absorbed dose"). Moreover, while tissue-absorbed doses are related to the administered activity, clinical studies have demonstrated that the administered activity alone is generally *not* a reliable predictor of radiation effect, either therapeutic or toxic.

▨ Absorbed dose

The absorbed dose, D, is perhaps the most widely used and biologically meaningful quantity for expressing radiation dose. Subject to a number of modifying factors, it is probably the best predictor of radiation effect, that is, of the probability and/or severity of the effect. Absorbed dose is defined as follows:

$$D \equiv \frac{\overline{dE}}{dm},$$ (Eq. 8.1)

where $\overline{dE}$ = the mean energy imparted by ionizing radiation to matter

and dm = the mass of matter to which the energy is imparted.

The SI unit of absorbed dose is the gray (1 Gy = 1 J/kg) and the conventional unit is the rad (1 rad = 100 erg/g); 1 Gy equals 100 rad and 1 rad equals 1 cGy (or 10 mGy).

▨ Linear energy transfer

The quality as well as the quantity of absorbed dose of radiation is an important determinant of the frequency and/or severity of radiogenic effects. The "quality" of a radiation is related to the microscopic spatial distribution of its energy-deposition events (ionizations), determined by the mass, charge, and energy (i.e., velocity) of the charged particles comprising the radiation or, in the case of x-rays, γ-rays, and neutrons, the charged particles produced by the radiation. Sparsely ionizing radiations such as x- and γ-rays and intermediate- to high-energy electrons and β-rays are characterized as "low-quality" radiations, while densely ionizing radiations such as low-energy electrons (Auger electrons), protons, neutrons, and α-rays are typically characterized as "high-quality" radiations. Importantly, for the same absorbed dose, the frequency and/or severity of radiogenic biologic effects are generally less for sparsely ionizing, low-quality radiations than for densely ionizing, high-quality radiations.

The quality of radiation is quantitatively characterized by the "linear energy transfer, L" or LET:

$$\text{LET} \equiv \frac{dE}{dl}, \qquad \text{(Eq. 8.2)}$$

where dE is the energy lost by radiation in traversing a distance of dl.

The LET of x-, γ-, and β-rays and conversion electrons is typically of the order of 1 keV/μm; for neutrons and protons it is 10 keV/μm; and for α-rays it is 100 keV/μm (Table 8.1). The actual value of LET for a given radiation is dependent on its energy and is therefore not fixed.

Relative biologic effectiveness

As noted above, for the same absorbed dose, the frequency and/or severity of radiogenic biologic effects are generally less for low-LET than for high-LET radiations. The influence of radiation quality on the frequency and/or severity of biologic effects historically has been quantified by the "relative biologic effectiveness, RBE(A)" of radiation "A" (Fig. 8.1):

$$\text{RBE}(A) \equiv \frac{D_{\text{reference}}}{D_A}, \qquad \text{(Eq. 8.3)}$$

where $D_{\text{reference}}$ = the absorbed dose of reference radiation (typically a widely available low-LET radiation such as cobalt-60 [^{60}Co] γ-rays) required to produce a specific expressed biologic effect

and D_A = the absorbed dose of radiation A required to produce the same specific, quantitative biologic effect with all pertinent parameters maintained as identical as possible except the radiation itself.

Because the relative RBE represents a ratio of absorbed doses, it is a dimensionless quantity.

Table **8.1**	**Physical properties of nuclear radiations**						
Radiation	Structure	Energy, E	Range, R, or Mean Free Path, MFP, in Soft Tissue	Typical LET[a] (kev/μm)	Radiation Weighting Factor, w_R[b]	Typical RBE[c]	Application
Penetrating (p) radiations							
x-ray	Photon	Up to 100 keV	5–10 cm	1	1	1	External imaging
γ-ray	Photon	100–1000 keV	10–20 cm	1	1	~1	External imaging
Nonpenetrating (np) radiations							
β-ray[d]	Negatron, e⁻	50–2000 keV	0.05–5 mm	1	1	~1	Therapy of macroscopic tumors
Conversion electron	Negatron, e⁻	10–500 keV	0.01–1 mm	1–5	1	~1	Therapy of macroscopic tumors
Auger electron	Negatron, e⁻	0.1–1 keV	1–500 nm	5–25	1	5–10 if intranuclear	Therapy, potentially, of single cells if localized in nucleus
α-ray	He nucleus	5–10 MeV	50–100 μm	50–100	20	5–20 if on or in cells	Therapy of single cells or microscopic cell clusters

[a]The actual LET of a given radiation depends on its energy; the LET values presented are representative values for each type of radiation.
[b]Assigned by International Commission on Radiation Units and Measurements (ICRU) for radiation protection purposes.
[c]The actual RBE of a given radiation depends on the specific biologic effect; the RBE values presented are representative values for various deterministic effects for each type of radiation.
[d]Positrons, emitted as positive β-rays, have the same track characteristics as negative β-rays. However, because there are two penetrating 511-keV annihilation γ-rays, which result from positron emission, positrons are not useful therapeutically due to the excessive irradiation of non target (normal) tissues.
LET, linear energy transfer; RBE, relative biologic effectiveness.

FIGURE 8.1 Representation of the dependence of RBE on LET for deterministic effects, specifically in vitro killing of human kidney (T_1) cells. Curves 1 (14.3 cGy), 2 (104 cGy), 3 (192 cGy), and 4 (340 cGy) correspond to cell survivals of 80%, 20%, 5%, and 0.5%, respectively, illustrating the dependence of RBE not only on LET but also on the quantitatively defined biologic effect. High-LET radiation results in a decreasing RBE with decreasing cell survival. As illustrated in the accompanying schematic diagram, as LET increases to approximately 100 keV/μm (typical of α-rays) the average spacing of radiation-induced ionizations (or "hits"), indicated by the asterisks, equals the average separation of the two strands of DNA comprising the double helix, maximizing the likelihood of induction of double-strand DNA damage and thus demonstrable biologic damage *per unit energy deposited*. That, in turn, results in a maximal value of RBE. As the LET continues to increase, the spacing of ionization becomes less than the DNA strand separation, resulting in even greater energy deposition and therefore absorbed dose but with *no* further increase in the likelihood of biologic damage. Beyond approximately 100 keV/μm, the RBE decreases with increasing LET. (Adapted from Refs. 4 and 5).

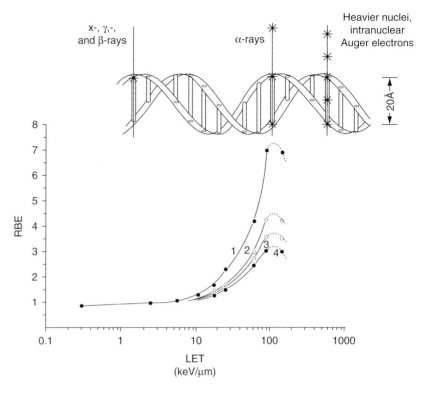

Equivalent dose

For radiation protection purposes, a simplified version of the RBE, the "radiation weighting factor, w_R," has been devised for expressing the relative effectiveness of different radiation in inducing low-level stochastic effects, namely germ-cell mutation and carcinogenesis, which are of greatest practical concern in occupational and diagnostic applications of radiation (6). The so-called "equivalent dose, ED," is related to the radiation weighting factor and the absorbed dose (6):

$$ED \equiv w_R \cdot D \qquad \text{(Eq. 8.4)}$$

The SI unit of equivalent dose is the sievert (Sv) and the conventional unit is the rem; 1 Sv equals 100 rem and 1 rem equals 1 cSv (10 mSv). The values of the radiation weighting factor, w_R, a dimensionless quantity, have been assigned as follows: 1 for x-, γ-, and β-rays; 5 to 10 for neutrons and protons; and 20 for α-rays (3,7).

Unlike the situation for stochastic effects, no well-defined formalism and associated special named quantities have been widely adopted for deterministic effects, which are the effects of greatest clinical concern in radiation therapy, including internal radionuclide therapy. Some scientific organizations have recommended that the RBE for specific deterministic effects be used to weight the absorbed dose for high LET (8). Currently, however, with no special named unit for absorbed doses weighted by deterministic RBE values, there has been some confusion regarding a biologically meaningful expression of dose values related to deterministic effects. The growth in therapeutic use of α-emitting radionuclides (9,10) as well as the advent of proton and other high-LET charged particle beam therapies (11,12) has highlighted the need for such a special named quantity applicable to deterministic effects. Several solutions have been proposed to address this need. For example, the NCRP has proposed the unit gray-equivalent (Gy-Eq) for an RBE-weighted absorbed dose (13). In 2007, the International Commission on Radiological Protection (ICRP) proposed the use of gray (Gy) for the unit of the RBE-weighted absorbed dose for deterministic biologic effects (14). In proton-beam therapy, the term "equivalent dose" has been used with units of gray-equivalent (GyE) or cobalt gray-equivalent (CGE) (15–17). A joint International Atomic Energy Agency (IAEA)–ICRU working group (18) recently proposed the quantity isoeffective dose (D_{IsoE}), expressed in units of Gy and defined as the product of absorbed dose (D) and an isoeffective weighting factor, w_{IsoE}. This weighting factor is defined to account for all the factors that could influence the clinical deterministic effects associated with a given absorbed dose. In radionuclide therapy, this would include, but would not be limited to, the radiation type, dose rate, and the spatial distribution of absorbed dose. The reference irradiation condition for determining w_{IsoE} was defined to be photons delivered at 2 Gy per fraction and five daily fractions per week, the time–dose–fractionation regimen commonly used in therapeutic external-beam radiation dosimetry. The MIRD Committee has recently recommended that the isoeffective-dose formalism be adopted for use in therapeutic nuclear medicine. To avoid confusion and to parallel the formalism established for stochastic effects, the MIRD Committee has further recommended that the isoeffective dose be expressed in a new special named unit, the barendsen (Bd), in recognition of GW Barendsen's seminal contributions to the radiobiology of high LET (8). No such quantity or unit has yet been universally adopted, however.

NATURE OF INTERNAL RADIONUCLIDE DOSIMETRY

Internal radionuclide therapy is the administration of unsealed sources of radioactivity designed to elicit a therapeutic response as a result of the irradiation of a target tissue. Radiation dosimetry for internally distributed, unsealed radionuclides differs fundamentally from that for external beam radiation therapy (XRT) or brachytherapy. For the latter two forms of radiation therapy, the treatment plan (i.e., the number, position, angulations, and "on" time of the radiation beams in XRT (19–22) and the number, activity, and distribution of the sealed sources in brachytherapy (23–26)) is ultimately based on *measured* absorbed-dose distributions in water-filled or other tissue-equivalent phantoms and is designed to deliver prescribed doses to a target volume or selected reference points therein and do not exceed empirically determined tolerance doses to surrounding normal tissues. Absorbed doses for internal radionuclides are *calculated*, not measured, and are based on a number of simplifying assumptions, most notably that of a standardized anatomic model which may or may not accurately approximate any particular patient. To the extent that individual patients deviate kinetically as well as anatomically from the respective kinetic and anatomic averages, population-averaged dose estimates will be inaccurate. Dr. Robert Loevinger, one of the originators of the MIRD schema (see the section "The MIRD Schema"), has cautioned that ". . . there is in principle no way of attaching a numerical uncertainty to the profound mismatch between the patient and the model (the totality of all assumptions that enter into the dose calculation). The extent to which the model represents in some meaningful way a patient, or a class of patients, is always open to question, and it is the responsibility of the clinician to make that judgment." (27). Inherently, therefore, dosimetry for internal radionuclides is generally less accurate and less precise than that for XRT or brachytherapy. Overall, when time–activity measurements are optimized and dose calculations adapted to the actual anatomy of individual patients, the uncertainty in absorbed-dose estimates is probably of the order of 20% to 30% (28–30). Because of the small risk–benefit ratios associated with *diagnostic* radiopharmaceuticals, such uncertainties in tissue dose estimates for individual patients are unimportant in diagnosis. With *therapeutic* radiopharmaceuticals, however, the risk–benefit ratios are dramatically larger and one must bear in mind these rather substantial uncertainties when planning radionuclide therapy on a patient-specific dosimetric basis.

A further consideration in internal radionuclide dosimetry is the spatial scale of a given dosimetric analysis (31–36). This ranges from macroscopic volumes such as the total body and whole organs and tumors (conventional dosimetry, sometimes also known as macrodosimetry) to macroscopic but smaller scale suborgan or subtumor volumes or even multicell clusters (small-scale dosimetry) to single-cell and subcellular volumes (cell-level dosimetry or microdosimetry) to subnuclear and even molecular volumes (nanodosimetry). In microdosimetry and, in particular, nanodosimetry, the stochastic (i.e., statistical) nature of radiation energy deposition is such that local doses may deviate widely from the average radiation dose. At the larger spatial scales of conventional and even small-scale dosimetry, energy deposition is largely a deterministic phenomenon (i.e., there is little statistical variation) and the average dose is therefore a reasonably reliable metric of the local dose. Note that the average dose, a deterministic quantity, may nonetheless vary considerably over a particular organ or tumor due to nonuniform distribution of activity within that tumor or organ. This is fundamentally different, however, from variation among local radiation doses due to the stochastic (statistical) nature of energy deposition in subnuclear and molecular volumes. In clinical practice, only conventional dosimetry and, to a lesser extent, small-scale dosimetry are generally considered.

CURRENT FORMS OF INTERNAL RADIONUCLIDE THERAPY

Therapeutic radiopharmaceuticals may be structurally simple (ions) to complex (antibodies) entities consisting of or labeled with a radionuclide. Such radiopharmaceuticals may be in solution or in the form of a colloid or suspension and may be administered systemically, locally, or regionally.

Historically, radioiodine therapy of thyroid disease, including hyperthyroidism as well as localized and metastatic thyroid cancer, has been the most active and successful area of radionuclide therapy, largely resulting from the high, rapid, and long-retained uptake of iodine in thyroid tissue, and low-level, rapidly eliminated uptake in extrathyroidal tissues. Although radioiodine therapy of thyroid disease remains the most widely used form of radionuclide therapy, there are a number of newer and/or less frequently applied radionuclide therapies (37–39). These include systemic therapies such as

- Radioimmunotherapy (therapy with radiolabeled antibodies or other immune fragments) of cancer
- Phosphorus-32 (^{32}P)-chromic phosphate therapy of myeloproliferative diseases (most notably polycythemia vera)
- *Meta*-iodine-131-iodobenzylguanidine (^{131}I-MIBG) therapy of neuroendocrine cancers (including pheochromocytomas and neuroblastomas)
- Radiolabeled peptide (indium-111 (^{111}In)-, yttrium-90 (^{90}Y)-, or lutecium-177 (^{177}Lu)-octreotide or octreotate) therapy of carcinoid and other tumors overexpressing cell-surface receptors (somatostatin receptors)
- Palliative radionuclide therapy of bone pain secondary to skeletal metastases using bone-seeking radiopharmaceuticals such as ^{32}P-orthophosphate, strontium-89 (^{89}Sr)-strontium chloride, ^{90}Y-yttrium citrate, rhenium-186

(^{186}Re)- or rhenium-188 (^{188}Re)-rhenium hydroxyethyli-dene diphosphonate (HEDP), samarium-153 (^{153}Sm)- or ^{177}Lu- ethylenediamine tetramethylene phosphonate (EDTMP), and tin-117m (^{117m}Sn) stannic diethylenetri-amine pentaacetate DTPA

as well as local/regional therapies such as

- Intracavitary (peritoneum, pleura, or pericardium) radioimmunotherapy and radiocolloid therapy of malignant effusions and/or ascites using ^{32}P, ^{90}Y, ^{86}Re, and gold-198 (^{198}Au) colloids
- Intrahepatic artery radioembolic therapy (^{131}I- or ^{188}Re-Lipiodol or ^{90}Y-microspheres (SIR-Spheres) of liver tumors
- Intracystic radiocolloid therapy, principally using ^{32}P-chromic phosphate, of cystic intracranial tumors
- Intrathecal radioimmunotherapy and radiocolloid (^{32}P and ^{198}Au) therapy of leptomeningeal tumors
- Intra-articular radiocolloid therapy (known as radiation synovectomy, synoviorthesis, or synoviolysis) of benign joint diseases (inflammatory arthritides) using chromium-51 (51Cr)-, ^{186}Re-, or ^{198}Au-colloid, ^{90}Y-yttrium citrate or silicate, samarium-153 (^{153}Sm)-hydroxyapatite, and erbium-169 (^{169}Er)-citrate

In systemic therapy, a therapeutic radionuclide is administered either enterally or parenterally (typically intravenously) and is thus distributed throughout the body via circulatory, secretory, metabolic, and/or excretory processes. In this way, some activity is deposited in all tissues of the body and thus each tissue irradiates and is irradiated by all other tissues of the body. In regional therapy, the therapeutic radionuclide is introduced directly into a specific space or region of the body and is thus mechanically deposited into or on the target region. In this way, specificity of dose delivery and the therapeutic index is maximized. In general, there is little or no leakage of the radionuclide from the target tissue and little systemic distribution of the radiopharmaceutical.

■ RADIOISOTOPE SOURCES FOR INTERNAL RADIONUCLIDE THERAPY

Selection of the optimum radionuclide(s) is clearly critical for successful therapy. Although difficult to generalize, dosimetric considerations can provide several guidelines for the selection of appropriate therapeutic radionuclides (40–42). Table 8.1 summarizes the pertinent physical properties of nuclear radiations in radionuclide therapy and Table 8.2 summarizes the physical properties of specific radionuclides that have been or may be used therapeutically.

If possible, the physical half-life of the radionuclide should be several fold longer than the uptake half-time but substantially shorter than the clearance half-time of the radiopharmaceutical in the target tissue (41,42). In this way, the residence time in the tumor and therefore the absorbed dose to the target tissue will be maximized while those for nontarget tissues will be minimized. In principle, because

of the dose rate effect (the *inverse* relation between radiobiologic effect and absorbed dose rate (45)), therapeutic radionuclides with an *excessively* long physical half-life (of weeks to months or longer) may be radiobiologically undesirable. In practice, however, even such long-lived radionuclides may still be therapeutically effective. For example, ^{89}Sr-strontium chloride, with a physical half-life of 50.5 days, is effective in palliating bone pain resulting from skeletal metastases (46–48). Further, some authors have argued that there is, in fact, a dose rate–related therapeutic *advantage* to longer lived radionuclides (49).

Because self-irradiation generally contributes the largest component of absorbed dose to a target region such as a tumor, a therapeutic radionuclide should emit principally nonpenetrating (particulate) radiations such as β-rays, Auger electrons, conversion electrons, and/or α-rays (to maximize self-irradiation of the target region) and relatively little penetrating radiation such as x- and γ-rays (to minimize irradiation of nontarget regions) (40–42). Such nonpenetrating radiation must nonetheless be sufficiently penetrating to actually irradiate target-cell nuclei, the critical radiobiologic region within the cell (50). For treatment of macroscopic disease (dimensions of the order of millimeters or larger), β-rays (negatrons) and energetic conversion electrons, with ranges in soft tissue of 0.1 to 10 mm, are the nuclear radiations of choice. Such radiations are sufficiently penetrating that even if all of the cells within the target volume do *not* localize the radiopharmaceutical (certain cells within a tumor do not express the targeted antigen) β-ray "cross-fire" may still deliver a therapeutically effective dose to all cells within the target volume. Although the energies, ranges, and track characteristics of positrons (positive β-rays) are similar to those of negatrons (negative β-rays), the former are not useful therapeutically: the two highly penetrating 511-keV annihilation γ-rays that result from positron emission travel long distances within the body and thus irradiate normal tissues while contributing little to irradiation of the target tissue.

For treatment of single cells (leukemia) and of microscopic cell clusters (clinically occult micrometastases), α-rays are almost ideal (9,51–53). Such radiations have ranges, approximately 10 to 60 μm, of the order of the radius of one to six mammalian cells, delivering almost their entire dose to the cell in or on which the α-ray emitter localizes. Moreover, the high LET and RBE of α-rays means that only relatively few—perhaps as few as one to several—α-ray tracks must pass through a cell nucleus in order to inactivate it. There is, however, virtually no cross-fire contribution with α-ray emitters and cells that do not localize the α-ray–emitting radiopharmaceutical are likely to avoid therapeutic irradiation and survive. A potential confounding consideration with at least some α-ray emitters (radium-223, ^{223}Ra), actinium-225 (^{225}Ac), and thorium-227 (^{227}Th) is the presence of radioactive, α-ray–emitting progeny, particularly, longer lived progeny (54,55); bismuth-213 (^{213}Bi), on the other hand, has no long-lived α-ray–emitting progeny and results in emission of only a single α-ray. Emission of

Table **8.2**   Physical properties of therapeutic radionuclides (43)

Radionuclide	Physical Half-Life	Particle Range in Soft Tissue[a] (mm)	"Imaging" x- or γ-Ray Energy (keV)	Mean Energy Per Disintegration, Δ (MeV) Nonpenetrating (np) Radiations, Δ_p	Penetrating (p) Radiations, Δ_{np}	Δ_{np}-to-Δ_p Ratio
β-Ray/electron emitters						
Phosphorus-32	14.3 days	1.85	—[b]	0.695	0[b]	—[a]
Phosporus-33	25.3 days	0.21	—[b]	0.076	0[b]	—[a]
Scandium-47	3.35 days	0.30	159	0.162	0.109	1.49
Copper-67	2.58 days	0.30	185	0.150	0.115	1.30
Strontium-89	50.5 days	2.03	—[b]	0.585	0[b]	—[b]
Yttrium-90	2.67 days	2.24	—[b]	0.933	0[b]	—b[a]
Palladium-109	13.7 hours	0.91	88	0.438	0.011	37.3
Tin-117m	13.8 days	0.22	159	0.162	0.158	1.03
Iodine-131	8.04 days	0.40	364	0.192	0.382	0.50
Samarium-153	1.94 days	0.53	103	0.270	0.064	4.20
Dysprosium-165	2.33 hours	1.97	95	0.447	0.027	16.7
Holmium-166	1.12 days	2.75	81	0.696	0.030	23.2
Erbium-169	9.40 days	0.13	—[b]	0.104	0[b]	—[b]
Lutetium-177	6.65 days	0.28	139, 208	0.148	0.035	4.23
Rhenium-186	3.72 days	0.92	137	0.336	0.021	16.2
Rhenium-188	17.0 hours	2.43	155	0.779	0.061	12.8
Gold-198	2.70 days	0.90	412	0.328	0.403	0.81
Gold-199	3.14 days	0.16	158	0.145	0.096	1.51
α-Ray emitters						
Astatine-211	7.21 hours	0.060		α-rays, 2.50 β-rays, 0.0059 Total, 2.51	0.037	67.6
Bismuth-212	60.6 months	0.062		α-rays 2.22 β-rays, 0.505 Total, 2.73	0.104	26.3
Bismuth-213	45.6 months	0.046		α-rays 0.125 β-rays 0.444 Total 0.569	0.128	4.44
Radium-223	11.4 days	0.058		α-rays 5.77 β-rays, 0.078 Total, 5.85	0.141	41.5
Radium-224	3.66 days	0.058		α-rays 5.78 β-rays, 0.0023 Total, 5.78	0.0104	556

[a]For β-rays, ranges were either taken from Ref. 41 or calculated by Cole's range–energy relation (44) using the mean β-ray energy. For α-rays, ranges were either taken from Ref. 41 or calculated by energy-dependent linear scaling based on the α-ray ranges given in the foregoing reference.
[b]Indicates a radionuclide that emits little or no x- or γ-radiations (i.e., penetrating radiations).

an α-ray results in a 50 to 100 nm recoil of the daughter nucleus sufficiently energetic to disrupt chemical bonds and to thus separate the daughter atoms from the parent radiopharmaceutical. Short-lived progeny will not have sufficient time to redistribute significantly and their dose distributions will likely approximate that of the parent. The biodistribution of a longer lived daughter and any subsequent progeny, however, will depend upon the site of decay of the parent radiopharmaceutical as well as their respective physical, chemical, and biologic properties (53). For example, [213]Bi, the longest lived daughter of ^{225}Ac, concentrates in the kidneys and ^{223}Ra, the daughter of ^{227}Th, localizes in bone. Dosimetric analyses for α-ray–emitting radionuclides must therefore account for the biodistribution of both the parent and any long-lived radioactive progeny.

Auger electrons are among the least penetrating nuclear radiations, with ranges in soft tissue of less than 1 μm, but with LETs and RBEs comparable to those of α-rays—but only if the Auger electron emitter localizes within the nucleus or, more specifically, within the DNA (56–59) (Fig. 8.1). Otherwise, little to none of the Auger electron dose is actually delivered to the cell nucleus. Auger electron–emitting radioligands (such as ^{125}I-tamoxifen) that bind to intranuclear receptors (i.e., estrogen receptors in breast cancers) have thus been investigated in preclinical models (60).

It is often desirable in practice that a therapeutic radionuclide either itself emits some penetrating radiations (x- and/or γ-rays) in sufficient abundance and of suitable energy for external imaging and time–activity measurements or has another radioisotope that emits such imageable radiations. For example, injection of ^{85}Sr (which emits an imageable 514-keV γ-ray [98% abundance]) with the "non-imageable" pure β-ray emitter ^{89}Sr, used in the form of strontium chloride for palliation of bone pain secondary to skeletal metastases, makes possible quantitative imaging-based time–activity measurements of radiostrontium (61,62). On the other hand, ^{32}P, used in the form of orthophosphate for the treatment of polycythemia vera, emits only a highly energetic β-ray and there does not exist an x- or γ-ray–emitting radioisotope of suitable half-life for quantitative imaging-based time–activity measurements of radiophosphorus; positron-emitting ^{30}P, for example, has a half-life of only 2.5 minutes. Nonetheless, the high-energy ^{32}P β-particle will undergo approximately 2% bremsstrahlung ("braking radiation") energy loss interactions in water/soft tissue and, like other radionuclides that emit high-energy β-rays (^{89}Sr (63) and ^{90}Y (64)), the resulting radiation (x-rays) can be scintigraphically counted and imaged (63–66). Alternatively, for pure β-particle–emitting radionuclides for which a suitable x- or γ-ray–emitting radioisotope does not exist, chemical homologs of the therapeutic radiopharmaceutical labeled with an x- or γ-ray–emitting radionuclide may be used. For example, ^{111}In-labeled antiferritin antibody has been used for quantitative imaging-based radiation dosimetry of antiferritin antibody labeled with the pure β-ray emitter ^{90}Y for treatment of hepatoma (67).

The use of *pure* β-ray–emitting radionuclides simplifies certain radiation safety issues in radionuclide therapy (63). For energies (no greater than ~1 MeV) used in such therapy, electrons have maximum ranges in water/soft tissue of only several millimeters and thus would be completely absorbed by the patient's tissues, effectively eliminating any external radiation hazard. However, a small portion of the β-ray energy will be lost as *bremsstrahlung* (i.e., radiative energy losses), resulting in the emission of generally low-energy photon radiation. For example, the high-energy ^{32}P

β-ray will undergo approximately 2% *bremsstrahlung* energy loss interactions in water/soft tissue yielding an energy spectrum with a broad maximum of approximately 70 keV (68). In practice, therefore, for the relatively low β-ray energies encountered in radionuclide therapy, the low abundance and energy of associated *bremsstrahlung* makes the external radiation hazard insignificant. Accordingly, there is no need to isolate or otherwise limit access to patients who have received radionuclide therapy with a pure β-ray emitter. Standard universal precautions are generally adequate for such patients.

In practice, besides the foregoing dosimetric considerations (Table 8.2), the selection of a therapeutic radionuclide depends, of course, on the availability and cost of the radionuclide and the chemical preparation and stability, particularly in vivo, of the radiopharmaceutical.

■ DOSE PRESCRIPTION ALGORITHMS FOR INTERNAL RADIONUCLIDE THERAPY

"Dose" (actually, administered activity) prescription algorithms for radionuclide therapy can generally be classified as follows (69–71):

■ Fixed administered activity—all patients receive the same administered activity (i.e., mCi, mCi/kg, mCi/m^2)
■ Maximum tolerated dose (MTD)—patients receive an individualized administered activity projected to deliver the maximum tolerated absorbed dose(s) (i.e., Gy) to the critical, or dose-limiting, normal tissue(s)
■ Prescribed tumor-absorbed dose—patients receive an individualized administered activity projected to deliver a prescribed therapeutic absorbed dose to the tumor (or other target tissue)

The fixed-administered activity approach is patient independent and does not require any kinetic or other patient measurements. It is therefore the simplest, most convenient, and least expensive approach. The MTD and prescribed tumor-absorbed dose approaches are patient specific, generally requiring the following in advance of the actual therapy administration: administration of a tracer (or "scout") activity (typically 1 to 5 mCi) of the therapeutic radiopharmaceutical or a suitable (imageable) surrogate; serial total body, organ, blood, and/or tumor activity measurements (by imaging or direct sampling and counting); determination of the absorbed dose per unit administered activity (Gy/mCi) to the dose-limiting normal tissue(s) and/or to the tumor; and calculation of the actual therapeutic administered to deliver either the MTD to the dose-limiting normal tissue or the prescribed therapeutic absorbed dose to the tumor. In the MTD approach, typically only one to several normal tissues will be at significant risk, that is, likely to receive absorbed doses approaching their respective tolerance dose. For ^{131}I-iodine treatment of metastatic thyroid cancer, for example, the therapeutic administered activity is that calculated to deliver no more than 200 cGy to blood (as a surrogate for bone marrow) (72). In radioimmunotherapy of non-Hodgkin B-cell lymphoma with ^{131}I-labeled anti-B1 anti-CD20 monoclonal antibody, on the other hand, the therapeutic administered activity is that delivering a dose of 75 cGy to the total body (again as a surrogate for bone marrow) (73,74). For [188]Re-labeled Lipiodol administered via the hepatic artery for treatment of liver cancer, the liver, lung, and red marrow, with tolerance absorbed doses (based on XRT experience) of 3000 cGy to liver, 1200 cGY to lung, and 150 cGy to red marrow, are the dose-limiting normal tissues (75). It should be recognized that characterizing maximum tolerated dose (MTD) as such is somewhat of a misnomer: as generally used in clinical practice, it does not actually correspond to an MTD dose value rigorously derived from dose-escalation studies but rather an empirically determined "safe" normal tissue dose.

In contrast to the fixed administered activity approach, patient-specific dosimetry is time-consuming for both patients and staff, labor intensive, and logistically demanding, requiring measurement for individual patients of pertinent organ and tumor volumetrics and kinetics (i.e., time–activity data) for a tracer administration of the therapeutic radiopharmaceutical or a suitable surrogate. There is also a perception, perhaps, that internal radionuclide dosimetry is currently not accurate or precise enough to serve as a basis for planning therapy. And there is currently no universally applied approach to patient-specific dosimetry for radionuclide therapy, with practitioners who perform such dosimetry typically employing some institution-specific protocol. Further, for internal radionuclides (and in contrast to XRT), an impression has persisted that there is a lack of reliable dose-toxicity data for normal tissues and perhaps even fewer dose–response data for tumors, dampening motivation among practitioners to pursue patient-specific dosimetry. Administration of a fixed activity to all patients thus remains a widely used approach to radionuclide therapy. There is mounting evidence, however, that increasingly accurate and precise methods for internal radionuclide dosimetry coupled with more discriminating measures of radiation effect warrant dosimetry-based individualized therapy (76–79). Sgouros, for example, recently reviewed the growing literature documenting clinically useful correlations between the radiation dose to at-risk normal tissues and therapy-limiting toxicities (myelosuppression in the case of RIT and nephrotoxicity in the case of radiopeptide therapy of neural-crest tumors) and between the dose to tumors and therapeutic responses, concluding, "The perception that individualized dosimetry has not been successful in predicting response or toxicity in patients is outdated." (Sgouros GS, private communication).

■ THE MIRD SCHEMA

The methodology most widely used for internal dose calculations in medicine, including age- and gender-specific reference data for human anatomy and body composition, remains that developed by the MIRD of the Society of Nuclear Medicine (SNM), generally referred to as the

"MIRD schema" or "MIRD formalism" (27,35,80–82). The ICRP has developed a similar methodology and similar reference data (83).

The MIRD schema, including notation, terminology, mathematical methodology, and reference data, has been disseminated in the form of the collected MIRD pamphlets and associated publications (27,35,80–82). With the publication of ORNL/TM-8381/V1-7 (84), age- and gender-specific body habitus other than the original 70-kg adult anthropomorphic model ("Standard Man") (85) are now incorporated into the MIRD schema. In addition, several computerized versions of the MIRD schema, including *MIRDOSE* (86), now superseded by *OLINDA* (87), have been developed. Like *MIRDOSE*, *OLINDA* includes the capability of providing self-irradiation absorbed doses to spherical tumors, modeled as unit-density spheres. In addition, if patient-specific organ masses are known, *OLINDA* can provide organ mass-adjusted absorbed-dose estimates.

As it is applied to *diagnostic* radiopharmaceuticals, its traditional application, the MIRD schema implicitly assumes that activity and cumulated activity are uniformly distributed within source regions—normal organs—and that radiation energy is uniformly deposited within target. Of course, the MIRD formalism can actually accommodate source and target regions of virtually any spatial scale and thus can be used, for example, to derive dose distributions within organs. Moreover, dosimetry for diagnostic radiopharmaceuticals is generally based on (a) average time–activity data in animal models and/or in a small cohort of human subjects and (b) as noted above, age- and gender-specific "average" models of human anatomy (84). As generally applied, the MIRD schema does *not* incorporate tumors as either source or target regions.

Calculation of the absorbed dose to an organ of the body from an internally distributed radionuclide is based on two conceptually straightforward quantities: the number of nuclear transitions (decays) that occur in an organ or other source region over the time period of interest (usually from the time of administration to "infinite" time, i.e., until complete decay of the radionuclide) and the amount of energy deposited in an organ or other target region per nuclear transition per unit mass of the organ. In practice, however, the calculation of internal absorbed dose requires knowledge of a number of factors and rests on a number of assumptions, including the anthropomorphic models of the "standard" human body and its major internal organs. Among the required data are the following:

- The amount of radioactivity administered—the administered activity
- The rate of radioactive decay of the administered radionuclide—the physical half-life (or decay constant)
- The types of radiation emitted by the decaying radionuclide and their frequencies and energies of emission—the equilibrium dose constant
- The fraction of the administered activity that localizes in each tissue or organ (i.e., "source region")—the uptake or, more completely, the time–activity function

- The length of time the radioactive material resides in each tissue or organ—the effective half-time—as derived from the time–activity function
- The total number of decays (nuclear transitions) that occur in each tissue or organ (or source region)—the cumulated activity
- The fraction of radiation energy that is absorbed in the tissue or organ itself as well as in other tissues and organs (or "target regions")—the absorbed fractions
- The mass of each tissue or organ (target region)

The basic calculation in the MIRD schema, yielding the *mean* absorbed dose $\overline{D}(r_k \leftarrow r_h)$ to target region r_k from the activity (cumulated activity) in source region r_h:

$$\overline{D}(r_k \leftarrow r_h) = \frac{\widetilde{A}_h \sum_i \Delta_i \phi_i(r_k \leftarrow r_h)}{M_k}, \quad \text{(Eq. 8.5a)}$$

$$= \widetilde{A}_h \sum_i \Delta_i \phi_i(r_k \leftarrow r_h), \quad \text{(Eq. 8.5b)}$$

$$= \widetilde{A}_h S(r_k \leftarrow r_h), \quad \text{(Eq. 8.5c)}$$

where $\widetilde{A}_h$ = the cumulated activity in source region r_h; that is, the total number of decays in source region r_h

M_k = the mass of target region r_k

Δ_i = the mean energy emitter per decay (formerly known as the equilibrium dose constant) for radiation i (43)

$= 2.13 n_i \overline{E}_i$ g-rad/μCi-h, (Eq. 8.6)

n_i = the frequency (relative intensity) of radiation i; that is, the number emitted per disintegration

$\overline{E}_i$ = the average energy (in MeV) per disintegration of radiation i

$\phi_i(r_k \leftarrow r_h)$ = the absorbed fraction in target region r_k for radiation i emitted in source region r_h; that is, the fraction of energy of radiation i emitted in source region r_h that is absorbed in target region r_k (84)

$\phi_i(r_k \leftarrow r_h)$ = the *specific* absorbed fraction in target region r_k for radiation i emitted in source region r_h; that is, the fraction of energy of radiation i emitted in source region r_h that is absorbed per unit mass in target region r_k (84)

$$= \frac{\phi_i(r_k \leftarrow r_h)}{M_k}, \quad \text{(Eq. 8.7)}$$

and $S(r_k \leftarrow r_h)$ = the radionuclide-specific S factor for target region r_k and source region r_h; that is, the absorbed dose to target region r_k per unit cumulated activity in source region r_h (88)

$$= \frac{\sum_i \Delta_i \phi_i(r_k \leftarrow r_h)}{M_k}. \quad \text{(Eq. 8.8)}$$

The various quantities in Equations 8.5a to 8.7 are illustrated in Figure 8.2.

An important simplification of absorbed dose calculations was introduced by combining the radionuclide-specific equilibrium dose constant Δ_i, the source region to target region absorbed fraction $\phi_i(r_k \leftarrow r_h)$, and the target region mass M_k into a single quantity, the S factor, as defined by Equation 8.8 (88). As a result, given the cumulated activity $\widetilde{A}_h$ in a given source region r_h, one can use the tabulated S factors to yield, by multiplication, the absorbed dose contribution $\overline{D}(r_k \leftarrow r_h)$ to a target region r_k from a target region r_h. Besides computationally simplifying the determination of absorbed dose, the S factor conceptually clarified this task by isolating all non–time-dependent and, largely, non–biology-dependent dosimetric factors into a single parameter.

The *total* mean absorbed dose $\overline{D}(r_k)$ to target region r_k is then calculated by summing the absorbed dose contributions from all source regions r_h:

$$\overline{D}(r_k) = \sum_h \frac{\widetilde{A}_h \sum_i \Delta_i \phi_i(r_k \leftarrow r_h)}{M_k} \quad \text{(Eq. 8.9a)}$$

FIGURE 8.2 Illustration of the relationship between source and target regions and of related quantities for internal radionuclide dosimetry based on the MIRD schema. See text for further explanation of the symbols and quantities.

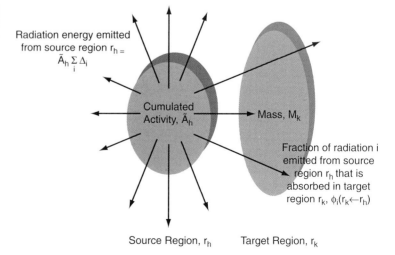

Radiation energy emitted from source region $r_{h} = \widetilde{A}_h \sum_i \Delta_i$

Cumulated Activity, $\widetilde{A}_h$

Mass, M_k

Fraction of radiation i emitted from source region r_h that is absorbed in target region r_k, $\phi_i(r_k \leftarrow r_h)$

Source Region, r_h Target Region, r_k

$$= \sum_{h} [\widetilde{A}_h \sum_{i} \Delta_i \phi_i (r_k \leftarrow r_h)] \qquad \text{(Eq. 8.9b)}$$

$$= \sum_{h} [\widetilde{A}_h S(r_k \leftarrow r_h)] \qquad \text{(Eq. 8.9c)}$$

■ INPUT DATA FOR PATIENT-SPECIFIC DOSIMETRY: ORGAN AND TUMOR MASSES AND TIME–ACTIVITY DATA

▓ Organ and tumor masses

The most practical and accurate approach to patient-specific organ and tumor volumetrics are high-resolution anatomic imaging modalities—either computed tomography (CT) or magnetic resonance imaging (MRI) (Fig. 8.3) (89). To determine masses of the tumor bed organ plus the tumor(s), regions of interest (ROIs) may be drawn around the entire organ, circumscribing the tumor(s) as well as the normal organ parenchyma. ROIs can then be drawn specifically around the individual tumors to determine their respective masses. The normal organ parenchyma mass can be calculated by subtracting the combined masses of the individual tumors from the mass of the entire organ (including tumor[s]). In general, organ volumetrics for patient-specific dosimetry is required for only the tumor-bearing organ and, at most, perhaps several "at-risk" normal organs. For other normal organs, the masses and S factors, etc., for the standard anatomic models may be used for individual patients; that is, organ volumetrics are not required for most normal organs for patient-specific dosimetry.

▓ Organ, tumor, and total-body time–activity data

Serial measurements of activities in normal organs, tumor(s), and the total body can be performed by planar gamma camera imaging, single-photon emission computed tomography (SPECT), or positron emission tomography (PET) (90). Three-dimensional imaging modalities such as SPECT and PET provide more accurate estimates of activities in situ by eliminating the confounding effect of counts

from activity in source regions surrounding the structure of interest (91,92). Further, with the introduction of SPECT-CT (93–95) and PET-CT (96–98) devices, activity distributions can be accurately correlated with anatomy, including abnormal anatomy, and tumor and normal organ masses can be measured in conjunction with activity measurements. Although notable advances have recently been made in quantitative SPECT (99), conventional (i.e., rotating-gamma camera) SPECT remains relatively insensitive and slow, typically requiring a 20- to 40-minute acquisition per bed position. Whole-body SPECT, requiring 2 to 3 hours, would therefore be prohibitively slow. In addition, propagation of statistical uncertainty (i.e., "noise") in the image reconstruction process generally results in rather mottled ("noisy") tomography images, degrading the precision of SPECT-based activity measurements. PET, on the other hand, offers better spatial resolution, higher sensitivity, and generally more accurate and precise activity quantization than SPECT (100) and quantitative whole-body PET scans can be completed in 30 minutes or less. However, other than [86]Y and [124]I, positron-emitting isotopes of the therapeutic β-ray emitters ^{90}Y and ^{131}I, respectively, positron-emitting isotopes of therapeutic radionuclides are not generally available. Thus, planar gamma camera imaging remains the best practical option for in vivo activity quantization in most cases.

Conjugate-view planar gamma camera imaging for activity measurements in normal organs, tumor(s), and the total body is best performed using a dual-detector large field-of-view (LFOV) system with whole-body scanning capability (Fig. 8.4A). A crystal thickness of at least 3/8 in. (9 mm) is required and ½ in. (12 mm) preferred in order to have sufficient intrinsic sensitivity for the photon emissions of all potential therapeutic radionuclides, up to and including the 364-keV γ-ray of [131]I. Implicit in the measurement of normal organ, tumor, and total body time–activity data is the capability of performing ROI analyses. Such measurements require an isotope-specific system calibration factor (in count rate per unit activity [cps/MBq]) and corrections for scatter (i.e., small-angle Compton scatter) and attenuation of x- and γ-rays emitted in vivo (101). Such corrections remain somewhat challenging, however. With the recent introduction (commercially) of combined SPECT-CT scanners, attenuation corrections may become more practical and more reliable (94,102,103).

A simplified, first-order approach to calculation of organ, tumor, and total-body activities uses the patient himself as a calibration standard and thus may minimize inaccuracies related to the lack of explicit scatter and attenuation corrections. In this approach (Fig. 8.4B), the patient undergoes a conjugate-view whole-body scan shortly after the tracer administration (at time 0) but *before* the first postadministration void or bowel movement. For each patient, the net (background-subtracted) geometric mean count rate for the total body for this initial scan thus corresponds to 100% of the administered activity. This scan is typically performed at ½ to 1 hour postadministration to

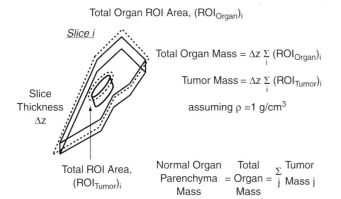

FIGURE 8.3 Estimation of organ and tumor masses for patient-specific dosimetry by tomography imaging (CT or MRI). As noted, it is assumed that the tissue mass density, ρ, is 1 g/cm^3.

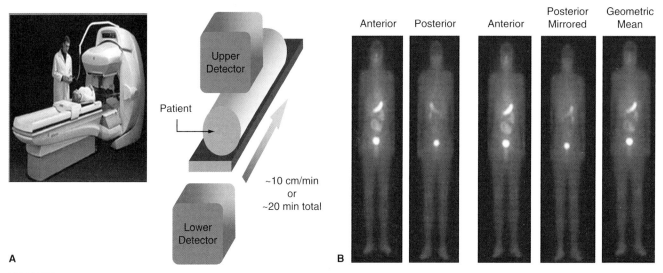

FIGURE 8.4 (A) Dual-detector whole-body gamma camera scanning (conjugate-view imaging) for measurement of organ, tumor, and total-body activities. For serial measurements, the *same* scan speed, scan length, and detector separation should be used for all scans. (B) Illustrative conjugate-view gamma camera whole-body scans of a thyroid cancer patient at approximately 2 hours postadministration of a 5-mCi tracer of ^{131}I-iodide. The "Posterior Mirrored" images represent the posterior image reversed about the vertical (longitudinal) axis of the patient to bring it into alignment with the anterior image prior to forming the geometric mean image (Equation 8.10). (Please see Color Insert).

allow some dispersion of the activity throughout the body, so that the effects of scatter and attenuation are grossly the same for this initial scan as for subsequent scans of the patient. For the time "0" and each subsequent conjugate-view whole-body scan, the posterior (lower-detector) image is "mirrored" to align it with the anterior upper-detector image. The geometric mean image is then formed to eliminate, in first order, the distance dependence of the detected count rate:

$$\frac{\text{Geometric mean}}{\text{image}} = \sqrt{\frac{\text{Upper detector}}{\text{image}} \times \frac{\text{Lower detector}}{\text{image}}}$$

(Eq. 8.10)

At any subsequent time t postadministration, the activity (*not* corrected for radioactive decay to the time of administration) in organ or tumor r_h expressed as percentage of the administered activity may then be calculated from the time t and time 0 geometric mean images as follows:

$$\begin{array}{l} \text{\% of administered} \\ \text{activity in organ or} \\ \text{tumor } r_h \text{ at time } t \end{array} = \frac{N_h[\bar{C}_h - (\bar{C}_{BG})_h]}{N_{TB}[\bar{C}_{TB}(0) - (\bar{C}_{BG})_{TB}(0)]} \times 100\%,$$

(Eq. 8.11)

where N_h = the total number of pixels in the ROI for organ or tumor r_h

N_{TB} = the total number of pixels in the ROI for the total body (TB)

$\bar{C}_h$ = the mean counts per pixel in the ROI for organ or tumor r_h at time t

$(\bar{C}_{BG})_h$ = the mean counts per pixel in the background ROI for organ or tumor r_h at time t

$\bar{C}_{TB}(0)$ = the mean counts per pixel in the ROI for total body at time 0 (i.e., within 1 hour

of administration of the activity but *before* the first postadministration void or other excretion of activity)

and $(\bar{C}_{BG})_{TB}(0)$ = the mean counts per pixels in the background ROI for the total body at time 0

Blood and bone marrow time–activity data

The bone marrow, specifically, the hematopoietic tissue, is highly radiosensitive and is often the dose-limiting normal tissue in radionuclide therapy. Quantization of activity in red marrow for dosimetry is problematic; however, it is a widely distributed source region that cannot be directly sampled except by biopsy. Moreover, there may be wide variability in activity concentrations among marrow sites (104), and biopsy and counting of activity in a marrow sample are therefore prone to sampling error. A more practical approach is based on peripheral blood sampling and counting of a weighed blood sample in a scintillation well counter calibrated for the therapeutic radionuclide. A blank (background) tube and independently assayed standard of the therapeutic radionuclide (with an activity of ~1 μCi or less to avoid prohibitive dead-time counting losses) should also be counted to convert gross to net count rates and net count rates to activities, respectively. The patient's hematocrit must also be measured. Importantly, for radiopharmaceuticals that do *not* localize on or in blood or marrow cells (102), the activity concentration in blood extracellular fluid (i.e., plasma) equals the activity concentration in red marrow extracellular fluid at equilibrium (which is the only source of activity in marrow for such radiopharmaceuticals). Therefore, the red marrow activity concentration can be calculated as follows (105,106):

$$\text{Activity concentration } (\mu Ci/g) \text{ in red marrow} = \frac{\frac{\text{Red marrow extracellular fluid fraction}}{1-\text{Hematocrit}}}{\times \text{Activity concentration } (\mu Ci/g) \text{ in blood}} \quad \text{(Eq. 8.12)}$$

For the purposes of radionuclide dosimetry, the American Association of Physicists in Medicine (AAPM) has recommended a value of 0.4 for the red marrow extracellular fluid fraction (106), while Sgouros has recommended a value of 0.2 (105).

The total activity in red marrow may then be calculated using the Reference Man or Reference Woman anthropomorphic models for male or female patients (84,85), respectively, and scaling by the patient's total-body mass:

$$\begin{aligned}\text{Patient activity } (\mu Ci) \text{ in red marrow} &= \text{Concentration } (\mu Ci/gm) \text{ in red marrow} \\ &\times \text{Total mass (g) of red marrow} \times \frac{\text{Patient total-body mass (kg)}}{\frac{\text{Reference man or woman}}{\text{Total-body mass (kg)}}}, \end{aligned} \quad \text{(Eq. 8.13)}$$

where the total-body mass is 73.7 kg and the total mass of red marrow is 1500 g for the Reference Man model and the total-body mass is 56.8 kg and the total mass of red marrow is 1300 g for the Reference Woman model.

An alternative approach to the estimation of red marrow activity is based on quantitative conjugate-view imaging, where an ROI is drawn around a marrow-rich area such as the lumbar vertebrae (106,107). For radiopharmaceuticals that localize specifically in red marrow (i.e., antibodies that cross-react with antigens expressed on hematopoietic cells), the foregoing blood-based method for estimation of marrow activity is not reliable because, for such radiopharmaceuticals, the total activity in marrow is due to that bound to or within cells as well as that in the marrow extracellular fluid (108). For such radiopharmaceuticals, therefore, an imaging-based method must be used. The activity concentration in the total-body marrow is then assumed to be equal to that measured in the region analyzed. To obtain this concentration from imaging, the volume of the selected marrow region must be determined, using, for example, CT or MRI (31).

However determined, the activity in red marrow (Equation 8.13) can then be converted to percentage of administered activity as follows:

$$\text{\% of administered activity in red marrow} = \frac{\text{Activity } (\mu Ci) \text{ in red marrow}}{\text{Administered activity } (\mu Ci)} \times 100\% \quad \text{(Eq. 8.14)}$$

CUMULATED ACTIVITIES FOR PATIENT-SPECIFIC DOSIMETRY

Once time–activity data for a particular patient have been measured, the cumulated activity, or time integral of activity, $\tilde{A}_h$, in a given source region r_h is calculated by integration from the time of administration of the radiopharmaceutical ($t = 0$) to the time of its complete elimination or decay ($t = \infty$) of the effective time–activity function, $(A_e)_h(t)$:

$$\tilde{A}_h = \int_0^\infty (A_e)_h(t)dt. \quad \text{(Eq. 8.15)}$$

The effective time–activity function, $(A_e)_h(t)$, incorporates both the physical decay constant of the radionuclide and its biologic disappearance constant(s).

Despite the complexity of the multiple underlying biologic processes, the time–activity data of most radiopharmaceuticals generally can be represented by an *exponential* function:

$$A_h(t) = \sum_j (A_h)_j e^{-[(\lambda_e)_h]_j t}, \quad \text{(Eq. 8.16)}$$

where $(A_h)_j$ = the (extrapolated) activity at time $t = 0$ for the jth exponential component of the time–activity function in source region r_h

and $[(\lambda_e)_h]_j$ = the effective clearance constant of the jth exponential component of the time–activity function in source region r_h; that is, the fraction per unit time of activity eliminated for the jth exponential component of the time–activity function in source region r_h

As noted, the parameter, $[(\lambda_e)_h]_j$, is actually the "effective (e)" clearance constant because it includes the effects of *both* biologic clearance and physical (radioactive) decay:

$$[(\lambda_e)_h]_j = \lambda_p + [(\lambda_b)_h]_j, \quad \text{(Eq. 8.17)}$$

where λ_p = the physical decay constant of the radionuclide

and $[(\lambda_b)_h]_j$ = the biologic clearance constant of the jth exponential component of the time–activity function in source region r_h; that is, the fraction per unit time of activity biologically eliminated for the jth exponential component of the time–activity function in source region r_h

For each exponential component, the half-life (or half-time), T, is related to its corresponding clearance constant:

$$T = \frac{\ln 2}{\lambda}, \quad \text{(Eq. 8.18a)}$$

$$= \frac{0.693}{\lambda}. \quad \text{(Eq. 8.18b)}$$

The effective half-time, $[(T_e)_h]_j$, of the jth exponential component of the time–activity function in source region r_h includes the effects of both the biologic and physical half-lives:

$$[(T_e)_h]_j = \cfrac{1}{\cfrac{1}{T_p} + \cfrac{1}{[(T_b)_h]_j}}, \qquad \text{(Eq. 8.19a)}$$

$$= \frac{T_p[(T_b)_h]_j}{T_p + [(T_b)_h]_j}, \qquad \text{(Eq. 8.19b)}$$

where T_p = the physical half-life of the radionuclide
and $[(T_b)_h]_j$ = the biologic half-time of the jth exponential component of the time–activity function in source region r_h

Integration of the time–activity function, $A_h(t) = \sum_j (A_h)_j\, e^{-[(\lambda_e)_h]_j t}$, in source region r_h (Equation (8.9) yields the cumulated activity in source region r_h:

$$\tilde{A}_h = \sum_j \frac{(A_h)_j}{[(\lambda_e)_h]_j} \qquad \text{(Eq. 8.20a)}$$

$$= 1.44 \sum_j (A_h)_j[(T_e)_h]_j \qquad \text{(Eq. 8.20b)}$$

The quantity cumulated activity is sometimes replaced by the residence time, τ_h, equivalent to the cumulated activity per unit administered activity in source region r_h (80):

$$\tau_h = \frac{\tilde{A}_h}{AA} \qquad \text{(Eq. 8.21)}$$

$$= 1.44 \sum_j \frac{(A_h)_j}{AA}[(T_e)_h]_j \qquad \text{(Eq. 8.22)}$$

$$= 1.44 \sum_j (f_h)_j[(T_e)_h]_j \qquad \text{(Eq. 8.23)}$$

where   AA = the administered activity
     $(f_h)_j$ = the (extrapolated) fraction of the administered activity at time $t = 0$ for the jth exponential component of the time–activity function in source region r_h

and $1.44 = \dfrac{1}{\ln(2)}$.

Therefore,

$$\tilde{A}_h = AA\tau_h \qquad \text{(Eq. 8.24)}$$

Numerous curve-fitting programs are available that can be used to fit time–activity data (i.e., percent of administered activity vs. time postadministration) to such an exponential function (i.e., Equation 8.8). Such programs are generally based on iteratively adjusting the function parameters, $(A_h)_j$ and $[(\lambda_e)_h]_j$, to minimize the sum of the squared differences between the measured data and the corresponding calculated (i.e., fitted) value. Such a sum-of-square minimization, or "least squares," algorithm can also be implemented with EXCEL (Microsoft, Redmond, WA) (109,110). Analytic integration of the time–activity function (Equation 8.8) then yields the cumulated activity in source region r_h (see Equations 8.15a and 8.15b). Alternatively, time–activity data may also be integrated numerically (by some adaptation of the trapezoidal rule or Simpson's rule) up to the last measured

datum (A_n at time t_n postadministration) and analytically thereafter, conservatively assuming elimination of the radionuclide by physical decay only. An advantage of numerical integration is its generality: it is adaptable to nonmonotonic time–activity curves and no assumptions are introduced regarding the analytic form of the time–activity curve. On the other hand, a disadvantage of the assumption of radionuclide elimination by physical decay only following the last measurement is that it results in a systematic overestimation, perhaps substantial, of the overall area under the time–activity curve (the cumulated activity).

It is difficult to formulate general recommendations for kinetic measurements, that is, for the number, spacing, and overall duration of measurements for each source region, for radionuclide dosimetry. For curve-fitting purposes, the so-called "degree of freedom," which is equal to the number of measurements minus the number of fitted parameters, should be at least one. Thus, for a one-component fit (with two fitted parameters, the intercept and clearance constant), at least three activity measurements should be obtained; for a two-component fit (with four fitted parameters, the intercept and clearance constant for each of the two components), at least five activity measurements should be obtained. In practice, however, time–activity data are often fit without the requisite number of measurements. For numerical integration, there is no such rigorously definable criterion. Practically, it is recommended to perform at least four activity measurements per source region, with the earliest performed no later than approximately 1 hour postadministration and the latest performed with no more than 25%, and preferably no more than 10%, of the non–decay-corrected activity remaining in the source region. As described previously, the "early" (≤ 1 hour) prevoid and pre–bowel-movement total-body activity scan is required to define the total-body net count rate corresponding to 100% of the administered activity.

ADAPTATION OF THE MIRD SCHEMA TO PATIENT-SPECIFIC DOSIMETRY

The standard anatomic models—ranging from the 3.4-kg Reference Newborn to the 70-kg Reference Man (Table 8.3) (84)—used in the MIRD schema represent normal, population-averaged human anatomy and thus do not include tumors. The schema can nonetheless be adapted to patient-specific normal organ dosimetry for planning radionuclide therapy (77,90,111). Not surprisingly, the most important quantitative adjustment for organ dosimetry in this adaptation involves the tumor-bearing organ(s). The schema can also be adapted, at least grossly, to incorporate tumors and tumor dosimetry (111). Together with the foregoing approaches to acquisition of the requisite time–activity data and calculation of cumulated activities, the dose calculation algorithm that follows illustrates the essential elements of a practical, systematic approach to patient-specific dosimetry for internal radionuclide therapy. It also represents a widely applicable algorithm, requiring only a

Table **8.3**   **The organs (source and target regions) and organ masses of the age-dependent standard anatomic models (phantoms) used in the MIRD schema (84,85)**

Organ	Mass (g) of Organ in Each Phantom					
	Newborn (3.4 kg)[a]	**Age 1 (9.8 kg)**	**Age 5 (19 kg)**	**Age 10 (32 kg)**	**Age 15-Adult Female (55–58 kg)**	**Adult Male (70 kg)**
Adrenals	5.83	3.52	5.27	7.22	10.5	16.3
Brain	352	884	1.260	1.360	1.410	1.420
Breasts, including skin	0.205	1.10	2.17	3.65	407	403
Breasts, excluding skin	0.107	0.732	1.51	2.60	361	351
Gallbladder contents	2.12	4.81	19.7	38.5	49.0	55.7
Gallbladder wall	0.408	0.910	3.73	7.28	9.27	10.5
GI tract						
LLI contents	6.98	18.3	36.6	61.7	109	143
LLI wall	7.98	20.6	41.4	70.0	127	167
SI contents and wall	52.9	138	275	465	838	1.100
Stomach contents	10.6	36.2	75.1	133	195	260
Stomach wall	6.41	21.8	49.1	85.1	118	158
ULI contents	11.2	28.7	57.9	97.5	176	232
ULI wall	10.5	27.8	55.2	93.4	168	220
Heart contents	36.5	72.7	134	219	347	454
Heart wall	25.4	50.6	92.8	151	241	316
Kidneys	22.9	62.9	116	173	248	299
Liver	121	292	584	887	1.400	1.910
Lungs	50.6	143	290	453	651	1.000
Ovaries	0.328	0.714	1.73	3.13	10.5	8.71
Pancreas	2.80	10.3	23.6	30.0	64.9	94.3
Remaining tissue	2.360	6.400	13.300	23.100	40.000	51.800
Skin	118	271	538	888	2.150	3.010
Spleen	9.11	25.5	48.3	77.4	123	183
Testes	0.843	1.21	1.63	1.89		39.1
Thymus	11.3	22.9	29.6	31.4	28.4	20.9
Thyroid	1.29	1.78	3.45	7.93	12.4	20.7
Urinary bladder contents	12.4	32.9	64.7	103	160	211
Urinary bladder wall	2.88	7.70	14.5	23.2	35.9	47.6
Uterus	3.85	1.45	2.70	4.16	79.0	
Whole body	3.600	9.720	19.800	33.200	56.800	73.700

[a] Total phantom weight.

conventional gamma camera. Although its nomenclature is rather daunting and its computations tedious, this algorithm is conceptually straightforward and can be implemented using a spreadsheet program such as EXCEL (109). Importantly, however, this approach has not been widely used in practice and has not been validated and yields only first-order estimates of absorbed doses. In fact, to the extent that patient-specific dosimetry is actually performed, the algorithms employed remain largely institution specific.

Organ dosimetry

For organ "non-self" irradiation (source region r_h ≠ target region r_k), S factors are relatively insensitive to organ (i.e., source and target region) size and shape. Therefore, unless the source and/or target regions are *grossly* abnormal (due to the presence of *massive* tumor), Reference Man (or Reference Woman) S factors may be applied to specific patients for calculating the organ and tumor nonself absorbed dose contribution:

$$\text{Patient } S(r_k \leftarrow r_h) \approx \text{Reference Man } S(r_k \leftarrow r_h). \quad \text{(Eq. 8.25)}$$

The "nonself-organ" contributions to the organ r_k dose, $\sum_{h \neq k} D(r_k \leftarrow r_h)$, therefore becomes:

$$\sum_{h \neq k} D(r_k \leftarrow r_h) = \sum_{h \neq k} \tilde{A}_h \cdot S(r_k \leftarrow r_h). \quad \text{(Eq. 8.26)}$$

For the dose contribution to an organ and tumor from activity in the "rest of body," that is, activity not explicitly assigned to specific source regions, Reference *muscle* S factors may be used:

$$\text{Patient } S(r_k \leftarrow \text{Rest of body})$$
$$\approx \text{Reference Man } S(r_k \leftarrow \text{Muscle}). \quad \text{(Eq. 8.27)}$$

The rest-of-body dose contribution to the organ r_k dose, $D(r_k \leftarrow \text{Rest of body})$, therefore becomes:

$$D(r_k \leftarrow \text{Rest of body}) \approx \tilde{A}_{\text{Rest of body}}$$
$$\times \text{Patient } S(r_k \leftarrow \text{Rest of body}), \quad \text{(Eq. 8.28)}$$

where

$$\tilde{A}_{\text{Rest of body}} = \text{the rest-of-body cumulated activity}$$
$$= \tilde{A}_{\text{TB}} - \sum_h \tilde{A}_h, \quad \text{(Eq. 8.29)}$$

where $\tilde{A}_{\text{TB}}$ = the total-body cumulated activity.

For "self" irradiation of organ r_k (i.e., source region r_h = target region r_k), adaptation of the MIRD schema is more complicated. First, the self-irradiation S factor can be separated into its nonpenetrating (np) and penetrating (p) radiation components:

$$S(r_k \leftarrow r_k) = S_{\text{np}}(r_k \leftarrow r_k) + S_p(r_k \leftarrow r_k), \quad \text{(Eq. 8.30)}$$

where $S(r_k \leftarrow r_k)$ = the total self-irradiation S factor for organ r_k

$S_{\text{np}}(r_k \leftarrow r_k)$ = the self-irradiation S factor for nonpenetrating radiations for organ r_k

and $S_p(r_k \leftarrow r_k)$ = the self-irradiation S factor for penetrating radiations for organ r_k

Because of the limited ranges (much shorter than the dimensions of typical human organs) of nonpenetrating radiations in tissue, such radiations are completely absorbed within the organ in which they are emitted and self-irradiation absorbed fractions for such radiations are therefore uniformly 1 ($\phi_{\text{np}}(r_k \leftarrow r_k) = 1$). The self-irradiation S factor for nonpenetrating radiations, $S_{\text{np}}(r_k \leftarrow r_k)$, thus varies in inverse proportion to the organ mass, M_k, and the patient-specific S factor for nonpenetrating radiations, Patient $S_{\text{np}}(r_k \leftarrow r_k)$, is simply:

$$\text{Patient } S_{\text{np}}(r_k \leftarrow r_k) = \frac{\Delta_{\text{np}}}{\text{Patient } M_k}, \quad \text{(Eq. 8.31)}$$

where Δ_{np} = the total mean energy per decay for nonpenetrating radiations,

$$= \sum_i (\Delta_{\text{np}})_i, \quad \text{(Eq. 8.32)}$$

where $(\Delta_{\text{np}})_i$ = the total mean energy per decay for nonpenetrating radiation i

The patient-specific self-irradiation S factor for penetrating radiations, Patient $S_p(r_k \leftarrow r_k)$, can be calculated based on the defining equation of the S factor and the approximation that the self-irradiation absorbed fraction for penetrating radiation i, $(\phi_p)_i(r_k \leftarrow r_k)$, generally increases as the cube root (⅓ power) of the mass, M_k, of the organ (90):

$$\text{Patient } S_p(r_k \leftarrow r_k) = \frac{\sum_i (\Delta_i)_p \text{ Reference Man } (\phi_i)_p(r_k \leftarrow r_h)}{\text{Reference Man } M_k}$$
$$\times \left[\frac{\text{Patient } M_k}{\text{Reference Man } M_k} \right]^{1/3} \quad \text{(Eq. 8.33)}$$

Importantly, while a useful approximation, Equation 8.33 is not accurate for all body regions (e.g., red marrow) or radionuclides (90,112).

Substituting the Equations 8.32 and 8.33 into Equation 8.30 then yields the total patient-specific self-irradiation S factor for organ r_k:

$$\text{Patient } S(r_k \leftarrow r_k) = \frac{\Delta_{\text{np}}}{\text{Patient } M_k}$$
$$+ \frac{\sum_i (\Delta_i)_p \text{ Reference Man } (\phi_i)_p(r_k \leftarrow r_k)}{\text{Reference Man } M_k}$$
$$\times \left[\frac{\text{Patient } M_k}{\text{Reference Man } M_k} \right]^{1/3} \quad \text{(Eq. 8.34)}$$

For a normal (non–tumor-bearing) organ, the self-irradiation absorbed doses for penetrating and nonpenetrating radiations—$D_p(r_h \leftarrow r_h)$ and $D_{\text{np}}(r_h \leftarrow r_h)$, respectively—to organ r_k (Fig. 8.5) are therefore:

$$D_{\text{np}}(r_k \leftarrow r_k) = \text{Patient } S_{\text{np}}(r_k \leftarrow r_k)$$
$$\times [\text{Patient organ } r_k \text{ cumulated activity}], \text{(Eq. 8.35)}$$

$$D_p(r_k \leftarrow r_k) = \text{Patient } S_p(r_k \leftarrow r_k)$$
$$\times [\text{Patient organ } r_k \text{ cumulated activity}]. \text{(Eq. 8.36)}$$

For a tumor-bearing organ (Fig. 8.5A), the self-irradiation organ absorbed dose (the absorbed dose to the organ's *normal parenchyma*) from penetrating radiations includes contributions from activity in both the normal organ parenchyma and from tumor within the organ. Assuming, based on the long (multicentimeter) path lengths of penetrating radiations, that the dose from such radiations to the normal parenchyma within a tumor-bearing organ would be the same as that for the total (i.e., normal parenchyma and tumor) being *uniformly* distributed between the parenchyma and tumor(s) (Fig. 8.5B):

$$D_p(r_k \leftarrow r_k) = \text{Patient } S_p(r_k \leftarrow r_k)$$
$$\times \left[\begin{array}{l} \text{Total (parenchyma + tumor)} \\ \text{organ } r_k \text{ cumulated activity} \end{array} \right]. \text{(Eq. 8.37)}$$

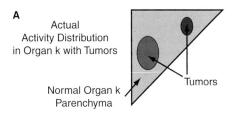

A
Actual
Activity Distribution
in Organ k with Tumors

Tumors

Normal Organ k
Parenchyma

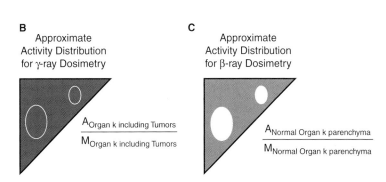

B
Approximate
Activity Distribution
for γ-ray Dosimetry

$$\frac{A_{\text{Organ } k \text{ including Tumors}}}{M_{\text{Organ } k \text{ including Tumors}}}$$

C
Approximate
Activity Distribution
for β-ray Dosimetry

$$\frac{A_{\text{Normal Organ } k \text{ parenchyma}}}{M_{\text{Normal Organ } k \text{ parenchyma}}}$$

FIGURE 8.5 **(A)** Hypothetical distribution of activity (and cumulated activity) in normal organ *k* parenchyma and in two tumors. The intensity of the shading reflects the relative activity (and cumulated activity). **(B)** The activity concentration in the entire organ (including tumor), equal to the ratio of the total organ activity (*including* that in tumors) to the total organ mass (*including* that of tumors), assumed for self-irradiation γ-ray dosimetry. **(C)** The activity concentration in the normal organ parenchyma, equal to the ratio of the normal organ parenchyma activity (*excluding* that in tumors) to the normal organ parenchyma mass (*excluding* that of tumors), assumed for self-irradiation normal organ parenchyma β-ray dosimetry (111).

In contrast, the self-irradiation organ absorbed dose from nonpenetrating radiations is contributed only by activity in its normal parenchyma because such radiations emitted in macroscopic tumors are completely absorbed within the tumors themselves; that is, such radiations cannot penetrate into the surrounding normal parenchyma (Fig. 8.5 C):

$$D_{\text{np}}(r_k \leftarrow r_k) = \text{Patient } S_{\text{np}}(r_k \leftarrow r_k)$$
$$\times \begin{bmatrix} \text{Normal parenchyma only} \\ \text{organ } r_k \text{ cumulated activity} \end{bmatrix}. \quad \text{(Eq. 8.38)}$$

The total self-irradiation absorbed dose to organ r_k is then simply the sum of the self-irradiation absorbed dose contributions from penetrating and nonpenetrating radiations:

$$D(r_k \leftarrow r_k) = D_{\text{p}}(r_k \leftarrow r_k) + D_{\text{np}}(r_k \leftarrow r_k). \quad \text{(Eq. 8.39)}$$

Summing all of the dose contributions, the total dose to organ r_k normal parenchyma, $D(r_k)$, for the activity administered becomes:

$$D(r_k) = D(r_k \leftarrow r_k) + \sum_{h \neq k} D(r_k \leftarrow r_h)$$
$$+ D(r_k \leftarrow \text{Rest of body}). \quad \text{(Eq. 8.40)}$$

If the maximum tolerated dose to organ r_k normal parenchyma is MTD(r_k) (from Refs. (113) and (114)), the maximum tolerated activity (i.e., administered activity) for target region r_k normal parenchyma, MTA(r_k), is:

$$\text{MTA}(r_k) = \frac{\text{MTD}(r_k)}{\dfrac{D(r_k)}{\text{Administered activity}}}. \quad \text{(Eq. 8.41)}$$

The patient-specific maximum tolerated activity, MTA, is then the minimum among the MTA (r_k) values.

Tumor dosimetry

Tumor dosimetry is *not* a component of the MTD approach to radionuclide therapy or of the MIRD schema. Nonetheless, tumor-absorbed doses can be estimated, at least grossly, using data already required for normal-tissue dosimetry and the dimensions of the tumor(s) measured by CT or MRI. First, one calculates the tumor self-irradiation dose:

$$D(\text{Tumor} \leftarrow \text{Tumor}) = D_{\text{p}}(\text{Tumor} \leftarrow \text{Tumor})$$
$$+ D_{\text{np}}(\text{Tumor} \leftarrow \text{Tumor}), \quad \text{(Eq. 8.42a)}$$
$$= \frac{0.0346 \cdot \Gamma \cdot \bar{g} \cdot \widetilde{A}_{\text{Tumor}}}{\text{Tumor mass}} + \frac{\Delta_{\text{np}}}{\text{Tumor mass}} \cdot \widetilde{A}_{\text{Tumor}}, \quad \text{(Eq. 8.42b)}$$

where

$D(\text{Tumor} \leftarrow \text{Tumor})$ = the tumor-to-tumor absorbed dose

$D_{\text{p}}(\text{Tumor} \leftarrow \text{Tumor})$ = the tumor-to-tumor absorbed dose for penetrating (p) radiations

$D_{\text{np}}(\text{Tumor} \leftarrow \text{Tumor})$ = the tumor-to-tumor absorbed dose for nonpenetrating (np) radiations

$$= \frac{0.0346 \cdot \Gamma \cdot \bar{g} \cdot \widetilde{A}_{\text{Tumor}}}{\text{Tumor mass}}, \quad \text{(Eq. 8.43)}$$

Γ = the specific γ-ray constant (rad-cm^2/mCi-h) for the therapeutic radionuclide (see Table 8.4 for a compilation of specific γ-ray constants (115))

$\bar{g}$ = the mean geometric factor (70,116)

Table 8.4 Specific (γ-ray constants, Γ, in R-cm²/mCi-h for selected radionuclides (115)

Nuclide	Γ	Nuclide	Γ	Nuclide	Γ
Actinium-227	−2.2	Gold-198	2.3	Potassium-43	5.6
Antimony-122	2.4	Gold-199	−0.9	Radium-226	8.25
Antimony-124	9.8	Hafnium-175	−2.1	Radium-228	−5.1
Antimony-125	−2.7	Hafnium-181	−3.1	Rhenium-186	−0.2
Arsenic-72	10.1	Indium-114m	−0.2	Rubidium-86	0.5
Arsenic-74	4.4	Iodine-124	7.2	Ruthenium-106	1.7
Arsenic-76	2.4	Iodine-125	−0.7	Scandium-46	10.9
Barium-131	3.0	Iodine-126	2.5	Scandium-47	0.56
Barium-133	−2.4	Iodine-130	12.2	Selenium-75	2.0
Barium-140	12.4	Iodine-131	2.2	Silver-110m	14.3
Beryllium-7	−0.3	Iodine-132	11.8	Silver-111	−0.2
Bromine-82	14.6	Iridium-192	4.8	Sodium-22	12.0
Cadmium-115m	−0.2	Iridum-194	1.5	Sodium-24	18.4
Calcium-47	5.7	Iron-59	6.4	Strontium-85	3.0
Carbon-11[c]	5.9	Krypton-85	−0.04	Tantalum-182	6.8
Cerium-141	0.35	Lanthanum-140	11.3	Tellurium-121	3.3
Cerium-144	−0.4	l.utetium-177	0.09	Tellurium-132	2.2
Cesium-134	8.7	Magnesium-28	15.7	Thulium-170	0.025
Cesium-137	3.3	Manganese-52	18.6	Tin-113	−1.7
Chlorine-38	8.8	Manganese-54	4.7	Tungsten-185	−0.5
Chromium-51	0.16	Manganese-56	8.3	Tungsten-187	3.0
Cobalt-56	17.6	Mercury-197	−0.4	Uranium-234	−0.1
Cobalt-57	0.9	Mercury-203	1.3	Vanadium-48	15.6
Cobalt-58	5.5	Molybdenum-99	1.8	Xenon-133	0.1
Cobalt-60	13.2	Neodymium-147	0.8	Ytterbium-175	0.4
Copper-64	1.2	Nickel-65	−3.1	Yttrium-88	14.1
Europium-152	5.8	Niobium-95	4.2	Yttrium-91	0.01
Europium-154	−6.2	Osmium-191	−0.6	Zinc-65	2.7
Europium-155	−0.3	Palladium-109	0.03	Zirconium-95	4.1

$$= \frac{\Delta_{np}}{\text{Tumor mass}} \times \tilde{A}_{\text{Tumor}}, \quad \text{(Eq. 8.44)}$$

$$= 3\,\pi\,r, \quad \text{(Eq. 8.45)}$$

and $\quad r =$ the radius (cm) of the tumor if spherical or

$$= \sqrt[3]{a \cdot b \cdot c}, \quad \text{(Eq. 8.46)}$$

where $\quad a, b, c =$ the orthogonal half-dimensions (in cm) of the tumor if nonspherical

Additional contributions to the tumor dose are from activity in the surrounding normal organ parenchyma in the organ r_k in which the tumor is located, in other organs, and in the rest of the body; these contributions are due only to penetrating radiations emitted within these respective source regions. The contributions to the tumor dose from activity in other organs and in the rest of the body are equal to the dose from other organs and from the rest of the body, respectively, to the organ in which the tumor is located. The total tumor dose for a tumor located in organ r_k, $D(\text{tumor})r_k$ is therefore:

$$D(\text{tumor})r_k = D(\text{Tumor} \leftarrow \text{Tumor}) + D_p(r_k \leftarrow r_k)$$

$$+ \sum_h D(r_k \leftarrow r_h) + D(r_k \leftarrow \text{Rest of body}), \quad \text{(Eq. 8.47)}$$

where

$D(\text{Tumor} \leftarrow \text{Tumor}) =$ the tumor-to-tumor absorbed dose
$D_p(r_k \leftarrow r_k) =$ the organ r_k to organ r_k penetrating radiation dose

$\Sigma_h D(r_k \leftarrow r_h) =$ the "nonself-organ" contributions to the organ r_k dose

and

$D(r_k \leftarrow \text{Rest of body}) =$ the rest-of-body dose contribution to the organ r_k dose

■ NONUNIFORM DOSE DISTRIBUTIONS IN INTERNAL RADIONUCLIDE DOSIMETRY

In the foregoing dosimetric analysis, only average organ and tumor absorbed doses were considered. Implicit in this analysis, therefore, are the assumptions that activities and cumulated activities are uniformly distributed in source regions and radiation energy is uniformly deposited in target regions. Scintigraphic imaging modalities (planar gamma camera imaging, SPECT, and even PET) often do not have sufficient spatial resolution to discern the heterogeneity of intraorgan and intratumor activity distributions (117). Normal-tissue toxicity and tumor therapeutic response, however, may not correlate with *average* doses even when based on individualized kinetics. O'Donoghue (118), for example, has modeled the impact of dose nonuniformity (117,119) on radiocurability of tumors and has shown that tumor response is poorer (tumor cell survival is greater) as dose nonuniformity increases, with a substantial fraction of tumor cells receiving sublethal doses. The tumor will therefore not regress even if the average tumor dose is sufficiently high to induce a significant therapeutic response, if the tumor were uniformly irradiated to that same average dose (as is very nearly the case in XRT and brachytherapy). Clinically predictive *average* dose–response curves may be difficult to derive in the face of such nonuniformity. Thus, in addition to patient-specific dosimetry, the issue of spatial nonuniformity of dose has become increasingly important at both the macroscopic (80,117,120–143) and microscopic (58,144–163) levels.

There are at least three approaches to the calculation of macroscopic nonuniform dose distributions (80) and these include dose-point kernel convolution, Monte Carlo simulation, and voxel *S* factors. The dose-point kernel has perhaps been the most widely used of these approaches (121,122,125,126,164), primarily because of the demanding computational requirements of Monte Carlo simulation and the limited availability of voxel *S* factors. A dose-point kernel is the radial distance-dependent absorbed dose about an isotropic point source in an infinite homogeneous medium, typically a soft tissue–equivalent medium such as water. With the wider availability of high-speed desktop computers and of compatible simulation codes, the use of Monte Carlo analysis has increased (123,124,165). Monte Carlo–based dosimetry can more accurately account for tissue variations in mass density and atomic number as well as edge effects that may be important at the periphery of the body and at soft tissue–lung and soft tissue–bone interfaces (124). For example, if the relevant distribution data were available (e.g., by autoradiography of biopsy specimens),

Monte Carlo analysis might be applicable to normal lung dosimetry in radioiodine treatment of metastatic thyroid cancer, particularly in the setting of dosimetrically problematic miliary disease. This method remains computationally time-consuming (124). Tabulations of voxel *S* factors, conceptually equivalent to voxel source kernels (the mean absorbed dose to a target voxel per radioactive decay in a source voxel), both of which are contained in an infinite homogeneous soft tissue medium, are available (80,120). In contrast to dose-point kernel– and Monte Carlo–based techniques, the voxel *S* factor method does not require specialized computer facilities and is relatively fast, and thus may emerge as the practical method of choice for calculation of macroscopic nonuniform dose distributions.

■ SUMMARY

Radiation dosimetry deals with the determination of the amount and the spatial and temporal distribution of energy deposited in matter by ionizing radiation. Internal radionuclide radiation dosimetry specifically deals with the deposition of radiation energy in tissue due to a radionuclide within the body. However, unlike external radiation dose (which can often be measured), internal radiation dose must be calculated. Internal radionuclide radiation dosimetry has evolved over more than 60 years from relatively simple approaches to those with a high level of sophistication. This chapter has reviewed technical aspects, basic concepts, and practical computational approaches to internal radiation dosimetry for radionuclide therapy. Although conceptually straightforward, the nomenclature presented is daunting and the computations tedious. Importantly, beginning with ROI-derived organ and tumor masses (from CT or MRI) and organ, tumor, and total-body activities (from gamma camera imaging) as input data, virtually all of the calculations can be performed with an EXCEL spreadsheet. Further, all necessary reference data (e.g., Reference Man organ masses, equilibrium dose constants, *S* factors, etc.) are readily available and can be incorporated into such a spreadsheet to largely automate the dose-calculation process.

■ REFERENCES

1. ICRU. *Radiation Quantities and Units. International Commission on Radiation Units and Measurements (ICRU) Report 33.* Bethesda, MD: International Commission on Radiation Units and Measurements (ICRU); 1980.
2. ICRU. *Fundamental Quantities and Units for Ionizing Radiation. International Commission on Radiation Units and Measurements (ICRU) Report 60.* Bethesda, MD: International Commission on Radiation Units and Measurements (ICRU); 1998.
3. NCRP. *SI Units in Radiation Protection and Measurements. National Council on Radiation Protection and Measurements (NCRP) Report 82.* Bethesda, MD: National Council on Radiation Protection and Measurements (NCRP); 1985.
4. Barendsen GW. The relationships between RBE and LET for different types of lethal damage in mammalian cells: biophysical and molecular mechanisms. *Radiat Res.* 1994;139(3):257–270.
5. Barendsen GW, Walter HM, Fowler JF, et al. Effects of different ionizing radiations on human cells in tissue culture. III. Experiments with cyclotron-accelerated alpha-particles and deuterons. *Radiat Res.* 1963;18:106–119.

6. ICRP. *Relative Biological Effectiveness (RBE), Quality Factor (Q), and Radiation Weighting Factor (w_R)*. *International Commission on Radiological Protection (ICRP) Publication 92*. London: Elsevier; 2003.

7. Meinhold CB. Quantities and units in radiation protection. *Radiat Prot Dosimetry*. 1995;60:343–346

8. Sgouros G, Howell RW, Bolch WE, et al. MIRD Commentary: proposed name for a dosimetry unit applicable to deterministic biological effects—the barendsen (Bd). *J Nucl Med*. 2009;50(3):485–487.

9. Mulford DA, Scheinberg DA, Jurcic JG. The promise of targeted {alpha}-particle therapy. *J Nucl Med*. 2005;46(suppl 1):199S–204S.

10. Sgouros G. Alpha-particles for targeted therapy. *Adv Drug Deliv Rev*. 2008;60(12):1402–1406.

11. Greco C. Particle therapy in prostate cancer: a review. *Prostate Cancer Prostatic Dis*. 2007;10(4):323–330.

12. Pijls-Johannesma M, Grutters JP, Lambin P, et al. Particle therapy in lung cancer: where do we stand? *Cancer Treat Rev*. 2008;34(3):259–267.

13. NCRP. *Radiation Protection Guidance for Activities in Low-earth Orbit. National Council on Radiation Protection and Measurements (NCRP) Report 132*. Bethesda, MD: National Council on Radiation Protection and Measurements (NCRP); 2000.

14. ICRP. 2007 Recommendations of the International Commission on Radiological Protection. International Commission on Radiological Protection (ICRP) Publication 103. *Annals of the ICRP*. 2007;37:1–332.

15. Fitzek MM, Thornton AF, Rabinov JD, et al. Accelerated fractionated proton/photon irradiation to 90 cobalt gray equivalent for glioblastoma multiforme: results of a phase II prospective trial. *J Neurosurg*. 1999;91(2):251–260.

16. Marucci L, Niemierko A, Liebsch NJ, et al. Spinal cord tolerance to high-dose fractionated 3D conformal proton-photon irradiation as evaluated by equivalent uniform dose and dose volume histogram analysis. *Int J Radiat Oncol Biol Phys*. 2004;59(2):551–555.

17. Trofimov A, Nguyen PL, Coen JJ, et al. Radiotherapy treatment of early-stage prostate cancer with IMRT and protons: a treatment planning comparison. *Int J Radiat Oncol Biol Phys*. 2007;69(2):444–453.

18. Wambersie A, Hendry JH, Andreo P, et al. The RBE issues in ion-beam therapy: conclusions of a joint IAEA/ICRU working group regarding quantities and units. *Radiat Prot Dosimetry*. 2006;122:463–470.

19. Hendee W, Ibbott G. *Radiation Therapy Physics*. 2nd ed. St Louis, MO: Mosby; 1996.

20. Mould R. *Radiotherapy Treatment Planning. Medical Physics Handbook 14*. Bristol, England: Adam Hilger Ltd/Hospital Physicists' Association; 1985.

21. Stanton R, Stinson D, Shahabi S. *An Introduction to Radiation Oncology Physics*. Madison, WI: Medical Physics Publishing; 1992.

22. Demidecki AJ, Williams LE, Wong JY, et al. Considerations on the calibration of small thermoluminescent dosimeters used for measurement of beta particle absorbed doses in liquid environments. *Med Phys*. 1993;20(4):1079–1087.

23. Anderson L. Dosimetry for interstitial radiation therapy. In: Hilaris B, ed. *Handbook of Interstitial Brachytherapy*. New York: Memorial Sloan-Kettering Cancer Center; 1975:87–115.

24. Espenan GD, Nelson JA, Fisher DR, et al. Experiences with high dose radiopeptide therapy: the health physics perspective. *Health Phys*. 1999;76(3):225–235.

25. Germano G, Erel J, Kiat H, et al. Quantitative LVEF and qualitative regional function from gated thallium-201 perfusion SPECT. *J Nucl Med*. 1997;38(5):749–754.

26. Hanson W. Brachytherapy source strength: Quantities, units, and standards. In: Williamson J, Thomadsen B, Nath R, eds. *Brachytherapy Physics*. Madison, WI: Medical Physics Publishing Co; 1995.

27. Loevinger R. The MIRD Perspective. In: Adelstein S, Kassis A, Burt R, eds. *Dosimetry of Administered Radionuclides*. Washington, DC: American College of Nuclear Physicians/Department of Energy; 1989:29–43.

28. Stabin MG. Radiopharmaceuticals for nuclear cardiology: radiation dosimetry, uncertainties, and risk. *J Nucl Med*. 2008;49(9):1555–1563.

29. Stabin MG. Uncertainties in internal dose calculations for radiopharmaceuticals. *J Nucl Med*. 2008;49(5):853–860.

30. Stabin MG, Siegel JA, Sparks RB. Sensitivity of model-based calculations of red marrow dosimetry to changes in patient-specific parameters. *Cancer Biother Radiopharm*. 2002;17(5):535–543.

31. Sgouros G. Toward patient-friendly cell-level dosimetry. *J Nucl Med*. 2007;48(4):496–497.

32. Stabin MG, Howell RW, Colas-Linhart NC. Modeling radiation dose and effects from internal emitters in nuclear medicine: from the whole body to individual cells. *Cell Mol Biol (Noisy-le-grand)*. 2001;47(3):535–543.

33. Rossi H. Microscopic energy distributions in irradiated manner. In: Attix F, Roesch W, Tochlin E, eds. *Radiation Dosimetry*. Vol I. New York: Academic Press; 1968:43–92.

34. Rossi HH, Zaider M. The biophysical stage of radiation carcinogenesis. *Health Phys*. 1988;55(2):257–263.

35. Howell RW. The MIRD schema: from organ to cellular dimensions. *J Nucl Med*. 1994;35(3):531–533.

36. Roeske JC, Aydogan B, Bardies M, et al. Small-scale dosimetry: challenges and future directions. *Semin Nucl Med*. 2008;38(5):367–383.

37. Bombardieri E, Buscombe J, Lucignani G, et al. eds. *Advances in Nuclear Oncology: Diagnosis and Therapy*. London: Informa Healthcare; 2007.

38. Harbert J, ed. *Nuclear Medicine Therapy*. New York: Thieme Medical Publishers; 1987.

39. Knox SJ. Systemic radiation therapy. *Semin Radiat Oncology*. 2000; 10:71–167.

40. Kassis AI. Therapeutic radionuclides: biophysical and radiobiologic principles. *Semin Nucl Med*. 2008;38(5):358–366.

41. Wessels BW, Meares CF. Physical and chemical properties of radionuclide therapy. *Semin Radiat Oncol*. 2000;10(2):115–122.

42. Wessels BW, Rogus RD. Radionuclide selection and model absorbed dose calculations for radiolabeled tumor associated antibodies. *Med Phys*. 1984;11(5):638–645.

43. Eckerman KF, Endo A. *MIRD: Radionuclide Data and Decay Schemes*. 2nd ed. Reston, VA: Society of Nuclear Medicine; 1989.

44. Cole A. Absorption of 20-eV to 50,000-eV electron beams in air and plastic. *Radiat Res*. 1969;38:7–33.

45. NCRP. *Influence of Dose and Its Distribution in Time on Dose-Response Relationships for Low-LET Radiations. NCRP Report No 64*. Bethesda, MD: National Council on Radiation Protection and Measurements (NCRP); 1980:64.

46. McEwan AJ, Amyotte GA, McGowan DG, et al. A retrospective analysis of the cost effectiveness of treatment with Metastron (89Sr-chloride) in patients with prostate cancer metastatic to bone. *Nucl Med Commun*. 1994;15(7):499–504.

47. McEwan AJ, Amyotte GA, McGowan DG, et al. A retrospective analysis of the cost effectiveness of treatment with Metastron in patients with prostate cancer metastatic to bone. *Eur Urol*. 1994;26(suppl 1):26–31.

48. Porter AT. Strontium-89 (Metastron) in the treatment of prostate cancer metastatic to bone. *Eur Urol*. 1994;26(suppl 1):20–25.

49. Howell RW, Goddu SM, Rao DV. Application of the linear-quadratic model to radioimmunotherapy: further support for the advantage of longer-lived radionuclides. *J Nucl Med*. 1994;35(11):1861–1869.

50. Warters RL, Hofer KG, Harris CR, et al. Radionuclide toxicity in cultured mammalian cells: elucidation of the primary site of radiation damage. *Curr Top Radiat Res Q*. 1978;12(1–4):389–407.

51. Allen BJ. Clinical trials of targeted alpha therapy for cancer. *Rev Recent Clin Trials*. 2008;3:185–191.

52. McDevitt MR, Sgouros G, Finn RD, et al. Radioimmunotherapy with alpha-emitting nuclides. *Eur J Nucl Med*. 1998;25(9):1341–1351.

53. Sgouros G, Roeske JC, McDevitt MR, et al. MIRD Pamphlet No. 22: radiobiology and dosimetry of alpha-particle emitters for targeted radionuclide therapy. *J Nucl Med*. 2010;51(2):311–328.

54. Sgouros G. Long-lived alpha emitters in radioimmunotherapy: the mischievous progeny. *Cancer Biother Radiopharm*. 2000;15(3):219–221.

55. Welch MJ. Potential and pitfalls of therapy with alpha-particles. *J Nucl Med*. 2005;46(8):1254–1255.

56. Kassis AI, Adelstein SJ. 5-[125I]Iodo-2'-deoxyuridine in the radiotherapy of solid CNS tumors in rats. *Acta Oncol*. 1996;35(7):935–939.

57. Kassis AI, Fayad F, Kinsey BM, et al. Radiotoxicity of an 125I-labeled DNA intercalator in mammalian cells. *Radiat Res*. 1989;118(2):283–294.

58. Kassis AI, Fayad F, Kinsey BM, et al. Radiotoxicity of 125I in mammalian cells. *Radiat Res*. 1987;111(2):305–318.

59. Kassis AI, Guptill WE, Taube RA, et al. Radiotoxicity of 5-[125I]iodo-2'-deoxyuridine in mammalian cells following treatment with 5-fluoro-2'-deoxyuridine. *J Nucl Biol Med*. 1991;35(3):167–173.

60. Bloomer WD, McLaughlin WH, Milius RA, et al. Estrogen receptor-mediated cytotoxicity using iodine-125. *J Cell Biochem*. 1983;21(1):39–45.

61. Blake GM, Zivanovic MA, McEwan AJ, et al. Strontium-89 therapy: strontium kinetics and dosimetry in two patients treated for metastasising osteosarcoma. *Br J Radiol*. 1987;60(711):253–259.

62. Breen SL, Powe JE, Porter AT. Dose estimation in strontium-89 radiotherapy of metastatic prostatic carcinoma. *J Nucl Med*. 1992;33(7):1316–1323.

63. Zanzonico PB, Binkert BL, Goldsmith SJ. Bremsstrahlung radiation exposure from pure beta-ray emitters. *J Nucl Med*. 1999;40(6):1024–1028.

64. Simon N, Feitelberg S. Scanning bremsstrahlung of yttrium-90 microspheres injected intra-arterially. *Radiology*. 1967;88(4):719–724.

65. Ott RJ, Flower MA, Jones A, et al. The measurement of radiation doses from P32 chromic phosphate therapy of the peritoneum using SPECT. *Eur J Nucl Med.* 1985;11(8):305–308.

66. Siegel JA, Zeiger LS, Order SE, et al. Quantitative bremsstrahlung single photon emission computed tomographic imaging: use for volume, activity, and absorbed dose calculations. *Int J Radiat Oncol Biol Phys.* 1995;31(4):953–958.

67. Leichner PK, Akabani G, Colcher D, et al. Patient-specific dosimetry of indium-111- and yttrium-90-labeled monoclonal antibody CC49. *J Nucl Med.* 1997;38(4):512–516.

68. Balachandran S, McGuire L, Flanigan S, et al. Bremsstrahlung imaging after 32P treatment for residual suprasellar cyst. *Int J Nucl Med Biol.* 1985;12(3):215–221.

69. Thomas SR. Options for radionuclide therapy: from fixed activity to patient-specific treatment planning. *Cancer Biother Radiopharm.* 2002; 17:71–82.

70. Zanzonico P, Brill A, Becker D. Radiation dosimetry. In: Wagner H, Szabo Z, Buchanan J, eds. *Principles of Nuclear Medicine.* 2nd ed. Philadelphia: WB Saunders Comp; 1995:106–134.

71. Zanzonico PB. Internal radionuclide radiation dosimetry: a review of basic concepts and recent developments. *J Nucl Med.* 2000;41(2): 297–308.

72. Benua R, Cicale N, Sonenberg M. The relation of radioiodine dosimetry to results and complications in the treatment of metastatic thyroid cancer. *Am J Roentgenol.* 1962;87:171–182.

73. Kaminski MS, Zasadny KR, Francis IR, et al. Radioimmunotherapy of B-cell lymphoma with [131I]anti-B1 (anti-CD20) antibody. *N Engl J Med.* 1993;329(7):459–465.

74. Zasadny K, Gates V, Fisher S, et al. Correlation of dosimetric parameters with hematological toxicity after radioimmunotherapy of non-Hodgkin's lymphoma with I-131 anti-B1. Utility of a new parameter: "Total body dose-lean" (Abstract). *J Nucl Med.* 1995;36:214.

75. Zanzonico PB, Divgi C. Patient-specific radiation dosimetry for radionuclide therapy of liver tumors with intrahepatic artery rhenium-188 lipiodol. *Semin Nucl Med.* 2008;38(2):S30–S39.

76. Stabin MG. Radiotherapy with internal emitters: what can dosimetrists offer? *Cancer Biother Radiopharm.* 2003;18(4):611–617.

77. Stabin MG. Update: the case for patient-specific dosimetry in radionuclide therapy. *Cancer Biother Radiopharm.* 2008;23(3):273–284.

78. Siegel JA, Stabin MG, Brill AB. The importance of patient-specific radiation dose calculations for the administration of radionuclides in therapy. *Cell Mol Biol (Noisy-le-grand).* 2002;48(5):451–459.

79. Siegel JA, Yeldell D, Goldenberg DM, et al. Red marrow radiation dose adjustment using plasma FLT3-L cytokine levels: improved correlations between hematologic toxicity and bone marrow dose for radioimmunotherapy patients. *J Nucl Med.* 2003;44(1):67–76.

80. Bolch WE, Bouchet LG, Robertson JS, et al. MIRD pamphlet No. 17: the dosimetry of nonuniform activity distributions—radionuclide S values at the voxel level. Medical Internal Radiation Dose Committee. *J Nucl Med.* 1999;40(1):11S–36S.

81. Loevinger R, Budinger T, Watson E, et al. *MIRD Primer for Absorbed Dose Calculations.* Revised ed.. New York: Society of Nuclear Medicine; 1991.

82. Bolch WE, Eckermna KF, Shouros G, et al. MIRD Pamphlet No 21: a generalized schema for radiopharmacaeutical dosimetry: standardization of nomenclature. *J Nucl Med.* 2009;50(3):477–484.

83. ICRP. *Radiation Dose to Patients from Radiopharmaceuticals.* International Commission on Radiological Protection (ICRP) Publication No. 53. Oxford: International Commission on Radiological Protection; 1983.

84. Cristy M, Eckerman K. *Specific Absorbed Fractions of Energy at Various Ages from Internal Photon Sources (I-VII).* Oak Ridge National Laboratory Report ORNL/TM-8381/V1-7. Springfield, VA: National Technical Information Service, Department of Commerce; 1987.

85. Snyder W, Ford M, Warner G Jr. Estimates of absorbed fractions for monoenergetic photon sources uniformyly distributed in various organs of a heterogeneous phantom. MIRD Pamphlet No. 5. *J Nucl Med.* 1969;10(suppl 3):5–52.

86. Stabin MG. MIRDOSE: personal computer software for internal dose assessment in nuclear medicine. *J Nucl Med.* 1996;37(3):538–546.

87. Stabin MG, Sparks RB, Crowe E. OLINDA/EXM: the second-generation personal computer software for internal dose assessment in nuclear medicine. *J Nucl Med.* 2005;46(6):1023–1027.

88. Snyder W, Ford M, Warner G, et al. *"S," Absorbed Dose Per Unit Cumulated Activity for Selected Radionuclides and Organs. Medical Internal Radiation Dose (MIRD) Pamphlet No 11.* New York: Society of Nuclear Medicine; 1975.

89. Prasad SR, Jhaveri KS, Saini S, et al. CT tumor measurement for therapeutic response assessment: comparison of unidimensional, bidimensional, and volumetric techniques initial observations. *Radiology.* 2002;225(2):416–419.

90. Stabin MG, Brill AB. State of the art in nuclear medicine dose assessment. *Semin Nucl Med.* 2008;38(5):308–320.

91. Zanzonico P. Technical requirements for SPECT: instrumentation, data acquisition and processing, and quality control. In: Kramer EL, Sanger JJ, eds. *Clinical SPECT Imaging.* New York: Raven Press; 1995:7–41.

92. Zanzonico P. Positron emission tomography: a review of basic principles, scanner design and performance, and current systems. *Semin Nucl Med.* 2004;34(2):87–111.

93. Israel O, Godlsmith SJ, eds. *Hybrid SPECT/CT: Imaging in Clinical Practice.* New York: Taylor & Francis; 2006.

94. O'Connor MK, Kemp BJ. Single-photon emission computed tomography/computed tomography: basic instrumentation and innovations. *Semin Nucl Med.* 2006;36(4):258–266.

95. Roach PJ, Schembri GP, Ho Shon IA, et al. SPECT/CT imaging using a spiral CT scanner for anatomical localization: impact on diagnostic accuracy and reporter confidence in clinical practice. *Nucl Med Commun.* 2006;27(12):977–987.

96. Beyer T, Townsend DW, Blodgett TM. Dual-modality PET/CT tomography for clinical oncology. *Q J Nucl Med.* 2002;46(1):24–34.

97. Beyer T, Townsend DW, Brun T, et al. A combined PET/CT scanner for clinical oncology. *J Nucl Med.* 2000;41(8):1369–1379.

98. Schoder H, Erdi Y, Larson S, et al. PET/CT: a new imaging technology in nuclear medicine. *Eur J Nucl Med Mol Imaging.* 2003;30(10):1419–1435.

99. Sgouros G, Frey E, Wahl R, et al. Three-dimensional imaging-based radiobiological dosimetry. *Semin Nucl Med.* 2008;38(5):321–334.

100. Abdulhathi MB, Al-Salam S, Kassis A, et al. Unusual presentation of cervical cancer as advanced ovarian cancer. *Arch Gynecol Obstet.* 2007;276(4):387–390.

101. King M, Farncombe T. An overview of attenuation and scatter correction of planar and SPECT data for dosimetry studies. *Cancer Biother Radiopharm.* 2003;18(2):181–190.

102. Willowson K, Bailey DL, Baldock C. Quantitative SPECT reconstruction using CT-derived corrections. *Phys Med Biol.* 2008;53(12):3099–3112.

103. Patton JA, Turkington TG. SPECT/CT physical principles and attenuation correction. *J Nucl Med Technol.* 2008;36(1):1–10.

104. Sgouros G, Jureidini IM, Scott AM, et al. Bone marrow dosimetry: regional variability of marrow-localizing antibody. *J Nucl Med.* 1996;37(4):695–698.

105. Sgouros G. Bone marrow dosimetry for radioimmunotherapy: theoretical considerations. *J Nucl Med.* 1993;34(4):689–694.

106. Siegel J, Wessels B, Watson E, et al. Bone marrow dosimetry and toxicity in radioimmunotherapy. *Antibody Immunoconj Radiopharm.* 1990;3: 213–223.

107. Siegel JA, Lee RE, Pawlyk DA, et al. Sacral scintigraphy for bone marrow dosimetry in radioimmunotherapy. *Int J Rad Appl Instrum B.* 1989;16(6):553–559.

108. Sgouros G, Stabin M, Erdi Y, et al. Red marrow dosimetry for radiolabeled antibodies that bind to marrow, bone, or blood components. *Med Phys.* 2000;27(9):2150–2164.

109. Herzog H, Zilken H, Niederbremer A, et al. Calculation of residence times and radiation doses using the standard PC software Excel. *Eur J Nucl Med.* 1997;24(12):1514–1521.

110. Furhang EE, Larson SM, Buranapong P, et al. Thyroid cancer dosimetry using clearance fitting. *J Nucl Med.* 1999;40(1):131–136.

111. Bernal P, Raoul JL, Stare J, et al. International Atomic Energy Agency-sponsored multination study of intra-arterial rhenium-188-labeled lipiodol in the treatment of inoperable hepatocellular carcinoma: results with special emphasis on prognostic value of dosimetric study. *Semin Nucl Med.* 2008;38(2):S40–S45.

112. Siegel JA, Stabin MG. Mass scaling of S values for blood-based estimation of red marrow absorbed dose: the quest for an appropriate method. *J Nucl Med.* 2007;48(2):253–256.

113. MIRD/Dose estimate report no. 8. Summary of current radiation dose estimates to normal humans from 99mTc as sodium pertechnetate. *J Nucl Med.* 1976;17(1):74–77.

114. Adam WE, Clausen M, Hellwig D, et al. Radionuclide ventriculography (equilibrium gated blood pool scanning)—its present clinical position and recent developments. *Eur J Nucl Med.* 1988;13(12):637–647.

115. Schlein B, Terpilak MS, eds. *The Health Physics and Radiological Health Handbook.* Olney, MD: Nucleon Lectern Associates; 1984.

116. Marinelli L, Quimby E, Hine G. Dosage determination with radioactive isotopes. I. Fundamental dosage formulae. *Nucleonics.* 1948;2:56–66.

117. Humm JL, Cobb LM. Nonuniformity of tumor dose in radioimmunotherapy. *J Nucl Med.* 1990;31(1):75–83.

118. O'Donoghue JA. Implications of nonuniform tumor doses for radioimmunotherapy. *J Nucl Med.* 1999;40(8):1337–1341.

119. Humm JL, Macklis RM, Bump K, et al. Internal dosimetry using data derived from autoradiographs. *J Nucl Med.* 1993;34(10):1811–1817.

120. Akabani G, Hawkins W, Eckblade M, et al. Patient-specific dosimetry using quantitative SPECT imaging and three-dimensional discrete fourier transform convolution. *J Nucl Med.* 1997;38:308–314.

121. Erdi AK, Wessels BW, DeJager R, et al. Tumor activity confirmation and isodose curve display for patients receiving iodine-131-labeled 16.88 human monoclonal antibody. *Cancer.* 1994;73(3 suppl):932–944.

122. Erdi AK, Yorke ED, Loew MH, et al. Use of the fast Hartley transform for three-dimensional dose calculation in radionuclide therapy. *Med Phys.* 1998;25(11):2226–2233.

123. Furhang EE, Chui CS, Kolbert KS, et al. Implementation of a Monte Carlo dosimetry method for patient-specific internal emitter therapy. *Med Phys.* 1997;24(7):1163–1172.

124. Furhang EE, Chui CS, Sgouros G. A Monte Carlo approach to patient-specific dosimetry. *Med Phys.* 1996;23(9):1523–1529.

125. Giap HB, Macey DJ, Bayouth JE, et al. Validation of a dose-point kernel convolution technique for internal dosimetry. *Phys Med Biol.* 1995;40(3):365–381.

126. Giap HB, Macey DJ, Podoloff DA. Development of a SPECT-based three-dimensional treatment planning system for radioimmunotherapy. *J Nucl Med.* 1995;36(10):1885–1894.

127. Howell RW, Rao DV, Sastry KS. Macroscopic dosimetry for radioimmunotherapy: nonuniform activity distributions in solid tumors. *Med Phys.* 1989;16(1):66–74.

128. Humm JL. Dosimetric aspects of radiolabeled antibodies for tumor therapy. *J Nucl Med.* 1986;27(9):1490–1497.

129. Kolbert KS, Sgouros G, Scott AM, et al. Implementation and evaluation of patient-specific three-dimensional internal dosimetry. *J Nucl Med.* 1997;38(2):301–308.

130. Koral KF, Lin S, Fessler JA, et al. Preliminary results from intensity-based CT-SPECT fusion in I-131 anti- B1 monoclonal-antibody therapy of lymphoma. *Cancer.* 1997;80(12 suppl):2538–2544.

131. Koral KF, Zasadny KR, Kessler ML, et al. CT-SPECT fusion plus conjugate views for determining dosimetry in iodine-131-monoclonal antibody therapy of lymphoma patients. *J Nucl Med.* 1994;35(10):1714–1720.

132. Kwok CS, Bialobzyski PJ, Yu SK, et al. Effect of tissue inhomogeneity on dose distribution of point sources of low-energy electrons. *Med Phys.* 1990;17(5):786–793.

133. Kwok CS, Irfan M, Woo MK, et al. Effect of tissue inhomogeneity on beta dose distribution of 32P. *Med Phys.* 1987;14(1):98–104.

134. Kwok CS, Prestwich WV, Wilson BC. Calculation of radiation doses for nonuniformity distributed beta and gamma radionuclides in soft tissue. *Med Phys.* 1985;12(4):405–412.

135. Leichner PK, Kwok CS. Tumor dosimetry in radioimmunotherapy: methods of calculation for beta particles. *Med Phys.* 1993;20(2 pt 2):529–534.

136. Mird-dose estimate report no. 2. Summary of current radiation dose estimates to humans from 66Ga-, 68Ga-, and 72Ga-citrate. *J Nucl Med.* 1973;14(10):755–756.

137. Liu A, Williams LE, Lopatin G, et al. A radionuclide therapy treatment planning and dose estimation system. *J Nucl Med.* 1999;40(7):1151–1153.

138. Ljungberg M, Strand SE. Dose planning with SPECT. *Int J Cancer Suppl.* 1988;2:67–70.

139. Mayer R, Dillehay LE, Shao Y, et al. A new method for determining dose rate distribution from radioimmuno- therapy using radiochromic media. *Int J Radiat Oncol Biol Phys.* 1994;28(2):505–513.

140. Sgouros G, Barest G, Thekkumthala J, et al. Treatment planning for internal radionuclide therapy: three-dimensional dosimetry for nonuniformly distributed radionuclides. *J Nucl Med.* 1990;31(11):1884–1891.

141. Sgouros G, Chiu S, Pentlow KS, et al. Three-dimensional dosimetry for radioimmunotherapy treatment planning. *J Nucl Med.* 1993;34(9):1595–1601.

142. Uchida I, Yamada Y, Oyamada H, et al. Calculation algorithm of three-dimensional absorbed dose distribution due to in vivo administration of nuclides for radiotherapy. *Kaku Igaku.* 1992;29(11):1299–1306.

143. Wessels BW, Yorke ED, Bradley EW. Dosimetry of heterogeneous uptake of radiolabeled antibody for radioimmunotherapy. *Front Radiat Ther Oncol.* 1990;24:104–108.

144. Adelstein S, Kassis A, Sastry K. Cellular vs organ approaches to dose estimates. In: Schlafke-Stelson A, Watson E, eds. *Proceedings of the Fourth International Radiopharmaceutical Dosimetry Symposium (Conf-85113 (DE86010102)).* Oak Ridge, TN: US Dept of Energy and Oak Ridge Associated Universities; 1986:13–25.

145. Adelstein SJ, Kassis AI. Radiobiologic implications of the microscopic distribution of energy from radionuclides. *Int J Rad Appl Instrum B.* 1987;14(3):165–169.

146. Goddu S, Howell R, Bouchet L, et al. *MIRD Cellular S Factors: Self-Absorbed Dose per Unit Cumulated Activity for Selected Radionuclides and Monoenergetic Electrons and Alpha Particle Emitters Incorporated into Different Cell Compartments.* Reston, VA: Society of Nuclear Medicine; 1997.

147. Goddu SM, Howell RW, Rao DV. Calculation of equivalent dose for Auger electron emitting radionuclides distributed in human organs. *Acta Oncol.* 1996;35(7):909–916.

148. Goddu SM, Rao DV, Howell RW. Multicellular dosimetry for micrometastases: dependence of self-dose versus cross-dose to cell nuclei on type and energy of radiation and subcellular distribution of radionuclides. *J Nucl Med.* 1994;35(3):521–530.

149. Griffiths GL, Govindan SV, Sgouros G, et al. Cytotoxicity with Auger electron-emitting radionuclides delivered by antibodies. *Int J Cancer.* 1999;81(6):985–992.

150. Humm JL, Howell RW, Rao DV. Dosimetry of Auger-electron-emitting radionuclides: report no. 3 of AAPM Nuclear Medicine Task Group No. 6. [Erratum in: *Med Phys.* 1995;22(11 pt 1):1837]. *Med Phys.* 1994;21(12):1901–1915.

151. Humm JL, Macklis RM, Lu XQ, et al. The spatial accuracy of cellular dose estimates obtained from 3D reconstructed serial tissue autoradiographs. *Phys Med Biol.* 1995;40(1):163–180.

152. Humm JL, Roeske JC, Fisher DR, et al. Microdosimetric concepts in radioimmunotherapy. *Med Phys.* 1993;20(2 pt 2):535–541.

153. Kassis AI, Adelstein SJ. Chemotoxicity of indium-111 oxine in mammalian cells. *J Nucl Med.* 1985;26(2):187–190.

154. Kassis AI, Adelstein SJ, Haydock C, et al. Radiotoxicity of 75Se and 35S: theory and application to a cellular model. *Radiat Res.* 1980;84(3):407–425.

155. Kassis AI, Adelstein SJ, Haydock C, et al. Thallium-201: an experimental and a theoretical radiobiological approach to dosimetry. *J Nucl Med.* 1983;24(12):1164–1175.

156. Macklis RM, Lin JY, Beresford B, et al. Cellular kinetics, dosimetry, and radiobiology of alpha-particle radioimmunotherapy: induction of apoptosis. *Radiat Res.* 1992;130(2):220–226.

157. Makrigiorgos GM, Adelstein SJ, Kassis AI. Limitations of conventional internal dosimetry at the cellular level. *J Nucl Med.* 1989;30(11):1856–1864.

158. Makrigiorgos GM, Ito S, Baranowska-Kortylewicz J, et al. Inhomogeneous deposition of radiopharmaceuticals at the cellular level: experimental evidence and dosimetric implications. *J Nucl Med.* 1990;31(8):1358–1363.

159. O'Donoghue JA. Strategies for selective targeting of Auger electron emitters to tumor cells. *J Nucl Med.* 1996;37(4 suppl):3S–6S.

160. O'Donoghue JA, Wheldon TE. Targeted radiotherapy using Auger electron emitters. *Phys Med Biol.* 1996;41(10):1973–1992.

161. Wrenn ME, Howells GP, Hairr LM, et al. Auger electron dosimetry. *Health Phys.* 1973;24(6):645–653.

162. Yorke ED, Williams LE, Demidecki AJ, et al. Multicellular dosimetry for beta-emitting radionuclides: autoradiography, thermoluminescent dosimetry and three-dimensional dose calculations. *Med Phys.* 1993;20(2 pt 2):543–550.

163. Zalutsky MR, Stabin MG, Larsen RH, et al. Tissue distribution and radiation dosimetry of astatine-211-labeled chimeric 81C6, an alpha-particle-emitting immunoconjugate. *Nucl Med Biol.* 1997;24(3):255–261.

164. Erdi AK, Erdi YE, Yorke ED, et al. Treatment planning for radioimmunotherapy. *Phys Med Biol.* 1996;41(10):2009–2026.

165. Tagesson M, Ljungberg M, Strand SE. A Monte-Carlo program converting activity distributions to absorbed dose distributions in a radionuclide treatment planning system. *Acta Oncol.* 1996;35(3):367–372.

Small-Scale Dosimetry and Microdosimetry

John C. Roeske, Bulent Aydogan, Manuel Bardiès, and John L. Humm

■ INTRODUCTION

When combined with a suitable targeting agent, radionuclides emitting particulate radiation (alpha particles, beta particles, or Auger electrons) offer the potential of delivering high doses to individual tumor cells while minimizing the volume of normal tissue irradiated (1–8). The dosimetry of these particulate emitters, however, is challenging due to the small scale on which the dose must be specified. For beta particles, this scale is on the order of millimeters, while for alpha particles the energy deposited must be estimated on a scale of microns (9,10). For shorter range emissions, such as Auger electrons, the scale of calculation is within the cell itself (11). These scales are all comparable to the range of the respective charged particles.

While the radionuclide decay processes and physical characteristics of energy deposition for each of these emitters are well known, the biologic aspects associated with dosimetry on this scale have a high degree of variability (12,13). In particular, two parameters are required for accurate dose calculation: the source distribution as a function of time and the cellular target geometry (14,15). As demonstrated in Chapter 8, planar imaging and single photon emission computed tomography (SPECT) imaging can be used to quantify the activity on a macroscopic level. At the current resolution of these imaging systems (millimeter to centimeter), small-scale dose estimates are not meaningful. Likewise, the target/tumor geometry is difficult to visualize in vivo at the microscopic level as the tissues of interest can range from individual cells to small micrometastatic clusters. Clearly, these are not visible with current clinical imaging modalities (such as magnetic resonance [MR], photon emission tomography [PET], or computed tomography [CT]).

Despite these limitations, small-scale and microdosimetry techniques provide valuable insight (16,17). As will be shown, these methods can provide the basis for designing clinical trials as well as interpreting clinical outcomes. After a brief discussion of the medical internal radiation dose (MIRD) methodology, techniques will be described for calculating dose from beta, alpha, and Auger emitters. For each methodology, the calculational techniques will be discussed, as well as their limitations.

■ MIRD

The estimate of absorbed radiation dose from internal emitters is required to assess the radiation risk associated with the administration of radiopharmaceuticals for medical applications. In 1965, the MIRD Committee was formed to provide an accurate estimate of patient dose from radiopharmaceuticals administered for diagnostic studies. At that time, it had been acknowledged that the assumption of a uniform distribution of activity throughout the body was not accurate, and there was a pressing need for a unified approach to performing organ-level dosimetry for internal emitters. As a result, the committee published "MIRD Pamphlet No. 1" describing a robust calculation method for absorbed dose from internally deposited radionuclides (18). This formalism reduced the complex nature of the absorbed dose calculation into a relatively simple form. The schema was originally published in 1968 (18), revised in 1976 (19), and republished with comprehensive examples as the *MIRD Primer* in 1988 and 1991 (20). Recently, "MIRD Pamphlet No. 21" (21) introduced a generalized schema for radiopharmaceutical dosimetry to accomplish two major goals: (a) to standardize nomenclature used in absorbed dose calculations and to restate the MIRD formalism for the assessment of absorbed dose "in a manner consistent with the needs of both the nuclear medicine and the radiation protection communities" and (b) to introduce dosimetric quantities such as *equivalent dose* and *effective dose* into the MIRD formalism for estimating potential risks of stochastic effects from nuclear medicine procedures (21). In addition, the need for dosimetric quantities to estimate deterministic effects from targeted radionuclide therapy was also discussed.

The MIRD schema combines the biologic distribution and clearance data of radiopharmaceuticals with the physical properties of radionuclides to calculate absorbed dose. This calculation thus relates the activity in a source organ to the dose deposited in the target organ (18). In the MIRD schema, the mean absorbed dose, $\overline{D}$, within the kth target from the ith source is defined as

$$\overline{D} = \widetilde{A}_i \sum_j \Delta_j \frac{\phi_j(k \leftarrow i)}{m_k}. \qquad \text{(Eq. 9.1)}$$

In this equation, $\widetilde{A}_i$ is the cumulated activity from the ith source, Δ_j is the mean energy emitted per nuclear transition from the jth transition, ϕ_j is the absorbed fraction (representing the fraction of energy emitted from the ith source, which is absorbed by the kth target), and m_k is the mass of the target (18–20). At the organ level, ϕ_j has values between 0 and 1 for penetrating radiations (photons) and typically 1 for nonpenetrating radiations (e.g., alpha particles, Auger electrons, and beta particles). However, as will be discussed in the next sections, a nonpenetrating radiation value of $\phi_j < 1$ may be required for small-scale dose calculations.

The MIRD equation can be further simplified by combining all physical data into a single parameter known as the S value. This parameter represents the mean dose deposited per unit of cumulated activity (18–20). Thus, the mean absorbed dose to the kth organ from the ith source, based on the MIRD schema, can be written as

$$\overline{D} = \sum \widetilde{A}_i S(k \leftarrow i). \qquad \text{(Eq. 9.2)}$$

Equation (9.2) can subsequently be rearranged as

$$\overline{D} = A_0 \tau_i \sum S(k \leftarrow i), \qquad \text{(Eq. 9.3)}$$

where τ_i is the residence time in source organ i. The residence time represents the "average" or "effective" life of the initial activity (A_0) in the source organ. Note that τ accounts for both physical decay and biologic removal from the source organ (18–20).

The publication of S value tables for a wide range of source/target organs and radionuclides has provided a simplified and consistent methodology for internal dosimetry calculations. "MIRD Pamphlet No. 11" provided tables of S values for a large number of radionuclides and source/target pairs (22). Subsequently, Stabin and Siegel introduced dose factors, an equivalent quantity to the S value, and provided tables for an even larger number of radionuclides (23). One of the advantages of the MIRD approach is that new tables can be published as updated decay data and phantom geometries become available, without changing the formalism.

Small-scale dosimetry

The mean absorbed dose deposited in individual organs is important in estimating the risk or biologic effect. However, the average dose at the organ or voxel level is less meaningful when using highly precise targeting methods that employ radionuclides with short-range emissions. For example, the mean tumor dose does not correlate well with the biologic effects observed with Auger electron emitters (24,25). For these classes of radionuclides, the absorbed dose should be calculated on a scale comparable to the range of their emissions.

Fortunately, the MIRD methodology is sufficiently general such that it can be applied to any dimension (organs to subcellular structures) (26,27). When planar imaging was primarily used, the MIRD method was used to estimate doses at the organ level (28–32). With the advent of PET and SPECT, suborgan dose calculations were possible (33,34).

Technological advances in these modalities to increase the spatial resolution have made dosimetry at the voxel level more relevant. "MIRD Pamphlet No. 17" provided tabulated S values for 3- and 6-mm voxels from a nonuniform activity distribution for the most commonly used radionuclides (35). Additionally, S values were also published for 0.1-mm voxels for I-131. Here, the activity distribution would be obtained from autoradiographic studies (35). This work has subsequently been expanded to voxel phantoms for internal dosimetry (36). A comparison of internal radiation doses estimated by "MIRD Pamphlet No. 17" and voxel techniques for a family of realistic phantoms was published in 2000 (37).

The MIRD schema was extended in 1997 to provide cellular S values allowing for the calculation of dose at this level (38). The geometry for these calculations consisted of a cell nucleus, which was modeled as a homogeneous, concentric sphere within a spherical cell (38). The MIRD cell model is shown in Figure 9.1. Highlighted are the principal compartments—the nucleus, cytoplasm, and cell surface. Here R_C and R_N represent the radii of the cell and nucleus, respectively. In the MIRD tables, these range in value from 3 to 10 μm and from 1 to 9 μm, respectively. Cellular S values for alpha- and beta-particle emitters were published for various source/target pairs including cell/cell, cell surface/cell, nucleus/nucleus, cytoplasm/nucleus, and cell surface/nucleus. In addition, S values were also published for monoenergetic electrons and alpha particles such that they can be used to compute S values for radionuclides that were not included in the report.

Cellular S values can be calculated using analytical methods or Monte Carlo (MC) techniques. In general, both methods yield similar results. Comparison of the mean doses calculated using an analytical approach (38) versus MC (39) for monoenergetic electrons demonstrated agreement to within 4%. In 2008, Champion et al. compared S values based on MC calculations using the CELLDOSE program with those obtained through analytical methods (40). Their calculated S values were on average about 4% less than those calculated by Goddu et al. (38) and on average about 6% greater than those by Bardiès and Chatal (41), thus demonstrating good overall agreement.

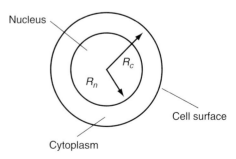

FIGURE 9.1 Schematic diagram of the MIRD cellular model used for calculation of the S value (adapted from Ref. (38)). In this model, R_N and R_C represent the radii of the nucleus and cell, respectively. The three source compartments—nucleus, cytoplasm, and cell surface—are highlighted.

Assumptions and limitations of MIRD dose calculations

The accuracy of small-scale MIRD calculations is limited by the ability to quantify the activity in each compartment, physical data including the number of particles emitted per disintegration, their type and energy and energy loss in tissue, and the geometry of the source and target regions. Quantification of the absolute activity in subcellular compartments is very difficult and as such is considered to be one of the major sources of error and/or uncertainty in small-scale dosimetry. However, the uncertainties in the physical parameters, and their subsequent effect on the S value, are well documented and will be discussed.

The rate of energy loss by a charged particle is often quantified by the stopping power (9–11). Hence, the stopping power data used in the calculations may have a considerable effect on the S values. There are a number of stopping power data available for electrons, positrons, and alpha particles in the literature (9–11,42–44). For electrons, the MIRD cellular S values report (38) uses Cole's empirical fit to experimental data (11). A comparison of S values calculated using Cole's data versus International Commission on Radiation Units and Measurements (ICRU) (9) stopping powers for monoenergetic electrons and positrons showed a difference of less than 7%. For alpha particles, the MIRD report uses the ICRU stopping powers (10) due to the international standing of these tables. However, S value differences of up to 40% were noted when comparing ICRU stopping powers versus Kaplan's data (38).

Absorbed dose estimations to very small volumes such as cellular and subcellular structures are also limited by the method used to account for escaping secondary electrons. Restricted stopping powers can be used to account for this energy loss. Typically, a cutoff energy of 10 to 20 keV would be used for cellular dimensions (38). For alpha particles, the stopping powers and the restricted stopping powers do not differ significantly in the energy range of 3 to 10 MeV (10). However, the difference can be substantial for high-energy electrons (38). In a comparison of S values based on unrestricted stopping powers versus the OREC (Oak Ridge electron transport code) (45) MC code, which follows every primary and secondary electron, only small differences were noted for electron energies less than 100 keV (38). However, the S values tended to be 10% to 25% lower for particle energies greater than 100 keV (38).

The tabulated S values provided by the MIRD committee (38) assume that cells can be adequately represented by a spherical geometry. However, cells in tissue tend to deviate from this idealized case. The OREC MC code was used to compare S values for spherical versus ellipsoidal target volumes (38). It was observed that the shape only marginally influenced the self-absorbed dose to nucleus, that is, when nucleus was both the source and the target for beta particles with energies less than 100 keV. However, up to a 14% difference was noted due to cell shape for beta particles with higher energies. When the activity was localized in the cytoplasm or on the cell surface, the nuclear S values differed considerably, particularly when the cell became elongated and electron energies were less than 10 keV. For example, the ratio of $S(N \leftarrow Cs)$ values ($S_{sphere}/S_{ellipsoid}$) was 0.085 for 5 keV electrons when cell was represented as an elongated ellipsoid (38).

It should be noted that the cellular S values represent the mean *self*-absorbed doses received by individual cells and hence do not include cross fire effects due to activity on neighboring cells. The cross fire contribution must be estimated separately. Moreover, within a population of cells, the dose to an individual cell will depend on many factors including its size and geometry, as well as the local distribution of activity. Hence, the dose variation within a group of cells as a function of position may be required for a meaningful correlation between the calculated dose and the biologic end point. Thus, many have questioned whether the mean absorbed dose to cell is an appropriate measure to infer biologic response in targeted therapy (26,27,39,46,47). Use of mean self-absorbed dose to an individual cell or at a particular point also assumes that charged particle equilibrium (CPE) conditions are satisfied with respect to the number of types of particle entering and exiting a calculation volume (48). For low-LET (linear energy transfer) radiation, a large number of decays are required to deposit a considerable dose, and hence this condition is generally satisfied (48). However, this assumption may not be valid when there is a very inhomogeneous cellular uptake or the cellular absorbed dose is low (49). CPE conditions may not be satisfied for alpha particles where only a few cellular decays are required to inactivate a single cell (50). In these cases, stochastic methods may be required. These and other dosimetric challenges specific to various emission types will be discussed in the following sections.

BETA EMITTERS

Beta emitters have a long history of use for targeted radiotherapy (1). The most commonly used beta emitters in this context are ^{131}I and ^{90}Y (2). However, several other beta emitters are currently proposed or being considered for therapy (51,52). Beta decay (negatron decay) occurs when the nucleus with atomic number Z and mass number A is transformed into one with atomic number $Z + 1$ and mass number A, and results in the emission of an electron and an antineutrino (53). Because the decay energy is shared between the beta particle and the antineutrino, the resultant beta particles have a spectrum of energies ranging from 0 to $E_{\beta max}$, where $E_{\beta max}$ is the energy of the transition. Typically, $E_{\beta max}$ is on the order of hundreds of kiloelectron volts. This energy corresponds to a maximum range of a few millimeters in water.

^{90}Y ($E_{\beta max} = 2.2$ MeV) is the most energetic beta emitter considered for targeted radiotherapy, and its maximum range is approximately 1.1 cm in water. Berger defined the 90-percentile distance, x_{90}, as the distance at which 90% of the energy is absorbed ("MIRD Pamphlet No. 7") (54). For ^{90}Y, this distance is 0.517 cm, indicating that most of the electrons in the beta spectrum are concentrated at a much lower energy. Therefore, the entire beta spectrum must be taken into account in beta emitter absorbed dose calculations. Use of the maximum or mean values can lead to erroneous results. For example, differences of up to 47% in the *S* value were observed when using the mean energy versus the complete beta particle spectrum (38).

Traditionally, beta particles are treated as nonpenetrating radiation, that is, $\phi = 1$. However, when the size of the target volume is on the same order as the maximum range of the beta particle emission, a value of $\phi < 1$ will occur with a significant fraction of the energy escaping the targeted volume. Moreover, the absorbed dose within the target volume will vary with position, and hence the mean absorbed dose as obtained from a MIRD calculation is less meaningful. In general, there are two methods for calculating positional variation in absorbed dose from beta emitters. The first is an analytical approach where the source distribution is modeled as a series of "point sources." Each contributes dose to the point in question weighted by the distance, the activity of the point source, and dose point kernel (DPK). The DPK provides the variation of the absorbed dose (or the absorbed fraction of energy) at a distance from an isotropic monoenergetic point source of electrons, in a homogeneous medium (usually water) (55,56). The DPK will have either an analytical or a tabulated form. The second approach is MC modeling of radiation transport and energy deposition. Unlike the DPK approach, MC calculations are not restricted to a homogeneous medium, and hence can take into account the density and composition of individual tissues.

■ Calculation approaches

If the medium of interest is of uniform density and composition, then the absorbed dose varies only as a function of the distance to the emission point. Following the superposition principle, the absorbed dose at a point is expressed as a convolution integral (57):

$$D(\vec{r}) = \int f(\vec{r} - \vec{r}')a(\vec{r}')\mathrm{d}r'^3, \qquad \text{(Eq. 9.4)}$$

where $f(\vec{r} - \vec{r}')$ is the DPK and $a(\vec{r}')$ is the intensity of the source per unit volume. The evaluation of the convolution integral through analytical methods is difficult even for simple geometries. Therefore, numerical integration methods are often used. Thus, Equation 9.4 is replaced by a summation with discrete volume elements:

$$D(x,y,z) = \sum_{x,y,z} a(x',y',z')f(x - x',y - y',z - z')$$
$$\Delta x' \Delta y' \Delta z', \qquad \text{(Eq. 9.5)}$$

where the primed variables represent the source position and the unprimed variables represent the location of the calculation point in a Cartesian coordinate system. For a three-dimensional source distribution without any symmetry, the computational time can be significant.

Hence, the fast Fourier transform (58) or fast Hartley transform (59) algorithms can be used to improve the speed of such calculations.

The input to Equations 9.4 and 9.5, the DPK, can be obtained from a variety of sources—measurements (60), calculations (55), or MC codes (61,62). The DPK can be monoenergetic, or specific to a particular radionuclide by integrating over the beta spectrum. The beta DPK, in terms of both measurement and mathematical formulation, can be traced back to Loevinger and Holt (63). Using planar sources consisting of beta emitters, the electron fluence was measured as a function of polystyrene thickness between the source and the detector. The DPK was obtained by differentiating the absorbed dose versus distance from the source and dividing by the square of the distance. Loevinger's mathematical formulation of the DPK included both a primary term (represented as an exponential) and a scatter term (consisting of a linear exponential). While this early form fit the data reasonably well over the beta-particle range, it underestimated the absorbed dose near the point of emission.

Spencer (64) provided an analytical solution to the radiation transport equation for monoenergetic electrons. This solution used the method of moments and the continuous slowing down approximation (CSDA) in which a particle is assumed to lose energy continuously during its trajectory. Due to the nature of these approximations, Spencer's solution did not take into account the production of secondary electrons. However, the results were used by Berger (55) and Cross and Williams (60) to compile DPK tables for a variety of beta emitters of clinical importance.

An alternative method for the generation of DPK involves the use of MC codes (65,66). Prestwich et al. (65) use the MC method to generate DPK for various radionuclides of interest in radioimmunotherapy. Simpkin and Mackie (66) used the EGS4 code to generate various DPK in water. While they demonstrated some minor disagreement with the DPK produced by Prestwich et al. (65), due to differences in sampling, they noted good agreement with Berger's data (55). In a comparison of DPK, Fujimori et al. (67) observed generally good agreement between their own kernels and those generated by Berger, Cross, and Prestwich. Other MC codes have been used more recently to generate DPK, and again the general conclusion is that most current DPK agree reasonably well (68).

MC codes are also used in cases where the medium has a nonuniform density and composition. In these cases, the DPK approach is not valid and a full simulation of the radiation transport is required. Two areas where MC is receiving increased attention are bone marrow and small-animal dosimetry.

Bone marrow cavities have been previously modeled by Cloutier and Watson (69) as 400-μm spheres surrounded by 70 μm thick shells representing the bone walls. The absorbed fractions and subsequent *S* factor produced using this model have been used for many years. Electron-absorbed fractions for bone and marrow compartments in an adult male were developed by Whitwell and Spiers (70). These data were used to calculate *S* factors in "MIRD Pamphlet No. 11" (22). The ICRP (71) later produced absorbed fractions derived partly from these previous studies. However, these calculations did not take into account the backscatter at the bone–soft tissue interface, which has been proven to be important (72). A newer dosimetric model proposed by Eckerman and Stabin (32,73) was incorporated into MIRDOSE3. Using the EGS4 code (74), Bouchet et al. (75) used more recent data on regional bone and marrow mass to calculate absorbed fractions. A revision to the model was published, which resolved the differences between these approaches (76) and were implemented in the OLINDA/EXM computer code (77).

In many preclinical studies, small-animal experiments are often performed to evaluate the efficacy of a targeted radiotherapy approach. Using biopsy or tissue samples, the activity can be counted and absorbed dose estimates can be performed. Because the organs and tumors within the mouse may be on the order of or less than the maximum range of the beta emission, a standard MIRD calculation assuming $\phi = 1$ may prove inaccurate. As such, Hui et al. (78) proposed a simple murine model in 1994. With improved small-animal imaging, several models have been published based on micro-CT or MR studies (79–84). These models can be categorized as either equation based or voxel based.

In Stabin et al.'s study, micro-CT was used to obtain voxel-based mouse and rat models (82). Each of these data sets had submillimeter sampling. Using the Monte Carlo N-Particle Transport code, a full MC radiation transport was implemented (85). In this study, absorbed fractions were calculated for 12 photon and electron energies within the various identified source organs. Additionally, absorbed fractions were also calculated for common beta emitters including ^{90}Y, ^{111}In, ^{131}I, and ^{188}Re. In a related study, Bitar et al. compared the results obtained with a full MC-absorbed dose calculation versus the standard MIRD approximation with $\phi = 1$ (86). For ^{188}Re, the absorbed dose within a

xenografted tumor was 39% to 69% lower using MC versus the assumption that all energy is absorbed within the target. These results indicate the necessity of improved calculational models for small-animal dosimetry.

A recent study (87) by Boutaleb et al. emphasized the point that dosimetric results rely on the animal model chosen and that geometric variations observed between animal strains could not be corrected for by using a simple mass-scaling factor (as is usually the case at the clinical level). Indeed, the fact is that in targeted radiotherapy, absorbed dose in organ sources (i.e., organ/tissues that concentrate the radiopharmaceutical) is mostly due to beta radiation (the gamma contribution to the absorbed dose being usually an order of magnitude less than the beta contribution). In clinical dosimetry, since organ/tissue dimensions markedly exceed the maximum range of the most energetic electrons, one can safely assume that all beta radiations are nonpenetrating. This explains why, for mean absorbed doses in organs, the mass scaling of *S* factors can be accepted as a first-order approximation (88). In contrast, the mass scaling does not bring satisfactory results in a situation where a significant amount of the emitted energy escapes the source region (i.e., when beta particles cannot be considered as nonpenetrating radiation), as is the case for small-animal dosimetry.

■ Example

Consider a spherical source of radius R_s, where all radioactivity is located on the surface. This situation corresponds to the case of radiolabeled antibodies that bind to the target surface (cell, or spherical cell cluster). In this example, the sphere and surrounding media are considered as water equivalent. The absorbed fraction in the sphere was calculated using the approach presented by Bardiès and Chatal (41).

Figure 9.2 shows a plot of the mean absorbed fraction as a function of the sphere's radius for various beta-particle emitters. In this case, the mean absorbed fraction tends

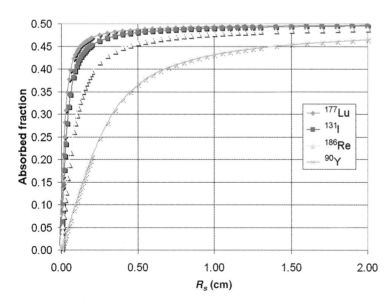

FIGURE 9.2. Absorbed fraction in spheres labeled on the surface for increasing source sphere radius R_s.

toward 0.5 as the source radius R_s increases. For a small sphere, most of the energy emitted on the surface is lost (i.e., absorbed outside of the sphere). However, for a large sphere, that is, when particle range becomes negligible relative to the spherical radius, a maximum of half of the emitted energy is absorbed in the sphere (the situation tends to that of a semi-infinite plane). This behavior is observed for every beta emitter, but the convergence in 0.5 will be observed first for low-energy emitters. Indeed, $E_{\beta mean}(^{177}Lu) < E_{\beta mean}(^{131}I) < E_{\beta mean}(^{186}Re) < E_{\beta mean}(^{90}Y)$.

In addition, using the absorbed fraction and the emitted energy, it is possible to calculate the mean absorbed dose per disintegration (S value). For a 2 cm radius sphere, this will lead to values of 3.48×10^{-13}, 4.54×10^{-13}, 7.97×10^{-13}, and 2.11×10^{-12} GyBq^{-1}s^{-1}, respectively, for ^{177}Lu, ^{131}I, ^{186}Re, and ^{90}Y. Note that for a 2 cm radius sphere, the S values increase with $E_{\beta mean}$ (this is expected since most absorbed fractions are equal to or near 0.5).

However, for the same geometry, for a much smaller sphere (e.g., a 20 μm radius sphere), the results are reversed. The S values are 3.15×10^{-5}, 2.47×10^{-5}, 1.98×10^{-5}, and 9.93×10^{-6} GyBq^{-1}s^{-1}, respectively, for ^{177}Lu, ^{131}I, ^{186}Re, and ^{90}Y. That is, low-energy emitters deposit more energy in small spheres.

This concept is further illustrated in Figure 9.3, which represents the absorbed fraction in a 5 μm radius sphere, concentric to the source sphere of radius R_s. For small source spheres ($R_s < 50$ μm), the absorbed fraction for low-energy beta emitters is greater than that of high-energy beta emitters. Furthermore, above 50 to 100 μm, because of the limited range of electrons, no energy is absorbed in the central target sphere. This means that even though the mean absorbed fraction in the sphere (and mean S value) is different from zero, the center of the sphere will not be irradiated at all.

From a radiobiologic point of view, the consequences are that the mean absorbed dose can be misleading if the spatial spread around the mean is elevated: absorbed dose gradients should be taken into account when reporting beta-absorbed doses. These absorbed dose gradients can be calculated—as in the former example—using a macrodosimetric approach (i.e., by calculating mean absorbed doses rather than specific energies) by considering small volumes where the spatial fluctuations around the mean dose are likely to be small.

■ ALPHA PARTICLES

A number of recent studies have described both the in vitro and in vivo application of alpha-particle emitters (3–6, 89–91). Alpha-particle decay generally occurs in high atomic number (Z) radionuclides and results in the emission of a helium nucleus (charge = 2+). Additionally, a gamma emission often accompanies the decay, which may be useful for imaging (53). Most alpha particles have initial energies of 3 to 9 MeV. Unlike beta emitters, alpha-particle energies are discrete. Similar to other charged particles, alpha particles have a defined range beyond which little or no energy is deposited. Typically, this range is 40 to 90 μm in tissue. Thus, alpha particles will irradiate only those cells in which they are in direct contact, or cells that are directly neighboring the point of emission. In addition to the attractive physical properties of alpha particles, they also provide radiobiologic advantages such as having a high LET and independence from dose rate and oxygen effects (92).

Alpha-particle dosimetry can be approached through two different methodologies. The MIRD method, as discussed previously in this chapter (in the section MIRD), can be used to estimate the average dose to cellular targets (38). However, the average dose often does not provide an accurate estimate of the energy imparted to individual cellular targets. This feature of alpha-particle dosimetry can be understood by considering a simple schematic diagram (Fig. 9.4). In this figure, cells are irradiated in a uniform solution of alpha-particle emitters. Some cell nuclei are hit directly by an alpha particle, and these deposit a significant amount of energy. Other cell nuclei are not hit at all, or are merely grazed by the alpha particle. In these cases, little or no direct energy is deposited. Lastly, some cells will receive multiple hits from alpha particles that can occur in any of the previous combinations. Based on this example, the traditional concepts of average absorbed dose break down, and the stochastic distribution of energy deposited must be considered. The field of microdosimetry was developed to address these issues (93).

Microdosimetry was proposed by Rossi as a study of the stochastic nature of energy deposition in small targets (94). Originally, microdosimetry was applied to quantify the stochastic distribution of energy deposited by external ionizing radiation. Later this theory was adapted to internally deposited radionuclides (95), fast neutrons (96), protons, and electrons (97). The principles of microdosimetry were later used by Fisher to study the stochastic distribution of energy deposited in cell nuclei by ^{212}Bi (98). Subsequently, Stinchcomb and Roeske modified Roesch's equations for the

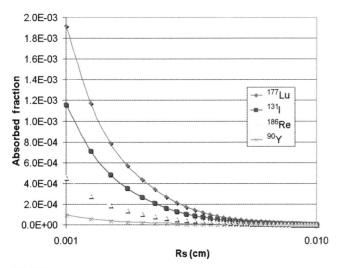

FIGURE 9.3 Absorbed fraction in a central target sphere (radius = 5 μm) from source spheres (radius R_s) labeled on the surface.

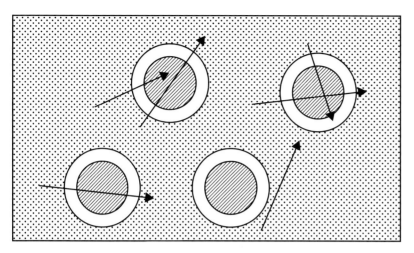

FIGURE 9.4 Schematic diagram illustrating the stochastic variations in the number of hits and in the energy deposited within cell nuclei from alpha-particle emitters. The alpha-particle tracks, represented by lines with arrows, intersect the cell nuclei (*shaded circles*) and deposit energy proportional to their track length. In certain cases, some cells receive no hits whatsoever. Adapted from Roeske and Humm (101).

specific case of antibodies labeled with short-lived alpha emitters (99).

In radiotherapy, absorbed dose is a fundamental quantity. The microdosimetric analogue of absorbed dose is specific energy. Like absorbed dose, specific energy represents the energy deposited per unit mass. However, unlike absorbed dose, specific energy is a stochastic quantity. Thus, it does not have a single value, but rather it has a spectrum of values. The single-event spectrum represents the probability distribution for exactly one alpha particle energy deposition event in a target. Alternatively, the multiple hit spectrum represents the distribution for N events. The multiple-event spectrum (for N hits) may be determined by convolving the single-event spectrum $N - 1$ times (94). Kellerer (100) developed a method to efficiently determine the multiple-event spectrum through the use of Fourier transforms. An additional quantity, the lineal energy (energy per unit path length through the target), is also used to present microdosimetry data (93).

Both the single-event and multiple-event spectra may be calculated using either analytical or MC methods (99,101). Analytical methods are broadly classified as those that rely on a mathematical formulation for the distribution of path lengths through the target volume. Based on this distribution, the single-event spectrum can be determined. Multiple-event spectra are determined by convolving the single-event spectrum as described earlier in the text. An alternative method is MC simulation. In this approach, the path of individual alpha particles is simulated based on random emission. For those alpha particles that intersect the target (often the nucleus), the MC code may simulate each interaction along the particle's path (102). Since alpha particles can be approximated to travel in straight lines, simplifications such as using the rate of energy loss per unit path length can be applied to determine the amount of energy deposited. Based on CSDA, these energies are extracted from range–energy tables that are available for a variety of materials (10,42,103). As a number of researchers have published range–energy tables, the choice of a particular table is not critical. Stinchcomb and Roeske (99)

compared specific energy distributions using Janni's range–energy tables (104) for protons (appropriately scaled for alpha particles) to Walsh's data (105). They observed only 1% to 7% differences in the mean specific energies. In general, MC methods provide greater flexibility than the analytical approach. For a more detailed description of the MC approach applied to alpha particles, see Roeske and Hoggarth (106).

Microdosimetric applications for alpha emitters

Once microdosimetric spectra are generated, through either MC or analytical means, the next question becomes "how to use these spectra?" The most basic approach is to consider these spectra as a more accurate characterization of the energy deposited. However, additional information can be obtained by combining these spectra with a biologic model (such as cell survival). For a multiple-event spectrum, the surviving fraction can be expressed as follows (99,101):

$$S(\bar{z}) = \int_0^\infty f(z) e^{-z/z_0} dz, \qquad \text{(Eq. 9.6)}$$

where $f(z)$ represents the fraction of cells receiving specific energies between z and $z + dz$, and $\exp(-z/z_0)$ is the fraction of cells that survive. Use of this survival model assumes that the cells are independent (no bystander effects) and that intratrack interactions dominate intertrack interactions. That is, unlike low-LET irradiation, there is no quadratic term in the exponent. For single-event spectra, it can be shown that the surviving fraction is given by the following equation (99,101):

$$S(\bar{z}) = \exp[- \langle n \rangle \{1 - T_1(z_0)\}], \qquad \text{(Eq. 9.7)}$$

where $<n>$ is the average number of hits to the cell nucleus and $T_1(z_0)$ is the Laplace transform of the single-event spectrum. In both cases, the same value of z_0 is used, and the equations generate the same surviving fraction for the same source–target configuration.

It is important to note that z_0 is not the same as D_0, which is obtained from the slope of the cell survival curve (99,101). Rather z_0 is a more fundamental quantity depending only on the radiation type and energy. D_0 is related to z_0 although it has folded into it the source–target geometry effects (99,101). To understand this concept, consider a cell in which all alpha-particle decays occur in the nucleus versus the same cell where all of the decays occur on the cell surface. In both cases, z_0 is the same; however, D_0 may differ because the specific energy spectra will differ between the two geometries due to differences in where the decays occur. Combining specific energy distributions with a model for cell survival has yielded both theoretical predictions of cell survival and experimental analysis to determine the value of z_0. Each of these will be described separately.

One of the first published studies on the application of microdosimetry for targeted alpha-particle irradiation can be attributed to Fisher (98). In this study, it was demonstrated that the specific energy deposited in the cell nucleus is highly nonuniform. As the concentration of alpha-particle emitters increases, the specific energy distribution appears to be normally distributed with a relatively large standard deviation. Most of the cells receive specific energies that can differ significantly from the average dose. Moreover, a fraction of the cells are not hit by alpha particles at all. In the absence of bystander effects, these cells can decrease the overall therapeutic effectiveness of therapy. Building upon one of the basic geometries of Fisher, Humm combined microdosimetric calculations with a model of cell survival to estimate the surviving fraction of cells within a tumor and cells located a short distance away from a capillary (107). In both geometries a uniform distribution of ^{211}At-labeled antibody was considered. Despite having average doses that were nearly the same, both cells had a significant variation in expected cell survival. This variation was due to differences in the specific energy spectra for cells within the tumor versus those outside the capillary. In particular, a significant fraction of the cells outside the capillary received no alpha-particle hits (cells farther from the capillary having a higher fraction receiving no hits). This study demonstrated the importance of the source–target geometry and indicated the need to include stochastic effects in modeling cell survival. Since this time, a number of studies have built on the previous works. Stinchcomb and Roeske (108) analyzed the effect of cell shape and size on expected cell survival. They demonstrated that the size of the target had a greater impact on the specific energy spectrum (and hence cell survival) than the shape. Palm et al. (109) performed microdosimetric calculation for ^{211}At and its daughter products as they diffused from the decay site. Kvinnsland et al. (110) examined the use of mean activity distribution and its effects on specific energy distributions. In general, these studies indicate the importance of accurately characterizing the source/target geometry in alpha-particle microdosimetry.

Kennel et al. (111) and Charlton (112) separately modeled multicellular spheroids. Unlike the previous studies where a single specific energy spectrum was used for the population, spheroids have a specific energy distribution that varies with depth inside the spheroid. Thus, three-dimensional modeling of the specific energy distribution, as well as the source distribution as a function of time, is required. Moreover, because the cells are in a closed-pack geometry, the use of Equation 9.6 is not as applicable. Rather, second-order processes, such as bystander effects, should be taken into account in these models. While these processes are more difficult to model, the ongoing refinement of cell survival models is currently an important research endeavor (113).

Complicated source–target geometry is bone marrow. The marrow cavities possess a complex geometry, and the presence of bone introduces density heterogeneity into the calculation. Charlton et al. (114) calculated microdosimetric spectra and subsequent cell survival based on geometries from human marrow samples for two different radionuclides—^{149}Tb and ^{211}At. These simulations indicated that for targeted decays, ^{149}Tb was five times more effective than ^{211}At when compared on a hit-by-hit basis. This enhancement was due to the lower energy of ^{149}Tb resulting in a higher LET of the incident alpha particles. Akabani and Zaltusky (115) addressed this issue by using histologic bone marrow samples. Using MC simulation, they estimated cell survival by folding in the specific energy spectra with a model of cell survival. This study demonstrated that the energy deposited from activity distributed on the cell surface was more lethal than from hits due to decays in the extracellular fluid (interstitium). Recently, small-scale imaging techniques (micro-CT and MR) have been used to obtain a more detailed geometry of the skeletal microstructure (116,117). As these imaging data are incorporated into microdosimetric calculations, further refinements of these results are expected.

▪ Example

As an example, consider ^{212}Bi, an alpha-particle emitter considered for therapy, uniformly distributed on the surface of spherical cells. These cells have a diameter of 12 μm and a nuclear diameter of 8 μm. ^{212}Bi has two alpha-particle decay branches. Direct decay occurs 36% of the time resulting in the emission of a 6.05 MeV alpha particle. The remaining 64% of the time, the isotope decays through a beta emission resulting in ^{212}Po. This radionuclide subsequently decays by producing an 8.78 MeV alpha particle (53).

In order to simulate the specific energy spectrum, an MC calculation was used (99,106). Briefly, the sources are uniformly distributed over the cell surface. Random numbers are generated to determine the energy of the alpha particle based on the previously described decay scheme. Next, a series of random numbers are generated to determine the directional path of the alpha particle and whether it will intersect the nucleus. If the alpha particle intersects the nucleus, the equations for a straight line are solved to determine the entrance and exit points. Using stopping power data, the energy deposited by each traversal is calculated

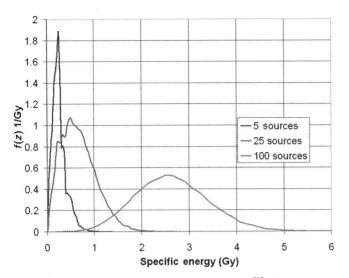

FIGURE 9.5 Specific energy spectra for 5, 25, and 100 ^{212}Bi decays on the surface of a cell with a nuclear diameter of 8 μm and a cellular diameter of 10 μm.

and summed. This process is repeated for all emitters on the cell surface. Since this simulation represents only one possible outcome, the process is repeated many times in an attempt to observe all possible outcomes. In this example, a total of 10^5 simulations were performed.

The results of this analysis are shown in Figure 9.5 for the cases of 5, 25, and 100 sources distributed on the cell surface. The curves are normalized such that the area under the curve is unity. A number of features are apparent in these spectra. For the case of only a few sources on the cell surface, the specific energy spectrum has a characteristic "triangular" shape. Moreover, a significant fraction of cells receive zero alpha-particle hits, and thus have zero specific energy deposited. These are represented by the vertical line along the y-axis. For 5, 25, and 100 surface decays, the fractions of cells recording zero events are 0.51, 0.033, and 0.00003, respectively. As the number of decays increase, the spectrum shape approaches a normal (Gaussian) distribution in accordance with the central limit theorem. The average doses received by these cells are 0.134, 0.674, and 2.71 Gy for 5, 25, and 100 sources, respectively. It is important to note that many cells receive specific energies that deviate significantly from the mean values.

For comparison, a MIRD calculation is also performed for this geometry. Based on Goddu et al. (38), the S values for ^{212}Bi and ^{212}Po are 0.0117 and 0.0238 Gy/Bq s, respectively. These S values consider only the alpha-particle component since it contributes significantly more dose than the other emissions (beta and gamma emissions). To obtain the overall S value, each value is weighted by the decay mode and summed to yield the S value. The S value of ^{212}Bi already takes into account the decay weighting, while the ^{212}Po S value is multiplied by 0.64. The resultant S value is 0.0269 Gy/Bq s. The average doses are 0.135, 0.673, and 2.69 Gy for 5, 25, and 100 sources, respectively. These values compare favorably with those generated by the MC calculation. However, the MC calculation provides additional insight

into the fraction of cells that are not hit, as well as the variation in specific energy deposited in individual cells.

■ AUGER ELECTRONS

Auger electron emitters have been used in a number of preclinical and clinical studies using delivery systems that directly target tumor cells (7,118–122). Auger electrons are emitted by radionuclides that decay through electron capture or internal conversion. Electron capture is a process whereby the nucleus captures an inner shell electron and a proton is transformed into a neutron (53). This process competes with positron emission where a proton is transformed into a neutron with the emission of a positron. Internal conversion is a way for an excited nucleus to return to the ground state by the ejection of an electron with energy equal to the residual nuclear excitation energy minus the binding energy of the inner shell orbiting electron (53). Both decay modes produce an inner shell electron vacancy that initiates a cascade of atomic shell transitions in which a number of low-energy Auger, Coster–Kronig, and super-Coster–Kronig electrons are liberated. These electrons have emission energies corresponding to the differences in the binding shell energies involved in the transition.

In nuclear medicine, radionuclides that decay through electron capture or internal conversion are commonly used in radiotracer studies. These include ^{67}Ga, ^{99m}Tc, ^{123}I, and ^{201}Tl. Because of the low energies associated with the electrons, it was assumed that these radionuclides would result in inconsequential radiation doses. However, when these radionuclides are attached to delivery systems that result in direct targeting of DNA, the radiobiologic damage produced by these low-energy electrons is similar to that produced by high-LET radiation. This damage was first identified in studies by Ertl, Feinendegen, and Heiniger (123) and Hofer and Hughes (124) using ^{125}I-labeled thymidine precursor iododeoxyuridine (^{125}IUdR). They independently observed that the cell survival curves appeared similar to those produced by alpha-particle emitters. In other studies, comparison of the absorbed dose to the cell nucleus from intranuclear decays demonstrated that ^{131}I deposited more dose than ^{125}I. However, ^{125}I produced significantly higher levels of cell kill than ^{131}I on a per-decay basis (125,126). Charlton and Booz (127) simulated the atomic relaxation of ^{125}I and demonstrated that on average 21 electrons are emitted per decay. These electrons deposited a significant amount of energy within a few nanometers of the decay site. Charlton subsequently demonstrated through simulation that the ionization density surrounding the ^{125}I decay is larger than that produced by an alpha particle. These calculations provided a physical explanation to the radiobiologic observations.

The therapeutic advantages of Auger emitters have been discussed by Daghighian et al. (128) and Behr et al. (129). Unlike other classes of radionuclides (alpha and beta emitters), the extremely short range of the Auger electrons significantly limits the dose delivered to normal tissue. Clinically,

Welt et al. (130) administered activities in excess of 29 GBq (800 mCi) of ^{125}I-labeled A33 antibody to patients and did not observe a dose-limiting toxicity. Because of the short range, the cell cytoplasm shields the DNA from emissions occurring on the cell surface. For antibodies that bind to the cell surface, and are subsequently internalized into the nucleus of tumor cells, Auger electron delivery provides an enhanced therapeutic ratio. However, for Auger electron therapy to be successful, the radionuclide needs to be internalized by each tumor cell, thus presenting a severe limitation.

The dosimetry of Auger electrons requires two components. First the spectrum of low-energy electrons has to be determined based on the electron vacancies and considering all possible pathways of filling these vacancies. Next, the energy deposited must be evaluated on a scale comparable to the range of these electrons, which is often the nanometer scale.

Electron spectra

An Auger electron transition may occur when an electron from a higher orbital shell fills an inner shell vacancy. When the energy gained from this transition is transferred and used to liberate an electron, from a higher orbital, this is referred to as an Auger electron process. The net result is the filling of one vacancy and the creation of two new vacancies. There is considerable stochastic variability in the way these vacancies are created. The number and energies of Auger electrons vary between individual disintegrations. This process is governed by inner shell transition probabilities. However, depending on the atomic number of the radionuclide, the number of possible de-excitation pathways through an atom can number in the hundreds. Charlton and Booz (127) were the first to use MC simulation to model these decay processes. Their original study modeled the spectrum produced from the decay of ^{125}I. Since that time, spectra have been calculated for a number of radionuclides (131).

The MC simulation of this process has been described previously (101,127). Briefly, a random number is used to select an inner shell vacancy according to the probabilities of capture within each of the respective orbitals (K, L1, L2, L3, etc.). The probabilities for all transitions to this vacancy are normalized to 1, where each allowed transition is weighted by its respective probability according to values for radiative (132) and nonradiative (133) transitions. These data are determined from quantum mechanical calculations of oscillator strengths. A second random number is then used to select one of these transitions, according to their respective weights. The new electron occupancy of the orbitals is recorded, and the next innermost shell vacancy is selected. This process then repeats until all of the vacancies have shifted to the outermost shells (the lowest energy state), and further transitions are no longer possible. The result of each simulation is an Auger and Coster–Kronig electron spectra.

In the previous implementation, the energy of the emitted electrons was calculated using the $Z/Z + 1$ approximation

(134). This approach uses a weighted ratio of the binding energies between the parent and daughter atoms. However, the binding energies of the electron orbitals change when there are multiple vacancies. The $Z/Z + 1$ approximation is strictly valid only for the first Auger transition, and hence the Auger electrons calculated by this approach are based only on approximate binding energies. A more accurate calculation of the electron energy states utilizes the Dirac–Fock computer codes developed by Desclaux (135). Pomplun et al. (136) solved the electron energy estimation by using an elaborate precalculated look-up table for the most frequent multielectron vacancy configurations.

Simulation of a large number of individual atomic de-excitations results in an output of multiple individual Auger electron and x-ray spectra. Each spectrum represents one stochastic example of a single atomic de-excitation. The data from 10,000 of these individual spectra can be used to calculate a frequency-weighted average Auger electron emission spectrum. Note that the use of an average emission spectrum for dosimetry calculations removes the highly stochastic nature from radionuclides such as ^{125}I. Dosimetric estimates to different compartments of the cell have been performed using the average Auger electron spectrum. It is important to note that the results are the same as when multiple individual Auger electron spectra are used. However, the stochastics of individual spectra may be pertinent if cellular inactivation is dependent on an energy deposition threshold or when detailed modeling of energy deposition in DNA is undertaken.

Dose calculations

In order to perform dose calculations for these radionuclides, it is first necessary to obtain the Auger and Coster–Kronig electron spectra, as described previously. Methods to perform dosimetric calculations based on these spectra are provided by Howell (131) and Humm et al. (137). Using such individual electron spectra, MC methods have been used to simulate the energy deposition events as each electron traverses through water, using cross-section data for water vapor (scaled to tissue density), where data is available down to 10 eV. The simulation begins by generating a random number and determining the distance traversed by the electron in accordance with its mean free path (which is a function of electron energy). The coordinates of the electron interactions are recorded as well as the local energy deposited. In addition, the directional cosines of the primary electron and any delta rays are also recorded. The energy deposition events are summed within concentric spherical sites around the point of emission to obtain energy (or specific energy) as a function of radius.

Alternatively, the energy deposition pattern may be superimposed upon a geometric model defining the spatial location of each atom in the DNA molecule. Currently, there is insufficient information to directly model the electron interactions within DNA. Zaider et al. (138) have described an MC code that simulates the interaction of electrons with

DNA using more realistic cross-sectional data obtained from quantum mechanical calculations of the dielectric response function of polycytidine (and polycytidine and Guanine stacks) contained within a condensed water moiety (139). The geometrical models of the DNA began as simple block segments consisting of a central cylindrical core, to represent the nucleotide pairs, surrounded by a rotating semi-annulus on each side interlocking to tightly enclose the central nucleotide cylinder, representing individual DNA strands (140). This model has been used to calculate the local deposition of energy for a number of radionuclides (141). One of the applications of this approach is in the estimation of threshold energy for DNA strand break. Using data from Martin and Haseltine (142) along with the stochastic energy deposition around ^{125}I incorporated in a geometric model of DNA, it was estimated that this threshold energy was 17.5 eV. To improve statistics, the process was repeated for the same individual Auger spectrum 10 times. The result was a substantial variability in the local energy deposition, which added another layer of stochastic variability to the data. It is important to appreciate that such models are simple compared to the true tertiary structure of the DNA molecules and the electron interactions within it.

More recent studies based on higher resolution and precision DNA strand break damage, which includes the influence of the radical scavenger dimethyl sulfoxide, have been conducted by Nikjoo et al. (143). This model incorporates the creation of water radical production and diffusion of the radiochemical species relative to the target strands. Furthermore, advances to the DNA model, which includes a chemical representation, can be used to determine the particular atom in closest proximity to the energy deposition (8,144,145).

While these models represent simplifications, overall they are extremely useful and provide a wealth of information on the stochastics of microscopic energy transport and energy deposition. In particular, the stochastics are important for predicting DNA damage because any threshold model of strand break damage does not bear a linear relationship to the mean energy deposition.

The stochastic effects of Auger electron emitters and the high-LET effects are relevant within a few nanometers of the decay site, since most Auger and Coster–Kronig electrons have ranges of this order. Therefore, for Auger sources that decay at the extracellular locations (as is the case for most diagnostic tracers used in nuclear medicine), concerns of high LET and the consequent radiotoxicity effects are unwarranted. However, the extreme short-range effects of Auger electron emitters do pose a new problem in assessing the dosimetry of novel radiopharmaceuticals. Humm et al. (137) and Goddu et al. (146) have recommended some guidelines for their evaluation, which requires the initial determination of the partition of the agent into extracellular, cell surface bound, intracellular, intranuclear, and appended to the DNA.

Many dosimetric calculations with Auger electron–emitting radionuclides do not require such advanced calculations but can reliably use the cellular S factors. Radionuclides that emit Auger electrons are in widespread clinical use in nuclear medicine. Absorbed dose calculations for such radionuclides are based on tabulated S-factor calculations, based on organ biodistribution data ascertained from imaging. The utility of these dosimetric estimates relies on the nonselective intranuclear incorporation of these agents (147). Cellular S factors for the former four compartments have been calculated by Goddu et al. (146,148) for a number of electron capture and internal conversion decaying radionuclides. The average radiation dose to the nucleus (or other compartment) can be determined by the piecewise addition of each contribution, based on experimental determination of the relative compartmental partitions. If a fraction of the radionuclide carrier becomes intracellular, intranuclear, and most importantly DNA associated, then the biologically effective dose increases. A method used to calculate equivalent dose for Auger electron–emitting radionuclides given a nonuniform cellular distribution of organ uptake is given by Goddu et al. (146). Whereas for most applications associated with non-DNA-targeting Auger-emitting radionuclides, the usage of average electron spectrum to calculate cellular doses is adequate and appropriate; difficulties can arise when estimating DNA strand break damage based on average spectra rather than the full stochastics of the individual decay spectra. The reader is referred to the example of Charlton (149) for further details.

Example

The following example is based on Example 1 from the *MIRD Cellular S Values* report (38). Consider a sample of 10^8 cells labeled with 25 µCi of ^{111}In-oxide that is injected intravenously. The cells have a diameter of 12 µm, and a nuclear diameter of 10 µm. The biologic clearance of this compound is 57 hours, and approximately 90% of the activity is localized to the cell nucleus. The goal is to estimate the dose to the cell nucleus.

As a first step, the cumulative activity per cell needs to be estimated. With a physical half-life of 67.9 hours, the effective half (T_{eff}) is 31 hours. By dividing the total activity by the number of cells and multiplying by 1.44 T_{eff}, the cumulative activity per cell can be determined. In this case, the cumulative activity per cell is $(1.44 \times 31)(25 \text{ µCi})/10^8$. With proper unit conversion, the cumulative activity per cell is 1.49×10^3 Bq s per cell. Using the MIRD approach, the cellular S values with the nucleus and cytoplasm as the source compartment are 1.48×10^{-3} and 2.20×10^{-4}, respectively, for the case where the nucleus is the target. By partitioning the activity in each compartment, based on the biodistribution, the absorbed dose to the nucleus is $(1.49 \times 10^3 \text{ Bq s})(0.9 \times 1.48 \times 10^{-3} + 0.1 \times 2.20 \times 10^{-4}) = 2.02$ Gy.

For decays located close to the DNA, the energy deposition within the critical target for cellular inactivation may be significant and may consequently result in a biologic effect that is incommensurate with the absorbed dose to the

FIGURE 9.6 The energy deposited as a function of distance from an In-111 source.

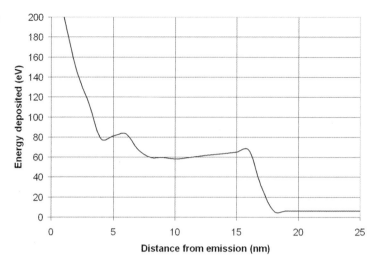

cell nucleus. To illustrate this concept, we model the energy absorbed on the nanometer scale using the approach described by Humm et al. (137). In this approach, Cole's range–energy relationships are used to estimate the energy deposited within concentric spherical shells. The average spectra obtained from Howell et al. (131) are used in conjunction with this calculation. Figure 9.6 shows the resultant energy deposition versus distance. For points close to the point of emission, the energy deposited is on the order of hundreds of electron volts. As the distance increases beyond 20 nm, the energy deposited is less than 10 eV. This example demonstrates the importance of characterizing the subcellular distribution of Auger electron emitters relative to critical targets within the nucleus.

SUMMARY

In this chapter, we have briefly summarized the calculation methods and challenges associated with the dosimetry of Auger electron, alpha-particle, and beta-particle emitters. In each case, specialized techniques have been developed to characterize the energy deposited by these emissions. It is important to note that in many cases, the MIRD approach may be sufficient to provide absorbed dose estimates. However, no matter which approach is used, there are two fundamental quantities that need to be established: the source/target geometry and the activity distribution as a function of time. Without the accurate characterization of either of these, the dose estimates obtained using these approaches will be of little value.

A question that is often asked is, "What is the clinical role of small-scale dosimetry?" In particular, both the source/target geometry and the activity distribution are difficult to estimate on a small scale in the clinical setting. As such, many centers rely on macroscopic dosimetry based on current nuclear medicine imaging technology. However, small-scale dosimetry can play an important role in preclinical studies. Based on in vitro and in vivo data from animals, combined with high-resolution small-animal imaging

devices, the essential elements for accurate small-scale dose calculations are available. Given the high costs associated with performing a clinical trial, small-scale dosimetry combined with preclinical data can guide these trials and assist in their intelligent design. Moreover, small-scale dosimetry may be able to explain clinical failures, and point the direction for overcoming these obstacles.

REFERENCES

1. Chatal JF, Hoefnagel CA. Radionuclide therapy. *Lancet.* 1999;354 (9182):931–935.
2. Wagner HN, Wiseman GA, Marcus CS, et al. Administration guidelines for radioimmunotherapy of non-Hodgkin's lymphoma with 90Y-labeled anti-CD20 monoclonal antibody. *J Nucl Med.* 2002;43(2):267–272.
3. Jurcic JG, Larson SM, Sgouros G, et al. Targeted alpha particle immunotherapy for myeloid leukemia. *Blood.* 2002;100:1233–1239.
4. Allen BJ, Tian Z, Rizvi S, et al. Preclinical studies of targeted alpha therapy for breast cancer using 213Bi-labelled-plasminogen activator inhibitor type 2. *Br J Cancer.* 2003;88:944–950.
5. Allen BJ, Raja C, Rizvi S, et al. Intralesional targeted alpha therapy for metastatic melanoma. *Cancer Biol Ther.* 2005;4:1318–1324.
6. Nilsson S, Larsen RH, Fossa SD, et al. First clinical experience with alpha-emitting radium-223 in the treatment of skeletal metastases. *Clin Cancer Res.* 2005;11:4451–4459.
7. Adelstein SJ, Kassis AI, Bodei L, et al. Radiotoxicity of iodine-125 and other auger-electron-emitting radionuclides: background to therapy. *Cancer Biother Radiopharm.* 2003;18:301–316.
8. Nikjoo H, Girard P, Charlton DE, et al. Auger electrons—a nanoprobe for structural, molecular and cellular processes. *Radiat Prot Dosimetry.* 2006;122(1–4):72–79.
9. ICRU. Stopping Powers for Electrons and Positrons. ICRU Report 37. Bethseda, MD: International Commission on Radiation Units and Measurements; 1984.
10. ICRU. Stopping Powers and Ranges for Protons and Alpha Particles. ICRU Report 49. Bethseda, MD: International Commission on Radiation Units and Measurements; 1993.
11. Cole A. Absorption of 20-eV to 50,000-eV electron beams in air and plastic. *Radiat Res.* 1969;38(1):7–33.
12. Bischof DA. The role of nuclear medicine in the treatment of non-Hodgkins lymphoma (NHL). *Leuk Lymphoma.* 2003;44(suppl 4):S29–S36.
13. Kletting P, Bunjes D, Reske SN, et al. Improving anti-CD45 antibody radioimmunotherapy using a physiologically based pharmacokinetic model. *J Nucl Med.* 2009;50(2):296–302.
14. Lampinen JS, Valimaki PJ, Kuronen AA, et al. Cluster models in cellular level electron dose calculations. *Acta Oncol.* 1999;38(3):367–372.

15. Flynn AA, Pedley RB, Green AJ, et al. The nonuniformity of antibody distribution in the kidney and its influence on dosimetry. *Radiat Res.* 2003;159(2):182–189.

16. DeNardo GL, Juweid ME, White CA, et al. Role of radiation dosimetry in radioimmunotherapy planning and treatment dosing. *Crit Rev Oncol Hematol.* 2001;39(1–2):203–218.

17. Brans B, Bodel L, Giammarile F, et al. Clinical radionuclide therapy dosimetry: the quest for the "Holy Gray". *Eur J Nucl Med Mol Imaging.* 2007;34(5):772–786.

18. Loevinger R, Berman M. A formalism for calculation of absorbed dose from radionuclides. *Phys Med Biol.* 1968;13:205–217.

19. Loevinger R, Berman M. *A Revised Schema for Calculating the Absorbed Dose from Biologically Distributed Radionuclides.* MIRD Pamphlet No. 1. Revised ed. New York, NY: Society of Nuclear Medicine; 1976.

20. Loevinger R, Budinger TF, Watson EE. *MIRD Primer for Absorbed Dose Calculations.* Revised ed. New York, NY: The Society of Nuclear Medicine; 1991.

21. Bolch WE, Eckerman KF, Sgouros G, et al. MIRD Pamphlet No. 21: a generalized schema for radiopharmaceutical dosimetry-standardization of nomenclature. *J Nucl Med.* 2009;50(3):477–484.

22. Snyder WS, Ford MR, Warner GG. "S," *Absorbed Dose per Unit Calculated Activity for Selected Radionuclides and Organs*: MIRD Pamphlet No. 11. New York, NY: The Society of Nuclear Medicine; 1975.

23. Stabin MG, Siegel JA. Physical models and dose factors for use in internal dose assessment. *Health Phys.* 2003;85:294–310.

24. Kassis AI, Howell RW, Sastry KSR, et al. Positional effects of Auger decays in mammalian cells in culture. In: Baverstock KY, Charlton DE, eds. *DNA Damage by Auger Emitters.* London: Taylor & Francis; 1988:1–14.

25. Sastry KSR, Howell RW, Rao DV, et al. Dosimetry of Auger-emitters: physical and phenomenological approaches. In: Baverstock KF, Charlton DE, eds. *DNA Damage by Auger Emitters.* London: Taylor & Francis; 1988:27–38.

26. Kassis AI. The MIRD approach: remembering the limitations. *J Nucl Med.* 1992;33:781–782.

27. Howell RW. The MIRD schema: from organ to cellular dimensions. *J Nucl Med.* 1994;35:531–533.

28. Bouchet LG, Bolch WE, Weber DA, et al. MIRD Pamphlet No. 15: radionuclide *S* values in a revised dosimetric model of the adult head and brain. *J Nucl Med.* 1999;40:62S–102S.

29. Mardirossian G, Tagesson M, Blanco P, et al. A new rectal model for dosimetry applications. *J Nucl Med.* 1999;40:1524–1531.

30. Ceccarelli C, Canale D, Battisti P, et al. Testicular function after ^{131}I therapy for hyperthyroidism. *Clin Endocrinol.* 2006;65:446–452.

31. Bouchet LG, Bolch WE, Howell RW, et al. *S* values for radionuclides localized within the skeleton. *J Nucl Med.* 2000;41:189–212.

32. Eckerman KF, Stabin MG. Electron absorbed fractions and dose conversion factors for marrow and bone by skeletal regions. *Health Phys.* 2000;78(2):199–214.

33. Bouchet LG, Bolch WE, Blanco HP, et al. MIRD Pamphlet No. 19: absorbed fractions and radionuclide *S* values for six age-dependent multiregion models of the kidney. *J Nucl Med.* 2003;44:1113–1147.

34. McAfee JG. Problems in evaluating the radiation dose for radionuclides excreted by the kidneys. In: Cloutier R, Edwards CL, Snyder WS, eds. *Medical Radionuclides: Radiation Dose and Effects.* Oak Ridge, TN: Atomic Energy Commission; 1969;271–294.

35. Bolch WE, Bouchet LG, Robertson JS, et al. MIRD Pamphlet No. 17: the dosimetry of nonuniform activity distributions-radionuclide *S* values at the voxel level. *J Nucl Med.* 1999;40(1):11S–36S.

36. Zankl M, Petoussi-Henss N, Fill U, et al. The application of voxel phantoms to the internal dosimetry of radionuclides. *Radiat Prot Dosimetry.* 2003;105:539–548.

37. Smith T, Petoussi-Henss N, Zankl M. Comparison of internal radiation doses estimated by MIRD and voxel techniques for a "family" of phantoms. *Eur J Nucl Med.* 2000;27:1387–1398.

38. Goddu SM, Howell R, Bouchet L, et al., eds. *MIRD Cellular S Values: Self-Absorbed Dose per Unit Cumulated Activity for Selected Radionuclides and Monoenergetic Electron and Alpha Particle Emitters Incorporated into Different Cell Compartments.* Reston, VA: Society of Nuclear Medicine; 1997.

39. Hindorf C, Emfietzoglou D, Linden O, et al. Internal microdosimetry for single cells in radioimmunotherapy of B-cell lymphoma. *Cancer Biother Radiopharm.* 2005;20:224–230.

40. Champion C, Zanotti-Fregonara P, Hindie E. CELLDOSE: a Monte Carlo code to assess electron dose distribution—*S* values for ^{131}I in spheres of various sizes. *J Nucl Med.* 2008;49:151–157.

41. Bardiès M, Chatal JF. Absorbed doses for internal radiotherapy from 22 beta-emitting radionuclides: beta dosimetry of small spheres. *Phys Med Biol.* 1994;39:961–981.

42. Ziegler JF. *TRIM: The Transport of Ions in Matter.* Yorktown, NY: IBM; 1992.

43. Palmer RBJ, Akhavan-Rezaynat A. Range–energy relations and stopping power in water, water vapour and tissue equivalent liquid for alpha particles over the energy range of 0.5 to 8 MeV. In: Booz H, Ebert HG, eds. *Proceedings of the Sixth Symposium on Microdosimetry,* Vol. II. London: Harwood Academic Publishers; 1978:739–759.

44. Kaplan I. *Nuclear Physics.* Reading, PA: Addison-Wesley; 1963.

45. Wright NA, Magee JL, Hamm RN, et al. Calculations of physical and chemical reactions produced in irradiated water containing DNA. *Radiat Prot Dosimetry.* 1985;13:133–136.

46. Sgouros G. Toward patient-friendly cell-level dosimetry. *J Nucl Med.* 2007;48:496–497.

47. Bolch WE. Alpha-particle emitters in radioimmunotherapy: new and welcome challenges to medical internal dosimetry. *J Nucl Med.* 2001;42:1222–1224.

48. Attix FH. *Introduction to Radiological Physics and Radiation Dosimetry.* New York: Wiley; 1986.

49. Makrigiorgos GM, Ito S, Baranowska-Kortylewicz J, et al. Inhomogeneous deposition of radiopharmaceuticals at the cellular level: experimental evidence and dosimetric implications. *J Nucl Med.* 1990;31: 1358–1363.

50. Roeske JC, Stinchcomb TG. The average number of alpha-particle hits to the cell nucleus required to eradicate a tumor cell population. *Phys Med Biol.* 2006;51:N179–N186.

51. Mausner LF, Srivastava SC. Selection of radionuclides for radioimmunotherapy. *Med Phys.* 1993;20(2 Pt 2):503–509.

52. Wessels BW, Rogus RD. Radionuclide selection and model absorbed dose calculations for radiolabeled tumor associated antibodies. *Med Phys.* 1984;11(5):638–645.

53. Weber DA, Eckerman KF, Dillman LT, et al. *MIRD: Radionuclide Data and Decay Schemes.* New York: The Society of Nuclear Medicine; 1989.

54. Berger MJ. MIRD Pamphlet No. 7: distribution of absorbed doses around point sources of electrons and beta particles in water and other media. *J Nucl Med.* 1971;12:5–23.

55. Berger MJ. Beta-ray dosimetry calculations with the use of point kernels. In: Cloutier RJ, Edwards CL, Snyder WS, eds. *Medical Radionuclides: Radiation Dose and Effects.* Washington, DC: US Atomic Energy Commission; 1970:63–86.

56. Bardiès M, Kwok C, Sgouros G. Dose point-kernels for radionuclide dosimetry. In: Zaidi H, Sgouros G, eds. *Therapeutic Applications of Monte Carlo Calculations in Nuclear Medicine.* Bristol & Philadelphia: IOP; 2003:158–174.

57. Roeske JC, Chen GTY, Atcher RW, et al. Modeling of dose to tumor and normal tissue from intraperitoneal radioimmunotherapy with alpha and beta emitters. *Int J Radiat Oncol Biol Phys.* 1990;19:1539–1548.

58. Roberson PL, Ten Haken RK, McShan DL, et al. Three-dimensional tumor dosimetry for radioimmunotherapy using serial autoradiography. *Int J Radiat Oncol Biol Phys.* 1992;24(2):329–334.

59. Akabani G, Hawkins WG, Eckbladenor MB, et al. Patient-specific dosimetry using quantitative SPECT imaging and three-dimensional discrete Fourier transform convolution. *J Nucl Med.* 1997;38(2): 308–334.

60. Cross WG, Williams G. *Tables of Beta Dose Distributions.* Chalk River, ON: Atomic Energy of Canada Limited; 1967.

61. Berger MJ. Monte Carlo calculation of the penetration of diffusion of fast charged particles. In: Alder B, ed. *Methods in Computational Physics.* New York: Academic Press; 1963:135–215.

62. Berger MJ. *Improved Point Kernels for Electrons and Beta-Ray Dosimetry.* Gaithersburg, MD: National Bureau of Standards; 1973.

63. Loevinger R, Holt JG. Internally administered radioisotopes. In: Hine GJ, Brownell GL, eds. *Radiation Dosimetry.* New York: Academic Press; 1956:801–873.

64. Spencer LV. Theory of electron penetration. *Phys Rev.* 1955;98: 1597–1615.

65. Prestwich WV, Nunes J, Kwok CS. Beta dose point kernels for radionuclides of potential use in radioimmunotherapy. *J Nucl Med.* 1989;30(6):1036–1046.

66. Simpkin DJ, Mackie TR. EGS4 Monte Carlo determination of the beta dose kernel in water. *Med Phys.* 1990;17(2):179–186.

67. Fujimori K, Fisher DR, Weinstein JN. Integrated microscopic-macroscopic pharmacology of monoclonal antibody radioconjugates: the radiation dose distribution. *Can Res.* 1991;51:4821–4827.

68. Ferrer L, Chouin N, Bitar A, et al. Implementing dosimetry in GATE: dose-point kernel validation with GEANT4 4.8.1. *Cancer Biother Radiopharm.* 2007;22(1):125–129.

69. Cloutier RJ, Watson EE. Radiation dose from isotopes in the blood. In: Cloutier RJ, Edwards CL, Snyder WS, eds. *Medical Radionuclides: Radiation Dose and Effects.* Oak Ridge, TN: U.S. Atomic Energy Commission; 1970.

70. Whitwell JR, Spiers FW. Calculated beta-ray dose factors for trabecular bone. *Phys Med Biol.* 1976;21(1):16–38.

71. ICRP. *Limits for Intakes of Radionuclides by Workers. ICRP Publication 30.* New York: Pergamon Press; 1979.

72. Kwok CS, Bialobzyski PJ, Yu SK. Effect of tissue inhomogeneity on dose distribution of continuous activity of low-energy electrons in bone marrow cavities with different topologies. *Med Phys.* 1991;18:533–541.

73. Stabin MG, Eckerman K. Dose conversion factors for marrow and bone by skeletal regions. *J Nucl Med.* 1994;35:112.

74. Nelson WR, Hirayama H, Rogers DW. *The EGS4 Code System.* Stanford, CA: Stanford Linear Accelerator Center; 1985.

75. Bouchet LG, Bolch WE, Howell RW, et al. S values for radionuclides localized within the skeleton. *J Nucl Med.* 2000;41:189–212.

76. Stabin MG, deLuz LC. Evolution and status of bone and marrow dose models. *Cancer Biother Radiopharm.* 2002;17(4):427–433.

77. Stabin MG, Sparks RB, Crowe E. OLINDA/EXM: the second-generation personal computer software for internal dose assessment in nuclear medicine. *J Nucl Med.* 2005;46(6):1023–1027.

78. Hui TE, Fisher DR, Kuhn JA, et al. A mouse model for calculating cross-organ beta doses from yttrium-90-labeled immunoconjugates. *Cancer.* 1994;73(3 suppl):951–957.

79. Hindorf C, Ljungberg M, Strand SE. Evaluation of parameters influencing S values in mouse dosimetry. *J Nucl Med.* 2004;45(11):1960–1965.

80. Miller WH, Hartmann-Siantar C, Fisher D, et al. Evaluation of beta-absorbed fractions in a mouse model for 90Y, 188Re, 166Ho, 149Pm, 64Cu, and 177Lu radionuclides. *Cancer Biother Radiopharm.* 2005;20(4):436–449.

81. Kolbert KS, Watson T, Marte C, et al. Murine S factors for liver, spleen, and kidney. *J Nucl Med.* 2003;44(5):784–791.

82. Stabin MG, Peterson TE, Holburn GE, et al. Voxel-based mouse and rat models for internal dose calculations. *J Nucl Med.* 2006;47(4):655–659.

83. Bitar A, Lisbona A, Thedrez P, et al. A voxel-based mouse for internal dose calculations using Monte Carlo simulations (MCNP). *Phys Med Biol.* 2007;52(4):1013–1025.

84. Larsson E, Strand SE, Ljundberg M, et al. Mouse S-factors based on Monte Carlo simulations in the anatomical realistic Moby phantom for internal dosimetry. *Cancer Biother Radiopharm.* 2007;22(3):438–442.

85. Briesmeister JF. *MCNP—A General Monte Carlo Code for Neutron and Photon Transport.* Los Alamos, NM: Los Alamos National Laboratory; 1997.

86. Bitar A, Lisbona A, Bardiès M. S-factor calculations for mouse models using Monte-Carlo simulations. *Q J Nucl Med Mol Imaging.* 2007;51:343–351.

87. Boutaleb S, Pouget J.-P, Hindorf C, et al. Impact of mouse model on pre-clinical dosimetry in targeted radionuclide therapy. *Proc IEEE* 97. 2009;12:2076–2085.

88. Divoli A, Chiavassa S, Ferrer L, et al. Effect of patient morphology on dosimetric calculations for internal irradiation as assessed by comparisons of Monte-Carlo versus conventional methodology. *J Nucl Med.* 2009;50(2):316–323.

89. Zalutsky MR, Stabin MG, Larsen RH, et al. Tissue distribution and radiation dosimetry of astatine-211-labeled chimeric 81C6, an alpha-particle-emitting immunoconjugate. *Nucl Med Biol.* 1997;24:255–251.

90. Couturier O, Faivre-Chauvet A, Filippovich IV, et al. Validation of 213Bi-alpha radioimmunotherapy for multiple myeloma. *Clin Cancer Res.* 1999;5:3165s–3170s.

91. Sgouros G, Ballangrud AM, Jurcic JG, et al. Pharmacokinetics and dosimetry of an alpha-particle emitter labeled antibody: ^{213}Bi-HuM195 (Anti-CD33) in patients with leukemia. *J Nucl Med.* 1999;40(11):1935–1946.

92. Hall EJ. *Radiobiology for the Radiologist.* Philadelphia, PA: Lippincott Williams & Wilkins; 2000.

93. Polig E. Dosimetry of alpha-emitters in bone. *Radiat Environ Biophys.* 1980;17:374.

94. Rossi HH. Microdosimetric energy distribution in irradiated matter. In: Attix FH, Roesch WC, eds. *Radiation Dosimetry. Volume I: Fundamentals.* New York: Academic Press; 1968.

95. Roesch WC. Microdosimetry of internal sources. *Radiat Res.* 1977;70:494–510.

96. Booz J, Coppola M. In: Booz J, Ebert HG, Eickel R, et al., eds. *Proceedings of the Fourth Symposium on Microdosimetry.* Pallanza, Italy: EUR 5112 d-e-f 983-1000; 1974:983–1000.

97. Wilson WE, Paretzke HG. Calculation of ionization frequency distributions in small sites. *Radiat Res.* 1980;81:326–335.

98. Fisher DR. The microdosimetry of monoclonal antibodies labeled with alpha emitters. In: Schlafke-Stelson AT, Watson EE, eds. *Proceedings of the Fourth International Radiopharmaceutical Dosimetry Symposium.* Oak Ridge, TN: Oak Ridge Associated Universities; 1985.

99. Stinchcomb TG, Roeske JC. Analytic microdosimetry for radioimmunotherapeutic alpha emitters. *Med Phys.* 1992;19(6):1385–1393.

100. Kellerer AM. In: Ebert HG, ed. *Proceedings of the Fourth Symposium on Microdosimetry.* Brussels: EUR 4452 d-e-f 107-34; 1970.

101. Roeske JC, Humm JL. Microdosimetry of targeted radionuclides. In: Zaidi H, Sgouros G, eds. *Therapeutic Applications of Monte Carlo Calculations in Nuclear Medicine.* Bristol: Institute of Physics Publishing; 2003.

102. Incerti S, Gault N, Habchi C, et al. A comparison of cellular irradiation techniques with alpha particles using the Geant4 Monte Carlo simulation toolkit. *Radiat Prot Dosimetry.* 2006;122:327–329.

103. Ziegler JF. The stopping and range of ions in solids. In: *Ion Implantation: Science and Technology.* San Diego: Academic Press; 1988.

104. Janni JF. *Calculation of Energy Loss, Range, Path Length, Straggling, Multiple Scattering and the Probability of Inelastic Nuclear Collisions for 0.1 to 1000 MeV Protons.* Technical Report No. AFWL-TR-65-150. Washington, DC; 1966.

105. Walsh PJ. Stopping power and range of alpha particles. *Health Phys.* 1970;19:312–316.

106. Roeske JC, Hoggarth M. Alpha-particle Monte Carlo simulation for microdosimetric calculations using a commercial spreadsheet. *Phys Med Biol.* 2007;52(7):1909–1922.

107. Humm JL. A microdosimetric model of astatine-211 labeled antibodies for radioimmunotherapy. *Int J Radiat Oncol Biol Phys.* 1987;13:1767–1773.

108. Stinchcomb TG, Roeske JC. Survival of alpha particle irradiated cells as a function of the shape and size of the sensitive target (nucleus). *Radiat Prot Dosimetry.* 1995;62(3):157–164.

109. Palm S, Humm JL, Rundqvist R, et al. Microdosimetry of astatine-211 single-cell irradiation: role of daughter polonium-211 diffusion. *Med Phys.* 2004;31(2):218–215.

110. Kvinnsland Y, Stokke T, Aurilien E. Radioimmunotherapy with alpha-particle emitters: microdosimetry of cells with heterogeneous antigen expression and with various diameters of cells and nuclei. *Radiat Res.* 2001;155:288–296.

111. Kennel SJ, Stabin M, Roeske JC, et al. Radiotoxicity of bismuth-231 bound to membranes of monolayer and spheroid cultures of tumor cells. *Radiat Res.* 1999;151:244–256.

112. Charlton DE. Radiation effects in spheroids of cells exposed to alpha emitters. *Int J Radiat Biol.* 2000;76(11):1555–1564.

113. Smilenov LB, Hall EJ, Bonner WM, et al. A microbeam study of DNA double-strand breaks in bystander primary human fibroblasts. *Radiat Prot Dosimetry.* 2006;122(1–4):256–259.

114. Charlton DE, Salmon PL, Utteridge TD. Monte Carlo/numerical treatment of alpha-particle spectra from sources buried in bone and resultant doses to surface cells. *Int J Radiat Biol.* 1998;73(1):89–92.

115. Akabani G, Zalutsky MR. Microdosimetry of astatine-211 using histological images: application to bone marrow. *Radiat Res.* 1997;148:599–607.

116. Rajon DA, Jokisch DW, Patton PW, et al. Voxel effects within digital images of trabecular bone and their consequences on chord-length distributions measurements. *Phys Med Biol.* 2002;47(10):1741–1759.

117. Hunt JG, Watchman CJ, Bolch WE. Calculation of absorbed fractions to human skeletal tissues due to alpha particles using Monte Carlo and 3-D chord-based transport techniques. *Radiat Prot Dosimetry.* 2007;127:223–226.

118. Mariani G, Di Sacco S, Volterrani D, et al. Tumor targeting by intra-arterial infusion of 5-[123I]iodo-2'-deoxyuridine in patients with liver metastases from colorectal cancer. *J Nucl Med.* 1996;37(4 suppl):22S–25S.

119. Chiou RK, Dalrymple GV, Baranowska-Kortylewicz J, et al. Tumor localization and systemic absorption of intravesical instillation of radio-iodinated iododeoxyuridine in patients with bladder cancer. *J Urol.* 1999;162(1):58–62.

120. Kassis AI, Adelstein SJ, Mariani G. Radiolabeled nucleoside analogs in cancer diagnosis and therapy. *J Nucl Med.* 1996;40(3):301–319.

121. DeSombre ER, Hughes A, Hanson RN, et al. Therapy of estrogen receptor-positive micrometastases in the peritoneal cavity with Auger electron-emitting estrogens—theoretical and practical considerations. *Acta Oncol.* 2000;39(6):659–666.

122. Karagiannis TC, Lobachevsky PN, Martin RF. Cytotoxicity of an 125I-labelled DNA ligand. *Acta Oncol.* 2000;39(6):681–685.

123. Ertl HH, Feinendegen LE, Heiniger HJ. Iodine-125, a tracer in cell biology: physical properties and biological aspects. *Phys Med Biol.* 1970;15(3):447–456.

124. Hofer KG, Hughes WL. Radiotoxicity of intranuclear tritium, 125 iodine and 131 iodine. *Radiat Res.* 1971;47(1):94–101.

125. Chan PC, Lisco E, Lisco S, et al. Cell survival and cytogenetic responses to 125I-UdR in cultured mammalian cells. *Curr Top Radiat Res Q.* 1978;12(1–4):426–435.

126. Hofer KG. Radiation biology and potential therapeutic applications of radionuclides. *Bull Cancer.* 1980;67(3):343–353.

127. Charlton DE, Booz J. A Monte Carlo treatment of the decay of 125I. *Radiat Res.* 1981;87(1):10–23.

128. Daghighian F, Barendswaard E, Welt S, et al. Enhancement of radiation dose to the nucleus by vesicular internalization of iodine-125-labeled A33 monoclonal antibody. *J Nucl Med.* 1996;37:1052–1057.

129. Behr TM, Behe M, Lohr M, et al. Therapeutic advantages of Auger electron- over beta-emitting radiometals or radioiodine when conjugated to internalizing antibodies. *Eur J Nucl Med.* 2000;27(7):753–765.

130. Welt S, Scott AM, Divgi CR, et al. Phase I/II study of iodine 125-labeled monoclonal antibody A33 in patients with advanced colon cancer. *J Clin Oncol.* 1996;14(6):1787–1797.

131. Howell RW. Radiation spectra for Auger-electron emitting radionuclides: report No. 2 of AAPM Nuclear Medicine Task Group No. 6. *Med Phys.* 1992;19(6):1371–1383.

132. Salem SI, Panossian SL, Krause RA. Experimental K and L relative X-ray emission rates. *Atom Data Nucl Data.* 1974;14:91–109.

133. Chen MH, Crasemann B, Mark H. Relativistic radiationless transition probabilities for atomic K and L shells. *Atom Data Nucl Data.* 1979;24:13–37.

134. Chung MF, Jenkins LH. Auger electron energies of the outer shell electrons. *Surf Sci.* 1970;22:479–485.

135. Desclaux JP. A multi-configuration relativistic Dirac-Fock program. *Comput Phys Commun.* 1976;9:31–45.

136. Pomplun E, Booz K, Charlton DE. A Monte Carlo simulation of Auger electron cascades. *Radiat Res.* 1987;111:553–552.

137. Humm JL, Howell RW, Rao DV. Dosimetry of Auger-electron-emitting radionuclides: report no. 3 of AAPM Nuclear Medicine Task Group No. 6. *Med Phys.* 1994;21(12):1901–1915.

138. Zaider M, Fung A, Bardash M. Charged-particle transport in biomolecular media: the third generation. *Basic Life Sci.* 1994;63:77–91.

139. Grobelsek-Vracko M, Zaider M. A study of the excited states in cytosine and guanine stacks in the Hartree-Fock and exciton approximations. *Radiat Res.* 1994;138(1):18–25.

140. Buchegger F, Perillo-Adamer F, Dupertius YM, et al. Auger radiation targeted into DNA: a therapy perspective. *Eur J Nucl Med Mol Imaging.* 2006;33(11):1352–1363.

141. Humm JL, Charlton DE. A new calculational method to assess the therapeutic potential of Auger electron emission. *Int J Radiat Oncol Biol Phys.* 1989;17:351–360.

142. Martin RF, Haseltine WA. Range of radiochemical damage to DNA with decay of iodine-125. *Science.* 1981;213(4510):896–898.

143. Nikjoo H, Martin RF, Charlton DE, et al. Modelling of Auger-induced DNA damage by incorporated 125I. *Acta Oncol.* 1996;35(7):849–856.

144. Terrissol M, Pomplun E. A nucleosome model for the simulation of DNA strand break experiments. *Basic Life Sci.* 1994;63:243–250.

145. Terrissol M, Edel S, Pomplun E. Computer evaluation of direct and indirect damage induced by free and DNA-bound iodine-125 in the chromatin fibre. *Int J Radiat Biol.* 2004;80(11–12):905–908.

146. Goddu SM, Howell RW, Rao DV. Calculation of equivalent dose for Auger electron emitting radionuclides distributed in human organs. *Acta Oncol.* 1996;35(7):909–916.

147. ICRU. Absorbed-Dose Specification in Nuclear Medicine. International Commission of Radiation Units. ICRU Report 67. Ashford,UK: Nuclear Technology Publishing; 2002.

148. Goddu SM, Rao DV, Howell RW. Cellular dosimetry: absorbed fractions for monoenergetic electron and alpha particle sources and S-values for radionuclides uniformly distributed in different cell compartments. *J Nucl Med.* 1994;35(2):303–316.

149. Charlton DE. Comments on strand breaks calculated from average doses to the DNA from incorporated isotopes. *Radiat Res.* 1988;114(1):192–197.

Radiation Safety for Radionuclide Therapy

Bruce Thomadsen, William Erwin, and Firas Mourtada

When a therapeutic quantity of radioactivity has been systemically administered, the care and management of the patient must account for the fact that the patient has effectively become a sealed but "leaky" radioactive source. The amount of radiation exposure received from such a source may be potentially high enough to warrant radiation protection measures, dependent upon a number of factors. First, and foremost, is the radionuclide itself (its half-life, emission types [γ-, β-, α-, x-ray] and energies, and the amount of radioactivity administered) (1). Secondly is the route of administration (oral, intravenous, intra-arterial, intratumoral, interstitial, intracavitary) and biologic characteristics of the carrier molecule or pharmaceutical to which the radionuclide is attached (uptake and clearance rates, and route(s) of excretion from the body). Other important considerations are whether the patients are able to care for themselves; whether the patient will be treated on an inpatient or outpatient basis; and special circumstances, such as therapy for pediatric patients. Depending upon these factors, different populations of individuals are destined to be more or less at risk for exposure; those populations being hospital or clinic personnel (both radiation and nonradiation workers), family and friends (including those providing care for the patient, such as parents of a child or caregivers of an elderly person), coworkers, and the population at large. The primary role of the medical physicist, health physicist, or radiation safety officer (RSO) with respect to radioactive patients is to provide guidance on (a) the handling and release of such patients (including those who expire while still radioactive above background); (b) handling of radioactive contaminations and waste; (c) application of radiation protection principles; and (d) relevant U.S. Nuclear Regulatory Commission (NRC) or Agreement State rules and regulations, as well as applicable institutional radiation safety policies and procedures. The physicist or RSO may also be called upon to perform specific dose or dose equivalent measurements or calculations, such as those related to a medical event (e.g., the administration of the incorrect material or wrong amount, or using an unintended route of administration) or contamination, when a patient may be released to the general public (see "Patient Release Criteria"), or dose equivalent received during a posttherapy medical event (e.g., adverse response to the treatment, radioactive patient "code," radioactive cadaver). The overall goal in the management of the radioactive patient is to keep radiation exposures to others as low as

reasonably achievable (ALARA) and below limits set forth by regulatory bodies, as well as minimizing the probability of radioactivity contaminations.

The two treatment paradigms for therapy with internally administered radiopharmaceuticals are inpatient and outpatient. The inpatient paradigm includes patients admitted for therapy but released when the radiation exposure to any other person is estimated to be no greater than that allowed by law and good practice; and therapy performed as an outpatient procedure, where the patient must then be admitted to the hospital while being radioactive, whether or not for reasons related to the therapy. As a consequence, the management of the radioactive inpatient must account for dose equivalent to hospital personnel, other nearby nonradioactive inpatients, and visiting relatives, friends, and caregivers. The outpatient paradigm includes patients released immediately after administration of the radioactivity, as well as those not admitted but held in isolation for a period of time after administration until the dose equivalent rate allows release, for example, until the voiding of a significant amount of the administered radionuclide, either with or without specific radiation safety instructions. The management of the radioactive outpatient is therefore concerned primarily with minimizing radiation exposure to others besides hospital or clinic personnel.

■ BASIC RADIATION PROTECTION DOSIMETRIC UNITS

Radiation protection is concerned with two situations: preventing acute injury, called deterministic effects, and carcinogenesis, called a stochastic effect. The doses of concern for carcinogenesis fall much below those for tissue damage, so deterministic effects pose little hazard. Cataract formation, a deterministic effect, is an exception with a threshold on the order of that of carcinogenic effects. The dose limits are discussed further in the text. The amount of radiation a person receives from a source depends upon several factors. Three important factors are the amount of source material, the amount of radiation emitted per unit amount, and the energy of the radiation coming from a source. These characterize the radiation source. While there are several methods to specify the amount of radioactive material, *activity*, the number of radionuclide atoms undergoing transition (decay) per unit time, is the most common "nomenclature" that is used to indicate the amount of radiation that is present or administered for radionuclide therapy. The unit for activity is becquerel (Bq), which is equal to one decay per second. As 1 Bq is a very small activity, more often source strengths fall in the regions of megabecquerel (MBq = 10^6 Bq) or gigabecquerel (GBq = 10^9 Bq), and sometimes terabecquerel (TBq = 10^{12} Bq). An older unit still encountered in the literature, the curie (Ci) equals 3.7×10^{10} transitions per second. Since 1 Ci is a very large amount of radioactivity, radionuclide sources might be specified in terms of millicuries (1 mCi = 10^{-3} Ci ≈ 27 × the strength in GBq).

For the same activity, different radionuclides emit different numbers of photons. Some radionuclides emit several photons for each transition, while others almost never emit one. A greater number of photons emitted results in more radiation to someone exposed. The energy of the photons plays two roles in the dose equivalent. One deals with penetration of shielding, as discussed in the section "Basic Radiation Protection for External Exposures: Time/Distance/Shielding." Energy also affects the dose equivalent to persons since as the energy increases, the nature of the interactions between the radiation and the matter changes and, thus also, the absorbed dose to a person exposed. Photons themselves do little to affect the medium through which they pass. A photon interacts with one atom and gives rise to an electron (or an electron and a positron), and that charged particle then interacts with thousands of atoms as it transfers its kinetic energy to the medium mostly through ionization. Thus, the deposition of energy in the matter is a two-step process: transfer of energy from the photon to a charged particle followed by that charged particle delivering the energy to the medium. The amount of energy per mass of the radiation transfers to the medium in that first interaction forms *kerma* (*k*inetic *e*nergy *r*eleased in *ma*tter), and then the energy absorbed per mass of the medium is *dose*. Both of these processes depend on the energy of the radiation and the atomic number of the medium. A useful quantity in radiation protection is the *kerma rate constant*,[a] $(\Gamma_\delta)_K$, which gives the kerma rate at a distance from a unit strength source,

$$\dot{K} = \frac{(\Gamma_\delta)_K A}{r^2}. \qquad \text{(Eq. 10.1)}$$

This equation and the definition of $(\Gamma_\delta)_K$ specify that all space is a vacuum except for the very small amount of air at the point of measurement. In a medium of an atomic number Z, a constant, c_k, gives the dose resulting from a kerma, K, for a given energy, E, of photons:

$$D = c_k (E, Z) K. \qquad \text{(Eq. 10.2)}$$

Both kerma and dose carry the units gray (Gy), which is equal to 1 joule/kg.

The discussion above applies only to photons. Charged particles of interest, electrons and alpha particles, do not go through the intermediary step of kerma but produce dose directly. Because alpha emitters have such a short range in tissue, these concepts have little utility and will be discussed separately.

Dose still is not the quantity of interest but requires adjustment for the type of radiation. Chapter 6 introduced the concept of relative biologic effectiveness (RBE), that is, equal doses of different types of radiation produce different effects. In radiation protection the RBE takes a simpler form than in radiotherapy proper and goes by the name *quality factor*, Q, in older literature or *radiation weighting factor*, w_r, in more recent works. Multiplying the dose by the radiation weighting factor gives the *equivalent dose*, H, in units of sieverts (Sv—which, interestingly, also equals 1 joule/kg),

$$H = w_r D. \qquad \text{(Eq. 10.3)}$$

The radiation weighting factor recognizes that some radiation, such as alpha particles, produces much more tissue damage per unit dose than photon radiation. The equivalent dose expresses the dose in terms of the carcinogenic potential, if the dose was delivered by moderate energy photons. Radiation protection dosimetry accepts accuracy of 20% because uncertainties often prevent more detailed determinations, so the radiation weighting factors (2) take on very rough values, as in Table 10.1. The table shows that all photons and most electrons have the same radiation weighting factor. This follows the mechanism of delivering dose for photons where they first transfer their energy to electrons. Auger electrons form a special case. With their very low energy, they move relatively slowly and transfer energy much more densely than electrons with energies above 20 keV, that is, most electrons encountered. If incorporated into the cell nucleus, they produce greater effects, and thus have a higher w_r value. For a given energy, the massive alpha particles move a fraction of the speed of an electron, and thus have much more time to transfer energy to matter, giving them a large radiation weighting factor. Equation 10.3 is applied to a single type of radiation. Because many radionuclides emit more than one type of radiation, the equivalent dose is the sum of the contributions of each type

Table **10.1** Radiation weighting factors (2)	
Radiation Type	**Radiation Weighting Factor, w_r**
Photons, electrons, positrons, Auger electrons (not in the cell nucleus)	1
Auger electrons in the cell nucleus or particularly on the DNA	4 or 20 respectively[a]
Alpha particles	20

[a] The ICRP recommends case-by-case analysis for Auger electrons in the cell nucleus, with values for w_r dependent on the analysis. These are suggested values only.

---

[a]The interested reader should consult Attix. 1. Attix F. *Introduction to Radiological Physics and Radiation Dosimetry*. New York, NY: John Wiley and Sons; 1986.

Table **10.2**	Tissue weighting factors (2)
Organ or Tissues (Each)	**Tissue Weighting Factor, w_t**
Red bone marrow, colon, lung, stomach, breast, remainder tissues (taken as a group: adrenals, extrathoracic tissues, gallbladder, heart, kidneys, lymph nodes, muscle, oral mucosa, pancreas, prostate or uterus, small intestine, spleen, thymus)	0.12
Gonads	0.08
Bladder, esophagus, liver, thyroid	0.04
Bone surface, brain, salivary glands, skin	0.01

to the absorbed dose multiplied by its weighting factor, giving

$$H = \sum_{i=\text{type}}^{\text{all types}} w_{r,i} D_i. \qquad \text{(Eq. 10.4)}$$

Table 6.1 in Chapter 6 provides values for the equivalent dose rate at a distance of 1 m from a 1-GBq source due to the photons emitted for a number of potentially interesting radionuclides.

The volume of the body irradiated strongly influences the expected effects and allowed limits for the radiation dose equivalent, recognized by the weighting of radiation doses by *tissue weighting factors*, w_t. These factors reflect the relative likelihood of carcinogenesis resulting from radiation to these organs at risk. Table 10.2 gives values for w_t.

Effective dose, E, is intended to relate to the probability of carcinogenesis, where

$$E = \sum_{\text{tissues}}^{\text{all}} w_t H. \qquad \text{(Eq. 10.5)}$$

Effective dose is measured in sieverts (Sv). Effective doses sum over internal and external exposures. The concept of the simple addition of the components of effective dose, yielding the total, inherently assumes that the probability of cancer formation relates to the effective dose linearly with no threshold, a hypothesis not well supporting in science but one that simplifies writing regulations. Permissible dose equivalents in most locales are in terms of effective dose. Table 10.3 gives some values for allowed permissible dose equivalents (3).

■ BASIC RADIATION PROTECTION FOR EXTERNAL EXPOSURES: TIME/DISTANCE/SHIELDING

Radiation safety amounts to two principles: reduce the exposure to radiation external to the body and avoid internal radioactive contamination. This section addresses the first of these principles: reducing the exposure from sources external to the body. Persons involved with radionuclide treatments encounter radiation from the source material before infusion into the patient, from radiation escaping the patient after infusion, and from the patient's body fluids. Assuming that the amount of radioactive material is fixed and necessary for the task or resulting from the therapy, the following three tools help reduce the exposure.

▓ Time

Dose and dose equivalent depend linearly on the duration of exposure. Usually, the situation becomes more complex than simply multiplying a dose by a time because, through movement, the dose rate varies continually. *Integrating dosimeters*, devices that respond to dose and accumulate a wearer's total dose for a period, allow assessment of dose

Table **10.3**	Permissible dose equivalents: recommendations of the ICRP (2) and regulations of the U.S. Nuclear Regulatory Commission (3)	
Category	**ICRP Recommendation**[a]	**U.S. NRC Regulation**
Occupational		
Whole body (effective dose)	20 averaged over 5-year periods	50
Lens of eye	150	150
Skin	500	500
Hands and feet	500	500 as for any individual organ
Unborn child	1 mSv over term	5
General public		
Effective dose	1	1
Lens of eye	15	
Skin	50	

All values are in mSv/year except as noted. The ALARA principle is usually applied to plan exposures so as to remain a factor of 10 below these values.
[a]Abstracted; for the complete set of regulations see Ref. 2 (Table 8).

equivalent. However, in principle, reducing the time exposed to radiation reduces the dose.

Distance

Dose and dose equivalent depend on the square of the distance from a point source, that is, $D \propto 1/r^2$. Thus, doubling the distance from the source reduces the dose by a factor of four. Thus, increasing distance provides a great reduction in the exposure to persons working around a source. For sources such as a line or a volume, the relation becomes more complicated, but far enough from a source (at a distance about twice the length of a line source) the radiation closely follows the inverse square relationship.

Shielding

Materials placed between the radiation source and the people working with it reduce the dose. Such material is referred to as *shielding*. For a narrow beam of monoenergetic photons, materials reduce the dose equivalent exponentially, that is, $D \propto e^{-\mu\tau}$, where τ is the thickness of the material (e.g., in cm) and μ the linear attenuation coefficient for the material and the energy of the photons (in this case in cm^{-1}). The attenuation coefficient gives the fraction of the beam removed per unit thickness of the material. A useful quantity is the thickness of material required to reduce the dose in half, called the half-value layer (HVL), $T_{1/2}$, where

$$T_{1/2} = \frac{-\ln(1/2)}{\mu}. \qquad \text{(Eq. 10.6)}$$

For broad beams, the relationship becomes more complicated, but still mostly follows the exponential format but with a smaller value for μ. For beams with a wider spectrum of energies, μ increases with the thickness at first, settling into a stable value usually after about two HVLs. No thickness of material eliminates the entire beam, but some thickness reduces the exposure sufficiently to make it safe to work with the source.

Beta particles also follow exponential attenuation for a while, but then, with a thickness equal to the maximum range of the betas, they stop and no longer expose someone behind the material. Most often, shielding for beta radiation uses a thickness just greater than the maximum range. Plastics form the materials of choice because of their low atomic number. Betas interacting with high–atomic number materials produce more bremsstrahlung photons that become harder to shield than the original betas. A thickness of 2 cm (3/4 in.) of acrylic will shield for all the beta emitters likely encountered for targeted radionuclide therapy.

Alpha emitters do not follow exponential attenuation but do have a range beyond which no alpha particles emerge. As discussed in Chapter 6, this range is extremely short. Almost any shielding will eliminate the exposure from alpha particles, including paper or a plastic syringe wall. Because the alpha particles cannot penetrate the dead layer of skin cells, they pose little hazard, except for extremely large exposures.

■ BASIC SAFETY FOR LIQUID RADIONUCLIDES

Protection from contamination that might be taken into the body was the second principle presented in the section "Basic Radiation Protection For External Exposures." For most of the agents used in radionuclide therapy, radioactive contamination forms a larger hazard than external exposure from the source. This is not always the case. Take, for example, treatment with 29 GBq (800 mCi) of ^{131}I, where the external exposure allows only very short times for staff to work in the room. For the most part, however, radioactive contamination would be of greater concern. The reason for the greater concern follows from the discussion of protection from external exposure: if the radionuclide were internal to the body, the distance would be close to zero, giving very high doses to the nearby cells. While the expectation would be that a person working with these radionuclides would likely receive some external exposure, they should take in no radioactive contamination.

Radioactive contamination enters the body by three routes: ingestion, inhalation, and absorption. The first route, *ingestion* of radioactive material, usually occurs by handling something with the radionuclide on it and then touching the mouth or nose, or transfer to food or cosmetics such as lipstick. It could also occur by touching smoking material with a contaminated hand, but then the smoke probably poses a greater hazard. The radioactive contamination may come from excreta, vomit, blood, sweat, or tears. The patient may then contaminate anything in the room that they touch. Prevention of ingestion entails keeping a barrier between the radioactive material and all personnel. Examples include wearing gloves and water-impermeable gowns when in the presence of the materials. After working with the radioactive material, washing hands thoroughly with soap and water is mandatory (alcohol disinfectants do nothing to remove radioactive contamination from hand.). When leaving the room of a patient under treatment with radionuclides, checking hands, feet, and the rest of the body with a radiation detector provides the first warning of contamination that could be ingested. The detector must be adequate to the task however. For example, most radiation detectors used in a hospital will not detect alpha particles, and many have insufficient sensitivity to detect small, but important, levels of photon- or beta-emitting contamination. A medical or health physicist should be involved in establishing the safety procedures for these treatments and selecting the proper detectors.

The second route of intake is *inhalation* of airborne contamination. Preventing inhalation of airborne molecules presents serious problems. Surgical masks and masks used for tuberculosis patients may prevent breathing in organisms but do not block molecules, which would require "heavy duty" filter systems such as those designed for gas warfare. Given the difficulty in providing a barrier to airborne contamination, prevention becomes key, particularly keeping body fluids from aerosolizing. Closing the lid of the toilet after patient use helps, as does having male patients sit on the toilet while urinating. Sodium iodide labeled with a radioactive isotope of iodine forms a particular hazard due to vaporization.

The third route is *absorption*, direct passage through the skin or mucosa. As with prevention of ingestion, prevention entails avoiding contact with radioactive materials. In addition to gloves and gowns, when the possibility of splashing body fluids exists, face shields should be worn. None of the precautions differs significantly from universal precautions.

■ RULES FOR SAFE RADIONUCLIDE ADMINISTRATION

General rules for working with radionuclides are very important. Consistent with sections "Basic Radiation Protection for External Exposures: Time/Distance/Shielding" and "Basic Safety for Liquid Radionuclides," the goals are to reduce external radiation dose equivalent and prevent intake of radioactive contamination. The rules for minimizing radiation dose equivalents while working with radionuclide-labeled pharmaceuticals may be summarized as follows:

1. Wear gloves, gown, and shoe covers when going into the patient's room, and face shield if body fluids may be encountered.
2. Wear your radiation monitors (body and, if provided, finger or extremity).
3. Work behind shielding whenever possible and at the greatest distance compatible with the task.
4. Work quickly, but not so quickly as to make mistakes.
5. Avoid handling the unshielded source material if at all possible.
6. Leave gloves and gown in the trash receptacle in the room when leaving.
7. Monitor yourself for radioactivity with the detector selected by the medical physicist either at the doorway just before leaving the room or just past a designated threshold.
8. Wash hands after being in the room before eating or applying cosmetics.
9. Should radioactive contamination be found during monitoring after leaving the room:
   a. Do not move beyond the edge of the room where the monitoring is done.
   b. Call someone to help you.
   c. Remove contaminated articles and place in the radioactive waste receptacle.
   d. If the skin is contaminated, wash with mild soap and copious amounts of water, repeating until monitoring levels are background or the reading stops decreasing. There are special washing preparations for removal of radioactive contamination (usually foaming cleaners), which should be available near the patient's room.

■ MANAGING RADIOACTIVE INPATIENTS

Radiation considerations discussed in this section include (a) assessment of patient admission to the type of room that is required, (b) room preparation for housing the radioactive patient, (c) radiation exposure from direct contact with the radioactive inpatient, by hospital personnel, (d) visitors, and (e) emergency procedures.

The first radiation safety consideration for management of an inpatient receiving internal radionuclide therapy is to assess whether the patient may be admitted to a regular hospital room with standard radiation safety precautions provided to the patient and clinic staff, or the patient must be admitted to an area dedicated to housing highly radioactive patients. Such a dedicated area may be a hospital clinic (possibly designed as a controlled radiation area) containing rooms with adequate radiation shielding; or a regular hospital room, with rooms and areas adjacent, above, and below possibly remaining vacant or having restricted access after the therapeutic administration, until the dose equivalent rate drops below that level allowed to members of the public. Patients treated internally with radionuclides that are effectively pure beta emitters (e.g., ^{90}Y, ^{89}Sr, ^{32}P) may be admitted to a regular hospital room, as the external dose equivalent rates remain well below regulatory limits and, thus, require no special radiation protection measures, such as shielding. Protection against radioactive contamination appropriate for the amounts of radioactivity typically administered still would apply (4,5). The overwhelming majority of the energy emitted from these radionuclides is absorbed internally, but with a small fraction exiting the patient as a result of bremsstrahlung x-ray production. Measurements of patients treated with such radionuclides have demonstrated dose equivalent rates and total dose equivalents that are orders of magnitude below those requiring anything beyond standard precautions (5).

The dose equivalent rates from patients treated with radionuclides that also have nonnegligible photon yields (e.g., ^{131}I, ^{153}Sm, ^{166}Ho) will necessarily be much higher than those for pure beta emitters for the same amount of radioactivity. These rates are often well above the minimum, requiring active radiation safety and protection measures (dependent upon the amount of radioactivity administered) (6–8). For both inpatients and outpatients, this affects the duration of confinement before release either with or without radiation safety instructions (see "Patient Release Criteria"). Facilities designed specifically for internal radionuclide therapy with such radionuclides have the advantage of incorporating models of dose equivalent rates and total annual dose equivalents in the design phase, to achieve limited dose equivalent rates and total dose equivalents in various controlled and uncontrolled areas. Usual design targets in the United States include keeping the radiation levels below 5 mSv/year to occupationally exposed persons in controlled areas. This calculation makes assumptions on the number of patients treated each year and the activities and radionuclides used for those patients. The design also addresses nonradiation workers and the general public (including other nonradioactive patients) in uncontrolled areas, keeping their doses below 1 mSv/year, including assumptions on the time that those areas might be occupied. In the United States, there is also a limit on the dose rate of 0.02 mSv in any 1 hour to a person continually present 30 cm from the wall in the rooms adjacent to a radioactive patient's room; however, the annual limits almost always prove to be more restrictive.

Once a decision has been made to admit a patient for internal radionuclide therapy, the first radiation safety consideration is where the patient will be admitted. As stated earlier, standard precautions and "no isolation of," or "restricted access to," are warranted for a patient treated with pure beta-emitting radionuclides. The only exceptions might be either an extremely high amount of administered radioactivity or significant risk of exposure from contaminations from bodily fluid such as blood or excreta, or vomitus (especially skin exposure from direct contact). The opposite is generally true for gamma- or x-ray–emitting radionuclides. Unless the activity administered is low enough for dose equivalents to be below acceptable limits and the dose equivalent rate and total dose equivalent levels are considered safe, the patient must be isolated and access restricted. In addition, either specially shielded rooms (9,10), corner rooms with two exterior-facing walls, or patient rooms with adjacent areas of low occupancy are preferable for additional reduction in the exposure to others. Any room used for such purposes must be private and have its own private bathroom. Regardless of the facilities used, radioactive material and/or radiation area cautionary signage must be posted in appropriate locations according to regulatory requirements. The signs at the door to the patient's room would carry the radiation symbol and the wording, "Caution, Radioactive Material" and either "Caution Radiation Area" if the dose equivalent rate 30 cm from the patient falls between 0.05 and 1 mSv/h or "Caution, High Radiation Area" if the dose equivalent rate exceeds 1 mSv/h. Areas outside of the patient's room with dose equivalent rates greater than 0.02 mSv/h must be controlled and closed to entry by members of the public.

Once the room for admission has been reserved, the second radiation safety consideration is preparation of the room to house the radioactive inpatient. Preparations should begin ahead of time for containment of possible contaminations. Disposable, plastic-backed, absorbent paper should be secured in strategic locations where contaminations are likely to occur. Separate plastic or plastic-line containers for removal and storage of both disposal and nondisposal items used by the patient, and which might become contaminated, should be placed in the room. Surveying for and removal of contaminated items should be performed on a daily basis. Patients who are continent and ambulatory should be instructed to flush the toilet several (typically three) times after each use. If dose equivalent rates from collected urine from an incontinent or nonambulatory catheterized patient are anticipated to be unacceptably high,

keeping the collection bags in an appropriately shielded and labeled container at the patient's bedside during use, for later disposal, may be warranted. Alternatively, shielding the urine bag and running the drainage tube through a pump and into the toilet, running the pump periodically, reduces the exposure from the urine and minimizes the handling. Measurement of the maximum dose equivalent rate at 1 m from the patient with a calibrated survey meter should be made at least once daily, beginning immediately after administration of the radioactivity. These data can be used to determine when the patient can be released from the hospital, when specific radiation safety precautions may be replaced with standard precautions if the patient is remaining in the hospital, or as reference data for improving radiation safety and protection policies and procedures. This information may also be used for designing future dedicated facilities and for prospective radiation exposure studies for future therapies utilizing the same or different amounts of the same radionuclide, and either the same or a different pharmaceutical. Upon release of the patient from the room, all radioactively contaminated items should be removed, a radiation survey performed with a sensitive meter, wipes taken of surfaces and counted to assess possible contamination, and an assessment from a radiation safety standpoint whether and when the room can be made available for next use.

The third consideration is radiation exposure from access to and direct contact with the radioactive inpatient by hospital personnel. As always, the principles of time, distance, and shielding should be employed to control such access and contact, with much tighter controls required for nonradiation versus radiation workers. If personnel generally considered nonradiation workers (e.g., doctors, nurses, and technicians not normally working in radiologic departments) are dedicated to providing care for radioactive patients, then their dose equivalents may exceed the corresponding regulatory limit (1 mSv/year) and consideration should be given to reclassifying them as radiation workers, which has much higher occupational dose equivalent limits (see Table 10.3). This change in status requires specialized training in radiation safety, the wearing of radiation measurement badges, and ongoing monitoring and documentation of their radiation dose equivalent. The care given to the radioactive patient should not differ substantially from usual and customary, but the patient should be informed in advance regarding possible radiation safety precautions that will be undertaken, to avoid misinterpretation of these measures as reflecting a lack of concern on the part of caregivers. Minimizing exposure under these conditions can be accomplished by observing standard precautions; providing direct contact care expeditiously and wearing proper protective equipment; and entering the room only when necessary and communicating verbally with the patient at a distance (and possibly behind a radiation barrier). It is also prudent to instruct food service, housekeeping, and other ancillary personnel regarding access and to minimize the amount of time spent in the patient's room. Telemetry reduces the need to enter the room to perform checks of vital signs.

The desire of family and friends to visit a patient when radiation safety precautions are in effect must be taken into account, especially if the duration of confinement is expected to be long. Certain individuals must necessarily be excluded from visitation during this time, namely, those under the age of 18 and pregnant or nursing females (except under extraordinary conditions, e.g., when directly involved in caregiving, or visiting a dying patient). Those who are allowed to visit must not be permitted entry without first registering their presence with the clinic and receiving radiation safety instructions. Limitations on the frequency and duration of each visit should be established, and the use of portable radiation shields considered, in order to keep the dose equivalent to these individuals ALARA and below the 1-mSv limit for members of the public. Designated, nonpregnant, and nonnursing adult caregivers given specific radiation safety training and instructions may be allowed a dose limit of 5 mSv annually. The NRC has recently published guidance on requesting exemptions from these limits, under circumstances where it is deemed in the best interest of a patient such as a small child undergoing inpatient internal radionuclide therapy, to allow certain family members or friends direct involvement in providing care (8). The dose equivalent such caregivers receive is neither involuntary (unlike that of members of the general public) nor occupational. The NRC has recognized that a relaxed dose equivalent limit somewhere between the 1-mSv member-of-the-public and the 50-mSv occupational limits should be specified for these individuals, to be determined on a case-by-case basis, and furthermore has recommended a default limit of 20 mSv for such exemptions.

In any medical setting, the patient may require emergent care for cardiac or respiratory arrest, choking, seizures, or similar situations. Most often, the amounts of radiation members of the resuscitation team would receive from such activities would not be excessive. However, patients with large amounts of photon-emitting radionuclides can deliver dose equivalents above normal regulatory limits. For life-saving situations, the limits do not apply, but the safety of the facility's staff requires planning for such contingencies beforehand, establishing a protocol and practicing the procedures before patient treatments begin. The protocol would detail who performs what functions and where they would be during the procedure. Working through the details in practice sessions helps to incorporate safety procedures, such as the use of shielding or distance, into the process. All of the persons potentially involved need training and education in radiation safety to reduce the fear often associated with encounters with radiation. Pregnant women should not participate in resuscitations involving patients where the room is posted with a "Caution, Radiation Area" sign. Table 10.4 shows a hypothetical example of how long a staff member could work 20 cm from a patient who received ^{131}I-labeled metaiodobenzylguanidine (MIBG)

Table **10.4**	Time to reach the annual maximum allowed dose (50 mSv) during a resuscitation involving a patient receiving ^{131}I-labeled MIBG							
Time Since Injection (h)	**Initial Amount Injected (mCi)**							
	100	200	300	400	500	600	700	800
0	9	5	3	3	2	2	2	1
2	9	5	3	3	2	2	2	1
4	10	5	3	3	2	2	2	2
8	11	5	4	3	2	2	2	2
12	12	6	4	3	3	2	2	2
18	15	7	5	4	3	3	2	2
24	18	9	6	5	4	4	3	3
36	24	12	8	7	5	5	4	4
48	36	18	12	10	8	7	6	6
60	38	19	13	11	8	7	6	6
72	40	20	13	11	9	8	7	6
84	41	21	14	12	9	8	7	6

1. Half the injected activity is excreted linearly over the first 24 hours, and a quarter over the next 24 hours. After that, the activity decreases with a half-life of 8 days.

2. The distance is assumed to be 20 cm from the patient and the dose equivalent at that distance follows an inverse square relationship.

3. Due to the larger patient size with higher doses, the patient absorbs 10% of the radiation for injections of 400 and 500 mCi, 15% for 600 and 700 mCi, and 20% for 800 mCi.

4. Dose equivalent constant equals 0.0022 mSv/(mCi h).

before exceeding the annual, occupational dose equivalent limits. Such a table should be calculated to guide the training and planning for these events. If resuscitation would be expected to exceed the annual occupational limit, the persons listed who would be called should be volunteers. This last provision becomes very difficult to assure in practical situations, particularly in facilities performing frequent, high-activity procedures, and becomes a matter for institutional policy.

More detailed coverage of the topic of managing radioactive patients can be found in the Report No. 155 of the National Council on Radiation Protection and Measures (5). That report provides a thorough and up-to-date guidance regarding all aspects of radiation safety and protection (programs and practices) related to internal radionuclide therapy.

■ PATIENT RELEASE CRITERIA

A patient undergoing internal radionuclide therapy may be released from radiation confinement by a radioactive materials licensee, when the dose to the maximally exposed individual (the person likely to receive the most radiation, typically, the sleeping partner or primary caregiver) is estimated not to exceed the limit set forth by the appropriate radiation safety regulatory agency (e.g., NRC or Agreement State). The values used in this section are those from the U.S. NRC. The currently accepted limits for total, or cumulative, dose equivalent (expressed in effective dose equivalent units, EDE) are 1 mSv for release without any instructions other than standard precautions, and 5 mSv with specific radiation safety instructions, including those intended to keep the cumulative dose to the special-case populations of pregnant women, nursing infants, children, as well as, members of the general public, below 1 mSv (4,5). One caveat to release above the 1-mSv limit is that the patient must be capable of following the instructions given. Such patients should be identified prior to therapy. If a licensee wishes to release a patient above the 1-mSv limit, written documentation of the dose equivalent calculation model upon which the release is based, as well as written instructions for the patient (and any family members/caregivers), is required.

There are three basic external dose calculation models that can be applied to the release of radioactive patients: administered activity, measured dose rate, and patient-specific (4). While each of these models makes certain assumptions regarding dose rate over time and cumulative dose, they are all based on the same fundamental dose-describing equations:

$$d(t) = \frac{24 \cdot \Gamma \cdot A \cdot E \cdot f(t) \cdot e^{-0.693t/T_\mathrm{P}}}{r^2} \quad \text{(Eq. 10.7)}$$

and

$$D(t) = \frac{24 \cdot \Gamma \cdot A \cdot E}{r^2} \cdot \int_{T_r}^{t} f(t) \cdot e^{-0.693t/T_\mathrm{P}} \, dt, \quad \text{(Eq. 10.8)}$$

where $d(t)$ = dose rate at time t, $D(t)$ = cumulative dose from time of release, T_r, to time t (days), Γ = radionuclide-specific γ-ray, or, for pure beta emitters, bremsstrahlung, dose constant (μSv-m^2/MBq-h),[b] A = the activity at the time of injection, called the administered activity (MBq), E = occupancy factor that gives the duration a person may be in the presence of the radiation, $f(t)$ = biologic fraction of the administered activity remaining in the patient at time t, T_p = physical half-life of the radionuclide (days), r = distance (cm or m). The 24 converts h^{-1} to d^{-1}.

These equations account for all factors that contribute to external dose equivalent: the dose equivalent rate for the given radionuclide; the administered activity and the fraction retained as a function of time; the distance from the radiation source; and the fraction of time spent at that distance.

The simplest and most conservative of the three models is release based on administered activity. This model assumes physical decay only; no patient self-attenuation; $r = 1$ m; $E = 1$ for $T_p \leq 1$ day or 0.25 for $T_p > 1$ day; and cumulative dose from $t = 0$ onward until complete decay, giving $D(\infty)$. The conservative occupancy factors effectively assume the maximally exposed person spends either the entire time ($T_p \leq 1$ day) or 6 h/day ($T_p > 1$ day) over the period of time the exposure occurs at 1 m from the patient. The NRC does not require instructions for patients released using this model, *unless* the release is not immediate and thus based on retained rather than administered activity or the patient is breast-feeding (described later in this section). The calculation of $D(\infty)$ and thus the activity at which a patient can be released is straightforward. Furthermore, published tables of release activities for both 1-mSv and 5-mSv limits for many therapy radionuclides, such as Table 10.5 (4), eliminate the need for even those simple calculations.

Alternatively, release can be based on a measurement of dose rate at 1 m, $\dot{d}_0$. This model requires more effort than release based solely on activity, since one or more measurements of dose rate from the patient must be made, and also requires release documentation. On the other hand, the dose-rate model simplifies the dose equivalent equations, as it can combine effectively all the factors except E into one, and account for self-attenuation of the radiation by the patient, giving

$$d(t) = \frac{24 \, \dot{d}_0 \, E \, f(t) \, e^{-0.693t/T_{1/2}}}{r^2}. \quad \text{(Eq. 10.9)}$$

and

$$D(t) = \frac{24 \, \dot{d}_0 \, E}{r^2} \int_{T_r}^{t} f(t) \, e^{-0.693t/T_{1/2}} \, dt. \quad \text{(Eq. 10.10)}$$

---

[b]Many radiation detectors still display older units of roentgens (R), in which case a Γ in R-cm^2/mCi-h with the appropriate energy-dependent R to dose equivalent conversion would be used.

Table **10.5** Activities and dose rates for authorizing patient release for various radionuclides (4)						
	Activities Below Which Patients May Be Released				**Dose Rates at 1 m Below Which Patients May Be Released**	
	Total Dose Equivalent					
	For 1 mSv		**For 5 mSv**		**For 1 mSv**	**For 5 mSv**
Radionuclide	**GBq**	**mCi**	**GBq**	**mCi**	**mSv/h**	**mSv/h**
Ag-111	3.8	104	19	520	0.016	0.08
Au-198	0.7	18.6	3.5	93	0.042	0.21
Cr-51	0.96	26	4.8	130	0.004	0.02
Cu-64	1.68	46	8.4	230	0.054	0.27
Cu-67	2.8	78	14	390	0.044	0.22
Ga-67	1.74	48	8.7	240	0.036	0.18
I-123	1.2	32	6	160	0.052	0.26
I-125	0.05	1.4	0.25	7	0.002	0.01
I-131	0.24	6.6	1.2	33	0.014	0.07
In-111	0.48	13	2.4	65	0.04	0.2
Re-186	5.6	154	28	770	0.03	0.15
Re-188	5.8	158	29	790	0.04	0.2
Sc-47	2.2	62	11	310	0.034	0.17
Se-75	0.0178	0.4	0.089	2	0.001	0.005
Sm-153	5.2	140	26	700	0.06	0.3
Sn-177m	0.22	5.8	1.1	29	0.008	0.04
Tl-201	3.2	86	16	430	0.038	0.19
Yb-169	0.074	2	0.37	10	0.004	0.02

Thus, patients may be releasable at a higher activity and/or an earlier point in time than that based solely on administered activity, due to the use of a patient self-attenuated (or "effective") dose-rate constant. Published tables of the 1-mSv and 5-mSv release dose rates for the various therapeutic radionuclides, such as Table 10.5, are also available for the worst-case assumption of physical decay only (i.e., no biologic clearance, $f(t) = 1$) (4).

Patient-specific external dose calculation, while more complex and requiring more effort than that based on either administered activity or measured dose rate, provides the least restrictive and most realistic model for release. Both an effective dose-rate constant and effective (biologic and physical) clearance of the radionuclide from the body, $f(t)'$, can be incorporated into the calculation of dose rate and cumulative dose on a case-by-case basis (6), so the equations become

$$d(t) = \frac{24\,\dot{d}_0\,E\,f(t)'}{r^2}. \qquad \text{(Eq. 10.11)}$$

and

$$D(t) = \frac{24\,\dot{d}_0\,E}{r^2}\int_{T_r}^{t} f(t)'dt. \qquad \text{(Eq. 10.12)}$$

The dose rate, $\dot{d}_0$, can be that measured on each individual patient, and the effective clearance can be based on either a direct estimate for each individual patient or an accepted model of clearance for the particular radiopharmaceutical (nonstandard occupancy factors, E, may also be utilized in certain instances). The result is a more appropriate and personalized release from radiation confinement and duration of postrelease instructions for each individual patient. Two primary examples of the patient-specific release model are radioactive iodine (RAI) therapy of thyroid cancer and radioimmunotherapy of non–Hodgkin B-cell lymphoma with ^{131}I-radiolabeled ibritumomab (BEXXAR, GlaxoSmithKline). A three-compartment model (circulating, thyroidal, and extrathyroidal) for RAI patient release has been published (4,7):

$$d(t) = \frac{24\,X\,E_1(0.8)\,e^{-0.693t/T_P}}{r^2},$$

for an initial nonvoid interval, T_{nv} $\qquad$ (Eq. 10.13)

$$d(t) = \frac{24\,X\,E_2\,e^{-0.693T_{nv}/T_P}}{r^2}\{f_1\,e^{-0.693t/T_1} + f_2(e^{-0.693t/T_2}\},$$

from T_{nv} onward $\qquad\qquad$ (Eq. 10.14)

Table **10.6**	Default values for the extrathyroidal and thyroidal compartment fractions and effective half-lives (Equations 10.14 and 10.15) (4)			
	Extrathyroidal		Thyroidal	
	f_1	T_1 (d)	f_2	T_2 (d)
Hyperthyroidism	0.20	0.32	0.80	5.2
Thyroid cancer (postthyroidectomy)	0.95	0.32	0.05	7.3

$$D(\infty) = \frac{34.6\,X}{r^2}\{E_1\,(0.8)T_p\,(1 - e^{-0.693T_{nv}/T_P})$$
$$+ E_2(f_1T_1 + f_2T_2)e^{-0.693T_{nv}/T_P}\}, \quad \text{(Eq. 10.15)}$$

where the dose rate at 1 m, X, can be either $\Gamma \times A$ or $\dot{d}_0$. Equation 10.13 represents the circulating compartment with an assumed circulating fraction = 0.8 and default value for $T_{nv} = 0.33$ days; the occupancy factors are 0.75 (E_1) and 0.25 (E_2); and default values for the extrathyroidal and thyroidal compartment fractions and effective half-lives are given in Table 10.6 (3). Calculations specific to BEXXAR (employing measured dose rate and effective half-life derived from the dosimetric study) have been developed (11), and are contained in its customer site training manual:

$$d(t) = \dot{d}_0\,(0.75)\,e^{-0.693t/T_P}$$
for an initial 3-h nonvoid interval,   (Eq. 10.16)

$$d(t) = \dot{d}_0\,(0.25)\,e^{-0.693(3)/T_P}\,e^{-t/\tau_{tb}}$$
from 3 hours onward,   (Eq. 10.17)

$$D(\infty) = 0.25\,\dot{d}_0\,\{8.95 + 0.99\tau_{tb}\}, \quad \text{(Eq. 10.18)}$$

where the distance is 1 m, 0.75 and 0.25 are occupancy factors, and τ_{tb} is the total body residence time (1.443 $\times$ effective half-life). The BEXXAR method furthermore employs a line-source model ($2/r$) rather than the conventional point-source model ($1/r^2$) for the patient when computing the dose at distances closer than 1 m, for example, for the sleeping partner (12).

The calculated total EDE (TEDE), in principle, should also include that from internal dose equivalent (so-called committed EDE, CEDE), in addition to the external component (so-called deep-dose equivalent, DDE); TEDE = DDE + CEDE. However, it is generally accepted that the internal component will be typically one or more orders of magnitude smaller than the external dose (an exception would be that for a nursing infant of a radioactive breast-feeding mother, discussed later in this section). The CEDE can be safely ignored if it is anticipated to be less than 10% of the DDE. Otherwise, the formula for estimating the CEDE is $A \times F \times C$, where A = administered activity (Bq), F = fractional intake, and C = dose conversion factor (Sv/Bq) for the given radiopharmaceutical and intake pathway (inhalation, digestion, skin). Typical values for F are 10^{-5} and 10^{-6} (4,7). Values for C usually come from the package insert for the radiopharmaceutical.

The list of radiation safety precautions to be taken, which is provided to a patient released with an estimated cumulative dose to another person above the 1-mSv limit, relates to restrictions in the following lifestyle categories:

- Travel
- Use of a bathroom
- Sleeping with others
- Time spent near other adults, children, and pregnant women
- Time spent in public places
- Work
- Breast-feeding (nursing mothers)

The time that precautions in each category are in effect will generally be unique and specific to each individual patient, and will be dependent upon the release model utilized. Occupancy factors, standard (or "index") distances, and dose limits specific to each category are employed; and, as indicated earlier, the duration will be the longest for release based on administered activity, and (generally) shortest for release based on patient-specific dose calculations. Default values for E, r, and TEDE to use for calculating time of release and duration of precautions for various categories and persons have been adopted and are shown in Table 10.7 (4,5). In addition, generalized operational equations for calculating time (postadministration) when a patient may be released and durations for sleeping

Table **10.7**	Values for occupancy factors, standard distances, and dose limits for use in calculation of release limits			
Category/Person		**E**	**r (m)**	**TEDE (mSv)**
Nonsleeping/Adult (children/pregnant women)		0.25	1	5 (1)
Sleeping/Nonpregnant (pregnant) partner		0.33	0.3	5 (1)
Holding children		0.2	0.3	1
Public places, work		0.33	1	1

alone, avoiding children and pregnant women, refraining from holding children, and avoiding public places and delaying returning to work have been published (13). Formulas were derived for both single and multiple exponential clearance models, as well as those for calculating the duration of sleeping alone in order to keep the total awake plus sleeping dose to the partner below the limit, for the case of both a nonpregnant and pregnant sleeping partner (a not-so-straightforward calculation).

Ideally, the released patient travels alone from the health care facility to their domicile. However, quite often either a family member/caregiver is a transportation provider or traveling companion, or the patient travels by means of public transportation. Travel restrictions should be determined on a case-by-case basis, based on calculations incorporating the mode and duration of travel, the time spent with and distances from other individuals during the trip, and the corresponding external dose limits. If being transported by automobile, the patient should be instructed to maximize their distance from traveling companion(s) with greater than 1 m recommended (5), and avoid, if possible, traveling with their sleeping partner/most exposed person, children, or pregnant women. Furthermore, due to the current state of heightened radiologic security at transportation depots and international border crossings, providing patients with documentation supporting the fact that they have been treated with a radioactive substance is highly recommended, in case they set off radiation detectors and are interrogated by the authorities at those checkpoints.

The duration over which the patient is instructed to have sole use of a bathroom should be based upon when the excretion of radioactivity is anticipated to be complete. Instructions to flush the toilet several times, as well as thoroughly rinse the shower, bath, or sink, after each use during that time should be given. As alluded to earlier, the number of nights of sleeping alone must take into account the dose anticipated to be received by the sleeping partner while both are awake, as well as, whether or not the sleeping partner is pregnant. When the patient is allowed to return to work should take into consideration whether the patient spends a lot of time in close proximity to coworkers and/or clients (e.g., if the patient is a surgeon, pediatrician, or day care worker).

Breast-feeding is contraindicated immediately after the administration of a therapeutic quantity of radioactivity to a nursing mother. There exists a probability that a significant fraction of the internally administered radiopharmaceutical will be secreted via lactation and thus be transferred to the nursing infant. The resultant internal dose received by the infant through ingestion will be much higher than that for an adult for the same amount of radioactivity due to much smaller organ and total body masses, and as a consequence may be significantly higher than 1 mSv. Furthermore, if the infant is receiving the milk directly from the mother's breast (as opposed to consuming pumped breast milk later from a bottle), the child will be in very close

proximity to the source of radiation for the duration of each feeding and may receive a substantial external dose as well. The period of discontinuation of breast-feeding can be calculated using the above formulas for the external and internal TEDE components, with appropriate parameter values and the 1-mSv TEDE limit. If the dose to the lactating breast itself is anticipated to be unacceptably high, lactation must be discontinued prior to therapy, for example, 4 to 6 weeks for RAI, which is known to collect in the lactating breast. If the calculated discontinuation period is on the order of, or greater than, the remaining time the infant would be nursing, permanent cessation should be considered (4,5). In some cases, viable options are pumping the breast milk in advance of the therapy for later bottle feeding, or after therapy and storing it until the radioactivity decays to an acceptable level, at which time it could be used.

Lastly, radioactive patient release criteria have historically been based upon the assumption of infrequent exposure of individuals to such radiation, in particular family members/caregivers. The NRC, in recognition of the increasing number of applications and frequency of administration of radiopharmaceuticals (both diagnostic and therapeutic), has recently clarified their guidelines with regard to the dose limits for patient release. Specifically, the dose limits specified are implicitly total per year and not per occurrence (14). A consequence of the increasing use of internal radionuclide therapy is the probability that a particular individual may receive exposure from multiple radioactive patients per annum. The multiple exposures may originate from the same person who receives repeat treatments in one 12-month period (either fractionated therapy of the same agent or therapies with different agents), or from two or more persons (family members, coworkers, etc.) who were treated within 1 year. Therefore, when it is known that a patient will be receiving multiple therapies over a period of 1 year or less, it is advisable to adopt the principle of exposure budgeting, whereby the dose limits for each release are scaled such that the total annual doses do not exceed the regulatory limits.

■ REFERENCES

1. Attix F. *Introduction to Radiological Physics and Radiation Dosimetry*. New York, NY: Wiley; 1986.
2. ICRP. Report 103: The 2007 Recommendations of the International Commission on Radiological Protection. Orlando, FL: International Commission on Radiological Protection; 2007.
3. U.S. Nuclear Regulatory Commission. 10 Code of Federal Regulations Part 20, Subparts C and D. Washington, DC; 2009.
4. U.S. Nuclear Regulatory Commission. Consolidated Guidance about Materials Licenses: NUREG 1556 Vol. 9. Washington, DC: Division of Industrial and Medical Nuclear Safety, Office of Nuclear Material Safety and Safeguards; 2002.
5. NCRP. Report 155: Management of Radionuclide Therapy Patients. Bethesda, MD: National Council on Radiation Protection and Management; 2006.
6. Al-Haj AN, Lagarde CS, Lobriguito AM. Patient parameters and other radiation safety issues in 131I therapy for thyroid cancer treatment. *Health Phys*. 2007;93:656–666.
7. Siegel JA, Marcus CS, Stabin MG. Licensee over-reliance on conservatisms in NRC guidance regarding the release of patients treated with 131I. *Health Phys*. 2007;93:667–677.

8. U.S. Nuclear Regulatory Commission. Requesting Exemption from the Public Dose Limits for Certain Caregivers of Hospital Patients: Regulatory Information Summary 2006-18. Washington, DC: Office of Nuclear Material Safety and Safeguards; 2006.

9. Thomadsen B, van de Geijn J, Buchler D, et al. Fortification of existing rooms used for brachytherapy patients. *Health Phys.* 1983;45:607–615.

10. Gitterman M, Webster EW. Shielding hospital rooms for brachytherapy patients: design, regulatory and cost/benefit factors. *Health Phys.* 1984;46:617–625.

11. Siegel JA, Kroll S, Regan D, et al. A practical methodology for patient release after tositumomab and (131)I-tositumomab therapy. *J Nucl Med.* 2002;43:354–363.

12. Siegel JA, Marcus CS, Sparks RB. Calculating the absorbed dose from radioactive patients: the line-source versus point-source model. *J Nucl Med.* 2002;43:1241–1244.

13. Zanzonico PB, Siegel JA, St Germain J. A generalized algorithm for determining the time of release and the duration of post-release radiation precautions following radionuclide therapy. *Health Phys.* 2000;78:648–659.

14. U.S. Nuclear Regulatory Commission. Dose limit for patient release under 10 CFR 35.75: Regulatory Information Summary 2008-07. Washington, DC: Office of Federal and State Materials and Environmental Management Programs; 2008.

Tumor Microenvironment and Delivery Strategies

Employing SEREX for Identification of Targets for Anticancer Targeted Therapy

Doo-Il Jeoung

■ INTRODUCTION

The identification of tumor antigens is essential for the development of anticancer therapeutic vaccines and clinical diagnosis of cancer. SEREX (serologic analysis of recombinant cDNA expression libraries) has been used to identify such tumor antigens by screening sera of patients with cDNA expression libraries. More than 2000 antigens have been discovered by SEREX. This review provides information on the application of SEREX for identification of tumor-associated antigens (TAAs) for the development of anticancer therapeutics.

■ SEREX (SEROLOGIC ANALYSIS OF RECOMBINANT cDNA EXPRESSION LIBRARY)

Sahin and his colleagues (1) have introduced a method for the identification of tumor antigens recognized by autologous serum immunoglobulin G (IgG) of cancer patients. This method, termed SEREX, has led to the identification of a series of tumor antigens with relevance to the diagnosis and therapy of cancer. So far, more than 2000 different antigens have been defined by SEREX analysis (Cancer Immunome database: http://www2.licr.org/CancerImmunomeDB). The recent development of a new approach to dissect the humoral immune response to cancer established a comprehensive picture of the immune repertoire against human cancer antigens. SEREX allows for a systematic and unbiased search for cancer-specific antigens and immunogenic proteins based on their reactivity with autologous patient serum.

SEREX-defined antigens showing cancer-restricted seroreactivity offer a range of opportunities for cancer diagnosis and disease monitoring, and perhaps immunotherapy. As opposed to methods used to assess serum antigen concentrations, such as prostate-specific antigen (PSA) or CA125 blood tests, assays for cancer-restricted seroreactivity measure serum titers of tumor-specific antibodies. SEREX analysis of renal cancer (2), colon cancer (3), gastric cancer (4), and breast cancer (5) have led to the identification of 13, 32, 12, and 40 different antigens, respectively, which react exclusively with sera from cancer patients, but not with sera from healthy controls.

In addition to the serologic definition of human tumor antigens, there has been a revolution in the structural identification of human tumor antigens. These antigens are recognized by the cellular immune system. Pioneering work of Hunt et al. (6) has initiated a method to identify peptide/protein antigens recognized by autologous cytotoxic T cells (cytotoxic T lymphocytes [CTLs]) and a variety of new antigens have been identified by this technique.

■ SEREX METHOD

The SEREX approach offers following features: (a) the use of tumor specimens restricts the analysis to genes that are expressed by the tumor cells in vivo; (b) the use of patient serum allows for the identification of multiple antigens; (c) the screening is restricted to antigens, against which, patients have raised high-titer antibody responses.

SEREX (Fig. 11.1) employs a bacteriophage recombinant cDNA expression library prepared from tumor tissues, tumor cell lines, and testis tissues. The use of tumor cell lines for SEREX analysis has benefits, including the absence of contaminating normal cell types invariably present in tumor specimens, and the elimination of B cells that give rise to false-positive IgG-expressing clones in the expression library. The cDNA expression library is used to transduce *Escherichia coli*. The recombinant protein library is then induced and transferred to nitrocellulose membranes. These membranes are then incubated with diluted (1:100 to 1:1000) extensively preabsorbed pooled serum from the autologous patient. Clones reactive with high-titer antibodies are identified using an enzyme (alkaline phosphatase-conjugated secondary antibody) specific for human IgG. Positive clones are then subjected to DNA sequencing. Sequence information of DNA insert can be used to determine expression profile of the transcript and to evaluate the incidence of antibody responses to the respective antigens. SEREX has been widely used in identifying antigens in patients with solid tumors (7), and autoimmune disease, including systemic sclerosis, systemic lupus erythematosus, and Sjogren syndrome (8–10). Many antigens identified by SEREX have also been identified by many other investigators working on different cancers. This led us to believe that there may

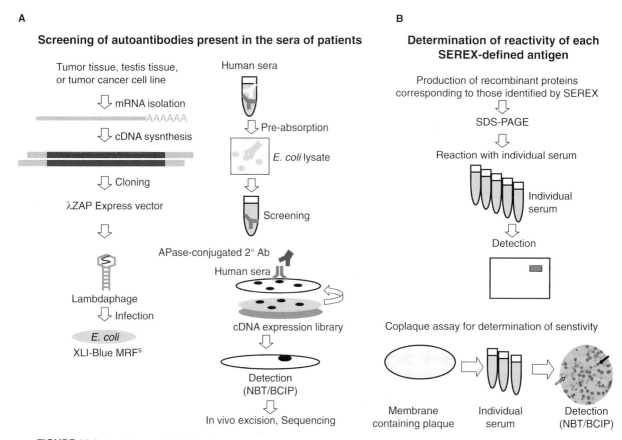

FIGURE 11.1 Identification of SEREX-defined antigens and its subsequent clinical application for diagnosis. **A:** Construction of cDNA expression library. cDNA expression libraries are made from tumor tissues, tumor cell lies, or testis tissues. For this, 5 μg of poly (A)$^+$ RNA was converted into cDNA by reverse transcriptase. Thus, obtained cDNA library is cloned into λ ZAP expression vector. Each library usually consists of 2×10^6 primary recombinants, on average. A total of 5×10^5 of these recombinants are used for immunoscreening. Each of these recombinant cDNA libraries is transformed into *Escherichia coli* to yield a recombinant cDNA expression library. cDNA expression libraries are screened with pooled sera of patients with cancers. Immune reactive clones are selected by reacting nitrocellulose membrane containing recombinant clones with pooled sera of patients with cancers followed by incubation with alkaline phosphatase-conjugated secondary antibody. Selected clones are subjected to in vivo excision and sequencing to determine identity of each immune reactive clone. **B:** Sensitivity and specificity of each clone is determined by incubating each clone with individual serum of cancer patients or healthy controls.

be defined number of antigens recognized by the immune systems of patients with cancers, collectively referred to as cancer "immunome."

CLASSIFICATION OF THE SEREX-DEFINED ANTIGENS

Cancer-restricted recognition suggests common origins of immunogenicity, such as gene mutation or aberrant expression, indicating that serologic methods of gene discovery can be used to identify molecules of etiologic relevance to cancer. In the past 20 years, SEREX has been applied to a range of tumor types, including melanoma (11), hepatocellular carcinoma (12), esophageal cancer (13), lung cancer (14,15), sarcoma (16), and gastric cancer (17,18). A number of SEREX-defined antigens can be classified into one of the following categories: differentiation antigens, mutational antigens, overexpressed antigens, and cancer/testis (CT) antigens.

Mutational antigens

Several mutational antigens have been isolated by SEREX. Tumor suppressor gene p53 has been identified by SEREX of ovarian cancer (5). In the case of colon cancer, a single-base substitution of p53 (A to G) was identified, confirming this mutation as the basis for the observed immunogenicity. Other examples of mutational antigens in colon cancer were AD034, with a 32-bp frameshift mutation (19), and CDX2, with a single-base frameshift mutation (20). Three genes coding for products identified by SEREX are clustered in chromosome 3p21, a region long known to be a hot spot of genetic aberrations in many cancer types and postulated to harbor tumor suppressor genes (21,22). Two of the three genes, NY-REN-9 and NY-REN-10, were derived from renal carcinoma and correspond to LUCA-15 and gene 21, respectively (2). The third gene, NY-LU-12, isolated from lung cancer, was identical to gene 16, which maps to the telomere break point of a small cell lung cancer line, NCI-H740 (15).

Differentiation antigens

Differentiation antigens are expressed in tumors in a lineage-specific pattern, but also in normal cells of the same origin. The classic example of a differentiation antigen recognized by SEREX is the melanocyte-specific protein tyrosinase (1). Other examples include NY-BR-1 in breast cancer (23) and glial fibrillary acidic protein in glioma (24).

Amplified or overexpressed antigens

Many SEREX-defined genes are overexpressed in cancer. Amplified or overexpressed antigens identified include carbonic anhydrase XII in breast (25), eIF-4 gamma (26) in lung cancer, AKT1 (27), and HER-2/neu (16) in breast cancer. Several mechanisms can account for amplified expression of gene products in cancer, including gene amplification (e.g., eIF-4 gamma), increased steady-state mRNA (e.g., KOC3), and increased protein stability (e.g., p53) (28).

Cancer/testis antigens

Certain CT gene families contain multiple members (e.g., MAGEA, GAGE1) as well as splice variants (e.g., XAGE1a, XAGE1b). CT antigens share the following characteristics: (a) predominant expression in testis, but generally not in other normal somatic tissues; (b) gene activation and mRNA expression in a wide range of human tumor types; (c) existence of multigene families; and (d) with rare exception, localization of coding genes to chromosome X. Table 11.1 shows partial list of CT antigens identified by various methods, including SEREX (1,11,13,17,29–33). The frequent expression of CT antigens in various types of tumors is an exception to the general rule that CT antigens predominate in testis. It suggests that the CT antigens, most of them with unknown function at present, are a distinct group of proteins in terms of their regulation and possibly their biologic function.

Immunogenicity of SEREX-defined antigens

Immunogenicity of SEREX-defined antigens can be ascribed to several mechanisms: gene activation, mutation, amplification, overexpression, or expression of abnormal splice variants. The antibody responses to CT antigens are related to the abnormal expression of these antigens in cancer that are usually expressed only in germ cells. Reportedly, abnormal expression of CT antigens has been closely related with demethylation of promoters of these CT antigens (34,35).

Abnormal antigen expression is also found in paraneoplastic syndromes affecting central nervous system. These syndromes result from autoimmune recognition of neural antigens aberrantly expressed by nonneural cancers, and specific autoantibodies are often found to be associated with specific tumor types (36).

Mutation forms the basis for the immunogenicity of SEREX-defined antigens. Examples include CDX2 and p53 (5,20). In the case of mutation, it is quite possible that the resulting antibodies recognize wild type. Therefore, sequencing of the independent clones from the same library is required. Many examples of autoantibodies to overexpressed proteins in cancers have been identified by SEREX. This indicates that immune system responds well to quantitative as well as qualitative changes in antigen expression.

RECOGNITION OF SEREX-DEFINED ANTIGENS

Growing evidence suggests that the immune system interacts with tumor cells during the course of the disease. The general properties of cancer antigens are described in Figure 11.2 and these include the following principles: (a) cancer antigens

Table **11.1**	Examples of cancer/testis antigens		
CT Antigen Family	**No. of Genes**	**Chromosome**	**Detection**
IMAGE	16	Xq28	CD8$^+$, Ab
BAGE	2	Unknown	CD8$^+$
GAGE	9	Xp11	CD8$^+$
SSX	>5	Xp11	Ab
NY-ESO-1	2	Xq28	Ab, CD8$^+$, RDA
SCP-1	3	P12-pB	Ab
MAGE-C1	1	Xq26	Ab, RDA
CTP11	1	Unknown	Ab
SAGE	1	lp	Ab
cTAGE-1	1	Xq27	Ab, RDA
CAGE	1	Xp22	Ab

Note: This is a partial list of CT antigens identified by various methods.
Ab, identification of cancer/testis antigens by SEREX; CT, cancer/testis; RDA, representational difference analysis.

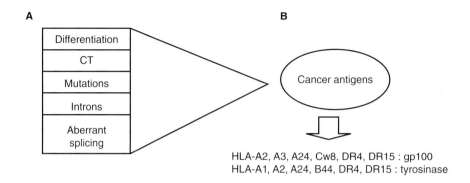

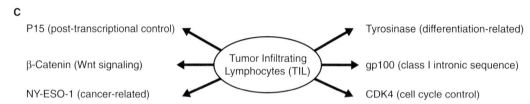

FIGURE 11.2 Properties of SEREX-defined tumor-associated antigens (TAA). **A:** Caner antigens can arise from differentiation antigens, cancer/testis antigens, mutant antigens, intronic sequences, and splicing variants. **B:** A single cancer antigen contains various epitopes that can be presented on many different alleles of HLA molecules. **C:** A single cancer patient usually develops immune response to multiple antigens.

contain epitopes binding to various human leukocyte antigen (HLA) alleles and (b) tumor infiltrating T lymphocytes (TIL) contain various cancer antigens. Large numbers of TIL from tumors have been shown to greatly increase T-cell populations capable of recognizing cancer antigens (37,38). The presence of TIL is associated with better prognosis in individual patients, indicating that TIL recognize specific antigens expressed by the tumor (Fig. 11.2). Before the identification of TAA by SEREX, conventional immunotherapy mainly focused on immunization with either autologs or allogeneic cancer cells or cancer cell extracts (Fig. 11.3). This approach is not effective because of minute amount of cancer antigens present in the intact cells. It also causes autoimmunity since many of the antigens overexpressed in tumors are also expressed in normal cells. Various approaches had been tried

to increase the immunogenicity of tumor cells, including injection of tumor cells along with adjuvants, or transducing cells with genes encoding cytokines such as tumor necrosis factor, interferon-γ, or granulocyte-macrophage colony-stimulating factor. However, these approaches have not been successful in generating T cells that recognize intact tumor cells. Cancer antigens identified by SEREX have offered new approaches to the development of anticancer therapeutic vaccines (Fig. 11.3). Tumor cells express antigens that can be recognized by the host's immune system. These TAAs can be injected into cancer patients in an attempt to induce a systemic immune response that may result in the destruction of the cancer growing in different body tissues.

Studies on experimental animals showed that cellular immunity rather than humoral response was responsible for

FIGURE 11.3 Vaccine approaches to the treatment of cancer patients. Numbers in parentheses denote references.

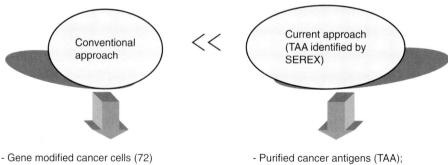

rejection of transplanted tumors or tissues. Identification of antigens recognized by CD8$^+$ CTL cells have been achieved by transfecting cDNA libraries from tumor cells into the target cells with appropriate HLA molecules, and then using antitumor cells to identify such transfectants (39,40). Once the gene is identified, the region encoding the antigenic peptide can be narrowed down by transfecting gene fragments. The synthetic peptides were then made and tested for recognition by the original tumor-specific CTL clone. Alternatively, peptides eluted from the surface of tumor cells are pulsed onto antigen-presenting cells, such as dendritic cells (DC), and tested for reactivity with specific antitumor lymphocytes (41,42).

SEREX has been used to identify cancer antigens that are recognized by CD8$^+$ T cells (CTL). Both CD8$^+$ cytotoxic T cells (CTL) and CD4$^+$ T-helper cells recognize antigens presented as small peptides in HLA. CD8$^+$ CTL cells recognize peptides of 8 to 10 amino acids presented on class I HLA. Peptides recognized by CTL are digested in proteosomes and presented via the endoplasmic reticulum. Experimental evidence in mice suggests that the effectiveness of CD8$^+$ T cells is dependent on factors from CD4$^+$ T-helper cells. Peptides recognized by CD4$^+$ T-helper cells are derived from extracellular proteins presented on class II HLA. HLA allelic variant binds only a subset of peptides that share conserved amino acid residues at fixed positions (43). The peptide–HLA complex is recognized by the T-cell receptor (TCR) on the surface of T lymphocytes. In addition to directly contacting the HLA molecule, other peptide residues are available to establish a direct contact with the TCR (44). Thus, whether a TAA peptide elicits a T-cell response is governed both by the ability of the peptide to bind the presenting HLA allele and by the resulting affinity of the peptide–HLA complex for the TCR.

T cell–defined TAAs include (a) differentiation antigens, which are expressed in a lineage-related manner and are detected in the normal counterpart of neoplastic tissue; (b) tumor-restricted antigens, which are expressed only on neoplastic cells; and (c) mutated antigens. Tumor-restricted antigens encompass both shared antigens of different origin and unique antigens. For unique TAAs (45–48), the immunogenic peptide includes a mutated amino acid sequence that confers immunogenicity through the exposure of an altered non–self-epitope.

It was not until 1991 that the first report describing the cloning of a gene encoding a human TAA, the melanoma antigen-1 (MAGE-1), was published (11). The identification of its nonamer peptide, which is recognized by HLA-A1-restricted CTLs, was published the following year (49). This T-cell epitope cloning technique was further employed to identify tumor antigens, such as BAGE and GAGE gene family (32,33). These antigens are typical of CT antigens in that their expression in normal tissues is restricted to testis and ovary while these antigens are widely expressed in various tumor tissues. Most of the tumor antigens recognized by CD8$^+$ T cells have been derived from melanomas.

With regard to gastric cancer, peptides from SEREX-defined antigens were able to induce HLA-specific CTL responses, indicating their potential uses as cancer vaccines in certain patients with gastric cancer (50). These CT antigens are likely to be oncogenes, in that they are expressed only in testis among normal tissues, an immune-privileged site, and widely expressed in various tumor tissues. Therefore, these CT antigens are ideal targets for the development of anticancer therapeutic vaccines.

The differentiation antigens comprise group of antigens that are recognized by CTL. These include tyrosinase (51), MEL-1 (52), and gp100 (53). Epitopes from differentiation antigens often exhibit low affinities for HLA molecules. Identification of class II HLA-restricted cancer antigens was made possible by fusing cDNA libraries to invariant chain sequence to guide the transfected proteins into the class II presentation pathways (54).

Mutated antigens are another group of TAAs. The p53 gene is the most commonly mutated gene in human tumors. According to several studies, peptides derived from p53 induced CTL response in vitro (55).

Examples of the antigens (32,33,46,47,53,56–72) recognized by CD8$^+$ CTL cells and presented on class I HLA molecules are shown in Table 11.2. Examples of the antigens (54,57,73–78) recognized by CD4$^+$ T-helper cells are also shown in Table 11.2.

Identification of TAA peptides expressed by different human tumors provides the basis for vaccination or active immunotherapy. Immunization studies using these TAA peptides have been relatively successful in generating high levels of T cells against cancer antigens (79,80).

The advantages of using peptide-based vaccines include (a) the simplicity of peptide administration in a clinical setting; (b) the possibility of treating only those patients whose tumors express the cognate epitopes, thus avoiding the useless immunization of patients whose tumors are TAA negative; and (c) the availability of in vitro or ex vivo assays that can assess patients' immune response to vaccine epitopes.

Although multitudes of T cell–defined TAA epitopes are now available for potential clinical application as vaccines, they are still of limited clinical use for the majority of cancers. Problems include (a) most of the available TAAs are expressed by melanoma, whereas relatively few TAA epitopes have been characterized in other tumors; (b) most of the already known TAA epitopes are recognized by only a few HLA alleles that are widely represented in the Caucasian population, leaving few epitopes available for recognition by T cells of subjects with less frequent HLA alleles; and (c) the majority of TAA epitopes are derived from normal proteins for which immune tolerance may prevent immunogenicity. Most T-cell responses require repeated in vitro stimulation with TAA epitopes (81,82) and show limited immunogenicity when used as vaccines for cancer patients (83,84). Therefore, most of the TAA peptides have elicited insufficient immune response to control cancer growth.

Table **11.2**	Examples of SEREX-defined antigens recognized by human T cells		
Antigen	**Reference**	**Antigen**	**Reference**
I. Class I—restricted antigens recognized by CD8⁺ T cells			
Differentiation antigens		**Cancer-testes antigens**	
MEL-1	(47)	MAGE-1	(59)
gp100(pmel-17)	(56)	MAGE-2	(60)
Tyrosinase	(46)	MAGE-3	(61)
Tyrosinase-related protein 1	(53)	MAGE-12	(62)
Tyrosinase-related protein 2	(57)	BAGE	(63)
Melanocyte-stimulating hormone receptor	(58)	GAGE	(32)
		NY-ESO-1	(33)
Mutated antigens		**Mutated antigens**	
CDK-4	(64)	α-Fetoprotein	(68)
Caspase-8	(65)	G-250	(69)
KIAA0205	(66)	Telomerase catalytic protein	(70)
HLA-A2-R	(67)	CEA	(71)
		P53	(72)
I. Class II—restricted antigens recognized by CD4⁺ lymphocytes			
Epitopes from nonmutated proteins		**Epitopes from mutated proteins**	
gp100	(73)	Triose-phosphate isomerase	(77)
MAGE-3	(74)	CDC-27	(57)
Tyrosinase	(75)	LDLR-FUT	(54)
NY-ESO-1	(76)		

The immunogenicity of TAA peptides can be increased by altering amino acid residues at positions that anchor the peptide to the appropriate HLA molecules (85). This modification induces a qualitatively and quantitatively improved T-cell response without changing the HLA-binding affinity or stability. This variant presumably improves immunogenicity through a more efficient interaction with the TCR.

The strategy of modifying TAA peptides to enhance antitumor T-cell responses represents a new way for the development of anticancer therapeutic vaccines.

Often, peptide vaccine alone does not give rise to sufficient immune responses to control cancer growth. Modified peptide from the gp100 (gp100:209-217), when used along with interleukin-2, led to significantly higher regression rate than when peptide alone was administered (86).

IMMUNOTHERAPY EMPLOYING DENDRITIC CELLS PRESENTING TAAS

The goal of active immunotherapy concerning tumors is to use tumor antigens to prime specific antitumor immunity by generating effector cells such as CTL to lyse tumor cells. DC are antigen-presenting cells that have the function of presenting antigens, including TAAs, to naive T cells in lymph nodes. DC have specialized characteristics that make them efficient at capturing, presenting antigens, and activating T cells. The generation of tumor-specific T cells against TAA-derived peptides requires a phase of "antigen presentation" by cells expressing HLA class I molecules (i.e., the antigen-presenting cells), of which the most efficient appear to be DC (87). They express high levels of HLA class I and II antigens in addition to various immunomodulatory molecules that are essential for cancer immunotherapy. For immunotherapy, DC are pulsed with TAA-derived peptides, tumor cell lysates, or naked DNA. DC can be fused to tumor cells to induce antitumor immune responses (88). The efficacy of DC-based vaccination against tumor growth can be substantially improved by combining the injection of TAA-loaded DC with the administration of cytokines such as interleukin-12 (89).

Immunotherapy employing DC has been successfully used in the treatment of various cancers, including gastric cancer, melanoma, colon cancer, and non-Hodgkin lymphoma. DC pulsed with peptides derived from Her-2/neu and MAGE-3 to immunize cancer patients yielded encouraging results in clinical trials (90,91).

■ EMPLOYING SEREX PRINCIPLE FOR TARGETED THERAPIES FOR PROSTATE CANCER

Prostate cancer is currently the most commonly diagnosed malignancy, and the second leading cause of cancer-related death in men, in the United States. There is a great deal of interest in the development of molecularly targeted approaches to the treatment of cancer, including prostate cancer. Immunotherapies represent a class of molecularly targeted approaches to cancer therapy that can be broadly classified into passive and active types of treatments. Passive approaches generally involve the infusion of monoclonal antibodies with specificity to a desired target antigen or adoptive immunotherapy with antigen- or tumor-specific lymphocytes. Vaccines represent an active immunotherapeutic approach in which the goal is to elicit, rather than exogenously supply, antigen-specific antibodies or lymphocytes.

Prostate cancer represents an excellent target for antibody-based therapies for several reasons: (a) the prostate is a non-vital organ, thereby allowing targeting of tissue-specific antigens; (b) prostate cancer metastases predominantly involve lymph nodes and bones, locations that receive high levels of circulating antibodies; (c) prostate cancer metastases are typically small in volume, allowing good antibody access and penetration; and (d) the PSA serum marker provides a means for the early detection of metastases and the monitoring of therapeutic efficacy.

SEREX approach has been employed to identify prostate cancer antigens by screening sera of patients with prostate cDNA expression library. Identified antigens were then evaluated in a larger panel of 62 subjects with prostatitis and 71 male controls, to prioritize antigens recognized selectively in the prostatitis population (92). Of note, a dominant antigen that we identified, MAD-Pro-34, was identical to the nucleolar protein identified by Fossa et al. (93), which suggested that this may in fact be a naturally recognized antigen of the prostate that could be further characterized as a vaccine antigen. The therapeutic potential of this antigen is being investigated.

■ TARGETS FOR THE TREATMENT OF PROSTATE CANCER

Prostate-specific membrane antigen (PSMA), also known as glutamate carboxy-peptidase II, has been proven to be an excellent target of prostate cancer, because it is (a) primarily expressed in the prostate, (b) abundantly expressed as protein at all stages of the disease, (c) upregulated in androgen-resistant or metastatic disease, (d) present at the cell surface but not released into the circulation, (e) associated with enzymatic activity, and (f) internalized after antibody binding by receptor-mediated endocytosis (94). Previously identified cell surface antigens such as PSMA and prostate stem cell antigen have been in various stages of clinical development for antibody-based treatments. Immunotherapy approaches using anti-PSMA antibodies conjugated with a toxin (95) or

radionuclides, such as ^{90}Y, ^{177}Lu (96,97), have been initiated (also see Chapter 31). PSMA-derived peptides have been used to activate DC to induce prostate cancer cell lysis (98). Using this technique, a phase II study was performed on 33 hormone-refractory metastatic prostate cancer patients. There were six partial and two complete responders (98). In another trial, by the same group, involving 37 prostate cancer patients with a local disease recurrence following primary treatment, 1 complete response and 10 partial responses were identified (99). Responses were associated with an increase in PSMA-specific cellular reactivity and overall cellular reactivity (100). Preclinical and clinical trials have been encouraging. Radiolabeled monoclonal antibody to the extracellular domain of PSMA demonstrated efficient targeting to both bone and soft-tissue lesions and led to objective antitumor responses in a subset of patients as measured by reductions in PSA levels and tumor burden. Early-stage vaccine trials showed that anti-PSMA immune responses can be generated without toxicity in prostate cancer patients. In addition to antibody and vaccine approaches, other PSMA-targeted modalities such as PSMA-directed T-bodies and diabodies were addressed and PSMA enzymatic activity was targeted for the development of prodrugs. Thus far, targeting PSMA has demonstrated only limited success. For the development of therapeutics against prostate cancer, the identification of novel prostate cancer antigens by using SEREX may be necessary. These novel prostate cancer antigens may eventually serve as targets for radioimmunotherapy and/or immunotherapy.

■ REFERENCES

1. Sahin U, Türeci ö, Schmitt H, et al. Human neoplasms elicit multiple specific immune responses in the autologous host. *Proc Natl Acad Sci U S A.* 1995;92:11810–11813.
2. Scanlan MJ, Gordan JD, Williamson B, et al. Antigens recognized by autologous antibody in patients with renal-cell carcinoma. *Int J Cancer.* 1999;83:456–464.
3. Scanlan MJ, Welt S, Gordon CM, et al. Cancer-related serological recognition of human colon cancer: identification of potential diagnostic and immunotherapeutic targets. *Cancer Res.* 2002;62:4041–4047.
4. Wang Y, Gu Q, Liu B, et al. Perspectives of SEREX-defined antigens in diagnosis and immunotherapy for gastric cancer. *Cancer Biol Ther.* 2004;3:806–811.
5. Scanlan MJ, Gout I, Gordon CM, et al. Humoral immunity to human breast cancer: antigen definition and quantitative analysis of mRNA expression. *Cancer Immun.* 2001;1:4.
6. Hunt DF, Henderson RA, Shabanowitz J, et al. Peptides presented to the immune system by the murine class II major histocompatibility complex molecule I-Ad. *Science.* 1992;255:1261–1263.
7. Chen YT, Gure AO, Tsang S, et al. Identification of multiple cancer/testis antigens by allogeneic antibody screening of a melanoma cell line library. *Proc Natl Acad Sci U S A.* 1998;95:6919–6923.
8. Jeoung DI, Lee E, Lee S, et al. Autoantibody to DNA binding protein B as a novel serologic marker in systemic sclerosis. *Biochem Biophys Res Commun.* 2002;299:549–554.
9. Lim Y, Lee DY, Lee S, et al. Identification of autoantibodies associated with systemic lupus erythematosus. *Biochem Biophys Res Commun.* 2002;295:119–124.
10. Uchida K, Akita Y, Matsuo K, et al. Identification of specific autoantigens in Sjogren's syndrome by SEREX. *Immunology.* 2005;116:53–63.
11. Boon T, Coulie PG, Van den Eynde BJ, et al. Human T cell responses against melanoma. *Annu Rev Immunol.* 2006;24:175–208.

12. Takashima M, Kuramitsu Y, Yokoyama Y, et al. Proteomic analysis of autoantibodies in patients with hepatocellular carcinoma. *Proteomics.* 2006;6:3894–3900.

13. Chen YT, Scanlan M, Sahin U, et al. A testicular antigen aberrantly expressed in human cancers detected by autologous antibody screening. *Proc Natl Acad Sci U S A.* 1997;94:1914–1918.

14. Okada T, Akada M, Fujita T, et al. A novel cancer testis antigen that is frequently expressed in pancreatic, lung, and endometrial cancers. *Clin Cancer Res.* 2006;12:191–197.

15. Güre AO, Altorki NK, Stockert E, et al. Human lung cancer antigens recognized by autologous antibodies: definition of a novel cDNA derived from the tumor suppressor gene locus on chromosome 3p21.3. *Cancer Res.* 1998;58:1034–1041.

16. Lee SY, Obata Y, Yoshida M, et al. Immunomic analysis of human sarcoma. *Proc Natl Acad Sci U S A.* 2003;100:2651–2656.

17. Cho B, Lim Y, Lee DY, et al. Identification and characterization of a novel cancer/testis antigen gene CAGE. *Biochem Biophys Res Commun.* 2002;292:715–726.

18. Obata Y, Takahashi T, Sakamoto J, et al. SEREX analysis of gastric cancer antigens. *Cancer Chemother Pharmacol.* 2000;46:S37–S42.

19. Line A, Slucka Z, Stengrevics A, et al. Characterisation of tumour-associated antigens in colon cancer. *Cancer Immunol Immunother.* 2002;51:574–582.

20. Ishikawa T, Fujita T, Suzuki Y, et al. Tumor-specific immunological recognition of frameshift-mutated peptides in colon cancer with microsatellite instability. *Cancer Res.* 2003;63:5564–5572.

21. Kok K, Naylor SL, Buys CH. Deletions of the short arm of chromosome 3 in solid tumors and the search for suppressor genes. *Adv Cancer Res.* 1997;71:27–92.

22. van den Berg A, Hulsbeek MF, de Jong D, et al. Major role for 3p21 region and lack of involvement of the t(3;8) breakpoint region in the development of renal cell carcinoma suggested by loss of heterozygosity analysis. *Genes Chrom Cancer.* 1996;15:64–72.

23. Jager D, Stockert E, Gure AO, et al. Identification of a tissue-specific putative transcription factor in breast tissue by serological screening of a breast cancer library. *Cancer Res.* 2001;61:2055–2061.

24. Schmits R, Cochlovius B, Treitz G, et al. Analysis of the antibody repertoire of astrocytoma patients against antigens expressed by gliomas. *Int J Cancer.* 2002;98:73–77.

25. Watson PH, Chia SK, Wykoff CC, et al. Carbonic anhydrase XII is a marker of good prognosis in invasive breast carcinoma. *Br J Cancer.* 2003;88:1065–1070.

26. Brass N, Heckel D, Sahin U, et al. Translation initiation factor eIF-4gamma is encoded by an amplified gene and induces an immune response in squamous cell lung carcinoma. *Hum Mol Genet.* 1997;6: 33–39.

27. van Nimwegen MJ, Huigsloot M, Camier A, et al. Focal adhesions kinase and protein kinase B cooperate to suppress doxorubicin-induced apoptosis of breast tumor cells. *Mol Pharmacol.* 2006;70:1330–1339.

28. Reich NC, Oren M, Levine AJ. Two distinct mechanisms regulate the levels of a cellular tumor antigen, p53. *Mol Cell Biol.* 1983;3:2143–2150.

29. Traversari C, van der Bruggen P, Van den Eynde B, et al. Transfection and expression of a gene coding for a human melanoma antigen recognized by autologous cytolytic T lymphocytes. *Immunogenetics.* 1992;35:145–152.

30. Costa FF, Le Blanc K, Brodin B. Concise review: cancer/testis antigens, stem cells, and cancer. *Stem Cells.* 2007;25:707–711.

31. Tureci O, Sahin U, Zwick C, et al. Identification of a meiosis-specific protein as a member of the class of cancer/testis antigens. *Proc Natl Acad Sci U S A.* 1998;95:5211–5216.

32. Boel P, Wildmann C, Sensi ML, et al. BAGE: a new gene encoding an antigen recognized on human melanoma by cytolytic T lymphocytes. *Immunity.* 1995;2:167–175.

33. Van den Eynde B, Peeters O, De Backer O. A new family of genes coding for an antigen recognized by autologous cytolytic T lymphocytes on a human melanoma. *Exp Med.* 1995;182:689–698.

34. Vatolin S, Abdullaev Z, Pack SD, et al. Conditional expression of the CTCF-paralogous transcriptional factor BORIS in normal cells results in demethylation and derepression of MAGE-A1 and reactivation of other cancer-testis genes. *Cancer Res.* 2005;65:7751–7762.

35. Sigalotti L, Fratta E, Coral S, et al. Intratumor heterogeneity of cancer/testis antigens expression in human cutaneous melanoma is methylation-regulated and functionally reverted by 5-aza-2'-deoxycytidine. *Cancer Res.* 2004;64:9167–9171.

36. Posner JB. Paraneoplastic syndromes: a brief review. *Ann N Y Acad Sci.* 1997;835:83–90.

37. Muul LM, Spiess PJ, Director EP, et al. Identification of specific cytolytic immune responses against autologous tumor in humans bearing malignant melanoma. *J Immunol.* 1987;138:989–995.

38. Itoh K, Platsoucas CD, Balch CM. Autologous tumor-specific cytotoxic T lymphocytes in the infiltrate of human metastatic melanomas. Activation by interleukin 2 and autologous tumor cells, and involvement of the T cell receptor. *J Exp Med.* 198;168:1419–1441.

39. Boon T, Coulie OG, Van den Eynde B. Tumor antigens recognized by T cells. *Immunol Today.* 1997;18:267–268.

40. Rosenberg SA. A new era for cancer immunotherapy based on the genes that encode cancer antigens. *Immunity.* 1999;10:281–287.

41. Hunt DF, Henderson RA, Shabanowitz J, et al. Characterization of peptides bound to the class I MHC molecule HLA-A2.1 by mass spectrometry. *Science.* 1992;255:1261–1263.

42. Calhoun RF, Naziruddin B, Enriquez-Rincon F, et al. Evidence for cytotoxic T lymphocyte response against human lung cancer: reconstitution of antigenic epitope with peptide eluted from lung adenocarcinoma MHC class I. *Surgery.* 2000;128:76–85.

43. Falk K, Rotzschke O, Stevanovic S, et al. Allele-specific motifs revealed by sequencing of self-peptides eluted from MHC molecules. *Nature.* 1991;351:290–296.

44. Bjorkman PJ. MHC restriction in three dimensions: a view of T cell receptor/ligand interactions. *Cell.* 1997;89:167–170.

45. Somasundaram R, Swoboda R, Caputo L, et al. Human leukocyte antigen-A2-restricted CTL responses to mutated BRAF peptides in melanoma patients. *Cancer Res.* 2006;66(6):3287–3293.

46. Robbins PF, El-Gamil M, Li YF, et al. A mutated beta-catenin gene encodes a melanoma-specific antigen recognized by tumor infiltrating lymphocytes. *J Exp Med.* 1996;183:1185–1192.

47. Chiari R, Foury F, De Plaen E, et al. Two antigens recognized by autologous cytolytic T lymphocytes on a melanoma result from a single point mutation in an essential housekeeping gene. *Cancer Res.* 1999; 59:5785–5792.

48. Takenoyama M, Baurain JF, Yasuda M, et al. A point mutation in the NFYC gene generates an antigenic peptide recognized by autologous cytolytic T lymphocytes on a human squamous cell lung carcinoma. *Int J Cancer.* 2006;118(8):1992–1997.

49. Traversari C, van der Bruggen P, Luescher IF, et al. A nonapeptide encoded by human gene MAGE-1 is recognized on HLA-A1 by cytolytic T lymphocytes directed against tumor antigen MZ2-E. *J Exp Med.* 1992;176:1453–1457.

50. Kono K, Rongcun Y, Charo J, et al. Identification of HER2/neu-derived peptide epitopes recognized by gastric cancer-specific cytotoxic T lymphocytes. *Int J Cancer.* 1998;78:202–208.

51. Maczek C, Berger TG, Schuler-Thurner B, et al. Differences in phenotype and function between spontaneously occurring melan-A-, tyrosinase- and influenza matrix peptide-specific CTL in HLA-A*0201 melanoma patients. *Int J Cancer.* 2005;115(3):450–455.

52. Walton SM, Gerlinger M, de la Rosa O, et al. Spontaneous CD8 T cell responses against the melanocyte differentiation antigen RAB38/NY-MEL-1 in melanoma patients. *J Immunol.* 2006;177(11):8212–8218.

53. Liu G, Ying H, Zeng G, et al. HER-2, gp100, and MAGE-1 are expressed in human glioblastoma and recognized by cytotoxic T cells. *Cancer Res.* 2004;64(14):4980–4986.

54. Wang RF, Wang X, Atwood AC, et al. Cloning genes encoding MHC class II-restricted antigens: mutated CDC27 as a tumor antigen. *Science.* 1999;284:1351–1354.

55. Ichiki Y, Takenoyama M, Mizukami M, et al. Simultaneous cellular and humoral immune response against mutated p53 in a patient with lung cancer. *J Immunol.* 2004;172:4844–4850.

56. Griffioen M, Borghi M, Schrier PI, et al. Detection and quantification of CD8(+) T cells specific for HLA-A*0201-binding melanoma and viral peptides by the IFN-gamma-ELISPOT assay. *Int J Cancer.* 2001;93:549–555.

57. Wang RF, Robbins PF, Kawakami Y, et al. Identification of a gene encoding a melanoma tumor antigen recognized by HLA-A31-restricted tumor-infiltrating lymphocytes. *Exp Med.* 1995;181: 799–804.

58. Prins RM, Odesa SK, Liau LM. Immunotherapeutic targeting of shared melanoma-associated antigens in a murine glioma model. *Cancer Res.* 2003;63(23):8487–8491.

59. Salazar-Onfray F, Nakazawa T, Chhajlani V, et al. Synthetic peptides derived from the melanocyte-stimulating hormone receptor MC1R can stimulate HLA-A2-restricted cytotoxic T lymphocytes that recognized naturally processed peptides on human melanoma cells. *Cancer Res.* 1997;57(19):4348–4355.

60. Ottaviani S, Zhang Y, Boon T, et al. A MAGE-1 antigenic peptide recognized by human cytolytic T lymphocytes on HLA-A2 tumor cells. *Cancer Immunol Immunother*. 2005;54(12):1214–1220.

61. Tahara K, Takesako K, Sette A, et al. Identification of a MAGE-2-encoded human leukocyte antigen-A24-binding synthetic peptide that induces specific antitumor cytotoxic T lymphocytes. *Clin Cancer Res*. 1999;5:2236–2241.

62. Lonchay C, van der Bruggen P, Connerotte T, et al. Correlation between tumor regression and T cell responses in melanoma patients vaccinated with a MAGE antigen. *Proc Natl Acad Sci U S A*. 2004;101(2):14631–14638.

63. Figueiredo DL, Mamede RC, Proto-Siqueira R, et al. Expression of cancer testis antigens in head and neck squamous cell carcinoma. *Head Neck*. 2006;28:614–619.

64. Zhao Y, Zheng Z, Robbins PF, et al. Primary human lymphocytes transduced with NY-ESO-1 antigen-specific TCR genes recognize and kill diverse human tumor cell lines. *J Immunol*. 2005;174:4415–4423.

65. Palmowski MJ, Lopes L, Ikeda Y, et al. Intravenous injection of a lentiviral vector encoding NY-ESO-1 induces an effective CTL response. *J Immunol*. 2004;172:1582–1587.

66. Benlalam H, Linard B, Guilloux Y, et al. Identification of five new HLA-B* 3501-restricted epitopes derived from common melanoma-associated antigens, spontaneously recognized by tumor-infiltrating lymphocytes. *J Immunol*. 2003;171(11):6283–6289.

67. Steitz J, Buchs S, Tormo D, et al. Evaluation of genetic melanoma vaccines in cdk4-mutant mice provides evidence for immunological tolerance against autochthonous melanomas in the skin. *Int J Cancer*. 2006;118:373–380.

68. Adrain C, Murphy BM, Martin SJ. Molecular ordering of the caspase activation cascade initiated by the cytotoxic T lymphocyte/natural killer (CTL/NK) protease granzyme B. *J Biol Chem*. 2005;280:4663–4673.

69. Gueguen M, Patard JJ, Gaugler B, et al. An antigen recognized by autologous CTLs on a human bladder carcinoma. *J Immunol*. 1998; 160:6188–6194.

70. Brandle D, Brasseur F, Weynants P, et al. A mutated HLA-A2 molecule recognized by autologous cytotoxic T lymphocytes on a human renal cell carcinoma. *J Exp Med*. 1996;183:2501–2508.

71. Butterfield LH, Koh A, Meng W, et al. Generation of human T-cell responses to an HLA-A2.1-restricted peptide epitope derived from alpha-fetoprotein. *Cancer Res*. 1999;59:3134–3142.

72. Vonderheide RH, Hahn WC, Schultze JL, et al. The telomerase catalytic subunit is a widely expressed tumor-associated antigen recognized by cytotoxic T lymphocytes. *Immunity*. 1999;10:673–679.

73. Lepage S, Lapointe R. Melanosomal targeting sequences from gp100 essential for MHC class II-restricted endogenous epitope presentation and mobilization to endosomal compartments. *Cancer Res*. 2006; 66:2423–2432.

74. Zhang Y, Renkvist N, Sun Z, et al. A polyclonal anti-vaccine CD4 T cell response detected with HLA-DP4 multimers in a melanoma patient vaccinated with MAGE-3.DP4-peptide-pulsed dendritic cells. *Eur J Immunol*. 2005;35(4):1066–1075.

75. Sugita S, Takase H, Taguchi C, et al. Ocular infiltrating CD4+ T cells from patients with Vogt-Koyanagi-Harada disease recognized human melanocyte antigens. *Invest Ophthalmol Vis Sci*. 2006;47(6):2547–2554.

76. Jager E, Karbach J, Gnjatic S, et al. Recombinant vaccinia/fowlpox NY-ESO-1 vaccines induce both humoral and cellular NY-ESO-1 specific immune responses in cancer patients. *Proc Natl Acad Sci U S A*. 2006;103(39):14453–14458.

77. Sundberg EJ, Sawicki MW, Southwood S, et al. Minor structural changes in a mutated human melanoma antigen correspond to dramatically enhanced stimulation of a CD4+ tumor-infiltrating lymphocyte line. *J Mol Biol*. 2002;319(2):449–461.

78. Pieper R, Christian RE, Gonzales MI, et al. Biochemical identification of a mutated human melanoma antigen recognized by CD4(+) T cells. *J Exp Med*. 1999;189(5):757–766.

79. Khong HT, Yang JC, Topalian SL, et al. Immunization of HLA-A*0201 and/or HLA-DPbeta1*04 patients with metastatic melanoma using epitopes from the NY-ESO-1 antigen. *J Immunother*. 2004;27(6):472–477.

80. Rosenberg SA, Yang JC, Schwartzentruber DJ, et al. Immunologic and therapeutic evaluation of a synthetic peptide vaccine for the treatment of patients with metastatic melanoma. *Nat Med*. 1998;4(3):321–327.

81. Rivoltini L, Kawakami Y, Sakaguchi K, et al. Induction of tumor-reactive CTL from peripheral blood and tumor-infiltrating lymphocytes of melanoma patients by in vitro stimulation with an immunodominant peptide of the human melanoma antigen MART-1. *J Immunol*. 1995;154:2257–2265.

82. Salgaller ML, Afshar A, Marincola FM, et al. Recognition of multiple epitopes in the human melanoma antigen gp100 by peripheral blood lymphocytes stimulated in vitro with synthetic peptides. *Cancer Res*. 1995;55:4972–4979.

83. Marchand M, van Baren N, Weynants P, et al. Tumor regressions observed in patients with metastatic melanoma treated with an antigenic peptide encoded by gene MAGE-3 and presented by HLA-A1. *Int J Cancer*. 1999;80:219–230.

84. Weber JS, Hua FL, Spears L, et al. A phase I trial of an HLA-A1 restricted MAGE-3 epitope peptide with incomplete Freund's adjuvant in patients with resected high-risk melanoma. *J Immunother*. 1999;22:431–440.

85. Rivoltini L, Squarcina P, Loftus DJ, et al. A superagonist variant of peptide MART1/Melan A27-35 elicits anti-melanoma CD8+ T cells with enhanced functional characteristics: implication for more effective immunotherapy. *Cancer Res*. 1999;59:301–306.

86. Rosenberg SA, Yang JC, Schwartzentruber DJ, et al. Impact of cytokine administration on the generation of antitumor reactivity in patients with metastatic melanoma receiving a peptide vaccine. *J Immunol*. 1999;163(3):1690–1695.

87. Greenberg PD. Adoptive T cell therapy of tumors: mechanisms operative in the recognition and elimination of tumor cells. *Adv Immunol*. 1991;49:281–355.

88. Gong J, Nikrui N, Chen D, et al. Fusions of human ovarian carcinoma cells with autologous or allogeneic dendritic cells induce antitumor immunity. *J Immunol*. 2000;165(3):1705–1711.

89. Grohmann U, Bianchi R, Ayroldi E, et al. A tumor-associated and self antigen peptide presented by dendritic cells may induce T cell anergy in vivo, but IL-12 can prevent or revert the anergic state. *J Immunol*. 1997;158:3593–3602.

90. Fay JW, Palucka AK, Paczesny S, et al. Long-term outcomes in patients with metastatic melanoma vaccinated with melanoma peptide-pulsed CD34(+) progenitor-derived dendritic cells. *Cancer Immunol Immunother*. 2006;55(10):1209–1218.

91. Kono K, Takahashi A, Sugai H,et al. Dendritic cells pulsed with HER-2/neu-derived peptides can induce specified T-cell responses in patients with gastric cancer. *Clin Cancer Res*. 2002;8(11):3394–3400.

92. Dunphy EJ, Eickhoff JC, Muller CH, et al. Identification of antigen-specific IgG in sera from patients with chronic prostatitis. *J Clin Immunol*. 2004;24:492–501.

93. Fossa A, Siebert R, Aasheim HC, et al. Identification of nucleolar protein No55 as a tumour-associated autoantigen in patients with prostate cancer. *Br J Cancer*. 2000;83:743–749.

94. Ghosh A, Heston WD. Tumor target prostate specific membrane antigen (PSMA) and its regulation in prostate cancer. *J Cell Biochem*. 2004;91:528–539.

95. Fracasso G, Bellisola G, Cingarlini S, et al. Anti-tumor effects of toxins targeted to the prostate specific membrane antigen. *Prostate*. 2002;53: 9–23.

96. Bander NH, Trabulsi EJ, Kostakoglu L, et al. Targeting metastatic prostate cancer with radiolabeled monoclonal antibody J591 to the extracellular domain of prostate specific membrane antigen. *J Urol*. 2003;170:1717–1721.

97. Bander NH, Milowsky MI, Nanus DM, et al. Phase I trial of [177] lutetium-labeled J591, a monoclonal antibody to the prostate-specific membrane antigen, in patients with androgen-independent prostate cancer. *J Clin Oncol*. 2005;23:4591–4601.

98. Murphy GP, Tjoa BA, Simmons SJ, et al. Infusion of dendritic cells pulsed with HLA-A2-specific prostate-specific membrane antigen peptides: a phase II prostate cancer vaccine trial involving patients with hormone-refractory metastatic disease. *Prostate*. 1999;38: 73–78.

99. Murphy GP, Tjoa BA, Simmons SJ, et al. Phase II prostate cancer vaccine trial: report of a study involving 37 patients with disease recurrence following primary treatment. *Prostate*. 1999;39:54–59.

100. Salgaller ML, Lodge PA, McLean JG, et al. Report of immune monitoring of prostate cancer patients undergoing T-cell therapy using dendritic cells pulsed with HLA-A2-specific peptides from prostate-specific membrane antigen (PSMA). *Prostate*. 1998;35:144–151.

12

Kinetics of Antibody Penetration into Tumors

Greg M. Thurber

■ INTRODUCTION

Chemotherapy remains the primary method of treating cancer that has metastasized to different parts of the body. These agents typically kill rapidly dividing cells, which include cells in the hair follicles, gastrointestinal tract, and bone marrow. The aim of radioimmunotherapy (RIT) is to deliver ionizing radiation specifically to cancer cells while sparing healthy tissues. The concept is straightforward; a radioisotope is attached to a cancer-specific antibody that is injected systemically in the bloodstream, localizes in the tumor, and decays over time. This enables the targeting of cancer cells that are subclinical or too small for efficient external beam radiation. In practice, however, it has been difficult to achieve substantial clinical results, particularly for solid tumors.

The reasons why RIT remains a challenge are several-fold; however, many of the causes trace back to one fundamental issue—delivery. The transport and uptake of antibodies in tumors is slow and heterogeneous. Of the total amount of antibody injected intravenously, very little reaches the tumor. A large portion remains circulating in the plasma or taken up in normal tissues, irradiating and killing healthy cells over time. It is therefore difficult to obtain a positive therapeutic window since the dose to normal tissues can be high relative to tumor tissue. The amount that does enter the tumor is spread very unevenly in the tissue for several reasons. First, the tumor vasculature remains the primary method of uptake in large tumors. Therefore, necrotic regions that lack functional vessels are completely devoid of antibody. While dead cells in these regions do not need to be targeted, hypoxic cells in the border regions may escape therapy and repopulate the tumor. Second, antibodies bind their targets much faster than they diffuse through tissue. This means that even in well-vascularized regions, only cells adjacent to blood vessels are targeted. Regions just a few cell diameters away often remain untargeted (1,2).

The low level of uptake in tumors affects all types of RIT. Ideally, the uptake and subsequent dose to a tumor would be large enough to kill the most resistant cancer cells, while the dose to normal tissues would be low enough to spare the most sensitive healthy cells. In practice, while leukemias and lymphomas can be fairly radiosensitive, other malignancies are more resistant (3). Given the radiosensitivity of

the bone marrow (and other healthy tissues), it is difficult to achieve a positive therapeutic window.

The effect of the uneven distribution of antibodies on RIT is dependent on the type of radioisotope used. With radioisotopes that have a short range, such as alpha emitters and Auger electron emitters, the distribution can have a major impact on efficacy. Cells lying outside the range of radiation will completely escape therapy. For low-linear energy transfer (low-LET) radioisotopes, such as yttrium-90 that has a range of several millimeters, heterogeneity around vessels will have less of an impact. The long range compensates for the distribution and spreads the dose more evenly over the tissue, targeting cells more distal to vessels and in necrotic regions. Ultimately, the low levels of antibodies in the tumor still limit the total delivered dose. Using radioisotopes with such long ranges also has its drawbacks. When targeting single cancer cells or small clusters, the majority of the localized dose may be absorbed by the surrounding healthy tissues (4). While beyond the scope of this chapter, the biologic effects of low and high LET radiation are also significantly different (5).

This chapter will discuss the uptake and distribution of antibodies in tumor tissue. Although the term "antibody" will be used throughout the chapter, the analysis is identical for smaller antibody fragments of the immunoglobulin G (IgG) molecule (Fab, $F(ab')_2$, scFv), larger antibody conjugates, and other engineered binding proteins; only the actual rates differ. The properties of these molecules, such as rates of diffusion and plasma clearance, and their effect on targeting are discussed.

The process of antibody localization is highly complex with many factors contributing to the distribution (6). Imagine an antibody delivered intravenously into the bloodstream. The agent must flow through the vasculature to the site of the tumor, extravasate across the tumor blood vessel wall, diffuse between the cells in the tissue, and bind the target. Meanwhile, the drug is being cleared from the circulation, and the antibody that does reach the tumor can be internalized and degraded by the cancer cells. Each one of these processes is influenced by many factors and will be discussed in turn. However, to obtain a broad perspective of the process, it is useful to compare the different steps to determine which factor contributes most to poor uptake.

Consider an analogy: the process of writing a manuscript. The writer sits down at a computer and turns on the power. It may take 10 seconds for the computer to activate. Writing the actual document then takes 3 hours of typing and editing, followed by 20 seconds to run the spell checker. Finally, the document is saved in less than a second. The entire process takes 3 hours, 0 minutes, and 31 seconds to complete, but clearly the writing and editing step had the slowest rate and required the longest amount of time. Even with significant variability in each step (a slow computer could take a minute to activate, and a fast writer may complete a draft in an hour), writing predominates as the rate-limiting step. A basic knowledge of these rates can be very useful in understanding the process as a whole.

These same concepts hold for tumor targeting. For macromolecules in tumors, the steps are blood flow to the tumor, extravasation across the blood vessel wall, diffusion in the tissue, and binding to the target. Blood flow occurs on the order of minutes, extravasation takes hours, diffusion occurs in minutes, and binding is completed in several seconds. All these rates can significantly affect the distribution of antibody in the tumor, but they do not all have a major impact on the total amount localized in the tissue. Extravasation across the blood vessel wall is the rate-limiting step in uptake, analogs to the writing step discussed earlier. All of these processes and their impact on tumor targeting will be discussed in turn.

TRANSPORT

Antibodies are transported in tumors by two main methods: convection and diffusion. Convection of material in a fluid, such as antibodies in a tumor, occurs from the movement of that liquid. This flow occurs when there is a difference in pressure; the fluid is forced from an area of high pressure to that of low pressure, such as blood in the cardiovascular system. With a constant velocity, the distance an antibody travels is directly proportional to the time. Therefore, it is a relatively efficient method of transport over long distances. The flux of antibodies (number of antibodies crossing an area per time) is

$$\text{Flux}_{\text{convection}} = \nu_{\text{fluid}}[\text{Ab}], \qquad \text{(Eq. 12.1)}$$

where ν is the fluid velocity and $[\text{Ab}]$ is the antibody concentration.

Diffusion occurs due to random Brownian motion of molecules in a liquid. Thermal energy causes the molecules to move in random directions such that over time, a net movement of molecules occurs from a highly concentrated region to a less concentrated region. Diffusion follows Fick's law:

$$\text{Flux}_{\text{diffusion}} = D \frac{\Delta[\text{Ab}]}{\Delta x}, \qquad \text{(Eq. 12.2)}$$

where D is the diffusion coefficient (units = area/time) and $\Delta[\text{Ab}]/\Delta x$ is the change in antibody concentration over the change in distance (gradient of antibody concentration).

Brownian motion is random, so the distance an antibody diffuses is proportional to the square root of time; in order to diffuse twice the distance, it takes four times as long. Diffusion over large distances therefore becomes exceedingly slow.

STEPS IN TARGETING

Tumor targeting of systemically delivered antibodies occurs in a series of steps (Fig. 12.1). An intravenously injected dose of antibody distributes relatively quickly throughout the systemic circulation (7), and a portion of that flow is directed to the tumor vasculature. For micrometastases that have not yet developed their own blood supply, the blood vessels in the surrounding normal tissue supply the antibody. The antibody must then exit the vasculature, entering the interstitial space. The antibody is transported from the site of extravasation to the target antigen, typically by diffusion. Finally, the antibody binds its target, such as a cell surface receptor. Each one of these steps can impact the localization of antibody.

Blood flow

An antibody drug enters the tumor by flowing through the vasculature. Blood flow in tumors, however, is very heterogeneous (6). In healthy tissue, a steady pressure gradient from the arterial end to venous end of a vessel maintains a consistent flow. This flow is disrupted in tumor tissue by several mechanisms. The poorly formed tumor vessels contain many bifurcations, closed loops, and blunt ends, increasing the geometric resistance to flow. High permeability caused by vascular endothelial growth factor (VEGF) and other signals allows fluid to leak from the vessels,

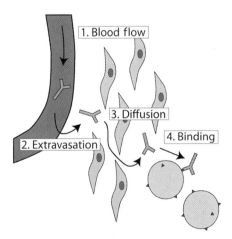

FIGURE 12.1 Systemically delivered antibodies encounter four major transport steps in tumor targeting. First, they must flow into the tumor blood vessels from the general circulation. Next, they extravasate across the tumor blood vessel wall. Once they are in the interstitial space (stroma), they diffuse to the target site (parenchyma; tumor cells). This may involve diffusion through the stroma with no binding sites (as illustrated) or through tissue that may already be saturated with antibodies (no free binding sites). Finally, when the antibody reaches an unbound target, it binds to the antigen.

increasing the hematocrit and therefore the viscosity of the blood. This fluid increases the interstitial pressure in tumors, which can disrupt the normal pressure gradients in the vessel, slowing down flow and diverting it to the periphery. Smooth muscle regulation of flow by arterioles is also disrupted in tumors, and due to solid stress, some vessels may operate in a partially collapsed state, transiently opening and closing. The inflammatory environment of the tumor may cause leukocytes to stick to the vessel walls, partially or fully occluding flow.

Blood flow can have a significant impact on the distribution of oxygen in tumors. Transient hypoxia can result from intermittent disruptions in flow by the mechanisms listed earlier. The impact on antibody targeting is lower, however. The transient opening and closing of vessels occurs on a time scale of minutes (8), and if the antibody is maintained in the systemic circulation during this time, it will enter the vessel once it reopens. The time required to deliver antibody to the tumor vasculature can be calculated by measuring the blood flow. The time for blood flow is (9)

$$\text{Blood flow time} = \frac{1}{Q(1 - \text{Ht})},\quad \text{(Eq. 12.3)}$$

where Q is the flow rate of blood in the tumor (volume of whole blood per volume of tumor per time) and Ht is the hematocrit. The extravasation rate of an IgG is very slow compared to measured flow rates, so typically the permeability has a greater impact on uptake.

Extravasation

Antibody that enters the tumor circulation must exit the vascular compartment to bind cancer cell–associated antigens. Although some small molecules, like oxygen and lipophilic agents, are able to diffuse into and across cells, hydrophilic molecules like proteins cannot easily penetrate the plasma membrane. These molecules transport between endothelial cells, across fenestrate, or through endothelial vesicles. Although the physical distance that the molecules must travel across the endothelial cells is small, less than 1 μm, these cells block much of the area for transport. The overall rate can be measured by experiment, but it is difficult to distinguish between diffusion and convection across the vessel wall. Therefore, the rate is often given as an effective permeability, which may contain diffusion and convection contributions (10).

The time associated with extravasation is determined by the surface area of blood vessels and the rate at which antibody crosses it. This is defined by the permeability, where the flux of antibodies crossing the vessel wall is

$$\text{Flux}_{\text{transcapillary}} = P\Delta[\text{Ab}],\quad \text{(Eq. 12.4)}$$

where P is the permeability of the vessel (11) and ΔAb is the difference in antibody concentration between the plasma and interstitium. The time it takes for antibody to enter a volume of tumor is therefore

$$\text{Extravasation time} = \frac{V}{PS},\quad \text{(Eq. 12.5)}$$

where P is the permeability and S/V is the blood vessel surface area to tumor volume ratio. This S/V ratio is a measure of the extent of vascularization of the tumor; necrotic regions may have a very low S/V ratio and other regions may be hypervascularized (12).

Interstitial transport

Once antibody exits the vessel, it will be carried by fluid flow and diffuse into different regions of the tumor. First, convection will be discussed.

The classic picture of convection in normal tissue is given by the Starling equation. The high pressure in the upstream region of blood vessels causes fluid to leak out of the vessels (convection), and if unchecked, this fluid would cause local edema. However, healthy vessel walls are not very permeable to macromolecules, so the concentration of protein builds up along the length of the vessel. This causes an increase in oncotic pressure, and by the end of the vessel, this pressure is larger than the fluid (hydrostatic) pressure. The high concentration of macromolecules in the blood causes a net flow of water from the surrounding tissue back into the vessels. Most of the fluid that initially left the vessels is resorbed in this manner. The remainder of fluid flows into the lymphatic vessels. These closed end, low-pressure vessels help transport excess fluid from the tissue, maintaining local fluid balance (13).

Two major differences exist concerning the flow of fluid, when comparing normal tissues to tumors. The first is the absence of functional lymphatics. This may exist because of poor lymphangiogenesis in tumors and as the result of solid pressure from rapidly dividing cancer cells preventing the formation of these structures. While the lymphatic system plays a large role in the development of local metastases (14), much of this may occur through vessels at the tumor periphery and the role of fluid flow in tumors is quite limited. This is detrimental to tumor uptake of macromolecules, since a functioning lymphatic system would help drain fluid and therefore increase convection/extravasation in the tumor. The second difference in the tumor is the increased permeability of vessels to both fluid and macromolecules. One of the major causes of this permeability is VEGF, which is also known as vascular permeability factor (15) and is typically overexpressed in tumors.

VEGF is often known for its role in angiogenesis, driving the formation of new blood vessels. However, its role in modulating permeability is equally important. The downstream effects of VEGF signaling include the formation of fenestrations in the blood vessels and disruption of cell–cell adhesion, allowing fluid, small molecules, and macromolecules to cross the "endothelial barrier" more easily. The higher fluid permeability causes more fluid to escape into the surrounding interstitium. No oncotic pressure difference exists to resorb fluid back into the bloodstream, since the vessels are now highly permeable to macromolecules. The lymphatic system that would normally carry away excess fluid does not exist. The result is a buildup of fluid in the interstitium and elevated interstitial pressure (16). Only near the edges of the tumor is fluid able to leak from the vessels and flow out of the tumor. Even in this area, measurements of fluid velocity are slow, approximately 0.1 to 0.2 µm/s (17).

As a result of this elevated interstitial pressure, the pressure in the blood vessels is close to the interstitial pressure in the surrounding tissue. This has several implications. First, since differences in pressure cause convection, the lack of fluid flow means diffusion dominates transport in the tumor. Second, blood flow can be disrupted and erratic, since the pressure that normally drives flow is disorganized. Finally, the vessels are more susceptible to collapse from the elevated interstitial pressure. This is not due to the fluid pressure from the surrounding tissue, since that fluid originated in the vessels. It is most likely due to solid stress from the rapidly dividing cancer cells. Normally, the higher fluid pressure inside the vessel could resist this solid stress; however, that force is minimal with the elevated interstitial pressure, leaving little to resist the crowding of the cancer cells (18).

Convection currents within the tissue are small compared to the rate of diffusion, so interstitial transport is mainly driven by diffusive movement. Similarly, for a prevascular metastasis, there are no blood vessels in the tissue, so diffusion controls uptake. Using Fick's law, diffusion into a spherical metastasis can be calculated, and the majority of uptake occurs by the time:

$$\text{Diffusion time} \approx \frac{R^2}{D\varepsilon}, \qquad \text{(Eq. 12.6)}$$

where R is the distance antibody must diffuse, D is the diffusion coefficient between the cells, and ε is the void fraction, the space the antibody has available to diffuse. This time scale does not take into account antigen binding, so it provides an estimate for diffusion in a region with no binding sites. Since the scaling is true for different geometries, the above time accounts for diffusion into a metastasis or outward from a blood vessel (Fig. 12.2A, B). The differences between targeting vascularized tumors and prevascular metastases will be discussed later.

Binding

Binding results when an antibody collides with its target and the interaction is energetically favorable. This rate depends on the concentration of antibodies in solution, the number of targets, and the intrinsic association rate for the binding interaction.

The dose of antibody required to saturate a tumor is very large, on the order of hundreds of micrograms for mice and hundreds of milligrams for humans. This has been shown both theoretically (19) and experimentally (20,21). For radiolabeled proteins, the tracer doses are many orders of magnitude lower, well below saturation. The number of binding

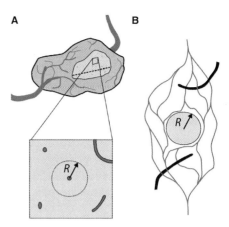

FIGURE 12.2 Antibodies are able to target both vascularized tumors and prevascular metastases. When targeting vascularized tumors **(A)**, the distance an antibody penetrates is measured outside of tumor capillary, up to the half distance with the surrounding vessels. For micrometastases **(B)**, antibodies diffuse inward from the surrounding vessels, and the distance an antibody must penetrate is the radius of the spherical cluster of tumor cells. Blood vessels are shown in grey and lymphatic vessels are shown in black. Vascularized tumors typically lack intact lymphatic vessels.

sites in the tumor therefore far outnumbers the number of antibodies. In this case, the time for an individual antibody to bind to an antigen is

$$\text{Binding time} = \frac{1}{k_{on}[Ag]}, \qquad \text{(Eq. 12.7)}$$

where k_{on} is the association rate, and $[Ag]$ is the antigen concentration. For most high-affinity antibodies and multivalent interactions, internalization occurs faster than dissociation, so binding is essentially irreversible (22). In this case, only association affects binding. The affect of affinity (and dissociation) is discussed in a later section.

■ TARGETING DISCUSSION

The four major steps in targeting all occur with the characteristic times given earlier. While there is extensive variability in all these steps, the magnitude of the time provides insight into the manner in which antibodies penetrate into tumors. For example, if blood flow is much slower than extravasation, antibody will leave the tumor vascular compartment much faster than blood flows into the tumor to replace it (a high extraction fraction). This results in a "flow limited" regime. If blood flow is much faster than extravasation, then antibodies are replaced as fast as they leave the vasculature. Therefore, the plasma concentration is not depleted and most of the antibody that flows into the tumor vascular compartment flows back out of the tumor in the blood (low extraction fraction). This is a "transfer limited" regime (9). Since these rates have been studied in tumors, sample times are shown for each of the steps (Table 12.1).

Blood flow is often measured in the clinic by small molecules that rapidly extravasate from the blood. These molecules have an extraction fraction close to 1, so all the agents

Table **12.1**	**Typical parameters in antibody targeting**		
Symbol	**Parameter**	**Typical Value**	**Note**
$[Ab]_{plasma,0}$	Dose, initial plasma concentration	Varies	10 μg IgG dose in mouse = ~30 nM
R_{cap}	Average tumor capillary radius	8 μm (5–15 μm)	R_{cap} and R_{Krogh} define the blood vessel surface area to tumor volume ratio
R_{Krogh}	Average radius of tissue surrounding tumor capillary	75 μm (20–150 + μm)	Necrosis lowers the surface area available for targeting
K_d	Antibody dissociation constant	10^{-12}–10^{-6} M	IgGs are often 1–10 nM
D	Antibody diffusion coefficient	IgG ~ 14 $μm^2/s$ (5–50 $μm^2/s$)	Dependent on molecule size
P	Tumor capillary permeability	IgG ~ 3×10^{-9} m/s (1–150×10^{-9} m/s)	Rate-limiting step in uptake Dependent on molecule size
$[Ag]$	Tumor antigen concentration	100 nM–1 μM	Depends on Ag/cell and cell packing density
ε	Tumor void fraction	IgG ~ 0.1–0.3 (0.05–0.5)	Dependent on molecule size, cell packing
k_e	Internalization/degradation rate	2×10^{-4}–2×10^{-6} per s	Related to properties of target
A, B, k_α, k_β	Clearance parameters	Minutes to weeks	Dependent on size, charge, FcRn interactions, etc.
V_{plasma}	Plasma volume	~2 mL mouse ~3 L human	Species/weight dependent
Q	Blood flow rate	2×10^{-2}–2×10^{-4} per s	Highly variable

IgG, immunoglobulin G.

entering the tissue from the blood exit into the interstitial space. At early times, the agent does not have time to leave the interstitium, so the uptake rate is approximately equal to the blood flow into the organ. While there is significant variability in the data, blood flow values in mice and humans are typically on the order of 3×10^{-3}/s (23–25). Taking into account the hematocrit (since this is flow of whole blood, and agents are typically measured as the plasma concentration), the characteristic time for blood flow is approximately 10 minutes.

Blood vessel permeability is more difficult to measure in the clinic. Often it is measured as the permeability surface area product and back calculated after measuring the blood vessel surface area. Several labs have measured the permeability in tumor xenografts, often using window chambers (10,11,23). For an IgG, a typical value for the permeability is 3×10^{-7} cm/s. The surface area of vessels is also highly heterogeneous, both between different tumors and even within different regions of the same tumor. These values can range from 10 to 200 cm^2/cm^3 or more (23,26,27). While the distribution of these vessels is chaotic in the tumor, an understanding of the value of this ratio can be obtained by looking at a "typical" Krogh cylinder. The Krogh cylinder was first used to examine the transport of oxygen in tissue and consists of a single blood vessel surrounded by a cylinder of tissue (28). The radius of that cylinder is equal to the half distance between adjacent blood vessels. For a typical vessel:

$$\frac{S}{V} \approx \frac{2\pi R_{cap}L}{\pi R_{Krogh}^2 L} = \frac{2R_{cap}}{R_{Krogh}^2}, \quad \text{(Eq. 12.8)}$$

where R_{cap} is the radius of the capillary, L is the length of the capillary, and R_{Krogh} is the half distance between vessels

or the radius tissue around the capillary (Fig. 12.3). For a typical value of 50 cm^2/cm^3 for the surface area (S) to volume (V) ratio and a capillary radius of 8 μm, R_{Krogh} is 57 μm, or about 100 μm between vessels. This value is in reasonable agreement with experimental data (29). With an S/V ratio of 50 cm^2/cm^3 and permeability of 3×10^{-7} cm/s, the characteristic time for extravasation is roughly 18 hours.

Distances for diffusion vary greatly in tumors due to the chaotic formation of the neovasculature. While the above average distance between vessels helps provide insight into the S/V ratio, in reality there is a broad distribution of distances between vessels. The maximum distance for viable cells is dictated by oxygen transport, and typically 95% of

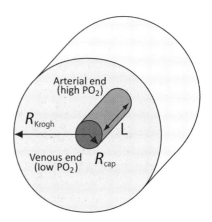

FIGURE 12.3 Diagram of a Krogh cylinder (not drawn to scale). R_{Krogh} is the radius of the tissue cylinder surrounding a typical vessel (approximately half the distance between vessels), and R_{cap} is the radius of the capillary. L is the approximate length of a capillary from arterial to venous end. The PO_2 is the partial pressure of oxygen in mm Hg.

viable cells are within 100 μm of a vessel. Diffusion coefficients depend on the molecular weight, but for a typical IgG, a value of 10 μm²/s is accurate. Using the distance of 57 μm from above and a void fraction of 0.23 for an IgG, the time to diffuse (without binding) this length (Equation 12.6) is about 24 minutes.

The final step in targeting is antibody binding. Regardless of the affinity, the association rates for protein–protein binding are typically around 10^5 per M/s (30). Antigen concentration depends on the cellular density in the tumor and number of binding sites per cell. For a highly expressed cancer antigen with 10^6 binding sites per cell and cellular density of 5×10^8 cells/mL, this would be 830 nM. The characteristic time for binding (Equation 12.7) is 12 seconds. For a moderate expression level of 10^5 antigen sites per cell, the binding time is approximately 2 minutes.

Much of the behavior of antibodies can be discerned from these time scales. The analysis indicated that blood flow takes 10 minutes, extravasation 18 hours, diffusion 24 minutes, and binding 12 seconds. First, blood flow is typically much faster than extravasation. This means the concentration of antibody is not depleted along the length of a typical tumor vessel, and the extraction fraction is very small. This has been shown both theoretically (16) and experimentally (31). Second, diffusion away from the capillary wall occurs much faster than the rate at which antibodies extravasate. This process results in the antibody concentration just outside the blood vessel being much smaller than what is in the plasma, so the tumor cells are exposed to a level well below the plasma concentration. With the high levels of antigen present in tumors, binding occurs within a few seconds, much faster than diffusion through the tissue. The antibody therefore binds the first antigen it encounters and does not penetrate the tissue until the binding sites near the vessel are saturated. Finally, of all the steps, extravasation is by far the slowest. This is the major limitation in the uptake of antibodies.

It is important to note that extravasation is limiting uptake in these tumors even with the increased permeability of tumor vessels. This step is often overlooked because of the well-known "high permeability" of tumor vessels. However, this rate is *high* relative to normal vessels, but *low* compared to the other steps in targeting (i.e., blood flow, interstitial transport, binding).

The above analysis was done without considering antibody dose, but the relative rates are fairly independent of dose. Doubling the antibody concentration in the blood will double the amount flowing into the tumor per milliliter of blood, double the rate of extravasation across the vessel wall, increase in the flux of antibodies diffusing through the tissue twofold, and result in twice the antibody binding its target.

It is important to keep in mind the heterogeneity present in tumors. For example, although the average tumor blood flow time is 10 minutes, the range of times can vary from 2 minutes to 3 hours (24). These parameters are usually not independent of each other, however. For example, a tumor with very few vessels may have poor blood flow and large distances between vessels, but the surface area of these vessels will also be low, increasing extravasation time as well. Variations in permeability (e.g., from VEGF levels), diffusion coefficients (e.g., extracellular matrix density), and binding (e.g., antigen expression levels) also exist. Due to the stochastic and heterogeneous nature of tumors, there are likely some regions where the general trends do not hold true. However, for the majority of regions within a tumor, this analysis is valid.

The analysis of time scales takes a first pass look at the steps limiting antibody targeting of tumors. However, over time, the few antibodies that do extravasate can build up within the tissue. In order to understand the maximum accumulation in the tumor and the distribution in the tissue, it is necessary to look at antibody clearance.

CLEARANCE

Transport carries antibodies into the tumor from the systemic circulation. There are two major clearance mechanisms that oppose the uptake of antibodies. The first is systemic clearance from the plasma and normal tissues in the body. Once the antibody is cleared from the blood in the tumor circulation and surrounding tissue, no more agent can enter the tumor. The second major clearance mechanism results from cellular internalization and degradation. After the antibody has bound its target, high-affinity binders typically do not dissociate before being internalized (22). After internalization, the antibody may be degraded and lost from the cell.

Systemic clearance

Target-independent clearance

After an intravenous injection, antibody-based drugs distribute in the plasma followed by exchange with interstitial fluid in normal tissues. For an IgG molecule, clearance from the circulation is slow, with beta phase clearance half-lives of several days (19). The exchange with normal tissues and elimination are often well described by a biexponential decay, with the faster alpha phase describing redistribution and the beta phase marking elimination from the body.

$$[Ab]_{plasma} = [Ab]_{plasma,\,0}(A \cdot e^{-k_\alpha t} + B \cdot e^{-k_\beta t}), \quad \text{(Eq. 12.9)}$$

where $[Ab]_{plasma}$ is the antibody plasma concentration, $[Ab]_{plasma,0}$ is the initial concentration after a bolus dose, and A and B are the fractions of alpha and beta phase clearance. k_α and k_β are alpha and beta phase rate constants where the half-lives are

$$t_{1/2,\alpha} = \frac{\ln(2)}{k_\alpha} \quad t_{1/2,\beta} = \frac{\ln(2)}{k_\beta} \quad A + B = 1. \quad \text{(Eq. 12.10)}$$

An antibody's long circulation time results from exclusion from renal filtration and salvage recycling by FcRn (32). Whole IgG molecules are not significantly filtered by the kidney, since they are larger than the 60 to 70 kDa size for glomerular filtration (33). Antibody fragments and other binding proteins below this size exhibit half-lives in mice of minutes to a couple hours as they are quickly filtered by the kidney, whereas larger proteins are primarily cleared by the liver. Nonspecifically, pinocytosed antibodies bind FcRn receptors expressed on many cell types, recycling the IgG back to the surface. Their catabolism is relatively diffuse with a major component from the reticuloendothelial system.

Target-dependent clearance

For some antibodies, binding to the antigen can cause significant plasma clearance. This has been termed "target-mediated drug disposition" or TMDD (34). This can occur by binding and internalization of the antibody on normal tissues or tumor cells expressing the antigen. TMDD effects are most pronounced when the target binding is large relative to the dose. Therefore, these effects are most significant with low doses, large volume disease, and target expression on normal tissues. Since RIT agents are often delivered at low doses, this can be significant. TMDD effects have been described for antibodies binding epidermal growth factor receptor, CD4, and CD11a (35).

▧ Local clearance

Internalization on tumor cells can affect the clearance from the plasma, but it exerts a more direct effect on the local distribution and retention in a tumor. Once an antibody reaches the tumor, a variety of processes are involved in clearing it from the tissue (Fig. 12.4). These include intravasation and

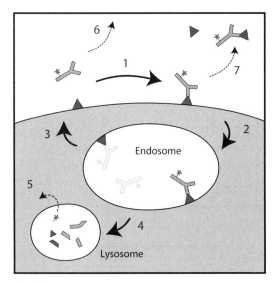

FIGURE 12.4 Local clearance of antibodies occurs by several processes. The most common route for high-affinity antibodies is through internalization *(solid arrows)*. The antibody first binds to the antigen *(1)* and is then internalized into endosomes *(2)*.The antibody can then be recycled along with the antigen *(3)* or directed to lysosomes *(4)*. Upon degradation, the label can be trapped in the cell for extended periods or diffuse back out of the cell and leave the tumor *(5)*. For lower affinity antibodies, a significant fraction remains unbound in the tissue and can be lost from the tumor *(6)*. Some antigens are shed in the interstitial space, and antibodies can bind previously shed antigen or be shed in this bound state *(7)*.

loss from the tumor surface for unbound antibody and (more slowly) for an antibody bound to shed antigen, protease degradation in the interstitial space, and internalization and degradation of the antibody by the tumor cells. For most high-affinity antibodies, internalization/degradation is the most important route.

Antibodies that are bound to their antigen typically traffic with their target on the surface of cells. They can be internalized in minutes to hours by clathrin-coated pit-mediated uptake, or days for more stable antigens (35). Uptake may occur relatively quickly (e.g., an hour) for a signaling receptor, but the antibody can be recycled back to the surface along with the receptor (36). Even cells that lack a transmembrane domain, such as carcinoembryonic antigen (CEA), will be internalized simply by constitutive membrane turnover during a long time period (37). In fact, for persistence on the cell surface, the target must often be held at the membrane surface, as exemplified by the association with tight junctions (38).

Internalized antibodies eventually end up in lysosomes where the protein is degraded. At this point, the protein function is lost; however, especially for RIT, it is the radioactive tag that is relevant for delivering the dose. Depending on the isotope, the tag may remain trapped in the lysosomes for an extended period of time. This is typical for isotopes like indium. However, some isotopes, particularly iodine, can dissociate from the antibody (dehalogenation) and diffuse back out of the cell and leave the tumor (22,39).

▧ LIMITED DISTRIBUTION OF ANTIBODIES

The relative rates of transport to the tumor and clearance determine the maximum amount of tumor localization and the distribution within the tissue. Faster transport and slower clearance will increase the maximum uptake while also increasing the distance antibodies penetrate in the tissue. For example, uptake increases steadily with increasing dose until saturation of the tumor, when all targets are bound by antibody. At this point, the maximum penetration distance is reached, where all cells are targeted. Further increases in transport, such as increasing the dose above saturation, may increase the amount of unbound antibody in the tumor, but this will be cleared quickly due to the lack of available binding sites. While such doses may be possible with unlabeled (cold) antibody, radiolabeled antibodies are far too toxic to deliver at these concentrations. At subsaturating doses, two possible mechanisms for limited uptake exist.

▧ Plasma clearance faster than transport

Clearance from the plasma plays a central role in determining the amount of localized radiation and depth of penetration for many therapeutic and imaging antibodies and their fragments. Proteins less than approximately 60 kDa are rapidly filtered by the kidney, quickly lowering the available antibody in the plasma for localization. For this reason, many fragments accumulate to very low levels, often 1% to

2 % ID/g. Note that since % ID/g (percentage injected dose per gram of tissue) is normalized to the dose, it is not a measure of the amount of antibody in the tissue but rather the efficiency of uptake. While this low efficiency decreases the dose delivered to the tumor, it is often advantageous in some applications.

For imaging, rapid clearance from the blood removes background radiation, allowing earlier imaging times with higher tumor to background ratios (40). It may also spare some healthy tissues such as the bone marrow by removing radioactivity from the blood. Unfortunately, the injected radioactivity must go somewhere, and it often localizes in the kidneys. Radiolabeled proteins that are filtered in the kidney are taken up in the proximal tubule, broken down for recycling of the amino acids, and irradiation of the kidneys occurs. Dosing with cationic amino acids helps block this uptake, but there is still significant accumulation in this organ (41). Although iodine has the ability to diffuse out of the cells after degradation, this same phenomenon can occur in the tumor, countering increases in tumor to kidney ratios.

The penetration depth of antibodies in tumor tissue is a function of the plasma clearance. When binding is much faster than diffusion, as shown earlier, the penetration depth of antibodies in tumor tissue can be solved exactly. The fast binding rate immobilizes the antibody immediately, but once this region is saturated, more antibody diffuses deeper into the tissue. The result is a moving saturation "front" of antibodies entering the tissue. For a tumor spheroid, the time of saturation is (42)

$$t_{\text{sat}} = \frac{R^2([Ag]/\varepsilon)}{6D[Ab]_{\text{surf}}}, \quad \text{(Eq. 12.11)}$$

where R is the radius of the spheroid, $[AG]$ is the antigen concentration/tumor volume (nM), and $[Ab]_{\text{surf}}$ is the concentration of antibody in the surrounding media. At this time, the saturation front reaches the center of the sphere. This is analogs to a micrometastasis but with a constant surface concentration. To take into account the clearance from the plasma, the clearance time is

$$t_{\text{clearance}} = \left(\frac{A}{k_\alpha} + \frac{B}{k_\beta} \right). \quad \text{(Eq. 12.12)}$$

For a single exponential clearance:

$$t_{\text{clearance}} = \frac{t_{1/2, \text{ clearance}}}{\ln(2)}, \quad \text{(Eq. 12.13)}$$

where $t_{1/2,\text{clearance}}$ is the blood half-life and $\ln(2) = 0.693$.

The maximum distance of antibody penetration is based on the ratio between penetration times and clearance times. In this manner, a dimensionless number called the clearance modulus is defined (19):

$$\Gamma \equiv \frac{R^2([Ag]/\varepsilon)}{D[Ab]_{\text{surf}}((A/k_\alpha) + (B/k_\beta))} \approx \frac{t_{\text{sat}}}{t_{\text{clearance}}}. \quad \text{(Eq. 12.14)}$$

This number has no units, but the magnitude describes a fundamental ratio in targeting. If the value of this ratio is

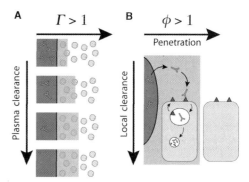

FIGURE 12.5 **Two major mechanisms exist for limited distribution of antibodies in tumor tissue.** Since binding rates are faster than diffusion, antibodies associate with the first available antigen before diffusing deeper into the tissue. As the antibody is cleared from the blood, fewer antibodies extravasate into the interstitium until there are no more free antibodies to penetrate deeper into the tissue **(A)**. For antibodies with long half-lives, such as immunoglobulin G molecules, or multiple doses, this is typically not a problem. However, if the rate at which antibodies enter the tissue is equal to the rate that the cells internalize them, no free antibodies exist to penetrate deeper in the tissue **(B)**.

greater than 1, then the time required to penetrate the distance R is greater than the amount of time antibody is present, and the distance will not be reached (Fig. 12.5A). If the value is less than 1, then antibody will penetrate to the distance R before it is cleared from the system. $[Ab]_{\text{surf}}$ is the concentration surrounding a micrometastasis imbedded in normal tissue, but for solid tumors, as discussed later, it is dependent on the permeability of the blood vessel.

The shape factor of 6 appears in the denominator for the exact solution of a high-affinity antibody in a sphere, but this dimensionless number will be generalized to low-affinity antibodies and penetration around a capillary in a later section, so the shape factor is dropped in the general scaling analysis.

The clearance modulus relates the cumulative exposure of the tumor to antibody versus the penetration distance. This is valid for clearance rates other than biexponential decay from the blood. In this case,

$$\Gamma \equiv \frac{R^2([Ag]/\varepsilon)}{D(\text{AUC}_{\text{surf}})}, \quad \text{(Eq. 12.15)}$$

where AUC is the area under the curve of the surface concentration versus time plot. This allows scaling in cases of TMDD, constant antibody infusions, or multiple doses. It should also be noted that this value depends on the observation time. An IgG often localizes in a tumor over days, so the cumulative exposure will not be sufficient to reach the maximum distance after only a few hours.

Antibody fragments, such as F(ab')$_2$, Fab, and scFvs, are cleared quickly enough from the plasma that significant penetration often does not occur. In this case, the moving antibody front is "frozen" in time after all the available free antibody binds its target. IgG molecules have very long circulation times in the blood, however, so k_α and k_β are generally small enough that $\Gamma < 1$. In this case, it is not the clearance from the plasma that limits uptake but rather local clearance in the tumor.

Local clearance faster than transport

Antibodies have long half-lives in the plasma, and they are often delivered in multiple doses, maintaining an elevated plasma concentration for extended periods of time. In this case, the exposure should eventually target all cells in the absence of local clearance. However, if a portion of the cells internalize and degrade the antibody at the same rate it enters the tumor, other cells will never be exposed to antibody and therefore remain untargeted.

Similar to the clearance modulus, a dimensionless number defines the distance antibody can penetrate before being cleared locally by the tissue. This is based on the endocytosis rate of the target:

$$t_{\text{endocytosis}} = \frac{1}{k_e} = \frac{t_{1/2,\text{endocytosis}}}{\ln(2)}, \quad \text{(Eq. 12.16)}$$

where k_e is the internalization rate constant and $t_{1/2,\text{endocytosis}}$ is the half-life of antibody on the cell surface.

The ratio of antibody penetration to cellular internalization is defined as a Thiele modulus (19):

$$\varphi^2 \equiv \frac{k_e R^2([\text{Ag}]/\varepsilon)}{D[\text{Ab}]_{\text{surf}}} \approx \frac{t_{\text{sat}}}{t_{\text{endocytosis}}}. \quad \text{(Eq. 12.17)}$$

Similar to the clearance modulus, the values must be defined in units that cancel, and if the magnitude of the group is greater than one, antibody will be internalized faster than it can penetrate to the distance R (Fig. 12.5B). If the value is less than one, then targeting will reach this distance. Historically, the Thiele modulus on the left hand side is squared, since this is the form originally used to describe diffusion and reaction of chemicals in catalyst pellets (43). The surface concentration for a micrometastasis is equal to the surrounding normal tissue concentration, but for the penetration outside of a blood vessel in vascularized tumors, it is dependent on the permeability.

MICROMETASTASES VERSUS VASCULARIZED TUMORS

Antibodies are used to treat both micrometastases and bulk tumors (44). So far, the penetration into tumor tissue has been discussed as a function of the surface concentration, $[\text{Ab}]_{\text{surf}}$. In vitro, this concentration is simply the concentration in the bulk fluid or in the media surrounding a tumor spheroid. In vivo, the surface concentration is a function of the steps in transport. For micrometastases (small clumps of tumor cells that are imbedded in normal tissue but have not yet recruited their own neovasculature), the only uptake is from their outer surface, but for vascularized tumors, the primary source is the blood vessels. The surface concentration is very different at these two interfaces.

For a vascularized tumor, $[\text{Ab}]_{\text{surf}}$ is the concentration of antibody just outside the blood vessel (after extravasation). This is related to the plasma concentration by the blood flow and extravasation rate. As shown earlier, blood flow is much faster than extravasation of antibodies, so the concentration in the tumor blood vessels is similar to the bulk plasma.

Extravasation of hydrophilic macromolecules (e.g., antibodies) is extremely slow. This results in a drastic decrease in antibody concentration moving from the tumor blood vessel to the interstitium. Like cars backing up behind a bottleneck in the highway, the concentration of antibody remains high in the plasma. Once the cars are through the bottleneck, they speed away, increasing the distance between them. Since diffusion is much faster than extravasation, the same phenomenon occurs, and the concentration of antibodies outside of the vessel is much lower. The ratio of these two rates, extravasation and diffusion, provides an estimate of the concentration drop across the blood vessel wall. It describes the rate of antibody entering the perivascular region from the blood and leaving by diffusion. This ratio is another dimensionless number known as the Biot number (35). Using Equations 12.5, 12.6, and 12.8:

$$\text{Bi} \equiv \frac{2PR_{\text{cap}}}{D\varepsilon} = \frac{\text{Diffusion time}}{\text{Extravasation time}}. \quad \text{(Eq. 12.18)}$$

The surface concentration is a function of the Biot number and blood concentration:

$$[\text{Ab}]_{\text{surf}} \approx \frac{[\text{Ab}]_{\text{plasma}}}{1 + (1/\text{Bi})}. \quad \text{(Eq. 12.19)}$$

For a very large Biot number, the surface concentration is roughly equal to the concentration in the plasma. For values much less than 1, the surface concentration is roughly

$$[\text{Ab}]_{\text{surf}} \approx \text{Bi}[\text{Ab}]_{\text{plasma}}. \quad \text{(Eq. 12.20)}$$

For an IgG, a typical value for the Biot number is

$$\text{Bi} = \frac{2(3 \times 10^{-7}\text{cm/s})(8 \times 10^{-4}\text{cm})}{(1 \times 10^{-7}\text{cm}^2/\text{s})(0.2)} = 0.02. \quad \text{(Eq. 12.21)}$$

This means the concentration outside the blood vessel is only 2% of what is in the plasma. For a 1 μM plasma level, the tumor cells in the interstitium are only exposed to a 20 nM concentration. The drop of almost two orders of magnitude is a major reason why targeting vascularized tumors is such a difficult task. The concentrations injected are much higher than the concentrations exposed to the tumor cells.

The situation is different for micrometastases. Here, the antibody originates from vessels surrounding the metastasis and enters the normal tissue where there are no targets to bind. Without targets to immobilize the antibody, it can diffuse to the surface of the metastasis from many surrounding vessels. While the supply from an individual vessel may be low (due to the lower permeability of healthy vessels), the number of vessels compensates for this difference. In addition, VEGF and other factors secreted by the tumor cells may increase the permeability of these surrounding vessels. Given the relatively fast rates of diffusion, the antibody concentration is not significantly depleted near the surface of the metastasis. While the exchange of antibody between the capillaries and interstitium of the normal tissue is organ dependent (e.g., blood–brain barrier effects) and antibody dependent (e.g., size and charge), the concentration in the healthy interstitium not typically orders of magnitude lower than the plasma. In this case, the surface concentration is approximately

$$[Ab]_{surf} \approx \frac{\kappa}{\lambda}[Ab]_{plasma,} \qquad (Eq.\ 12.22)$$

where κ is the plasma to normal tissue exchange rate and λ is the lymphatic (normal tissue to blood) exchange rate. Often, this ratio is approximately 1 (45).

The higher concentration of antibody in the surrounding tissue is one reason micrometastases are easier to target than vascularized tumors. In general, smaller tumors are easier to target for several reasons, such as antibody uptake from the tumor surface, better vascularization in smaller tumors (increased S/V), and lack of necrotic regions.

It is worth mentioning that since antibodies are used to treat leukemias and lymphomas, free cancer cells floating in the blood can be targeted directly. They do not have transport issues with tumor blood flow, extravasation, or diffusion. The high concentrations in the blood simply bind to the cell surface. There are other issues in this scenario, such as competition with "cold" antibody and lower probability of having a decay path traverse the nucleus. However, as far as targeting, there are fewer obstacles.

SURFACE UPTAKE VERSUS VASCULAR UPTAKE

So far, localization in a tumor has been discussed in terms of the heterogeneity around blood vessels. However, histological examination reveals heterogeneities on larger length scales as well. Implicit in the discussion on vascular uptake is that areas of high vessel density will have higher uptake than areas with few or no blood vessels. These necrotic areas, often present in the center of the tumor due to vascular collapse, are often surrounded by more vascularized, proliferating tissue (12). The result in imaging is typically a "rim sign" with higher uptake at the outside of the tumor (Fig. 12.6A), and this is a

common mechanism for peripheral uptake in larger tumors (~1 cm or greater).

Smaller tumors and metastases can also have uptake from the surface. This is the same mechanism as a micrometastasis where antibodies diffuse in from the surrounding tissue, but it can occur even after the tumor becomes vascularized (Fig. 12.6B). However, as the tumor grows larger, the relative uptake from the surface becomes less important. For example, an antibody that diffuses and binds 100 μm inward from the surface of a tumor that is 10 cm across targets a negligible fraction of cells. However, penetrating 100 μm into a 2-mm-diameter tumor can target over 25% of the cells. This type of surface uptake in small, vascularized tumors has been observed experimentally (46,47).

A third mechanism for higher uptake near the surface occurs from increased permeability. The rate that antibodies exit the blood vessels is very slow. Near the periphery of the tumor, however, the interstitial pressure can drop as fluid leaks out of the surface of the tumor. With higher vascular pressure than interstitial pressure, fluid extravasates from the vessel, carrying antibody with it (Fig. 12.6C). The result is a higher effective permeability for vessels near the surface (16). This outward convection can also counter the inward diffusion, mentioned previously.

TUMOR CLEARANCE: AFFINITY AND SHED ANTIGEN

Most antibodies, after binding cell surface receptors, are internalized into the cell and end up in the lysosomes. Loss of the intact protein can occur fairly quickly by degradation in the lysosomes or more slowly for fluorescent or radiolabeled tags. However, there are cases where tumor clearance can be dominated by other processes, such as unbound antibody (especially for low-affinity antibodies) or binding to shed antigen. Increased local clearance by these mechanisms can lower the amount of uptake in the tumor.

Affinity plays several roles in determining antibody uptake and distribution. The affinity is often characterized by the dissociation constant, K_d. The K_d for a "true" monovalent interaction (where there is one binding site per target

A   B   C

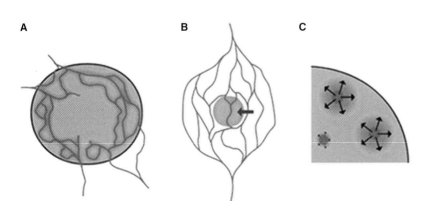

FIGURE 12.6 Several mechanisms exist for higher peripheral uptake in tumors, depending on the tumor size. For larger tumors (greater than 1 cm), central necrosis is common **(A)**. For very small tumors, only several millimeters or less in diameter, diffusion inward from the surface can significantly contribute to the uptake **(B)**. If the interstitial pressure drops near the surface of the tumor, convection may allow more antibody to extravasate, increasing the effective permeability near the surface **(C)**, which was first simulated in a 1-cm-diameter tumor.

and one binding site per antibody, such as a Fab fragment) in a tumor is

$$K_{\mathrm{d}} = \frac{([Ab]/\varepsilon)([Ag]/\varepsilon)}{([B]/\varepsilon)} = \frac{k_{\mathrm{off}}}{k_{\mathrm{on}}}, \quad (\text{Eq. } 12.23)$$

where $[B]$ is the bound antibody–antigen complex concentration at equilibrium, and k_{off} is the dissociation rate constant. The void fraction appears since the concentrations are based on the overall tissue volume, but the interaction is only occurring in the space between cells. The K_{d} for biomolecular interactions varies by many orders of magnitude, but typically IgG antibodies have affinities on the order of 1 nM.

When half of the target is bound by antibody (the unbound antigen concentration equals the bound complex concentration), the K_{d} is equal to the free antibody concentration. In practice, the concentration at half maximum binding is often reported as the K_{d}, even for interactions that are multivalent. This is relatively common, since IgG molecules are bivalent. This "effective" K_{d} is dependent on the intrinsic affinity of the interactions as well as the target concentration on the surface of the cell (48).

For most antibodies, binding occurs much faster than diffusion, leading to rapid binding on the cell surface. With high-affinity antibodies, the rate of internalization is much faster than dissociation, so the antibody is permanently immobilized by the cell. This is also true for most multivalent interactions. Although the individual interactions may be weak, all binding sites must dissociate at the same time for the protein to be completely free in solution for diffusion. With the antibody permanently immobilized, penetration only occurs by additional antibodies diffusing deeper into the tissue (Fig. 12.7A).

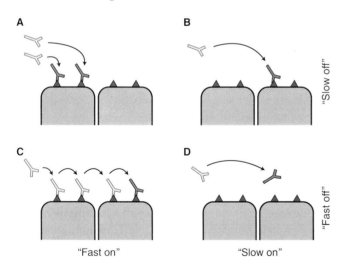

FIGURE 12.7 Antibodies that bind and diffuse through tissue can exhibit four different qualitative behaviors. For high-affinity antibodies, the molecules associate quickly and are internalized before dissociating, so the antibodies saturate cell layer after layer (A). For low target concentrations, slow association rates, or smaller molecules with faster diffusion coefficients, the molecule can diffuse farther in the tissue before binding (B). Low-affinity antibodies that are able to quickly dissociate from their target will diffuse farther in the tissue, although they can be lost from the tumor when unbound (C). For antibodies that bind slowly and dissociate quickly, little remains bound to the target and they act as nonbinding antibodies (D).

The binding rate for antibodies is dependent on the target concentration and the association rate. The antigen concentration is fairly high for most cancer antigens, since many of them are upregulated in the tumor. However, targets with much lower antigen concentration will take longer to bind. This would allow antibody to diffuse farther in the tissue, giving a more even distribution (Fig. 12.7B). The drawback of this scenario is fewer antibodies bind each cell.

While the association rates of antibodies are very similar, the dissociation rate can vary by orders of magnitude, depending on the affinity (30). If the antibody is able to dissociate quickly, it can diffuse deeper into the tissue (Fig. 12.7C). The dissociation rate, which determines the length of time for each "jump" and the association rate, which determines the distance the antibody will diffuse before binding, dictate the distance of penetration. This distance is therefore a function of affinity. The result can be combined with the clearance and Thiele modulus to give parameters that describe both high- and low-affinity antibodies:

$$\Gamma \equiv \frac{R^2([Ag]/\varepsilon)}{D([Ab]_{\mathrm{surf}} + K_{\mathrm{d}})((A/k_\alpha) + (B/k_\beta))}$$
$$\varphi^2 \equiv \frac{k_{\mathrm{e}}R^2([Ag]/\varepsilon)}{D([Ab]_{\mathrm{surf}} + K_{\mathrm{d}})}. \quad (\text{Eq. } 12.24)$$

For a high-affinity antibody, the K_{d} is much smaller than the dose, and the results are the same as above. For low-affinity antibodies, the affinity is weak enough that a significant amount of antibody can dissociate and penetrate deeper in the tissue. For this to occur, the K_{d} must be much higher than $[Ab]_{\mathrm{surf}}$.

The Thiele and clearance modulus describe penetration around individual vessels as a function of affinity, but it also helps to look at the role of affinity in the tumor as a whole. Since binding and diffusion take place within minutes inside a tumor, typically a local equilibrium develops in the tissue. Since the large doses required to saturate a tumor are rarely used, the target concentration is higher than the antibody concentration in the interstitium. In this case, it can be assumed that the antigen concentration is relatively unchanged. Combined with Equation 12.23, the fraction of antibody in a tumor that is bound to antigen is

$$[B] = \frac{([Ag]/\varepsilon)}{K_{\mathrm{d}} + ([Ag]/\varepsilon)}[Ab]_{\mathrm{total}}. \quad (\text{Eq. } 12.25)$$

With antigen concentrations in the hundreds of nM and K_{d} values often single digit nM or below, the vast majority of antibody is bound to its target in the tumor. However, once the affinity starts approaching the concentration of target in the tumor, a significant fraction of antibody will remain unbound in the tissue. The unbound antibody is able to intravasate back into the blood or leaves the surface of the tumor. This is one down-side to lowering affinity: there is reduced retention in the tumor (1,49). The other potential drawback is local cell coverage. Extravasation of the antibody across the blood vessel wall is not a function of affinity, so equal amounts reach the tissue. High-affinity antibodies saturate the cells close to the blood vessel, while lower affinity antibodies spread out more in the tissue. For example, a high-affinity antibody may saturate the entire surface of 10% of the tumor cells, whereas a lower affinity antibody may target every cell but only label 10% of the surface antigen. The impact depends on the desired effect. If the antibody is labeled with an alpha emitter, it is unnecessary to target 10^5 antibodies per cell. If, however, the antibody is blocking signaling or initiating antibody-dependent cellular cytotoxicity (ADCC), the low level of binding may be insufficient for the desired effect (48,50). For radioisotopes with a longer range, such as Y-90, a higher affinity is better. There is little benefit to more homogeneous distribution and the high affinity will ensure maximum retention in the tumor.

The fourth case of a slow-binding, rapidly dissociating antibody is not discussed (Fig. 12.7D). Due to the slow-on and fast-off rates, little target is bound, and the protein behaves as a nonbinding antibody.

Experiments with antibodies that bind the same epitope with varying affinity have helped elucidate the impact on tumor localization (1,49). The effect of shed antigen on antibody localization is more difficult to control in vivo. There are several antigens that are known to be shed from the cell surface, such as CEA, MUC-1, CA 19-9, mesothelin, and high molecular weight melanoma-associated antigen and some of these are monitored in the plasma for tumor recurrence. Antibodies will bind to the antigen in the plasma, lowering the number of free antibodies that can target the tumor. The concentrations are often well below the antibody dose in the plasma, in which case this plasma binding has a minimal effect on targeting. However, these complexes may get taken up in the liver, altering the biodistribution.

Shed antigen often has a larger impact on local clearance. When targeting an antigen that is shed, antibodies entering the tumor interstitium may bind antigen on the cell surface followed by shedding of the complex, or they may bind previously shed antigen that builds up in the interstitial spaces of the tumor. An antibody–antigen complex that is no longer bound to the cell surface is free to diffuse throughout the tumor and intravasate. For example, an IgG at 150 kDa that binds CEA at 180 kDa increases to over 300 kDa in size. The molecular weight of the complex is increased, which lowers diffusion and intravasation rates, but large complexes (and even nanoparticles) are still able to cross the capillary wall. The rate that the complex leaves the tumor may be slower than an unbound antibody, but it can still leave. This antibody loss decreases the amount of localization in the tumor by preventing binding to antigen that is anchored in a cell membrane. Furthermore, it can have a dramatic pharmacodynamic impact if the antibody must be internalized for efficacy, such as with immunotoxins (51). Experiments have shown that in some cases, the majority of antibody is bound to shed antigen, not the cell surface (52).

COLD DOSING

"Cold" antibody that does not contain an actively decaying isotope plays a role in antibody targeting. This can either be due to deliberate dosing of unlabeled antibody (53) or simply the fact that it is not possible to conjugate 100% of an antibody with active radioisotope. For this discussion, it will be assumed that the radiolabeling procedure has not affected the binding affinity of the antibody, which can be verified prior to administration.

An initial dose of cold antibody is often delivered to reduce uptake in healthy tissues. The idea is that the cold antibody will bind easily accessible sites in healthy tissues prior to administration of the radiolabeled dose. Large volumes of healthy tissue may form a significant sink relative to the amount of radiolabeled antibody injected, but the low concentration in these tissues can be easily saturated. Although permeability of healthy vessels is lower than tumor vessels, the vascular density (S/V) is more uniform, blood flow is significantly better, and normal interstitial convection can carry antibody to all healthy cells. The lower concentrations of antigen in healthy tissues are saturated quickly, while poor transport in tumors prevents the entire antigen mass from being targeted. Blocking sites in healthy tissue sometimes increases the blood half-life of the radiolabeled antibody, slowing clearance and increasing uptake in the tumor.

Blocking of the binding sites on healthy cells will not be complete. For instance, although cells in the blood may be near saturation after a cold dose, the radiolabeled antibody may be able to compete off some of the cold antibody. Similarly, any internalization or shedding will reduce the amount of cold antibody on the surface, and recycling or synthesis provides fresh antigen.

Cold antibody may play another important role in targeting. The penetration distance in tissue (given by the clearance modulus and Thiele modulus) is dependent on the antibody dose, not the activity. Antibodies saturate cells layer by layer, regardless of whether they contain a radioisotope. By increasing the antibody dose and delivering the same amount of activity (i.e., lower specific activity), the antibody will penetrate farther into the tissue. For isotopes with a short range in tissue, this may provide an advantage in targeting more cells. Similar to affinity, while this increases penetration, it will lower the concentration of radioisotope on the targeted cells due to the increased cold antibody. If the cold antibody is dosed well above tumor saturation levels, the total amount of radiolabeled antibody in the tumor will be significantly reduced.

PERSPECTIVES

Two areas of research that have gained more attention recently are antiangiogenic treatments and pretargeting. Both have an impact on RIT strategies, so each will be discussed briefly.

While antiangiogenic treatments have been shown to normalize the vasculature and improve blood flow, these techniques are not likely to improve the *pharmacokinetics* of antibodies. The reason is that vascular normalization reduces the permeability of blood vessels to macromolecules (54), slowing down the rate-limiting step of uptake. It also lowers the surface area of blood vessels, decreasing the area for exchange. It is likely to work best for small molecule agents that are blood flow limited by improving this aspect of transport. However, although the pharmacokinetics of antibodies may get worse with these therapies, it is not possible to predict the *pharmacodynamic* effects. For instance, improved oxygenation may help make the radiation dose from RIT more effective or improve ADCC.

A major problem in RIT is that very little of the administered dose reaches the tumor, and there must be a way to remove the unlocalized radiation from the patient. Pretargeting is one way to avoid long-term exposure of healthy tissue from radiolabeled IgGs and renal uptake of systemically delivered fragments. This strategy works by using a slowly localizing antibody that has the potential to bind a radioisotope (a hapten, chelated metal, etc.). Unlocalized antibody is either cleared naturally or artificially using clearing agents (55). A small molecule radiolabeled secondary agent is then delivered that can quickly be taken up in the tumor and bind to the pretargeted antibody. Due to its small size, the small molecule is rapidly cleared from the plasma by kidney filtration. Since it is not attached to a protein, it avoids renal resorption and clears via the urine. While this technique has shown promise (56–58), one of the challenges is developing better procedures for delivery in animals and patients. The increased number of choices (absolute and relative doses of each agent, waiting interval, etc.) makes development more difficult. Models and experiments examining the optimal delivery setup and an increase in the quality of agents will further improve this strategy. Ultimately, a significant improvement in the morbidity and mortality of patients will be required to justify the added complexity of the technique.

CONCLUSIONS

The distribution and uptake of antibodies in tumor tissue depends on the various rates of transport in the body. In general, the slow rate of extravasation from tumor blood vessels limits the amount of antibody taken up in the tumor. Plasma clearance and local clearance in the tumor work against transport to reduce the maximum uptake and penetration distances in the tissue. This makes obtaining a positive therapeutic index challenging. Since binding rates are much faster than diffusion, the antibodies localize outside of functional vessels, leaving distal cells and necrotic regions untargeted. This can be detrimental to RIT with radioisotopes that have a short range, such as alpha emitters and Auger electron emitters.

An understanding of the rates that dictate antibody localization can be used to aid in experimental design, scale from animals to humans, interpret experimental results,

and design better agents. The predictive nature of these mechanistic insights, combined with experimental feedback, will continue to facilitate hypothesis-driven research.

Acknowledgments

Special thanks are extended to Dane Wittrup for helpful comments on the chapter and the Wittrup lab, where much of this analysis was conducted.

REFERENCES

1. Adams G, Schier R, McCall A, et al. High affinity restricts the localization and tumor penetration of single-chain Fv antibody molecules. *Cancer Res.* 2001;61:4750–4755.
2. Dennis MS, Jin HK, Dugger D, et al. Imaging tumors with an albumin-binding Fab, a novel tumor-targeting agent. *Cancer Res.* 2007; 67(1):254–261.
3. Goldenberg DM. Targeted therapy of cancer with radiolabeled antibodies. *J Nucl Med.* 2002;43(5):693–713.
4. vanDieren EB, Plaizier M, vanLingen A, et al. Absorbed dose distribution of the Auger emitters Ga-67 and I-125 and the beta-emitters Cu-67, Y-90, I-131, and Re-186 as a function of tumor size, uptake, and intracellular distribution. *Int J Radiat Oncol Biol Phys.* 1996;36(1):197–204.
5. Hall E, Giaccia A. *Radiobiology for the Radiologist.* 6th ed. Philadelphia, PA: Lippincott Williams & Wilkins; 2006.
6. Jain RK. Transport of molecules, particles, and cells in solid tumors. *Annu Rev Biomed Eng.* 1999;01:241–263.
7. Tofts PS. Modeling tracer kinetics in dynamic Gd-DTPA MR imaging. *J Magn Reson Imaging.* 1997;7(1):91–101.
8. Chaplin DJ, Olive PL, Durand RE. Intermittent blood-flow in a murine tumor—radiobiological effects. *Cancer Res.* 1987;47(2):597–601.
9. Tofts PS, Brix G, Buckley DL, et al. Estimating kinetic parameters from dynamic contrast-enhanced T-1-weighted MRI of a diffusable tracer: standardized quantities and symbols. *J Magn Reson Imaging.* 1999; 10(3):223–232.
10. Dreher MR, Liu WG, Michelich CR, et al. Tumor vascular permeability, accumulation, and penetration of macromolecular drug carriers. *J Natl Cancer Inst.* 2006;98(5):335–344.
11. Yuan F, Leunig M, Berk DA, et al. Microvascular permeability of albumin, vascular surface-area, and vascular volume measured in human adenocarcinoma Ls174t using dorsal chamber in SCID mice. *Microvasc Res.* 1993;45(3):269–289.
12. Ahlstrom H, Christofferson R, Lorelius L. Vascularization of the continuous human colonic cancer cell line LS 174 T deposited subcutaneously in nude rats. *APMIS.* 1988;96:701–710.
13. Swartz MA. The physiology of the lymphatic system. *Adv Drug Deliv Rev.* 2001;50(1–2):3–20.
14. Swartz MA, Skobe M. Lymphatic function, lymphangiogenesis, and cancer metastasis. *Microsc Res Tech.* 2001;55(2):92–99.
15. Weis SM, Cheresh DA. Pathophysiological consequences of VEGF-induced vascular permeability. 2005;437(7058):497–504.
16. Baxter L, Jain RK. Transport of fluid and macromolecules in tumors: 1. Role of interstitial pressure and convection. *Microvasc Res.* 1989; 37:77–104.
17. Butler TP, Grantham FH, Gullino PM. Bulk transfer of fluid in interstitial compartment of mammmary-tumors. *Cancer Res.* 1975;35(11): 3084–3088.
18. Boucher Y, Jain RK. Microvascular pressure is the principal driving force for interstitial hypertension in solid tumors: implications for vascular collapse. *Cancer Res.* 1992;52:5110–5114.
19. Thurber GM, Zajic SC, Wittrup KD. Theoretic criteria for antibody penetration into solid tumors and micrometastases. *J Nucl Med.* 2007;48(6):995–999.
20. Blumenthal RD, Fand I, Sharkey RM, et al. The effect of antibody protein dose on the uniformity of tumor distribution of radioantibodies—an autoradiographic study. *Cancer Immunol Immunother.* 1991;33(6): 351–358.
21. Fenwick J, Philpott G, Connett J. Biodistribution and histological localization of anti-human colon cancer monoclonal antibody (MAb) 1A3: the influence of administered MAb dose on tumor uptake. *Int J Cancer.* 1989;44:1017–1027.

22. Mattes MJ, Griffiths G, Diril H, et al. Processing of antibody-radioisotope conjugates after binding to the surface of tumor cells. *Cancer.* 1994; 73:787–793.

23. Graff BA, Bjornaes I, Rofstad EK. Macromolecule uptake in human melanoma xenografts. relationships to blood supply, vascular density, microvessel permeability and extracellular volume fraction. *Eur J Cancer.* 2000;36(11):1433–1440.

24. Mullani NA, Herbst RS, O'Neil RG, et al. Tumor blood flow measured by PET dynamic imaging of first-pass 18F-FDG uptake: a comparison with 15O-labeled water-measured blood flow. *J Nucl Med.* 2008; 49(4):517–523.

25. Vaupel P, Kallinowski F, Okunieff P. Blood-flow, oxygen and nutrient supply, and metabolic microenvironment of human-tumors—a review. *Cancer Res.* 1989;49(23):6449–6465.

26. Hilmas D, Gillette E. Morphometric analyses of the microvasculature of tumors during growth and after X-irradiation. *Cancer.* 1974;33: 103–110.

27. Solesvik OV, Rofstad EK, Brustad T. Vascular structure of five human malignant melanomas grown in athymic nude mice. *Br J Cancer.* 1982;46(4):557–567.

28. Krogh A. The number and distribution of capillaries in muscles with calculations of the oxygen pressure head necessary for supplying the tissue. *J Physiol.* 1919;52(6):409–415.

29. Baker J, Lindquist K, Huxham L, et al. Direct visualization of heterogeneous extravascular distribution of trastuzumab in human epidermal growth factor receptor type 2 overexpressing xenografts. *Clin Cancer Res.* 2008;14(7):2171–2179.

30. Schier R, McCall A, Adams GP, et al. Isolation of picomolar affinity anti-c-erbB-2 single-chain Fv by molecular evolution of the complementarity determining regions in the center of the antibody binding site. *J Mol Biol.* 1996;263(4):551–567.

31. Heijn M, Roberge S, Jain RK. Cellular membrane permeability of anthracyclines does not correlate with their delivery in a tissue-isolated tumor. *Cancer Res.* 1999;59(17):4458–4463.

32. Ghetie V, Ward ES. Transcytosis and catabolism of antibody. *Immunol Res.* 2002;25(2):97–113.

33. Deen WM, Lazzara MJ, Myers BD. Structural determinants of glomerular permeability. *Am J Physiol Renal Physiol.* 2001;281(4): F579–F596.

34. Mager DE. Target-mediated drug disposition and dynamics. *Biochem Pharmacol.* 2006;72(1):1–10.

35. Thurber GM, Schmidt MM, Wittrup KD. Antibody tumor penetration: transport opposed by systemic and antigen-mediated clearance. *Adv Drug Deliv Rev.* 2008;60(12):1421–1434.

36. Austin CD, De Maziere AM, Pisacane PI, et al. Endocytosis and sorting of ErbB2 and the site of action of cancer therapeutics trastuzumab and geldanamycin. *Mol Biol Cell.* 2004;15(12):5268–5282.

37. Schmidt MM, Thurber GM, Wittrup KD. Kinetics of anti-carcinoembryonic antigen antibody internalization: effects of affinity, bivalency, and stability. *Cancer Immunol Immunother.* 2008;57(12):1879–1890.

38. Ackerman ME, Chalouni C, Schmidt MM, et al. A33 antigen displays persistent surface expression. *Cancer Immunol Immunother.* 2008;57(7): 1017–1027.

39. Ferl GZ, Kenanova V, Wu AM, et al. A two-tiered physiologically based model for dually labeled single-chain Fv-Fc antibody fragments. *Mol Cancer Ther.* 2006;5(6):1550–1558.

40. Wu AM, Senter PD. Arming antibodies: prospects and challenges for immunoconjugates. *Nat Biotechnol.* 2005;23(9):1137–1146.

41. Flynn AA, Pedley RB, Green AJ, et al. The nonuniformity of antibody distribution in the kidney and its influence on dosimetry. *Radiat Res.* 2003;159(2):182–189.

42. Graff CP, Wittrup KD. Theoretical analysis of antibody targeting of tumor spheroids: importance of dosage for penetration, and affinity for retention. *Cancer Res.* 2003;63(6):1288–1296.

43. Thiele EW. Relation between catalytic activity and size of particle. *Ind Eng Chem.* 1939;31(7):916–920.

44. Romond EH, Perez EA, Bryant J, et al. Trastuzumab plus adjuvant chemotherapy for operable HER2-positive breast cancer. *N Engl J Med.* 2005;353(16):1673–1684.

45. Sung C, Vanosdol WW. Pharmacokinetic comparison of direct antibody targeting with pretargeting protocols based on streptavidin-biotin binding. *J Nucl Med.* 1995;36(5):867–876.

46. Fidarova EF, El-Emir E, Boxer GM, et al. Microdistribution of targeted, fluorescently labeled anti carcinoembryonic antigen antibody in metastatic colorectal cancer: implications for radioimmunotherapy. *Clin Cancer Res.* 2008;14(9):2639–2646.

47. Shockley TR, Lin JK, Nagy JA, et al. Spatial-distribution of tumor-specific monoclonal-antibodies in human-melanoma xenografts. *Cancer Res.* 1992;52(2):367–376.

48. Tang Y, Lou J, Alpaugh RK, et al. Regulation of antibody-dependent cellular cytotoxicity by IgG intrinsic and apparent affinity for target antigen. *J Immunol.* 2007;179(5):2815–2823.

49. Thurber GM, Wittrup KD. Quantitative spatiotemporal analysis of antibody fragment diffusion and endocytic consumption in tumor spheroids. *Cancer Res.* 2008;68:3334–3341.

50. Schoeberl B, Eichler-Jonsson C, Gilles ED, et al. Computational modeling of the dynamics of the MAP kinase cascade activated by surface and internalized EGF receptors. *Nat Biotechnol.* 2002;20(4):370–375.

51. Zhang YJ, Xiang LM, Hassan R, et al. Immunotoxin and taxol synergy results from a decrease in shed mesothelin levels in the extracellular space of tumors. *Proc Natl Acad Sci U S A.* 2007;104(43):17099–17104.

52. Lin K, Nagy JA, Xu HH, et al. Compartmental distribution of tumor-specific monoclonal-antibodies in human-melanoma xenografts. *Cancer Res.* 1994;54(8):2269–2277.

53. Hernandez M, Knox S. Radiobiology of radioimmunotherapy: targeting CD20 B-cell antigen in non-Hodgkin's lymphoma. *Int J Radiat Oncol Biol Phys.* 2004;59(5):1274–1287.

54. Tong R, Boucher Y, Kozin S, et al. Vascular normalization by vascular endothelial growth factor receptor 2 blockade induces a pressure gradient across the vasculature and improves drug penetration in tumors. *Cancer Res.* 2004;64:3731–3736.

55. Subbiah K, Hamlin DK, Pagel JM, et al. Comparison of immunoscintigraphy, efficacy, and toxicity of conventional and pretargeted radioimmunotherapy in CD20-expressing human lymphoma xenografts. *J Nucl Med.* 2003;44(3):437–445.

56. Goldenberg DM, Sharkey RM, Paganelli G, et al. Antibody pretargeting advances cancer radioimmunodetection and radioimmunotherapy. *J Clin Oncol.* 2006;24(5):823–834.

57. Pagel J, Orgun N, Hamlin D, et al. A Comparative analysis of conventional and pretargeted radioimmunotherapy of B-cell lymphomas by targeting CD20, CD22, and HLA-DR singly and in combinations. *Blood.* 2009;113:4903–4913.

58. Sharkey R, Karacay H, Johnson C, et al. Pretargeted versus directly targeted radioimmunotherapy combined with anti-CD20 antibody consolidation therapy of non-Hodgkin lymphoma. *J Nucl Med.* 2009;50(3):444–453.

13

Modulation of Biologic Impediments for Radioimmunotherapy of Solid Tumors

Maneesh Jain, Sukhwinder Kaur, and Surinder K. Batra

◼ INTRODUCTION

Antibody-based radiopharmaceuticals have revolutionized cancer diagnosis and some antibodies conjugated to therapeutic radioisotopes have been immensely successful in the treatment of hematologic malignancies. However, despite its immense potential, the clinical success of radioimmunotherapy (RIT) for solid tumors has been modest. The large molecular size of immunoglobulins (IgGs) results in prolonged serum half-life, which causes dose-limiting radiotoxicity to nontarget organs; and poor diffusion rates, which result in poor tumor penetration and uptake. Although antibody engineering has facilitated the generation of a variety of small–molecular weight antibody fragments with improved pharmacokinetics and tumor penetration, the clinical application of the engineered antibody fragments for RIT of solid tumors is compromised by their suboptimal tumor uptake and short tumor residence time. There is an increasing realization that optimization of the molecular size of the antibodies alone is not sufficient for clinical success of RIT. Unlike hematologic malignancies, radiolabeled antibodies encounter several impediments in solid tumors on their way to target antigen expressed before reaching their target antigens on tumor cell surface. These include inefficient perfusion in large tumors, permeability of vascular endothelium, elevated interstitial fluid pressure (IFP) in tumors, decreased macromolecular diffusion in tumor stroma, and heterogeneous antigen expression. With improved understanding and appreciation of the biologic impediments encountered in solid tumors, the new approaches for the optimization of RIT of such tumors involve modulation of these barriers with the use of biologic modifiers. This chapter outlines ongoing efforts for improving the uptake, distribution, and retention of antibody-based radiopharmaceuticals in solid tumors by targeting the aforementioned biologic impediments with biologic and pharmaceutical modulators.

Due to their exquisite specificity for their cognate antigen, antibodies have long been envisaged as excellent vehicles for specific delivery of therapeutic agents like drugs, toxins, enzymes, and radioisotopes to the disease site. RIT is an attractive therapeutic approach involving the utilization of antibodies to target cytotoxic radionuclides to tumors in

an antigen-specific manner. The two Food and Drug Administration–approved radiolabeled antibodies Bexxar and Zevalin have been very successful in the RIT of hematologic malignancies, particularly lymphoma (1–3). Due to its ability to target both known and occult metastatic sites, RIT is an attractive approach for solid tumors. Monoclonal antibodies (MAbs) directed against several tumor antigens like carcinoembryonic antigen (CEA), tumor-associated glycoprotein 72 (TAG-72), and prostate-specific membrane antigen successfully deliver imaging radionuclides to solid tumors and are being effectively used as imaging agents in the clinics (4–7). Therapeutic radionuclide-conjugated antibodies against the aforementioned antigens and several others, like mucin 1, mesothelin, and CD 56 are in clinical trials for treating a variety of solid tumors (3). However, only limited clinical success of RIT for solid tumors has been achieved due to insufficient tumor localization. It is estimated that as low as 0.001% to 0.01% of the administered antibody localizes in the tumors and poor pharmacokinetics of intact antibodies causes myelotoxicity preclude dose escalation (8–10). For improving the clinical efficacy of RIT for solid tumors, significant research efforts are being directed to enhance the uptake and retention of radiolabeled antibodies in the tumor and minimize the exposure of nontarget tissues.

Several factors including undesirable pharmacokinetics, poor tumor uptake, and high immunogenicity of intact antibodies have resulted in the limited success of the RIT of solid tumors. Antibodies exhibit remarkable serum stability and their molecular weight of 150 kDa is well above the "cutoff" for renal excretion. Thus, radiolabeled antibodies have poor pharmacokinetics leading to long circulation times that causes dose-limiting radiotoxicity to the nontarget tissues. Unlike hematologic malignancies where the target antigen is easily accessible, the targeting of solid tumors with macromolecules, such as antibodies, is compromised by their slow diffusion rates and long distances of diffusion in poorly vascularized tumors. In normal tissues, macromolecular transport is driven primarily by convection that results from the pressure gradients between the IFP and the microvascular pressure (MVP) (Fig. 13.1). However, the increased "leakiness" of tumor vasculature, due to structural and functional abnormalities and the absence of functional lymphatic

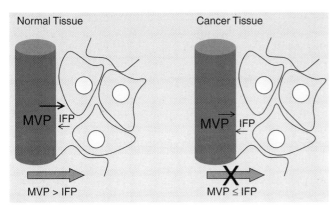

FIGURE 13.1 The driving forces for the macromolecular transport in normal and tumor tissues. Macromolecular transport is driven by the pressure gradient between microvascular pressure (MVP) and tissue interstitial fluid pressure (IFP). In normal tissues, MVP is higher than the IFP and macromolecules are transported from the microvessels to the tissue interstitium along this pressure gradient. In tumor tissues, the structural and functional insufficiencies in the tumor vasculature and absence of a functional lymphatic system result in decreased MVP and elevated IFP. This results in the lowering or complete elimination of the pressure gradient and macromolecular transport is compromised in tumor tissues. Macromolecules may still move into the tumor interstitium along a concentration gradient, a process termed as diffusion. Diffusion, however, tends to be a very slow process, where millimeter movement is measured in days.

system in tumor, results in reduced MVP and elevated IFP (11–13). As a result, the pressure gradients that drive the macromolecular transport are lower or completely eliminated in the tumor tissue, thereby impairing the uptake of radiolabeled antibodies (Fig. 13.1). Further, it is compelling to believe that most RIT regimens should require dose fractionation which involves repeated administration of intact IgGs. This leads to the generation of human antiglobulin antibody responses which result in enhanced elimination of antibodies during repeat administration, thereby limiting the frequency of dose administration (14).

Most of the aforementioned undesirable characteristics of intact IgGs that limit their clinical application for solid tumor RIT result from their large size. The modular structure of IgGs allows for their modification in several ways without compromising their specific antigen binding. Antibody engineering has facilitated the generation of various smaller antibody fragments like mono-, di-, and tetravalent single-chain Fvs (scFvs), diabodies, minibodies with a size range between 30 and 120 kDa (15–19). The small engineered antibodies exhibit rapid clearance rates from the serum and normal tissues as compared to intact IgGs, thereby reducing the radiotoxicity to nontarget tissues. Further, due to their smaller size and enhanced diffusion rates, antibody fragments exhibit rapid accretion and improved distribution in the tumor, thereby increasing the homogeneity of radiation dose deposition within tumors. The impact of antibody engineering on the pharmacokinetics, biodistribution, and immunogenicity has been the subject of several review articles (15,20–22). However, despite the improved pharmacokinetics, engineered antibodies exhibit much lower absolute tumor uptake and shorter tumor residence

time than that of intact IgGs and thus have lower efficacy in RIT. Several alternative approaches like pretargeting and combined modality RIT have considerably improved the efficacy of RIT of solid tumors in clinics. The underlying principles, experimental strategies, and clinical application of these approaches have been adequately reviewed elsewhere (3,23–29). However, even with these advanced strategies, the uptake, retention, and distribution of the antibody-based radiopharmaceuticals remain suboptimal due to inherent biologic impediments in solid tumors.

In solid tumors, there are formidable physiologic barriers which radiolabeled antibodies must overcome prior to reaching their target antigen on the tumor cells. After intravenous administration, the radiolabeled antibody has to extravasate the vascular endothelium and diffuse through the tumor stroma in order to reach the tumor cells. Further, heterogeneities in tumor perfusion and antigen expression result in heterogeneous distribution of radiolabeled antibodies within the tumor. This improved understanding and appreciation of such key physical and physiologic barriers has resulted in the next wave of optimization of RIT employing biologic modifiers to modulate the tumor microenvironment for enhancing the tumor uptake, retention, and therapeutic efficacy of radiolabeled antibodies. Some of the important determinants that have been manipulated for improving the uptake of radiolabeled antibodies include tumor blood flow, vascular permeability, structure and composition of tumor stroma, and tumor IFP. The purpose of this chapter is to discuss various approaches for RIT optimization that involve the use of biologic modifiers targeting these obstructive forces of solid tumors.

Modulation of tumor vascular flow

Tumor vasculature is characterized by structural and functional anomalies as compared to normal vasculature. Tumor blood vessels are poorly interconnected, tortuous, and irregularly shaped with areas of dilation and constriction that result in turbulent and inefficient blood flow in the tumor tissue (11,30,31). Further, the tumor blood vessels are hyperpermeable due to discontinuous endothelial lining, abnormal pericytes, and basement membrane and lack smooth muscle (31,32). The hyperpermeable nature of the tumor vessels and the absence of functional lymphatic system lead to elevated IFP in the tumors. Elevated IFP and inefficient vascular blood flow in the tumor tissue are the primary causes of poor uptake and heterogeneous distribution of macromolecules, including radiolabeled antibodies (12,33,34). The poor blood supply in the tumor also results in hypoxia which in turn contributes to the radioresistance of tumor cells. Thus, targeted modulation of tumor blood flow can not only improve the uptake and distribution of radiolabeled antibodies in the tumors but also enhance the radiosensitivity of tumor cells. Tumor vascular flow can be selectively enhanced by vasoactive agents like angiotensin II, by physical means such as hyperthermia, or by normalization of tumor vessels by antiangiogenic agents.

Angiotensin II

Angiotensin II (ATII) is a vasoactive peptide that has exhibited some promise in improving the uptake of radiolabeled antibodies in solid tumors. Systemic administration of ATII induces widespread hypertension by causing arteriolar constriction. However, due to the absence of smooth muscle in the tumor vasculature, the tumor blood vessels remain unaffected, thereby resulting in increased blood flow and enhanced fluid filtration across tumor vessels.

Continuous infusion of ATII increased the uptake of ^{111}In-DTPA–labeled MAb A7 in colon carcinoma xenografts; although no change in the tumor-to-normal tissue ratios was observed (35). However, tumor–to–normal tissue ratios improved when ATII was infused over a shorter time scale of 0.5 to 3 hours (36). In order to further improve the tumor biodistribution of radiolabeled antibodies, the use of ATII has been explored in combination with enalapril, a kininase inhibitor which may increase the concentration of bradykinin in tumors with the resulting extravasation of antibodies into tumor tissue. The combination resulted in further improvement of tumor uptake and more uniform intratumoral distribution of ^{111}In-DTPA-A7 (37) which consequently translated into enhanced therapeutic efficacy of ^{131}I-A7 as evident by an increase in tumor quadrupling time (38). The effect of periodic and continuous ATII administration on tumor uptake of specific (anti-TAG-72 MAb CC49) and nonspecific IgG was also studied in LS174T colon carcinoma xenografts (39). Both periodic and chronic infusion of ATII resulted in 40% enhancement in the uptake of specific antibody, while the tumor uptake of a nonspecific antibody was unaffected. It was argued that periodic ATII administration enhances fluid filtration across tumor vasculature resulting in the extravasation of antibodies across the vascular wall. While the nonspecific antibodies, due to the lack of specific binding in the extravascular space, can cross the vessel wall in both directions, the transport of high-affinity antibodies is unidirectional as the molecules that extravasate are trapped in the tumor tissue due to specific binding to the cognate antigen (39).

ATII administration was also demonstrated to improve the uptake of radioiodinated Fab fragment of an antibody directed against alkaline phosphatase–related antigen in osteosarcoma xenografts (40). The genetically engineered fusion protein of divalent scFv of MAb CC49 with an intrinsic ATII peptide sequence was recently generated. In the fusion protein, the specific antigen-binding affinity of scFv or the biologic activity of ATII was unperturbed (41). Although the addition of ATII did not improve the absolute tumor uptake of the scFv, the peptide–scFv fusion protein exhibited a more homogenous intratumoral distribution compared to the unmodified scFv.

Vascular Normalization

Due to imbalance of pro- and antiangiogenic factors in tumor tissue, the tumor vasculature is characterized by the presence of tortuous, dilated, hyperpermeable, and poorly organized blood vessels. These structural and functional abnormalities in the tumor vasculature cause elevated IFP and result in inefficient and heterogeneous distribution of radiopharmaceuticals in the tumor. Emerging evidence suggests that antiangiogenic agents, such as antibodies directed against vascular endothelial growth factor (VEGF) or its receptor VEGFR2, result in transient normalization of tumor vasculature (31). The normalized vessels are less tortuous with decreased vessel diameter, have thinner basement membrane and increased pericyte coverage, and exhibit reduced permeability (31,42). During this so-called "normalization window," there is a lowering of tumor IFP and improved delivery and distribution of chemotherapeutic agents (43). The effect of VEGF inhibitor AG-01376 on the distribution of extravasated antibodies was recently studied by confocal microscopy (44). The antiangiogenic treatment resulted in overall decrease in antibody accumulation in the tumor due to the pruning of tumor vasculature. However, there was enhanced transport of antibodies from the surviving "normalized" blood vessels and anti-E-cadherin antibodies were able to label the surface of the tumor cells. Antibodies accumulated in the sleeves of basement membrane left behind by the regressing vessels which possibly serve as the preferred routes of distribution in tumors (44). Vascular normalization also reduces tumor hypoxia, hence is an effective means to reduce the radioresistance of tumor cells. Pretreatment with anti-VEGRF2 antibody DC101 resulted in enhanced efficacy of radiation therapy in the glioblastoma xenograft model (42). Taking into account the improved uptake of antibodies and enhanced radiosensitivity following vascular normalization, future studies are warranted to determine if antiangiogenic agents can improve the efficacy of RIT for solid tumors.

Modulation of vascular permeability

In solid tumors, to reach the target antigen expressed on tumor cells, radiopharmaceuticals have to cross through vascular endothelium. However, due to tight junctional contacts, extravasation of macromolecules across vascular endothelium is highly restricted and tightly regulated. However, some vasoactive agents are capable of altering the permeability of vascular endothelium and overcome its obstructive effects. Several such agents, including cytokines like interleukin-2 and tumor necrosis factor alpha, VEGF, and activated complement 5a, have been used to improve tumor uptake of radiolabeled antibodies in both clinical and experimental studies.

Interleukin-2

Interleukin-2 (IL-2) is a pleiotropic cytokine that mediates both immune and nonimmune functions. IL-2 is involved in the activation and proliferation of lymphocytes and other immune cells, and the recruitment and activation of lymphokine-activated killer cells. Due to these immunomodulatory effects, IL-2 has been used for the treatment of melanoma and renal cell carcinoma. In addition to its immunomodulatory roles, IL-2 induces enhanced vascular permeability. IL-2 results in the release of nitric oxide in the local tissue microenvironment which in turn acts on endothelial cells causing them to round up and develop microfenestrations that allow the fluid to leak into the surrounding tissue (45). Due to its ability to enhance vascular permeability, IL-2 has been used to improve the uptake of radiolabeled antibodies in several studies. Pretreatment with free IL-2 resulted in enhanced tumor uptake of ^{99m}Tc-labeled anti-CEA MAb; however, nontargeted delivery of IL-2 resulted in generalized enhancement of vasopermeability, thus, enhanced antibody uptake was observed also in nontarget tissues (46). Coupling IL-2 to tumor-specific antibodies in subsequent studies allowed for localized enhancement of vascular permeability resulting in nearly fourfold increased uptake in tumor as compared to unconjugated antibody administered alone or following pretreatment with free IL-2 (47). Targeting IL-2 to various tumor compartments resulted in similar enhancement in vascular permeability (45,48–50). Conjugation of IL-2, either chemically or genetically, to antibodies directed toward tumor vasculature (antifibronectin MAb TV-1), tumor cell surface (anti–B-cell lymphoma MAb Lym-1 and anti-TAG-72 MAb B72.1), or necrotic regions (anti-DNA MAb TNT) induced similar levels of vasopermeability in various tumor types including prostate, colon, lung, and lymphomas. In these studies the tumor uptake of tracer antibodies was enhanced by two- to fourfold following pretreatment with IL-2 conjugates in a dose- and time-dependent manner (45,48–50). The vasopermeability induced by IL-2–antibody conjugates was abrogated by NOS inhibitor 1-NMA, thus suggesting the involvement of nitric oxide (45).

In a recent study, a linear stretch of 37 amino acids (residues 22 to 58) in the IL-2 was found to retain the entire vasopermeability activity of IL-2 but was devoid of its cytokine and receptor-binding functions (51). This was subsequently termed as permeability-enhancing peptide (PEP) and the corresponding synthetic peptide exhibited maximal activity in dimeric form. Pretreatment with PEP–antibody conjugates targeting Lym-1 and TNT resulted in fourfold enhancement in the tumor uptake of radioiodinated tracer TNT MAb which is similar to that obtained with intact IL-2–containing conjugates (51). Further, pretreatment with a fusion protein containing a PEP dimer with NHS76, a third-generation TNT MAb directed against nuclear debris in necrotic regions of the tumors, resulted in 4.4-fold increase in the accumulation of ^{125}I-labeled tracer MAb B72.3 in LS174T tumors (52).

Tumor Necrosis Factor α

Tumor necrosis factor α (TNF-α) is another cytokine capable of enhancing the vascular permeability. Although the underlying mechanism remains poorly understood, TNF-α has demonstrated enhanced uptake of drugs and macromolecules, including radiolabeled antibodies, in solid tumors. In search for a better vasoactive agent, Khawali et al. compared the effect of seven vasoactive immunoconjugates (IL-1 β,

IL-2, TNF-α, physalaemin, leukotriene B4, histamine, and bradykinin) on the uptake of the ^{125}I-labeled TNT-1 F(ab)$_2$ fragment in ME-180 human cervical carcinoma xenografts (53). Among these immunoconjugates, TNF-α was the second most (after IL-2) effective vasoactive agent resulting in enhanced uptake of radioiodinated TNT-1 F(ab)$_2$ in tumor xenografts (53). Coadministration of TNF-α with ^{125}I-labeled antibody–carboxypeptidase G2 conjugate improved the tumor uptake of antibody–enzyme conjugate in murine thymoma (54). Likewise, intratumorally administered TNF-α enhanced the vascular permeability by eight- to tenfold and resulted in a threefold increase in the uptake of intravenously administered radioiodinated anti-CEA MAb in colon carcinoma xenografts (55). The effect of TNF-α on the tumor uptake of the specific and nonspecific IgG was compared (56). As early as 1 hour, a 2.6-fold increase in the tumor uptake of specific antibody was observed in response to TNF-α. High antibody levels in the tumor were sustained and the tumor levels of was nearly 30% higher at day 3 as compared to control. In contrast, the tumor uptake of nonspecific antibody increased transiently by TNF-α treatment (56). However, in addition to enhancing the tumor uptake, TNF-α treatment simultaneously enhanced the accumulation of radiolabeled antibody in the nontarget tissues (54–56).

Complement 5a

Complement 5a (C5a) is an anaphylatoxin generated as a cleavage product of complement C5 protein during the activation of serum complement pathway and is capable of enhancing vascular permeability. C5a recruits and activates neutrophils which in turn act on adherens junctions of vascular endothelial cells thus modulating the vascular permeability (57,58). A conformationally constrained peptide agonist of C5a, C5aAP was demonstrated to improve the efficacy of RIT of xenografts derived from LS174T colon carcinoma cell line (59). C5aAP increased the tumor uptake of radioiodinated anti-TAG-72 MAb B72.3 in a dose-dependent manner and was most effective when preadministered in fractionated doses 3 to 6 hours prior to the radioimmunoconjugate (59). However, despite increasing the uptake of radiolabeled antibodies in the tumors, C5aAP failed to improve the tumor–to–normal tissue ratios since the increase in vascular permeability was not restricted to the tumor only. Nonetheless, the benefit of C5aAP was evident in the therapy studies involving ^{131}I-labeled B72.3, where C5aAP treatment resulted in an increase in the tumor quadrupling time.

Vascular Endothelial Growth Factor

Vascular endothelial growth factor (VEGF) is one of the most critical angiogenic factors that affect various characteristics of endothelial cells, like the expression of cell surface adhesion molecules, endothelial cell survival, proliferation, and overall vascular permeability. Due to the overexpression of VEGF receptors in tumors and the involvement of VEGF signaling in tumor neovasculariztion, both VEGF and anti-VEGF antibodies are being investigated for cancer therapy. VEGF is a potential targeting agent and has been used for delivering toxins and thus inhibiting tumor growth in preclinical studies (60–63). VEGF is also an important molecule capable of modulating the vascular permeability to enhance macromolecular uptake. To exploit the ability of VEGF to enhance vascular permeability, fusion proteins containing VEGF and an scFv L19 recognizing ED-B domain of fibronectin (a tumor vasculature specific marker) were generated (64). However, the accumulation of scFv–VEGF fusion protein in the tumor was similar to that of unmodified. Antiangiogenic strategies targeting VEGF signaling pathway have demonstrated to augment the uptake of drugs and antibodies in the tumor (42–44). However, this observed enhancement of drug and antibody uptake in such approaches is believed to be mediated by the normalization of tumor vasculature and was discussed in detail in the previous section.

Stromal barriers and their modulation

Therapeutic agents including antibodies, after extravasating from the tumor vasculature, have to diffuse through tumor stroma in order to reach the target tumor cells. Tumor stoma is composed of nonmalignant supporting tissue such as connective tissue, blood vessels, stromal cells, including fibroblasts, dendritic cells, macrophages, lymphocytes, and endothelial cells; and an extracellular matrix (ECM) that consists of a protein network (mainly collagen) embedded in a hydrophilic gel–containing glycosaminoglycans (GAGs) and proteoglycans. Tumor stroma differs from that of normal tissues due to modified composition of the ECM, increased microvessel density, the presence of fibroblasts with an "activated" phenotype, and an infiltration of inflammatory cells. Macromolecular transport in the interstitium is facilitated by interstitial convection that is driven by pressure gradients between MVP and IFP and hydraulic conductivity (12,34) (Fig. 13.1). As mentioned earlier, inefficiencies in the vascular flow and aberrant vascular permeability are the major factors contributing to high IFP in the tumors and their modulation is an effective way to lower the IFP and increase MVP, and thus increase the transvascular pressure gradient. There is growing evidence that tumor stroma also contributes to high IFP in the tumors and targeting the involved signaling pathways is an attractive means to modulate tumor IFP. Hydraulic conductivity in the tumor tissue is dependent on the interstitial space, composition, and structure of stromal components (65). IFP and hydraulic conductivity in the interstitium inversely correlate with the collagen and GAG content in the ECM (33,65–67). Further, increased collagen content contributes to the mechanical stiffness of the tumor tissue and results in poor penetration of the macromolecules (68). In contrast to collagen, hyaluronan content directly correlates with the diffusion coefficient of macromolecules in the tumor tissues (68–70). Thus, both the cellular components and ECM of the tumor stroma are critical determinants of macromolecular

transport and their modulation can potentially improve the uptake of antibody-based radiopharmaceuticals.

PDGF Inhibitors

Platelet-derived growth factor (PDGF) is one of the key regulators of IFP in normal connective tissues where it acts by triggering signaling pathways via PDGF receptors (PDGFR) expressed on the stromal cells. Inhibition of PDGF signaling in tumors has been shown to decrease the tumor IFP and improve the tumor uptake of chemotherapeutic agents (71). A series of studies has recently demonstrated the utility of the PDGFR-β inhibitor STI571 (also known as Gleevec, imatinib mesylate) in improving the uptake of radiolabeled MAbs and efficacy of RIT (72–74). In colon carcinoma xenografts derived from LS174T cells, STI571 treatment resulted in 50% lowering of tumor IFP and increased the tumor uptake of anti-TAG-72 MAb B72.3 by 2.4 times (72). The increased uptake of radiolabeled antibody in response to the inhibition of PDGF signaling improved the therapeutic efficacy of ^{131}I-B72.3 as indicated by the increase in the tumor doubling time from 19 to nearly 40 days (72). Similarly, in pancreatic cancer xenografts derived from SW1990 cells, inhibition of PDGFR-β signaling resulted in nearly 30% lowering of tumor IFP that was associated with increased tumor uptake of anti-TAG-72 MAb CC49 (74). The tumor doubling times increased from 13 to 26.3 days in the groups treated with the inhibitor (74). However, in prostate cancer xenografts, the inhibition of PDGFR-β signaling did not result in significant lowering of tumor IFP but still appeared to improve the efficacy of RIT possibly due to lower expression of the receptor in the stromal cells (73). There was marginal increase in the tumor uptake of radiolabeled MAb CC49 following treatment with STI571 in a dose-dependent manner (73). However, inhibition of PDGFR-β resulted in significant inhibition of HIF1-α, a transcription factor that is a critical regulator of hypoxia-associated genes (73). The improved efficacy of RIT following PDGFR-β inhibition was attributed to both oxygen-dependent (lower IFP) and oxygen-independent pathways regulated by HIF1-α (73). Although PDGFR-β inhibition appears to positively augment the efficacy of RIT in multiple tumor models, the underlying operative mechanisms appear to differ in various tumor types. These differences could be due to the differences in cell types that express PDGFR-β (stromal cells vs. tumor cells) or due to the differences in the upstream or downstream signaling networks, or differences in the tissue of origin. Thus, a detailed characterization of the underlying mechanisms is warranted prior to the clinical translation of this approach.

Collagenase and Hyaluronidase

Collagen and hyaluronan are important components of the ECM and several studies have suggested that modulating collagen and hyaluronan by enzymatic treatment can improve the access, uptake, and diffusion of antibodies into the tumor. Pretreatment with collagenase resulted in about twofold increase in the diffusion rate of nonbinding IgG in the tumor interstitium (68). In osteosarcoma xenografts, collagenase treatment decreased both IFP and MVP with differing kinetics, thereby causing transient increase in the transcapillary gradient that resulted in the increased uptake, diffusion, and penetration of osteosarcoma-specific MAb TP-3 (75). Similarly, regional administration of hyaluronidase caused transient lowering of IFP in both subcutaneous and orthotopic osteosarcoma xenografts (76) and periodic injection of the enzyme increased the tumor uptake of radioiodinated TP-3 by 70% (77). In contrast, the uptake of nonspecific antibody was decreased by 20% in the tumor and liver with hyaluronidase suggesting that the treatment resulted in increased specificity of the MAb for tumor (77). Choi et al. compared the effect of collagenase and hyaluronidase treatment on the penetration of antibodies in metastatic ovarian carcinoma xenografts implanted in the abdominal wall of rats (78). Treatment of the tumor surface with collagenase resulted in substantial lowering of tumor IFP, while no significant change was observed following hyaluronidase treatment. In contrast to the observations in the osteosarcoma model, collagenase treatment resulted in increased uptake and penetration of both specific and nonspecific radioiodinated antibodies. In collagenase-treated tumors, the concentrations of radioiodinated trastuzumab and nonspecific mouse IgG at the tumor surface were nearly twofold higher, while the mean distance of penetration increased nearly fourfold (78). However, hyaluronidase treatment had no effect on the transport and penetration of the radioiodinated antibodies (78). The differences in the response to both hyaluronidase and collagenase treatment in osteosarcoma and ovarian cancer models could be due to the differences in the experimental modals, origin of tumors, properties of the antibodies used, or manner of enzyme and radioconjugate administration. A recent study compared the effect of collagenase and hyaluronidase on the tumor uptake of macromolecules (fluorescent-labeled MAb TP-3) and small drug (liposome-encapsulated doxorubicin) in the osteosarcoma model by confocal microscopy (79). The degradation of collagen network was found to improve the delivery of IgG, while hyaluronidase treatment had higher impact on the tumor distribution of doxorubicin (79). Thus, all these preclinical studies suggest that modulation of collagen in the tumor stroma is a promising way to improve the uptake of radiolabeled antibodies. However, the use of collagenase in a clinical setting may not be a viable option because it is known to promote metastasis of various tumors. Moreover, systemically administered collagenase would act similarly on collagen in the tumor stroma and that expressed in normal tissues, thereby resulting increased uptake in nontarget tissues. Therefore, alternative agents capable of modulating collagen content in tumor stroma need to be explored. Relaxin is a pleiotropic peptide hormone primarily produced in the ovary and placenta during pregnancy. Relaxin inhibits collagen synthesis and secretion in fibroblasts and upregulates matrix metalloproteases and is thus involved in collagen remodeling (80). Brown et al. demonstrated that administration of relaxin, via osmotic pumps, increased the

collagen turnover in the tumor. The remodeled tumor matrix exhibited a more porous structure and weaker diffusive hindrance, thereby improving the diffusion coefficient of IgG in HSTS26T-derived sarcoma xenografts (81).

Cell penetration for improved uptake and retention

The eventual target of antibody-based radiopharmaceutical is the tumor cell. The radiolabeled antibody has to bind to the antigen expressed on the tumor cell, or in the ECM in close proximity to the tumor cells. Internalization of radiolabeled antibodies can have a positive effect on the efficacy of RIT by increasing the overall accumulation of radiolabeled antibodies and improving the tumor residence time of radioimmunoconjugates. Further, cell penetration will increase the relevance of alpha emitter–based radiopharmaceuticals because in order to obtain maximum tumor cell death, the resulting radionuclide decay should occur in close proximity to the cell nucleus due to the very short path length of alpha particles. Cell-penetrating peptides (CPPs) are a new class of modifiers capable of delivering cargoes of varying size across biologic membranes in a cell- and energy-independent manner (82–84). Most CPPs are derived from naturally occurring protein sequences. TAT peptide derived from HIV TAT protein and penetratin derived from *Drosophila* antennapedia protein are two of the most studied and well-characterized CPPs (82–84). Initial studies showed that TAT conjugation resulted in improved uptake and retention of antibody fragments in the tumor cells in vitro (85,86). However, when analyzed in vivo, TAT conjugation resulted in increased uptake of antibody fragments in liver and spleen and a significant decrease in tumor uptake, thus abolishing the tumor-targeting properties of the antibody fragments (86). Our recent studies indicate that coadministration of CPPs with radiolabeled fragments of anti-TAG-72 MAb CC49 can have potential benefits for RIT of solid tumors (87). Without altering the pharmacokinetics and biodistribution in nontarget tissues, CPPs resulted in improved tumor retention and homogenous distribution of radiolabeled antibody fragments in the tumor (87). However, a generalized increase in antibody uptake is observed in the nontarget tissues when increased amounts of CPPs are used. Thus, the optimal CPP/antibody ratios need to be carefully determined since the advantage of CPPs in biodistribution ceases at higher concentration of CPPs (87). In addition to the optimal antibody: CPP ratios, the choice of CPPs can be critical. Considerable difference in distribution and retention in various tissues was observed when the nonbinding antibody fragments were modified by three different CPPs, namely TAT, Rev, and penetratin (88). Studies have also tried to exploit internalization as a means to target intracellular antigens for RIT where cell penetration will precede antigen recognition (89). However, for an approach using RIT, specific targeting has to be achieved first followed by internalization which can be a means to trap the targeted immunoconjugate in the tumor cells. In a recent article, the various factors that need to be considered prior to the exploitation of CPPs in improving RIT have been discussed (90).

Although internalization of radiopharmaceuticals by CPPs has potential advantages, internalization of radioimmunoconjugates can result in the rapid loss of radioactivity following degradation of the tumor cells. Therefore, conjugation chemistry used to enhance the intracellular stability of the radiopharmaceuticals is greatly needed. Some promising methods and reagents have been developed by Zalutsky and coworkers to address these issues. Anti-HER2/neu MAbs, radioiodinated using N-succinimidyl-5-iodo-3-pyridinecarboxylate or tyramine cellobiose, exhibited 2.3 to 3.0 times higher intracellular radioiodine activity than iodogen-labeled antibodies in vitro (91). Similarly, an internalizing EGFRvIII MAb L8A4 radioiodinated via positively charged D-amino acid peptide (D-KRYRR) showed higher accumulation in glioblastoma xenografts as compared to the directly labeled antibody (92). A new radiolabeled prosthetic group, N^{ε}-(3[^{125}I]iodobenzoyl)-Lys-^{5}-N^{α}-maleimido-Gly^1-GEEEK ([^{125}I]IB-Mal-D-GEEEK) was synthesized and conjugated to internalizing L8A4. The antibody radioiodinated with [^{125}I]IB-Mal-D-GEEEK exhibited nearly 15-fold increase in the internalized radioactivity in tumor cells in vitro than directly labeled antibody (93).

CONCLUSION AND PERSPECTIVES

RIT has progressed significantly since the development of MAbs and has emerged as a clinically viable approach for the treatment of hematologic malignancies. In contrast, despite the availability of numerous tumor-specific antigens, RIT of solid tumors has garnered only limited success due to the various biologic impediments discussed in this chapter. Although advances in molecular biology technologies have resulted in the generation of genetically engineered antibodies with altered pharmacokinetics, effector functions, and immunogenicity, the uptake of these antibodies into solid tumors remains suboptimal. Various optimization strategies have been described that target the biologic impediments inherent to solid tumors. These studies have been performed using various antigen–antibody pairs in different tumor models with varying degree of success. Most of these studies have been limited to animal models and several concerns need to be addressed before these approaches can be tested in clinics. Due to its short half-life, ATII treatment will require continuous intravenous infusion (for the entire duration when the antibody is in circulation), which is difficult to perform in humans. Cytokines are useful agents used to modulate vascular permeability, but they lack target specificity. Similarly, agents targeting tumor stroma, like collagenase and hyaluronidase lack specificity and cannot distinguish their targets in normal and cancer tissues and would lead to harmful side effects if administered in patients. In order to exploit cell penetration as a means to improve the efficacy of RIT, new labeling methodologies and reagents need to be developed and the correct

balance between the cell-penetrating activity and specific antigen binding needs to be determined. Nevertheless, multiple preclinical studies have improved our understanding of the various biologic impediments that macromolecular radiopharmaceuticals encounter in solid tumors. These studies have also demonstrated that the biologic impediments of solid tumors can be modulated to improve the uptake, distribution, and retention of radiopharmaceuticals. Future studies should be directed toward finding clinically acceptable ways of overcoming these barriers and improve the efficacy of RIT for solid tumors in patients.

Acknowledgments

The authors are supported, in parts, by NIH grants R03 CA 139285, UO1 CA111294, RO1 CA 133774, RO1 CA 131944, and RO1 CA78590.

REFERENCES

1. DeNardo GL, Sysko VV, DeNardo SJ. Cure of incurable lymphoma. *Int J Radiat Oncol Biol Phys.* 2006;66(2 suppl):S46–S56.
2. Macklis RM. Iodine-131 tositumomab (Bexxar) in a radiation oncology environment. *Int J Radiat Oncol Biol Phys.* 2006;66(2 suppl):S30–S34.
3. Koppe MJ, Postema EJ, Aarts F, et al. Antibody-guided radiation therapy of cancer. *Cancer Metast Rev.* 2005;24(4):539–567.
4. Ghesani M, Belgraier A, Hasni S. Carcinoembryonic antigen (CEA) scan in the diagnosis of recurrent colorectal carcinoma in a patient with increasing CEA levels and inconclusive computed tomographic findings. *Clin Nucl Med.* 2003;28(7):608–609.
5. Manyak MJ. Capromab Pendetide immunoscintigraphy: connecting the dots for prostate cancer imaging. *Cancer Biother Radiopharm.* 2000;15(2):127–130.
6. Doerr RJ, Abdel-Nabi HH. OncoScint CR103 imaging in the surgical management of patients with colorectal cancer. *Targ Diagn Ther.* 1992;6:89–109.
7. Goldenberg DM. Perspectives on oncologic imaging with radiolabeled antibodies. *Cancer.* 1997;80(12 suppl):2431–2435.
8. Goldenberg DM. Advancing role of radiolabeled antibodies in the therapy of cancer. *Cancer Immunol Immunother.* 2003;52(5):281–296.
9. Mach JP, Carrel S, Forni M, et al. Tumor localization of radiolabeled antibodies against carcinoembryonic antigen in patients with carcinoma: a critical evaluation. *N Engl J Med.* 1980;303(1):5–10.
10. Verhaar-Langereis MJ, Zonnenberg BA, de Klerk JM, et al. Radioimmunodiagnosis and therapy. *Cancer Treat Rev.* 2000;26(1):3–10.
11. Carmeliet P, Jain RK. Angiogenesis in cancer and other diseases. *Nature.* 2000;407(6801):249–257.
12. Jain RK. Transport of molecules in the tumor interstitium: a review. *Cancer Res.* 1987;47(12):3039–3051.
13. Padera TP, Kadambi A, di TE, et al. Lymphatic metastasis in the absence of functional intratumor lymphatics. *Science.* 2002;296(5574):1883–1886.
14. Mirick GR, Bradt BM, DeNardo SJ, et al. A review of human antiglobulin antibody (HAGA, HAMA, HACA, HAHA) responses to monoclonal antibodies. Not four letter words. *Q J Nucl Med Mol Imaging.* 2004;48(4):251–257.
15. Batra SK, Jain M, Wittel UA, et al. Pharmacokinetics and biodistribution of genetically engineered antibodies. *Curr Opin Biotechnol.* 2002;13(6):603–608.
16. Adams GP, Schier R, McCall AM, et al. Prolonged in vivo tumour retention of a human diabody targeting the extracellular domain of human HER2/neu. *Br J Cancer.* 1998;77(9):1405–1412.
17. Hu S, Shively L, Raubitschek A, et al. Minibody: a novel engineered anti-carcinoembryonic antigen antibody fragment (single-chain Fv-CH3) which exhibits rapid, high-level targeting of xenografts. *Cancer Res.* 1996;56(13):3055–3061.
18. Pavlinkova G, Beresford GW, Booth BJ, et al. Pharmacokinetics and biodistribution of engineered single-chain antibody constructs of MAb CC49 in colon carcinoma xenografts. *J Nucl Med.* 1999;40(9):1536–1546.

19. Goel A, Colcher D, Baranowska-Kortylewicz J, et al. Genetically engineered tetravalent single-chain Fv of the pancarcinoma monoclonal antibody CC49: improved biodistribution and potential for therapeutic application. *Cancer Res.* 2000;60(24):6964–6971.
20. Russeva MG, Adams GP. Radioimmunotherapy with engineered antibodies. *Expert Opin Biol Ther.* 2004;4(2):217–231.
21. Huhalov A, Chester KA. Engineered single chain antibody fragments for radioimmunotherapy. *Q J Nucl Med Mol Imaging.* 2004;48(4):279–288.
22. Adams GP, Weiner LM. Monoclonal antibody therapy of cancer. *Nat Biotechnol.* 2005;23(9):1147–1157.
23. DeNardo GL, Schlom J, Buchsbaum DJ, et al. Rationales, evidence, and design considerations for fractionated radioimmunotherapy. *Cancer.* 2002;94(4 suppl):1332–1348.
24. Sharkey RM, Goldenberg DM. Perspectives on cancer therapy with radiolabeled monoclonal antibodies. *J Nucl Med.* 2005;46(suppl 1):115S–127S.
25. DeNardo SJ, DeNardo GL. Targeted radionuclide therapy for solid tumors: an overview. *Int J Radiat Oncol Biol Phys.* 2006;66(2 suppl):S89–S95.
26. Pohlman B, Sweetenham J, Macklis RM. Review of clinical radioimmunotherapy. *Expert Rev Anticancer Ther.* 2006;6(3):445–461.
27. Boerman OC, van Schaijk FG, Oyen WJ, et al. Pretargeted radioimmunotherapy of cancer: progress step by step. *J Nucl Med.* 2003;44(3):400–411.
28. Goldenberg DM, Sharkey RM, Paganelli G, et al. Antibody pretargeting advances cancer radioimmunodetection and radioimmunotherapy. *J Clin Oncol.* 2006;24(5):823–834.
29. Sharkey RM, Goldenberg DM. Advances in radioimmunotherapy in the age of molecular engineering and pretargeting. *Cancer Invest.* 2006;24(1):82–97.
30. Dvorak HF. Rous-Whipple Award Lecture. How tumors make bad blood vessels and stroma. *Am J Pathol.* 2003;162(6):1747–1757.
31. Jain RK. Normalization of tumor vasculature: an emerging concept in antiangiogenic therapy. *Science.* 2005;307(5706):58–62.
32. Morikawa S, Baluk P, Kaidoh T, et al. Abnormalities in pericytes on blood vessels and endothelial sprouts in tumors. *Am J Pathol.* 2002;160(3):985–1000.
33. Jain RK, Baxter LT. Mechanisms of heterogeneous distribution of monoclonal antibodies and other macromolecules in tumors: significance of elevated interstitial pressure. *Cancer Res.* 1988;48(24 pt 1):7022–7032.
34. Jain RK. Barriers to drug delivery in solid tumors. *Sci Am.* 1994;271(1):58–65.
35. Kinuya S, Yokoyama K, Konishi S, et al. Effect of induced hypertension with angiotensin II infusion on biodistribution of 111In-labeled monoclonal antibody. *Nucl Med Biol.* 1996;23(2):137–140.
36. Kinuya S, Yokoyama K, Yamamoto W, et al. Short-period-induced hypertension could improve tumor-to-nontumor ratios of radiolabeled monoclonal antibody. *Nucl Med Biol.* 1997;24(6):547–551.
37. Kinuya S, Yokoyama K, Yamamoto W, et al. Persistent distension and enhanced diffusive extravasation of tumor vessels improved uniform tumor targeting of radioimmunoconjugate in mice administered with angiotensin II and kininase inhibitor. *Oncol Res.* 1998;10(11–12):551–559.
38. Kinuya S, Yokoyama K, Kawashima A, et al. Pharmacologic intervention with angiotensin II and kininase inhibitor enhanced efficacy of radioimmunotherapy in human colon cancer xenografts. *J Nucl Med.* 2000;41(7):1244–1249.
39. Netti PA, Hamberg LM, Babich JW, et al. Enhancement of fluid filtration across tumor vessels: implication for delivery of macromolecules. *Proc Natl Acad Sci USA.* 1999;96(6):3137–3142.
40. Nakamoto Y, Sakahara H, Saga T, et al. A novel immunoscintigraphy technique using metabolizable linker with angiotensin II treatment. *Br J Cancer.* 1999;79(11–12):1794–1799.
41. Wittel UA, Jain M, Goel A, et al. Engineering and characterization of a divalent single-chain Fv angiotensin II fusion construct of the monoclonal antibody CC49. *Biochem Biophys Res Commun.* 2005;329(1):168–176.
42. Winkler F, Kozin SV, Tong RT, et al. Kinetics of vascular normalization by VEGFR2 blockade governs brain tumor response to radiation: role of oxygenation, angiopoietin-1, and matrix metalloproteinases. *Cancer Cell.* 2004;6(6):553–563.
43. Tong RT, Boucher Y, Kozin SV, et al. Vascular normalization by vascular endothelial growth factor receptor 2 blockade induces a pressure gradient across the vasculature and improves drug penetration in tumors. *Cancer Res.* 2004;64(11):3731–3736.
44. Nakahara T, Norberg SM, Shalinsky DR, et al. Effect of inhibition of vascular endothelial growth factor signaling on distribution of extravasated antibodies in tumors. *Cancer Res.* 2006;66(3):1434–1445.
45. Hornick JL, Khawli LA, Hu P, et al. Pretreatment with a monoclonal antibody/interleukin-2 fusion protein directed against DNA enhances the delivery of therapeutic molecules to solid tumors. *Clin Cancer Res.* 1999;5(1):51–60.
46. Nakamura K, Kubo A. Effect of interleukin-2 on the biodistribution of technetium-99m-labelled anti-CEA monoclonal antibody in mice bearing human tumour xenografts. *Eur J Nucl Med.* 1994;21(9):924–929.
47. Nakamura K, Kubo A. Biodistribution of iodine-125 labeled monoclonal antibody/interleukin-2 immunoconjugate in athymic mice bearing human tumor xenografts. *Cancer.* 1997;80(12 suppl):2650–2655.
48. Epstein AL, Khawli LA, Hornick JL, et al. Identification of a monoclonal antibody, TV-1, directed against the basement membrane of tumor vessels, and its use to enhance the delivery of macromolecules to tumors after conjugation with interleukin 2. *Cancer Res.* 1995;55(12):2673–2680.
49. Hu P, Hornick JL, Glasky MS, et al. A chimeric Lym-1/interleukin 2 fusion protein for increasing tumor vascular permeability and enhancing antibody uptake. *Cancer Res.* 1996;56(21):4998–5004.
50. LeBerthon B, Khawli LA, Alauddin M, et al. Enhanced tumor uptake of macromolecules induced by a novel vasoactive interleukin 2 immunoconjugate. *Cancer Res.* 1991;51(10):2694–2698.
51. Epstein AL, Mizokami MM, Li J, et al. Identification of a protein fragment of interleukin 2 responsible for vasopermeability. *J Natl Cancer Inst.* 2003;95(10):741–749.
52. Khawli LA, Hu P, Epstein AL. NHS76/PEP2, a fully human vasopermeability-enhancing agent to increase the uptake and efficacy of cancer chemotherapy. *Clin Cancer Res.* 2005;11(8):3084–3093.
53. Khawli LA, Miller GK, Epstein AL. Effect of seven new vasoactive immunoconjugates on the enhancement of monoclonal antibody uptake in tumors. *Cancer.* 1994;73(3 suppl):824–831.
54. Melton RG, Rowland JA, Pietersz GA, et al. Tumour necrosis factor increases tumour uptake of co-administered antibody-carboxypeptidase G2 conjugate. *Eur J Cancer.* 1993;29A(8):1177–1183.
55. Folli S, Pelegrin A, Chalandon Y, et al. Tumor-necrosis factor can enhance radio-antibody uptake in human colon carcinoma xenografts by increasing vascular permeability. *Int J Cancer.* 1993;53(5):829–836.
56. Rowlinson-Busza G, Maraveyas A, Epenetos AA. Effect of tumour necrosis factor on the uptake of specific and control monoclonal antibodies in a human tumour xenograft model. *Br J Cancer.* 1995;71(4):660–665.
57. Kurizaki T, Abe M, Sanderson SD, et al. Role of polymorphonuclear leukocytes, nitric oxide synthase, and cyclooxygenase in vascular permeability changes induced by C5a agonist peptides. *Mol Cancer Ther.* 2004;3(1):85–91.
58. Tinsley JH, Wu MH, Ma W, et al. Activated neutrophils induce hyperpermeability and phosphorylation of adherens junction proteins in coronary venular endothelial cells. *J Biol Chem.* 1999;274(35):24930–24934.
59. Kurizaki T, Okazaki S, Sanderson SD, et al. Potentiation of radioimmunotherapy with response-selective peptide agonist of human C5a. *J Nucl Med.* 2002;43(7):957–967.
60. Veenendaal LM, Jin H, Ran S, et al. In vitro and in vivo studies of a VEGF121/rGelonin chimeric fusion toxin targeting the neovasculature of solid tumors. *Proc Natl Acad Sci USA.* 2002;99(12):7866–7871.
61. Olson TA, Mohanraj D, Roy S, et al. Targeting the tumor vasculature: inhibition of tumor growth by a vascular endothelial growth factor-toxin conjugate. *Int J Cancer.* 1997;73(6):865–870.
62. Wild R, Ramakrishnan S, Sedgewick J, et al. Quantitative assessment of angiogenesis and tumor vessel architecture by computer-assisted digital image analysis: effects of VEGF-toxin conjugate on tumor microvessel density. *Microvasc Res.* 2000;59(3):368–376.
63. Wild R, Dhanabal M, Olson TA, et al. Inhibition of angiogenesis and tumour growth by VEGF121-toxin conjugate: differential effect on proliferating endothelial cells. *Br J Cancer.* 2000;83(8):1077–1083.
64. Halin C, Niesner U, Villani ME, et al. Tumor-targeting properties of antibody-vascular endothelial growth factor fusion proteins. *Int J Cancer.* 2002;102(2):109–116.
65. Aukland K, Nicolaysen G. Interstitial fluid volume: local regulatory mechanisms. *Physiol Rev.* 1981;61(3):556–643.
66. Weinberg PD, Carney SL, Winlove CP, et al. The contributions of glycosaminoglycans, collagen and other interstitial components to the hydraulic resistivity of porcine aortic wall. *Connect Tissue Res.* 1997;36(4):297–308.

67. Swabb EA, Wei J, Gullino PM. Diffusion and convection in normal and neoplastic tissues. *Cancer Res.* 1974;34(10):2814–2822.

68. Netti PA, Berk DA, Swartz MA, et al. Role of extracellular matrix assembly in interstitial transport in solid tumors. *Cancer Res.* 2000;60(9):2497–2503.

69. Pluen A, Boucher Y, Ramanujan S, et al. Role of tumor-host interactions in interstitial diffusion of macromolecules: cranial vs. subcutaneous tumors. *Proc Natl Acad Sci USA.* 2001;98(8):4628–4633.

70. de Lange Davies C, Berk DA, Pluen A, et al. Comparison of IgG diffusion and extracellular matrix composition in rhabdomyosarcomas grown in mice versus in vitro as spheroids reveals the role of host stromal cells. *Br J Cancer.* 2002;86(10):1639–1644.

71. Pietras K. Increasing tumor uptake of anticancer drugs with imatinib. *Semin Oncol.* 2004;31(2 suppl 6):18–23.

72. Baranowska-Kortylewicz J, Abe M, Pietras K, et al. Effect of platelet-derived growth factor receptor-beta inhibition with STI571 on radioimmunotherapy. *Cancer Res.* 2005;65(17):7824–7831.

73. Kimura Y, Inoue K, Abe M, et al. PDGFRbeta and HIF-1alpha inhibition with imatinib and radioimmunotherapy of experimental prostate cancer. *Cancer Biol Ther.* 2007;6(11):1763–1772.

74. Baranowska-Kortylewicz J, Abe M, Nearman J, et al. Emerging role of platelet-derived growth factor receptor-beta inhibition in radioimmunotherapy of experimental pancreatic cancer. *Clin Cancer Res.* 2007;13(1):299–306.

75. Eikenes L, Bruland OS, Brekken C, et al. Collagenase increases the transcapillary pressure gradient and improves the uptake and distribution of monoclonal antibodies in human osteosarcoma xenografts. *Cancer Res.* 2004;64(14):4768–4773.

76. Brekken C, Bruland OS, de Lange DC. Interstitial fluid pressure in human osteosarcoma xenografts: significance of implantation site and the response to intratumoral injection of hyaluronidase. *Anticancer Res.* 2000;20(5B):3503–3512.

77. Brekken C, Hjelstuen MH, Bruland OS, et al. Hyaluronidase-induced periodic modulation of the interstitial fluid pressure increases selective antibody uptake in human osteosarcoma xenografts. *Anticancer Res.* 2000;20(5B):3513–3519.

78. Choi J, Credit K, Henderson K, et al. Intraperitoneal immunotherapy for metastatic ovarian carcinoma: resistance of intratumoral collagen to antibody penetration. *Clin Cancer Res.* 2006;12(6):1906–1912.

79. Erikson A, Tufto I, Bjonnum AB, et al. The impact of enzymatic degradation on the uptake of differently sized therapeutic molecules. *Anticancer Res.* 2008;28(6A):3557–3566.

80. Samuel CS. Relaxin: antifibrotic properties and effects in models of disease. *Clin Med Res.* 2005;3(4):241–249.

81. Brown E, McKee T, diTomaso E, et al. Dynamic imaging of collagen and its modulation in tumors in vivo using second-harmonic generation. *Nat Med.* 2003;9(6):796–800.

82. Lindgren M, Hallbrink M, Prochiantz A, et al. Cell-penetrating peptides. *Trends Pharmacol Sci.* 2000;21(3):99–103.

83. Lundberg P, Langel U. A brief introduction to cell-penetrating peptides. *J Mol Recognit.* 2003;16(5):227–233.

84. Vives E. Present and future of cell-penetrating peptide mediated delivery systems: "is the Trojan horse too wild to go only to Troy?". *J Control Release.* 2005;109(1–3):77–85.

85. Anderson DC, Nichols E, Manger R, et al. Tumor cell retention of antibody Fab fragments by an attached HIV TAT protein-derived peptide. *Biochem Biophys Res Commun.* 1993;194(2):876–884.

86. Niesner U, Halin C, Lozzi L, et al. Quantitation of the tumor-targeting properties of antibody fragments conjugated to cell-permeating HIV-1 TAT peptides. *Bioconjug Chem.* 2002;13(4):729–736.

87. Jain M, Chauhan SC, Singh AP, et al. Penetratin improves tumor retention of single-chain antibodies: a novel step toward optimization of radioimmunotherapy of solid tumors. *Cancer Res.* 2005;65(17):7840–7846.

88. Kameyama S, Horie M, Kikuchi T, et al. Effects of cell-permeating peptide binding on the distribution of 125I-labeled fab fragment in rats. *Bioconjug Chem.* 2006;17(3):597–602.

89. Hu M, Chen P, Wang J, et al. (123)I-labeled HIV-1 tat peptide radioimmunoconjugates are imported into the nucleus of human breast cancer cells and functionally interact in vitro and in vivo with the cyclin-dependent kinase inhibitor, p21(WAF-1/Cip-1). *Eur J Nucl Med Mol Imaging.* 2007;34(3):368–377.

90. Jain M, Venkatraman G, Batra SK. Cell-penetrating peptides and antibodies: a new direction for optimizing radioimmunotherapy. *Eur J Nucl Med Mol Imaging.* 2007;34(7):973–977.

91. Zalutsky MR, Xu FJ, Yu Y, et al. Radioiodinated antibody targeting of the HER-2/neu oncoprotein: effects of labeling method on cellular processing and tissue distribution. *Nucl Med Biol.* 1999;26(7):781–790.

92. Foulon CF, Reist CJ, Bigner DD, et al. Radioiodination via D-amino acid peptide enhances cellular retention and tumor xenograft targeting of an internalizing anti-epidermal growth factor receptor variant III monoclonal antibody. *Cancer Res.* 2000;60(16):4453–4460.

93. Vaidyanathan G, Alston KL, Bigner DD, et al. Nepsilon-(3-[*I]Iodobenzoyl)-Lys5-Nalpha-maleimido-Gly1-GEEEK ([*I]IB-Mal-D-GEEEK): a radioiodinated prosthetic group containing negatively charged D-glutamates for labeling internalizing monoclonal antibodies. *Bioconjug Chem.* 2006;17(4):1085–1092.

Pretargeted Radioimmunotherapy

Robert M. Sharkey and David M. Goldenberg

■ INTRODUCTION

One of the earliest forms of targeted therapy was the use of radiolabeled antibodies, starting in the early 1950s (1–5). By today's standards, the materials and tools that these investigators worked with were crude. Tumor-associated antigens would not be discovered for another 15 years. The methods to purify antibodies (then only polyclonal antisera existed) were just being developed, and therefore mixtures of specific- and irrelevant-binding immunoglobulins were used. Relatively few radionuclides were available, having questionable purity; and methods for binding them to proteins were only beginning to be developed (mostly radioiodination). Yet, when one reads the literature from that era, it is inspiring how the insights of that generation are echoed in the discoveries of today.

In the 1950s and 1960s, only a few groups were involved in this line of investigation, but then interest faded, in part, because the concept was not yet applicable to human studies. With the discoveries in the 1960s of human oncofetal, tumor-associated antigens, such as alpha-fetoprotein, beta-human choriogonadotrophin, and carcinoembryonic antigen (CEA) (6), new targets for human tumors became available. When a human colonic tumor cell line, being propagated serially in hamsters, was found to express CEA (7), this marked the beginning of our group's journey into the application of radiolabeled antibodies for cancer detection and therapy (8–11), and the exploitation of human tumor xenograft for the in vivo testing of radiolabeled antibodies.

While this road has been long, it has also been very rewarding to see the efforts of so many investigators confirm and build on the work of the pioneers who first laid the foundation of targeting radionuclides (12). Like any scientific pursuit, there have been periods of promise and disappointment, yet today there are still many opportunities for antibody-targeted radionuclides in cancer therapy, and perhaps even therapy of infectious diseases (13). In this chapter, we review a technology known as pretargeting that has evolved over the past 10 years, and discuss how this technology could very well be the next leading edge approach for targeted radionuclide therapy.

■ THE PROBLEM WITH DIRECTLY RADIOLABELED ANTIBODIES

Since its inception, it was evident that while antibodies (i.e., IgG) could selectively localize in a tissue or tumor, it often took several days for this process to occur and to reveal that this uptake was specific for the intended target over nontargeted tissues (tumor/nontumor ratio), or that this uptake was more selective than an irrelevant immunoglobulin (localization ratio or index) (9,10). It appears that there are several reasons for this slow accretion of antibody into a tumor. First, immunoglobulins are relatively large molecules (IgG ~150 kDa) that are designed to remain in the circulation for extended periods of time. Therefore, the radioactivity coupled to antibodies remains primarily in the circulation, often masking the uptake in the tumor for several days before the concentration in the blood is cleared sufficiently to allow visualization of that bound in the target tissue. Second, the vascular physiology of tumors makes them more permeable to macromolecules than a number of other tissues (14–16), and thus, it can also take several days before selective binding of the antibody in the tumor can be identified over that of an irrelevant immunoglobulin present in the vascular and extravascular space of the tumor. The lengthy residence time in the blood provides a slow, sustained supply of antibody to the tumor, allowing for a slow but steady increase in the amount of antibody retained in the tumor. For example, in xenografted tumors in mice, maximum accretion of an IgG can take 2 to 3 days, with tumor/blood ratios only marginally favoring the tumor over this period. However, the sustained concentration in the blood continually exposes the sensitive red marrow to radiation, resulting in dose-limiting hematologic toxicity. This situation seriously limits the therapeutic prospects for IgG-targeted radionuclides, unless the tumor is as sensitive to radiation as the bone marrow, which is the case with hematologic malignancies, such as non-Hodgkin lymphoma, the only cancer where a radioconjugate has been approved for therapeutic use (17). However, for the vast number of solid tumors that are more resistant to radiation, there are real challenges for an IgG-targeted radionuclide to deliver a sufficient dose to kill the tumor before being limited by the sensitivity of the bone marrow. Indeed, even in clinical trials where myeloablative doses of radiolabeled IgG have been given with bone marrow/stem cell support, clinical responses have been unsatisfactory (17). For this reason, many studies are now turning to using radiolabeled antibodies for the treatment of more localized and compartmentalized disease (18).

IgG is a relatively large molecule, with just a small portion responsible for binding to an antigen, the complementarity-determining regions (CDR). This structure allows the molecule to be segmented into progressively smaller fragments through enzymatic digestion that will form a 100-kDa bivalent-binding structures ($F(ab')_2$), which can then be reduced to 50-kDa monovalent Fab' fragments. In part because of their smaller size, but also because of the removal of the Fc portion of the IgG that contains moieties to control the recycling of immunoglobulins (neonatal Fc receptor; FcRn) (18), these structures clear much faster from the blood, allowing better visualization at an earlier time. Indeed, today, molecular engineering is able to dissect an antibody down to even smaller fragments and tether together the variable light and heavy chains that contain the basic framework structures that hold the CDRs in their three-dimensional form that will bind to the antigen. These 25-kDa single-chain Fv or scFv fragments have become a building block on which many new structures have been built (19–21), but a number of new structure types are also being synthesized that have antibody-like binding abilities and are even smaller in size (22).

Smaller targeting structures have the advantage of (a) rapidly leaving the confines of the blood vessels, (b) being capable of moving into the extravascular space where most solid tumors exist, and (c) being less impeded by the imbalance in the interstitial pressure within tumors, which lack a well-structured vasculature and lymphatic vessel network that properly draws fluids through the tumor (23). However, the faster a molecule clears from the blood, the fewer opportunities it has to find its way to the tumor's blood supply, which represents a small fraction of the total vascular/extravascular fluid in the body. Thus, there is often a negative relationship between how much targeting construct is accreted by the tumor and the residence time in the blood. While the faster clearance from the blood reduces myelotoxicity, allowing progressively higher amounts of radioactivity to be administered, often the increase in administered activity is not sufficient to offset the lower level of delivery of radioactivity to the tumor. Nevertheless, a few preclinical studies have shown improved responses with antibody fragments as compared to the same IgG, with most studies focusing on the use of radioiodinated antibodies (24–33). The key reason as to why the rapid delivery of radioactivity can enhance responses, even if the total amount is somewhat lower, is related to a higher radiation dose rate over the early delivery periods (27). Unfortunately, the smaller fragments often have a more rapid washout due to the lower binding avidity of a monovalent-binding fragment. However, even under these conditions, if the residence time of the targeting agent is appropriately balanced with the physical half-life of the radionuclide, the therapeutic response could be optimized. Meares and his group have suggested that the residence time in the tumor might be enhanced through specific modifications in the binding ligand that would enable selective covalent binding of the ligand once it is locked in place; however, at this time, this approach has been possible when such a suitable receptor is transfected into the target cells (34–38). Others have discovered that binding small molecules to albumin bestows

extended serum half-lives, thereby improving tumor uptake (39–43).

All of these new structures are being developed in an attempt to circumvent the fundamental physiologic manner that the body uses to clear these structures—a process that continues to challenge their therapeutic prospects. The body removes agents primarily by two pathways, through renal filtration with urinary elimination or by hepatobiliary filtration with elimination through the intestinal tract. Molecular size largely governs the route of elimination, with molecules ≤60 kDa being capable of filtration through the kidneys, with other factors, such as hydrophobicity and charge, playing a role. There may also be natural or synthetic complementary structures that can result in the recognition of a molecule in a given tissue that could remove it from the circulation, such as binding to galactose or Fc-binding receptors in the liver (44–48).

Radioactive elements also have discrete elimination pathways. The liver and reticuloendothelial tissues alone sequester most of the radiometals. Some radiometals will become associated with plasma proteins, while some portion will bind to the cortical bone, and the remainder will be filtered and captured by the kidneys or eliminated in the urine. Somewhat unique is radioiodine, which can find its way into thyroid hormones and result in retention in the thyroid. Radioiodine may also be absorbed into other tissues such as salivary glands and the parietal cells of the stomach.

When a radionuclide is stably attached to a molecule, its elimination path will be governed first by that molecule. Most engineered antibody constructs are stable in serum, albeit disulfide bonds can be reduced, which destabilizes the construct (49). Radiometals bound to antibodies through a chelate also can be susceptible to some level of transchelation, with the radionuclide usually being captured by one of the metal-binding serum proteins (50–57). However, the vast majority of the radionuclide in most radioimmunoconjugates is firmly bound to the antibody, and therefore the fate of the radionuclide is shared with the antibody. Antibodies are usually transported inside cells, where they are catabolized. Radiometals often remain firmly bound to the chelate, and these chelate–radionuclide complexes are usually unable to be transported out of the cell (e.g., residualized) (58,59). Molecules that contain directly radioiodinated tyrosine residues are not retained by the cell (nonresidualizing), and are typically expelled as monoiodotyrosine, which is eliminated primarily in the urine, feces, or sweat.

While the basic size and structure of an antibody can be changed, inevitably only a small portion of the product is taken up by the tumor, with the vast majority eventually being eliminated by one of these two pathways. This leaves us with a few fundamental principles that govern how a given antibody form will behave when it is directly conjugated to the radionuclide. As discussed already, proteins that remain in the circulation for extended periods usually lead to the highest tumor uptake, but the continued exposure of the sensitive bone marrow limits the amount of a radioimmunoconjugate that can be given. As mentioned previously, modifying the amino acid composition of the FcR-binding structures on the Fc portion of an IgG can reduce its time in the blood. Agents that remain in the blood for extended periods can be eliminated by administering a clearing agent, such as a "second" antibody (anti-antibody or an anti-idiotype antibody), but the complexes that are formed are filtered from the blood by the liver or the spleen (60–62). This causes a substantial increase in activity in these tissues, and unless the radioactivity is quickly eliminated, the risk of increased toxicity to these tissues might be unacceptable. Other techniques that enable selective cleavage of a radiometal–chelate complex from an antibody by enzymes in the liver are helpful for radiolabeled IgG, but the magnitude in the reduction was also not sufficient to allow therapeutically effective doses to be administered (63–67). The radiolabeled antibody can also be removed by extracorporeal absorption methods. With this technique, the patient's serum is passed through a filter that will selectively remove the antibody, with current methods exploring the use of avidin-coated resins to capture a radiolabeled biotinylated antibody (68–70). This method is an improvement over removal by a second antibody, since the radioactivity is eliminated from the body rather than being deposited in other tissues, and further refinements of this method suggests that it might be possible to eliminate the activity from the body with minimal losses in tumor uptake. However, the radiolabeled antibody still needs to remain in the body for at least 1 to 2 days to allow time for optimal tumor accretion before it is removed from the blood. Nevertheless, improvements in tumor/blood ratios have been observed, warranting further investigation.

Molecules with shorter retention in the blood are often removed by renal filtration. A significant problem occurs when these molecules pass through the proximal tubules in the renal cortex, where these cells trap radiometals, while radioiodine from directly radioiodinated proteins will be flushed out. Since the vast majority of the injected product, for these rapidly clearing agents, is eliminated through the renal system, the retention in the kidneys most often exceeds that in the tumor by a substantial margin (often >5:1). Renal uptake can be tempered to some degree by administering positively charged amino acids or other techniques (71–73). These methods might reduce renal uptake by 30% to 50%, but even this amount may not be sufficient to raise tumor/kidney ratios to a favorable level for therapeutic consideration.

In summary, the main attribute of directly radiolabeled antibodies is their stability, a property we encourage, yet one that places real limitations on our ability to deliver the therapeutic dose required for clinically meaningful antitumor responses, except for those most radiosensitive tumors. So how can we deliver a radionuclide to a tumor so that it will clear from the blood very quickly, reducing risks of hematologic toxicity, yet is able to localize in the tumor at a level similar to what is achieved with a slower clearing radiolabeled IgG?

■ THE PRINCIPLES OF PRETARGETING USING A BISPECIFIC ANTIBODY AND A RADIOLABELED HAPTEN

If binding the radionuclide stably to an antibody carrier creates so many challenges in finding just the right form of antibody and radionuclide for a given application, another option would be to separate the two compounds. Immunochemical procedures often use different types of two- to three-step bridging methods to amplify signal detection, but could these same principles be applied to amplify the targeting of the radionuclide to tumors in vivo? This is precisely the premise behind the pretargeting procedure first conceptualized by Reardan et al. (74). This group described the development of antibodies to different chelates loaded with metals, and further envisioned a process where a new type of antibody, known as a bispecific monoclonal antibody (bsMAb), could be prepared that had the capacity to bind to a target antigen, as well as having the additional capacity to bind to the chelate–metal complex. As mentioned earlier, elemental radionuclides have their own unique distribution properties, but when a radiometal is bound by a chelate its biodistribution is altered, with the majority being eliminated very quickly in the urine. Thus, these small chelate–metal complexes equilibrate throughout the body's total fluidic volume rapidly, entering the extravascular space within minutes of their injection, where they can be trapped by the antichelate-binding arm of the bsMAb that is bound to the tumor. Within just a few hours, there is very little residual activity remaining in tissues, but the portion of the radionuclide–chelate complex trapped by the antichelate antibody that is attached to the tumor by the bsMAb provides a significant contrast enhancement. Over a few years, this new technology culminated in the first clinical trials using a bsMAb prepared by chemically coupling an anti-CEA Fab' fragment to another Fab' that bound an EDTA derivative (EOTUBE) that was radiolabeled with ^{111}In (75). Patients were given 20 to 40 mg of the bsMAb, and when it had cleared from the blood (4 days later), 25 nmol of ^{111}In-EOTUBE was given with 0.1 to 5.0 mg of the bsMAb. The rationale for premixing the ^{111}In-EOTUBE with the bsMAb was to slow the chelate's clearance from the blood, giving it more time to localize in the tumor (EOTUBE-bsMAb half-life was about 8.8 minutes) (75). Once in the tumor, the dissociated EOTUBE could then be bound by the bsMAb prelocalized to malignant tissue. The ^{111}In-EOTUBE had a distribution half-life in the blood of 2.6 hours and an elimination half-life of 28 hours, with a mean volume of distribution of 9.7 L, all illustrating that the ^{111}In-EOTUBE distributed quickly in the total fluidic volume. Tumors could be detected within 2 to 3 days, and in a few cases, metastatic colon cancer in the liver was detected based on a higher uptake than in the normal liver. This was a significant accomplishment, since clinical studies at this time with an ^{111}In-labeled anti-CEA IgG most often only revealed lesions in the liver as "cold" spots, meaning that the uptake in the normal liver was higher than that in the tumor. This illustrates the natural clearing process of the IgG though the liver, a process that captures more of the antibody than the cancers in the liver. Thus, this study clearly showed pretargeting had a distinct advantage over direct targeting, providing higher tumor/blood and tumor/tissue ratios than a directly radiolabeled IgG.

Another group of investigators from Immunotech (Marseille, France), who were also focusing on the use of bsMAbs for pretargeting cancer, made an important discovery that significantly enhanced the localization of the chelate–radiometal complex. LeDoussal et al. (76) found that by tethering two haptens on a short peptide linker, the retention of hapten–peptide (HP) in the tumor was enhanced when compared to a monovalent agent. Thus, the divalent nature of the radiolabeled HP led to an *affinity enhancements system* (AES). Since its initial reporting, other groups have reported similar improvements in pretargeting when a divalent hapten was used (77,78). Figure 14.1 illustrates the bsMAb-pretargeting process.

Immunotech SA, Marseille, France performed an extensive number of preclinical and clinical studies, mostly focusing on the pretargeting of a divalent compound using two DTPAs linked to a tyrosine–lysine (TL) peptide, which enabled the HP to be radiolabeled with ^{111}In (via binding to DTPA) for initial imaging studies and then ^{131}I (via the tyrosine residue in the peptide) for therapy. The bsMAb most studied was composed of a murine anti-CEA (F6) Fab' chemically conjugated to the Fab' of a murine antibody, 734, that bound indium-loaded DTPA (79). This system was used to target a number of different CEA-producing tumors, including colorectal, small cell lung cancer, and medullary thyroid cancer (MTC) (80–89). Clinical studies with the ^{131}I-labeled HP provided additional evidence that pretargeting could deliver as much activity to tumors as a directly radiolabeled anti-CEA antibody, but with lower tissue uptake (82,87,90), and preclinical studies confirmed this therapeutic advantage in animal models representing these different cancer types (83,85,86,88,89,91,92). Although clinical trials were limited to initial phase I testing, a retrospective review of two phase I pretargeted radioimmunotherapy (PT-RAIT) clinical trials, in MTC using the ^{131}I-HP, found that a subgroup of patients whose calcitonin levels (a sensitive and specific tumor marker for MTC) doubled within 2 years had a significant survival advantage over a similar contemporaneous group of untreated patients. This remarkable success in a highly radioresistant disease was attributed to the finding that many of these patients had micrometastatic bone/bone marrow involvement (93), which was detected in pretargeted imaging studies in 20 of 29 patients. In fact, the overall 10-year survival for those patients with bone marrow involvement, as identified by the imaging study at the time of treatment, was significantly longer than patients without marrow involvement.

The clinical testing of the bsMAb-pretargeting procedure was largely limited because the bsMAb was of murine origin, and patients naturally developed an antimouse antibody response. Our group collaborated with the group in France to pursue additional clinical studies using a chemically prepared Fab' × Fab' bsMAb using a humanized anti-CEA paired with the murine anti-DTPA antibody. The initial experience found that tumors were best visualized when bsMAb doses of 50 or 100 mg/m^2 were given 7 days prior to ~100 nmol of the ^{131}I-di-DTPA-TL hapten–peptide (94). In a compromise to obtain faster clearance of the radiolabeled HP without reducing tumor uptake, it was determined that 40 mg/m^2 (400 nmol/m^2) of the bsMAb given 5 days in advance of the ^{131}I-HP (~60 nmol/m^2) was optimal. Under these conditions, the bsMAb's molar concentration in the blood was reduced to 10 nM at the time the HP was given. Therefore, the molar concentration of the bsMAb was about fourfold less than the molar concentration that the HP would have been (assuming the moles of peptide instantly distribute in the plasma volume), thereby reducing the chance for complexation with residual bsMAb in the blood. Radiation-absorbed doses to the tumors ranged from 0.5 to 12.6 Gy/GBq (~2 to 47 cGy/mCi). Interestingly, hematologic toxicity

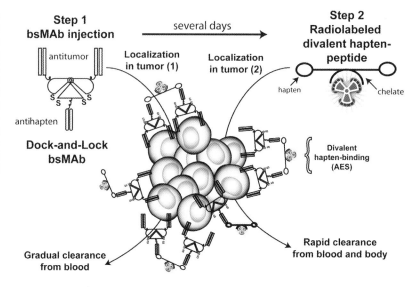

FIGURE 14.1 Bispecific pretargeting procedure. The bsMAb is injected and then over several days it will localize in the tumor and clear from the blood. The bsMAb shown in this example is based on the Dock-and-Lock method for preparing recombinant bsMAb (see Fig. 14.3) that has two binding arms; one for the tumor and the other for the hapten. Once the molar concentration of the bsMAb is low enough, the radiolabeled hapten–peptide is given. The hapten–peptide has two haptens for more stable binding within the tumor, perhaps by crosslinking two adjacent bsMAb through a process known as the affinity-enhancement system (AES). The peptide portion usually contains four to five D-amino acids with a single chelator bound to one of the amino acids that is used to capture the radionuclide.

was dose limiting under these conditions, particularly in the MTC patients, where escalation was limited to 1.8 GBq/m^2 (~50 mCi/m^2), while a dose of 2.9 GBq/m^2 (~75 mCi/m^2) was not yet dose limiting for non-MTC patients (95). Unlike earlier studies performed with the murine bsMAb, where most patients developed an antimouse antibody response, among 12 patients, only one developed an antimouse response, but four developed antibody responses to the humanized anti-CEA portion of the bsMAb.

■ NEXT GENERATION bsMAb-PRETARGETING AGENTS

Over the past 25 years, molecular engineering has changed how antibodies are prepared, and bsMAbs used for pretargeting are no exception. We have examined several different constructs for pretargeting, starting with bispecific diabodies that had monovalent binding to the target antigen and hapten, then triabodies with divalent binding to the tumor and monovalent binding to the hapten, and finally a novel process for joining multiple antibody forms called the Dock-and-Lock (DNL) method (96–98) (Fig. 14.2). For pretargeting, a tri-Fab structure has been pursued, since earlier studies with chemically prepared antitumor × antihapten bsMAb (e.g., IgG × Fab' vs. F(ab')$_2$ × Fab' and Fab' × Fab') indicated that a bsMAb with divalent binding to the tumor is preferred over a structure with monovalent binding to the tumor, but it was also important that the bsMAb clear at a reasonably rapid rate from the blood (99). The bsMAb needs only to have monovalent hapten binding, since the divalency of the HP provides enhanced avidity.

Bispecific antibody-pretargeting systems have almost always relied on the ability of the bsMAb to clear from the blood naturally, which in animals usually has taken 1 to 2 days for a 100 kDa Fab' × Fab' bsMAb, and 4 to 5 days in humans (95,100). Although the tri-Fab bsMAbs have the same molecular weight as an IgG (~157 kDa), they too clear very rapidly from the blood, with less than 1% per gram of the injected product remaining in the blood within 1 day (98,101–103). HPLC studies found the tri-Fab bsMAbs were stable in serum in vitro and in vivo, with no evidence of dissociation to their primary Fab structures. Thus, we believe their rapid clearance is at least partially due to an absence of an Fc. We also noted considerable differences in their tissue distribution when radiolabeled with radioiodine or [111]In (102).

Because they clear so quickly, their uptake in the tumor is much lower than that of an IgG, reaching a maximum level within 6 hours (101). The protein dose can be increased to load the tumor with progressively higher amounts of the bsMAb. This is one of several key elements of a pretargeting procedure, that is, the need to place a sufficient amount of a surrogate binding protein (i.e., the bsMAb) in the tumor to capture the radiolabeled HP. It is not essential to administer antigen-saturating amounts of the bsMAb, but it is important to have enough bsMAb in the tumor to maximize the amount of radiolabeled HP captured. We defined this relationship as the bsMAb/peptide mole ratio, a ratio that takes into account the amount of moles of the bsMAb that will be injected with a prescribed amount of radiolabeled HP (104). Most xenograft model systems that we have examined achieve the highest tumor uptake when 10- to 20-fold more moles of bsMAb than moles of HP were injected. Typically, ~1% to 4% of the bsMAb will be bound per gram tumor at the time the radiolabeled HP is administered, and this can result in between 10% and 30% per gram of the HP being captured in the tumor. On a mole basis, this averages to be 1 mol of HP per 1 to 2 mol of bsMAb. Since the bsMAb has monovalent hapten binding and the HP is divalent, under optimal conditions each bsMAb in the tumor is occupied with an HP.

When one considers how fast the radiolabeled HP clears from the blood and body, one has to consider pretargeting to be highly efficient binding system. Indeed, O'Connor and Bale (105) estimated that only about 15% of the IgG that is able to recirculate in the blood over several days will ever

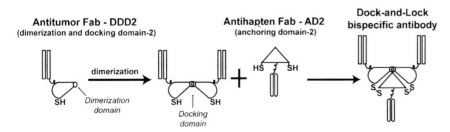

Antitumor Fab - DDD2
(dimerization and docking domain-2)

dimerization

SH   *Dimerization domain*

SH   SH   *Docking domain*

Antihapten Fab - AD2
(anchoring domain-2)

HS   SH

Dock-and-Lock bispecific antibody

FIGURE 14.2 Bispecific antibodies based on the Dock-and-Lock procedure. The Fd portion of the antitumor Fab is linked to a short peptide used to tether to what is referred to as a dimerization-docking-domain (DDD) that is derived from the regulatory subunits of the human cAMP-dependent protein kinase. This amino acid sequence was modified to insert a cysteine residue in a strategic location (DDD2). The antitumor Fab-DDD2 constructs naturally form noncovalent dimers, with the resulting complex forming a docking domain capable of binding the AD sequence (derived from the A-kinase anchor proteins) that is linked to the Fd portion of the antihapten Fab. The AD is a specially modified sequence with two cysteine residues inserted on either end of the sequence to form the AD2. When the antitumor-DDD2 is mixed with the antihapten-AD2, the molecules naturally form 157 kDa complex with a specific orientation that places the cysteine residues in position that allows for the formation of covalent disulfide bonds.

pass through a tumor. In all likelihood, the exceptionally fast HP clearance might only allow a single pass. Dynamic imaging studies showed the HP penetrates the tumor within 5 minutes, with maximum accretion occurring within 30 to 60 minutes, and at least 60% is in the urine in just 1 hour (106). In contrast, over the same hour, a radiolabeled Fab' showed very little movement into the tumor. Thus, because the radiolabeled HP traverses the vascular space efficiently, and by ensuring there is enough bsMAb accessible for capturing the small amount of HP that ultimately reaches the tumor, pretargeting creates a large therapeutic window within an hour that is sustained over several days.

Another key element in the optimization of a pretargeting procedure is the timing of the radiolabeled HP injection. The HP binds to the bsMAb's antihapten binding arm. If the HP is injected when there is an excess amount of bsMAb in the blood, there would be preferential binding of the HP to the bsMAb in the blood. As discussed earlier, the first preclinical and clinical pretargeting studies were performed under conditions to encourage complex formation between a monovalent, radiolabeled hapten, and the antihapten antibody or bsMAb as a means of slowing the blood clearance of the radiolabeled hapten (75,107). When LeDoussel et al. (76) first described the affinity-enhancement concept, they emphasized differences between the binding of the divalent hapten within the tumor, where the proximity of two antibodies on a cell surface might lead to cross-linking that increased the residence time in the tumor, as opposed to monovalently bound complexes formed in the blood that would dissociate rapidly. Thus, with the bsMAb-pretargeting procedure, there is a level at which one can allow the radiolabeled HP to interact with the bsMAb in the blood. In our preclinical experience, we observed the highest tumor uptake occurred when the radiolabeled HP's injection was delayed until the bsMAb had cleared to less than 1% per gram in the blood (100,104). When the concentration exceeded this level, blood concentrations increased and eventually tumor uptake also decreased. If the interval is extended too long, then there is a risk that the concentration of the bsMAb in the tumor will decrease to a less optimal level for capturing the radiolabeled HP. It should be strongly emphasized that even under less than optimal pretargeting conditions, tumor/nontumor ratios are still often much better than a directly radiolabeled antibody.

The relationships between a bsMAb and an HP should be expressed according to their molar concentrations, since this will allow better extrapolation across a wider range of blood volumes (e.g., mouse to man). We estimate the HP's molar concentration in the blood at the instant it is injected by assuming 100% is distributed in the total vascular volume, which is calculated to be 7% of the animal's body weight. We found that if the bsMAb's molar concentration is 10-fold lower than the molar concentration of the HP, then the HP will clear at a rate similar to that when given in the absence of a prior bsMAb injection. As this ratio decreases (i.e., higher bsMAb concentrations), the HP's clearance

gradually slows. The precise concentration of bsMAb in the blood that would impede the targeting of the radiolabeled HP will depend on the affinity of the hapten–antihapten interaction, but at the usual 10^{-9} M affinity constants for antibodies, the HP is never permanently bound to the bsMAb in the blood. Therefore, it would likely take large amounts of the bsMAb in the blood to slow the HP's clearance to equal that of the bsMAb. In our estimation, the full benefit of a pretargeting procedure will occur when the radiolabeled HP is allowed to clear quickly enough so that hematologic toxicity is not dose limiting, so it is best to minimize the bsMAb concentration in the blood before administering the radiolabeled HP.

The final key element of a pretargeting procedure is to maximize the specific activity (e.g., Ci/mmol) of the radiolabeled HP, since this will dictate the amount of radioactivity delivered to the selected target site. The lower the specific activity, the less radioactivity delivered per unit of HP captured. As mentioned earlier, the optimum moles of bsMAb administered are linked to the moles of HP administered, and therefore one would need to increase the bsMAb dose to capture HP labeled at a lower specific activity. However, this might not always be possible, as illustrated in the examples shown in Figure 14.3. In the first example (A), the HP is labeled at a maximum specific activity of 3 mCi/nmol, and we assumed the maximum tolerated dose in a mouse is 1.0 mCi. Thus, 3 nmol of the HP is administered, and in our typical situation, 20-fold more moles of the bsMAb (60 nmol) would be given to optimize tumor targeting. We assumed that if 2%-injected dose per gram of the bsMAb was localized in the tumor at the time the radiolabeled HP is given, 1.2 nmol of bsMAb would be available. We further assumed that the antigen in the tumor is fully saturated at this bsMAb dose. We then project that ~0.6 nmol or 20% injected dose per gram (1 mol divalent HP for each mole bsMAb) is captured in the tumor, delivering 0.2 mCi/g tumor. If the specific activity of the radiolabeled HP were reduced 10-fold (example B), then 30 nmol of the HP would need to be injected to administer 1.0 mCi of radiolabeled HP. If the bsMAb dose were increased to 600 nmol in order to maintain the same bsMAb/peptide mole ratio as in the first example, in the same tumor model, we would still only have the maximum ability to bind 1.2 nmol, or only 0.2% of the injected bsMAb dose. Thus, when 30 nmol of the radiolabeled HP are injected, the maximum binding capacity would likely remain at 0.6 nmol, and therefore only 2% of the injected dose of the radiolabeled HP would be bound, with only 0.02 mCi of activity delivered to the tumor. However, in a tumor with greater antigen expression (example C), the percent uptake and activity delivered to the tumor could be fully restored even with an HP prepared at the lower specific activity, so long as more bsMAb were given and its percent uptake remained the same.

This simple example can also serve to illustrate other fundamental principles affecting pretargeting. First, the maximum tolerated radioactivity dose will be defined by the uptake and clearance rate of the HP from the blood and

A **If antigen content/cell = 1.2 nmol, at a high specific activity with a saturating bsMAb dose:**

Bispecific antibody		Radiolabeled hapten-peptide (HP)			
Injected dose	Fraction bound	HP specific activity	HP injected	Radioactivity injected	Fraction bound
60 nmol	2%	3 nmol/mCi	3 nmol	1 mCi	20%

Resulting in:	bsMAb bound	HP bound	Radioactivity targeted
	1.2 nmol	0.6 nmol	0.2 mCi

B **If antigen content/cell = 1.2 nmol, but the specific activity was tenfold lower, when the same amount of activity is administered (the HP and bsMAb dose would need to be increased proportionally), less radioactivity is delivered.**

Bispecific Antibody		Radiolabeled hapten-peptide (HP)			
Injected dose	Fraction bound	HP specific activity	HP injected	Radioactivity injected	Fraction bound
600 nmol	0.2%	0.3 nmol/mCi	30 nmol	1 mCi	2%

Resulting in:	bsMAb bound	HP bound	Radioactivity targeted
	1.2 nmol	0.6 nmol	0.02 mCi

C **But, if antigen content/cell = 12 nmol, then even at a tenfold lower specific activity, by increasing bsMAb dose proportional to HP dose:**

Bispecific Antibody		Radiolabeled hapten-peptide (HP)			
Injected dose	Fraction bound	HP specific activity	HP injected	Radioactivity injected	Fraction bound
600 nmol	2%	0.3 nmol/mCi	30 nmol	1 mCi	20%

Resulting in:	bsMAb bound	HP bound	Radioactivity targeted
	12 nmol	0.6 nmol	0.2mCi

FIGURE 14.3 The effect of HP-specific activity and antigen content on HP targeting.

tissues. This clearance rate is defined by the molar relationship of the bsMAb and HP in the blood. Since the moles of the radiolabeled HP would be fixed at this maximum radioactivity dose, and since the moles of bsMAb administered to optimize the capture of this amount of HP would be within a defined range, optimizing pretargeting essentially revolves around knowing how much HP will be given at the maximum radioactivity dose tolerated.

Nearly all of the hapten-binding systems described in the literature have been based on antibodies that bind to a metal–chelate complex, such as indium-loaded EOTUBE or indium-loaded DTPA (75,76,79,107–110). These antibodies are often very specific for the metal–chelate complex, and while a given chelate can bind other metals, often the binding affinity of the antichelate antibody is optimized for the specific metal–chelate complex (74,111). Since not all radiometals are bound stably by a single chelate, this creates a situation where a unique antichelate antibody might be suitable for one radionuclide, but not another. In order to circumvent this situation, it would be better to have the antihapten antibody bind to a compound that was not integrally involved in the binding of the radionuclide. With the hapten portion of the HP involved only with the binding to the antihapten antibody, the peptide portion could be modified to allow the optimal binding for any radionuclide. LeDoussal et al. first worked with an anti-DNP (dinitrophenol) antibody with divalent DNP-peptide structures that contained either DTPA for binding indium or a tyrosine residue for radioiodination (76). However, they then switched to an antihapten antibody developed against indium-loaded DTPA cyclic anhydride and a peptide prepared by attaching two DTPA moieties to a TL peptide (79). This change may have been prompted by tissue cross-reactivity problems with an anti-DNP antibody, a problem that needs to be carefully considered when developing any antibody for in vivo targeting. This antihapten-binding system became their cognomen for clinical development. However, this group also studied another antihapten antibody; one that was developed in a project that was investigating immunoassays for the detection of histamine. As one can imagine, histamine, a natural component of many mammalian species, is not immunogenic, and thus a variety of derivatives of histamine were developed, and an antibody to one of these derivatives, histamine–succinyl–glycine (HSG), was selected for use in pretargeting. Figure 14.4 illustrates the advantages of the HSG binding system. This antibody (679) had an acceptable affinity to HSG (e.g., $\sim 10^{-9}$ M), but a very weak affinity to histamine (112,113). Pretargeting studies with a variety of radioiodinated derivatives were examined (86,113), and later, a number of other peptides containing two HSG residues were developed for use with other radionuclides, including ^{99m}Tc, ^{111}In, ^{90}Y, ^{177}Lu, ^{124}I, ^{68}Ga, and ^{18}F (106,114–120). Thus, this type of hapten system opened the possibility for a more universally adaptable HP configuration that conceivably could be used with any type of imaging or therapeutic compound. Preclinical studies required for clinical testing have indicated no tissue binding associated with the anti-HSG

FIGURE 14.4 **Advantages of the HSG antihapten binding system.** An antichelate antibody is prepared by immunizing animals with a given chelate usually preloaded with a specific metal. The antibody developed from this immunization will be very specific for that chelate, binding other chelates with less affinity if at all (**A**). As is often the case, the chelate is best used with a given radiometal, and thus there could be a very restricted number of chelate–metal complexes that could be used to bind the antihapten antibody (**B**). In the HSG system, HSG is not involved in binding the radionuclide (**C**), and with bsMAb using the anti-HSG antibody, the HP can be synthesized with any number of different chelates, needing only to have two HSG residues to ensure bsMAb binding (**D**).

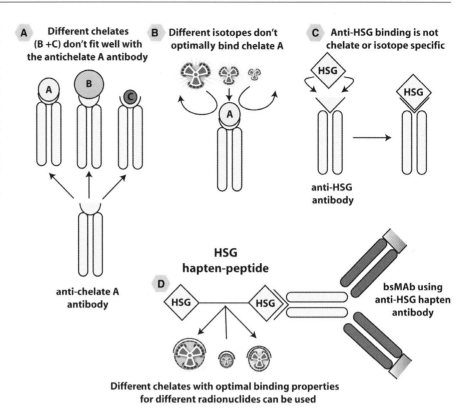

antibody, and peptides containing HSG do not have histamine-like pharmacologic activity.

Directly radiolabeled peptides that bind to cell receptors have made considerable progress in imaging and therapy, but a pretargeting system might offer an advantage. For example, slight modifications to a peptide in an effort to introduce a moiety for binding a radionuclide might adversely affect the peptide's binding to the receptor or alter its physiochemical properties, leading to a less favorable biodistribution or targeting. Indeed, the intrinsic structure of a receptor-binding peptide might not have ideal biodistribution properties, perhaps having high uptake in the liver or kidneys. In a pretargeting setting, the amino acids that comprise the peptide portion of the HP can be modified to compensate for binding ligands that might lead to increased hydrophobicity that would likely cause considerable hepatic uptake. The main criterion for the pretargeted HP is that the peptide needs to have at least two HSG residues in an easily accessible configuration that will allow for cross-linking bsMAb localized on the surface of the target cell. Thus, as long as an antibody could be manufactured, specific to the receptor, a pretargeting system could be developed where the radiolabeled HP might have better overall targeting properties (i.e., target uptake and less background) than a receptor-binding peptide. In the situation where the antigen or receptor is found in the serum, pretargeting systems might also be expected to have an advantage over a directly radiolabeled antibody or peptide. The formation of immune complexes usually results in elevated hepatic uptake, particularly with radiometal-labeled antibody. Since the bsMAb is

not radiolabeled, complexes formed with circulating antigen may be removed by the liver, and as long as they are processed before the HP is given, liver uptake of the radiolabeled HP will remain low.

The primary challenge to the concept of pretargeting is the need for the pretargeted agent to remain accessible (e.g., on the surface or within the interstitial space of the tumor) over the course of time required to allow the agent to clear from the blood. While most bsMAb-pretargeting procedures have waited for several days for the bsMAb to clear, other pretargeting procedures have successfully incorporated a clearing step that is designed to remove the pretargeted agent from the blood after allowing enough time for the agent to localize in the tumor (121). Even bsMAb procedures can benefit from a clearing step (122,123), but because this approach requires the development of another agent whose use would also need to be optimized, a clearing step should be reserved for those situations where it is found to be essential. For example, pretargeting procedures that utilize streptavidin/avidin and biotin incorporate a clearing step because the ultra-high affinity between these agents would result in highly stable complexes in the blood that could reduce the targeting quality.

If the binding of a bsMAb to the antigen results in its internalization, the quality of targeting could be reduced. While internalizing targets might not be the most ideal for pretargeting, acceptable targeting can be achieved. For example, we previously reported the rapid internalization of an antibody that binds to EGP-1 (also known as Trop 2 and GA733-1), designated RS7 (124,125). A tri-Fab bsMAb

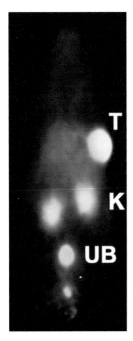

FIGURE 14.5 **Imaging of the PC3 human prostate cancer cell line pretargeted with RS7 tri-Fab bsMAb and ^{68}Ga-labeled HP.** A nude mouse bearing a subcutaneous PC3 xenograft was injected with the RS7 tri-Fab bsMAb and then 16 hours later, received an intravenous injection of the ^{68}Ga-HP. One hour later, the animal was imaged. This figure shows a posterior coronal slice in the plane of the tumor *(T)* that also captures the activity transiting through in the kidneys *(K)* into the urinary bladder *(UB).* (Please see Color Insert).

based on RS7 antitumor and anti-HSG binding was developed and successfully used to localize a radiolabeled HP to a prostate cancer cell line (Fig. 14.5). Others using a different type of pretargeting agent to CD22, an antigen found on human lymphoma cells and known to internalize when bound by anti-CD22 antibodies, found this pretargeting system was less satisfactory than an anti-CD20 pretargeting agent that would not be readily internalized (126), and it was clearly inferior when used for therapy against three different human lymphoma cell lines (127). However, since the affinity of the anti-CD22 antibody was nearly 10-fold lower than the anti-CD20 antibody and CD22 expression of the cell lines was much lower (126,127), it is uncertain what role internalization of the anti-CD22 pretargeted agent might have had in these determinations. Nevertheless, while targeting procedures would most likely benefit from having more abundant and more accessible targets, these experiences suggest that each system should be evaluated to determine the possibility that a pretargeting procedure will be suitable.

It is also important to keep in mind the role that tumor physiology plays in defining the localization of any targeting compound. Studies by van Schaijk et al. (128) in three renal carcinoma models with an ^{111}In-hapten(DTPA)-peptide pretargeted by an anti-G250 bsMAb (an IgG produced by a quadroma) clearly showed pretargeting was subject to the same types of physiologic limitations as other targeted molecules. One tumor cell line with an antigen density of just 4000 copies per cell had the highest uptake of the pretargeted ^{111}In-HP when compared to two other cell lines with 80,000 and 600,000 copies. However, the vascular permeability was threefold higher in this tumor, and it had the highest density of blood vessels all contained within the thin outer rim of the xenograft that had a large necrotic core. Although this cell line had the highest uptake within 1 to 4 hours of the HP injection, it also had the fastest washout, reducing from 300% injected dose per gram to 100% by 24 hours. These tumor cell lines also appeared to have different internalization rates as measured by the differences in the uptake between an [125]I- and ^{111}In-labeled anti-G250 IgG, albeit the cell line with the highest tumor uptake also appeared to have the same level of internalization as one of the other cell lines, so this was not likely an overarching issue in this model system. Nevertheless, this study provided a number of insightful studies that illustrate the complexities all targeting systems face (129).

The HSG-based bsMAb-pretargeting system has been examined in at least five different model systems directed against CEACAM5 (96–98,104,106,115,118,119,130,131), colon-specific antigen-p (CSAp) (115), CD20 (102,103,132), a pancreatic mucin (antibody PAM4) (101,133), neural cell adhesion molecule (NCAM) (86), and as mentioned earlier, a new system targeting EGP-1. In non-Hodgkin lymphoma and in colorectal and pancreatic cancers, pretargeting has shown exceptional localization for improved imaging and therapy. The therapeutic advantage is derived primarily from two perspectives. First, the area under the curve (AUC) for the red marrow is very low when compared to a directly radiolabeled IgG, allowing for substantially higher doses of ^{90}Y-activity to be given (e.g., 0.7 to 0.9 mCi for a pretargeted HP vs. 0.15 mCi for a directly radiolabeled IgG) (102,130,133). At the maximum tolerated dose, the AUC for the tumor is often 1.3- to 1.5-fold higher in the pretargeting-treated animals compared to the directly radiolabeled IgG. However, another key advantage is that the radiation is deposited in the tumor in minutes, with maximum accrual within 1 hour. This means the radiation is immediately localized in the tumor providing a two- to threefold higher dose rate than a directly radiolabeled IgG (121). Tumor uptake may stay at this level for 1 day, but we usually observe a decrease of ~30% to 50% over each subsequent day. Therefore, while pretargeting delivers the radiation quickly, its rate of dissociation is often faster than that of a whole IgG that can take 1 to 3 days to reach maximum levels in the tumor, but in some model systems, the radioactivity delivered by an IgG can remain at this level for several days. As with any targeting system, careful matching of the physical half-life of the radionuclide with the residence time in the tumor will lead to more optimal therapy. Additionally, we have found that weekly fractionation of the pretargeted therapy with a ^{90}Y-HP can improve responses as compared to a single treatment (133). In this regard, use of a humanized bsMAb construct will be important in the future use of pretargeted therapy.

STREPTAVIDIN-BASED PRETARGETING SYSTEMS

While the pretargeting concept started with bsMAbs, soon, the ultra-high affinity avidin/streptavidin and biotin system was introduced. Avidin–biotin pretargeting systems, as first introduced by Hnatowich et al. (134), have several key attractions. First, the binding affinity of avidin or streptavidin for biotin, which at 10^{-15} M was five- to sixfold higher than that of an antibody for a hapten, results in a highly stable radiolabeled biotin–streptavidin complex. Second, streptavidin and avidin have four biotin-binding sites, which translate into more radioactivity that could be bound per mole of streptavidin than with the HP system. Pretargeting based on this approach could be configured in a number of different ways, but two systems have dominated. One approach used a streptavidin-conjugated antitumor antibody for pretargeting radiolabeled biotin. Another procedure used a biotin-conjugated antitumor antibody as the primary pretargeting agent, followed by the administration of streptavidin or avidin. The streptavidin would bind to the biotin-IgG in the tumor, providing a bridge for binding the subsequently administered radiolabeled biotin.

A key element of each of these pretargeting approaches is the use of a "clearing" agent that is designed to reduce the amount of the primary targeting agent from the blood. This introduction was largely a consequence of the exceptional high binding affinity of biotin for streptavidin. Even the smallest amount of the streptavidin–IgG in the blood would be a magnet for the radiolabeled biotin, and unlike the bsMAb–hapten system, the complexes formed in the blood would likely not dissociate, and therefore the radioactivity would circulate with the half-life of the IgG conjugate. This method, which was developed by NeoRx during the late 1990s into early 2000s, initially used human serum albumin conjugated to galactose and biotin as the clearing agent. The biotin would bind to the streptavidin conjugate in the blood to form complexes, but as an added measure to reduce the possibility that the albumin–biotin conjugate would also enter the tumor and bind to the pretargeted IgG–streptavidin conjugate, galactose was coupled to the albumin. Galactose conjugation ensured the albumin–biotin would be rapidly cleared into the liver, since there are galactose receptors on the hepatocytes (135). Conditions were devised where the streptavidin–IgG conjugate was cleared 2 to 3 days after its injection, which allowed ample time for the conjugate to achieve maximum uptake in the tumor (136). One to two days later, after the complexes had been processed in the liver, the radiolabeled biotin was given. Figure 14.6 illustrates the components and process used in this pretargeting procedure.

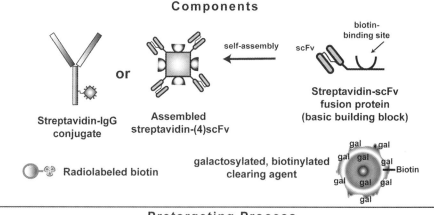

FIGURE 14.6 Streptavidin–biotin pretargeting procedure using a streptavidin-conjugated antibody or fusion protein and radiolabeled biotin. This procedure initially used a chemical conjugate of streptavidin and the antibody, but later, streptavidin fusion proteins were used. The pretargeting procedure starts with the injection of the streptavidin fusion protein, which is subsequently cleared by a synthetic agent that contains galactose residues for hepatic clearance and biotin to capture the fusion protein. Once the fusion protein is cleared from the blood, radiolabeled biotin is given. While a portion of the radiolabeled biotin will bind to the pretargeted fusion protein, the majority is cleared from the blood and body by urinary excretion.

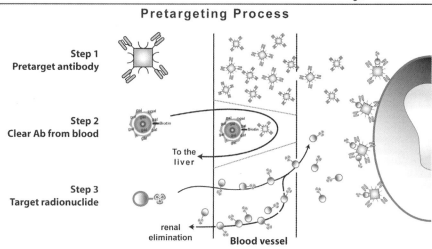

Although the ability of pretargeting to provide higher tumor/nontumor ratios as compared to a directly radiolabeled IgG had been established previously with the bsMAb-pretargeting method, Axworthy et al. were the first to show that they could achieve a similar uptake of radiolabeled biotin in the tumor with their two-step pretargeting approach (137,138). This was an exciting, yet provocative finding, since prior experience with progressively smaller antibody fragments had shown that as the size of the antibody got smaller with faster blood clearance, tumor uptake decreased ~10-fold when compared to IgG. Yet, here was a method using radiolabeled biotin that cleared much faster from the blood than any antibody fragment, but it had the ability to deliver the same fractional amount of the injected dose as compared to a directly radiolabeled IgG. While we are not entirely sure what fraction of the radiolabeled biotin or HP actually passes through a given tumor, as discussed earlier, its rapid and thorough equilibration in the extravascular space efficiently delivers the small molecule to the tumor cells bearing the pretargeted capturing agent. This pretargeting method, like the bsMAb approach, enhanced antitumor responses compared to the directly radiolabeled IgG in several tumor models (138).

The other avidin/biotin method also included a clearing step, but in this case, avidin was given to remove the biotinylated IgG from the blood. Unlike the bacterial-derived streptavidin, avidin from mammalian sources are glycosylated and naturally cleared quite quickly from the blood into the liver (139). Streptavidin had a somewhat longer half-life in the blood, and therefore was used as the "bridging agent." Thus, 1 to 2 days after injecting the biotinylated IgG, avidin was administered as a clearing agent and then a few hours later the streptavidin was given. The next day, radiolabeled biotin was given. This procedure also produced excellent targeting results, superior to that of a directly radiolabeled IgG (139–141).

While streptavidin-based pretargeting systems benefit from the strong binding of biotin for streptavidin and a bsMAb–HP pretargeting technique gains from having a divalent hapten, both systems are bound in the tumor by an antibody, and thus the residence time of the radioactivity in the tumor will depend on the weakest link. Streptavidin-based approaches are also susceptible to endogenous biotin, which is particularly problematic in studies in mice that have a high concentration of biotin in their blood (142,143); however, the lower concentration of biotin in the blood of humans does not appear to have an impact on this pretargeting method (144).

Both avidin/biotin pretargeting procedures have been studied extensively in patients. The NeoRx method focused on an IgG–streptavidin conjugate that used an antibody, NR-LU-10, that bound to most solid tumors. This antibody was later found to bind to an antigen known as EpCAM (also known as CO-17-1A or epithelial glycoprotein-2), which had cross-reactivity with normal bowel and kidneys (145). Investigators carefully optimized the pretargeting system, evaluating the best dose of the antibody conjugate, the

clearing agent and radiolabeled biotin, as well as the timing of various conditions (136,146). A phase I therapy trial using ^{90}Y-biotin found dose-limiting gastrointestinal toxicity at 140 mCi/m^2, with intense localization of large intestine, and declared the MTD to be 110 mCi/m^2 (147). A phase II therapy trial in advanced colorectal cancer was performed using the optimal pretargeting conditions with 110 mCi/m^2 of the ^{90}Y-biotin, but with an overall response rate of just 8% (2/25 PR) and a free-from progression duration of 16 weeks, additional clinical studies were not pursued (145). This study also highlighted one of the major concerns for pretargeting procedures that employ streptavidin, namely the immunogenicity of this bacterial protein. In the phase II study that used the murine NR-LU-10-streptavidin–IgG conjugate, all patients developed an antistreptavidin response within 4 to 5 weeks.

More recent preclinical and clinical studies with this approach have focused on the use of streptavidin–scFv fusion proteins (148–155). Streptavidin consists of four polypeptide chains. The fusion protein tethers a single scFv on the streptavidin polypeptide chain, and when it self-assembles, the molecule has four scFv binding arms to the tumor antigen with a fully functional streptavidin capable of binding four biotins. A new synthetic clearing agent containing galactose, to assist in hepatic clearance, and biotin for capturing the streptavidin fusion protein was also introduced, replacing the albumin conjugate. Two constructs have been examined clinically, one targeting CD20 for therapy of non-Hodgkin lymphoma and another targeting TAG-72 using the CC49-streptavidin fusion protein in colorectal cancer (156–158). In both indications, clinical testing was restricted primarily to an examination of conditions for optimal targeting.

Forero et al. (158) reported the initial clinical study with a streptavidin fusion protein that used a single-chain region of the murine B9E9 anti-CD20 monoclonal antibody (159). Patients were given 160 or 320 mg/m^2 of the fusion protein, and then 2 to 3 days later, they were given a synthetic clearing agent at a dose of 45 mg/m^2, followed 24 hours later with a co-injection of ^{111}In- (5 mCi) and ^{90}Y-DOTA-biotin (15 mCi/m^2). Biodistribution and tumor targeting of the B9E9 fusion protein was evaluated in several patients through the use of an ^{186}Re-labeled product. Most patients had bulky disease and had received numerous prior therapies. Severe hematologic toxicity occurred in 2 of 15 patients, but it was believed to be due to other nontreatment-related issues. Eleven patients had no hematologic toxicity. Three patients had an objective response (two complete responses lasting 91 and 325 days and a partial response lasting 297 days). Fewer patients developed an anti-antibody response to streptavidin than previously found with the chemical conjugate in colorectal cancer patients. However, prior clinical trials using murine monoclonal antibodies in previously treated lymphoma patients had indicated that these patients were less likely to develop an antimurine IgG response, suggesting their ability to elicit an antibody response is reduced. No specific correlative information concerning the tumor-localizing capability of the ^{186}Re-B9E9 fusion protein or ^{111}In-biotin was given, but images of two patients showed very clear and remarkable uptake in multiple lesions. Interestingly, the images did not appear to show intense uptake in the spleen, even though this is commonly found with directly radiolabeled anti-CD20 IgG, prompting the need to predose patients with an unlabeled IgG to reduce excessive uptake of the directly radiolabeled IgG. Radiation-absorbed doses to 20 tumors in 10 patients averaged 26 ± 4 cGy/mCi, but ranged from 2 to 69 cGy/mCi.

No additional clinical testing with this agent has been reported, but there have been a number of additional preclinical studies with this fusion protein and other chemically prepared or engineered scFv-streptavidin fusion proteins against CD20, CD22, or CD45 for targeting lymphoma (126,127,154,155,159–165). These preclinical studies have consistently revealed a superiority of pretargeting over directly radiolabeled antibodies, with anti-CD20 and anti-CD45 constructs generally having better targeting than an anti-CD22 construct. Preparations appear to be under way to bring the anti-CD45-streptavidin fusion protein to clinical testing, most likely in a myeloablative setting, since CD45 is expressed on a number of normal white blood cells (166).

Initial clinical testing of the CC49 anti-TAG-72-streptavidin fusion protein was also reported (156,157). Unlike the NR-LU-10 conjugate, this agent did not specifically direct the radiolabeled biotin to the intestines. Again, this trial was performed mainly to assess conditions for optimal targeting. The most important observation was tumor dosimetry that indicated three of nine patients had tumor/kidney radiation-absorbed dose ratios ≥5:1 (157). This ratio is important because if we assume renal toxicity was dose limiting and that the kidneys could tolerate 2000 cGy, then the tumors in these patients would have received a dose of ≥10,000 cGy, a level that would be expected to have some therapeutic response. Indeed, clinical trials with ^{90}Y-DOTA-TOC have indicated that renal doses of up to 2700 cGy can be tolerated as long as patient-specific renal dosimetry is performed (167–171). If pretargeting procedures are also limited by renal toxicity rather than hematologic toxicity, it may be possible to deliver ≥5000 cGy to tumors with a targeting radiation dose ratio of just 2:1.

Clinical studies using the pretargeting procedure with biotinylated antibodies have been studied primarily in ovarian and brain cancers. Both of these cancers are amenable for a more localized treatment (i.e., intraperitoneal and intracavity, respectively), but intravenous injections were used in the initial clinical studies. Figure 14.7 illustrates the materials and processes used in this pretargeting method.

For brain cancer treatment, a biotinylated murine antitenascin IgG was used, with the first trial performed in 48 patients with established disease, while the second trial focused on treating 37 patients after the primary lesion was resected (172,173). In both of these trials, the agents were administered systemically by intravenous infusion. In established disease, objective responses were observed in 12 of 48 patients (172). Patients were treated with 60, 70, or 80 mCi/m^2 of the ^{90}Y-biotin, and at the highest dose, 4/12

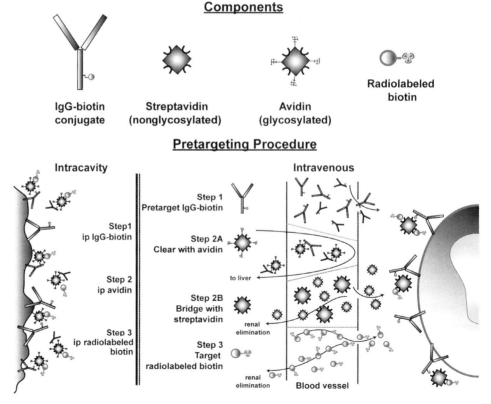

FIGURE 14.7 Streptavidin–biotin bridging-pretargeting procedure using a biotinylated antibody and radiolabeled biotin. Treatment starts with a biotinylated antitumor antibody. After giving 1 to 2 days to localize in the tumor, it is cleared from the blood using avidin, because its glycosylation is naturally recognized in the liver, pulling the complexes out of the blood. A few hours later, streptavidin is given, which circulates and binds to the antitumor antibody, while itself clearing quickly from the blood though renal elimination. The final step is the administration of the radiolabeled biotin. An intracavity treatment consists of the biotinylated antibody followed by avidin. There is no clearing step in this situation, since any biotinylated antibody not already bound to the tumor that would form complexes with avidin could subsequently bind the tumor and be involved in localizing the radiolabeled biotin.

patients had a grade IV hematologic toxicity, and thus this was considered the maximum tolerated dose. No notable nonhematologic toxicities were noted.

In the second study, all patients were treated with 60 mCi/m^2, and as expected, only grade I and II hematologic toxicity was observed in 42% of the patients, with the remaining patients having no hematologic toxicity (173). Eight patients with a primary diagnosis of glioblastoma multiforme were treated, and another 12 patients served as controls (patients assigned to control group because of insufficient expression of tenascin, history of allergic reactions, or because of lack of materials, and were otherwise given standard of care). At the time this report was published, 5/8 of the treated patients had died, while all of the control patients had died (significant median survival of 33.5 months for treated vs. 8 months for control). Since only 2 of the 11 treated patients with Grade III gliomas had died at the time of this reporting, the median survival could not be given, but the median disease-free interval was estimated to be 56 months. On the basis of an estimate for the median survival in the control group of 33 months, a significant improvement for the treated group was reported.

This same group of investigators also initiated trials using a locoregional-pretargeted treatment, alone and in combination with oral temozolomide (174,175). This treatment regimen consisted of an intracavity injection of 2 to 5 mg of biotinylated antitenascin IgG, followed 1 day later with an injection of avidin, which was followed 18 hours later with the ^{90}Y-biotin (15 to 30 mCi). This trial was designed to give at least two treatment cycles 8 to 10 weeks apart. Temozolomide (150 mg/m^2/d) was given for five consecutive days and repeated every 28 days as tolerated, but on average, two consecutive cycles of temozolomide were given with two cycles of pretargeted therapy. Thirty-eight patients received pretargeting alone and 35 received pretargeting with temozolomide. Overall, 75% of the patients had disease stabilization, but there was only a trend suggesting the combination achieved a better objective response. The median progression-free survival and overall survival for patients receiving the standard of care were 8 and 21 months, respectively. The group given pretargeted radioimmunotherapy alone had a median overall survival of just 17.5 months and a progression-free survival of 5 months. However, patients receiving the combined treatment had an overall and progression-free survival of 25 and 10 months, respectively, which represented a significant improvement over the nonrandomized control group.

In ovarian cancer, these same investigators initiated a trial using a mixture of three different biotinylated antibodies binding TAG-72 (B72.3), CEA, and an antifolate receptor antibody (MoV18). The antibodies (20 to 50 mg) were administered intraperitoneally, and 1 day later, avidin was injected intraperitoneally. The ^{90}Y-biotin was administered 24 hours later and given either intraperitoneally in patients with appropriate peritoneal distribution (as determined by a ^{99m}Tc-albumin scan) or intravenously if the activity was focal. ^{90}Y-activities varied from 10 to 100 mCi, but most

patients received between 30 and 60 mCi. Only 3 of 38 patients experienced grade III or IV hematologic toxicity. Bremsstrahlung images of the patients indicated the radioactivity was almost entirely confined to the peritoneal cavity, with evidence of focal uptake in tumors. Objective responses were generally seen in 5% to 10% of the patients irrespective of whether the ^{90}Y-biotin was given intraperitoneally or intravenously.

OLIGOMER/COMPLEMENTARY OLIGOMER PRETARGETING

This type of system uses the natural attraction of complementary, short-chain nucleic acids rather than proteins for pretargeting. This model system has examined a number of different synthetic compounds, including peptide nucleic acids and phosphorodiamidate morpholino oligomers (MORFs) (176–184). The MORF compounds are particularly interesting because their core structure is stable in vivo and their chemistries allow modifications for linking a variety of agents for binding radionuclides. For example, Liu et al. reported the ability to radiolabel an MAG$_3$-conjugated complementary MORF (cMORF) with ^{188}Re to a specific activity of 2 to 25 mCi/μg, and with a molecular weight of ~6.5 kDa, representing ~12 to 150 mCi/nmol (185). The use of polymeric forms of the pretargeted agent provides even greater loading capability (179,182). Liu et al. (186) subsequently reported a modest but significantly improved therapeutic response for their ^{188}Re-cMORF pretargeted with an anti-CEA IgG–MORF conjugate compared to untreated, unlabeled MORF–anti-CEA IgG and nonpretargeted ^{188}Re-MORF in nude mice bearing established LS174T human colon tumors. Additional pretargeting studies with this system were reported using an MORF-conjugated anti-TAG-72 antibody (B72.3) in nude mice bearing a human prostate cancer cell line (CWR22) (187). A comparison of the pretargeting of a ^{99m}Tc-cMORF to that of ^{111}In-B72.3 showed somewhat improved tumor/nontumor ratios 3 hours after the ^{99m}Tc-cMORF as compared to 3 days with the ^{111}In-IMP-288, but overall, tumor/nontumor ratios were not as robust as seen with other pretargeting methods in other model systems (e.g., tumor/blood was 0.7, tumor/liver was 2.4). This pretargeting system has not progressed to clinical testing at the time of this writing.

CONCLUDING REMARKS

Antibody targeting of radionuclides is one of the earliest selective therapies. While a one-step process with a directly radiolabeled antibody is the simplest approach, there is abundant preclinical evidence that other pretargeting procedures can be as, or more, therapeutically effective, and uniformly delivered with less toxicity. Thus, the effort required to optimize the treatment with these approaches is certainly warranted. Whether these procedures will be able to deliver the necessary benefit clinically remains to be proven. Animal models are indicating particularly promising results for pretargeted therapy of non-Hodgkin lymphoma (102,103, 164,165), an indication where directly radiolabeled antibodies have been successful in the clinic. Given some of the more recent clinical trials where directly radiolabeled antibodies are being given in conjunction with chemotherapeutic regimens that are limited by hematologic toxicity (188–195), the minimal red marrow exposure with pretargeting procedures could hold another advantage over the current use of the directly radiolabeled antibodies. Combining pretargeting with chemotherapy to improve responses in animal models of solid tumors has been reported (133,149,196). Therefore, pretargeted radioimmunotherapy is a promising technology with broad applications in oncology.

Acknowledgments

The authors thank our many colleagues who have contributed to the research efforts in pretargeting including Jacques Barbet, PhD, Professor Otto Boerman, PhD, Chien-Hsing Chang, PhD, Professor Jean-François Chatal, MD, Habibe Karacay, PhD, Professor Françoise Kraeber-Bodéré, MD, William J. McBride, PhD, and Edmund A. Rossi, PhD. The authors are supported in part from PHS grants P01 CA103985 and R01 CA107088.

REFERENCES

1. Pressman D. The zone of localization of antibodies. III. The specific localization of antibodies to rat kidney. *Cancer.* 1949;2:697–700.
2. Pressman D, Korngold L. The in vivo localization of anti-Wagner-osteogenic-sarcoma antibodies. *Cancer.* 1953;6:619–623.
3. Korngold L, Pressman D. The localization of antilymphosarcoma antibodies in the Murphy lymphosarcoma of the rat. *Cancer Res.* 1954;14:96–99.
4. Bale WF, Spar IL. Studies directed toward the use of antibodies as carriers of radioactivity for therapy. *Adv Biol Med Phys.* 1957;5:285–356.
5. Bale WF, Spar IL, Goodland RL. Experimental radiation therapy of tumors with I-131-carrying antibodies to fibrin. *Cancer Res.* 1960;20:1488–1494.
6. Gold P, Freedman SO. Specific carcinoembryonic antigens of the human digestive system. *J Exp Med.* 1965;122:467–481.
7. Goldenberg DM, Hansen HJ. Carcinoembryonic antigen present in human colonic neoplasms serially propagated in hamsters. *Science.* 1972;175:1117–1118.
8. Goldenberg DM, DeLand F, Kim E, et al. Use of radiolabeled antibodies to carcinoembryonic antigen for the detection and localization of diverse cancers by external photoscanning. *N Engl J Med.* 1978;298:1384–1386.
9. Primus FJ, Wang RH, Goldenberg DM, et al. Localization of human GW-39 tumors in hamsters by radiolabeled heterospecific antibody to carcinoembryonic antigen. *Cancer Res.* 1973;33:2977–2982.
10. Goldenberg DM, Preston DF, Primus FJ, et al. Photoscan localization of GW-39 tumors in hamsters using radiolabeled anticarcinoembryonic antigen immunoglobulin G. *Cancer Res.* 1974;34:1–9.
11. Primus FJ, Macdonald R, Goldenberg DM, et al. Localization of GW-39 human tumors in hamsters by affinity-purified antibody to carcinoembryonic antigen. *Cancer Res.* 1977;37:1544–1547.
12. Goldenberg DM, Sharkey RM, Barbet J, et al. Radioactive antibodies: selective targeting and treatment of cancer and other diseases. *Appl Radiol.* 2007;36:10–29.
13. Dadachova E, Casadevall A. Radioimmunotherapy of infectious diseases. *Semin Nucl Med.* 2009;39:146–153.
14. Jain RK. Physiological barriers to delivery of monoclonal antibodies and other macromolecules in tumors. *Cancer Res.* 1990;50:814s–819s.
15. Jain RK. Transport of molecules, particles, and cells in solid tumors. *Annu Rev Biomed Eng.* 1999;1:241–263.
16. Fukumura D, Jain RK. Tumor microenvironment abnormalities: causes, consequences, and strategies to normalize. *J Cell Biochem.* 2007;101:937–949.
17. Sharkey RM, Goldenberg DM. Perspectives on cancer therapy with radiolabeled monoclonal antibodies. *J Nucl Med.* 2005;46(suppl 1): 115S–127S.
18. Sharkey RM, Goldenberg DM. Use of antibodies and immunoconjugates for the therapy of more accessible cancers. *Adv Drug Deliv Rev.* 2008;60:1407–1420.
19. Batra SK, Jain M, Wittel UA, et al. Pharmacokinetics and biodistribution of genetically engineered antibodies. *Curr Opin Biotechnol.* 2002;13:603–608.
20. Olafsen T, Kenanova VE, Wu AM. Tunable pharmacokinetics: modifying the in vivo half-life of antibodies by directed mutagenesis of the Fc fragment. *Nat Protoc.* 2006;1:2048–2060.
21. Wu AM, Olafsen T. Antibodies for molecular imaging of cancer. *Cancer J.* 2008;14:191–197.
22. Sharkey RM, Goldenberg DM. Novel radioimmunopharmaceuticals for cancer imaging and therapy. *Curr Opin Investig Drugs.* 2008; 9:1302–1316.
23. Jain M, Venkatraman G, Batra SK. Optimization of radioimmunotherapy of solid tumors: biological impediments and their modulation. *Clin Cancer Res.* 2007;13:1374–1382.
24. Buchegger F, Pelegrin A, Delaloye B, et al. Iodine-131-labeled MAb F(ab')$_2$ fragments are more efficient and less toxic than intact anti-CEA antibodies in radioimmunotherapy of large human colon carcinoma grafted in nude mice. *J Nucl Med.* 1990;31:1035–1044.
25. Stein R, Blumenthal R, Sharkey RM, et al. Comparative biodistribution and radioimmunotherapy of monoclonal antibody RS7 and its F(ab')$_2$ in nude mice bearing human tumor xenografts. *Cancer.* 1994;73:816–823.
26. Adams GP, McCartney JE, Wolf EJ, et al. Optimization of in vivo tumor targeting in SCID mice with divalent forms of 741F8 anti-c-erbB-2 single-chain Fv: effects of dose escalation and repeated i.v. administration. *Cancer Immunol Immunother.* 1995;40:299–306.
27. Behr TM, Memtsoudis S, Sharkey RM, et al. Experimental studies on the role of antibody fragments in cancer radio-immunotherapy: influence of radiation dose and dose rate on toxicity and anti-tumor efficacy. *Int J Cancer.* 1998;77:787–795.
28. Pavlinkova G, Beresford GW, Booth BJ, et al. Pharmacokinetics and biodistribution of engineered single-chain antibody constructs of MAb CC49 in colon carcinoma xenografts. *J Nucl Med.* 1999;40: 1536–1546.
29. Behr TM, Behe M, Stabin MG, et al. High-linear energy transfer (LET) alpha versus low-LET beta emitters in radioimmunotherapy of solid tumors: therapeutic efficacy and dose-limiting toxicity of 213Bi-versus ^{90}Y-labeled CO17-1A Fab' fragments in a human colonic cancer model. *Cancer Res.* 1999;59:2635–2643.
30. Behr TM, Blumenthal RD, Memtsoudis S, et al. Cure of metastatic human colonic cancer in mice with radiolabeled monoclonal antibody fragments. *Clin Cancer Res.* 2000;6:4900–4907.
31. Behr TM, Behe M, Sgouros G. Correlation of red marrow radiation dosimetry with myelotoxicity: empirical factors influencing the radiation-induced myelotoxicity of radiolabeled antibodies, fragments and peptides in pre-clinical and clinical settings. *Cancer Biother Radiopharm.* 2002;17:445–464.
32. Berndorff D, Borkowski S, Sieger S, et al. Radioimmunotherapy of solid tumors by targeting extra domain B fibronectin: identification of the best-suited radioimmunoconjugate. *Clin Cancer Res.* 2005; 11:7053s–7063s.
33. Rogers BE, Roberson PL, Shen S, et al. Intraperitoneal radioimmunotherapy with a humanized anti-TAG-72 (CC49) antibody with a deleted CH2 region. *Cancer Biother Radiopharm.* 2005;20:502–513.
34. Chmura AJ, Orton MS, Meares CF. Antibodies with infinite affinity. *Proc Natl Acad Sci USA.* 2001;98:8480–8484.
35. Chmura AJ, Schmidt BD, Corson DT, et al. Electrophilic chelating agents for irreversible binding of metal chelates to engineered antibodies. *J Control Release.* 2002;78:249–258.
36. Butlin NG, Meares CF. Antibodies with infinite affinity: origins and applications. *Acc Chem Res.* 2006;39:780–787.
37. Meares CF. The chemistry of irreversible capture. *Adv Drug Deliv Rev.* 2008;60:1383–1388.
38. Miao Z, McCoy MR, Singh DD, et al. Cysteinylated protein as reactive disulfide: an alternative route to affinity labeling. *Bioconjug Chem.* 2008;19:15–19.

39. Muller D, Karle A, Meissburger B, et al. Improved pharmacokinetics of recombinant bispecific antibody molecules by fusion to human serum albumin. *J Biol Chem*. 2007;282:12650–12660.

40. Stork R, Muller D, Kontermann RE. A novel tri-functional antibody fusion protein with improved pharmacokinetic properties generated by fusing a bispecific single-chain diabody with an albumin-binding domain from streptococcal protein G. *Protein Eng Des Sel*. 2007;20:569–576.

41. Yazaki PJ, Kassa T, Cheung CW, et al. Biodistribution and tumor imaging of an anti-CEA single-chain antibody-albumin fusion protein. *Nucl Med Biol*. 2008;35:151–158.

42. Tijink BM, Laeremans T, Budde M, et al. Improved tumor targeting of anti-epidermal growth factor receptor Nanobodies through albumin binding: taking advantage of modular Nanobody technology. *Mol Cancer Ther*. 2008;7:2288–2297.

43. Tolmachev V, Orlova A, Pehrson R, et al. Radionuclide therapy of HER2-positive microxenografts using a ^{177}Lu-labeled HER2-specific Affibody molecule. *Cancer Res*. 2007;67:2773–2782.

44. Jain M, Kamal N, Batra SK. Engineering antibodies for clinical applications. *Trends Biotechnol*. 2007;25:307–316.

45. Werner RG, Kopp K, Schlueter M. Glycosylation of therapeutic proteins in different production systems. *Acta Paediatr Suppl*. 2007;96:17–22.

46. Beckman RA, Weiner LM, Davis HM. Antibody constructs in cancer therapy: protein engineering strategies to improve exposure in solid tumors. *Cancer*. 2007;109:170–179.

47. Tabrizi MA, Tseng CM, Roskos LK. Elimination mechanisms of therapeutic monoclonal antibodies. *Drug Discov Today*. 2006;11:81–88.

48. Sinclair AM, Elliott S. Glycoengineering: the effect of glycosylation on the properties of therapeutic proteins. *J Pharm Sci*. 2005;94:1626–1635.

49. Leung SO, Qu Z, Hansen HJ, et al. The effects of domain deletion, glycosylation, and long IgG3 hinge on the biodistribution and serum stability properties of a humanized IgG1 immunoglobulin, hLL2, and its fragments. *Clin Cancer Res*. 1999;5:3106s–3117s.

50. Bass LA, Wang M, Welch MJ, et al. In vivo transchelation of copper-64 from TETA-octreotide to superoxide dismutase in rat liver. *Bioconjug Chem*. 2000;11:527–532.

51. Rogers BE, Anderson CJ, Connett JM, et al. Comparison of four bifunctional chelates for radiolabeling monoclonal antibodies with copper radioisotopes: biodistribution and metabolism. *Bioconjug Chem*. 1996;7:511–522.

52. Xue LY, Noujaim AA, Sykes TR, et al. Role of transchelation in the uptake of ^{99m}Tc-MAb in liver and kidney. *Q J Nucl Med*. 1997;41:10–17.

53. Mardirossian G, Wu C, Hnatowich DJ. The stability in liver homogenates of indium-111 and yttrium-90 attached to antibody via two popular chelators. *Nucl Med Biol*. 1993;20:65–74.

54. Hnatowich DJ, Mardirossian G, Rusckowski M, et al. Directly and indirectly technetium-99m-labeled antibodies—a comparison of in vitro and animal in vivo properties. *J Nucl Med*. 1993;34:109–119.

55. Deshpande SV, Subramanian R, McCall MJ, et al. Metabolism of indium chelates attached to monoclonal antibody: minimal transchelation of indium from benzyl-EDTA chelate in vivo. *J Nucl Med*. 1990;31:218–224.

56. Paik CH, Eckelman WC, Reba RC. Transchelation of ^{99m}Tc from low affinity sites to high affinity sites of antibody. *Int J Rad Appl Instrum B*. 1986;13:359–362.

57. Ma D, Lu F, Overstreet T, et al. Novel chelating agents for potential clinical applications of copper. *Nucl Med Biol*. 2002;29:91–105.

58. Stein R, Govindan SV, Mattes MJ, et al. Improved iodine radiolabels for monoclonal antibody therapy. *Cancer Res*. 2003;63:111–118.

59. Govindan SV, Mattes MJ, Stein R, et al. Labeling of monoclonal antibodies with diethylenetriaminepentaacetic acid-appended radioiodinated peptides containing D-amino acids. *Bioconjug Chem*. 1999;10:231–240.

60. Goldenberg DM, Sharkey RM, Ford E. Anti-antibody enhancement of iodine-131 anti-CEA radioimmunodetection in experimental and clinical studies. *J Nucl Med*. 1987;28:1604–1610.

61. Sharkey RM, Primus FJ, Goldenberg DM. Second antibody clearance of radiolabeled antibody in cancer radioimmunodetection. *Proc Natl Acad Sci USA*. 1984;81:2843–2846.

62. Blumenthal RD, Sharkey RM, Snyder D, et al. Reduction by anti-antibody administration of the radiotoxicity associated with ^{131}I-labeled antibody to carcinoembryonic antigen in cancer radioimmunotherapy. *J Natl Cancer Inst*. 1989;81:194–199.

63. Haseman MK, Goodwin DA, Meares CF, et al. Metabolizable ^{111}In chelate conjugated anti-idiotype monoclonal antibody for radioimmunodetection of lymphoma in mice. *Eur J Nucl Med*. 1986;12:455–460.

64. Meares CF, McCall MJ, Deshpande SV, et al. Chelate radiochemistry: cleavable linkers lead to altered levels of radioactivity in the liver. *Int J Cancer Suppl*. 1988;2:99–102.

65. Peterson JJ, Meares CF. Enzymatic cleavage of peptide-linked radiolabels from immunoconjugates. *Bioconjug Chem*. 1999;10:553–557.

66. DeNardo GL, Kroger LA, Meares CF, et al. Comparison of 1,4,7,10-tetraazacyclododecane-N,N′,N″,N‴-tetraacetic acid (DOTA)-peptide-ChL6, a novel immunoconjugate with catabolizable linker, to 2-iminothiolane-2-[p-(bromoacetamido)benzyl]-DOTA-ChL6 in breast cancer xenografts. *Clin Cancer Res*. 1998;4:2483–2490.

67. Peterson JJ, Meares CF. Cathepsin substrates as cleavable peptide linkers in bioconjugates, selected from a fluorescence quench combinatorial library. *Bioconjug Chem*. 1998;9:618–626.

68. Chen JQ, Strand SE, Tennvall J, et al. Extracorporeal immunoadsorption compared to avidin chase: enhancement of tumor-to-normal tissue ratio for biotinylated rhenium-188-chimeric BR96. *J Nucl Med*. 1997;38:1934–1939.

69. Linden O, Kurkus J, Garkavij M, et al. A novel platform for radioimmunotherapy: extracorporeal depletion of biotinylated and ^{90}Y-labeled rituximab in patients with refractory B-cell lymphoma. *Cancer Biother Radiopharm*. 2005;20:457–466.

70. Martensson L, Nilsson R, Ohlsson T, et al. Reduced myelotoxicity with sustained tumor concentration of radioimmunoconjugates in rats after extracorporeal depletion. *J Nucl Med*. 2007;48:269–276.

71. Behr TM, Goldenberg DM, Becker W. Reducing the renal uptake of radiolabeled antibody fragments and peptides for diagnosis and therapy: present status, future prospects and limitations. *Eur J Nucl Med*. 1998;25:201–212.

72. Vegt E, van Eerd JE, Eek A, et al. Reducing renal uptake of radiolabeled peptides using albumin fragments. *J Nucl Med*. 2008;49:1506–1511.

73. van Eerd JEM, Vegt E, Wetzels JFM, et al. Gelatin-based plasma expander effectively reduces renal uptake of ^{111}In-octreotide in mice and rats. *J Nucl Med*. 2006;47:528–533.

74. Reardan DT, Meares CF, Goodwin DA, et al. Antibodies against metal chelates. *Nature*. 1985;316:265–268.

75. Stickney DR, Anderson LD, Slater JB, et al. Bifunctional antibody: a binary radiopharmaceutical delivery system for imaging colorectal carcinoma. *Cancer Res*. 1991;51:6650–6655.

76. Le Doussal JM, Martin M, Gautherot E, et al. In vitro and in vivo targeting of radiolabeled monovalent and divalent haptens with dual specificity monoclonal antibody conjugates: enhanced divalent hapten affinity for cell-bound antibody conjugate. *J Nucl Med*. 1989;30:1358–1366.

77. Goodwin DA, Meares CF, McTigue M, et al. Pretargeted immunoscintigraphy: effect of hapten valency on murine tumor uptake. *J Nucl Med*. 1992;33:2006–2013.

78. Boerman OC, Kranenborg MH, Oosterwijk E, et al. Pretargeting of renal cell carcinoma: improved tumor targeting with a bivalent chelate. *Cancer Res*. 1999;59:4400–4405.

79. Le Doussal JM, Gruaz-Guyon A, Martin M, et al. Targeting of indium 111-labeled bivalent hapten to human melanoma mediated by bispecific monoclonal antibody conjugates: imaging of tumors hosted in nude mice. *Cancer Res*. 1990;50:3445–3452.

80. Le Doussal JM, Chetanneau A, Gruaz-Guyon A, et al. Bispecific monoclonal antibody-mediated targeting of an indium-111-labeled DTPA dimer to primary colorectal tumors: pharmacokinetics, biodistribution, scintigraphy and immune response. *J Nucl Med*. 1993;34:1662–1671.

81. Chetanneau A, Barbet J, Peltier P, et al. Pretargeted imaging of colorectal cancer recurrences using an ^{111}In-labelled bivalent hapten and a bispecific antibody conjugate. *Nucl Med Commun*. 1994;15:972–980.

82. Bardies M, Bardet S, Faivre-Chauvet A, et al. Bispecific antibody and iodine-131-labeled bivalent hapten dosimetry in patients with medullary thyroid or small-cell lung cancer. *J Nucl Med*. 1996;37:1853–1859.

83. Gautherot E, Bouhou J, Le Doussal JM, et al. Therapy for colon carcinoma xenografts with bispecific antibody-targeted, iodine-131-labeled bivalent hapten. *Cancer*. 1997;80:2618–2623.

84. Barbet J, Peltier P, Bardet S, et al. Radioimmunodetection of medullary thyroid carcinoma using indium-111 bivalent hapten and anti-CEA × anti-DTPA-indium bispecific antibody. *J Nucl Med*. 1998;39:1172–1178.

85. Gautherot E, Le Doussal JM, Bouhou J, et al. Delivery of therapeutic doses of radioiodine using bispecific antibody-targeted bivalent haptens. *J Nucl Med*. 1998;39:1937–1943.

86. Hosono M, Hosono MN, Kraeber-Bodere F, et al. Two-step targeting and dosimetry for small cell lung cancer xenograft with anti-NCAM/antihistamine bispecific antibody and radioiodinated bivalent hapten. *J Nucl Med*. 1999;40:1216–1221.

87. Kraeber-Bodere F, Bardet S, Hoefnagel CA, et al. Radioimmunotherapy in medullary thyroid cancer using bispecific antibody and iodine 131-labeled bivalent hapten: preliminary results of a phase I/II clinical trial. *Clin Cancer Res*. 1999;5:3190s–3198s.

88. Kraeber-Bodere F, Faivre-Chauvet A, Sai-Maurel C, et al. Toxicity and efficacy of radioimmunotherapy in carcinoembryonic antigen-producing medullary thyroid cancer xenograft: comparison of iodine 131-labeled F(ab')2 and pretargeted bivalent hapten and evaluation of repeated injections. *Clin Cancer Res*. 1999;5:3183s–3189s.

89. Gautherot E, Rouvier E, Daniel L, et al. Pretargeted radioimmunotherapy of human colorectal xenografts with bispecific antibody and ^{131}I-labeled bivalent hapten. *J Nucl Med*. 2000;41:480–487.

90. Chatal JF, Faivre-Chauvet A, Bardies M, et al. Bifunctional antibodies for radioimmunotherapy. *Hybridoma*. 1995;14:125–128.

91. Hosono M, Hosono MN, Kraeber-Bodere F, et al. Biodistribution and dosimetric study in medullary thyroid cancer xenograft using bispecific antibody and iodine-125-labeled bivalent hapten. *J Nucl Med*. 1998;39:1608–1613.

92. Barbet J, Kraeber-Bodere F, Vuillez JP, et al. Pretargeting with the affinity enhancement system for radioimmunotherapy. *Cancer Biother Radiopharm*. 1999;14:153–166.

93. Mirallie E, Vuillez JP, Bardet S, et al. High frequency of bone/bone marrow involvement in advanced medullary thyroid cancer. *J Clin Endocrinol Metab*. 2005;90:779–788.

94. Kraeber-Bodere F, Faivre-Chauvet A, Ferrer L, et al. Pharmacokinetics and dosimetry studies for optimization of anti-carcinoembryonic antigen × anti-hapten bispecific antibody-mediated pretargeting of Iodine-131-labeled hapten in a phase I radioimmunotherapy trial. *Clin Cancer Res*. 2003;9:3973S–3981S.

95. Kraeber-Bodere F, Rousseau C, Bodet-Milin C, et al. Targeting, toxicity, and efficacy of 2-step, pretargeted radioimmunotherapy using a chimeric bispecific antibody and ^{131}I-labeled bivalent hapten in a phase I optimization clinical trial. *J Nucl Med*. 2006;47:247–255.

96. Rossi EA, Sharkey RM, McBride W, et al. Development of new multivalent-bispecific agents for pretargeting tumor localization and therapy. *Clin Cancer Res*. 2003;9:3886S–3896S.

97. Rossi EA, Chang CH, Losman MJ, et al. Pretargeting of carcinoembryonic antigen-expressing cancers with a trivalent bispecific fusion protein produced in myeloma cells. *Clin Cancer Res*. 2005;11:7122s–7129s.

98. Rossi EA, Goldenberg DM, Cardillo TM, et al. Stably tethered multifunctional structures of defined composition made by the dock and lock method for use in cancer targeting. *Proc Natl Acad Sci USA*. 2006;103:6841–6846.

99. Karacay H, Sharkey RM, McBride WJ, et al. Pretargeting for cancer radioimmunotherapy with bispecific antibodies: role of the bispecific antibody's valency for the tumor target antigen. *Bioconjug Chem*. 2002;13:1054–1070.

100. Karacay H, McBride WJ, Griffiths GL, et al. Experimental pretargeting studies of cancer with a humanized anti-CEA x murine anti-[In-DTPA] bispecific antibody construct and a [99m]Tc-/[188]Re-labeled peptide. *Bioconjug Chem*. 2000;11:842–854.

101. Gold DV, Goldenberg DM, Karacay H, et al. A novel bispecific, trivalent antibody construct for targeting pancreatic carcinoma. *Cancer Res*. 2008;68:4819–4826.

102. Sharkey RM, Karacay H, Litwin S, et al. Improved therapeutic results by pretargeted radioimmunotherapy of non-Hodgkin's lymphoma with a new recombinant, trivalent, anti-CD20, bispecific antibody. *Cancer Res*. 2008;68:5282–5290.

103. Sharkey RM, Karacay H, Johnson CR, et al. Pretargeted versus directly targeted radioimmunotherapy combined with anti-CD20 antibody consolidation therapy of non-Hodgkin lymphoma. *J Nucl Med*. 2009;50:444–453.

104. Sharkey RM, Karacay H, Richel H, et al. Optimizing bispecific antibody pretargeting for use in radioimmunotherapy. *Clin Cancer Res*. 2003;9:3897S–3913S.

105. O'Connor SW, Bale WF. Accessibility of circulating immunoglobulin G to the extravascular compartment of solid rat tumors. *Cancer Res*. 1984;44:3719–3723.

106. Sharkey RM, Cardillo TM, Rossi EA, et al. Signal amplification in molecular imaging by pretargeting a multivalent, bispecific antibody. *Nat Med*. 2005;11:1250–1255.

107. Goodwin DA, Meares CF, David GF, et al. Monoclonal antibodies as reversible equilibrium carriers of radiopharmaceuticals. *Int J Rad Appl Instrum B*. 1986;13:383–391.

108. Goodwin DA, Mears CF, McTigue M, et al. Monoclonal antibody hapten radiopharmaceutical delivery. *Nucl Med Commun*. 1986;7:569–580.

109. Le Doussal JM, Gautherot E, Martin M, et al. Enhanced in vivo targeting of an asymmetric bivalent hapten to double-antigen-positive mouse B cells with monoclonal antibody conjugate cocktails. *J Immunol*. 1991;146:169–175.

110. Goodwin DA, Meares CF, Watanabe N, et al. Pharmacokinetics of pretargeted monoclonal antibody 2D12.5 and [88]Y-Janus-2-(p-nitrobenzyl)-1,4,7,10-tetraazacyclododecanetetraacetic acid (DOTA) in BALB/c mice with KHJJ mouse adenocarcinoma: a model for ^{90}Y radioimmunotherapy. *Cancer Res*. 1994;54:5937–5946.

111. Feng X, Pak RH, Kroger LA, et al. New anti-Cu-TETA and anti-Y-DOTA monoclonal antibodies for potential use in the pre-targeted delivery of radiopharmaceuticals to tumor. *Hybridoma*. 1998;17:125–132.

112. Morel A, Darmon M, Delaage M. Recognition of imidazole and histamine derivatives by monoclonal antibodies. *Mol Immunol*. 1990;27:995–1000.

113. Janevik-Ivanovska E, Gautherot E, Hillairet de Boisferon M, et al. Bivalent hapten-bearing peptides designed for iodine-131 pretargeted radioimmunotherapy. *Bioconjug Chem*. 1997;8:526–533.

114. Gestin JF, Loussouarn A, Bardies M, et al. Two-step targeting of xenografted colon carcinoma using a bispecific antibody and [188]Re-labeled bivalent hapten: biodistribution and dosimetry studies. *J Nucl Med*. 2001;42:146–153.

115. Sharkey RM, McBride WJ, Karacay H, et al. A universal pretargeting system for cancer detection and therapy using bispecific antibody. *Cancer Res*. 2003;63:354–363.

116. Griffiths GL, Chang CH, McBride WJ, et al. Reagents and methods for PET using bispecific antibody pretargeting and ^{68}Ga-radiolabeled bivalent hapten–peptide–chelate conjugates. *J Nucl Med*. 2004;45:30–39.

117. Morandeau L, Benoist E, Loussouarn A, et al. Synthesis of new bivalent peptides for applications in the Affinity Enhancement System. *Bioconjug Chem*. 2005;16:184–193.

118. McBride WJ, Zanzonico P, Sharkey RM, et al. Bispecific antibody pretargeting PET (immunoPET) with an [124]I-labeled hapten–peptide. *J Nucl Med*. 2006;47:1678–1688.

119. McBride WJ, Sharkey RM, Karacay H, et al. A novel method of F-18 radiolabeling for PET. *J Nucl Med*. 2009;50:991–998.

120. Schoffelen R, Sharkey RM, Goldenberg DM, et al. Pretargeted immunoPET imaging of CEA-expressing tumors with a bispecific antibody and a [68]Ga- and ^{18}F-labeled hapten–peptide in mice with human tumor xenografts. *Mol Cancer Ther*. 2010;9(4):1019–1027.

121. Sharkey RM, Karacay H, Cardillo TM, et al. Improving the delivery of radionuclides for imaging and therapy of cancer using pretargeting methods. *Clin Cancer Res*. 2005;11:7109s–7121s.

122. Mirallie E, Sai-Maurel C, Faivre-Chauvet A, et al. Improved pretargeted delivery of radiolabelled hapten to human tumour xenograft in mice by avidin chase of circulating bispecific antibody. *Eur J Nucl Med Mol Imaging*. 2005;32:901–909.

123. Goldenberg DM, Sharkey RM, Paganelli G, et al. Antibody pretargeting advances cancer radioimmunodetection and radioimmunotherapy. *J Clin Oncol*. 2006;24:823–834.

124. Govindan SV, Stein R, Qu Z, et al. Preclinical therapy of breast cancer with a radioiodinated humanized anti-EGP-1 monoclonal antibody: advantage of a residualizing iodine radiolabel. *Breast Cancer Res Treat*. 2004;84:173–182.

125. Stein R, Govindan SV, Mattes MJ, et al. Targeting human cancer xenografts with monoclonal antibodies labeled using radioiodinated, diethylenetriaminepentaacetic acid-appended peptides. *Clin Cancer Res*. 1999;5:3079s–3087s.

126. Pantelias A, Pagel JM, Hedin N, et al. Comparative biodistributions of pretargeted radioimmunoconjugates targeting CD20, CD22, and DR molecules on human B-cell lymphomas. *Blood*. 2007;109:4980–4987.

127. Pagel JM, Orgun N, Hamlin DK, et al. A comparative analysis of conventional and pretargeted radioimmunotherapy of B-cell lymphomas by targeting CD20, CD22, and HLA-DR singly and in combinations. *Blood*. 2009;113:4903–4913.

128. van Schaijk FG, Oosterwijk E, Molkenboer-Kuenen JD, et al. Pretargeting with bispecific anti-renal cell carcinoma × anti-DTPA(In) antibody in 3 RCC models. *J Nucl Med*. 2005;46:495–501.

129. Sharkey RM. The direct route may not be the best way to home. *J Nucl Med*. 2005;46:391–394.

130. Karacay H, Brard PY, Sharkey RM, et al. Therapeutic advantage of pretargeted radioimmunotherapy using a recombinant bispecific antibody in a human colon cancer xenograft. *Clin Cancer Res*. 2005;11:7879–7885.

131. Sharkey RM, Karacay H, Vallabhajosula S, et al. Metastatic human colonic carcinoma: molecular imaging with pretargeted SPECT and PET in a mouse model. *Radiology*. 2008;246:497–507.

132. Sharkey RM, Karacay H, Chang CH, et al. Improved therapy of non-Hodgkin's lymphoma xenografts using radionuclides pretargeted with a new anti-CD20 bispecific antibody. *Leukemia*. 2005; 19:1064–1069.

133. Karacay H, Sharkey RM, Gold DV, et al. Pretargeted radioimmunotherapy of pancreatic cancer xenografts in nude mice: safety and efficacy alone and combined with gemcitabine. *J Nucl Med*. 2009; 50(12):2008–2016.

134. Hnatowich DJ, Virzi F, Rusckowski M. Investigations of avidin and biotin for imaging applications. *J Nucl Med*. 1987;28:1294–1302.

135. Mattes MJ. Biodistribution of antibodies after intraperitoneal or intravenous injection and effect of carbohydrate modifications. *J Natl Cancer Inst*. 1987;79:855–863.

136. Breitz HB, Weiden PL, Beaumier PL, et al. Clinical optimization of pretargeted radioimmunotherapy with antibody–streptavidin conjugate and ^{90}Y-DOTA-biotin. *J Nucl Med*. 2000;41:131–140.

137. Axworthy DB, Fritzberg AR, Hylarides MD, et al. Preclinical evaluation of an anti-tumor monoclonal antibody/streptavidin conjugate for pretargeted 90Y radioimmunotherapy in a mouse xenograft model. *J Immunother*. 1994;16:158.

138. Axworthy DB, Reno JM, Hylarides MD, et al. Cure of human carcinoma xenografts by a single dose of pretargeted yttrium-90 with negligible toxicity. *Proc Natl Acad Sci USA*. 2000;97:1802–1807.

139. Paganelli G, Malcovati M, Fazio F. Monoclonal antibody pretargeting techniques for tumour localization: the avidin-biotin system. International Workshop on Techniques for Amplification of Tumour Targeting. *Nucl Med Commun*. 1991;12:211–234.

140. Paganelli G, Magnani P, Zito F, et al. Three-step monoclonal antibody tumor targeting in carcinoembryonic antigen-positive patients. *Cancer Res*. 1991;51:5960–5966.

141. Paganelli G, Pervez S, Siccardi AG, et al. Intraperitoneal radiolocalization of tumors pre-targeted by biotinylated monoclonal antibodies. *Int J Cancer*. 1990;45:1184–1189.

142. Hnatowich DJ. The in vivo uses of streptavidin and biotin: a short progress report. *Nucl Med Commun*. 1994;15:575–577.

143. Sharkey RM, Karacay H, Griffiths GL, et al. Development of a streptavidin-anti-carcinoembryonic antigen antibody, radiolabeled biotin pretargeting method for radioimmunotherapy of colorectal cancer. Studies in a human colon cancer xenograft model. *Bioconjug Chem*. 1997;8:595–604.

144. Kalofonos HP, Rusckowski M, Siebecker DA, et al. Imaging of tumor in patients with indium-111-labeled biotin and streptavidin-conjugated antibodies: preliminary communication. *J Nucl Med*. 1990;31:1791–1796.

145. Knox SJ, Goris ML, Tempero M, et al. Phase II trial of yttrium-90-DOTA-biotin pretargeted by NR-LU-10 antibody/streptavidin in patients with metastatic colon cancer. *Clin Cancer Res*. 2000;6:406–414.

146. Breitz HB, Fisher DR, Goris ML, et al. Radiation absorbed dose estimation for ^{90}Y-DOTA-biotin with pretargeted NR-LU-10/streptavidin. *Cancer Biother Radiopharm*. 1999;14:381–395.

147. Murtha A, Weiden P, Knox S, et al. Phase I dose escalation trial of pretargeted radioimmunotherapy with ^{90}Yttrium. Proceedings of the annual meeting. *Am Soc Clin Oncol*. 1998;17:1687.

148. Zhang M, Zhang Z, Garmestani K, et al. Pretarget radiotherapy with an anti-CD25 antibody–streptavidin fusion protein was effective in therapy of leukemia/lymphoma xenografts. *Proc Natl Acad Sci USA*. 2003;100:1891–1895.

149. Graves SS, Dearstyne E, Lin Y, et al. Combination therapy with pretarget CC49 radioimmunotherapy and gemcitabine prolongs tumor doubling time in a murine xenograft model of colon cancer more effectively than either monotherapy. *Clin Cancer Res*. 2003; 9:3712–3721.

150. Lewis MR, Zhang J, Jia F, et al. Biological comparison of ^{149}Pm-, ^{166}Ho-, and ^{177}Lu-DOTA-biotin pretargeted by CC49 scFv-streptavidin fusion protein in xenograft-bearing nude mice. *Nucl Med Biol*. 2004;31: 213–223.

151. Cheung NK, Modak S, Lin Y, et al. Single-chain Fv-streptavidin substantially improved therapeutic index in multistep targeting directed at disialoganglioside GD2. *J Nucl Med*. 2004;45:867–877.

152. Sato N, Hassan R, Axworthy DB, et al. Pretargeted radioimmunotherapy of mesothelin-expressing cancer using a tetravalent single-chain Fv-streptavidin fusion protein. *J Nucl Med*. 2005;46: 1201–1209.

153. Buchsbaum DJ, Khazaeli MB, Axworthy DB, et al. Intraperitoneal pretarget radioimmunotherapy with CC49 fusion protein. *Clin Cancer Res*. 2005;11:8180–8185.

154. Pagel JM, Lin Y, Hedin N, et al. Comparison of a tetravalent single-chain antibody–streptavidin fusion protein and an antibody–streptavidin chemical conjugate for pretargeted anti-CD20 radioimmunotherapy of B-cell lymphomas. *Blood*. 2006;108:328–336.

155. Lin Y, Pagel JM, Axworthy D, et al. A genetically engineered anti-CD45 single-chain antibody–streptavidin fusion protein for pretargeted radioimmunotherapy of hematologic malignancies. *Cancer Res*. 2006;66:3884–3892.

156. Forero-Torres A, Shen S, Breitz H, et al. Pretargeted radioimmunotherapy (RIT) with a novel anti-TAG-72 fusion protein. *Cancer Biother Radiopharm*. 2005;20:379–390.

157. Shen S, Forero A, LoBuglio AF, et al. Patient-specific dosimetry of pretargeted radioimmunotherapy using CC49 fusion protein in patients with gastrointestinal malignancies. *J Nucl Med*. 2005;46:642–651.

158. Forero A, Weiden PL, Vose JM, et al. Phase 1 trial of a novel anti-CD20 fusion protein in pretargeted radioimmunotherapy for B-cell non-Hodgkin lymphoma. *Blood*. 2004;104:227–236.

159. Schultz J, Lin Y, Sanderson J, et al. A tetravalent single-chain antibody–streptavidin fusion protein for pretargeted lymphoma therapy. *Cancer Res*. 2000;60:6663–6669.

160. Pagel JM, Hedin N, Subbiah K, et al. Comparison of anti-CD20 and anti-CD45 antibodies for conventional and pretargeted radioimmunotherapy of B-cell lymphomas. *Blood*. 2003;101:2340–2348.

161. Pagel JM, Pantelias A, Hedin N, et al. Evaluation of CD20, CD22, and HLA-DR targeting for radioimmunotherapy of B-cell lymphomas. *Cancer Res*. 2007;67:5921–5928.

162. Subbiah K, Hamlin DK, Pagel JM, et al. Comparison of immunoscintigraphy, efficacy, and toxicity of conventional and pretargeted radioimmunotherapy in CD20-expressing human lymphoma xenografts. *J Nucl Med*. 2003;44:437–445.

163. Gopal AK, Press OW, Wilbur SM, et al. Rituximab blocks binding of radiolabeled anti-CD20 antibodies (Ab) but not radiolabeled anti-CD45 Ab. *Blood*. 2008;112:830–835.

164. Pagel JM, Hedin N, Drouet L, et al. Eradication of disseminated leukemia in a syngeneic murine leukemia model using pretargeted anti-CD45 radioimmunotherapy. *Blood*. 2008;111:2261–2268.

165. Press OW, Corcoran M, Subbiah K, et al. A comparative evaluation of conventional and pretargeted radioimmunotherapy of CD20-expressing lymphoma xenografts. *Blood*. 2001;98:2535–2543.

166. Green DJ, Pagel JM, Nemecek ER, et al. Pretargeting CD45 enhances the selective delivery of radiation to hematolymphoid tissues in nonhuman primates. *Blood*. 2009;114:1226–1235.

167. Valkema R, Pauwels S, Kvols LK, et al. Survival and response after peptide receptor radionuclide therapy with [^{90}Y-DOTA0,Tyr3]octreotide in patients with advanced gastroenteropancreatic neuroendocrine tumors. *Semin Nucl Med*. 2006;36:147–156.

168. Barone R, Borson-Chazot F, Valkema R, et al. Patient-specific dosimetry in predicting renal toxicity with ^{90}Y-DOTATOC: relevance of kidney volume and dose rate in finding a dose-effect relationship. *J Nucl Med*. 2005;46(suppl 1):99S–106S.

169. Valkema R, Pauwels SA, Kvols LK, et al. Long-term follow-up of renal function after peptide receptor radiation therapy with (90)Y-DOTA(0),Tyr(3)-octreotide and (177)Lu-DOTA(0), Tyr(3)-octreotate. *J Nucl Med*. 2005;46(suppl 1):83S–91S.

170. Pauwels S, Barone R, Walrand S, et al. Practical dosimetry of peptide receptor radionuclide therapy with ^{90}Y-labeled somatostatin analogs. *J Nucl Med*. 2005;46(suppl 1):92S–98S.

171. Bodei L, Cremonesi M, Ferrari M, et al. Long-term evaluation of renal toxicity after peptide receptor radionuclide therapy with ^{90}Y-DOTA-TOC and ^{177}Lu-DOTATATE: the role of associated risk factors. *Eur J Nucl Med Mol Imaging*. 2008;35:1847–1856.

172. Paganelli G, Grana C, Chinol M, et al. Antibody-guided three-step therapy for high grade glioma with yttrium-90 biotin. *Eur J Nucl Med*. 1999;26:348–357.

173. Grana C, Chinol M, Robertson C, et al. Pretargeted adjuvant radioimmunotherapy with yttrium-90-biotin in malignant glioma patients: a pilot study. *Br J Cancer*. 2002;86:207–212.

174. Bartolomei M, Mazzetta C, Handkiewicz-Junak D, et al. Combined treatment of glioblastoma patients with locoregional pre-targeted ^{90}Y-biotin radioimmunotherapy and temozolomide. *Q J Nucl Med Mol Imaging*. 2004;48:220–228.

175. Paganelli G, Bartolomei M, Ferrari M, et al. Pre-targeted locoregional radioimmunotherapy with ^{90}Y-biotin in glioma patients: phase I study and preliminary therapeutic results. *Cancer Biother Radiopharm*. 2001;16:227–235.

176. Rusckowski M, Qu T, Chang F, et al. Pretargeting using peptide nucleic acid. *Cancer*. 1997;80:2699–2705.

177. Wang Y, Chang F, Zhang Y, et al. Pretargeting with amplification using polymeric peptide nucleic acid. *Bioconjug Chem*. 2001;12:807–816.

178. Liu G, Mang'era K, Liu N, et al. Tumor pretargeting in mice using ^{99m}Tc-labeled morpholino, a DNA analog. *J Nucl Med*. 2002;43:384–391.

179. He J, Liu G, Zhang S, et al. Pharmacokinetics in mice of four oligomer-conjugated polymers for amplification targeting. *Cancer Biother Radiopharm*. 2003;18:941–947.

180. Liu G, Liu C, Zhang S, et al. Investigations of ^{99m}Tc morpholino pretargeting in mice. *Nucl Med Commun*. 2003;24:697–705.

181. Liu CB, Liu GZ, Liu N, et al. Radiolabeling morpholinos with ^{90}Y, ^{111}In, ^{188}Re and ^{99m}Tc. *Nucl Med Biol*. 2003;30:207–214.

182. He J, Liu G, Gupta S, et al. Amplification targeting: a modified pretargeting approach with potential for signal amplification-proof of a concept. *J Nucl Med*. 2004;45:1087–1095.

183. Liu G, He J, Dou S, et al. Pretargeting in tumored mice with radiolabeled morpholino oligomer showing low kidney uptake. *Eur J Nucl Med Mol Imaging*. 2004;31:417–424.

184. Liu G, Dou S, Yin D, et al. A novel pretargeting method for measuring antibody internalization in tumor cells. *Cancer Biother Radiopharm*. 2007;22:33–39.

185. Liu G, Dou S, He J, et al. Radiolabeling of MAG3-morpholino oligomers with ^{188}Re at high labeling efficiency and specific radioactivity for tumor pretargeting. *Appl Radiat Isot*. 2006;64:971–978.

186. Liu G, Dou S, Mardirossian G, et al. Successful radiotherapy of tumor in pretargeted mice by ^{188}Re-radiolabeled phosphorodiamidate morpholino oligomer, a synthetic DNA analogue. *Clin Cancer Res*. 2006;12:4958–4964.

187. Liu G, Dou S, Pretorius PH, et al. Pretargeting CWR22 prostate tumor in mice with MORF-B72.3 antibody and radiolabeled cMORF. *Eur J Nucl Med Mol Imaging*. 2008;35:272–280.

188. Perrotti AP, Niscola P, Boemi S, et al. Long-lasting remission of a relapsed large cell non-Hodgkin's lymphoma by Y90 ibritumomab tiuxetan as salvage therapy. *Tumori*. 2009;95:129–130.

189. Winter JN, Inwards DJ, Spies S, et al. Yttrium-90 ibritumomab tiuxetan doses calculated to deliver up to 15 Gy to critical organs may be safely combined with high-dose BEAM and autologous transplantation in relapsed or refractory B-cell non-Hodgkin's lymphoma. *J Clin Oncol*. 2009;27:1653–1659.

190. Jacobs SA, Swerdlow SH, Kant J, et al. Phase II trial of short-course CHOP-R followed by ^{90}Y-ibritumomab tiuxetan and extended rituximab in previously untreated follicular lymphoma. *Clin Cancer Res*. 2008;14:7088–7094.

191. Morschhauser F, Radford J, Van Hoof A, et al. Phase III trial of consolidation therapy with yttrium-90-ibritumomab tiuxetan compared with no additional therapy after first remission in advanced follicular lymphoma. *J Clin Oncol*. 2008;26:5156–5164.

192. Peyrade F, Triby C, Slama B, et al. Radioimmunotherapy in relapsed follicular lymphoma previously treated by autologous bone marrow transplant: a report of eight new cases and literature review. *Leuk Lymphoma*. 2008;49:1762–1768.

193. Zinzani PL, Tani M, Pulsoni A, et al. Fludarabine and mitoxantrone followed by yttrium-90 ibritumomab tiuxetan in previously untreated patients with follicular non-Hodgkin lymphoma trial: a phase II non-randomised trial (FLUMIZ). *Lancet Oncol*. 2008; 9:352–358.

194. Zinzani PL, Tani M, Fanti S, et al. A phase II trial of CHOP chemotherapy followed by yttrium 90 ibritumomab tiuxetan (Zevalin) for previously untreated elderly diffuse large B-cell lymphoma patients. *Ann Oncol*. 2008;19:769–773.

195. Krishnan A, Nademanee A, Fung HC, et al. Phase II trial of a transplantation regimen of yttrium-90 ibritumomab tiuxetan and high-dose chemotherapy in patients with non-Hodgkin's lymphoma. *J Clin Oncol*. 2008;26:90–95.

196. Kraeber-Bodere F, Sai-Maurel C, Campion L, et al. Enhanced antitumor activity of combined pretargeted radioimmunotherapy and paclitaxel in medullary thyroid cancer xenograft. *Mol Cancer Ther*. 2002;1:267–274.

Extracorporeal Techniques for Improving Radioimmunotherapy of Disseminated Malignant Tumors

Rune Nilsson, Michael Garkavij, Ola Linden, Katarina Sjögreen Gleisner,
Michael Ljungberg, Sven-Erik Strand, and Jan Tennvall

■ INTRODUCTION

Immunoconjugates used for radioimmunotherapy generally remain in the circulation for many days. As a consequence, toxicity to other organs prevents the administration of a sufficient amount of activity to obtain the absorbed dose required to eradicate metastases of malignant tumors. This chapter describes extracorporeal depletion. This increases the clearance rate of monoclonal antibodies (mAbs) from the circulation, allowing the problem of the low tumor-to-normal tissue ratio to be overcome, and reducing the toxicity to normal organs.

The technical aspects of extracorporeal affinity adsorption are discussed together with the evaluation of the method in experimental models and clinical studies. These studies confirm that extracorporeal affinity adsorption treatment (ECAT) can be used safely and efficiently to reduce the myelotoxicity associated with radioimmunotherapy, as well as the toxicity to other radiosensitive organs such as the lungs, kidneys, and liver. ECAT allows an increase in the administered activity without increasing the toxicity to normal tissue, thus increasing the absorbed dose to the tumor. ECAT has been studied in a syngeneic rat tumor model, in a nonhuman primate model, and in humans. In all cases, the application of extracorporeal depletion reduced the amount of nonspecific radiation to normal organs, allowing higher activities to be delivered.

Although considerable progress has been made in optimizing and improving radioimmunotherapy in the treatment of disseminated malignant tumors, the therapeutic value when treating solid tumors remains limited. In contrast to other neoplasms, such as leukemia and lymphoma, the interstitial pressure in solid tumors impedes molecular transport through the vessel wall and in the interstitium (1). In addition, the interstitium of solid tumors contains inflammatory cells, fibroblasts, and other accessory cells and enzymes, which also affect the delivery of immunoconjugates to the tumor (2). Immunoconjugates generally remain in the circulation for many days, penetrating the tumor slowly. This results in low tumor-to-blood (T/B) and tumor-to-normal tissue (T/N) ratios. As a consequence, toxicity to vital organs prevents the administration of the activity needed in terms of MBq or mCi to achieve the absorbed doses in terms of Gy or rad required to eradicate solid tumors. In order to overcome this problem, the ratio of accumulated radioactivity in tumors to radiosensitive normal tissue must be increased. Although damage to the marrow (the most radiosensitive tissue) can be successfully alleviated by hematopoietic cell transplantation, this is not the case with the other radiosensitive organs, such as the lungs, kidneys, intestines, and liver.

Increasing the clearance rate of mAbs has been proposed as a means of overcoming the problem of low T/N ratios, and reducing the toxicity in radiosensitive vital organs. This has been achieved by administering secondary antibodies, for example, anti-immunoglobulin (3) or anti-idiotypic antibodies (4). These secondary antibodies bind the circulating radiolabeled mAbs and form complexes that are rapidly trapped in the liver. The use of secondary antibodies thus efficiently eliminates radioactivity from the blood but introduces the problem of liver toxicity. A similar approach is the use of avidin to eliminate biotinylated antibodies; the avidin–antibody complex is also trapped in the liver, resulting in the same problem as the use of secondary antibodies (5–8).

One way of increasing the T/N ratio is pretargeting, which involves the administration of a so-called pretargeting antibody that binds to the tumor, before the delivery of the therapeutic agent, which in turn binds to the tumor-localizing antibody. The use of bispecific antibodies with hapten radionuclides in the treatment of tumors is a promising strategy (9). Pretargeting could perhaps be used in combination with extracorporeal adsorption to further increase the T/N ratio (Chapter 14).

Another method of removing radiolabeled antibodies is by extracorporeal depletion of mAbs from the circulation (10–14). In this chapter, we will specifically discuss ECAT. Theoretical simulations of extracorporeal affinity adsorption have indicated that the T/N activity ratio could be increased considerably (15). However, the results of plasmapheresis studies revealed some serious drawbacks regarding efficacy and safety. This prompted us to develop a safer and more efficient procedure, namely extracorporeal affinity adsorption. This process has been evaluated in a syngeneic rat tumor model (16–19), in a nonhuman primate model using macaque monkeys (20), and in human studies (21,22).

■ EXTRACORPOREAL AFFINITY ADSORPTION

▦ The principle of selectivity

Extracorporeal affinity adsorption is an attractive method for the selective removal of substances from the blood circulation, while allowing the simultaneous return of the purified blood to the patient, thus avoiding loss of essential blood components and eliminating the need for replacement solutions. During ECAT, the blood is circulated through an adsorbent, as illustrated in Figure 15.1. This consists of a matrix to which a substance that is selective for the component to be removed has been immobilized by covalent linkages. The immunoconjugate must have structural entities that allow it to bind to the adsorbent. These structural entities may be an integral part of the immunoconjugate, or may be artificially introduced to the immunoconjugate prior to administration to the patient. An example of the former is the use of immobilized antibodies directed against specific and assessable epitopes present on the monoclonal antibody itself. An extracorporeal system utilizing species-specific anti-immunoglobulin (antimouse IgG) directed against immunoconjugates based on mouse mAbs has been developed and tested clinically (13). However, it is difficult to use this principle of selection today as most mAbs in clinical use are humanized or fully human. This means that the immunoconjugate cannot be selectively recognized in the presence of endogenous human IgG. An alternative is to use anti-idiotypic antibodies that react with the antigen-binding epitopes on the monoclonal antibody. However, a specific anti-idiotypic monoclonal antibody and an adsorbent based in this anti-idiotype must be developed and approved for each immunoconjugate

of interest for human use. Also, circulating tumor antigens may bind to the immunoconjugate inhibiting the binding to the immobilized anti-idiotype, resulting in lower depletion efficiency.

Any generally applicable affinity adsorption device must be based on artificially introduced characteristics of the exogenous antibodies (immunoconjugate) in order to differentiate between the patient's own IgG and foreign IgG. This can be achieved by the conjugation of the immunoconjugate with affinity ligands. Such affinity ligands should exhibit high affinity as well as high selectivity toward a given receptor immobilized on the solid matrix. The affinity labeling of the immunoconjugate must not significantly alter the tumor-binding properties of the immunoconjugate or change the biodistribution in an undesirable way, nor should conjugation enhance the immunogenicity of the immunoconjugate. The linker between the affinity ligand and the immunoconjugate must be stable since the extracorporeal removal of circulating immunoconjugate will be dependent on the presence of accessible affinity ligand on the conjugate. Furthermore, the immobilized receptor must not interfere with blood through activation or inhibition of vital physiologic processes.

The system employing biotin as the affinity ligand in conjunction with avidin or streptavidin immobilized on the adsorbent fulfills most of the above criteria. Biotin is a water-soluble vitamin, usually classified as vitamin H, with a molecular weight of 244 kDa. It has a head region that binds to avidin, and a carboxyl tail that can be chemically modified to a linker that can bind to a protein, for example, a monoclonal antibody, without altering its ability to bind to avidin. Avidin is a 66-kDa glycoprotein obtained from hen's egg consisting of four identical subunits, each with a binding site for biotin (23,24). Biotin has an extremely high affinity to avidin (dissociation constant of 10^{-15} M), and in practical terms binding is irreversible. A very efficient affinity adsorbent can thus be produced by immobilizing avidin on a solid matrix. The strong binding results in very little

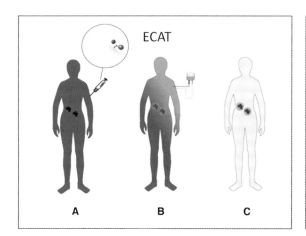
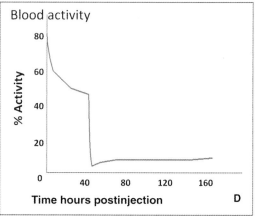

FIGURE 15.1 The use of extracorporeal depletion in radioimmunotherapy. **A:** The biotinylated radioimmunoconjugate is administered to the patient. **B:** After a suitable amount of time to allow uptake of the radioimmunoconjugate in the tumor, the radioimmunoconjugate circulating in the blood is removed by extracorporeal depletion. **C:** After depletion, a higher tumor-to-normal activity ratio is obtained, resulting in reduced side effects. **D:** Level of radioimmunoconjugate in the blood during treatment. (Please see Color Insert).

dissociation of bound biotinylated mAbs from the adsorbent, and the biotinylated conjugate in the blood passing through the adsorbent will be completely removed.

Conjugation of the monoclonal antibody

Three separate conjugation procedures are usually required to produce a biotinylated radioimmunoconjugate labeled with radiometals (e.g., ^{111}In, ^{90}Y, ^{177}Lu). First, the mAb is conjugated with a chelator (e.g., DTPA or DOTA) and then radiolabeled with the radionuclide. Finally, the radioimmunoconjugate is conjugated with biotin molecules. Methods for the conjugation of proteins, such as mAbs, with biotin have been thoroughly reviewed (25,26).

In cooperation with Professor Scott Wilbur at the University of Washington, Seattle, United States, we have developed a trifunctional chelator, as shown in Figure 15.2, which is composed of the biotin moiety and the radiolabeling moiety (DOTA) in a single molecule that also contains a reactive group for covalent linkage to the amine groups (lysine) on proteins (27). DOTA was chosen as the chelator because of the higher stability of the radiometal–chelate complex compared to DTPA, which often exhibits dissociation of the radiometal from the metal chelate (28,29). An aspartic acid moiety is incorporated next to the biotin moiety to block the endogenous biotin-cleaving enzyme biotinidase (30,31). By using this trifunctional reagent, one of the conjugation procedures can be omitted, and the unnecessary exposure of the mAb to various conjugation chemicals and conditions is minimized. Moreover, the heterogeneity of the radioimmunoconjugate is reduced, as identical numbers of biotin molecules and chelators are always present on each conjugate molecule, and a minimum number of conjugation reagents or moieties can be used.

To achieve sufficiently high binding to the avidin adsorbent, and therefore efficient depletion, without significantly changing the antigen-binding or tumor-targeting properties of the radioimmunoconjugate, the number of conjugated affinity ligands (biotin moieties) should be limited, but high enough to ensure that almost all the conjugate molecules carry at least one biotin residue. The optimal number varies for different mAbs and also depends on the conditions used

during extracorporeal removal, but two to three biotin residues per mAb has been shown to be appropriate for most mAbs studied to date.

The hemoadsorption system

Our group has developed an affinity adsorbent for the binding of biotinylated immunoconjugates based on avidin–agarose. The solid agarose matrix consists of beads of a cross-linked form of a polysaccharide polymer material. Initial animal studies showed that extracorporeal antibody removal from plasma was possible (32–34). Further studies showed that biotin–avidin binding could be performed in whole blood when the bead size was increased, to prevent the entrapment of blood cells during the passage of the blood through the adsorbent (16,35). However, the beads must not be too large as this will increase the diffusion distance in and out of the agarose beads, resulting in unfavorable binding kinetics and a reduction in efficiency, that is, a lower clearance rate. Extracorporeal depletion from whole blood is advantageous as no plasma separation is necessary. This simplifies the process, making it easier to use in the clinical setting. It is essential that no hemolysis takes place in the system and that blood clots are not formed in the adsorbent or the patient. Citrate is therefore added to the blood before it enters the adsorbent to inhibit the activation of plasmatic coagulation and the complement system. The optimal level of citrate and the hemocompatibility properties of the hemoadsorption system have been evaluated on human subjects (36). A hemoadsorption system using the same avidin–agarose adsorbent for extracorporeal depletion in nonhuman primates (macaque monkeys) has also been evaluated (20).

On the basis of the experience obtained from the animal studies, a hemoadsorption system for clinical use was developed. The system is based on the avidin–agarose adsorbent described above. The safety (22) and efficacy (21) of the hemoadsorption device in clinical use have been evaluated in humans, and approval and marketing authorization as a CE-labeled device have been obtained from the European authorities.

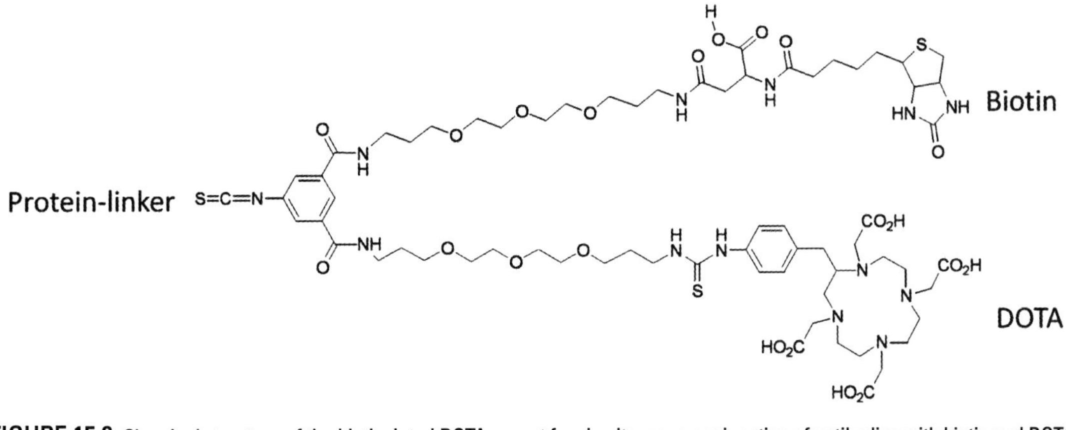

FIGURE 15.2 Chemical structure of the biotinylated DOTA regent for simultaneous conjugation of antibodies with biotin and DOTA.

ECAT STUDIES IN A SYNGENEIC RAT TUMOR MODEL

Our group at Lund University has been studying ECAT in rats since 1987. Most of the studies have been conducted using a syngeneic rat colon carcinoma tumor line (BN7005), grown in the immunocompetent Brown Norwegian (BN) strain. This inbred rat strain has a fully developed immune system, which we believe is important, as the interaction with, and influence on, the immune system during radioimmunotherapy is increasingly being regarded as important (37). Chemically induced rat colon carcinoma in syngeneic immunocompetent rat strains shares many characteristics with human colon adenocarcinomas, and is therefore a useful model to test new radioimmunotherapeutic concepts. The BN7005 tumor cell line expresses an epitope that is reactive with the blood group antigen Lewis Y on the cell surface. The BN rats also express this epitope in some radiosensitive organs, such as the gastrointestinal tract (esophagus, stomach, intestines, pancreas), hence mimicking the human situation (38). A chimeric (mouse/human) monoclonal IgG1 antibody, BR96 (Seattle Genetics Inc., Seattle, WA), binding the tumor-associated Lewis Y glycoprotein, was used as the targeting molecule in our experimental studies. The extracorporeal affinity adsorption system used for these rat studies is schematically illustrated in Figure 15.3. The adsorbent contains 1.5 mL avidin–agarose, and the entire extracorporeal volume is about 3.5 mL. The extracorporeal system and procedure have been described in detail by Martensson et al. (39).

Antibody conjugation

In several animal studies using different mAbs and different radionuclides (^{125}I, ^{188}Re, ^{111}In, ^{90}Y, ^{177}Lu,), we have shown that biotinylation of radiolabeled mAbs does not result in any major change in the pharmacokinetics or tissue distribution compared to nonbiotinylated radiolabeled mAbs (33,40). We have also shown that different mAbs conjugated with the biotinylated DOTA reagent have comparable pharmacokinetics (41).

Efficiency of extracorporeal depletion

Extracorporeal affinity adsorption is usually performed for 2 to 3 hours. During this time, the blood volume of the rat is processed about three times, and 90% to 95% of the radioimmunoconjugate circulating in the blood is removed. This is close to the theoretically possible removal when processing three volumes of blood (42). Therefore, it can be concluded that the adsorption process is very efficient.

The level of whole-body activity is generally reduced by 40% to 60%, and the radioactivity in the bone marrow, livers, kidneys, lungs, pancreas, and bowel directly after the completion of ECAT is similarly reduced, by 40% to 70% (16). Most of the reduction in the activity in the various organs results from the depletion of radioimmunoconjugates from the blood vessels in the organs, although there is some reduction in extravascular activity after redistribution to the blood.

Effects on tumor levels of radioimmunoconjugate

In our rat colon carcinoma model, the maximal uptake in tumor (percentage of injected activity per gram) was reached about 24 hours postinjection. Directly after the completion of ECAT, performed 24 hours postinjection, the activity in the tumor had decreased by 15% to 20%, which corresponds to the activity in the blood content of the tumor (19). In animals not subjected to ECAT, the tumor activity remained constant for 72 hours, while it decreased with time after completion of the procedure in animals subjected to ECAT (Fig. 15.4). This indicates that radioimmunoconjugates

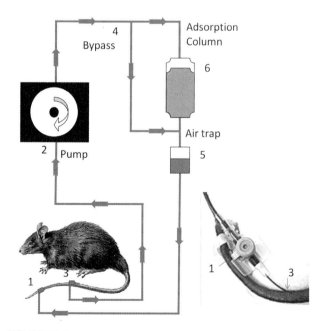

FIGURE 15.3 Illustration of ECAT in rats. A cannula is inserted into one of the lateral tail veins for the return of blood *(1)*, and this is connected to the extracorporeal system, regulated by a pump *(2)*. Another cannula is inserted into the ventral tail artery for blood access *(3)*. When the cannulae have been correctly inserted, the extracorporeal circulation is started in bypass mode *(4)*, that is, without the column connected. Once the circuit is filled with blood and any air bubbles in the circuit have been collected in the air trap *(5)*, the column *(6)* is connected to the circuit and affinity adsorption is started.

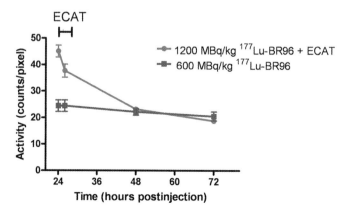

FIGURE 15.4 Activity accumulation in tumors after treatment with ^{177}Lu-labeled and biotinylated BR96 antibody. Rats were given 600 MBq/kg ^{177}Lu-BR96 without ECAT and 1200 MBq/kg ^{177}Lu-BR96 in combination with ECAT, at 24 hours postinjection.

continue to accumulate in tumors from the blood in rats not subjected to ECAT. In rats given ECAT, the decrease in activity in the tumor tissue is due to both radionuclide decay and redistribution of activity into the vascular volume.

Timing of ECAT postinjection

The kinetics governing the accumulation of the radioimmunoconjugate in the tumor and the blood must be known in order to determine the optimal time for ECAT. The optimal timing for ECAT is a compromise between minimizing the myelotoxicity resulting from exposure of the bone marrow (i.e., a short time after radioimmunoconjugate injection) and allowing a sufficient amount of radioimmunoconjugate to accumulate in the tumor tissue (i.e., a long time). We have investigated the effects of ECAT on the accumulation of radioimmunoconjugates at different times postinjection, using scintillation camera images (43). Subjecting the animals to ECAT 12 hours after the injection of radioimmunoconjugates considerably reduced the activity in tumors (34%), while the reduction was less 24 hours and 48 hours postinjection (both 18%). Imaging also demonstrated that the activity in the volume of blood in the tumors was approximately 33%, 17%, and 13% of the total activity in the tumor at 12, 24, and 48 hours postinjection, respectively. At 12 hours postinjection fewer radioimmunoconjugates have penetrated into the extravascular tumor tissue, and a greater fraction of the tumor activity is due to radioimmunoconjugates in the blood vessels of the tumor. This means that ECAT should be performed later, when the radioimmunoconjugates have accumulated in the tumor tissue. As expected, the timing of ECAT influenced the rate and degree of bone marrow recovery, with earlier recovery in animals subjected to ECAT early after injection (Fig. 15.5). The optimal time for ECAT in rats was thus found to be 24 hours postinjection. At this time, the T/B ratio of the accumulated activity (expressed as the area under the curve [AUC] when the activity was plotted against time postinjection) was maximal.

As most humanized and human mAbs exhibit a longer biologic half-life in the human circulation, the optimal time for ECAT in humans is probably later after injection. The physical half-life of the radionuclide used should also be sufficiently long, that is, corresponding to the biologic half-life of the antibody.

Reduction in dose-limiting toxicity

We have determined the maximal tolerable dose (MTD; defined here as the maximal tolerable activity per kilogram body weight) of the BR96 mAb labeled with ^{90}Y or ^{177}Lu in rats (44), in order to establish a platform for the investigation of the toxicity-reducing potential of ECAT. We have also compared the MTD of ^{90}Y- and ^{177}Lu-labeled immunoconjugates. Increasing activity levels of BR96 labeled with ^{90}Y or ^{177}Lu (MBq/kg body weight) were administered to groups of rats. Since myelotoxicity is generally dose-limiting in radioimmunotherapy, the toxic effect of the radioimmunoconjugates was evaluated by monitoring changes in blood parameters after injection. MTD was defined as the highest activity at which 100% of the animals survived without clinical signs of toxicity, such as infections, bleeding, or diarrhea, and a loss in body weight of less than 20%. The results showed a dose-dependent toxicity for both the radionuclides. In addition, this study showed that the MTD of ^{177}Lu-labeled BR96 was significantly higher than that of the corresponding ^{90}Y-labeled mAb.

The theoretical activities accumulated in the blood and tumor were calculated to predict the effect of ECAT on the myelotoxicity and tumor activity accumulation following radioimmunotherapy (43). Bone marrow dosimetry was not performed because neither the red marrow/blood ratio nor the appropriate S-values are known with sufficiently high accuracy. ECAT was simulated at different times postinjection, by reducing the blood activity to 5%, and calculating the AUC for tumor and blood activity, with the two labeling isotopes, ^{177}Lu and ^{90}Y. The T/B AUC ratio was then calculated after ECAT at each time. The results of these calculations were used

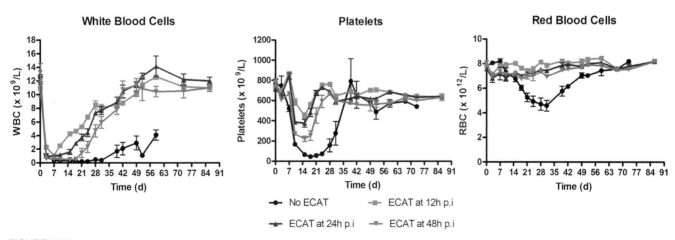

FIGURE 15.5 White blood cell counts, platelet counts, and red blood cell counts as a function of time after injection when rats were injected with 800 MBq/kg ^{177}Lu-labeled biotinylated BR96 antibody and subjected to ECAT 12, 24, and 48 hours after injection. Results from control animals (not subjected to ECAT) are also plotted.

to design the study presented by our group (18). In addition, the values obtained were used to estimate the extent to which it should be possible to increase the administered activity when radioimmunotherapy is combined with ECAT, and how different parameters, such as the timing of ECAT, and the half-life of the radionuclide, would affect this increase. The aim of the study was to evaluate the possibility of decreasing the myelotoxicity associated with radioimmunotherapy by performing ECAT after the administration of radioimmunoconjugate. The optimal combination of radionuclide and the time between injection of the radioimmunoconjugates and the subsequent ECAT was assessed in rats, taking into account both myelotoxicity and the activity in the tumor. Rats were injected with ^{177}Lu- or ^{90}Y-labeled antibody conjugate and the conjugate was subsequently removed from the circulation by ECAT at 12, 24, and 48 hours postinjection. Myelotoxicity was assessed by the analysis of blood parameters for 12 weeks. The effect of ECAT on the tumor activity concentration was evaluated in parallel by gamma camera imaging of rats injected with ^{111}In-labeled immunoconjugate.

Control animals, which were injected with activities corresponding to the maximal tolerable activity and not subjected to ECAT, displayed late-phase toxicity, resulting in acute weight loss combined with signs of dehydration, and had to be sacrificed 8 to 9 weeks after injection. No comparable late-phase toxicity or body weight loss was seen in animals subjected to ECAT. The control animals had not recovered in terms of leukocytes 2 months after injection, whereas all the rats subjected to ECAT showed complete recovery with regard to blood parameters within the same period. Myelotoxicity was thus significantly milder in animals subjected to ECAT than in the controls. The timing of ECAT influenced the rate and degree of bone marrow recovery; earlier recovery was seen in animals subjected to ECAT early postinjection. The toxicity-reducing effect of ECAT was more distinct in animals injected with ^{177}Lu-labeled mAbs than in animals injected with ^{90}Y-labeled mAbs, indicating that the physical half-life of the radionuclide is important for the toxicity-reducing potential of ECAT at a specific time. The longer range of the beta particle from ^{90}Y (maximum range 12 mm) compared to the shorter range of beta particles emitted from ^{177}Lu (maximum range 1.5 mm) also contributes to a higher absorbed dose in the bone marrow due to cross-dose from the surrounding tissue. This difference in toxic effect of cross-dose is more evident in small animals and less important in humans because of the greater distances between adjacent organs.

It was found that the MTD of ^{177}Lu-labeled BR96 could be doubled, and that of ^{90}Y-labeled BR96 increased 1.5 times, when radioimmunotherapy was combined with ECAT 24 hours postinjection.

Therapeutic effects of radioimmunotherapy in combination with ECAT

Groups of rats with a manifest tumor ($\sim 10 \times 15$ mm) treated with ^{177}Lu-biotin-BR96 at $2 \times$ MTD (1200 MBq/kg) in combination with ECAT at 24 hours postinjection were compared to rats treated with ^{177}Lu-biotin-BR96 at MTD (600 MBq/kg) without ECAT (19). Other groups of rats were treated with ^{90}Y-biotin-BR96 at $1.5 \times$ MTD (525 MBq/kg) in combination with ECAT at 24 hours postinjection, and were compared to rats treated with ^{90}Y-biotin-BR96 at MTD (350 MBq/kg) without ECAT. All rats treated with the radiolabeled immunoconjugates exhibited persistent, local, complete response within 16 days postinjection, regardless of the radionuclide or activity administered. Complete remission was defined as a tumor that had regressed completely and was not palpable for at least a week. Since complete remission was also achieved in the groups of animals given a lower activity and not subjected to ECAT, it was not possible to determine a dose-response relationship, and it was difficult to draw conclusions concerning the therapeutic benefit of ECAT. However, the use of ECAT made it possible to administer an activity twice the maximal tolerable without increased toxicity. A doubling in administered activity results in a higher absorbed dose to the tumor, which is generally correlated to increased therapeutic efficacy. The therapeutic effects seen are probably attributable to the more favorable "radiation sensitivity ratio" between tumor and bone marrow of rats than that of humans. The BN7005 cell line has an intermediate radiosensitivity; the survival fraction after exposure to 2-Gy low-LET radiation is 0.5 (unpublished data). These findings are also supported by a higher $LD_{50/60}$ (lethal dose for 50% to 60% of exposed individuals) in rodents than in humans. To discern a difference in therapeutic effects in rodents when using ECAT, suboptimal activities with respect to tumor effect must be administered.

Dosimetric aspects of ECAT in experimental animals

The radionuclides mentioned previously, commonly used for radioimmunotherapy, are beta emitters, and the range of beta particles is comparable to the size of the organs in experimental animals such as mice and rats. This means that there is a considerable cross-dose in these animals. Therefore, good geometric models of these species are required for reliable dosimetry. In humans, however, the range of beta particles is much shorter than the dimensions of the organs, and the self-dose to the organ dominates.

Simplified models of rats based on the geometrical shapes of the major organs have been developed by Hindorf et al. (45). In recent years, more anatomically realistic computer phantoms have been developed for simulation studies of small-animal microSPECT/microPET/microCT imaging. An example of these types of "computer phantoms" is the Moby phantom (46). Moby is based on NURB (non-uniform rational basis) spline surfaces that allow for considerable flexibility in defining the properties of a particular mouse, and produces transverse images of mice with arbitrary spatial resolution. The dimensions of the organs of the mouse are provided in an input file. The phantom is also dynamic in the sense that the transverse images can be created at different times during the respiratory and cardiac cycles.

Modifications can also be made to the shape, size, and locations of the internal organs in order to create mouse populations. Another simulation program, based on image data obtained using a dedicated small-animal computed tomography (CT) scanner, has recently been published (47).

It is also necessary to be able to calculate S-values for the small animals, since tabulated S-values are not generally available, as for humans. An S-value describes the absorbed dose in a target volume per unit activity in a source volume. The absorbed dose to the target can then be obtained by multiplying the residence time of the radionuclide in the source organ by the S-value for the particular source/target configuration. Examples of Monte Carlo programs in the public domain that can do this are the EGS (electron gamma shower) family of programs (EGS4 and EGSnrc), and Monte Carlo neutron protein crystallography (MCNPX). An important component in dosimetry is the measurement of time–activity curves for different organs in the animal. Until now, this has mainly been done using planar scintillation cameras or human single photon emission computed tomography (SPECT) systems with parallel-hole or pinhole collimators. However, the latter have a relatively poor spatial resolution in animal imaging. The development of commercial small-animal systems has been very rapid during the past 5 years, and systems are available today for both SPECT and positron emission tomography (PET) in combination with CT, which have a very high spatial resolution and the facility for coregistration of CT images. Both CT images and image fusion can be used for attenuation corrections and Monte Carlo–based three-dimensional (3D) dosimetry.

In our previous studies of the biokinetics in animals in association with ECAT, we used planar imaging with either parallel-hole collimators or pinhole collimators. The spatial resolution in these settings is about 5 mm with parallel-hole collimators and 2 mm with pinhole collimators. More detailed pharmacokinetic studies can be performed with higher-resolution methods such as microSPECT and microPET to obtain more accurate absorbed dose estimates from the biodistribution data. Single-pinhole SPECT was introduced in the 1990s (48,49). Small-animal SPECT systems allow the imaging of the anatomy of living mice with a spatial resolution of 50 to 200 μm. Today, state-of-the-art PET systems have a spatial resolution of 1.5 mm or better, which provides an adequate field of view for whole-body imaging of mice. With this new imaging technology, the optimization of ECAT will be possible using pharmacokinetic modeling and parametric imaging. For studies on the outcome of radioimmunotherapy, accurate dosimetry models should be used, taking into account S-values, the geometry of the animals, and cross-doses (50).

ECAT STUDIES IN A NONHUMAN PRIMATE MODEL

At the Fred Hutchinson Cancer Center in Seattle, United States, Nemecek and coworkers (20) applied ECAT to tumor-free macaques. One blood volume per hour was passed through an avidin–agarose adsorbent for 3 hours, 24 hours after an intravenous injection of [111]In- or ^{177}Lu–biotin–rituximab. Serial blood, bone marrow, and lymph node samples, gamma-camera images, and necropsy tissues were obtained to estimate the absorbed doses in organs of interest. As a result of ECAT, the radiation doses were reduced in analyzed organs: kidneys (49% ± 12%), liver (42% ± 10%), lungs (60% ± 6%), bone marrow (50% ± 15%), spleen (38% ± 10%), and lymph nodes (19% ± 3%), while the whole-body dose was reduced by 51% ± 16%. Despite the reduction in both target (spleen and lymph nodes) and nontarget tissues, therapeutic ratios were significantly higher in animals treated with ECAT than in the controls.

No abnormalities were observed in serum electrolytes, liver transaminases, creatinine, blood counts, serum complements, or coagulation panel tests at any point in time. No side effects attributable to the antibody or ECAT were found. Vital signs, general status, and blood coagulation were not affected by ECAT. The advantages of this model, compared to the rat tumor model, are that the bone marrow sensitivity and the body size are more similar to those of humans. The disadvantage is that the lymph nodes and spleen are used as surrogate CD20 targets, since the animals did not have any tumors. Flow cytometry measurements of cell suspensions showed 4% to 20% and 3% to 15% CD20-positive cells in macaque lymph nodes and spleen, respectively. Much better targeting is anticipated in human lymphoma patients, where 20% to 99% of lymph node cells are expected to express the CD20 antigen. Nemecek et al. (20) also suggested the study of cynomolgus monkeys infected with simian immunodeficiency virus, since these animals have increased expression of CD20-positive cells in lymphopoietic tissues, and most develop B-cell lymphoma with time.

ECAT STUDIES IN HUMANS

Extracorporeal affinity depletion system for clinical use

On the basis of the knowledge gained from the studies using the syngeneic rat tumor model, an affinity adsorption device for clinical use in humans was developed by Mitra Medical Technology AB, Lund, Sweden (Fig. 15.6). The adsorbent is based on the avidin–agarose matrix for the treatment of whole blood. In cooperation with Fresenius SE (Germany), the company developed a hemoadsorption monitor for the control and monitoring of the extracorporeal affinity adsorption process in humans. The system consists of an adsorption monitor with blood and anticoagulant pumps, and various pressure monitors used for monitoring of process and safety. The adsorbent and the hemoadsorption system have gained approval and marketing authorization from the authorities in Europe as a CE-labeled device for depletion of biotinylated substances from human whole blood.

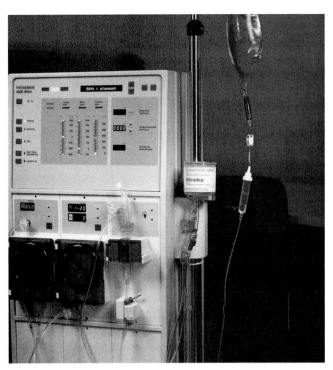

FIGURE 15.6 The hemoadsorption monitor (Fresenius Mitra 4008) and the avidin adsorbent (Mitradep) developed for clinical application of ECAT.

During ECAT, the blood flow rate is typically 60 to 80 mL/min; thus, three times the blood volume of the patient is processed in under 3 hours. Coagulation is prevented by a bolus dose of heparin to the patient, and continuous infusion of acid citrate dextrose solution (ACD-A) to the extracorporeal circuit. This is sufficient to overcome the thrombogenicity of the extracorporeal system, preventing thrombotic episodes and bleeding in the patients.

Evaluation of safety and efficiency

The safety and efficiency of hemoadsorption has been evaluated in humans (21,22). Eight patients with refractory B-cell lymphoma (all but one of whom had aggressive or mantle cell B-cell lymphoma), who had failed to respond to standard therapies, received infusions of 250 mg/m^2 nonconjugated rituximab, and 150 MBq ^{111}In–rituximab–biotin for immunoscintigraphy. A week later, the patients were treated with another 250 mg/m^2 rituximab followed by ^{111}In/^{90}Y–rituximab–biotin (11 to 15 MBq ^{90}Y/kg body weight). ECAT was performed 48 hours later. All eight patients showed tumor uptake. The mean depletion of ^{90}Y–rituximab–biotin after ECAT was 96% in whole blood, 49% in the whole body, 62% in the lungs, and 40% in the liver and kidneys. A further nine patients with relapsing B-cell lymphoma received 18 or 21 MBq/kg body weight without showing any dose-limiting toxicity, 1.5 × MTD for Zevalin (unpublished data). This dose-escalation study was unfortunately stopped due to economical problems for the company responsible for the clinical implementation.

During the same clinical investigation, the biocompatibility of the affinity adsorbent was evaluated (22). Blood components, plasma complement fragments, C3a and C5a, and plasma bradykinin were analyzed during ECAT and other laboratory tests were monitored during the study. Clinical observations made during ECAT indicated neither any signs of fatigue or exhaustion nor any significant differences noted in heart rate, systolic or diastolic blood pressure, or body temperature. No fever, shivering, chills, or respiratory difficulties were observed. The only severe clinical problem experienced was a catheter-related septicemia occurring in one patient. A slight decrease in blood hemoglobin was observed (8.3% compared to pretreatment values), but there were no signs of hemolysis. Some decrease in blood thrombocytes (11.4% of pretreatment values) and plasma albumin (14.3% of pretreatment values) was observed, but these could be explained by the dilution of the blood with normal saline and ACD-A during the procedure. The avidin adsorbent had no effect on the patient's blood cells, immunologic status, or plasma bradykinin level. This study confirmed the ability of ECAT to remove unbound radioactivity from the blood, and reduce the exposure of nontarget organs to radiolabeled mAbs in a clinical setting.

Implementing ECAT at the optimal time after administration of an internalizing antibody such as epratuzumab (humanized antiCD22) may allow the delivery of higher absorbed doses than is possible with conventional radioimmunotherapy, by the removal of residual, nonspecific unbound activity. Another alternative to improve therapeutic ratios is the use of antigens that are present at higher copy numbers in target tissues, such as CD45.

Dosimetry in patients treated with ECAT

Determination of the absorbed dose relies on an accurate calculation of the number of disintegrations during a specific period per unit administered activity, and data must be measured at a minimum of three points in time to fit an exponential function to the time–activity curve. For a patient not undergoing ECAT this period is normally from the time of injection to infinity. When ECAT is employed, two exponential functions must be fitted: one before ECAT and one after, and thus a minimum of six measurements must be made. The accuracy in the dosimetry is thus very dependent on the number of activity measurements. Dosimetry can be based on a two-dimensional (2D) imaging protocol using conjugate view–based planar scintillation camera images, or sequential SPECT measurements. The latter is advantageous as it is a 3D method, and the problems associated with planar methods, such as overlapping activity uptake, background contribution, and inaccuracies in attenuation and scatter corrections, can be avoided. The iterative reconstruction methods MLEM/OSEM with its possibility to include compensation for nonhomogeneous attenuation scatter in the patient and collimator response makes SPECT a truly quantitative method. However, the limited axial field of view in SPECT may present a problem when performing dosimetry for multiple organs. Combined SPECT/CT systems make 3D dosimetry possible for routine dosimetry protocols, by multiple time point SPECT/CT imaging. Since SPECT allows for suborgan dosimetry, a consistent delineation of volumes of interest (VOIs) in each of the SPECT/CT studies is essential. The CT information, coaligned to the SPECT studies based on hardware, can be used for VOI delineation in each time point image. If one single set of VOIs is to be used for all time points, then accurate image coregistration becomes necessary. The anatomical information in the CT studies can then be used to coregister the SPECT/CT studies from the different time points. Coregistered studies also allow for calculation of voxel-based time–activity curves for mapping of the 3D distribution of absorbed dose.

The dosimetry performed in the ECAT study in Lund (21) was based on the LundADose software (51). Planar-based dosimetry was performed for normal organs, whereas SPECT/CT was used for tumor dosimetry. One potential problem associated with ECAT, which must be considered, is that the circulating activity also contributes to the absorbed dose in tumors. This is of special importance for long-range beta-emitting radionuclides, such as ^{90}Y, which also irradiate the extravascular space. When applying ECAT to reduce the circulating blood activity, the absorbed dose to the tumor may also be reduced, requiring compensation by an increase in the activity administered in order to obtain the prescribed absorbed dose. The pharmacokinetics of ECAT can be evaluated and modeled with compartment analysis, and evaluated in all organs and tissues (15,52) to give a better understanding of the biokinetics. Using patient biokinetics data from pretherapy studies has shown the usefulness of compartment modeling to predict the biokinetics of radioimmunotherapy including the ECAT procedure (53). This gives the possibility of treatment planning with optimal choice of time for ECAT.

IMPROVING PRETARGETING WITH ECAT

Pretargeting has been shown to improve the T/B ratio in several preclinical trials and a few clinical studies (9). We have investigated whether ECAT could be used in combination with a pretargeting protocol, and evaluated the possibility of reducing the accumulation of radioactivity in radiosensitive organs (18). Rats were first injected with biotinylated BR96 antibodies and subjected to ECAT 24 hours postinjection to remove the antibodies from the circulation. The animals were then injected with ^{111}In–DOTA–streptavidin. In the third step, the animals were again subjected to ECAT after the injection of ^{111}In–DOTA–streptavidin to remove the DOTA–streptavidin from the circulation. In this ECAT the avidin–agarose column was coated with a biotin trimer to allow the selective adsorption of streptavidin from blood (54). The biodistribution and tumor-targeting capacity of DOTA–streptavidin were then determined.

Elimination of the biotinylated antibody by ECAT prior to the injection of DOTA–streptavidin increased the tumor targeting by 50%. In addition, the levels of DOTA–streptavidin in the liver and lymph nodes were reduced by 60%, which implies 4.3-fold and 3.8-fold increases in tumor/liver and tumor/lymph node ratios, respectively. ECAT was thus shown to be an efficient means of removing biotinylated antibodies, and would probably also be efficient in removing antibodies in other pretargeting strategies, for example, for clearance of streptavidin-conjugated antibody constructs. However, the use of ECAT to remove radiolabeled streptavidin does not seem to offer any advantage as the tumor accumulation was reduced to the same extent as in normal tissues. This was probably due to the fact that ECAT was performed too early, before maximal tumor penetration and binding of ^{111}In–DOTA–streptavidin had been achieved. A further delay of the ECAT would probably have resulted in higher tumor retention, but reduced depletion as the blood levels would have been lower. Because only 25% of the ^{111}In–DOTA–streptavidin was left in the blood 8 hours after injection, a further delay would minimize the activity-reducing potential of ECAT in blood and normal tissues.

SUMMARY

ECAT can safely and efficiently reduce myelotoxicity associated with radioimmunotherapy. By using ECAT, it is also possible to significantly reduce the toxicity in other radiosensitive vital organs, that is, the lungs, kidneys, and liver. ECAT allows higher levels of activity to be administered, with the aim of increasing the absorbed dose to the tumor, without increasing the toxicity. ECAT has been applied in a syngeneic rat tumor model, in a nonhuman primate model, and in human beings with corresponding results regarding the reduction in the amount of nonspecific radiation by extracorporeal depletion. ECAT also facilitates the delivery of higher activities of radiation by virtue of decreased toxicity to normal organs.

Acknowledgments

The ECAT studies in macaque monkeys were performed by OW Press and coworkers at the Fred Hutchinson Cancer Center, Seattle, United States. We would like to thank Dr. Peter Senter (Seattle Genetics, Seattle, WA) for kindly providing the monoclonal antibody BR96. We also acknowledge the contributions from all our former and present coworkers at the Department of Oncology, Department of Medical Radiation Physics at Lund University, and the Department of Oncology at Lund University Hospital. The research conducted by the authors has been supported by grants from the Swedish Research Council, the Swedish Cancer Society, the Swedish Medical Society, Mrs. Berta Kamprad's Foundation, Gunnar Nilsson's Foundation, the Lund University Medical Faculty Foundation, and the Lund University Hospital Fund.

■ REFERENCES

1. Jain RK. Delivery of molecular and cellular medicine to solid tumors. *Adv Drug Deliv Rev.* 2001;46(1–3):149–168.
2. Thurber GM, Schmidt MM, Wittrup KD. Antibody tumor penetration: transport opposed by systemic and antigen-mediated clearance. *Adv Drug Deliv Rev.* 2008;60(12):1421–1434.
3. Ullen A, Ahlstrom KR, Hietala SO, et al. Secondary antibodies as tools to improve tumor to non tumor ratio at radioimmunolocalisation and radioimmunotherapy. *Acta Oncol.* 1996;35(3):281–285.
4. Sandstrom P, Johansson A, Ullen A, et al. Idiotypic–anti-idiotypic antibody interactions in experimental radioimmunotargeting. *Clin Cancer Res.* 1999;5(10suppl):3073s–3078s.
5. Kobayashi H, Sakahara H, Hosono M, et al. Improved clearance of radiolabeled biotinylated monoclonal antibody following the infusion of avidin as a "chase" without decreased accumulation in the target tumor. *J Nucl Med.* 1994;35(10):1677–1684.
6. Marshall D, Pedley RB, Boden JA, et al. Clearance of circulating radioantibodies using streptavidin or second antibodies in a xenograft model. *Br J Cancer.* 1994;69(3):502–507.
7. Paganelli G, Stella M, Zito F, et al. Radioimmunoguided surgery using iodine-125-labeled biotinylated monoclonal antibodies and cold avidin. *J Nucl Med.* 1994;35(12):1970–1975.
8. Chen JQ, Strand SE, Tannvall J, et al. Extracorporeal immunoadsorption compared to avidin chase: enhancement of tumor-to-normal tissue ratio for biotinylated rhenium-188-chimeric BR96. *J Nucl Med.* 1997;38(12):1934–1939.
9. Goldenberg DM, Sharkey RM, Paganelli G, et al. Antibody pretargeting advances cancer radioimmunodetection and radioimmunotherapy. *J Clin Oncol.* 2006;24(5):823–834.
10. Wahl RL, Piko CR, Beers BA, et al. Systemic perfusion: a method of enhancing relative tumor uptake of radiolabeled monoclonal antibodies. *Int J Rad Appl Instrum B.* 1988;15(6):611–616.
11. Strand SE, Norrgren K, Ingvar C, et al. Plasmapheresis as a tool for enhancing contrast in radioimmunoimaging and modifying absorbed dose in radioimmunotherapy. *Med Phys.* 1989;16:465.
12. Nilsson R, Lindgren L, Lilliehorn P. Extracorporeal immunoadsorption therapy on rats. In vivo depletion of specific antibodies. *Clin Exp Immunol.* 1990;82(3):440–444.
13. Lear JL, Kasliwal RK, Feyerabend AJ, et al. Improved tumor imaging with radiolabeled monoclonal antibodies by plasma clearance of unbound antibody with anti-antibody column. *Radiology.* 1991;179(2):509–512.
14. DeNardo GL, Maddock SW, Sgouros G, et al. Immunoadsorption: an enhancement strategy for radioimmunotherapy. *J Nucl Med.* 1993;34(6):1020–1027.
15. Norrgren K, Strand SE, Ingvar C. Contrast enhancement in RIT and modification of the therapeutic ratio in RIT: a theoretical evaluation of simulated extracorporeal immunoadsorption. *Antibody Immunoconj Radiopharm.* 1992;5:61–73.
16. Garkavij M, Tennvall J, Strand SE, et al. Extracorporeal whole-blood immunoadsorption enhances radioimmunotargeting of iodine-125-labeled BR96-biotin monoclonal antibody. *J Nucl Med.* 1997;38(6):895–901.
17. Tennvall J, Garkavij M, Chen JQ, et al. Improving tumor-to-normal-tissue ratios of antibodies by extracorporeal immunoadsorption based on the avidin–biotin concept: development of a new treatment strategy applied to monoclonal antibodies murine L6 and chimeric BR96. *Cancer.* 1997;80(12suppl):2411–2418.
18. Martensson L, Nilsson R, Ohlsson T, et al. Improved tumor targeting and decreased normal tissue accumulation through extracorporeal affinity adsorption in a two-step pretargeting strategy. *Clin Cancer Res.* 2007;13(18 pt 2):5572s–5576s.
19. Martensson L, Nilsson R, Ohlsson T, et al. High-dose radioimmunotherapy combined with extracorporeal depletion in a syngeneic rat tumor model—evaluation of toxicity, therapeutic effect and tumor model. *Cancer Biother Radiopharm.* 2008;23(4):517 (Abstract 14, Twelfth Conference on Cancer Therapy with Antibodies and Immunoconjugates, Parsippany, NJ, October 16–18, 2008).
20. Nemecek ER, Green DJ, Fisher DR, et al. Extracorporeal adsorption therapy: a method to improve targeted radiation delivered by radiometal-labeled monoclonal antibodies. *Cancer Biother Radiopharm.* 2008;23(2):181–191.
21. Linden O, Kurkus J, Garkavij M, et al. A novel platform for radioimmunotherapy: extracorporeal depletion of biotinylated and ^{90}Y-labeled

22. Kurkus J, Nilsson R, Linden O, et al. Biocompatibility of a novel avidin–agarose adsorbent for extracorporeal removal of redundant radiopharmaceutical from the blood. *Artif Organs.* 2007;31(3):208–214.
23. Wilchek M, Bayer EA. Biotin-containing reagents. *Methods Enzymol.* 1990;184:123–138.
24. Wilchek M, Bayer EA. Introduction to avidin–biotin technology. *Methods Enzymol.* 1990;184:5–13.
25. Bayer EA, Wilchek M. Protein biotinylation. *Methods Enzymol.* 1990;184:138–160.
26. Wilchek M, Bayer EA. Applications of avidin–biotin technology: literature survey. *Methods Enzymol.* 1990;184:14–45.
27. Wilbur DS, Chyan MK, Hamlin DK, et al. Trifunctional conjugation reagents. Reagents that contain a biotin and a radiometal chelation moiety for application to extracorporeal affinity adsorption of radiolabeled antibodies. *Bioconjug Chem.* 2002;13(5):1079–1092.
28. Deshpande SV, DeNardo SJ, Kukis DL, et al. Yttrium-90-labeled monoclonal antibody for therapy: labeling by a new macrocyclic bifunctional chelating agent. *J Nucl Med.* 1990;31(4):473–479.
29. Liu S. Bifunctional coupling agents for radiolabeling of biomolecules and target-specific delivery of metallic radionuclides. *Adv Drug Deliv Rev.* 2008;60(12):1347–1370.
30. Wilbur DS, Hamlin DK, Chyan MK, et al. Biotin reagents for antibody pretargeting. 5. Additional studies of biotin conjugate design to provide biotinidase stability. *Bioconjug Chem.* 2001;12(4):616–623.
31. Wilbur DS, Hamlin DK, Chyan MK. Biotin reagents for antibody pretargeting. 7. Investigation of chemically inert biotinidase blocking functionalities for synthetic utility. *Bioconjug Chem.* 2006;17(6):1514–1522.
32. Norrgren K, Strand SE, Nilsson R, et al. Evaluation of extracorporeal immunoadsorption for reduction of the blood background in diagnostic and therapeutic applications of radiolabelled monoclonal antibodies. *Antibody Immunoconj Radiopharm.* 1991;4:907–914.
33. Norrgren K, Strand SE, Nilsson R, et al. A general, extracorporeal immunoadsorption method to increase the tumor-to-normal tissue ratio in radioimmunoimaging and radioimmunotherapy. *J Nucl Med.* 1993;34(3):448–454.
34. Garkavij M, Tennvall J, Strand SE, et al. Improving radioimmunotargeting of tumors: the impact of preloading unlabeled L6 monoclonal antibody on the biodistribution of 125I-L6 in rats. *J Nucl Biol Med.* 1994;38(4):594–600.
35. Garkavij M, Tennvall J, Strand SE, et al. Extracorporeal immunoadsorption from whole blood based on the avidin–biotin concept. Evaluation of a new method. *Acta Oncol.* 1996;35(3):309–312.
36. Bosch T, Lennertz A, Durh C, et al. Ex vivo biocompatibility of avidin–agarose: a new device for direct adsorption of biotinylated antibodies from human whole blood. *Artif Organs.* 2000;24(9):696–704.
37. Green DR, Ferguson T, Ziivtogel L, et al. Immunogenic and tolerogenic cell death. *Nat Rev Immunol.* 2009;9(5):353–363.
38. Sjogren HO, Isaksson M, Willner D, et al. Antitumor activity of carcinoma-reactive BR96-doxorubicin conjugate against human carcinomas in athymic mice and rats and syngeneic rat carcinomas in immunocompetent rats. *Cancer Res.* 1997;57(20):4530–4536.
39. Martensson L, Nilsson R, Sjogren HO, et al. A nonsurgical technique for blood access in extracorporeal affinity adsorption of antibodies in rats. *Artif Organs.* 2007;31(4):312–316.
40. Chen JQ, Strand SE, Sjogren HO, et al. Combination of biotinylation and indium-111 labeling with chelate SCN-Bz-CHX-A-DTPA for chimeric BR96: biodistribution and pharmacokinetic studies in colon carcinoma isografted rats. *Tumor Target.* 1996;2:66–75.
41. Wang Z, Martensson L, Nilsson R, et al. Blood pharmacokinetics of various monoclonal antibodies labeled with a new trifunctional chelating reagent for simultaneous conjugation with 1,4,7,10-tetraazacyclododecane-N,N',N'',N'''-tetraacetic acid and biotin before radiolabeling. *Clin Cancer Res.* 2005;11(19 pt 2):7171s–7177s.
42. Schindhelm K. Transport and kinetics in synthetic and immunospecific adsorption columns. *Artif Organs.* 1989;13(1):21–27.
43. Martensson L, Nilsson R, Ohlsson T, et al. Reduced myelotoxicity with sustained tumor concentration of radioimmunoconjugates in rats after extracorporeal depletion. *J Nucl Med.* 2007;48(2):269–276.
44. Martensson L, Wang Z, Nilsson R, et al. Determining maximal tolerable dose of the monoclonal antibody BR96 labeled with ^{90}Y or ^{177}Lu in rats: establishment of a syngeneic tumor model to evaluate means to improve radioimmunotherapy. *Clin Cancer Res.* 2005;11(19 pt 2):7104s–7108s.

rituximab in patients with refractory B-cell lymphoma. *Cancer Biother Radiopharm.* 2005;20(4):457–466.

45. Hindorf C, Ljungberg M, Strand SE. Evaluation of parameters influencing S values in mouse dosimetry. *J Nucl Med*. 2004;45(11):1960–1965.

46. Segars WP, Tsui BMW, Frey EC, et al. Development of a 4-D digital mouse phantom for molecular imaging research. *Mol Imaging Biol*. 2004;6(3):149–159.

47. Stabin MG, Peterson TE, Holburn GE, et al. Voxel-based mouse and rat models for internal dose calculations. *J Nucl Med*. 2006;47(4):655–659.

48. Strand SE, Ivanovic M, Erlandsson K, et al. High resolution pinhole SPECT for tumor imaging. *Acta Oncol*. 1993;32(7–8):861–867.

49. Weber DA, Ivanovic M, Franceschi D, et al. Pinhole SPECT: an approach to in vivo high resolution SPECT imaging in small laboratory animals. *J Nucl Med*. 1994;35(2):342–348.

50. Larsson E, Ljungberg M, Segars W, et al. Dosimetry for Norwegian rats based on Monte Carlo simulations using a realistic rat phantom and kinetics for ^{177}Lu- and ^{90}Y-BR96 monoclonal antibodies. *J Nucl Med*. 2009;50:1860.

51. Sjogreen K, Ljungberg M, Wingardh K, et al. The LundADose method for planar image activity quantification and absorbed-dose assessment in radionuclide therapy. *Cancer Biother Radiopharm*. 2005;20(1):92–97.

52. Strand SE, Zanzonico P, Johnson TK. Pharmacokinetic modeling. *Med Phys*. 1993;20(2 pt 2):515–527.

53. Nickel M, Strand SE, Linden O, et al. Development and evaluation of a pharmacokinetic model for prediction of radioimmunotherapy based on pretherapy data. *Cancer Biother Radiopharm*. 2009;24(1):111–122.

54. Wilbur DS, Pathare PM, Hamlin DK, et al. Biotin reagents for antibody pretargeting. 2. Synthesis and in vitro evaluation of biotin dimers and trimers for cross-linking of streptavidin. *Bioconjug Chem*. 1997;8(6):819–832.

Combined Modality Therapy: Relevance for Targeted Radionuclide Therapy

Fares Al-Ejeh and Michael P. Brown

■ INTRODUCTION

Inherent in the technology of targeted radionuclide therapy (TRT) is the promise of cure of occult and small-volume metastatic disease by tumor-selective delivery of radioactivity, which should thus limit normal tissue toxicity (1). Most clinical studies of TRT have used β-emitters, which have low linear energy transfer (LET) and are most effective in tissues with a high oxygen tension (2) such as small-volume metastases (3). Because of the exquisite specificity of monoclonal antibodies (mAbs), radioimmunotherapy (RIT) has been the most thoroughly investigated type of TRT. Even though antilymphoma mAb may deliver a tumor radiodose comparable with that of solid tumor antibody delivery systems (4), the intrinsic radiosensitivity of lymphoma ensures that RIT is effective clinically as a single modality treatment (5,6). In contrast, carcinoma responses to nonmyeloablative RIT are sporadic (7). According to tumor type, a number of extrinsic and intrinsic radioresistance factors variously contribute to the limited efficacy of TRT for solid tumors. Intrinsic radioresistance factors include epidermal growth factor receptor (EGFR) expression and deoxyribonucleic acid (DNA) repair capacity and extrinsic factors include abnormal tumor vasculature and hypoxia. However, a combined modality therapy (CMT) approach, which comprises a systemic therapeutic agent and TRT, could attenuate some of these radioresistance factors and increase the efficacy of TRT in solid tumors. Moreover, TRT itself may alter tumor dynamics sufficiently to either increase the efficiency of action of complementary therapeutic agents or expose other targets for drug action and/or TRT.

The most effective and acceptable of current cancer chemotherapy combinations tend to have non–cross-resistant mechanisms of action and nonoverlapping toxicity profiles and thus have the highest therapeutic ratio. In keeping with these principles, the rational design of CMT would favor the addition of drugs that exploit the defects peculiar to tumor tissue without reinforcing the normal tissue toxicity of TRT. Notwithstanding preclinical data in support of a particular CMT, clinical testing of CMT will always be required and will necessarily involve a more heterogeneous population of individuals than studied in many preclinical model systems. Unacceptable toxic interactions that limit the therapeutic ratio may only be discovered in clinical trials. Therefore, the emphasis of this chapter will be on CMT approaches that have been evaluated clinically and on studies that are clinically applicable in the short-to-medium term.

Rationale for combined modality therapy

The effectiveness of CMT using external beam radiotherapy (EBRT) and radiosensitizing chemotherapy for the treatment of locally advanced cancer is well known in routine clinical oncology practice. Although EBRT itself may have curative potential, the addition usually of concurrent cisplatin and/or 5-fluorouracil (5-FU) chemotherapy to EBRT enhances its efficacy by augmenting locoregional control rates and survival rates for many different types of locally advanced malignancies including those of anus, rectum, head and neck, lung, esophagus, stomach, and brain (8). It is important to note that in some of the clinical trials supporting the use of chemoradiotherapy, the incidence of distant metastases was reduced compared with radiation alone. These results could be interpreted to mean that chemotherapy delivered at radiosensitizing doses acted against systemic micrometastases either directly or indirectly via improved locoregional control (9), although the latter interpretation is preferred (8).

The increasing trend toward molecular subclassification of tumors is changing forever the cancer treatment paradigm based on at least two major premises. First, the "Achilles heel" known as oncogene addiction describes how amplification, translocation, or activating mutation of a key gene converts a signal transduction pathway to the dominant driver of cancer cell proliferation and survival (10). Second, synthetic lethality has emerged recently as a powerful concept to improve therapeutic index in clinical oncology. The concept originally arose from yeast genetics where if mutations in either one of two genes did not cause cell death, mutations in both genes did. When applied to cancer therapy, mutations in certain tumor suppressor or metabolic genes may cause tumor cells to rely for their

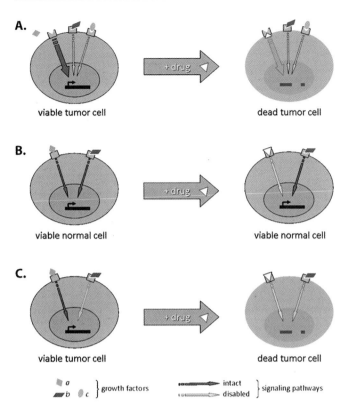

FIGURE 16.1 The therapeutic ratio of combined modality therapy may be improved either by exploiting cancer vulnerabilities such as oncogene addiction (A) or signaling pathway deficiencies adopting a synthetic lethal approach (B, C). A: The activity of the constitutively active "*a*" signaling pathway, which is ligand independent, drives tumor cell growth and proliferation. The contribution of "*b*" and "*c*" pathways to tumor cell growth and differentiation is minor. Thus, survival of tumor cells rather than normal cells is susceptible to specific inhibition of pathway "*a*" with a drug. B: Survival-promoting growth factors signal specifically via pathways "*a*" and "*b*" in normal cells. Therefore, drug-mediated inhibition of pathway "*a*" does not impair normal cell survival because pathway "*b*" remains operative. C: While survival-promoting pathway "a" is intact in tumor cells, pathway "b" is defective. Therefore, in the absence of pathway "*b*," drug-mediated inhibition of pathway "*a*" produces tumor cell death.

viability solely on a druggable mechanism, whereas normal cells depend on more than one mechanism to remain viable and so are little affected by the drug of interest (Fig. 16.1). Further, if the founding mutation in a tumor is not itself druggable, then the tumor may still be "set up for a fall" because it depends for its survival on a druggable mechanism (11,12).

It is worth noting here that a specific and measurable goal of CMT should be the eradication of tumor cells. Although specific drugs may augment radiation-induced apoptosis, apoptosis may not be the principal mode of radiation-induced tumor cell death. Other modes of cell death or inactivation such as autophagic cell death, mitotic catastrophe, and senescence may be more significant after clinical cancer therapy (13,14). A novel approach of combining RIT and cytotoxic chemotherapy to create new cell death targets may be employed to augment the effects of radiation cross fire and thus increase the tumor-absorbed dose of radiation (15).

Accordingly, this new treatment paradigm arising from knowledge of the tumor genotype provides the rationale for combining TRT with biologics or targeted therapeutics. First, the latter agents are often most effective when used in combination, either with the conventional cytotoxic agents that disrupt DNA or chromosomal replication or ionizing radiation. Second, the genomic instability of metastatic tumors ensures that new mechanisms of resistance will always evolve under the selection pressures of therapy to guarantee tumor survival. Therefore, better understanding of therapeutic resistance mechanisms may lead to treatment advances (16,17), although methods to improve delivery of TRT must still be pursued to enhance radiation-absorbed dose at sites of metastatic spread.

Biology of targeted radionuclide and combined modality therapy

Even if lessons are learned from the successes and limitations of conventional chemoradiotherapy, TRT is distinct from EBRT, and these differences will need to be taken into consideration when developing systemic CMT. High dose rate EBRT and low dose rate (LDR) TRT exert significantly different radiobiologic effects (1,2). The LDR of TRT itself (18) and the associated low-dose hyperradiosensitivity phenomenon (19–21) indicate that cytotoxic effects of TRT may be potentiated by pairing TRT with agents that interfere with DNA repair and/or cell cycle control (22). Furthermore, we anticipate that systemic CMT using LDR-TRT (18) and repeated small doses of radiosensitizing drugs would result in a concentration × time product that produces higher dose intensity.

The distribution and density of the tumor target antigen is another critical parameter that governs the efficacy of TRT by influencing the self-dose and cross-dose of the targeted radiation and thus the overall radiation-absorbed dose (23). TRT itself may compensate for the nonuniform distribution of targeted radiation within a tumor (24) via both the amplifying effects of radiation cross fire (25,26) and the in vivo bystander effects of LDR radiation, which produce unexpected potency (27). Then, in addition, incorporation of systemically administered cytotoxic or noncytotoxic agents into antigen-poor tumor cells may augment their susceptibility to the radiation-induced cytotoxicity of TRT (28). Finally, radiation dose rate may have differential effects on endothelial cells versus tumor cells and on mechanisms of apoptosis (29–33).

Ligand specificity largely determines tumor targeting in TRT and thus chemotherapy may be scheduled after TRT when the radionuclide has accumulated in tumor and mostly cleared from the body. Steel and Peckham proposed a theoretical framework for chemoradiotherapy, which included concepts of spatial cooperation, independent cell kill, protection of normal tissues, and enhanced tumor response. Spatial cooperation describes the independent operation of radiotherapy and chemotherapy each at fully active doses to treat local (in-field) and systemic (out-of-field) disease, respectively. Consequently, nonoverlapping toxicities would be produced (34). Moreover, in-field cooperation between radiation and chemotherapy is usually observed to be important for locoregional control and results from additive or supra-additive (synergistic) radiosensitizing interactions (9), which result from lowering of the radiation dose-response threshold (35). Importantly, as applied to systemic CMT, in-field cooperation may extend across the entire body and affect normal as well as tumor tissues.

In discussing systemic CMT, it is helpful to keep in mind the two-cell compartment model comprising tumor cells and their supporting stroma including the vasculature (36) as well as the five precepts of radiobiology. The five Rs, which also apply to TRT, are the repair of sublethal damage, the redistribution of cells in the cell cycle, the repopulation of cells during treatment, the reoxygenation of cells, and the intrinsic radiosensitivity of cells. As LDR-TRT encourages sublethal DNA repair and repopulation within tumors, it allows recovery in affected normal tissues by sublethal damage repair and repopulation of cells. Thus, the therapeutic gain of CMT may be particularly acute if tumor cell-specific defects in DNA repair and cell cycle checkpoints can be exploited to a synthetically lethal extent by combining LDR-TRT with DNA repair and cell cycle checkpoint inhibitors.

■ INTRINSIC TUMOR TARGETS OF COMBINED MODALITY THERAPY

▌ Conventional cytotoxic radiosensitizing agents

Antimetabolites

Antimetabolites such as 5-FU and gemcitabine have been tested clinically in conjunction with RIT. In short, both drugs act as DNA synthesis inhibitors and thus impair DNA repair after radiation. As nucleoside prodrugs, both are converted to nucleotide forms that prevent biosynthesis of deoxyribonucleotides for DNA replication: 5-FU by inhibiting thymidylate synthase (TS) and gemcitabine as a false substrate for DNA polymerases leading to early chain termination.

5-Fluorouracil As a fluorinated analogue of uracil, which is preferentially utilized by cancer cells, 5-FU becomes phosphorylated and incorporated into ribonucleic acid (RNA) to disrupt both ribosomal (rRNA) and messenger RNA (mRNA). Thymidine phosphorylase (TP) and thymidine kinase act in important catalysis steps to produce FdUMP, which in turn forms a stable ternary complex with TS thus inhibiting DNA synthesis by blocking thymidine incorporation. Together, these effects on normal RNA and DNA function promote cytotoxicity.

The radiosensitization and cytotoxicity mechanisms of 5-FU appear to be similar (28) because 5-FU is primarily a TS inhibitor. Even though 5-FU radiosensitization depends on preradiation exposure of cells to 5-FU as well as S phase progression, which reduces the repair of lethal DNA damage, the precise mechanisms of 5-FU–radiation interaction have not

been elucidated (37). Some studies suggest that radiation has a differential effect on tumors by increasing tumor cytotoxicity via 5-FU incorporation into RNA and DNA and decreasing tumor 5-FU clearance compared with normal tissues (38).

Maximal radiosensitizing effects of 5-FU in vitro occur at least 24 hours before and up to 48 hours after radiation exposure, which explains the enhanced clinical activity of continuous infusional 5-FU. However, although protracted infusional 5-FU given during radiotherapy decreases death rates by 31% in early-stage colorectal cancer patients, chemoradiotherapy is more toxic than radiotherapy alone with more acute and severe local reactions (37).

Nevertheless, RIT directed at the tumor cell surface carcinoembryonic antigen (CEA), which was combined with continuous infusional 5-FU over 5 days, did not appear to be more toxic than either modality alone in a phase I dose escalation study of 27 advanced colorectal cancer patients (4). Twenty-one patients received CMT with 13 patients receiving one cycle and 8 patients receiving two cycles of CMT. All patients were heavily pretreated and 19 patients had previously received 5-FU with 16 patients having had two or more courses of 5-FU. The RIT consisted of the intact chimeric immunoglobulin G1 (IgG1) mAb, T84.66, which was conjugated to ^{90}Y using the diethylenetriaminepentaacetic acid chelator. The starting dose of this radioconjugate was 16.6 mCi/m^2, which was the previously determined maximum tolerated dose (MTD). The 5-FU infusion was commenced 4 hours before the RIT and was designed to be active during the period of tumor targeting, which was optimal 48 to 72 hours after RIT. 5-FU was dose escalated in 100 mg/m^2/day increments to 1000 mg/m^2/day, which was close to its MTD. The final cohort received 20.6 mCi/m^2 of ^{90}Y-T84.66 with 5-FU 1000 mg/m^2/day. Up to three cycles of ^{90}Y-T84.66/5-FU every 6 weeks were planned.

Two dose-limiting toxicities (DLTs) of grade 4 thrombocytopenia and grade 4 mucositis were recorded and established the MTD of the CMT as 16.6 mCi/m^2 for ^{90}Y-T84.66 and 1000 mg/m^2/day for 5-FU, which are dose levels comparable with the MTD of each agent alone. Reversible hematologic toxicity (mainly neutropenia and thrombocytopenia) occurred in 19 of 21 patients with count nadirs 4 to 6 weeks after RIT. As a single agent, infusional 5-FU has a nonoverlapping toxicity profile of mucositis and hand–foot syndrome. Accordingly, in this CMT, the nonhematologic toxicities were low grade and characteristic of 5-FU.

Despite the favorable toxicity profile of this CMT, there were no objective tumor responses although 11 previously progressing patients developed stable disease lasting 3 to 8 months and one patient had a mixed response. The mean tumor dose of 13 gray (Gy) was comparable with that achieved in previous ^{90}Y-T84.66 monotherapy trials. The greatest tumor doses were observed in lesions less than 20 mL in volume and indicated that small-volume disease would most likely benefit from the CMT approach (4).

Capecitabine is an oral FU prodrug, which is converted to 5-FU by carboxylesterase, cytidine deaminase, and TP. TP catalyzes the final conversion step to 5-FU. In comparison with matched normal tissues, various types of tumor tissue preferentially express TP. During infusional 5-FU, concentrations of FU do not differ between tumor and normal tissues, whereas after capecitabine, FU concentrations in human tumor tissue are up to 3.2-fold higher than in normal tissue (39). Therefore, selective tumor conversion to FU may improve the therapeutic ratio of capecitabine, particularly since the toxicity profile of capecitabine is similar to that of infusional 5-FU. Radiation may induce expression of TP (40) although there are conflicting data (28). Currently, NSABP is conducting a phase III trial of preoperative capecitabine with radiotherapy in locally advanced rectal cancer after the feasibility of this approach was shown in earlier studies (41). Therefore, combining capecitabine with TRT in future clinical studies may be worthwhile.

The safety of TRT using ^{177}Lu-octreotate (LuTate) in combination with capecitabine has recently been reported (42). In this study, seven patients with inoperable somatostatin receptor–expressing gastroenteropancreatic neuroendocrine tumors (GEPNETs) were treated with 7.4-GBq LuTate and capecitabine (1650 mg/m²/day) for 14 days. None of the patients had hand–foot syndrome. As the most serious toxicities, one patient had grade 3 anemia and another patient had grade 3 thrombocytopenia. Although small in patient number, this study compares favorably with safety data from a series of 504 patients given single-agent LuTate for treatment of GEPNET. Here, grade 3 or 4 hematologic toxicity occurred in at least one of several treatments in 9.5% of patients (43). Consequently, a randomized phase III study of LuTate with or without capecitabine has commenced in patients with GEPNET (44).

Gemcitabine Gemcitabine is one of the most potent radiosensitizing drugs, and its mechanisms of radiosensitization differ from those of 5-FU. Although incorporation of false nucleotides into DNA is thought to be the primary mechanism of gemcitabine-induced cytotoxicity, inhibition of ribonucleotide reductase at low gemcitabine concentrations with consequent depletion of cellular pools of deoxyadenosine triphosphate mainly contributes to gemcitabine-induced radiosensitization (28,45). Maximal radiosensitization requires gemcitabine-induced accumulation of cells in S phase, which is when homologous recombination repair (HRR) is active (28). In vitro studies suggested that gemcitabine radiosensitizes base excision repair (BER)-deficient cells by interfering with HRR (46).

Gemcitabine is now considered standard of care for metastatic pancreatic cancer patients. Adjuvant gemcitabine chemotherapy produces a similar survival advantage to 5-FU in completely resected pancreatic cancer patients suggesting that it can eradicate preexisting micrometastatic disease (47). Although concurrent chemoradiotherapy using 5-FU remains the standard of care for locally advanced, unresectable disease, delivery of gemcitabine concurrently with radiotherapy is feasible in the adjuvant setting by using smaller radiation fields or lower systemic doses of gemcitabine (48). These data indicate that systemic delivery of radiation and radiosensitizing chemotherapy may be an encouraging approach to pancreatic cancer treatment particularly given that even subcytotoxic doses of gemcitabine can effectively lower the threshold for radiation-induced carcinoma cell death (28).

For example, the combination of a ^{90}Y-labeled radioimmunoconjugate of the hPAM4 mAb (clivatuzumab tetraxetan), which targets the mucin 1 (MUC1) antigen, with gemcitabine has been shown to be more active in human tumor xenograft models of pancreatic cancer than either modality of therapy alone (49,50). The combination of ^{90}Y-hPAM4 with gemcitabine has achieved orphan drug status with the Food and Drug Administration and has shown promising antitumor activity in a phase Ib trial. The therapy comprises 4-week cycles of weekly clivatuzumab tetraxetan followed 2 days later in each week by low-dose (200 mg/m²) gemcitabine. Half of the patients (5/10, 50%) showed evidence of disease shrinkage or stabilization and there was one dose-limiting episode of refractory grade 4 thrombocytopenia. RIT dose escalation is continuing (51).

Tubule-targeting drugs

The taxanes such as paclitaxel and docetaxel are microtubule stabilizers, which arrest cells during the G_2/M phase of the cell cycle, which is its most radiosensitive phase, and thus produce a potentially proapoptotic mitotic block (52,53,69). Consequently, taxanes are particularly useful in the management of p53-mutant cancers, which fail to arrest at the G1 cell cycle checkpoint after DNA damage (54). Paclitaxel inhibits the function of the antiapoptotic BCL-2 protein (55), which is overexpressed by many cancers and which can inhibit both P53-dependent and -independent cell death. The taxanes including paclitaxel have also been shown to have antiangiogenic effects particularly at low dose and in combination with ionizing radiation (56,57).

Preclinical studies The scheduling of paclitaxel with respect to RIT was determined empirically using the P53-mutant and BCL-2–overexpressing HBT 3477 human breast cancer xenograft model. The RIT was ^{90}Y-ChL6, which targets a membrane glycoprotein overexpressed on many adenocarcinomas. The 300- and 600-μg doses of paclitaxel were equivalent to human doses of 42 mg/m² and 84 mg/m² (58), respectively, and are considerably lower than the 175 to 200 mg/m² dose range used clinically. Neither paclitaxel nor a 9.6-MBq dose of ^{90}Y-ChL6 was curative. However, unlike paclitaxel alone, ^{90}Y-ChL6 alone produced tumor regression. The highest cure rate (88%) was obtained by giving 600-μg paclitaxel 48 hours after ^{90}Y-ChL6, whereas paclitaxel given before RIT was much less effective. Giving paclitaxel 48 hours after RIT has the advantage that its low molecular weight (mw 854 Da) enables rapid tumor penetration by the time that ^{90}Y-ChL6 (mw 150 kDa) has accumulated in the tumor (and by the time that it has dissipated in normal tissues) (53). In the PC3 human prostate tumor xenograft model, a 300-μg dose of paclitaxel interacted more effectively with a 2.78-MBq dose of ^{90}Y-ChL6 (at 50% of MTD) than a 600-μg dose of paclitaxel to produce a 67% rate of cure (59). In each tumor model, the expected myelotoxicity was no worse by combining RIT with a taxane. However, these studies did demonstrate that antitumor effects of CMT could critically depend on the timing of chemotherapy with RIT.

A ^{90}Y-conjugate of the humanized hu3S193 mAb (^{90}Y-hu3S193) directed against the oligosaccharide antigen, Lewis Y (Le^Y), which is found at high density (~4 × 10^6 antibody binding sites/cell) on the surface of carcinoma cells (60), was used with paclitaxel in the MCF7 human breast cancer xenograft model. A single 3.70-MBq dose of ^{90}Y-hu3S193 produced sustained complete remissions of subcutaneous tumor xenografts without evident toxicity. The 600-μg dose of paclitaxel itself was ineffective in this study. The 0.46-, 0.92-, and 1.85-MBq doses of ^{90}Y-hu3S193 given with paclitaxel produced dose-dependent tumor control, which was more effective than placebo, ^{90}Y-hu3S193 alone, or a ^{90}Y-labeled isotype control. However, unlike the single 3.70-MBq dose of ^{90}Y-hu3S193, none of the combined modality treatments resulted in tumor eradication (60).

Clinical studies RIT and paclitaxel together have been evaluated clinically in metastatic prostate and breast cancer patients using a phase I trial design and m170, a murine IgG1 mAb that recognizes aberrant glycosylation patterns of MUC-1 expressed abundantly by 90% of prostate and breast adenocarcinomas. Unlike in previous phase I clinical studies, the investigators conjugated m170 to ^{90}Y using a new cathepsin-cleavable peptide linker designed to accelerate liver clearance of radiometal. Nine prostate cancer patients of median age 70 years and with predominantly bone-only disease were enrolled. Eight heavily pretreated breast cancer patients of median age 53.5 years and with predominantly chest wall and/or nodal disease were enrolled. On day 0, patients received an imaging dose of ^{111}In-DOTA-pep-m170 and dosimetry was performed. Dosimetry studies indicated that liver was the nonmarrow organ that received the highest radiation dose but, in comparison with previous studies of the conventional linker, liver exposure was significantly less using the cathepsin-cleavable peptide linker and occurred without compromise of the tumor-directed dose.

Imaging studies identified known metastatic lesions in all patients who subsequently received therapy. On day 7, three prostate and four breast cancer patients received starting doses of ^{90}Y-DOTA-pep-m170 at 12 and 22 mCi/m^2, respectively. Breast cancer patients were started at a higher dose because of the results of previous high-dose RIT studies incorporating peripheral blood stem cell (PBSC) support. Thus, before RIT, all breast cancer patients had granulocyte colony-stimulating factor–stimulated PBSC collected and stored to be given in the event of prolonged grade 4 cytopenia(s) or neutropenic fever.

The second cohort of patients received CMT. Based on a schedule and dose with an optimal therapeutic ratio

previously determined in preclinical studies, patients received paclitaxel 75 mg/m^2 48 hours after the RIT dose. Three prostate and two breast cancer patients received CMT. Although the RIT infusions were tolerated well, myelosuppression was the predominant toxicity. The two breast cancer patients who received CMT had prolonged neutropenia or thrombocytopenia (more than 7 days) and were rescued with a PBSC transplant. These same two patients had transient tumor responses with less than 50% reduction in soft tissue disease lasting less than 1 month. Of the three prostate cancer patients who received CMT, two patients had grade 4 neutropenia, one lasting 1 day and the other 6 days. This latter patient and the remaining CMT patient had a 50% fall in prostate-specific antigen level lasting 2 months. Two of the prostate cancer patients who received RIT alone reported a reduction in bone pain, whereas the other treated prostate cancer patients had had minimal pretreatment tumor-related pain (61). Interestingly, ^{111}In-DOTA-pep-m170 dosimetry studies demonstrated 30% more tumor-accumulated radioactivity after the administration of both paclitaxel and ^{90}Y-DOTA-pep-m170. This statistically significant increase did not occur in normal tissues or in patients who received ^{90}Y-DOTA-pep-m170 alone and may result from antiangiogenic effects of paclitaxel (58). Dose escalation in the third and fourth cohorts was planned as 10 mCi/m^2 increments of ^{90}Y-DOTA-pep-m170 while keeping the paclitaxel dose constant. However, although the MTD had not been reached, this study was closed because of poor accrual (61).

In summary, of the two breast cancer patients treated with CMT, transient tumor responses occurred but PBSC transplantation was required to aid bone marrow recovery (61). Irrespective of the number of lines of cytotoxic chemotherapy that many advanced breast cancer patients receive, the therapeutic ratio of the CMT approach described here is less favorable than many of the approved cytotoxic agents for breast cancer.

Even if, as the investigators discussed for prostate cancer patients, the dose intensity of this particular CMT approach were to be escalated with PBSC support to an extrapolated liver tolerance level of 30 Gy, it is difficult to envisage that it would have a better therapeutic ratio than standard or other investigational systemic therapy for metastatic prostate cancer. Single-agent docetaxel is now standard first-line chemotherapy for advanced castration-resistant prostate cancer. In the pivotal phase III randomized controlled trial, for patients treated with mitoxantrone versus three-weekly docetaxel, extended follow-up indicated that docetaxel significantly prolonged median overall survival (16.3 vs. 19.2 months) (62) and significantly improved pain and quality of life (63). Even if it were possible to use this CMT approach to achieve durable partial or complete remissions in advanced breast or prostate cancer patients, previous experience using potentially curative PBSC transplantation for lymphoma illustrates the difficulties posed by bone marrow contamination with malignant cells (64). Finally, radium-223, which is a calcium-mimetic, is emerging as a stand-alone bone-targeted α-particle therapy that may prolong the survival of advanced castration-resistant prostate cancer patients with minimal myelotoxicity (65).

Signal transduction inhibitors

Ionizing radiation elicits a cytoprotective stress response

Ionizing radiation is an exogenous cell stressor that may induce a cytoprotective response in both normal and cancer cells. This stress response includes activation of cell surface receptor tyrosine kinases (RTKs), which engage branched signaling cascades to couple exogenous stimuli to endogenous cellular responses of proliferation and survival, which together may contribute to postradiotherapy-accelerated tumor cell repopulation and radioresistance (Fig. 16.2). The

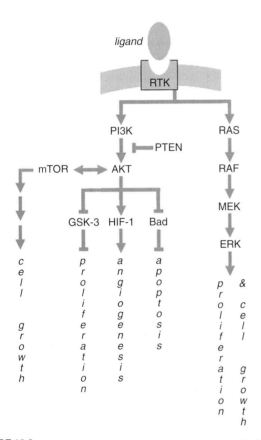

FIGURE 16.2 Schematic diagram illustrating major signal transduction pathways, which are present in both normal and cancer cells. These signaling pathways are normally activated by binding of ligands such as epidermal growth factor (EGF) or vascular endothelial growth factor (VEGF) to its cognate receptor tyrosine kinase (RTK). However, in cancer cells, genotypic alterations in key signaling molecules can deregulate normal functioning of these signaling pathways and promote malignant phenotypic changes such as enhanced cell growth, proliferation, and survival and angiogenesis. For example, somatic mutations in genes encoding signaling proteins such as RAS or RAF may act as "oncogene drivers" and thus constitutively activate the RAS/RAF/MEK/ERK signaling pathway in a "feed forward" manner (↓). Alternatively, deletion or silencing of a tumor suppressor gene such as PTEN can remove negative feedback (⊥) from the PI3K/AKT pathway and result in its constitutive activation. As described in Ref. 66, interactions between mTOR and PI3K/AKT pathways are complex (↔). (Adapted from Weinberg RA. *The Biology of Cancer*. New York, NY: Garland Science; 2007.)

clinically significant RTKs include ErbB receptor family members such as EGFR and HER2 in epithelial cells (reviewed in Ref. 67) and vascular endothelial growth factor receptor (VEGFR) and platelet-derived growth factor receptor isoforms, which regulate endothelial cell functions and angiogenesis (reviewed in Refs. 68 and 69). Together with their downstream signaling molecules, these receptors are the targets of many registered and investigational targeted therapeutics (Fig. 16.2).

Overall tumor radiosensitivity depends not only on the intrinsic radiosensitivity of tumor cells but also on the radiosensitivity of tumor microvasculature (70,71). Although higher doses of ionizing radiation (10 to 15 Gy) can have a lethal effect on tumor vasculature, lower doses (2 to 3 Gy) of ionizing radiation activate PI3K/AKT prosurvival pathways as part of the stress response to confer relative radioresistance (32). In an in vitro study, X-irradiation produced rapid (within minutes) and cell type–specific activation of AKT either via activation of EGFR in A431 human squamous carcinoma cells or of VEGFR in primary human umbilical vein endothelial cells and microvascular endothelial cells (72).

It is important to note that TRT delivers particulate ionizing radiation to tumors at a lower dose rate and in a more heterogeneous pattern than EBRT delivers photons. Interestingly, AKT activation in vitro was observed at least at a 1-Gy dose of X-irradiation (72), which is consistent with typical TRT dose rates of 1 Gy/h or less (18). Consequently, LDR-TRT may produce radiobiologic effects that differ from an equivalent low dose of EBRT delivered at a high dose rate. In addition, radiation dose rate–dependent responses of cells may differ in vascular compared with tumor cell compartments of tumors. In vivo studies that directly compare the radiobiology of high dose rate EBRT with LDR-TRT appear not to have been performed.

Radioresistance also occurs in response to low dose rate radioimmunotherapy

External γ-irradiation (15 Gy) of mice bearing syngeneic tumors activated the master angiogenic regulator, hypoxia inducible factor-1 (HIF-1), which led to upregulated expression of downstream angiogenic cytokines (73). In vivo studies using both syngeneic and xenogeneic tumor models inferred that radiation induced tumor cell secretion of VEGF. In turn, paracrine VEGF by tumors in vivo enhanced tumor radioresistance most likely via its prosurvival effects on tumor endothelial cells (70).

In studies of single-dose RIT in human tumor xenograft models, tumor microvascular and cytokine responses were analyzed. CEA- or epithelial glycoprotein-1–specific mAbs were labeled with ^{131}I and delivered at the MTD of approximately 0.25 mCi (9 MBq) per mouse. Tumor type–specific upregulation of proangiogenic factors such as VEGF, placental growth factor (PlGF), and angiopoietins 1 and 2 occurred 2 to 4 weeks after the RIT dose (74) and the angiogenic cytokine profile correlated with the relative resistance to RIT of the corresponding tumors (75). Within 3 weeks of the RIT dose, the vascular reaction to

RIT included significantly increased proliferation associated with tumor microvessels, increased microvessel density, and reduced pericyte coverage of microvessels, which are all changes consistent with increased intratumoral production of VEGF and/or PlGF (76).

These studies indicate that multiple cytokines and signaling pathways may be involved in the radioresistance of both tumor and endothelial cells. Thus, inhibition of multiple RTK may be more radiosensitizing than VEGFR blockade alone (77), which is of particular clinical relevance because registered multitargeted tyrosine kinase inhibitors (TKIs) such as sunitinib and sorafenib are among the most effective TKIs (78,79).

Epidermal growth factor receptor as a target

The most clinically promising new target for radiosensitization is the EGFR signaling pathway. EGFR is overexpressed in most cases of the common types of human carcinoma where signaling downstream of EGFR promotes the malignant phenotype by contributing to cellular proliferation, enhanced cellular survival, angiogenesis, and invasion. Signaling downstream of EGFR may be mediated by PI3K/AKT, RAS/RAF/MEK/ERK, PKC, and STAT pathways (80,81). Overexpression and activation of EGFR are associated with poor prognosis and radioresistance, which may be reversed by blockade of EGFR signaling using mAbs such as cetuximab, panitumumab, and pertuzumab or small-molecule TKIs such as gefitinib and erlotinib (80).

As an example of the cytoprotective response mediated by ionizing radiation, it has been shown that radiation can induce the phosphorylation and activation of EGFR and the processing and release of transforming growth factor-alpha, which mediated radioresistance in EGFR-overexpressing tumors such as head and neck squamous cell carcinoma (HNSCC) in part by accelerated tumor cell repopulation during radiotherapy (80,81). Inhibition of EGFR signaling can activate cell cycle arrest in G1, and combining EGFR inhibitors with radiation can augment cell cycle arrest and further reduce cell proliferation in comparison with either treatment alone (80). For example, combined in vitro treatment with cetuximab and radiation halted more human SCC cells in the relatively radiosensitive G1 and G2/M phases of the cell cycle while reducing the proportion of cells in the relatively radioresistant S phase (80,82). Cetuximab reduces postradiation repair of sublethal DNA damage (83). Cetuximab blocks radiation-induced nuclear import of EGFR, which in turn activates DNA-protein kinase (DNAPK), thus inhibiting DNA repair and postradiation cell survival (84). DNAPK is a key enzyme of the nonhomologous end joining (NHEJ) repair pathway responsible for repair of otherwise lethal DNA double-strand breaks (DSBs) (85). Both cetuximab and the EGFR TKI, gefitinib, may contribute to tumor regression by antiangiogenic effects manifest as reduced tumor vascularity (86) and reduced tumor expression of VEGF (83,86).

The most compelling data, however, come from a phase III randomized controlled trial of EBRT alone versus EBRT with cetuximab, which were used with curative intent in patients with locally advanced HNSCC. The addition of cetuximab to EBRT significantly improved both overall survival (49.0 vs. 29.3 months) and the median duration of locoregional control (24.4 vs. 14.9 months) (87) and this efficacy compared favorably with that observed for the addition of radiosensitizing chemotherapy to EBRT (88,89). The study was not sufficiently powered to determine if accelerated radiotherapy schedules improved efficacy (90), perhaps by limiting accelerated repopulation (80,91).

Interestingly, the similar incidence of distant metastases in the two groups (87) suggested that the survival advantage of CMT derived from a beneficial interaction between local radiotherapy and systemically administered cetuximab and had been supported by prior in vitro observations of reduced proliferation and increased apoptosis among HNSCC lines after combined treatment with radiotherapy and cetuximab (92). Aside from acneiform rash and infusion reactions, grade 3 or higher toxicities were not significantly increased by adding cetuximab to EBRT (87). In contrast, combining EBRT with radiosensitizing chemotherapy often accentuated severe toxicities such as mucositis (93). Therefore, the concurrent use of cetuximab dramatically enhanced the therapeutic gain of EBRT for locally advanced HNSCC.

It is important to note in this phase III study that a loading dose of cetuximab was given 1 week before commencement of EBRT (87). Patients who received concurrent chemoradiotherapy for locally advanced rectal adenocarcinoma using capecitabine as the radiosensitizing agent also received a loading dose of cetuximab 1 week before chemoradiotherapy as well as maintenance cetuximab during the chemoradiotherapy. Tumor biopsies were taken before and after the first treatment with cetuximab and showed significantly reduced tumor cell proliferation measured by Ki67 staining. Since the pathologic complete response (pCR) rate in this study was observed to be lower than the pCR rates found for preoperative chemoradiotherapy regimens that did not include cetuximab, it was postulated that growth arrest induced by prior cetuximab limited the cytotoxic and radiosensitizing potential of concurrent capecitabine (81). These data suggest that cetuximab may be more effective if given with radiotherapy alone or even extended as a monotherapy after concurrent use with radiotherapy (94).

Interactions between anti-EGFR therapy and radioimmunotherapy Will the combination of RIT and systemic anti-EGFR therapy have the same favorable therapeutic ratio as EBRT and cetuximab? Some preclinical data indicate that increased antitumor efficacy results from combining RIT and systemic anti-EGFR therapy. In the HBT 3477 human breast cancer xenograft model, cetuximab administered 24 hours before ^{90}Y-ChL6 caused cures and tumor shrinkage in 11% and 78% of mice, respectively. This compared with 0% cure rates, and 79% and 29% response rates for RIT and cetuximab, respectively. In contrast, when cetuximab was given 24 hours after RIT, the cure and response rates were 0% and 29%, respectively. Most striking, however, were schedule-dependent differences in mortality rates. Untreated animals or mice given cetuximab alone had an approximate mortality rate of 10%. For the administration of cetuximab 24 hours before RIT, the mortality rate of 80% compared with a mortality rate of 20% for cetuximab 24 hours after RIT. The authors speculated that cetuximab given after RIT had insufficient time to penetrate and radiosensitize tumors when significant radioactivity was present but enough time to radiosensitize normal tissues such as gut and liver where toxicity was lethal (95,96).

In spite of these results, which suggest that significant caution be exercised in any future clinical studies of RIT with cetuximab, later preclinical studies have not raised such safety concerns. The L19 human bivalent "small immunoprotein" (L19-SIP) is directed against the extra domain B (ED-B) of fibronectin and has been shown to bind selectively to the abluminal surface of tumor blood vessels (97). New tumor blood vessels express ED-B but not blood vessels of normal mature tissues (98). ED-B–expressing tumor blood vessels correlate with the aggressiveness of HNSCC (99). The efficacy of ^{131}I-labeled L19-SIP was evaluated in human tumor xenograft models of HNSCC with or without the addition of cetuximab. In addition to its radiosensitizing properties mediated by redistribution to the more radiosensitive G1 and G2/M phases of the cell cycle and reduced repair of sublethal DNA damage, cetuximab may also induce antiangiogenic effects via reduced tumor expression of VEGF (82). Mice received a single injection of ^{131}I-L19-SIP RIT at its MTD on day 0 or twice-weekly injections of cetuximab commencing on day 0 and continued for 4 weeks or the combination. In the FaDu HNSCC xenograft model, cetuximab alone had little impact on tumor growth, RIT itself was active, and the combination of RIT with cetuximab extended the period of tumor growth delay by almost one third and modestly prolonged the survival of tumor-bearing mice. In the HNX-OE HNSCC xenograft model, cetuximab was more active, whereas RIT alone had little activity. However, the combination of RIT with cetuximab markedly delayed tumor regrowth and almost doubled the number of surviving and tumor-bearing mice. No additional toxicity was observed in either model using the combination of cetuximab and RIT (99) and the improved therapeutic ratio supports clinical testing of this combination because the respective DLTs of cetuximab and RIT on epithelium and bone marrow do not overlap.

Additional reassuring preclinical safety data of RIT in combination with anti-EGFR therapy derive from studies of [90]Y- or ^{177}Lu-labeled radioimmunoconjugates of hu3S193 with the small-molecule EGFR TKI, AG1478 (100,101). Using the DU145 prostate cancer xenograft model, a subtherapeutic dose of AG1478 was commenced 4 hours after single escalating doses of ^{177}Lu-hu3S193 and continued on an intermittent schedule for 14 days. AG1478 reinforced apoptotic and cytotoxic effects mediated by ^{177}Lu-hu3S193 on DU145 cells in vitro. No additional toxicity of CMT was observed and all mice survived to the end of the study. In comparison with either modality alone, CMT produced the greatest reduction in tumor cell proliferation in vivo by day 14 and was associated with abrogation of EGFR phosphorylation. For reasons that are unclear, supra-additive antitumor effects of CMT using AG1478 were observed at lower doses of ^{177}Lu-hu3S193 but of CMT using docetaxel were greatest at the MTD of ^{177}Lu-hu3S193 (100). These data suggested that the antitumor activity of AG1478 combined with ^{177}Lu-hu3S193 prevented EGFR activation and tumor cell repopulation in the DU145 prostate tumor xenograft model (100). Similar safe and synergistic antitumor effects of ^{177}Lu-hu3S193 combined with a subtherapeutic dose of AG1478 were reported for the A431 squamous cell carcinoma xenograft model (101). A phase II trial of hu3S193 in refractory ovarian cancer is currently active (http://www.cancer.gov/clinicaltrials/RECEPTA-RCP-Ov-01.06). Together, these data again illustrate the vital importance of determining the safest schedules of CMT in preclinical models.

DNA damage repair and cell cycle inhibitors

Radiation-induced DNA lesions include base damage, single-strand breaks (SSBs), and DSBs. The sum of these lesions present at the time of cell division is the major contributor to radiation-induced lethality (102). Although frequent, base damage and SSB are rapidly repaired with high fidelity by the BER pathway thus preventing lethality. In contrast, DSB repair is rather slow and occurs by either error-free NHEJ or error-prone HRR (85). Most radiation-induced DNA damage is repaired by NHEJ during G1 of the cell cycle, or BER, but HRR also contributes during S and G2 in cycling cells (85,102,103). Unless they are repaired, DSBs result in nonreciprocal chromosomal translocations and subsequently mitotic catastrophe and cell death or senescence (13). That many tumors arise as the result of defective DNA repair provides the opportunity to target nonredundant DNA repair pathways in tumor cells, while completely proficient normal cells will survive in the presence of the DNA repair inhibitor (102). Moreover, many oncogene-driven tumors already carry a high burden of DNA damage associated with replicative stress, which is most evident at DNA replication forks (104). Thus, radiation adds to the tumor cell burden of unrepaired DNA lesions, which are lacking in normal cells. Given that tumor formation may also be promoted by cell cycle checkpoint defects, the time available for DNA repair in tumor cells is reduced (unlike in normal cells) and thus allows tumor cells to progress through the cell cycle with an accumulation of irreparable DNA damage.

Synthetic lethal approaches may increase the therapeutic index of combined modality therapy Most clinical RIT employs β-emissions, which, while sparsely ionizing, can induce apoptosis in leukemia cells after accumulation of irreversible DNA damage (105). However, radioresistance is more likely in carcinoma and is associated with repair of sublethal DNA damage, which presents a therapeutic opportunity if DNA repair mechanisms can be inhibited.

Some cancers have arisen primarily because of defects in DNA repair, for example, deficient HRR in cells that lack the genes for BRCA1 or BRCA2 and other proteins of the Fanconi anemia pathway (106,107).

The small-molecule poly(ADP) ribose polymerase-1 (PARP1) inhibitors are a promising new class of agent, which in HRR-defective tumor cells dramatically illustrate the synthetic lethality concept. Through an NAD-mediated reaction, PARP1 is an enzyme that provides a scaffold for BER effector proteins and its inhibition produces stalled replication forks. In HRR-defective cells, which are unable to repair this lesion, the replication forks collapse and produce lethality at 1000-fold lower concentrations than in HRR-proficient cells (106,108).

In a phase I study, the oral PARP1 inhibitor, olaparib, demonstrated antitumor activity but only in patients with known BRCA mutations (90). In subsequent phase II studies, the efficacy of olaparib was evaluated in heavily pretreated patients with BRCA-deficient breast or ovarian cancers and produced objective response rates of 41% (109) and 33% (110), respectively. In each study, olaparib was quite well tolerated without grade 3 or 4 hematologic toxicity (109,110). Significant myelotoxicity was not evident in early phase clinical studies of another PARP1 inhibitor, BSI-201, which indicates that in HRR-proficient bone marrow, PARP inhibition is not deleterious (111). The efficacy of BSI-201 combined with DSB-inducing chemotherapy in patients with triple-negative breast cancer (111), which has features of "BRCAness" including HRR repair defects (112,113), suggests that this synthetic lethal approach may be extended to other tumors with possible HRR defects (106,107). In conclusion, the apparent nonoverlapping toxicity profiles of PARP1 inhibitors and RIT provide a rationale for their combination.

Approximately 50% of tumors have defective function of the p53 tumor suppressor. Therefore, p53-deficient tumors lack a functional G1 checkpoint and depend on S/G2 checkpoints to arrest cells and allow time for DNA repair after DNA-damaging treatment. Checkpoint kinase 1 (CHK1) is a key regulator of S/G2 checkpoints. In tumor xenograft models, inhibition of CHK1 using the potent and selective small molecule, PF-00477736, enhanced antitumor activity of gemcitabine and was well tolerated. Thus, unlike in checkpoint-competent normal cells after gemcitabine treatment, PF-00477736 overrode the checkpoint defenses required to prevent tumor cells with stalled replication forks from prematurely entering mitosis with lethal DNA damage (28,114). CHK1 inhibitors also radiosensitize tumor cells and are being investigated with gemcitabine-induced radiosensitization (114).

In contrast, agents that lack selectivity for tumor-specific targets may not yield an improved therapeutic ratio in combination with RIT. For example, IC87361 is a specific small-molecule inhibitor of DNAPK, which participates in DSB repair by NHEJ. First, in a study of two types of tumor hosted by wild-type mice or DNAPK-deficient SCID mice, fractionated radiotherapy (21 Gy/7 fractions) delayed tumor growth, and to a significantly greater extent in SCID

hosts. In response to 3-Gy ionizing radiation in vitro, the clonogenic survival of SCID endothelial cells was reduced compared with wild-type endothelial cells and was associated with evidence of more DSBs. Similarly, after radiation, greater reduction in vascular length density (using the in vivo dorsal skinfold window model) was observed in SCID than in wild-type mice. Second, using IC87361 to inhibit DNAPK, these vascular effects were reproduced in wild-type endothelial cells and blood vessels but not in SCID tissues thus indicating the specificity of action of IC87361. IC87361 itself did not exert any cytotoxic effects on tumor or endothelial cells. Although these results indicate that radiosensitization of tumor endothelial cells had a greater impact on tumor growth than direct radiation-induced cytotoxicity of tumor cells, radiosensitization of normal tissues by up to threefold by IC87361 risks significant toxicity (33).

■ EXTRINSIC TUMOR TARGETS OF COMBINED MODALITY THERAPY

Targeting the tumor vasculature may be a potent therapeutic maneuver to improve the efficiency of TRT because tumor cell proliferation, survival, and metastasis depend critically on angiogenesis (115). Tumors grow because of new blood vessel formation largely driven by intratumoral production of VEGF. The vasculature of tumors is abnormal and characterized by vessels that are immature, tortuous, and leaky with blind ends and shunts and that cause variable and inefficient perfusion and raised interstitial pressure. Two major consequences of therapeutic significance arise. First, regional hypoxia develops and, via induction of HIF-1, further promotes formation of abnormal tumor vasculature (116). Hypoxic areas harbor radioresistant cells with higher metastasizing potential (117). Second, intratumoral penetration by macromolecules such as therapeutic antibodies is retarded because of large interstitial transport distances, high interstitial pressures that oppose inward diffusion of antibody, and heterogeneity of tumor blood flow that contributes to nonuniform antibody distribution even in well-perfused areas (118).

▨ Tumor endothelial cell signaling

As discussed in section "Ionizing radiation elicits a cytoprotective stress response," the tumor endothelial cell itself may also be the target of radiosensitizing therapeutic interventions. In addition to the known role of EGFR stimulation and ionizing radiation in activating the PI3K/AKT pathway, VEGF may also activate this pathway to promote endothelial cell survival. A 3-Gy treatment with X-irradiation activated AKT within minutes. Pharmacologic blockade of this pathway using a PI3K inhibitor in conjunction with radiation-induced apoptosis of tumor endothelial cells consequently destroyed tumor vasculature and delayed tumor growth significantly more than either treatment alone (32,119).

Questions concerning the overall toxicity of this approach await comprehensive testing of more selective inhibitors of the PI3K/AKT pathway (35). Another approach is to target components of the PI3K/AKT pathway further downstream. For example, ionizing radiation also activated mammalian target of rapamycin (mTOR) (Fig. 16.2). The combination of the mTOR inhibitor, everolimus, with radiotherapy delayed growth of glioma xenografts significantly more than either treatment alone. It was inferred that the antitumor activity of CMT resulted from reduced vascular density as radiosensitized tumor endothelial cells underwent apoptosis (120). Since regulatory authorities have recently approved everolimus and another mTOR inhibitor, temsirolimus, for treatment of metastatic renal cell carcinoma, tumor radiosensitization by pharmacologic inhibition of mTOR signaling is clinically testable.

Finally, it has been suggested that inhibition of signaling via the master transcription factor, HIF-1, which regulates multiple angiogenic cytokines, may be the most effective way to block endothelial cell radioresistance (73). Support for this approach was found in studies of tumor xenograft models, which showed potent radiosensitization with a selective inhibitor of HIF-1 (121). Importantly, selectively overcoming radiation-induced and HIF-1-mediated radioresistance of endothelial cells may improve the therapeutic ratio of CMT more than inhibition of endothelial cell survival signals such as PI3K/AKT activation, which risks radiosensitizing both normal and tumor tissues. In this respect, inhibition of HIF-1 was confined to tumor cells and prevented tumor cell secretion of angiogenic cytokines, which occurred strictly in concert with HIF-1 expression (73). In effect, targeting HIF-1 may recapitulate synthetic lethality and promote therapeutic gain if combined with TRT.

Tumor neovasculature

Although the effects of combination treatment with EBRT and tumor vasculature–normalizing antiangiogenic agents have been studied clinically (122,123), the effects of TRT on tumor vasculature and its interactions with antiangiogenic agents remain relatively underexplored (124). Nevertheless, a sound rationale exists for improving the therapeutic ratio of TRT if radiosensitization of the minor tumor vascular compartment selectively kills the vessels feeding large numbers of tumor cells thus overcoming overall tumor radioresistance (36,125).

The "small immunoprotein," L19-SIP, binds ED-B–expressing tumor blood vessels and thus directly targets the tumor neovasculature (97). Clinically significant antitumor activity has been observed after treatment of Hodgkin lymphoma patients with ^{131}I-L19-SIP (126). This construct has been evaluated in a phase I clinical trial of solid tumor patients and has demonstrated expected but transient myelosuppression and some clinical activity (127). Multicenter phase II clinical trials are underway (http://www.philogen.com) and may expand the potential for combining this RIT with other therapeutic modalities.

The vascular disrupting agent, combrestatin-A4-phosphate (CA4P), is a tubulin-binding agent. It preferentially depolymerizes cytoskeletal microtubules of tumor vascular endothelial cells and causes a vascular "shut down" and central tumor necrosis leaving behind a viable tumor rim that can repopulate the tumor (128,129). Tumor microdistribution studies of radiolabeled anti-CEA mAb demonstrated preferential location of mAb in viable areas of tumor containing the highest target antigen density (130). Therapeutic studies of human colorectal tumor xenografts showed that when CA4P was given 48 hours after administration of ^{131}I-labeled and CEA-specific A5B7 murine mAb, ^{131}I-A5B7 had achieved maximal levels of tumor accumulation and produced cures in five out of six mice unlike either treatment alone. The enhanced efficacy of CMT was thought to be due to the additive effects of tumor cell killing from the action of CA4P on the central portion of the tumor and of RIT on the peripheral rim; combined, CA4P induced a 90% increase in tumor accumulation of ^{131}I-A5B7 (128).

In initial clinical studies, the MTD for each agent was determined and myelosuppression was the DLT of ^{131}I-A5B7. One of the 10 colorectal cancer patients treated with ^{131}I-A5B7 alone achieved a partial response. No objective tumor response was found in patients given CA4P alone. Potential complementary clinical activity of each modality of treatment provided the rationale for a clinical trial of CMT. It was hypothesized that ^{131}I-A5B7 would prevent regrowth of the viable rim, whereas CA4P would treat poorly perfused, hypoxic, and consequently relatively radioresistant central tumor regions, which would be penetrated poorly by ^{131}I-A5B7 (130) mAb. An initial dose of CA4P was given within 14 days of the ^{131}I-A5B7 dose on day 1, subsequently on days 3 and 4 and then weekly for up to 7 weeks. Four of 10 evaluable patients accumulated ^{131}I-A5B7 to a level higher than that for all normal organs except lung. The starting dose of CA4P was 25% below the MTD and below the dose that reliably produced dynamic contrast-enhanced MRI–detected changes in tumor blood flow. Despite commencing ^{131}I-A5B7 at a dose also 25% below the MTD, two patients developed grade 4 neutropenia necessitating de-escalation of the ^{131}I-A5B7 dose by another 11%. The initial myelosuppression was attributed to the RIT and the CA4P dose was escalated to 10% below MTD. Nevertheless, two further patients developed grade 4 neutropenia and the trial was ceased. Of 10 patients evaluable by RECIST, none had a response although one patient had a fall in the level of a serum tumor marker.

In spite of promising preclinical data, the lack of efficacy in this CMT study was associated with unacceptable toxicity, which may partly be explained by the fact that most patients had two or more prior regimens of chemotherapy. After other factors such as red marrow dose and an effect of CA4P on the pharmacokinetics of ^{131}I-A5B7 were excluded, the heightened sensitivity of bone marrow to CMT may have resulted from an interaction between the two agents, which are each expected to have direct myelotoxic effects. Studies in a human colorectal tumor xenograft model demonstrated that ^{131}I-A5B7 was trapped within the tumor when clinically relevant doses of CA4P, which reduced tumor blood flow, were given 48 hours after ^{131}I-A5B7 (129). Therefore, the priming dose of CA4P, which was administered in the clinical study for pharmacokinetic purposes, may have impeded tumor retention of ^{131}I-A5B7 and thus contributed to the limited efficacy of CMT (131).

SELECTIVE TUMOR CELL DEATH AND ITS INTERACTIONS WITH TARGETED RADIONUCLIDE THERAPY

Of future interest for combination with TRT are the new classes of drugs, particularly proapoptotic agents, which are in preclinical and early clinical development. For example, ABT737 is a small-molecule drug, which acts as a BH3-mimetic to inhibit antiapoptotic proteins and which synergizes with radiation-induced death signals to promote cytotoxicity (132). The radiosensitizing effects of ABT737 are augmented in a lung cancer xenograft model by combination with the mTOR inhibitor, rapamycin, which induces autophagy (133). Other examples for which radiosensitizing effects have been demonstrated include proapoptotic receptor antagonists such as tumor necrosis factor–related apoptosis-inducing ligand (TRAIL) (134,135) or TRAIL-specific mAb (136), inhibitors of apoptosis (137,138), and epigenetic modifiers such as histone deacetylase (HDAC) inhibitors (139). For example, LBH589 is an oral HDAC inhibitor, which is in clinical development and which radiosensitizes non–small lung cancer cells to produce synergistic increases in radiation-induced tumor cell apoptosis and antitumor activity in vivo (140).

In addition to drug-induced and -selective enhancement of tumor cell death, selective targeting of dead tumor cells themselves may also improve the therapeutic ratio of CMT.

Rationale for a dead cancer cell target antigen

Although most antibody-based therapies for cancer are directed against cell surface antigens, selective immunotargeting of dead cancer cells may enable delivery of bystander or third-party killing to nearby viable tumor cells. We have discovered that La/SSB is a novel dead cancer cell antigen, which is expressed preferentially in a wide variety of tumor types after DNA-damaging anticancer treatment (59). During apoptosis, like many nuclear antigens, La undergoes caspase-mediated cleavage to release a 3-kDa C-terminal fragment that contains its nuclear localization signal. Consequently, during apoptosis, La translocates from nucleus to cytoplasm (141,142) where it is available for specific antibody binding in vitro (59). Dead cells eventually lose cell membrane integrity and dead cancer cells persist in vivo while apoptotic cells in normal tissues are cleared rapidly (143). It is important to remember that cancer cell "death features" are prominent among many cancers and may result from unfavorable tumor dynamics (144,145) and/or the effects of anticancer treatment (146,147). Our in vivo studies using murine subcutaneous transplantable tumor models showed that the La antigen in dead tumor cells

directed tumor-selective binding of radiolabeled mAb (148,149).

Other studies have identified dead cancer cells in vivo. Clinical and preclinical imaging and biodistribution studies using ProstaScint (^{111}In-labeled capromab pendetide) indicated that dead cancer cells were found among prostate cancer metastases in vivo. ProstaScint originated as the 7E11 mAb after immunization of mice with prostate-specific membrane antigen (PSMA)-expressing LNCaP human prostate cancer cells (150). The 7E11 epitope is in the cytoplasmic domain of PSMA, which is unavailable in viable cells (151,152). The 7E11 mAb detected four of six clinically imaged soft tissue lesions (153) and not more than two sites of disease in 7 of 11 patients with evaluable soft tissue or bone mets (154). In contrast, the J591 mAb, which recognizes the extracellular domain of PSMA, detected 13 of 18 extrahepatic soft tissue lesions (155). The tumor necrosis therapy (TNT1; Cotara) mAb binds histones and/or single-stranded DNA and localized in necrotic and degenerating areas of tumors. In a pivotal trial of ^{131}I-labeled TNT mAb in patients with advanced lung cancer, a 35% overall response rate was achieved (156) although survival was not apparently different from historical controls.

Role of the La/SSB antigen in cancer

La has an essential role in mammalian development where it is required for inner cell mass formation in the mouse blastocyst (157). La is a highly abundant and ubiquitously expressed ribonucleoprotein (RNP) and RNA-binding protein, which is located predominantly in the nucleus and especially in the nucleolus. La acts as a molecular chaperone for RNA polymerase III–generated transcripts such as transfer RNA (tRNA) and rRNA, which contribute to protein synthesis at ribosomes. Nucleoli, which are ribosome factories, are prominent in malignant cells (158). Moreover, nucleolar proteins and RNP are overexpressed and RNA polymerase III is overactive in cancer. In keeping with these findings, we found that La was overexpressed in cancer cells (59). La may also have a role in coupling transcription and translation (159), and thus La would be expected to have an obligatory function in the protein synthetic machinery of cancer cells.

Although La is an autoantigen in Sjogren syndrome and systemic lupus erythematosus where La-specific IgG is of high titer and high affinity, the autoantibodies are not pathogenic except in the rare instance of congenital heart block, which affects the fetuses of only 1% to 2% of pregnant women with serum autoantibodies (160).

Preclinical proof of concept for selective targeting of a dead cancer cell antigen

In vitro, we found that La-specific mAb binds dead cancer cells with high avidity in an antigen-specific, rapid, and saturable manner and, in particular, "loads" the cytoplasm of dead cancer cells. During apoptosis, La is preferentially cross-linked or "fixed" in malignant cell types by transglutaminase-2 and the La-specific mAb itself becomes cross-linked in dead cancer cells. Binding of La-specific mAb to dead cancer cells in vitro is "induced" in response to DNA-damaging agents (59), and in vivo tumor accumulation of La-specific mAb is augmented by DNA-damaging chemotherapy and is dose dependent and saturable (148).

La-directed radioimmunotherapy given after chemotherapy may further improve the therapeutic ratio

Antigen-specific tumor uptake of the La-specific DAB4 mAb was confirmed in the EL4 lymphoma model in which cyclophosphamide and etoposide chemotherapy briskly induce robust tumor cell apoptosis (161). Uptake of DAB4 by untreated tumors was significantly greater when compared with uptake of the Sal5 isotype control mAb of irrelevant specificity (20 ± 1 vs. 11 ± 2% ID/g). Chemotherapy significantly augmented tumor uptake (45 ± 1 vs. 18 ± 2% ID/g) in a dose-dependent manner. Delaying the administration of ^{111}In-DOTA-DAB4 until 24 hours after chemotherapy accelerated its tumor uptake and blood clearance and was associated with a significant reduction in normal organ uptake (less than 4% ID/g) (149). Tumor accumulation of DAB peaked at 90 ± 1% ID/g (corrected for radioactive decay) 72 hours after chemotherapy when levels of tumor cell death (70 ± 1% 7AAD$^+$ cells) also peaked. In addition, the number of apoptotic tumor cells containing activated caspase 3 and cleaved PARP1, which are markers of early and late apoptosis, respectively, increased directly with chemotherapy dose. As evidence of target antigen induction by DNA-damaging chemotherapy, the ex vivo binding of DAB4 per tumor cell increased steadily postchemotherapy and was maximum at 96 hours after chemotherapy (149). Therefore, an improved therapeutic ratio of La-directed RIT is possible because tumor accumulation of DAB4 is directly related to the amount of chemotherapy-induced target antigen, which is not available for binding to any significant extent in normal tissues.

La-directed radioimmunotherapy synergizes with chemotherapy to create new target antigens

The therapeutic efficacy of a ^{90}Y-labeled radioimmunoconjugate of DAB4 was compared with ^{90}Y-DOTA-Sal5. Only ^{90}Y-DOTA-DAB4 produced significant tumor growth delay, and higher doses (1.80 and 3.60 MBq) eradicated the subcutaneous implants of EL4 lymphoma. Surprisingly, the subcurative doses of ^{90}Y-DOTA-DAB4 (0.46 and 0.92 MBq) became curative when administered 24 hours after a subcurative dose of chemotherapy. The interaction was synergistic because the combination allowed a fourfold lower dose of DAB4-RIT to effect cure. Treated mice tolerated DAB4-RIT well with less than 5% acute weight loss and without evident chronic pathologic changes in a necropsy study (15). Interestingly, comparative biodistribution studies in the EL4 model using ^{111}In- and ^{90}Y-labeled DAB4 suggested that ^{90}Y-DOTA-DAB4 begat its own uptake in tumors. For the same radiodose of ^{111}In- and ^{90}Y-labeled DAB4, significantly

more ^{90}Y-DOTA-DAB4 accumulated in tumors than ^{111}In-DOTA-DAB4. Analyses of the tumor content of dead cells and of the ex vivo tumor cell binding of DAB4 indicated that the enhanced tumor accumulation of ^{90}Y-DOTA-DAB4 resulted from the creation of additional binding targets. Over the time course of tumor cell death, combination treatment produced significantly more tumor cell death and greater per tumor cell binding of DAB4 than either RIT or chemotherapy alone. In contrast, ex vivo EL4 tumor cell binding of TNT1 mAb was not induced by DNA-damaging treatment. Using treatment with nonionic detergent to detect protein–protein cross-linking in tumors in vivo, we found that combined modality RIT and chemotherapy promoted retention of tumor-bound radioactivity (15).

As expected in a carcinoma model, chemotherapy induced lower and clinically relevant levels of tumor cell apoptosis in the syngeneic Lewis lung carcinoma (LL2) model. Accordingly, the single-agent activity of ^{90}Y-DOTA-DAB4 in the LL2 model was modest because only the highest dose (3.6 MBq) significantly delayed LL2 tumor growth. However, administering 0.92-, 1.8-, and 3.6-MBq doses of ^{90}Y-DOTA-DAB4 24 hours after radiosensitizing cisplatin and gemcitabine chemotherapy produced significant growth retardation compared with either treatment alone (15).

Unexpectedly, we found that the same dose of radioactivity given as a ^{177}Lu-DOTA conjugate of DAB4 had comparable antitumor activity to ^{90}Y-DOTA-DAB4 (Al-Ejeh et al., unpublished data, 2010). We reasoned that the physical half-life of ^{177}Lu matched well the time in which the tumor retained ^{177}Lu-DOTA-DAB4. Moreover, we argue that as LL2 tumors shrink in response to chemotherapy, the short-range β-emissions of the more slowly decaying ^{177}Lu are deposited more often within the confines of the tumor than the longer-range β-emissions of ^{90}Y.

In studies of human tumor xenograft–bearing nude mice, we found that ^{90}Y-DOTA-DAB4 synergized with cisplatin and gemcitabine chemotherapy to prolong survival of mice bearing the pancreatic (PANC-1) and prostate (LNCaP) cancers. This effect was more pronounced in the p53 wild-type LNCaP model than in the p53-mutant PANC-1 model. Strikingly, ^{90}Y-DOTA-DAB4 when combined with chemotherapy extended the median survival time (MST) of LNCaP-bearing mice to 61 days, whereas the same radiodose of ^{90}Y-DOTA-7E11 given after chemotherapy produced an MST of 29 days. To explain these results, we contend that La-directed ^{90}Y-DOTA-DAB4 created more targets for further binding than did PSMA-directed ^{90}Y-DOTA-7E11 (15).

In summary, the La antigen is universal, high density, overexpressed in malignancy, "induced" in dead malignant cells by DNA-damaging therapy and available for binding after dead normal cells have been cleared, and durably retained within tumors. Arming DAB4 mAb with a β-emitting generates third-party killing via radiation cross fire, self-amplifying recruitment of DAB4, and prolonged intratumoral retention of DAB4 (15). Consequently, these properties of DAB4-β-RIT result in its synergy with cytotoxic doses of radiosensitizing drugs. The tumor-targeting ability of DAB4 may be extended by increasing the radioactive payload contained in attached nanoparticles (162). Our preclinical data have been sufficiently encouraging to prepare for a phase I clinical trial of ^{177}Lu-DOTA-DAB4 as APOMAB.

CONCLUSIONS

Although clinical trials of CMT may follow the traditional drug development route and include the usual study populations of unselected treatment-resistant patients, scientific rigor together with the prospect of improved safety and efficacy results should demand of CMT clinical investigators that patients be selected on the basis of a tumor genotype that confers probable susceptibility to a targeted therapeutic. Thus, the target characteristics of both the TRT and the agent to be used in combination will be defined. Tumor selectivity and the scheduling of individual CMT components will remain the critical determinants of the therapeutic ratio of CMT.

The remarkable curative potential of chemoradiotherapy for locally advanced carcinomas should provide a fillip to those who research and treat metastatic carcinomas. Clinical investigators should feel encouraged to investigate vigorously safe combinations of systemic agents that complement the mode of action of TRT and enhance its efficiency. In related fields of pure research or in the cross-fertilized fields of translational research, other scientists can pursue the mechanistic basis for therapeutically beneficial interactions in CMT.

REFERENCES

1. Flynn AA, Pedley RB, Green AJ, et al. Antibody and radionuclide characteristics and the enhancement of the effectiveness of radioimmunotherapy by selective dose delivery to radiosensitive areas of tumour. *Int J Radiat Biol*. 2002;78:407–415.
2. Kassis AI, Adelstein SJ. Radiobiologic principles in radionuclide therapy. *J Nucl Med*. 2005;46(suppl 1):4S–12S.
3. Shipley WU, Stanley JA, Steel GG. Tumor size dependency in the radiation response of the Lewis lung carcinoma. *Cancer Res*. 1975;35:2488–2493.
4. Wong JY, Shibata S, Williams LE, et al. A phase I trial of 90Y-anti-carcinoembryonic antigen chimeric T84.66 radioimmunotherapy with 5-fluorouracil in patients with metastatic colorectal cancer. *Clin Cancer Res*. 2003;9:5842–5852.
5. Wang M, Oki Y, Pro B, et al. Phase II study of yttrium-90-ibritumomab tiuxetan in patients with relapsed or refractory mantle cell lymphoma. *J Clin Oncol*. 2009;27:5213–5218.
6. Dancey G, Violet J, Malaroda A, et al. A phase I clinical trial of CHT-25 a 131I-labeled chimeric anti-CD25 antibody showing efficacy in patients with refractory lymphoma. *Clin Cancer Res*. 2009;15:7701–7710.
7. Sharkey RM, Goldenberg DM. Perspectives on cancer therapy with radiolabeled monoclonal antibodies. *J Nucl Med*. 2005;46(suppl 1):115S–127S.
8. Nyati MK, Morgan MA, Feng FY, et al. Integration of EGFR inhibitors with radiochemotherapy. *Nat Rev Cancer*. 2006;6:876–885.
9. Seiwert TY, Salama JK, Vokes EE. The concurrent chemoradiation paradigm—general principles. *Nat Clin Pract Oncol*. 2007;4:86–100.
10. Weinstein IB, Joe A. Oncogene addiction. *Cancer Res*. 2008;68:3077–3080.
11. Kaelin WG, Jr. The concept of synthetic lethality in the context of anticancer therapy. *Nat Rev Cancer*. 2005;5:689–698.
12. Brown MP, Buckley MF, Rudzki Z, et al. Why we will need to learn new skills to control cancer. *Intern Med J*. 2007;37:201–204.
13. Brown JM, Attardi LD. The role of apoptosis in cancer development and treatment response. *Nat Rev Cancer*. 2005;5:231–237.
14. Roninson IB, Broude EV, Chang BD. If not apoptosis, then what? Treatment-induced senescence and mitotic catastrophe in tumor cells. *Drug Resist Updat*. 2001;4:303–313.
15. Al-Ejeh F, Darby JM, Brown MP. Chemotherapy synergizes with radioimmunotherapy targeting La autoantigen in tumors. *PloS ONE*. 2009;4:e4630.
16. Merlo LMF, Maley CC. The role of genetic diversity in cancer. *J Clin Invest*. 2010;120:401–403.
17. Ellis LM, Hicklin DJ. Resistance to targeted therapies: refining anticancer therapy in the era of molecular oncology. *Clin Cancer Res*. 2009;15:7471–7478.
18. Carlsson J, Eriksson V, Stenerlow B, et al. Requirements regarding dose rate and exposure time for killing of tumour cells in beta particle radionuclide therapy. *Eur J Nucl Med Mol Imaging*. 2006;33:1185–1195.
19. Marples B, Wouters BG, Collis SJ, et al. Low-dose hyper-radiosensitivity: a consequence of ineffective cell cycle arrest of radiation-damaged G2-phase cells. *Radiat Res*. 2004;161:247–255.
20. Joiner MC, Marples B, Lambin P, et al. Low-dose hypersensitivity: current status and possible mechanisms. *Int J Radiat Oncol Biol Phys*. 2001;49:379–389.
21. Fernet M, Megnin-Chanet F, Hall J, et al. Control of the G2/M checkpoints after exposure to low doses of ionising radiation: implications for hyper-radiosensitivity. *DNA Repair*. 2009;9:48–57.
22. Marples B, Collis SJ. Low-dose hyper-radiosensitivity: past, present, and future. *Int J Radiat Oncol Biol Phys*. 2008;70:1310–1318.
23. Howell RW, Neti PV, Pinto M, et al. Challenges and progress in predicting biological responses to incorporated radioactivity. *Radiat Prot Dosimetry*. 2006;122:521–527.
24. Flynn AA, Green AJ, Pedley RB, et al. A model-based approach for the optimization of radioimmunotherapy through antibody design and radionuclide selection. *Cancer*. 2002;94:1249–1257.
25. Hartman T, Lundqvist H, Westlin JE, et al. Radiation doses to the cell nucleus in single cells and cells in micrometastases in targeted therapy with (131)I labeled ligands or antibodies. *Int J Radiat Oncol Biol Phys*. 2000;46:1025–1036.
26. Essand M, Gronvik C, Hartman T, et al. Radioimmunotherapy of prostatic adenocarcinomas: effects of 131I-labelled E4 antibodies on cells at different depth in DU 145 spheroids. *Int J Cancer*. 1995;63:387–394.
27. Xue LY, Butler NJ, Makrigiorgos GM, et al. Bystander effect produced by radiolabeled tumor cells in vivo. *Proc Natl Acad Sci USA*. 2002;99:13765–13770.
28. Shewach DS, Lawrence TS. Antimetabolite radiosensitizers. *J Clin Oncol*. 2007;25:4043–4050.
29. Fuks Z, Kolesnick R. Engaging the vascular component of the tumor response. *Cancer Cell*. 2005;8:89–91.
30. Rotolo JA, Maj JG, Feldman R, et al. Bax and Bak do not exhibit functional redundancy in mediating radiation-induced endothelial apoptosis in the intestinal mucosa. *Int J Radiat Oncol Biol Phys*. 2008;70:804–815.
31. Ch'ang HJ, Maj JG, Paris F, et al. ATM regulates target switching to escalating doses of radiation in the intestines. *Nat Med*. 2005;11:484–490.
32. Edwards E, Geng L, Tan J, et al. Phosphatidylinositol 3-kinase/Akt signaling in the response of vascular endothelium to ionizing radiation. *Cancer Res*. 2002;62:4671–4677.
33. Shinohara ET, Geng L, Tan J, et al. DNA-dependent protein kinase is a molecular target for the development of noncytotoxic radiation-sensitizing drugs. *Cancer Res*. 2005;65:4987–4992.
34. Steel GG, Peckham MJ. Exploitable mechanisms in combined radiotherapy-chemotherapy: the concept of additivity. *Int J Radiat Oncol Biol Phys*. 1979;5:85–91.
35. Kim DW, Huamani J, Fu A, et al. Molecular strategies targeting the host component of cancer to enhance tumor response to radiation therapy. *Int J Radiat Oncol Biol Phys*. 2006;64:38–46.
36. Camphausen K, Menard C. Angiogenesis inhibitors and radiotherapy of primary tumours. *Expert Opin Biol Ther*. 2002;2:477–481.
37. Rich TA, Shepard RC, Mosley ST. Four decades of continuing innovation with fluorouracil: current and future approaches to fluorouracil chemoradiation therapy. *J Clin Oncol*. 2004;22:2214–2232.
38. Lawrence TS, Tepper JE, Blackstock AW. Fluoropyrimidine–radiation interactions in cells and tumors. *Semin Radiat Oncol*. 1997;7:260–266.
39. Schuller J, Cassidy J, Dumont E, et al. Preferential activation of capecitabine in tumor following oral administration to colorectal cancer patients. *Cancer Chemother Pharmacol*. 2000;45:291–297.

40. Ishitsuka H. Capecitabine: preclinical pharmacology studies. *Invest New Drugs.* 2000;18:343–354.

41. Corvo R, Pastrone I, Scolaro T, et al. Radiotherapy and oral capecitabine in the preoperative treatment of patients with rectal cancer: rationale, preliminary results and perspectives. *Tumori.* 2003;89:361–367.

42. van EM, Krenning EP, Kam BL, et al. Report on short-term side effects of treatments with ^{177}Lu-octreotate in combination with capecitabine in seven patients with gastroenteropancreatic neuroendocrine tumours. *Eur J Nucl Med Mol Imaging.* 2008;35:743–748.

43. Kwekkeboom DJ, de Herder WW, Kam BL, et al. Treatment with the radiolabeled somatostatin analog [^{177}Lu-DOTA 0,Tyr3]octreotate: toxicity, efficacy, and survival. *J Clin Oncol.* 2008;26:2124–2130.

44. Kwekkeboom DJ, Kam BL, Essen MV, et al. Somatostatin receptor-based imaging and therapy of gastroenteropancreatic neuroendocrine tumors. *Endocr Relat Cancer* 2010;17:R53–R73.

45. Morgan MA, Parsels LA, Maybaum J, et al. Improving gemcitabine-mediated radiosensitization using molecularly targeted therapy: a review. *Clin Cancer Res.* 2008;14:6744–6750.

46. Wachters FM, Van Putten JW, Maring JG, et al. Selective targeting of homologous DNA recombination repair by gemcitabine. *Int J Radiat Oncol Biol Phys.* 2003;57:553–562.

47. Neoptolemos J, Buchler M, Stocken DD, et al. ESPAC-3(v2): a multicenter, international, open-label, randomized, controlled phase III trial of adjuvant 5-fluorouracil/folinic acid (5-FU/FA) versus gemcitabine (GEM) in patients with resected pancreatic ductal adenocarcinoma. *J Clin Oncol (Meeting Abstracts).* 2009;27:LBA4505.

48. Allen AM, Zalupski MM, Robertson JM, et al. Adjuvant therapy in pancreatic cancer: phase I trial of radiation dose escalation with concurrent full-dose gemcitabine. *Int J Radiat Oncol Biol Phys.* 2004;59:1461–1467.

49. Gold DV, Schutsky K, Modrak D, et al. Low-dose radioimmunotherapy ((90)Y-PAM4) combined with gemcitabine for the treatment of experimental pancreatic cancer. *Clin Cancer Res.* 2003;9:3929S–3937S.

50. Gold DV, Modrak DE, Schutsky K, et al. Combined 90Yttrium-DOTA-labeled PAM4 antibody radioimmunotherapy and gemcitabine radiosensitization for the treatment of a human pancreatic cancer xenograft. *Int J Cancer.* 2004;109:618–626.

51. Pennington K, Guarino MJ, Serafini AN, et al. Multicenter study of radiosensitizing gemcitabine combined with fractionated radioimmunotherapy for repeated treatment cycles in advanced pancreatic cancer. *J Clin Oncol (Meeting Abstracts).* 2009;27:4620.

52. Choy H, Akerley W, Glantz M, et al. Concurrent paclitaxel and radiation therapy for solid tumors. *Cancer Control.* 1996;3:310–318.

53. DeNardo SJ, Richman CM, Kukis DL, et al. Synergistic therapy of breast cancer with Y-90-chimeric L6 and paclitaxel in the xenografted mouse model: development of a clinical protocol. *Anticancer Res.* 1998;18:4011–4018.

54. Wahl AF, Donaldson KL, Fairchild C, et al. Loss of normal p53 function confers sensitization to Taxol by increasing G2/M arrest and apoptosis. *Nat Med.* 1996;2:72–79.

55. Haldar S, Basu A, Croce CM. Bcl2 is the guardian of microtubule integrity. *Cancer Res.* 1997;57:229–233.

56. Dicker AP, Williams TL, Iliakis G, et al. Targeting angiogenic processes by combination low-dose paclitaxel and radiation therapy. *Am J Clin Oncol.* 2003;26:e45–e53.

57. Grant DS, Williams TL, Zahaczewsky M, et al. Comparison of antiangiogenic activities using paclitaxel (taxol) and docetaxel (taxotere). *Int J Cancer.* 2003;104:121–129.

58. Miers L, Lamborn K, Yuan A, et al. Does paclitaxel (Taxol) given after ^{111}In-labeled monoclonal antibodies increase tumor-cumulated activity in epithelial cancers? *Clin Cancer Res.* 2005;11:7158s–7163s.

59. Al-Ejeh F, Darby JM, Brown MP. The La autoantigen is a malignancy-associated cell death target that is induced by DNA-damaging drugs. *Clin Cancer Res.* 2007;13:5509s–5518s.

60. Cullinane C, Dorow DS, Kansara M, et al. An in vivo tumor model exploiting metabolic response as a biomarker for targeted drug development. *Cancer Res.* 2005;65:9633–9636.

61. Richman CM, DeNardo SJ, O'Donnell RT, et al. High-dose radioimmunotherapy combined with fixed, low-dose paclitaxel in metastatic prostate and breast cancer by using a MUC-1 monoclonal antibody, m170, linked to indium-111/yttrium-90 via a cathepsin cleavable linker with cyclosporine to prevent human anti-mouse antibody. *Clin Cancer Res.* 2005;11:5920–5927.

62. Berthold DR, Pond GR, Soban F, et al. Docetaxel plus prednisone or mitoxantrone plus prednisone for advanced prostate cancer: updated survival in the TAX 327 study. *J Clin Oncol.* 2008;26:242–245.

63. Tannock IF, de WR, Berry WR, et al. Docetaxel plus prednisone or mitoxantrone plus prednisone for advanced prostate cancer. *N Engl J Med.* 2004;351:1502–1512.

64. Jacquy C, Soree A, Lambert F, et al. A quantitative study of peripheral blood stem cell contamination in diffuse large-cell non-Hodgkin's lymphoma: one-half of patients significantly mobilize malignant cells. *Br J Haematol.* 2000;110:631–637.

65. Nilsson S, Franzen L, Parker C, et al. Bone-targeted radium-223 in symptomatic, hormone-refractory prostate cancer: a randomised, multicentre, placebo-controlled phase II study. *Lancet Oncol.* 2007;8:587–594.

66. Weinberg RA. *The Biology of Cancer.* New York, NY: Garland Science; 2007.

67. Baselga J, Arteaga CL. Critical update and emerging trends in epidermal growth factor receptor targeting in cancer. *J Clin Oncol.* 2005;23:2445–2459.

68. Hsu JY, Wakelee HA. Monoclonal antibodies targeting vascular endothelial growth factor: current status and future challenges in cancer therapy. *BioDrugs.* 2009;23:289–304.

69. Ivy SP, Wick JY, Kaufman BM. An overview of small-molecule inhibitors of VEGFR signaling. *Nat Rev Clin Oncol.* 2009;6:569–579.

70. Gorski DH, Beckett MA, Jaskowiak NT, et al. Blockage of the vascular endothelial growth stress response increases the antitumor effects of ionizing radiation. *Cancer Res.* 1999;59:3374–3378.

71. Garcia-Barros M, Paris F, Cordon-Cardo C, et al. Tumor response to radiotherapy regulated by endothelial cell apoptosis. *Science.* 2003;300:1155–1159.

72. Zingg D, Riesterer O, Fabbro D, et al. Differential activation of the phosphatidylinositol 3'-kinase/Akt survival pathway by ionizing radiation in tumor and primary endothelial cells. *Cancer Res.* 2004;64:5398–5406.

73. Moeller BJ, Cao Y, Li CY, et al. Radiation activates HIF-1 to regulate vascular radiosensitivity in tumors: role of reoxygenation, free radicals, and stress granules. *Cancer Cell.* 2004;5:429–441.

74. Taylor AP, Osorio L, Craig R, et al. Tumor-specific regulation of angiogenic growth factors and their receptors during recovery from cytotoxic therapy. *Clin Cancer Res.* 2002;8:1213–1222.

75. Blumenthal RD, Sharkey RM, Kashi R, et al. Changes in tumor vascular permeability in response to experimental radioimmunotherapy: a comparative study of 11 xenografts. *Tumour Biol.* 1997;18:367–377.

76. Taylor AP, Rodriguez M, Adams K, et al. Altered tumor vessel maturation and proliferation in placenta growth factor-producing tumors: potential relationship to post-therapy tumor angiogenesis and recurrence. *Int J Cancer* 2003;105:158–164.

77. Ning S, Laird D, Cherrington JM, et al. The antiangiogenic agents SU5416 and SU6668 increase the antitumor effects of fractionated irradiation. *Radiat Res.* 2002;157:45–51.

78. Grimaldi AM, Guida T, D'Attino R, et al. Sunitinib: bridging present and future cancer treatment. *Ann Oncol.* 2007;18(suppl 6):vi31–vi34.

79. Gollob JA, Wilhelm S, Carter C, et al. Role of Raf kinase in cancer: therapeutic potential of targeting the Raf/MEK/ERK signal transduction pathway. *Semin Oncol.* 2006;33:392–406.

80. Sartor CI. Mechanisms of disease: radiosensitization by epidermal growth factor receptor inhibitors. *Nat Clin Pract Oncol.* 2004;1:80–87.

81. Debucquoy A, Haustermans K, Daemen A, et al. Molecular response to cetuximab and efficacy of preoperative cetuximab-based chemoradiation in rectal cancer. *J Clin Oncol.* 2009;27:2751–2757.

82. El-Emir E, Dearling JL, Huhalov A, et al. Characterisation and radioimmunotherapy of L19-SIP, an anti-angiogenic antibody against the extra domain B of fibronectin, in colorectal tumour models. *Br J Cancer.* 2007;96:1862–1870.

83. Huang SM, Harari PM. Modulation of radiation response after epidermal growth factor receptor blockade in squamous cell carcinomas: inhibition of damage repair, cell cycle kinetics, and tumor angiogenesis. *Clin Cancer Res.* 2000;6:2166–2174.

84. Dittmann K, Mayer C, Fehrenbacher B, et al. Radiation-induced epidermal growth factor receptor nuclear import is linked to activation of DNA-dependent protein kinase. *J Biol Chem.* 2005;280:31182–31189.

85. Meyn RE, Munshi A, Haymach JV, et al. Receptor signaling as a regulatory mechanism of DNA repair. *Radiother Oncol.* 2009;92:316–322.

86. Solomon B, Hagekyriakou J, Trivett MK, et al. EGFR blockade with ZD1839 ("Iressa") potentiates the antitumor effects of single and multiple fractions of ionizing radiation in human A431 squamous cell carcinoma. Epidermal growth factor receptor. *Int J Radiat Oncol Biol Phys.* 2003;55:713–723.

87. Bonner JA, Spencer SA. Postoperative radiotherapy in non-small-cell lung cancer warrants further exploration in the era of adjuvant

chemotherapy and conformal radiotherapy. *J Clin Oncol.* 2006;24: 2978–2980.

88. Pignon JP, Bourhis J, Domenge C, et al. Chemotherapy added to locoregional treatment for head and neck squamous-cell carcinoma: three meta-analyses of updated individual data. MACH-NC Collaborative Group. Meta-Analysis of Chemotherapy on Head and Neck Cancer. *Lancet.* 2000;355:949–955.

89. Argiris A. Update on chemoradiotherapy for head and neck cancer. *Curr Opin Oncol.* 2002;14:323–329.

90. Verel I, Visser GW, van Dongen GA. The promise of immuno-PET in radioimmunotherapy. *J Nucl Med.* 2005;46(suppl 1):164S–171S.

91. Perk LR, Visser GW, Vosjan MJ, et al. (89)Zr as a PET surrogate radioisotope for scouting biodistribution of the therapeutic radiometals (90)Y and (177)Lu in tumor-bearing nude mice after coupling to the internalizing antibody cetuximab. *J Nucl Med.* 2005;46:1898–1906.

92. Bonner JA, Raisch KP, Trummell HQ, et al. Enhanced apoptosis with combination C225/radiation treatment serves as the impetus for clinical investigation in head and neck cancers. *J Clin Oncol.* 2000;18:47S–53S.

93. Brizel DM. Radiotherapy and concurrent chemotherapy for the treatment of locally advanced head and neck squamous cell carcinoma. *Semin Radiat Oncol.* 1998;8:237–246.

94. Milas L, Fang FM, Mason KA, et al. Importance of maintenance therapy in C225-induced enhancement of tumor control by fractionated radiation. *Int J Radiat Oncol Biol Phys.* 2007;67:568–572.

95. Burke PA, DeNardo SJ, Miers LA, et al. Combined modality radioimmunotherapy. Promise and peril. *Cancer.* 2002;94:1320–1331.

96. DeNardo SJ, Kroger LA, Lamborn KR, et al. Importance of temporal relationships in combined modality radioimmunotherapy of breast carcinoma. *Cancer.* 1997;80:2583–2590.

97. Violet JA, Dearling JL, Green AJ, et al. Fractionated 131I anti-CEA radioimmunotherapy: effects on xenograft tumour growth and haematological toxicity in mice. *Br J Cancer.* 2008;99:632–638.

98. Wikstrom P, Damber J, Bergh A. Role of transforming growth factor-beta1 in prostate cancer. *Microsc Res Tech.* 2001;52:411–419.

99. Tijink BM, Neri D, Leemans CR, et al. Radioimmunotherapy of head and neck cancer xenografts using 131I-labeled antibody L19-SIP for selective targeting of tumor vasculature. *J Nucl Med.* 2006;47:1127–1135.

100. Kelly MP, Lee ST, Lee FT, et al. Therapeutic efficacy of ^{177}Lu-CHX-A"-DTPA-hu3S193 radioimmunotherapy in prostate cancer is enhanced by EGFR inhibition or docetaxel chemotherapy. *Prostate.* 2009;69:92–104.

101. Lee FT, Mountain AJ, Kelly MP, et al. Enhanced efficacy of radioimmunotherapy with 90Y-CHX-A"-DTPA-hu3S193 by inhibition of epidermal growth factor receptor (EGFR) signaling with EGFR tyrosine kinase inhibitor AG1478. *Clin Cancer Res.* 2005;11:7080s–7086s.

102. Jorgensen TJ. Enhancing radiosensitivity: targeting the DNA repair pathways. *Cancer Biol Ther.* 2009;8:665–670.

103. Jeggo P, Lobrich M. Radiation-induced DNA damage responses. *Radiat Prot Dosimetry.* 2006;122:124–127.

104. Di MR, Fumagalli M, Cicalese A, et al. Oncogene-induced senescence is a DNA damage response triggered by DNA hyper-replication. *Nature.* 2006;444:638–642.

105. Friesen C, Lubatschofski A, Kotzerke J, et al. Beta-irradiation used for systemic radioimmunotherapy induces apoptosis and activates apoptosis pathways in leukaemia cells. *Eur J Nucl Med Mol Imaging.* 2003; 30:1251–1261.

106. McCabe N, Turner NC, Lord CJ, et al. Deficiency in the repair of DNA damage by homologous recombination and sensitivity to poly(ADP-ribose) polymerase inhibition. *Cancer Res.* 2006;66:8109–8115.

107. Marsit CJ, Liu M, Nelson HH, et al. Inactivation of the Fanconi anemia/BRCA pathway in lung and oral cancers: implications for treatment and survival. *Oncogene.* 2004;23:1000–1004.

108. Farmer H, McCabe N, Lord CJ, et al. Targeting the DNA repair defect in BRCA mutant cells as a therapeutic strategy. *Nature.* 2005;434: 917–921.

109. Tutt A, Robson M, Garber JE, et al. Phase II trial of the oral PARP inhibitor olaparib in BRCA-deficient advanced breast cancer. *J Clin Oncol (Meeting Abstracts).* 2009;27:CRA501.

110. Audeh MW, Penson RT, Friedlander M, et al. Phase II trial of the oral PARP inhibitor olaparib (AZD2281) in BRCA-deficient advanced ovarian cancer. *J Clin Oncol (Meeting Abstracts).* 2009;27:5500.

111. O'Shaughnessy J, Osborne C, Pippen J, et al. Efficacy of BSI-201, a poly (ADP-ribose) polymerase-1 (PARP1) inhibitor, in combination with gemcitabine/carboplatin (G/C) in patients with metastatic triple-negative breast cancer (TNBC): results of a randomized phase II trial. *J Clin Oncol (Meeting Abstracts).* 2009;27:3.

112. Turner N, Tutt A, Ashworth A. Hallmarks of 'BRCAness' in sporadic cancers [review]. *Nat Rev Cancer.* 2004;4:814–819.

113. Cleator S, Heller W, Coombes RC. Triple-negative breast cancer: therapeutic options. *Lancet Oncol.* 2007;8:235–244.

114. Blasina A, Hallin J, Chen E, et al. Breaching the DNA damage checkpoint via PF-00477736, a novel small-molecule inhibitor of checkpoint kinase 1. *Mol Cancer Ther.* 2008;7:2394–2404.

115. Folkman J. Role of angiogenesis in tumor growth and metastasis. *Semin Oncol.* 2002;29:15–18.

116. Haugland HK, Vukovic V, Pintilie M, et al. Expression of hypoxia-inducible factor-1alpha in cervical carcinomas: correlation with tumor oxygenation. *Int J Radiat Oncol Biol Phys.* 2002;53(4): 854–861.

117. Hockel M, Vaupel P. Biological consequences of tumor hypoxia. *Semin Oncol.* 2001;28(2 suppl 8):36–41.

118. Jain RK. Physiological barriers to delivery of monoclonal antibodies and other macromolecules in tumors. *Cancer Res.* 1990;50:814s–819s.

119. Tan J, Geng L, Yazlovitskaya EM, et al. Protein kinase B/Akt-dependent phosphorylation of glycogen synthase kinase-3beta in irradiated vascular endothelium. *Cancer Res.* 2006;66:2320–2327.

120. Shinohara ET, Cao C, Niermann K, et al. Enhanced radiation damage of tumor vasculature by mTOR inhibitors. *Oncogene.* 2005;24: 5414–5422.

121. Schwartz DL, Powis G, Thitai-Kumar A, et al. The selective hypoxia inducible factor-1 inhibitor PX-478 provides in vivo radiosensitization through tumor stromal effects. *Mol Cancer Ther.* 2009;8:947–958.

122. Willett CG, Duda DG, Czito BG, et al. Targeted therapy in rectal cancer. *Oncology (Williston Park).* 2007;21:1055–1065.

123. Willett CG, Duda DG, di TE, et al. Complete pathological response to bevacizumab and chemoradiation in advanced rectal cancer. *Nat Clin Pract Oncol.* 2007;4:316–321.

124. Zhu H, Baxter LT, Jain RK. Potential and limitations of radioimmunodetection and radioimmunotherapy with monoclonal antibodies. *J Nucl Med.* 1997;38:731–741.

125. Denekamp J. Review article: angiogenesis, neovascular proliferation and vascular pathophysiology as targets for cancer therapy. *Br J Radiol.* 1993;66:181–196.

126. Sauer S, Erba PA, Petrini M, et al. Expression of the oncofetal ED-B-containing fibronectin isoform in hematologic tumors enables ED-B-targeted 131I-L19SIP radioimmunotherapy in Hodgkin lymphoma patients. *Blood.* 2009;113:2265–2274.

127. Del Conte G, Tosi D, Fasolo A, et al. A phase I trial of antifibronectin 131I-L19-small immunoprotein (L19-SIP) in solid tumors and lymphoproliferative disease. *J Clin Oncol (Meeting Abstracts).* 2008;26:2575.

128. Pedley RB, Hill SA, Boxer GM, et al. Eradication of colorectal xenografts by combined radioimmunotherapy and combretastatin A-4 3-O-phosphate. *Cancer Res.* 2001;61:4716–4722.

129. Lankester KJ, Maxwell RJ, Pedley RB, et al. Combretastatin A-4-phosphate effectively increases tumor retention of the therapeutic antibody, 131I-A5B7, even at doses that are sub-optimal for vascular shut-down. *Int J Oncol.* 2007;30:453–460.

130. Flynn AA, Boxer GM, Begent RH, et al. Relationship between tumour morphology, antigen and antibody distribution measured by fusion of digital phosphor and photographic images. *Cancer Immunol Immunother.* 2001;50:77–81.

131. Meyer T, Gaya AM, Dancey G, et al. A phase I trial of radioimmunotherapy with 131I-A5B7 anti-CEA antibody in combination with combretastatin-A4-phosphate in advanced gastrointestinal carcinomas. *Clin Cancer Res.* 2009;15:4484–4492.

132. Oltersdorf T, Elmore SW, Shoemaker AR, et al. An inhibitor of Bcl-2 family proteins induces regression of solid tumours. *Nature.* 2005; 435:677–681.

133. Kim KW, Moretti L, Mitchell LR, et al. Combined Bcl-2/mammalian target of rapamycin inhibition leads to enhanced radiosensitization via induction of apoptosis and autophagy in non-small cell lung tumor xenograft model. *Clin Cancer Res.* 2009;15:6096–6105.

134. Shankar S, Singh TR, Srivastava RK. Ionizing radiation enhances the therapeutic potential of TRAIL in prostate cancer in vitro and in vivo: intracellular mechanisms. *Prostate.* 2004;61:35–49.

135. Shankar S, Singh TR, Chen X, et al. The sequential treatment with ionizing radiation followed by TRAIL/Apo-2L reduces tumor growth and induces apoptosis of breast tumor xenografts in nude mice. *Int J Oncol.* 2004;24:1133–1140.

136. Straughn JM Jr., Oliver PG, Zhou T, et al. Anti-tumor activity of TRA-8 anti-death receptor 5 (DR5) monoclonal antibody in combination with chemotherapy and radiation therapy in a cervical cancer model. *Gynecol Oncol.* 2006;101:46–54.

137. Karikari CA, Roy I, Tryggestad E, et al. Targeting the apoptotic machinery in pancreatic cancers using small-molecule antagonists of the X-linked inhibitor of apoptosis protein. *Mol Cancer Ther.* 2007;6:957–966.

138. Zaffaroni N, Daidone MG. Survivin expression and resistance to anticancer treatments: perspectives for new therapeutic interventions. *Drug Resist Updat.* 2002;5:65–72.

139. Bolden JE, Peart MJ, Johnstone RW. Anticancer activities of histone deacetylase inhibitors. *Nat Rev Drug Discov.* 2006;5:769–784.

140. Geng L, Cuneo KC, Fu A, et al. Histone deacetylase (HDAC) inhibitor LBH589 increases duration of gamma-H2AX foci and confines HDAC4 to the cytoplasm in irradiated non-small cell lung cancer. *Cancer Res.* 2006;66:11298–11304.

141. Al-Ejeh F, Darby JM, Brown MP. The La autoantigen is a malignancy-associated cell death target that is induced by DNA-damaging drugs. *Clin Cancer Res.* 2007;13:5509s–5518s.

142. Rutjes SA, Utz PJ, van der Heijden A, et al. The La (SS-B) autoantigen, a key protein in RNA biogenesis, is dephosphorylated and cleaved early during apoptosis. *Cell Death Differ.* 1999;6:976–986.

143. Ayukawa K, Taniguchi S, Masumoto J, et al. La autoantigen is cleaved in the COOH terminus and loses the nuclear localization signal during apoptosis. *J Biol Chem.* 2000;275:34465–34470.

144. Wyllie AH, Kerr JF, Currie AR. Cell death: the significance of apoptosis [review]. *Int Rev Cytol.* 1980;68:251–306.

145. Leers MPG, Bjorklund V, Bjorklund B, et al. An immunohistochemical study of the clearance of apoptotic cellular fragments. *Cell Mol Life Sci.* 2002;59:1358–1365.

146. Larson CJ, Moreno JG, Pienta KJ, et al. Apoptosis of circulating tumor cells in prostate cancer patients. *Cytometry A.* 2004;62:46–53.

147. Chang J, Ormerod M, Powles TJ, et al. Apoptosis and proliferation as predictors of chemotherapy response in patients with breast carcinoma. *Cancer.* 2000;89:2145–2152.

148. Davis DW, Buchholz TA, Hess KR, et al. Automated quantification of apoptosis after neoadjuvant chemotherapy for breast cancer: early assessment predicts clinical response. *Clin Cancer Res.* 2003;9:955–960.

149. Al-Ejeh F, Darby JM, Pensa K, et al. In vivo targeting of dead tumor cells in a murine tumor model using a monoclonal antibody specific for the La autoantigen. *Clin Cancer Res.* 2007;13:5519s–5527s.

150. Al-Ejeh F, Darby JM, Tsopelas C, et al. APOMAB, a La-specific monoclonal antibody, detects the apoptotic tumor response to life-prolonging and DNA-damaging chemotherapy. *PLoS ONE.* 2009;4:e4558.

151. Horoszewicz JS, Kawinski E, Murphy GP. Monoclonal antibodies to a new antigenic marker in epithelial prostatic cells and serum of prostatic cancer patients. *Anticancer Res.* 1987;7:927–935.

152. Troyer JK, Beckett ML, Wright GL Jr. Location of prostate-specific membrane antigen in the LNCaP prostate carcinoma cell line. *Prostate.* 1997;30:232–242.

153. Smith-Jones PM, Vallabhajosula S, Navarro V, et al. Radiolabeled monoclonal antibodies specific to the extracellular domain of prostate-specific membrane antigen: preclinical studies in nude mice bearing LNCaP human prostate tumor. *J Nucl Med.* 2003;44:610–617.

154. Wynant GE, Murphy GP, Horoszewicz JS, et al. Immunoscintigraphy of prostatic cancer: preliminary results with 111In-labeled monoclonal antibody 7E11-C5.3 (CYT-356). *Prostate.* 1991;18:229–241.

155. Deb N, Goris M, Trisler K, et al. Treatment of hormone-refractory prostate cancer with 90Y-CYT-356 monoclonal antibody. *Clin Cancer Res.* 1996;2:1289–1297.

156. Bander NH, Trabulsi EJ, Kostakoglu L, et al. Targeting metastatic prostate cancer with radiolabeled monoclonal antibody J591 to the extracellular domain of prostate specific membrane antigen. *J Urol.* 2003;170:1717–1721.

157. Chen S, Yu L, Jiang C, et al. Pivotal study of iodine-131-labeled chimeric tumor necrosis treatment radioimmunotherapy in patients with advanced lung cancer. *J Clin Oncol.* 2005;23:1538–1547.

158. Park JM, Kohn MJ, Bruinsma MW, et al. The multifunctional RNA-binding protein La is required for mouse development and for the establishment of embryonic stem cells. *Mol Cell Biol.* 2006;26:1445–1451.

159. Ruggero D, Pandolfi PP. Does the ribosome translate cancer? *Nat Rev Cancer.* 2003;3:179–192.

160. Kenan DJ, Keene JD. La gets its wings. *Nat Struct Mol Biol.* 2004;11:303–305.

161. Rahman A, Isenberg DA. Systemic lupus erythematosus. *N Engl J Med.* 2008;358:929–939.

162. Zhao M, Beauregard DA, Loizou L, et al. Non-invasive detection of apoptosis using magnetic resonance imaging and a targeted contrast agent. *Nat Med.* 2001;7:1241–1244.

163. Thierry B, Al-Ejeh F, Majewsky P, et al. Immunotargeting of advanced functional nanostructures for MRI detection of apoptotic tumor cells [abstract]. *Adv Mater.* 2009;21:541–545.

The Delivery Construct: Maximizing the Therapeutic Ratio of Targeted Radionuclide Therapy

Ingrid J. G. Burvenich and Andrew M. Scott

TARGETED DELIVERY OF RADIONUCLIDES: WHEN DOES IT WORK?

To be effective, targeted radionuclide therapy (TRT) needs specific delivery of therapeutic radioisotopes to the tumor cells. Ideally, once injected into the body the delivery construct seeks the tumor cells and delivers the radioactive isotope to the target site with minimal toxicity to normal tissues. A classic example of TRT is the use of radioactive iodine (sodium-^{131}I) as a postsurgery treatment in papillary and follicular thyroid cancer (1–3). The aim of the postsurgery treatment in differentiated thyroid cancer is the selective irradiation of occult microscopic cancer foci, and ablation of any remaining normal thyroid tissue. The use of ^{131}I for postablative scanning allows detection of persistent or metastatic carcinoma; upon finding a focus of such persistent or metastatic carcinoma, it may also allow precise removal of such foci in selected cases (4). Achieving these goals leads to a decreased recurrence rate and, more importantly, an improved tumor-specific survival (5).

A key characteristic of an optimal delivery construct is its selective uptake by the targeted tumor tissue with minimal toxicity delivered to normal tissues. For ^{131}I, the selective accumulation of iodine by thyroid cells occurs in a process called iodide trapping. An ion pump called the sodium-iodide symporter actively cotransports sodium and iodide (I^-) across the basolateral membrane into thyroid epithelial cells and allows a radiotherapeutic dose to accumulate in the thyroid.

Another established example of TRT, used in the clinic, is radiolabeled metaiodobenzylguanidine (^{131}I-mIBG), a norepinephrine analog. ^{131}I-mIBG is actively transported into neuroblastoma cells by the norepinephrine transporter, although some passive diffusion has been noted (6). In the past 20 years, radiolabeled mIBG has been tested and used in the clinic mainly for the palliative treatment of neuroblastoma patients (7). More recently it has been included in combination with myeloablative therapy before bone marrow rescue or in combination with chemotherapy (8–10).

A number of different carriers have been investigated for the selective delivery of radioisotopes for cancer therapy. These agents include peptides, nucleotides, affinity proteins, antibodies, and nanostructures (e.g., liposomes, microparticles, nanoparticles, spheres, nanoshells, and minicells). Today, only four delivery agents are FDA-approved for targeted delivery of radionuclides (Table 17.1). Two of these drugs (SirSphere and TheraSphere) are administered via a catheter into the liver and are microparticles radiolabeled with ^{90}Y used for the treatment of hepatocellular carcinoma and hepatic metastases of colon cancer. The other two drugs (Zevalin and Bexxar) are radiolabeled antibodies used in the treatment of B-cell lymphoma and are administered systematically. An additional radioimmunotherapy approach (^{131}I-cTNT) has been recently approved for the treatment of lung cancer patients in China (11). Antibodies have dominated the research field of targeted delivery of radionuclides and represent the largest expanding group of delivery agents. After the approval of radioimmunotherapy in the treatment of non–Hodgkin lymphoma, investigators are optimizing the antibody construct and are trying different approaches to maximize the therapeutic index and broaden the use of the technology to treatment of solid tumors. Interestingly, although all delivery agents are under constant evolution either via improvement in technique or the discovery of novel entities, antibodies are also used in combination with the other agents to increase their specific delivery. In this chapter, we will overview the major steps taken to increase the therapeutic index in radioimmunotherapy using antibodies (Fig. 17.1). Most progress has been made in the field of genetic engineering of antibodies, and although mainly tested in preclinical studies, pretargeting strategies have now entered the clinical phase. In addition, the development of novel nanomedicine structures as delivery agents has benefited from employing antibodies to increase their specific delivery (10,12–51).

OPTIMIZING THE THERAPEUTIC INDEX BY ANTIBODY ENGINEERING

Two intact antibodies, Zevalin (murine, IgG1κ, ^{90}Y-labeled anti-CD20) and Bexxar (murine, IgG2λ, ^{131}I-labeled anti-CD20) are the only FDA-approved antibodies available for radioimmunotherapy of B-cell lymphoma. Clinical studies with Zevalin and Bexxar have now shown that targeted

Table **17.1**	Overview of different agents used in the delivery of radionuclides for cancer therapy			
Agent	**Radionuclide**	**Disease**	**Development Stage**	**Reference**
Norepinephrine analog				
MIBG	^{131}I	Neuroblastoma	Phase III	(10,12)
Peptides				
RGD peptides	^{90}Y, ^{177}Lu	Tumor-induced angiogenesis	Preclinical[a]	(13–21)
Octreotide	^{90}Y, ^{177}Lu	Neuroendocrine tumors	Phase II	
Biotin	^{90}Y	Breast cancer	Phase II	(22)
SHALs[b]	^{111}In	Lymphoma	Preclinical	(23,24)
Affibody	^{177}Lu	Solid tumors	Preclinical	(25,26)
Antibodies				
Intact	^{90}Y, ^{131}I	Lymphoma	FDA-approved	(27–35)
	^{131}I	Lung cancer	Approved in China	
	^{225}Ac	Leukemia	Phase I	
Intact and fragments	^{90}Y, ^{131}I	Solid tumors	Phase II–III	
	^{131}I	Liver cancer	Approved in China	
	^{177}Lu	Solid tumors	Phase II	
	^{213}Bi, ^{211}At, ^{225}Ac, ^{186}Re, ^{188}Re, ^{67}Cu	Solid tumors	Phase I–II	
Pretargeting	^{177}Lu	Solid tumors	Phase I	
Liposomes	^{225}Ac, ^{186}Re, ^{188}Re, ^{10}B	Solid tumors	Preclinical[c]	(36–40)
Nanoparticles	^{188}Re, ^{90}Y	Solid tumors	Preclinical[d]	(41,42)
Dendrimer	^{10}B, ^{188}Re	Solid tumors	Preclinical	(43,44)
Morpholinos	^{188}Re	Solid tumors	Preclinical	(45–47)
Spheres	^{90}Y	Hepatic lesions	FDA-approved	(48–51)

[a]Phase I for PET imaging.
[b]SHALs, selective high-affinity ligand.
[c]Phase I–II for delivery of drugs.
[d]Phase I for imaging applications.

radioactivity significantly improves the rate of objective responses in comparison to antibody alone (52,53). Both antibodies are monoclonal, of murine origin, and are immunoglobulin G (IgG) antibodies. Although there are five antibody classes (IgG, IgA, IgM, IgE, and IgD), IgG is the most studied antibody form in radioimmunotherapy with only a few IgM molecules being investigated in preclinical and clinical studies (54,55). Table 17.2 provides an overview of some active clinical trials in radioimmunotherapy as reported on the FDA clinical trial website (http://www.clinicaltrials.gov/).

IgGs are large glycoproteins of 150,000 Da. Their Y-shaped structure consists of two Fab (fragment antigen binding, ~50,000 Da) ends and an Fc fragment (crystallizable fragment, ~50,000 Da) (Fig. 17.1A). IgG antibodies are bivalent and each Fab binds its antigen with high specificity. Targeting an antigen with multiple repetitive epitopes or a cell with multiple receptors increases their functional affinity referred to as the avidity of antibodies. The Fc fragment

is responsible for Fcγ receptor binding, thereby recruiting cytotoxic effector functions and binding to the neonatal Fc receptor (FcRn) (56,57). Interaction with FcRn rescues IgGs from being degraded and gives them a long serum half-life (up to 3 to 4 weeks).

Highly specific recognition of the antigen targets and high-avidity binding make antibodies attractive candidates for delivery of radionuclides. Although high tumor uptake is often found in preclinical studies using mouse models, tumor uptake and tumor penetration have been the most challenging limitations of intact antibodies targeting solid tumors (58). Accretion into the tumor may be as low as 0.001% to 0.01% ID/g in patients, often resulting in tumor doses of less than 1500 cGy (59). Another limitation seen in preclinical and clinical studies is a higher radioresistance of solid tumors versus hematologic tumors (60–62).

The current status of radioimmunotherapy in several solid tumor types has been recently summarized for medullary thyroid carcinoma (63), breast cancer (32,64),

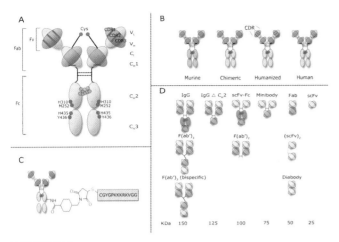

FIGURE 17.1 Antibody engineering: different strategies to improve the therapeutic index in radioimmunotherapy. **A:** Typical structure of a humanized IgG1 antibody. Following engineering strategies are presented: *Black dots*, mutations in amino acids involved in FcRn binding that influence the pharmacokinetics of the IgG; *CDR1–3*, murine CDRs grafted into a human IgG backbone to humanize the antibody; *Cys*, engineered cysteine residues for site-specific conjugation. **B:** Humanization strategies: *purple*, indicating the murine portion of the IgG and *blue*, indicating the human portion of the IgG. **C:** Introducing a nuclear localizing signal. **D:** Monospecific and bispecific fragments used in radioimmunotherapeutic strategies. Abbreviations: CDR, complementary-determining regions; C$_H$, constant domain heavy chain; C$_L$, constant domain light chain; Fc, crystallizable fragment; Fv, variable fragment. (Please see Color Insert).

ovarian cancer (32,65), renal and colorectal cancer (32), and head and neck carcinoma (66). Here the most important strategies in improving the therapeutic index when using radiolabeled antibodies will be reviewed.

Humanization

The original technology used to generate monoclonal antibodies (mAbs) for clinical applications was realized by Köhler and Milstein when they developed the hybridoma technology in 1975, thereby creating mAbs of murine origin (67). Herein, mouse hybridomas were generated from the fusion of immortalized myeloma cells with B cells from immunized mice. While these murine antibodies are very specific and proved excellent for use in immunohistochemical staining of histology sections and for drug discovery, once injected into humans, these antibodies induce a human antimouse antibody (HAMA) response. The murine origin of Bexxar and Zevalin is not so important in the area of delivering radionuclides for therapy of lymphoma, where the disease is characterized by decreased host immune recognition and a single dose is highly effective. With lymphoma, a single high dose of radioimmunotherapy is associated with high response rates due to the radiosensitivity of

Table **17.2**	**Examples of current radioimmunotherapy trials in solid tumors (http://www.clinicaltrials.gov)**						
Agent	**Action**	**Target**	**Radionuclide**	**Disease**	**Phase**	**Site/Sponsor**
hMN-14 × m679 (bispecific)	Pretargeting	CEA	^{177}Lu	Colorectal cancer	Phase I	RUNMC
J591 (humanized)	Single therapy	PSMA	^{177}Lu	Prostate cancer	Phase I/II	WMCCU
				Nonprostate cancer	Phase I	WMCCU
J591 (humanized)	Combination therapy	PSMA	^{177}Lu	Prostate cancer	Phase I/II	WMCCU
cT84.66 (chimeric)	Combination therapy	CEA	^{90}Y	Colorectal Cancer	Phase I	NCI
				Liver metastasis		
				NSCLC		
3F8 (murine)	Combination therapy	GD2	^{131}I	Neuroblastoma	Phase I	MSKCC, NCI
	Combination therapy	GC2	^{131}I	Brain and central nervous system tumors	Phase II	MSKCC, NCI
81C6 (murine, Neuradiab)	Combination therapy	tenascin	^{131}I	Glioblastoma	Phase III	Bradmer Pharmaceuticals
ch81C6 (chimeric)	Single therapy	tenascin	^{211}At	Brain tumors	Phase I/II	Duke University, NCI
m170 (murine)	Combination therapy	MUC1	^{90}Y	Breast cancer	Phase I	NCI
				Prostate cancer		
HMFG1 (murine)	Single therapy	MUC1	^{90}Y	Ovarian cancer	Phase III	NCI
cG250 (chimeric)	Single therapy	G250	^{90}Y	Renal cancer	Phase I	MSKCC, LICR
			^{177}Lu	Renal cancer	Phase I/II	RUNMC, LICR

Abbreviations: CEA, carcinoembryonic antigen; GD2, disialoganglioside; LICR, Ludwig Institute for Cancer Research; MSKCC, Memorial Sloan-Kettering Cancer Center; MUC1, mucin 1; NCI, National Cancer Institute; PSMA, prostate-specific membrane antigen; RUNMC, Radboud University Nijmegen Medical Centre; WMCCU, Weill Medical College of Cornell University.

lymphoma. However, effective solid tumor radioimmunotherapy may need repeated administration of nonimmunogenic antibodies. Patients who develop HAMA responses can no longer receive radiolabeled murine antibodies, because the antimouse antibodies in the blood would result in a complex that redistributes to the liver and spleen. This phenomenon also could result in clinical adverse symptoms. As a result, the fraction of radioactivity being delivered to the tumor is reduced (31). Two strategies have been used to reduce the immunogenicity of mAbs: production of antibody chimeras derived from both mouse and human DNA and the production of humanized or fully human antibodies (Fig. 17.1B).

Recombinant DNA techniques such as chimerization and humanization were the first techniques used to reduce the HAMA response. A chimeric antibody is created by linking the DNA segments encoding mouse variable regions (heavy-chain domain [V_H] and light-chain domain [V_L]) specific for the hapten/antigen of interest to the genes encoding constant domains (C_L, C_{H1}, C_{H2}, C_{H3}) of a human antibody (68,69). However, some of these antibodies are still able to induce a human antichimeric response. Interestingly, a chimeric tumor necrosis therapy antibody (^{131}I-cTNT) has been approved in China for the treatment of advanced lung cancer (11).

A next step in reducing the immunogenicity was to replace the complementarity-determining regions (CDR) of a human antibody by those of a defined specific murine antibody (70). The CDRs are six highly variable regions in the variable domains (three in V_L and three in V_H) and they contain the residues most likely to bind antigen. Therefore, the CDRs are usually retained in the humanized antibodies. Further replacement of key residues from the parent mouse antibody in the human framework is generally required to restore its original function or binding affinity (71,72). If too many back mutations are required, it might be optimal to keep the core and CDRs of the mouse variable domains, but replace the surface residues with those from a human sequence. This technique is called resurfacing or veneering (73,74). The xenogeneic CDRs of the humanized antibodies may evoke anti-idiotypic (anti-Id) response in patients. Further improvements to minimize the anti-Id response in patients are based on grafting only the specificity-determining residues onto the human frameworks, the CDR residues that are most crucial in the antibody–ligand interaction. This has successfully been done for the anticarcinoma mAb CC49 that specifically recognizes tumor-associated glycoprotein (TAG)-72 (75).

Later evolutions in genetic engineering made it possible to produce fully human antibodies either by phage display libraries or from transgenic mice. Phage display technology opened the pathway to fully human antibodies using large human Ig gene combinatorial libraries (76). In 1994, transgenic mice were described for the generation of fully human antibodies. These mice used for antigen immunization are transgenic for human Ig genes and have disrupted mouse Ig heavy-chain and Igκ light-chain loci (77,78). Further improve-

ments set out to recapitulate the human antibody response in mice by functional transplant of megabase human Ig loci (79), which led to the Xenomouse technology (80,81).

As nonimmunogenic humanized antibodies are necessary for repetitive administration in the treatment of solid tumors, compared with murine parental antibodies, these antibodies remain longer in the circulation, thereby increasing the hematologic toxicity of radiolabeled forms. Further optimization of pharmacokinetic properties of these nonimmunogenic antibodies might be a necessity before increase in therapeutic ratio for radioimmunotherapy can be clinically achieved in patients.

Antibody fragments

Therapeutically, targeting hematologic tumors has been more successful than targeting solid tumors. Challenges with targeting solid tumors are poor penetration of large tumors, low radiosensitivity, poor penetration through the vasculature by large proteins, and high interstitial pressure preventing homogenous distribution of the intact antibodies into the tumor (82,83). Also, the long antibody half-life causes the bone marrow typically to be the dose-limiting organ for radioimmunotherapy (33). To overcome these hurdles, several strategies have been used to optimize the delivery of antibodies for radioimaging and radiotherapy. At the same time, the appropriate choice of an isotope is crucial for a positive outcome. As described in Chapters 6, 18, 20, and 27, different radionuclides have different chemical and physical properties making them suitable for different volumes of disease (minimal disease or bulky disease) or different methods for delivery (cell surface receptor, internalizing receptor, nuclear targeting). Radionuclides with β-emissions travel millimeter distances and deposit their energy across several hundred cell diameters. They might be beneficial for targeting heterogenous tumors where not all cells express the target receptor. This is called the "cross-fire effect." On the other hand, radionuclides emitting α-particles travel 40 to 100 µm (5 to 10 cell diameters) and are more appropriate for micrometastatic disease or applications where single cells or small cell clusters are targeted. Auger emitters deposit their low energy over very short distances (less than 100 nm) and preferentially need to be delivered into the nucleus of target cells. Because the function of antibodies is separated in different domains, namely the Fab and Fc domain, the half-life of antibodies can be modified by fragmentation. This will potentially increase the therapeutic index and make the tumor uptake and penetration more suitable depending on the use of α-, β-, or Auger therapy.

Chemical fragments

Originally, fragmentation was performed by enzymatic digestions (papain or pepsin). In 1983, comparative in vivo studies of an intact ^{131}I-labeled anti–carcinoembryonic antigen (CEA) mAb and the associated F(ab')$_2$ and Fab fragments were reported for the first time. Radiolabeled fragments, in particular Fab, resulted in much higher tumor-to-background ratios and tumor detection, as determined by external scanning, than did the intact mAb in a model of nude mice grafted with a human colon carcinoma (84). Wahl et al. suggested F(ab')₂ was the better candidate for radioimmunotherapy as shown in a hamster colon carcinoma model (85). In a retrospective clinical study by Delaloye et al., an Fab was found to detect metastasis better in patients with colorectal cancer (86). It must also be noted that the absolute tumor uptake of antibody fragments is less than intact IgG. At present, only one radiolabeled Fab, Licartin (radioiodinated metuximab), has been approved for treatment of liver cancer in China (87).

Engineered fragments

In the last decade, antibody engineering has been utilized for optimizing antibody fragments for improved delivery of radionuclides. Examples of engineered fragments are presented in Figure 17.1D. Many in vivo studies have shown that reducing the size of an intact antibody changes its pharmacokinetics, increases the tumor penetration, advances the maximum tumor uptake to an earlier time point, and shifts the dose-limiting organ from bone marrow to other organs such as liver and kidneys (29,30,33,88).

The building block typically used for engineered antibody fragments is the scFv (single-chain variable fragment), a fragment where Ig heavy chain and light chain are covalently connected by a flexible peptide linker (89–92). Several scFvs have been evaluated for their specific in vivo tumor targeting of antigens such as TAG-72, CEA, and the HER2/neu receptor. They have demonstrated more rapid clearance and higher tumor-to-normal tissue ratios than the corresponding IgG or Fab fragments, although total tumor concentration may not always approach that of intact IgG (93–95). Furthermore, while penetration of scFv into a tumor from the vasculature (demonstrated with autoradiography) has been reported to be superior to that of corresponding intact IgG, F(ab')₂, or Fab (96), this finding is not always consistently found with a single infusion due to the short serum half-life of scFvs.

The next step was to modify the linkers and to identify other forms of antibodies, such as diabodies, triabodies, and tetrabodies (29,30,97–101); one of the easiest approaches for the production of dimeric scFvs is based on spontaneous formation of noncovalent dimers such as 50-kDa diabodies (102). Adams et al. described an improvement with in vivo tumor targeting using divalent forms of anti–neu-scFv with a C-terminal Gly₄Cys joined by a disulfide bond (94,103). Others have fused scFvs to protein domains capable of multimerization, for example, leucine zipper proteins (104), streptavidin (105), or the κ-constant region (106).

Radiolabeled small fragments (less than 60 kDa; e.g., scFv, diabodies, and sc(Fv)₂) show a short serum half-life because of direct filtration from the blood in the kidneys. They have excellent tumor-to-blood ratios, but limitations of these fragments are reduced accumulation in the tumor

and unfavorable tumor-to-kidney ratios when radiometals are used (107,108).

To increase tumor uptake, intermediately sized fragments have been generated (~80 kDa; e.g., anti–TAG-72 delta-CH2 (109), anti-CEA minibody (110), anti–extra domain B [ED-B] of fibronectin small immunoprotein [SIP] (111), antimindin/RG-1 (112)), and large multivalent fragments (100 to 150 kDa; e.g., anti-CC49 (sc(Fv)₂)₂ (98), anti-CEA scFv-Fc (113), and F(ab')₃-x (114,115)).

Considerable progress has been achieved in this field, with a diversity of antibody constructs with different targeting properties now available. Studies comparing different formats suggest that the larger antibody formats may be more suitable for radioimmunotherapy because of their higher tumor uptake, whereas the smaller formats may be more suitable for radiodiagnostic applications because of rapid blood clearance and higher tumor-to-background ratios. None of these engineered fragments is currently approved for clinical use in the United States or Europe and further clinical studies are required to determine which radionuclide would be most effectively matched with each of these constructs for optimal therapeutic response. An example of an engineered antibody fragment currently in clinical trial is ¹³¹I-L19-SIP (116). In this construct, the L19scFv is connected to the CH4 domain of the human IgE secretory isoform IgE-S2 by a short glycine–serine linker (117,118).

▌Bispecific fragments

A second class of fragments has been engineered to be multispecific. These bispecific antibodies (BsAbs) or multispecific antibodies are able of binding two or more different antigens. An example of a bispecific trivalent antibody is shown in Figure 17.1D. Originally, these antibodies were made by chemical crosslinking (119,120) or by fusion of two hybridomas (121–123). With the introduction of recombinant technology, the production efficiency of the molecules increased and different strategies are available to create these BsAbs, which vary in size and valency (95,124–126). The "dock-and-lock" modular system is one of the latest systems developed to create multivalent multispecific antibodies (34,127). Phase I and Phase II clinical studies using these pretargeting strategies are now in progress (Table 17.2).

BsAb fragments can also improve tumor targeting by the method of pretargeting. The key advantage of pretargeting strategies is that antibody localization to the tumor is separated from the delivery of the radionuclides, thereby enhancing the tumor-to-background ratios and increasing the administration dose and toxicity within the tumor (31). For a detailed background of the different pretargeting strategies refer to Chapter 14.

In pretargeting strategies, BsAbs are designed to use one or more binding sites to attach to the antigen (Fab or scFv) and the other binding site to a carrier hapten. Once the BsAb localizes at the tumor and clears from the blood and other normal tissues, the hapten carrying an imaging or therapeutic radionuclide is administered. The hapten either obtains high accretion and high tumor-to-background ratios because it only binds to the mAb localized in the tumor or it clears rapidly from the body. One example described by Moosmayer et al. showed that targeting of the ED-B of fibronectin (a marker of tumor angiogenesis) with AP39 × m679 and subsequent injection of a ^{90}Y-hapten–peptide showed an improvement of the therapeutic efficacy in solid tumors by greater than threefold compared to directly radiolabeled ^{131}I-L19-SIP (128).

Boron neutron capture therapy (BNCT) is another form of radionuclide pretargeting therapy where the use of BsAbs has been studied in an attempt to increase the therapeutic index. BNCT is based on the nuclear reaction (see Chapter 27) that occurs when boron-10 (^{10}B), a stable isotope, is irradiated with neutrons of the appropriate energy (thermal neutrons, n_{th}). Irradiation with thermal neutrons is accomplished with a suitable external neutron source and used directly for irradiation of the treatment volume, just as is performed with standard photon (x-ray) therapy. Boron-11, an unstable form, is then formed and undergoes instantaneous nuclear fission to produce high-energy α-particles and recoiling lithium-7 nuclei (^{10}B + n_{th} → [^{11}B] → α-particles +^{7}Li) (129). If enough ^{10}B is selectively delivered to tumor cells in amounts higher than in the surrounding normal tissues and enough low-energy thermal neutrons reach the treatment volume, then the tumor cells can be destroyed as a result of the ^{10}B(n, α) ^{7}Li capture reaction. Using mAbs as the delivery carrier would be challenging for this type of therapy. This is because heavy boron loads are required for adequate delivered doses to cancer cells. Antibody conjugation generally results in relatively low prodrug-to-antibody ratios and increasing the prodrug-to-antibody ratio could interfere with the antibody's immunoreactivity potentially resulting in lower tumor accumulation and higher liver uptake (130). To address these issues, BsAbs were successfully designed to bind to tumor-specific antigens and also recognize a hapten included on the boron-containing carborane constructs (131). For BNCT, other types of carriers, such as liposomes with high prodrug-to-carrier ratios have also been studied, both as passive and targeted delivery carriers (see "Immunoliposomes").

Altering pharmacokinetics—interaction with FcRn

The FcRn is an MHC class I-like protein that plays a role in perinatal transfer of IgG across the syncytiotrophoblast of the placenta. The binding of IgG to FcRn occurs in a pH-dependent manner. FcRn also plays a role in maintaining the serum levels of IgG and albumin, thereby preventing them from being degraded and giving both their long serum half-life. IgG:FcRn interaction modulation can be used to shorten the pharmacokinetics of antibodies used to deliver radionuclides (57).

The FcRn binding site on IgG has been mapped using a combination of site-directed mutagenesis, functional analyses, and x-ray crystallography (132–134). Several amino acids have been identified that when altered abrogate (I253, H310, H433, H435), reduce (Y436), or improve IgG binding (T250, M252, S254, T256, T307, E380, M428) to FcRn (57). Reducing the binding to FcRn has shown to reduce the serum half-life, and increasing the binding results in increasing the half-life (29,113,132).

Problems associated with IgG:FcRn interaction modulation are that it may reduce the delivery of the immunoconjugates to the tumor if serum half-life is reduced, it requires reengineering of each construct, and it requires regulatory approval for each new construct. Jaggi et al. suggest that a more general and feasible approach would be to pharmacologically block the binding of the conjugated antibody to FcRn. They showed enhanced blood and whole-body clearance by high-dose polyclonal IgG therapy (135). A disadvantage of this approach is that the antibody level of a patient may significantly fluctuate and it is hard to predict for each patient what effect that will have on the immune system or the extent to which reliable change in FcRn binding occurs.

Introducing labeling sites

Traditional radiochemistry modifies selected amino acids across the whole surface of an antibody, which can potentially cause instability or a loss in immunoreactivity. Radioiodination methods such as Iodogen use random tyrosine residues, whereas radiometal labeling strategies modify ε-amino groups of lysine residues randomly located at the surface of the antibody. Inactivity of small antibody formats following iodination (136,137) or steric hindrance caused when a large group is added to a lysine in or near the antigen-binding site (137,138) has been reported.

Protein engineering can be used to introduce specific radiolabel sites within the recombinant proteins allowing greater control near the labeling site and improved stoichiometry of the labeling site. An example of this is the use of His-tags originally introduced for purification of recombinant proteins using metal chelate affinity chromatography (139). Labeling His-tags in recombinant proteins with TcCO has been proven very efficient and stable, with neither transchelation nor loss of binding activity, although immunogenicity to His-tags can occur (140). This technology can be extended to $^{186/188}$Re for radiotherapy as well. However, although a commercial kit (Mallinckrodt, St. Louis) for the preparation of ^{99m}Tc tricarbonyl is now available, a procedure for the preparation of ^{188}Re tricarbonyl with a yield of over 90% has yet to be developed (141).

Alternatively, site-directed mutagenesis has been used to place cysteine (Cys) residues on the surface of proteins to provide reactive thiol groups for site-specific labeling of antibodies (142,143). In order to allow site-specific radiolabeling using thiol-specific reagents, Cys diabodies in which the C-terminal Cys residues form an interchain disulfide bridge can be reduced and conjugated for radiolabeling (144,145). C-terminally engineered Cys was also used to site-specifically radiolabel annexin V with ^{18}F for imaging apoptosis (146), and an anti-HER2 affibody molecule with [99m]Tc (147).

In a more recent approach, phage display was used to identify Cys substitution sites that provide thiol reactivity within the hu4D5Fab without compromising immunoreactivity (148). The selected substitution sites were located in either the heavy chain (HC-A114C) or the light chain (LC-V110C) of the Fab and these sites were used to create a THIOMAB (149). The HC-A114C was also used in an anti–mucin 16 (MUC16) antibody, and an improved therapeutic index was observed when the thiol sites were used for site-specific drug conjugation. Further studies are required to show whether this approach would also increase the therapeutic index in radioimmunotherapy.

Localizing peptides

So far, the majority of radiolabeled antibodies have targeted tumor-associated antigens and surface receptors. Intracellular targets within the cytoplasm or nucleus have not been generally accessible or utilized for antibody delivery. Recent studies have shown that cell-penetrating peptides or nuclear localizing peptide sequences (NLSs) can transport antibodies into the cytoplasm and the nucleus (150,151). This offers opportunities to increase the therapeutic ratio in the field of radionuclide therapy by using antibodies.

Perhaps, one of the most important new developments to emerge is the use of NLSs to direct antibodies, conjugated to Auger electron–emitting radionuclides, to the nucleus of cancer cells following their receptor-mediated internalization. This has successfully been performed in preclinical studies targeting acute myeloid leukemia and breast cancer. In the first study, the humanized anti-CD33 (HuM195), modified by adding NLS to HuM195 (152), showed an increase in nuclear translocation and cytotoxicity of ^{111}In-HuM195. The NLS is a 13-mer peptide, CGYG-*PKKKRKV*GG containing the NLS of SV-40 large T antigen (153) and was conjugated by maleimide-derivatized huM195 with the N-terminal Cys of the NLS peptides. Because of their nanometer-to-micrometer range (154), Auger electron emitters such as ^{111}In are most damaging to DNA if their decay occurs in close proximity to the cell nucleus (155).

Compared to β-particles such as ^{90}Y and ^{131}I that are often limited by myelotoxicity, this approach might also reduce the toxicity to normal tissues because the conjugates are potent and cytotoxic after entering the nucleus. It was also possible to increase the numbers of conjugated NLS without significantly reducing the affinity of the antibody so high doses might not be needed. A similar study using NLS-modified ^{111}In–anti-HER2/neu antibody (Trastuzumab) showed a doubling of in vivo nucleus uptake in MDA-MB-361 tumor-bearing mice 72 hours after injection (150).

■ ANTIBODIES TO ENHANCE THE DELIVERY OF RADIONUCLIDES IN NANOMEDICINE

Other carriers have been developed for the delivery of diagnostic and therapeutic agents. Nanostructures such as (immuno)liposomes, gold nanoparticles, polymeric micelles, dendrimers, carbon nanotubes (CNTs), semiconductor quantum dots, hydrogels, and minicells are nanoscale delivery systems that are currently under investigation (156). The principal use of nanostructures so far has been as a delivery tool for drugs, where the use of nanocarriers improves the therapeutic efficacy of chemotherapy by reducing the toxic side effects and providing a more selective delivery to the tumor. The delivery of these nanocarriers is nonspecific and takes advantage of the defective tumor vasculature in tumors, leaving gaps as large as 600 to 800 nm between adjacent endothelial cells. Another characteristic of tumors is their poor lymphatic drainage. Both characteristics result in an enhanced permeability and retention effect (157–160) that enables macromolecules and nanostructures to accumulate in the tumor.

Many nanocarriers have been used for the delivery of radioisotopes in nuclear imaging and radiotherapy of cancer (161). Most of these carriers are used in preclinical settings where they are being used as a reporting system for drug delivery or for imaging purposes. Many studies show that uptake by the reticuloendothelial system is often a limiting factor when using these particles to deliver radioisotopes. Some of the challenges for the use of nanostructures in nuclear medicine include the ideal half-life that allows a suitable imaging time window and high enough accumulation in target cells for therapeutic purposes and selective binding to target cells to increase local retention and an acceptable toxicity profile.

Several factors such as size, coating, and attached ligands affect the delivery of these nanocarriers, and more research is necessary to reliably modulate the effects on pharmacokinetics and biodistribution (162). The efficacy of nanostructures as radionuclide delivery systems can be enhanced by making them tumor specific via the attachment of various ligands. Antibodies and other proteins have been used for that purpose (Fig. 17.2). Increasing evidence from preclinical studies has revealed therapeutic efficacy using antibodies for targeted delivery of a variety of radionuclide nanostructures.

Immunoliposomes

Liposomes are self-assembling spherical vesicles formed by one or several concentric lipid bilayers. The size can vary from small (~100 nm) to large unilamellar vesicles (~200 to 800 nm) and can reach up to 5 μm for multilamellar vesicles (163). Promising therapeutic applications seen in the delivery of liposomal drugs such as Doxorubicin have sparked interest to further develop this delivery vehicle for other purposes. One of the limitations of the use of liposomes is their fast half-life and uptake by the reticuloendothelial

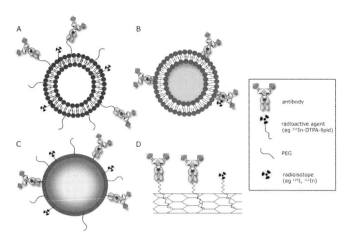

FIGURE 17.2 Targeted delivery of nanostructures using antibodies. **A:** Long-circulating immunoliposomes. **B:** Radioiodinated targeted minicells. **C:** Antibody-coated nanoparticles. **D:** Antibody-functionalized radiolabeled carbon nanotubes. (Please see Color Insert).

system, primarily in the liver. Several methods have been explored to extend the circulation time including coating the liposome surface with amphipathic polyethyleneglycols (PEGs) (164,165). Another modification is the use of surface-attached ligands, where antibodies have been the most widely used proteins. These antibody-conjugated liposomes (immunoliposomes), although demonstrating better tumor targeting, still showed high liver uptake. The next step in liposome development involved combining the properties of long-circulating liposomes and immunoliposomes, creating long-circulating immunoliposomes (166,167).

Radiotherapy with liposomes is still in its early testing stage. A promising radioneuclide currently under investigation is the use of actinium-225 (^{225}Ac) encapsulated in immunoliposomes. Immunoliposomes with encapsulated ^{225}Ac have been known to specifically target and become internalized by cancer cells (38,168). However, to enable therapeutic use of ^{225}Ac-containing liposomes, high activities of ^{225}Ac need to be stably encapsulated into liposomes, thereby overcoming the generally low specific activity of radiolabeled antibodies with ^{225}Ac (168–170). Current studies reporting on the adequate binding efficacy and specificity to cancer cells of immunoliposomes carrying ^{225}Ac suggest that these particles may be used for targeted α-therapy of micrometastatic disease. In vivo studies are still necessary to prove the usefulness of such an approach and whether immunoliposomes make better delivery systems than their radiolabeled antibody counterparts.

Other radioisotopes that have been encapsulated in liposomes are ^{186}Re and ^{188}Re (171), Radium-223 (^{223}Ra) and ^{224}Ra (39). A dosimetric assessment of tumor therapy using radiolabeled liposomes suggests that adequate tumor targeting and dose delivered to tumors may be achieved before normal tissue toxicity. Unlike the case with radioimmunotherapy, the dose-limiting organ is likely to be the liver and not the bone marrow, and strategies intended to reduce reticuloendothelial system accumulation are needed to further improve such a tumor-targeting approach (36,172).

A different approach is seen when using ^{10}B encapsulated in targeted liposomes (129,173,174). Targeted liposomes used for BNCT include boron-containing folate receptor–targeted liposomes (175), EGF-conjugated PEGylated liposome (176), Cetuximab-conjugated liposome (177), and transferrin-coupling pendant-type PEG liposomes (178).

Targeted minicells

Minicells are bacterially derived particles of 400 nm size (Fig. 17.2B). The use of minicells to deliver chemotherapeutics and siRNA has now been studied in several preclinical in vivo studies (179–181). The biodistribution of intravenously administered minicells bearing ^{125}I-labeled BsAbs was studied in nude mice bearing xenografts and clearly demonstrated that in contrast to nonspecifically targeted minicells, BsAbs-coated minicells are localized and concentrated in the tumor microenvironment. Targeting of radioiodinated BsAbs-coated minicells was compared to BsAbs alone and showed that 30% of the BsAbs-coated minicells was localized in the tumor at 2 hours, as compared to 3% of radioiodinated BsAbs alone (180).

Targeted nanoparticles

Nanoparticles are less than 1 μm-sized particles, made of polymeric, lipid, or inorganic material (Fig. 17.2C) (182). One of the advantages suggested with these nanoparticles is that when synthetized smaller than 100 nm, no surface modifications are necessary to evade the reticuloendothelial system. However, a recent review of Gaumet et al. warns about the need for precise size measurements when evaluating the biodistribution of nanoparticles (183).

Active targeting based on ligand–receptor or antibody–antigen interactions has been achieved with antibody-conjugated lipid nanoparticles to target the $\alpha_v\beta_3$ integrin to selectively deliver radionuclides (41,184) or with gold nanoparticles as radiosensitizers (185–187).

Carbon nanotubes

Single-wall CNTs are graphene cylinders of nanometer-range diameters and a length of several microns (188) (Fig. 17.2D). The feasibility of CNTs to deliver drugs, peptides, nucleic acids, and other loads has now been studied in several preclinical in vivo studies (189). Applications in delivery of radiolabeled CNTs in vivo have so far been limited to cancer imaging (190–194). A detailed description on the practicalities of functionalizing CNTs and conjugation with targeting ligands, including peptides and antibodies, and introducing radiolabels is provided in the review of Liu et al. (195).

Two main strategies have been used to modify CNTs to increase their solubility and biocompatibility: noncovalent coating of nanotubes using amphiphilic molecules (e.g., lipid–PEG) or covalent coating of nanotubes with various chemical groups (189,196). There are two reports on the biodistribution of two differently chemically functionalized nanotubes for delivery of radioisotopes. Wang et al. labeled the hydroxylated CNTs with radioactive ^{125}I atoms (197). Singh et al. chelated the ammonium-functionalized CNTs with diethylentriaminepentaacetic and labeled it with ^{111}In (190). Both studies demonstrate fast clearance of the nanotubes with little uptake in the liver and kidneys. This is different from the other nonmaterial that generally shows high uptake by the reticuloendothelial system.

In an attempt to establish targeted accumulation of CNTs in vivo, Liu et al. used PEG-functionalized nanotubes (191). Macrocyclic agent 1,4,7,10-tetraazacyclododecane-1,4,7,10-tetraacetic acid (DOTA) was attached to the termini of the PEG chains and used to conjugate positron-emitting radionuclide ^{64}Cu. Efficient targeting of integrin $\alpha_v\beta_3$-positive tumors was shown using arginine–glycine–aspartic acid (RGD) functionalization of the PEGylated CNTs. McDevitt et al. demonstrated the feasibility of using antibody-functionalized radiolabeled CNTs to specifically target the tumor (193).

Significant and specific tumor uptake have been shown both with RGD-functionalized and antibody-functionalized CNTs. However, it is not clear yet whether the use of CNTs for delivery of isotopes is an advantage over the use of the existing radiolabeled peptides and antibodies. In a direct comparison, McDevitt et al. showed that the ^{111}In-labeled Rituximab targeted better than the antibody-functionalized radiolabeled CNTs (193). In addition, the biodistribution studies reported by Wang et al. and Singh et al. revealed high liver and kidney uptake with CNTs free of RGD peptide or antibody (190,197).

Opportunities for CNTs as delivery constructs for radioisotopes are potentially with their use as delivery constructs of multiple copies of targeting agents. For example, a 200-nm-long CNT could hold more than a 100 available DOTA chelates and 6 intact antibodies per construct molecules. Therefore, CNT constructs could provide a means of significantly amplifying the diagnostic or therapeutic function of radionuclides. Assuming that a therapeutic radioisotope such as ^{225}Ac or ^{90}Y could be chelated, the specific delivery of a therapeutic payload to a cancer cell could be enabled. Further studies are necessary to understand the benefits of these CNTs for the delivery of radiotherapy.

CONCLUSIONS

A variety of parameters characterizing solid tumors are not usually observed in normal tissues or organs. These characteristics include high interstitial pressure, extensive angiogenesis, defective vascular architecture, poor lymphatic drainage, and high expression of cell surface receptors that are due to the expression of gene mutations or gene amplification in tumor cells. These parameters form the basis of optimization strategies to increase the delivery of radionuclides for radioimmunotherapy. With two radioimmunoconjugates

marketed for the treatment of non–Hodgkin lymphoma, antibodies represent the most studied class of molecules for the delivery of radionuclides in the treatment of solid tumors. In addition to the two intact murine antibodies used for lymphoma therapy, China has approved radioiodinated F(ab')$_2$ (Licartin) for the treatment of liver cancer and a radioiodinated chimeric tumor necrosis therapy mAb (^{131}I-cTNT) for the treatment of advanced lung cancer. This chapter has presented how antibody engineering strategies currently under preclinical and clinical investigations have increased the therapeutic index and hold promise for antibody-based cancer therapeutics of the future.

Acknowledgments

We appreciate the assistance of Rachael Canfield in designing the figures. We thank Dr Zhanqi Liu for helpful discussions.

REFERENCES

1. Schlumberger MJ. Papillary and follicular thyroid carcinoma. *N Engl J Med*. 1998;338:297–306.
2. Mazzaferri EL. An overview of the management of papillary and follicular thyroid carcinoma. *Thyroid*. 1999;9:421–427.
3. Sherman SI. Thyroid carcinoma. *Lancet*. 2003;361:501–511.
4. Verburg FA, Dietlein M, Lassmann M, et al. Why radioiodine remnant ablation is right for most patients with differentiated thyroid carcinoma. *Eur J Nucl Med Mol Imaging*. 2009;36:343–346.
5. Mazzaferri EL, Jhiang SM. Long-term impact of initial surgical and medical therapy on papillary and follicular thyroid cancer. *Am J Med*. 1994;97:418–428.
6. Tepmongkol S, Heyman S. 131I MIBG therapy in neuroblastoma: mechanisms, rationale, and current status. *Med Pediatr Oncol*. 1999;32:427–431; discussion 432.
7. Hoefnagel CA, den Hartog Jager FC, Taal BG, et al. The role of I-131-MIBG in the diagnosis and therapy of carcinoids. *Eur J Nucl Med*. 1987;13:187–191.
8. Mastrangelo S, Tornesello A, Diociaiuti L, et al. Treatment of advanced neuroblastoma: feasibility and therapeutic potential of a novel approach combining 131-I-MIBG and multiple drug chemotherapy. *Br J Cancer*. 2001;84:460–464.
9. DuBois SG, Matthay KK. Radiolabeled metaiodobenzylguanidine for the treatment of neuroblastoma. *Nucl Med Biol*. 2008;35(suppl 1):S35–S48.
10. Lessig MK. The role of 131I-MIBG in high-risk neuroblastoma treatment. *J Pediatr Oncol Nurs*. 2009;26:208–216.
11. Chen S, Yu L, Jiang C, et al. Pivotal study of iodine-131-labeled chimeric tumor necrosis treatment radioimmunotherapy in patients with advanced lung cancer. *J Clin Oncol*. 2005;23:1538–1547.
12. Garaventa A, Bellagamba O, Lo Piccolo MS, et al. 131I-metaiodobenzylguanidine (131I-MIBG) therapy for residual neuroblastoma: a mono-institutional experience with 43 patients. *Br J Cancer*. 1999; 81:1378–1384.
13. Heppeler A, Froidevaux S, Eberle AN, et al. Receptor targeting for tumor localisation and therapy with radiopeptides. *Curr Med Chem*. 2000;7:971–994.
14. Grotzinger C, Wiedenmann B. Somatostatin receptor targeting for tumor imaging and therapy. *Ann N Y Acad Sci*. 2004;1014:258–264.
15. Weiner RE, Thakur ML. Radiolabeled peptides in oncology: role in diagnosis and treatment. *BioDrugs*. 2005;19:145–163.
16. Kwekkeboom DJ, Mueller-Brand J, Paganelli G, et al. Overview of results of peptide receptor radionuclide therapy with 3 radiolabeled somatostatin analogs. *J Nucl Med*. 2005;46(suppl 1):62S–66S.
17. Kwekkeboom DJ, Teunissen JJ, Bakker WH, et al. Radiolabeled somatostatin analog [177Lu-DOTA0,Tyr3]octreotate in patients with endocrine gastroenteropancreatic tumors. *J Clin Oncol*. 2005;23:2754–2762.
18. Frilling A, Weber F, Saner F, et al. Treatment with (90)Y- and (177)Lu-DOTATOC in patients with metastatic neuroendocrine tumors. *Surgery*. 2006;140:968–976; discussion 976–977.

19. de Visser M, Verwijnen SM, de Jong M. Update: improvement strategies for peptide receptor scintigraphy and radionuclide therapy. *Cancer Biother Radiopharm.* 2008;23:137–157.

20. Tweedle MF. Peptide-targeted diagnostics and radiotherapeutics. *Acc Chem Res.* 2009;42:958–968.

21. Dijkgraaf I, Boerman OC, Oyen WJ, et al. Development and application of peptide-based radiopharmaceuticals. *Anticancer Agents Med Chem.* 2007;7:543–551.

22. Paganelli G, De Cicco C, Ferrari ME, et al. Intraoperative avidination for radionuclide treatment as a radiotherapy boost in breast cancer: results of a phase II study with (90)Y-labeled biotin. *Eur J Nucl Med Mol Imaging.* 2010;37:203–211.

23. Balhorn R, Hok S, Burke PA, et al. Selective high-affinity ligand antibody mimics for cancer diagnosis and therapy: initial application to lymphoma/leukemia. *Clin Cancer Res.* 2007;13:5621s–5628s.

24. Balhorn R, Hok S, DeNardo S, et al. Hexa-arginine enhanced uptake and residualization of selective high affinity ligands by Raji lymphoma cells. *Mol Cancer.* 2009;8:25.

25. Steffen AC, Almqvist Y, Chyan MK, et al. Biodistribution of 211At labeled HER-2 binding affibody molecules in mice. *Oncol Rep.* 2007;17:1141–1147.

26. Tolmachev V, Orlova A, Pehrson R, et al. Radionuclide therapy of HER2-positive microxenografts using a 177Lu-labeled HER2-specific Affibody molecule. *Cancer Res.* 2007;67:2773–2782.

27. Allen TM. Ligand-targeted therapeutics in anticancer therapy. *Nat Rev Cancer.* 2002;2:750–763.

28. Adams GP, Weiner LM. Monoclonal antibody therapy of cancer. *Nat Biotechnol.* 2005;23:1147–1157.

29. Wu AM, Senter PD. Arming antibodies: prospects and challenges for immunoconjugates. *Nat Biotechnol.* 2005;23:1137–1146.

30. Carter PJ. Potent antibody therapeutics by design. *Nat Rev Immunol.* 2006;6:343–357.

31. Sharkey RM, Goldenberg DM. Advances in radioimmunotherapy in the age of molecular engineering and pretargeting. *Cancer Invest.* 2006;24:82–97.

32. Boerman OC, Koppe MJ, Postema EJ, et al. Radionuclide therapy of cancer with radiolabeled antibodies. *Anticancer Agents Med Chem.* 2007;7:335–343.

33. Boswell CA, Brechbiel MW. Development of radioimmunotherapeutic and diagnostic antibodies: an inside-out view. *Nucl Med Biol.* 2007;34:757–778.

34. Sharkey RM, Goldenberg DM. Novel radioimmunopharmaceuticals for cancer imaging and therapy. *Curr Opin Investig Drugs.* 2008;9:1302–1316.

35. Deckert PM. Current constructs and targets in clinical development for antibody-based cancer therapy. *Curr Drug Targets.* 2009;10:158–175.

36. Emfietzoglou D, Kostarelos K, Sgouros G. An analytic dosimetry study for the use of radionuclide-liposome conjugates in internal radiotherapy. *J Nucl Med.* 2001;42:499–504.

37. Park JW, Hong K, Kirpotin DB, et al. Anti-HER2 immunoliposomes: enhanced efficacy attributable to targeted delivery. *Clin Cancer Res.* 2002;8:1172–1181.

38. Sofou S, Thomas JL, Lin HY, et al. Engineered liposomes for potential alpha-particle therapy of metastatic cancer. *J Nucl Med.* 2004;45:253–260.

39. Henriksen G, Schoultz BW, Michaelsen TE, et al. Sterically stabilized liposomes as a carrier for alpha-emitting radium and actinium radionuclides. *Nucl Med Biol.* 2004;31:441–449.

40. Sofou S. Radionuclide carriers for targeting of cancer. *Int J Nanomedicine.* 2008;3:181–199.

41. Li L, Wartchow CA, Danthi SN, et al. A novel antiangiogenesis therapy using an integrin antagonist or anti-Flk-1 antibody coated 90Y-labeled nanoparticles. *Int J Radiat Oncol Biol Phys.* 2004;58:1215–1227.

42. Chunfu Z, Jinquan C, Duanzhi Y, et al. Preparation and radiolabeling of human serum albumin (HSA)-coated magnetite nanoparticles for magnetically targeted therapy. *Appl Radiat Isot.* 2004;61:1255–1259.

43. Kobayashi H, Wu C, Kim MK, et al. Evaluation of the in vivo biodistribution of indium-111 and yttrium-88 labeled dendrimer-1B4M-DTPA and its conjugation with anti-Tac monoclonal antibody. *Bioconjug Chem.* 1999;10:103–111.

44. Barth RF, Wu G, Yang W, et al. Neutron capture therapy of epidermal growth factor (+) gliomas using boronated cetuximab (IMC-C225) as a delivery agent. *Appl Radiat Isot.* 2004;61:899–903.

45. Liu G, Dou S, He J, et al. Radiolabeling of MAG3-morpholino oligomers with 188Re at high labeling efficiency and specific radioactivity for tumor pretargeting. *Appl Radiat Isot.* 2006;64:971–978.

46. Liu G, Dou S, Mardirossian G, et al. Successful radiotherapy of tumor in pretargeted mice by 188Re-radiolabeled phosphorodiamidate morpholino oligomer, a synthetic DNA analogue. *Clin Cancer Res.* 2006;12:4958–4964.

47. Liu G, Dou S, He J, et al. Predicting the biodistribution of radiolabeled cMORF effector in MORF-pretargeted mice. *Eur J Nucl Med Mol Imaging.* 2007;34:237–246.

48. Carr BI. Hepatic arterial 90Yttrium glass microspheres (Therasphere) for unresectable hepatocellular carcinoma: interim safety and survival data on 65 patients. *Liver Transpl.* 2004;10:S107–S110.

49. King J, Quinn R, Glenn DM, et al. Radioembolization with selective internal radiation microspheres for neuroendocrine liver metastases. *Cancer.* 2008;113:921–929.

50. Riaz A, Salem R. Yttrium-90 radioembolization in the management of liver tumors: expanding the global experience. *Eur J Nucl Med Mol Imaging.* 2010;37:451–452.

51. Raoul JL, Boucher E, Rolland Y, et al. Treatment of hepatocellular carcinoma with intra-arterial injection of radionuclides. *Nat Rev Gastroenterol Hepatol.* 2010;7:41–49.

52. Witzig TE, Flinn IW, Gordon LI, et al. Treatment with ibritumomab tiuxetan radioimmunotherapy in patients with rituximab-refractory follicular non-Hodgkin's lymphoma. *J Clin Oncol.* 2002;20:3262–3269.

53. Davis TA, Kaminski MS, Leonard JP, et al. The radioisotope contributes significantly to the activity of radioimmunotherapy. *Clin Cancer Res.* 2004;10:7792–7798.

54. Schweitzer AD, Rakesh V, Revskaya E, et al. Computational model predicts effective delivery of 188-Re-labeled melanin-binding antibody to metastatic melanoma tumors with wide range of melanin concentrations. *Melanoma Res.* 2007;17:291–303.

55. Dadachova E, Revskaya E, Sesay MA, et al. Pre-clinical evaluation and efficacy studies of a melanin-binding IgM antibody labeled with 188Re against experimental human metastatic melanoma in nude mice. *Cancer Biol Ther.* 2008;7:1116–1127.

56. Woof JM, Burton DR. Human antibody-Fc receptor interactions illuminated by crystal structures. *Nat Rev Immunol.* 2004;4:89–99.

57. Roopenian DC, Akilesh S. FcRn: the neonatal Fc receptor comes of age. *Nat Rev Immunol.* 2007;7:715–725.

58. Burvenich I, Schoonooghe S, Cornelissen B, et al. In vitro and in vivo targeting properties of iodine-123- or iodine-131-labeled monoclonal antibody 14C5 in a non-small cell lung cancer and colon carcinoma model. *Clin Cancer Res.* 2005;11:7288–7296.

59. Goldenberg DM. Advancing role of radiolabeled antibodies in the therapy of cancer. *Cancer Immunol Immunother.* 2003;52:281–296.

60. Scott AM, Lee FT, Jones R, et al. A phase I trial of humanized monoclonal antibody A33 in patients with colorectal carcinoma: biodistribution, pharmacokinetics, and quantitative tumor uptake. *Clin Cancer Res.* 2005;11:4810–4817.

61. Chong G, Lee FT, Hopkins W, et al. Phase I trial of 131I-huA33 in patients with advanced colorectal carcinoma. *Clin Cancer Res.* 2005;11:4818–4826.

62. Scott AM, Tebbutt N, Lee FT, et al. A phase I biodistribution and pharmacokinetic trial of humanized monoclonal antibody Hu3s193 in patients with advanced epithelial cancers that express the Lewis-Y antigen. *Clin Cancer Res.* 2007;13:3286–3292.

63. Chatal JF, Campion L, Kraeber-Bodere F, et al. Survival improvement in patients with medullary thyroid carcinoma who undergo pretargeted anti-carcinoembryonic-antigen radioimmunotherapy: a collaborative study with the French Endocrine Tumor Group. *J Clin Oncol.* 2006;24:1705–1711.

64. DeNardo SJ. Radioimmunodetection and therapy of breast cancer. *Semin Nucl Med.* 2005;35:143–151.

65. Meredith RF, Buchsbaum DJ, Alvarez RD, et al. Brief overview of preclinical and clinical studies in the development of intraperitoneal radioimmunotherapy for ovarian cancer. *Clin Cancer Res.* 2007;13:5643s–5645s.

66. Nestor MV. Targeted radionuclide therapy in head and neck cancer. *Head Neck.* 2010;32:666–678.

67. Köhler G, Milstein C. Continuous cultures of fused cells secreting antibody of predefined specificity. *Nature.* 1975;256:495–497.

68. Morrison SL, Johnson MJ, Herzenberg LA, et al. Chimeric human antibody molecules: mouse antigen-binding domains with human constant region domains. *Proc Natl Acad Sci USA.* 1984;81:6851–6855.

69. Boulianne GL, Hozumi N, Shulman MJ. Production of functional chimaeric mouse/human antibody. *Nature.* 1984;312:643–646.

70. Jones PT, Dear PH, Foote J, et al. Replacing the complementarity-determining regions in a human antibody with those from a mouse. *Nature.* 1986;321:522–525.

71. Verhoeyen M, Milstein C, Winter G. Reshaping human antibodies: grafting an antilysozyme activity. *Science.* 1988;239:1534–1536.

72. Riechmann L, Clark M, Waldmann H, et al. Reshaping human antibodies for therapy. *Nature.* 1988;332:323–327.

73. Padlan EA. A possible procedure for reducing the immunogenicity of antibody variable domains while preserving their ligand-binding properties. *Mol Immunol.* 1991;28:489–498.

74. Pedersen JT, Henry AH, Searle SJ, et al. Comparison of surface accessible residues in human and murine immunoglobulin Fv domains. Implication for humanization of murine antibodies. *J Mol Biol.* 1994; 235:959–973.

75. Tamura M, Milenic DE, Iwahashi M, et al. Structural correlates of an anticarcinoma antibody: identification of specificity-determining residues (SDRs) and development of a minimally immunogenic antibody variant by retention of SDRs only. *J Immunol.* 2000;164:1432–1441.

76. Vaughan TJ, Williams AJ, Pritchard K, et al. Human antibodies with sub-nanomolar affinities isolated from a large non-immunized phage display library. *Nat Biotechnol.* 1996;14:309–314.

77. Green LL, Hardy MC, Maynard-Currie CE, et al. Antigen-specific human monoclonal antibodies from mice engineered with human Ig heavy and light chain YACs. *Nat Genet.* 1994;7:13–21.

78. Lonberg N, Taylor LD, Harding FA, et al. Antigen-specific human antibodies from mice comprising four distinct genetic modifications. *Nature.* 1994;368:856–859.

79. Mendez MJ, Green LL, Corvalan JR, et al. Functional transplant of megabase human immunoglobulin loci recapitulates human antibody response in mice. *Nat Genet.* 1997;15:146–156.

80. Green LL. Antibody engineering via genetic engineering of the mouse: XenoMouse strains are a vehicle for the facile generation of therapeutic human monoclonal antibodies. *J Immunol Methods.* 1999; 231:11–23.

81. Jakobovits A, Amado RG, Yang X, et al. From XenoMouse technology to panitumumab, the first fully human antibody product from transgenic mice. *Nat Biotechnol.* 2007;25:1134–1143.

82. Jain RK. Transport of molecules in the tumor interstitium: a review. *Cancer Res.* 1987;47:3039–3051.

83. Goldenberg DM. Targeted therapy of cancer with radiolabeled antibodies. *J Nucl Med.* 2002;43:693–713.

84. Buchegger F, Haskell CM, Schreyer M, et al. Radiolabeled fragments of monoclonal antibodies against carcinoembryonic antigen for localization of human colon carcinoma grafted into nude mice. *J Exp Med.* 1983;158:413–427.

85. Wahl RL, Parker CW, Philpott GW. Improved radioimaging and tumor localization with monoclonal F(ab')2. *J Nucl Med.* 1983;24: 316–325.

86. Delaloye B, Bischof-Delaloye A, Buchegger F, et al. Detection of colorectal carcinoma by emission-computerized tomography after injection of 123I-labeled Fab or F(ab')2 fragments from monoclonal anti-carcinoembryonic antigen antibodies. *J Clin Invest.* 1986;77: 301–311.

87. Nelson AL, Reichert JM. Development trends for therapeutic antibody fragments. *Nat Biotechnol.* 2009;27:331–337.

88. Holliger P, Hudson PJ. Engineered antibody fragments and the rise of single domains. *Nat Biotechnol.* 2005;23:1126–1136.

89. Bird RE, Hardman KD, Jacobson JW, et al. Single-chain antigen-binding proteins. *Science.* 1988;242:423–426.

90. Huston JS, Levinson D, Mudgett-Hunter M, et al. Protein engineering of antibody binding sites: recovery of specific activity in an anti-digoxin single-chain Fv analogue produced in Escherichia coli. *Proc Natl Acad Sci USA.* 1988;85:5879–5883.

91. Colcher D, Bird R, Roselli M, et al. In vivo tumor targeting of a recombinant single-chain antigen-binding protein. *J Natl Cancer Inst.* 1990;82:1191–1197.

92. Pluckthun A. Antibody engineering: advances from the use of Escherichia coli expression systems. *Biotechnology (NY).* 1991;9:545–551.

93. Milenic DE, Yokota T, Filpula DR, et al. Construction, binding properties, metabolism, and tumor targeting of a single-chain Fv derived from the pancarcinoma monoclonal antibody CC49. *Cancer Res.* 1991;51:6363–6371.

94. Adams GP, McCartney JE, Tai MS, et al. Highly specific in vivo tumor targeting by monovalent and divalent forms of 741F8 anti-c-erbB-2 single-chain Fv. *Cancer Res.* 1993;53:4026–4034.

95. Wu AM, Chen W, Raubitschek A, et al. Tumor localization of anti-CEA single-chain Fvs: improved targeting by non-covalent dimers. *Immunotechnology.* 1996;2:21–36.

96. Yokota T, Milenic DE, Whitlow M, et al. Microautoradiographic analysis of the normal organ distribution of radioiodinated single-chain Fv and other immunoglobulin forms. *Cancer Res.* 1993;53:3776–3783.

97. Goel A, Beresford GW, Colcher D, et al. Divalent forms of CC49 single-chain antibody constructs in Pichia pastoris: expression, purification, and characterization. *J Biochem.* 2000;127:829–836.

98. Goel A, Colcher D, Baranowska-Kortylewicz J, et al. Genetically engineered tetravalent single-chain Fv of the pancarcinoma monoclonal antibody CC49: improved biodistribution and potential for therapeutic application. *Cancer Res.* 2000;60:6964–6971.

99. Todorovska A, Roovers RC, Dolezal O, et al. Design and application of diabodies, triabodies and tetrabodies for cancer targeting. *J Immunol Methods.* 2001;248:47–66.

100. Hudson PJ, Souriau C. Engineered antibodies. *Nat Med.* 2003;9: 129–134.

101. Presta L. Antibody engineering for therapeutics. *Curr Opin Struct Biol.* 2003;13:519–525.

102. Holliger P, Prospero T, Winter G. "Diabodies": small bivalent and bispecific antibody fragments. *Proc Natl Acad Sci USA.* 1993; 90:6444–6448.

103. Huston JS, Adams GP, McCartney JE, et al. Tumor targeting in a murine tumor xenograft model with the (sFv')2 divalent form of anti-c-erbB-2 single-chain Fv. *Cell Biophys.* 1994;24–25:267–278.

104. Kostelny SA, Cole MS, Tso JY. Formation of a bispecific antibody by the use of leucine zippers. *J Immunol.* 1992;148:1547–1553.

105. Dubel S, Breitling F, Kontermann R, et al. Bifunctional and multimeric complexes of streptavidin fused to single chain antibodies (scFv). *J Immunol Methods.* 1995;178:201–209.

106. McGregor DP, Molloy PE, Cunningham C, et al. Spontaneous assembly of bivalent single chain antibody fragments in Escherichia coli. *Mol Immunol.* 1994;31:219–226.

107. Yazaki PJ, Wu AM, Tsai SW, et al. Tumor targeting of radiometal labeled anti-CEA recombinant T84.66 diabody and t84.66 minibody: comparison to radioiodinated fragments. *Bioconjug Chem.* 2001;12: 220–228.

108. Tahtis K, Lee FT, Smyth FE, et al. Biodistribution properties of (111)indium-labeled C-functionalized trans-cyclohexyl diethylene-triaminepentaacetic acid humanized 3S193 diabody and F(ab')(2) constructs in a breast carcinoma xenograft model. *Clin Cancer Res.* 2001;7:1061–1072.

109. Mueller BM, Reisfeld RA, Gillies SD. Serum half-life and tumor localization of a chimeric antibody deleted of the CH2 domain and directed against the disialoganglioside GD2. *Proc Natl Acad Sci USA.* 1990;87:5702–5705.

110. Hu S, Shively L, Raubitschek A, et al. Minibody: a novel engineered anti-carcinoembryonic antigen antibody fragment (single-chain Fv-CH3) which exhibits rapid, high-level targeting of xenografts. *Cancer Res.* 1996;56:3055–3061.

111. Borsi L, Balza E, Bestagno M, et al. Selective targeting of tumoral vasculature: comparison of different formats of an antibody (L19) to the ED-B domain of fibronectin. *Int J Cancer.* 2002;102:75–85.

112. Schneider DW, Heitner T, Alicke B, et al. In vivo biodistribution, PET imaging, and tumor accumulation of 86Y- and 111In-antimindin/RG-1, engineered antibody fragments in LNCaP tumor-bearing nude mice. *J Nucl Med.* 2009;50:435–443.

113. Kenanova V, Olafsen T, Crow DM, et al. Tailoring the pharmacokinetics and positron emission tomography imaging properties of anti-carcinoembryonic antigen single-chain Fv-Fc antibody fragments. *Cancer Res.* 2005;65:622–631.

114. Schott ME, Frazier KA, Pollock DK, et al. Preparation, characterization, and in vivo biodistribution properties of synthetically cross-linked multivalent antitumor antibody fragments. *Bioconjug Chem.* 1993;4:153–165.

115. Werlen RC, Lankinen M, Offord RE, et al. Preparation of a trivalent antigen-binding construct using polyoxime chemistry: improved biodistribution and potential for therapeutic application. *Cancer Res.* 1996;56:809–815.

116. Del Conte G, Tosi D, Fasolo A, et al. A phase I trial of antifibronectin 131I-L19-small immunoprotein (L19-SIP) in solid tumors and lymphoproliferative disease. *J Clin Oncol.* 2008;26:2575.

117. Tijink BM, Neri D, Leemans CR, et al. Radioimmunotherapy of head and neck cancer xenografts using 131I-labeled antibody L19-SIP for

selective targeting of tumor vasculature. *J Nucl Med.* 2006;47:
1127–1135.

118. El-Emir E, Dearling JL, Huhalov A, et al. Characterisation and
radioimmunotherapy of L19-SIP, an anti-angiogenic antibody against
the extra domain B of fibronectin, in colorectal tumour models. *Br J
Cancer.* 2007;96:1862–1870.

119. Glennie MJ, McBride HM, Worth AT, et al. Preparation and performance of bispecific F(ab' gamma)2 antibody containing thioether-
linked Fab' gamma fragments. *J Immunol.* 1987;139:2367–2375.

120. Stevenson GT, Pindar A, Slade CJ. A chimeric antibody with dual Fc
regions (bisFabFc) prepared by manipulations at the IgG hinge. *Anticancer Drug Des.* 1989;3:219–230.

121. Tiebout RF, van Boxtel-Oosterhof F, Stricker EA, et al. A human
hybrid hybridoma. *J Immunol.* 1987;139:3402–3405.

122. Hombach A, Jung W, Pohl C, et al. A CD16/CD30 bispecific monoclonal antibody induces lysis of Hodgkin's cells by unstimulated
natural killer cells in vitro and in vivo. *Int J Cancer.* 1993;55:830–836.

123. Renner C, Stehle I, Lee FT, et al. Targeting properties of an anti-
CD16/anti-CD30 bispecific antibody in an in vivo system. *Cancer
Immunol Immunother.* 2001;50:102–108.

124. Kontermann RE. Recombinant bispecific antibodies for cancer therapy. *Acta Pharmacol Sin.* 2005;26:1–9.

125. Das D, Suresh MR. Producing bispecific and bifunctional antibodies.
Methods Mol Med. 2005;109:329–346.

126. Shen J, Vil MD, Jimenez X, et al. Single variable domain antibody as
a versatile building block for the construction of IgG-like bispecific
antibodies. *J Immunol Methods.* 2007;318:65–74.

127. Rossi EA, Goldenberg DM, Cardillo TM, et al. Stably tethered multifunctional structures of defined composition made by the dock and
lock method for use in cancer targeting. *Proc Natl Acad Sci USA.*
2006;103:6841–6846.

128. Moosmayer D, Berndorff D, Chang CH, et al. Bispecific antibody pretargeting of tumor neovasculature for improved systemic radiotherapy of solid tumors. *Clin Cancer Res.* 2006;12:5587–5595.

129. Barth RF. A critical assessment of boron neutron capture therapy: an
overview. *J Neurooncol.* 2003;62:1–5.

130. Paxton RJ, Beatty BG, Varadarajan A, et al. Carboranyl peptide-
antibody conjugates for neutron-capture therapy: preparation,
characterization, and in vivo evaluation. *Bioconjug Chem.* 1992;
3:241–247.

131. Pak RH, Primus FJ, Rickard-Dickson KJ, et al. Preparation and properties of nido-carborane-specific monoclonal antibodies for potential
use in boron neutron capture therapy for cancer. *Proc Natl Acad Sci
USA.* 1995;92:6986–6990.

132. Kim JK, Firan M, Radu CG, et al. Mapping the site on human IgG for
binding of the MHC class I-related receptor, FcRn. *Eur J Immunol.*
1999;29:2819–2825.

133. Martin WL, West AP Jr, Gan L, et al. Crystal structure at 2.8 A of an
FcRn/heterodimeric Fc complex: mechanism of pH-dependent binding. *Mol Cell.* 2001;7:867–877.

134. Shields RL, Namenuk AK, Hong K, et al. High resolution mapping
of the binding site on human IgG1 for Fc gamma RI, Fc gamma RII,
Fc gamma RIII, and FcRn and design of IgG1 variants with improved
binding to the Fc gamma R. *J Biol Chem.* 2001;276:6591–6604.

135. Jaggi JS, Carrasquillo JA, Seshan SV, et al. Improved tumor imaging
and therapy via i.v. IgG-mediated time-sequential modulation of neonatal Fc receptor. *J Clin Invest.* 2007;117:2422–2430.

136. Nikula TK, Bocchia M, Curcio MJ, et al. Impact of the high tyrosine
fraction in complementarity determining regions: measured and predicted effects of radioiodination on IgG immunoreactivity. *Mol Immunol.* 1995;32:865–872.

137. Olafsen T, Bruland OS, Zalutsky MR, et al. Cloning and sequencing
of V genes from anti-osteosarcoma monoclonal antibodies TP-1 and
TP-3: location of lysine residues and implications for radiolabeling.
Nucl Med Biol. 1995;22:765–771.

138. Benhar I, Brinkmann U, Webber KO, et al. Mutations of two lysine
residues in the CDR loops of a recombinant immunotoxin that reduce
its sensitivity to chemical derivatization. *Bioconjug Chem.* 1994;5:
321–326.

139. Crowe J, Dobeli H, Gentz R, et al. 6xHis-Ni-NTA chromatography as
a superior technique in recombinant protein expression/purification.
Methods Mol Biol. 1994;31:371–387.

140. Waibel R, Alberto R, Willuda J, et al. Stable one-step technetium-99m
labeling of His-tagged recombinant proteins with a novel Tc(I)-
carbonyl complex. *Nat Biotechnol.* 1999;17:897–901.

141. Liu G, Hnatowich DJ. Labeling biomolecules with radiorhenium: a
review of the bifunctional chelators. *Anticancer Agents Med Chem.*
2007;7:367–377.

142. Lyons A, King DJ, Owens RJ, et al. Site-specific attachment to recombinant antibodies via introduced surface cysteine residues. *Protein
Eng.* 1990;3:703–708.

143. Stimmel JB, Merrill BM, Kuyper LF, et al. Site-specific conjugation on
serine right-arrow cysteine variant monoclonal antibodies. *J Biol
Chem.* 2000;275:30445–30450.

144. Li L, Olafsen T, Anderson AL, et al. Reduction of kidney uptake in
radiometal labeled peptide linkers conjugated to recombinant antibody fragments. Site-specific conjugation of DOTA-peptides to a Cys-
diabody. *Bioconjug Chem.* 2002;13:985–995.

145. Olafsen T, Cheung CW, Yazaki PJ, et al. Covalent disulfide-linked
anti-CEA diabody allows site-specific conjugation and radiolabeling
for tumor targeting applications. *Protein Eng Des Sel.* 2004;17:21–27.

146. Li X, Link JM, Stekhova S, et al. Site-specific labeling of annexin
V with F-18 for apoptosis imaging. *Bioconjug Chem.* 2008;19:
1684–1688.

147. Ahlgren S, Wallberg H, Tran TA, et al. Targeting of HER2-expressing
tumors with a site-specifically 99mTc-labeled recombinant affibody
molecule, ZHER2:2395, with C-terminally engineered cysteine. *J Nucl
Med.* 2009;50:781–789.

148. Junutula JR, Bhakta S, Raab H, et al. Rapid identification of reactive
cysteine residues for site-specific labeling of antibody-Fabs. *J Immunol
Methods.* 2008;332:41–52.

149. Junutula JR, Raab H, Clark S, et al. Site-specific conjugation of a cytotoxic drug to an antibody improves the therapeutic index. *Nat Biotechnol.* 2008;26:925–932.

150. Costantini DL, Chan C, Cai Z, et al. (111)In-labeled trastuzumab (Herceptin) modified with nuclear localization sequences (NLS): an Auger
electron-emitting radiotherapeutic agent for HER2/neu-amplified
breast cancer. *J Nucl Med.* 2007;48:1357–1368.

151. Kersemans V, Kersemans K, Cornelissen B. Cell penetrating peptides
for in vivo molecular imaging applications. *Curr Pharm Des.* 2008;
14:2415–2447.

152. Chen P, Wang J, Hope K, et al. Nuclear localizing sequences promote
nuclear translocation and enhance the radiotoxicity of the anti-CD33
monoclonal antibody HuM195 labeled with 111In in human myeloid
leukemia cells. *J Nucl Med.* 2006;47:827–836.

153. Weis K. Importins and exportins: how to get in and out of the nucleus.
Trends Biochem Sci. 1998;23:185–189.

154. Hofer KG, Harris CR, Smith JM. Radiotoxicity of intracellular 67Ga,
125I and 3H. Nuclear versus cytoplasmic radiation effects in murine
L1210 leukaemia. *Int J Radiat Biol Relat Stud Phys Chem Med.* 1975;
28:225–241.

155. Goddu SM, Howell RW, Rao DV. Cellular dosimetry: absorbed fractions for monoenergetic electron and alpha particle sources and
S-values for radionuclides uniformly distributed in different cell compartments. *J Nucl Med.* 1994;35:303–316.

156. Murday JS, Siegel RW, Stein J, et al. Translational nanomedicine:
status assessment and opportunities. *Nanomedicine.* 2009;5:251–273.

157. Matsumura Y, Maeda H. A new concept for macromolecular therapeutics in cancer chemotherapy: mechanism of tumoritropic accumulation of proteins and the antitumor agent smancs. *Cancer Res.*
1986;46:6387–6392.

158. Seymour LW. Passive tumor targeting of soluble macromolecules and
drug conjugates. *Crit Rev Ther Drug Carrier Syst.* 1992;9:135–187.

159. Maeda H, Wu J, Sawa T, et al. Tumor vascular permeability and the
EPR effect in macromolecular therapeutics: a review. *J Control Release.*
2000;65:271–284.

160. Maeda H, Sawa T, Konno T. Mechanism of tumor-targeted delivery
of macromolecular drugs, including the EPR effect in solid tumor and
clinical overview of the prototype polymeric drug SMANCS. *J Control
Release.* 2001;74:47–61.

161. Mitra A, Nan A, Line BR, et al. Nanocarriers for nuclear imaging and
radiotherapy of cancer. *Curr Pharm Des.* 2006;12:4729–4749.

162. Chithrani BD, Stewart J, Allen C, et al. Intracellular uptake, transport,
and processing of nanostructures in cancer cells. *Nanomedicine.*
2009;5:118–127.

163. Torchilin VP. Recent advances with liposomes as pharmaceutical carriers. *Nat Rev Drug Discov.* 2005;4:145–160.

164. Klibanov AL, Maruyama K, Torchilin VP, et al. Amphipathic polyethyleneglycols effectively prolong the circulation time of liposomes.
FEBS Lett. 1990;268:235–237.

165. Torchilin VP. Immunoliposomes and PEGylated immunoliposomes: possible use for targeted delivery of imaging agents. *Immunomethods.* 1994;4:244–258.

166. Torchilin VP, Klibanov AL, Huang L, et al. Targeted accumulation of polyethylene glycol-coated immunoliposomes in infarcted rabbit myocardium. *FASEB J.* 1992;6:2716–2719.

167. Blume G, Cevc G, Crommelin MD, et al. Specific targeting with poly(ethylene glycol)-modified liposomes: coupling of homing devices to the ends of the polymeric chains combines effective target binding with long circulation times. *Biochim Biophys Acta.* 1993;1149:180–184.

168. Sofou S, Kappel BJ, Jaggi JS, et al. Enhanced retention of the alpha-particle-emitting daughters of Actinium-225 by liposome carriers. *Bioconjug Chem.* 2007;18:2061–2067.

169. McDevitt MR, Ma D, Simon J, et al. Design and synthesis of 225Ac radioimmunopharmaceuticals. *Appl Radiat Isot.* 2002;57:841–847.

170. Ballangrud AM, Yang WH, Palm S, et al. Alpha-particle emitting atomic generator (Actinium-225)-labeled trastuzumab (herceptin) targeting of breast cancer spheroids: efficacy versus HER2/neu expression. *Clin Cancer Res.* 2004;10:4489–4497.

171. Hafeli U, Tiefenauer LX, Schbiger PA, et al. A lipophilic complex with 186Re/188Re incorporated in liposomes suitable for radiotherapy. *Int J Rad Appl Instrum B.* 1991;18:449–454.

172. Kostarelos K, Emfietzoglou D. Tissue dosimetry of liposome-radionuclide complexes for internal radiotherapy: toward liposome-targeted therapeutic radiopharmaceuticals. *Anticancer Res.* 2000;20:3339–3345.

173. Barth RF, Soloway AH, Goodman JH, et al. Boron neutron capture therapy of brain tumors: an emerging therapeutic modality. *Neurosurgery.* 1999;44:433–450; discussion 450–451.

174. Carlsson J, Kullberg EB, Capala J, et al. Ligand liposomes and boron neutron capture therapy. *J Neurooncol.* 2003;62:47–59.

175. Pan XQ, Zheng X, Shi G, et al. Strategy for the treatment of acute myelogenous leukemia based on folate receptor beta-targeted liposomal doxorubicin combined with receptor induction using all-trans retinoic acid. *Blood.* 2002;100:594–602.

176. Kullberg EB, Nestor M, Gedda L. Tumor-cell targeted epidermal growth factor liposomes loaded with boronated acridine: uptake and processing. *Pharm Res.* 2003;20:229–236.

177. Pan X, Wu G, Yang W, et al. Synthesis of cetuximab-immunoliposomes via a cholesterol-based membrane anchor for targeting of EGFR. *Bioconjug Chem.* 2007;18:101–108.

178. Maruyama K, Ishida O, Kasaoka S, et al. Intracellular targeting of sodium mercaptoundecahydrododecaborate (BSH) to solid tumors by transferrin-PEG liposomes, for boron neutron-capture therapy (BNCT). *J Control Release.* 2004;98:195–207.

179. MacDiarmid JA, Madrid-Weiss J, Amaro-Mugridge NB, et al. Bacterially-derived nanocells for tumor-targeted delivery of chemotherapeutics and cell cycle inhibitors. *Cell Cycle.* 2007;6:2099–2105.

180. MacDiarmid JA, Mugridge NB, Weiss JC, et al. Bacterially derived 400 nm particles for encapsulation and cancer cell targeting of chemotherapeutics. *Cancer Cell.* 2007;11:431–445.

181. MacDiarmid JA, Amaro-Mugridge NB, Madrid-Weiss J, et al. Sequential treatment of drug-resistant tumors with targeted minicells containing siRNA or a cytotoxic drug. *Nat Biotechnol.* 2009;27:643–651.

182. Wang X, Wang Y, Chen ZG, et al. Advances of cancer therapy by nanotechnology. *Cancer Res Treat.* 2009;41:1–11.

183. Gaumet M, Vargas A, Gurny R, et al. Nanoparticles for drug delivery: the need for precision in reporting particle size parameters. *Eur J Pharm Biopharm.* 2008;69:1–9.

184. Guccione S, Li KC, Bednarski MD. Vascular-targeted nanoparticles for molecular imaging and therapy. *Methods Enzymol.* 2004;386:219–236.

185. Hainfeld JF, Slatkin DN, Smilowitz HM. The use of gold nanoparticles to enhance radiotherapy in mice. *Phys Med Biol.* 2004;49:N309–N315.

186. Roa W, Zhang X, Guo L, et al. Gold nanoparticle sensitize radiotherapy of prostate cancer cells by regulation of the cell cycle. *Nanotechnology.* 2009;20:375101.

187. Jeong SY, Park SJ, Yoon SM, et al. Systemic delivery and preclinical evaluation of Au nanoparticle containing beta-lapachone for radiosensitization. *J Control Release.* 2009;139:239–245.

188. Iijima S. Helical microtubules of graphitic carbon. *Nature.* 1991;354:56–58.

189. Kostarelos K, Bianco A, Prato M. Promises, facts and challenges for carbon nanotubes in imaging and therapeutics. *Nat Nanotechnol.* 2009;4:627–633.

190. Singh R, Pantarotto D, Lacerda L, et al. Tissue biodistribution and blood clearance rates of intravenously administered carbon nanotube radiotracers. *Proc Natl Acad Sci USA.* 2006;103:3357–3362.

191. Liu Z, Cai W, He L, et al. In vivo biodistribution and highly efficient tumour targeting of carbon nanotubes in mice. *Nat Nanotechnol.* 2007;2:47–52.

192. McDevitt MR, Chattopadhyay D, Jaggi JS, et al. PET imaging of soluble yttrium-86-labeled carbon nanotubes in mice. *PLoS One.* 2007;2:e907.

193. McDevitt MR, Chattopadhyay D, Kappel BJ, et al. Tumor targeting with antibody-functionalized, radiolabeled carbon nanotubes. *J Nucl Med.* 2007;48:1180–1189.

194. Lacerda L, Ali-Boucetta H, Herrero MA, et al. Tissue histology and physiology following intravenous administration of different types of functionalized multiwalled carbon nanotubes. *Nanomedicine (Lond).* 2008;3:149–161.

195. Liu Z, Tabakman SM, Chen Z, et al. Preparation of carbon nanotube bioconjugates for biomedical applications. *Nat Protoc.* 2009;4:1372–1382.

196. Tasis D, Tagmatarchis N, Bianco A, et al. Chemistry of carbon nanotubes. *Chem Rev.* 2006;106:1105–1136.

197. Wang H, Wang J, Deng X, et al. Biodistribution of carbon single-wall carbon nanotubes in mice. *J Nanosci Nanotechnol.* 2004;4:1019–1024.

Therapeutic Ratios of Targeted Radionuclides

Amin I. Kassis

■ INTRODUCTION

Over the past century, the scientific and medical communities have been using radionuclides for therapy. However, the hope for employing unsealed sources continues to be mainly unrealized. The problem has three major components. The first has to do with the availability of radionuclides that have appropriate physical properties. The second involves the radiation biology of the decaying moiety. The third involves the identification of carrier molecules with which to target the radionuclide to the tumors. In the case of the radionuclide, one must consider its mode of decay, including the nature of the particulate radiations and their energies, its physical half-life, and its chemistry in relation to the carrier molecule. In the case of the carrier, one must define its stability and specificity; the biologic mechanisms that will bind it to the targeted cells, including the number of accessible sites and the affinity of the carrier to these sites, the stability of the receptor–carrier molecule complex, the distribution of the binding sites among cells (both targeted and nontargeted), the relationship of binding-site expression to the cell cycle, and the microenvironment of the target (for a tumor, its vascularity, vascular permeability, oxygenation, and microscopic organization and architecture). In addition, the outcome is dependent on certain biologic responses that are outlined below.

This chapter will emphasize the special features that characterize the radiobiologic effects consequent to the traversal of charged particles through mammalian cells and the state of knowledge concerning the use of these radionuclides to treat cancers. The current status of radionuclide-based therapies will also be summarized.

■ PARTICULATE RADIATION

▉ Energetic particles

In general, the distribution of therapeutic radiopharmaceuticals within a solid tumor is not homogeneous. This is mainly the result of (a) the inability of the radiolabeled molecules to evenly penetrate dissimilar regions within a solid tumor mass, (b) the high interstitial pressure of solid tumors, or (c) differences in the binding-site densities in tumor cells. In the case of radiopharmaceuticals labeled with energetic alpha-particle and beta-particle emitters (range of emitted particle being much greater than the diameter of the targeted cell), such nonuniformity will lead to dosimetric heterogeneities, that is, major differences in the absorbed doses to individual cells within the mass of the targeted tumor. Consequently, the mean absorbed dose will not be a good predictor of radiotherapeutic efficacy.

Alpha-particle emitters

Alpha-particle–emitting radionuclides are positively charged with a mass and charge equal to that of the helium nucleus, and their emission leads to a daughter nucleus that has two fewer protons and two fewer neutrons (Fig. 18.1). These particles have energies ranging from 5 to 9 MeV, travel in straight lines, and have a corresponding tissue range of approximately 5 to 10 mammalian cell diameters (Table 18.1). The LET (linear energy transfer, in keV/μm, which reflects energy deposition and, therefore, ionization density along the track of a charged particle) of these energetic and doubly charged (+2) particles is very high ($\sim$50 to 100 keV/μm) along most of their path before increasing to approximately 250 keV/μm toward the end (last $\sim$20 to 30 μm) of the track (Bragg peak) (Fig. 18.2). Consequently, the therapeutic efficacy of alpha-particle emitters depends on (a) the distance of the decaying atom from the targeted mammalian cell *nucleus*—vis-à-vis the probability of a nuclear traversal (Fig. 18.3) and (b) contribution of heavy ion recoil of the daughter atom, in particular when the alpha-particle emitter is covalently bound to nuclear deoxyribonucleic acid (DNA) (1). Of equal importance is the contribution(s) from the bystander effects and the magnitude of cross-fire dose (see "Beta-Particle Emitters") as this will vary considerably depending on the size of the labeled cell cluster and the fraction of cells labeled (2).

Beta-particle emitters

Beta particles are negatively charged electrons that are emitted from the nuclei of decaying radioactive atoms (1 electron/decay) with various energies (zero up to a maximum) and, thus, a distribution of ranges (Table 18.1). After their emission, the daughter nucleus has one more proton and one less neutron (see Fig. 18.1). As these particles traverse matter, they lose their kinetic energies and eventually (below 100 keV) follow a contorted path and come to a stop.

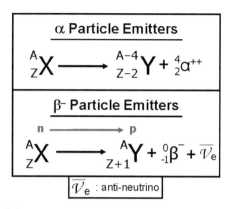

FIGURE 18.1 Schematic of emissions produced during decay of energetic particles (alpha and beta).

Because of their small mass, the recoil energy of the daughter nucleus is negligible. In addition, the LET of these energetic and negatively charged (1) particles is very low ($\sim$0.2 keV/μm) along their "up-to-a-centimeter" path (i.e., they are sparsely ionizing), except for the final few hundreds of nanometers at the end of the range (Fig. 18.4). Consequently, the therapeutic efficacy of radiopharmaceuticals labeled with energetic electron emitters predicates the presence of very high radionuclide concentrations on or within the targeted tissue. The long range of these emitted electrons leads to the production of cross-fire, a circumstance that negates the need to target every cell within the tumor, so long as *all* the cells are within the range of the decaying atoms. As with alpha particles, the probability of the emitted beta particle to traverse the targeted cell nucleus depends to a large degree on (a) the position of the decaying atom vis-à-vis the nucleus—specifically nuclear DNA—of the targeted tumor cell; (b) its distance from the tumor cell nucleus; and (c) the radius of the latter (see Fig. 18.3). Obviously, intranuclear localization of therapeutic radiopharmaceuticals is highly advantageous and, if possible, should always be sought.

■ Nonenergetic particles

During the decay of many radioactive atoms, a vacancy is commonly formed in the K shell as a consequence of electron capture (EC) and/or internal conversion (IC) (Fig. 18.5).

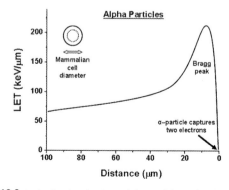

FIGURE 18.2 Ionization density along alpha-particle track as function of traversed distance.

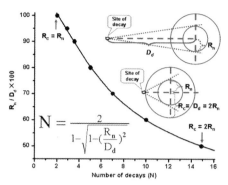

FIGURE 18.3 Number of radioactive atoms (*N*) required to ensure traversal of cell nucleus by one energetic particle. Nuclear radius to distance of decaying atom (percentage) is plotted as function of number of decays (assume 1 particle per decaying atom). R_c: cell radius; R_n: nuclear radius; D_d: distance of decaying atom from center of cell for one nuclear traversal (this must equal or be less than the particle range). Note that (i) when decaying atoms are on nuclear membrane, *two or more* radioactive atoms are needed for one nuclear traversal; (ii) when decaying atoms are localized on cell membrane and diameter of cell is twice that of nucleus, greater than 15 radioactive atoms are necessary to insure one nuclear traversal; and (iii) nuclear localization of radioactive atom is the only condition that will lead to one traversal per decaying atom.

Each such vacancy is rapidly filled by an electron dropping in from a higher shell, a process that leads to a cascade of atomic electron transitions and the movement of the vacancy to the outermost shell. These inner-shell electron transitions result in the emission of characteristic x-ray photons or an Auger, Coster–Kronig, or super Coster–Kronig monoenergetic electron (collectively called Auger electrons). Typically, an average of 5 to 30 Auger electrons, with energies ranging from a few eV to approximately 1 keV, are emitted per decaying atom (3). This also leaves the daughter atom with a high positive charge resulting in subsequent charge-transfer processes. The very low energies of Auger electrons have three major consequences: (a) most of these light, negatively (1) charged particles travel in contorted paths and their range in water is a few nanometers to approximately 0.5 μm (Table 18.1); (b) the LET of these particles is quite high ($\sim$4 to 26 keV/μm); and (c) multiple ionizations occur in the immediate vicinity of the decay site (Fig. 18.6) (4), reminiscent of those observed along the path of an alpha particle (3). An important consequence of the short electron range of Auger electrons is the need to position the radiopharmaceutical in very close proximity to the radiosensitive target (DNA) for radiotherapeutic effectiveness (5–7).

■ RADIOBIOLOGY

The deposition of energy by ionizing radiation is a random process. The energy absorbed by cells can induce molecular modifications that may lead to DNA alterations and cell death.

DNA is the principal target responsible for the radiation-induced biologic effects. A number of different lesions are produced (e.g., single-strand breaks, double-strand breaks [DSBs], base damage, DNA–protein cross-links, and multiply

Chapter 18 • Therapeutic Ratios of Targeted Radionuclides

Table 18.1	General characteristics of therapeutic radionuclides			
Decay	**Particles**	$E_{min}-E_{max}$	**Range**	**LET**[a]
α^{++} particle	He nuclei	5–9 MeV[b]	40–100 μm	~50–100 keV/μm
β^- particle	Energetic electrons	50–2300 keV[c]	0.05–12 mm	~0.2 keV/μm
EC/IC	Nonenergetic electrons	eV–keV[b]	2–500 nm	~4–26 KeV/μm

[a]Along most of the track.
[b]Monoenergetic.
[c]Average (>1% intensity); continuous distribution of energy.

damaged sites). Such lesions may be produced by the direct ionization of DNA (direct effect) or by the interaction of free radicals (mostly hydroxyl radicals produced in water molecules that diffuse ~5 nm) with DNA. Most of these lesions, however, are repaired with high fidelity.

The distribution of "ionizations" within the DNA structure and the type of lesions created depend on the nature of the incident particle and its energy. Alpha particles produce a high density along a linear path (Fig. 18.6, bottom); energetic beta particles, infrequent ionizations along a linear path (Fig. 18.6, top); low-energy electrons, frequent ionizations along an irregular path; and Auger cascades, clusters of high ionization density (Fig. 18.6, center). DSBs generated by high specific ionization (alpha particles and Auger-electron cascades) are less reparable than those created by more sparsely ionizing radiation.

Cellular responses

Clonal survival

When mammalian cells are exposed to ionizing radiation, their ability to undergo cell division indefinitely declines as a function of radiation dose. The shape of the survival curve (Fig. 18.7) depends on the density of ionizations. For densely ionizing radiation (alpha particles and Auger-electron cascades), the logarithmic response is linear ($\ln SF = \alpha D$), where SF is the survival fraction, α is the slope, and D is the absorbed dose. For sparsely ionizing irradiation (photons and energetic beta particles), the logarithmic response is linear-quadratic

($\ln SF = \alpha D + \beta D^2$) where α is the rate of cell kill by a single-hit mechanism, D is the dose delivered, and β equals the rate of cell kill by a double-hit mechanism. The βD^2 term is thought to represent accumulated and reparable damage. It is essential to note that the α-to-β ratio represents the dose at which cell killing by the linear and quadratic components is equal, that is, when $\alpha D = \beta D^2$ ($D = \alpha/\beta$; see Chapter 27). This type of survival curve is routinely seen when mammalian cells are exposed to low-LET radiation (e.g., x-rays, energetic beta particles, extranuclear Auger electrons).

Whereas it is clear that pharmaceuticals labeled with radionuclides whose decay results in a purely exponential decrease in cell survival (with every decay resulting in a corresponding decrease in survival) are preferable for radiotherapy, the exponential nature of both types of survival curve has important implications. In essence, it indicates that only very high doses will reduce the number of viable cancer cells in a macroscopic tumor to less than one, and that no dose will be sufficiently large to eradicate with certainty 100% of the clonogenic cells, especially since the magnitude of the dose will always be limited by normal tissue tolerance.

Division delay and programmed cell death

After irradiation, delay in the progression of dividing cells through their cell cycle is a well-documented phenomenon. It is reversible and the length of this delay is dose dependent. The delay occurs only at specific points in the cell cycle and is similar for both surviving and nonsurviving cells.

When cells are irradiated and DNA is damaged, the damage is sensed and various genes are activated. Cells held at checkpoints await repair of DNA and then proceed through the cell cycle. Alternatively, damage may be

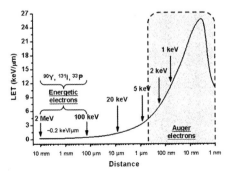

FIGURE 18.4 Linear energy transfer (LET), reflecting ionization density as function of distance, along tracks of energetic beta particles and Auger electrons.

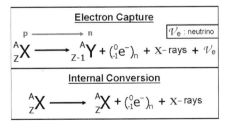

FIGURE 18.5 Schematic of emissions produced during electron capture (EC) and internal conversion (IC).

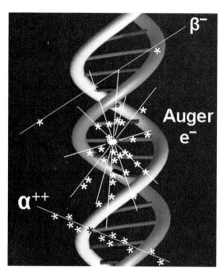

FIGURE 18.6 Ionization densities produced along track of energetic beta particles, Auger electrons, alpha particles.

nonreparable and the cells are induced to undergo programmed cell death or apoptosis. Lymphoid tumor cells are more likely to undergo apoptosis than epithelial cells, and this may account for the success of radioimmunotherapy in certain lymphomas. In epithelial cells, apoptosis appears to account for only a small portion of clonal cell death.

Oxygen enhancement ratios

Oxygen radiosensitizes mammalian cells to the damaging effects of radiation. Consequently, hypoxic cells can be up to threefold more radioresistant than well-oxygenated cells. The oxygen effect is maximal for low-ionization-density radiation (high-energy beta particles) and minimal for high-LET radiation (alpha particles, low-energy electrons including Auger-electron cascades).

Bystander effect

The term "bystander effect" is applied to the biologic responses of cells that neighbor irradiated cells but have not been irradiated themselves. Increased mutation rates and decreased survival rates have been reported. Originally observed with external alpha-particle beams in vitro, the phenomenon has been observed in vitro and in vivo (8–10). These observations have negated a central tenet of radiobiology that damage to cells is caused only by direct ionizations and/or free radicals generated as a consequence of the deposition of energy within the nuclei of mammalian cells. The importance of the bystander effect as an enhancer of radiotherapeutic efficacy is yet to be clearly determined.

Self-dose, cross-fire, and nonuniform dose distribution

When radionuclides are employed for therapy, cells may be irradiated by decays taking place on or within the targeted cells (self-dose) or in neighboring or distant cells (cross-fire). Because of geometric factors associated with linear paths, the self-dose from energetic alpha and beta particles is very dependent on their position on or within the tumor cell, whereas that for Auger-electron emitters depends on the proximity of the decaying atom to DNA.

In targeted radionuclide therapy, the distribution of radioactivity and, hence, the absorbed dose tend to be nonuniform. Consequently, higher doses are required to sterilize the targeted cells. Using mathematical modeling, Humm et al. (11,12) has calculated that the difference in dose needed for a similar decrease in survival fraction with uniform and nonuniform dose distributions of alpha-particle–emitting radionuclides is greater than that for energetic beta particles (Fig. 18.8). O'Donoghue (13) has also described a mathematical model that examines the impact of dose nonuniformity, as well as dose-rate effect, on therapeutic response. This model predicts that (a) as the absorbed dose distribution becomes less uniform, the surviving fraction increases for any mean absorbed dose; (b) a nonuniform dose distribution grows proportionately less effective as the absorbed dose increases; and (c) the difference in survival fraction resulting from uniform versus nonuniform doses is more pronounced as the radiosensitivity of tumor cells increases.

Half-life

Because many biologic responses to radiation are sensitive to dose rate as well as total dose, the physical half-life

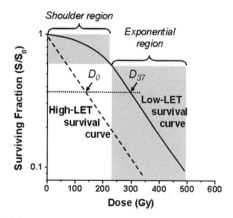

FIGURE 18.7 Survival of mammalian cells after high- and low-LET irradiation. With high-LET radiation (alpha and nonenergetic electrons) curve shows exponential decrease in survival, while with low-LET radiation (energetic electrons) curve exhibits a broad shoulder.

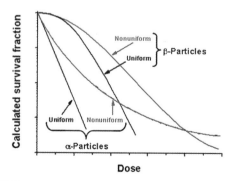

FIGURE 18.8 Schematic representation of relationship between mammalian cell survival and radionuclide distribution as function of dose. Curves for uniform irradiation with alpha and beta particles (black lines) and for nonuniform irradiation (gray lines).

Table **18.2**	Alpha-particle emitters: physical properties		
Radionuclide	E_{av} **(MeV)**[a]	R_{av} **(μm)**[b]	**Half-Life**
[211]At	6.79	60	7.2 hours
[212]Bi	7.80	75	61 minutes
[213]Bi	8.32	84	46 minutes
[223]Ra	5.64	45	11.43 days
[225]Ac	6.83	61	10 days

[a]Mean energy of alpha particles emitted per disintegration (15).
[b]Mean range of alpha particles calculated using second-order polynomial regression fit (16): $R = 3.87E + 0.75E^2 - 0.45$, where R is the range (μm) in unit density matter and E is the alpha-particle energy (MeV).

($T_{1/2P}$) of the radionuclide employed and the tumor and normal biologic half-life ($T_{1/2B}$) can be of consequence. For a radiopharmaceutical with an infinite residence time in a tumor or tissue, a radionuclide with a long physical half-life will deliver more decays than one with a short half-life if both have the same initial radioactivity. Moreover, there can be a striking difference in the time-dependent dose rate delivered by the two. If the number of radionuclide atoms per unit of tissue mass is n and the energy emitted (and absorbed) per decay is E, then the absorbed-dose rate is proportional to nE/T where T is the half-life. The ratio E/T is an important indicator of the intrinsic radiotherapeutic potency of the radionuclide (14). In general, for biologic reasons, higher dose rates delivered over shorter treatment times are more effective than lower dose rates delivered over longer periods. Thus, a radionuclide with a shorter half-life will tend to be more biologically effective than one with a similar emission energy but longer half-life. For example, when the same number of iodine-125 and iodine-123 atoms (covalently conjugated to a tumor-targeting agent) is bound to a tumor, their relative effectiveness depends on the tumor doubling time and the rate at which the radiopharmaceutical dissociates from the target. When both factors are very long, the longer-lived iodine-125 ($T_{1/2}$ = 60 days) is theoretically more effective; otherwise, the shorter-lived iodine-123 ($T_{1/2}$ = 13.3 hours) is preferred.

■ EXPERIMENTAL THERAPEUTICS

▨ Energetic particle emitters

Alpha emitters

The application of alpha-particle–emitting radionuclides as targeted therapeutic agents continues to be of interest. When these radionuclides selectively accumulate in targeted tissues (e.g., tumors), the resulting decay should lead to a highly localized energy deposition in the tumor cells and minimal irradiation of surrounding normal host tissues.

The investigation of the therapeutic potential of alpha-particle emitters has focused mainly on five radionuclides: astatine-211 ([211]At), bismuth-212 ([212]Bi), bismuth-213 ([213]Bi),

radium-223 ([223]Ra), and actinium-225 ([225]Ac) (Table 18.2). In vitro studies (17,18) have demonstrated that the decrease in mammalian cell survival after exposure to uniformly distributed alpha particles from such radionuclides is monoexponential but that, as predicted theoretically (12) and shown experimentally (1) after the decay of [211]At-labeled 5-astato-2'-deoxyuridine ([211]AtUdR), these curves develop a tail when the dose is nonuniform. Such studies have also indicated that the traversal of one to four alpha particles through a mammalian cell nucleus will kill the cell (1,17,18). In comparison, since the LET of negatrons emitted by the decay of energetic beta emitters used for tumor therapy is approximately 0.2 keV/μm (see Fig. 18.4), thousands of beta particles must traverse a cell nucleus for its sterilization.

Investigators have also assessed the therapeutic potential of alpha-particle emitters in tumor-bearing animals (19–23). For example, Bloomer and coworkers (19,20) have reported a dose-related prolongation in median survival when mice bearing an intraperitoneal murine ovarian tumor are treated with [211]At–tellurium colloid administered directly into the peritoneal cavity. Whereas this alpha-particle–emitting radiocolloid is curative without serious morbidity (Fig. 18.9), beta-particle–emitting radiocolloids (phosphorus-32, dysprosium-165, yttrium-90) are much less efficacious. In another set of in vivo studies examining the therapeutic efficacy of a [212]Bi-labeled monoclonal antibody, the radionuclide

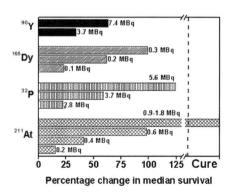

FIGURE 18.9 Percentage change in median survival of ovarian cancer-bearing mice treated with alpha- and beta-particle–emitting radiocolloids.

is most effective when used with a carrier that entails target specificity (21). Finally, a recent report by McDevitt and coworkers (23) has demonstrated that [225]Ac-labeled internalizing antibodies are therapeutically effective in mice bearing solid prostate carcinoma or disseminated lymphoma.

Beta emitters

Radionuclide-based tumor therapy has been carried out mainly with beta-particle emitters. Findings indicate that the exposure of cells in vitro to beta particles leads, in general, to survival curves that have a distinct shoulder and a D_0 of several thousand decays (24,25). Despite the rather low in vitro toxicity, these radionuclides continue to be pursued for targeted therapy. To a great extent, this is due to the availability and favorable characteristics of many energetic beta-particle–emitting isotopes (Table 18.3), including the irradiation of cells within the longer range (mm-to-cm) of the emitted electron particles (i.e., cross-fire). As mentioned in section "Beta-Particle Emitters," the main advantage of cross-fire is that it negates the necessity of the radiotherapeutic agents being present within each of the targeted cells, that is, it counteracts a certain degree of heterogeneity. However, to deliver an effective therapeutic dose to the targeted tissue, the following conditions must be met: (a) the radiotherapeutic agent must concentrate within foci throughout the targeted tumor mass; (b) the distances between these foci must be equal to or less than twice the maximum range of the emitted energetic beta particles; (c) the concentration of the radiotherapeutic agent within each focus must be sufficiently high to produce a cumulative cross-fire dose of 10,000 cGy or more to the surrounding targeted cells. Since dose is inversely proportional to the square of distance, the concentration of the therapeutic agent needed to deposit such cytocidal doses

rises many folds when the distance between the radioactive foci increases.

Experimentally, these predictions have been substantiated in various animal tumor-therapy studies. Investigators have assessed the therapeutic efficacy of ^{131}I-labeled monoclonal antibodies in rodents bearing subcutaneous tumors. Although a substantial proportion of cells within a tumor mass show reduced/no expression of the targeted antigen and, therefore, are not targeted by the radioiodinated antibody, ^{131}I-labeled antibodies that localize in high concentrations in tumors are therapeutically efficacious and can lead to total tumor eradication (27). Thus, even when iodine-131 is not so uniformly distributed within a tumor, the decay of this radionuclide can lead to sterilization of small tumors in mice so long as it is present in sufficiently high concentrations. Similar results have been reported with radiopharmaceuticals labeled with other beta-particle–emitting isotopes, in particular yttrium-90 (28–30) and copper-67 (31). An important outcome of these findings has been the recent successful introduction of [131]I- and ^{90}Y-labeled antibodies in the clinic (32,33).

▨ Nonenergetic particle emitters

The therapeutic potential of radionuclides that decay by EC and/or IC has, for the most part, been established with iodine-125. Studies with this and other Auger-electron–emitting radionuclides (Table 18.4) have shown that (a) multiple electrons are emitted per decaying atom; (b) the distances traversed by these electrons are mainly in the nanometer range; (c) the LET of the electrons is greater than 20-fold higher than that observed along the tracks of energetic (>50 keV) beta particles; and (d) many of the emitted electrons dissipate their energy in the immediate vicinity of the decaying atom and deposit 10^6 to 10^9 cGy/decay within a few-nanometer sphere around the decay site (5,6,35–37).

Table **18.3**	Beta-particle emitters: physical characteristics		
Radionuclide	**Half-Life**	E_β-(max) (keV)[a]	R_β-(max) (mm)[b]
[33]P	25.4 days	249	0.63
[177]Lu	6.7 days	497	1.8
[67]Cu	61.9 hours	575	2.1
[131]I	8.0 days	606	2.3
[186]Re	3.8 days	1077	4.8
[165]Dy	2.3 hours	1285	5.9
[89]Sr	50.5 days	1491	7.0
[32]P	14.3 days	1710	8.2
[166]Ho	28.8 hours	1854	9.0
[188]Re	17.0 hours	2120	10.4
[90]Y	64.1 hours	2284	11.3

[a]Maximum energy of beta particles emitted per disintegration.
[b]Range (μm) for electrons with $E = 0.02–100$ keV calculated using Cole's equation (4): $R = 0.043(E + 0.367)^{1.77} - 0.007$, whereas range (mm) for electrons with E (MeV) calculated using second-order fits (26): $R_{(0.1-0.5\ \text{MeV})} = 2.4E + 2.86E^2 - 0.14$ and $R_{(0.5-2.5\ \text{MeV})} = 5.3E + 0.0034E^2 - 0.93$.

Table **18.4**	Auger-electron emitters: physical properties			
		Total Electron Yield Per Decay		
Radionuclide (#)[a]	Half-Life	"Long" Range Electrons (%)	"Short" Range Electrons (%)	"Very Short" Range Electrons (%)
^{125}I (22)	60.5 days	20 (98%)	18 (86%)	8 (39%)
^{123}I (11)	13.3 hours	11 (98%)	10 (89%)	5 (40%)
^{77}Br (7)	57 hours	7 (100%)	6 (95%)	3 (51%)
^{111}In (17)	3 days	15 (98%)	14 (91%)	8 (53%)
^{195m}Pt (34)	4 days	33 (92%)	33 (79%)	7 (19%)
	Range:	<0.5 m	<100 nm	<2 nm
	LET[b]:	4–26	9–26	<18

[a]Average number of electrons emitted per decay.
[b]Fit of data by Cole (4).

From a radiobiologic perspective, the tridimensional organization of chromatin within the mammalian cell nucleus involves many structural level compactions (nucleosome, 30-nm chromatin fiber, chromonema fiber, etc.) whose dimensions are within the range of these high-LET (4 to 26 keV/μm), low-energy (1.6 keV), and short-range (150 nm) electrons. Therefore, the toxicity of Auger-electron–emitting radionuclides is expected to be quite high and to depend critically on close proximity of the decaying atom to DNA. These predictions have been substantiated by the results of in vitro studies that have shown that (a) the decay of Auger-electron emitters covalently bound to nuclear DNA leads to a monoexponential decrease in survival (6,37,38); (b) the resulting cell survival curves may or may not exhibit a shoulder when the decaying atoms are not covalently bound to nuclear DNA (34,39–41); and (c) in general, intranuclear decay accumulation is highly toxic (D_0 = ~100 to 500 decays/cell), whereas decay within the cytoplasm or extracellularly produces no extraordinary lethal effects and these survival curves resemble those observed with x-rays (having a distinct shoulder) (42,43).

The radiotoxicity of Auger-electron emitters has been examined in mammalian cells in vitro and in vivo. The survival of Chinese hamster V79 cells has been scored as a function of DNA-incorporated iodine-125 and compared with that of iodine-131 (24). Unlike the low-LET type of survival curve (with shoulder) obtained following the decay of beta-emitting iodine-131 in DNA, a high-LET curve (with no shoulder) is observed with iodine-125, and the slope of the iodine-125 curve is much steeper than that of the iodine-131 curve. Kassis et al. (43) have reported a mean relative biologic effectiveness (RBE) of 7.3 when the cumulated dose to the cell nucleus at 37% survival is compared with the corresponding value from 250-kVp x-rays for the same cell line. In contrast, the decay of iodine-125 in the cytoplasm, which is much less efficient at cell killing, has an RBE of about 1.3. Such results support the notion that the biologic effects of an Auger-electron emitter are strongly dependent on its intracellular localization, in particular its proximity to DNA.

The extreme degree of cytotoxicity observed with DNA-incorporated Auger-electron emitters has been exploited in experimental radionuclide therapy. In most of these in vivo studies, the thymidine analog 5-iodo-2'-deoxyuridine (IUdR) has been used (44–47), and the results have shown excellent therapeutic efficacy. For example, the injection of ^{125}IUdR into mice bearing an *intraperitoneal ascites* ovarian cancer has led to a 5-log reduction in tumor cell survival (44). Similar findings occur with ^{123}IUdR (45). Therapeutic doses of ^{125}IUdR injected *intrathecally* into rats with intrathecal tumors significantly delay the onset of paralysis, and the coadministration of methotrexate, an antimetabolite that enhances IUdR uptake by DNA-synthesizing cells, enhances substantially the therapeutic efficacy (Fig. 18.10) as exemplified by a 5- to 6-log tumor cell kill and the curing of approximately 30% of the tumor-bearing rats (46,47).

■ CHOICE OF VECTOR OR LIGAND

The choice of a chemical carrier in cancer therapy is of equal importance to that of the radionuclide. It is the properties of the former upon which targeted therapy depends. The selection of a suitable carrier molecule rests on many factors, including (a) biologic specificity and in vivo stability; (b) the mechanism(s) that lead to its binding to the targeted cells and the affinity of the carrier for the binding sites; and (c) the stability of the receptor–carrier complex thus formed.

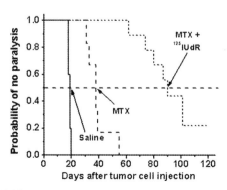

FIGURE 18.10 Induction of hind leg paralysis in rats by intrathecally growing tumor cells after various treatment protocols. Treatments include (A) saline; (B) methotrexate *(MTX)*; and (C) methotrexate plus ^{125}IUdR.

Obviously, the chemical properties of the carrier molecule must enable the conjugation of a therapeutic radionuclide without degradation of the intrinsic characteristics of the molecule.

PROPERTIES OF TARGETS

Important factors in the case of tumors are their accessibility, the number of binding sites, the distribution of binding sites among the targeted and nontargeted cells, and the expression of these binding sites during each phase of the cell cycle. The microscopic environment of the target, including tumor vascularity, vascular permeability, oxygenation, as well as its microscopic organization and architecture, is also extremely important (48,49).

To optimally target a radiopharmaceutical, the route of administration (e.g., intravenous, intralymphatic, intraperitoneal, intracerebral, intravesical, intrathecal, and intrasynovial) must also be considered. Some pathways may provide a mechanical means for maximizing tumor-to-nontumor ratios.

Lastly, specific activity (fraction of targeting molecules that are tagged with radioactive atoms) of the radiopharmaceutical should be taken into account, especially when receptors can be saturated easily and, therefore, weaker nonspecific binding to nontargeted cells can compete with the target. It should be noted that certain treatments are sometimes assisted by an antibody mass effect; for example, tumor uptake of radiolabeled antibodies can be enhanced by the addition of unlabeled immunoglobulin.

THE IDEAL THERAPEUTIC RADIOPHARMACEUTICAL

Under ideal conditions, a therapeutic radiopharmaceutical would be characterized by (a) very high specificity for tumor cells, (b) high affinity to tumor cells, (c) stability in blood in vivo (not catabolized/metabolized; if somewhat unstable, metabolism/catabolism half-life should be much greater than physical half-life ($T_{1/2P}$) of the radionuclide), (d) biologic half-life ($T_{1/2B}$) comparable with $T_{1/2P}$ of the radionuclide, (e) rapid targeting of tumor cells, (f) significant retention by tumor cells for period two- to threefold longer than the $T_{1/2P}$ of the radionuclide, (g) lack of catabolism by tumor cells, (h) minimal uptake and retention by normal tissues/cells, (i) rapid excretion from the body, (j) pharmacokinetics not altered by repeated injection, (k) efficient cell killing, that is, inefficient at causing other radiation-induced biologic effects (e.g., mutations, transformations), (l) less heterogeneity within tumor cell clusters than the range of emitted particles, (m) deposition of a therapeutic dose to *all* tumor cells, and (n) delivery of a toxic dose to tumor cells *prior to* deposition of the maximum tolerated dose in normal tissues.

The successful development of a therapeutic radiopharmaceutical necessitates the multistep matching of (a) the tumor and the carrier molecule, (b) the tumor and the radionuclide, (c) the carrier and the radionuclide (forming the radiopharmaceutical), and (d) the radiopharmaceutical

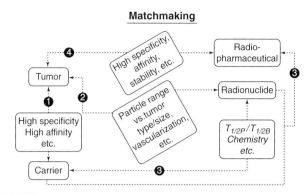

FIGURE 18.11 Matchmaking of tumor, radionuclide, targeting ligand, and radiopharmaceutical.

and the tumor (Fig. 18.11). During these successive steps, special attention must be paid to ensure the compatibility of the individual components. Once the matchmaking of the radiopharmaceutical has been completed, it is ready for being assessed further in vivo, first in tumor-bearing mice and then in human trials (Fig. 18.12).

CONCLUSIONS

A significant increase in our understanding of the dosimetry and therapeutic potential of various modes of radioactive decay has heightened the possibility of utilizing radiolabeled carriers in cancer therapy. Moreover, as a consequence of the great strides in genomics, the development of more precise targeting molecules is at hand. Further progress in the field of targeted radionuclide therapy is being made by the judicious design of radiolabeled molecules that match the physical and chemical characteristics of both the radionuclide and the carrier molecule with the clinical character of the tumor. Whereas significant improvement has been made in the treatment of highly radiosensitive hematologic tumors in humans, the radionuclide therapy of solid tumors remains a challenge.

In conclusion, (a) if sufficient uniformity of radiopharmaceutical distribution can be achieved within a tumor, α-particle and Auger-electron emitters will be practical for therapy and, in this situation, tumor size is irrelevant; (b) if radiopharmaceutical distribution within tumor is nonuniform, energetic beta-particle emitters will be more appropriate and, obviously, all tumor cells must be within the range

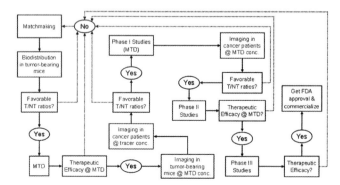

FIGURE 18.12 Scheme showing steps necessary for assessment of therapeutic potential of radiopharmaceuticals.

of the emitted particles; (c) targeted radionuclide therapy will rely increasingly on both the accessibility to various radionuclides, their availability in large quantities and at high specific activity, and the development of more specific carriers, hopefully provided by knowledge of genomics; and (d) dose specification must incorporate information on nonuniformity, RBE, and cellular localization of the therapeutic radionuclide.

■ REFERENCES

1. Walicka MA, Vaidyanathan G, Zalutsky MR, et al. Survival and DNA damage in Chinese hamster V79 cells exposed to alpha particles emitted by DNA-incorporated astatine-211. *Radiat Res.* 1998;150:263–268.
2. Goddu SM, Howell RW, Rao DV. Cellular dosimetry: absorbed fractions for monoenergetic electron and alpha particle sources and S-values for radionuclides uniformly distributed in different cell compartments. *J Nucl Med.* 1994;35:303–316.
3. Kassis AI. The amazing world of Auger electrons. *Int J Radiat Biol.* 2004;80:789–803.
4. Cole A. Absorption of 20-eV to 50,000-eV electron beams in air and plastic. *Radiat Res.* 1969;38:7–33.
5. Kassis AI, Adelstein SJ, Haydock C, et al. Radiotoxicity of ^{75}Se and ^{35}S: theory and application to a cellular model. *Radiat Res.* 1980;84:407–425.
6. Kassis AI, Adelstein SJ, Haydock C, et al. Lethality of Auger electrons from the decay of bromine-77 in the DNA of mammalian cells. *Radiat Res.* 1982;90:362–373.
7. Kassis AI, Sastry KSR, Adelstein SJ. Intracellular localisation of Auger electron emitters: biophysical dosimetry. *Radiat Prot Dosimetry.* 1985;13:233–236.
8. Xue LY, Butler NJ, Makrigiorgos GM, et al. Bystander effect produced by radiolabeled tumor cells in vivo. *Proc Natl Acad Sci USA.* 2002;99:13765–13770.
9. Kishikawa H, Wang K, Adelstein SJ, et al. Inhibitory and stimulatory bystander effects are differentially induced by iodine-125 and iodine-123. *Radiat Res.* 2006;165:688–694.
10. Boyd M, Ross SC, Dorrens J, et al. Radiation-induced biologic bystander effect elicited in vitro by targeted radiopharmaceuticals labeled with a-, b-, and Auger electron–emitting radionuclides. *J Nucl Med.* 2006;47:1007–1015.
11. Humm JL, Cobb LM. Nonuniformity of tumor dose in radioimmunotherapy. *J Nucl Med.* 1990;31:75–83.
12. Humm JL, Chin LM, Cobb L, et al. Microdosimetry in radioimmunotherapy. *Radiat Prot Dosimetry.* 1990;31:433–436.
13. O'Donoghue JA. The impact of tumor cell proliferation in radioimmunotherapy. *Cancer.* 1994;73:974–980.
14. ICRU. Absorbed-dose specification in nuclear medicine (ICRU Report 67). *J. ICRU.* 2002;2(1):1–110.
15. Kocher DC. *Radioactive Decay Data Tables: A Handbook of Decay Data for Application to Radiation Dosimetry and Radiological Assessments.* Springfield, VA: National Technical Information Center, US Department of Energy; 1981.
16. ICRU. *Stopping Powers and Ranges for Protons and Alpha Particles, Report 49.* Bethesda, MD: International Commission on Radiation Units and Measurements; 1993.
17. Kassis AI, Harris CR, Adelstein SJ, et al. The in vitro radiobiology of astatine-211 decay. *Radiat Res.* 1986;105:27–36.
18. Charlton DE, Kassis AI, Adelstein SJ. A comparison of experimental and calculated survival curves for V79 cells grown as monolayers or in suspension exposed to alpha irradiation from ^{212}Bi distributed in the growth medium. *Radiat Prot Dosimetry.* 1994;52:311–315.
19. Bloomer WD, McLaughlin WH, Neirinckx RD, et al. Astatine-211–tellurium radiocolloid cures experimental malignant ascites. *Science.* 1981;212:340–341.
20. Bloomer WD, McLaughlin WH, Lambrecht RM, et al. ^{211}At radiocolloid therapy: further observations and comparison with radiocolloids of ^{32}P, ^{165}Dy, and ^{90}Y. *Int J Radiat Oncol Biol Phys.* 1984;10:341–348.
21. Macklis RM, Kinsey BM, Kassis AI, et al. Radioimmunotherapy with alpha-particle–emitting immunoconjugates. *Science.* 1988;240:1024–1026.
22. Zalutsky MR, McLendon RE, Garg PK, et al. Radioimmunotherapy of neoplastic meningitis in rats using an alpha-particle-emitting immunoconjugate. *Cancer Res.* 1994;54:4719–4725.
23. McDevitt MR, Ma D, Lai LT, et al. Tumor therapy with targeted atomic nanogenerators. *Science.* 2001;294:1537–1540.
24. Chan PC, Lisco E, Lisco H, et al. The radiotoxicity of iodine-125 in mammalian cells. II. A comparative study on cell survival and cytogenetic responses to ^{125}IUdR, ^{131}IUdR, and ^{3}HTdR. *Radiat Res.* 1976;67:332–343.
25. Burki HJ, Koch C, Wolff S. Molecular suicide studies of ^{125}I and ^{3}H disintegration in the DNA of Chinese hamster cells. *Curr Top Radiat Res Q.* 1977;12:408–425.
26. ICRU. *Stopping Powers for Electrons and Positrons, Report 37.* Bethesda, MD: International Commission on Radiation Units and Measurements; 1984.
27. Esteban JM, Schlom J, Mornex F, et al. Radioimmunotherapy of athymic mice bearing human colon carcinomas with monoclonal antibody B72.3: histological and autoradiographic study of effects on tumors and normal organs. *Eur J Cancer Clin Oncol.* 1987;23:643–655.
28. Otte A, Mueller-Brand J, Dellas S, et al. Yttrium-90-labelled somatostatin-analogue for cancer treatment. *Lancet.* 1998;351:417–418.
29. Chinn PC, Leonard JE, Rosenberg J, et al. Preclinical evaluation of ^{90}Y-labeled anti-CD20 monoclonal antibody for treatment of non-Hodgkin's lymphoma. *Int J Oncol.* 1999;15:1017–1025.
30. Axworthy DB, Reno JM, Hylarides MD, et al. Cure of human carcinoma xenografts by a single dose of pretargeted yttrium-90 with negligible toxicity. *Proc Natl Acad Sci USA.* 2000;97:1802–1807.
31. DeNardo GL, Kukis DL, Shen S, et al. Efficacy and toxicity of ^{67}Cu-2IT-BAT-Lym-1 radioimmunoconjugate in mice implanted with human Burkitt's lymphoma (Raji). *Clin Cancer Res.* 1997;3:71–79.
32. Witzig TE. Yttrium-90-ibritumomab tiuxetan radioimmunotherapy: a new treatment approach for B-cell non-Hodgkin's lymphoma. *Drugs Today (Barc).* 2004;40:111–119.
33. Kaminski MS, Tuck M, Estes J, et al. ^{131}I-tositumomab therapy as initial treatment for follicular lymphoma. *N Engl J Med.* 2005;352:441–449.
34. Kassis AI, Fayad F, Kinsey BM, et al. Radiotoxicity of an ^{125}I-labeled DNA intercalator in mammalian cells. *Radiat Res.* 1989;118:283–294.
35. Kassis AI, Adelstein SJ, Haydock C, et al. Thallium-201: an experimental and a theoretical radiobiological approach to dosimetry. *J Nucl Med.* 1983;24:1164–1175.
36. Kassis AI, Sastry KSR, Adelstein SJ. Intracellular distribution and radiotoxicity of chromium-51 in mammalian cells: Auger-electron dosimetry. *J Nucl Med.* 1985;26:59–67.
37. Kassis AI, Sastry KSR, Adelstein SJ. Kinetics of uptake, retention, and radiotoxicity of ^{125}IUdR in mammalian cells: implications of localized energy deposition by Auger processes. *Radiat Res.* 1987;109:78–89.
38. Hofer KG, Hughes WL. Radiotoxicity of intranuclear tritium, ^{125}iodine and ^{131}iodine. *Radiat Res.* 1971;47:94–109.
39. Bloomer WD, McLaughlin WH, Weichselbaum RR, et al. Iodine-125-labelled tamoxifen is differentially cytotoxic to cells containing oestrogen receptors. *Int J Radiat Biol.* 1980;38:197–202.
40. Walicka MA, Ding Y, Roy AM, et al. Cytotoxicity of [^{125}I]iodoHoechst 33342: contribution of scavengeable effects. *Int J Radiat Biol.* 1999;75:1579–1587.
41. Yasui LS, Chen K, Wang K, et al. Using Hoechst 33342 to target radioactivity to the cell nucleus. *Radiat Res.* 2007;167:167–175.
42. Hofer KG, Harris CR, Smith JM. Radiotoxicity of intracellular ^{67}Ga, ^{125}I and ^{3}H: nuclear versus cytoplasmic radiation effects in murine L1210 leukaemia. *Int J Radiat Biol.* 1975;28:225–241.
43. Kassis AI, Fayad F, Kinsey BM, et al. Radiotoxicity of ^{125}I in mammalian cells. *Radiat Res.* 1987;111:305–318.
44. Bloomer WD, Adelstein SJ. 5-^{125}I-iododeoxyuridine as prototype for radionuclide therapy with Auger emitters. *Nature.* 1977;265:620–621.
45. Baranowska-Kortylewicz J, Makrigiorgos GM, Van den Abbeele AD, et al. 5-[^{123}I]iodo-2'-deoxyuridine in the radiotherapy of an early ascites tumor model. *Int J Radiat Oncol Biol Phys.* 1991;21:1541–1551.
46. Kassis AI, Dahman BA, Adelstein SJ. In vivo therapy of neoplastic meningitis with methotrexate and 5-[^{125}I]iodo-2'-deoxyuridine. *Acta Oncol.* 2000;39:731–737.
47. Kassis AI, Kirichian AM, Wang K, et al. Therapeutic potential of 5-[^{125}I]iodo-2'-deoxyuridine and methotrexate in the treatment of advanced neoplastic meningitis. *Int J Radiat Biol.* 2004;80:941–946.
48. Jain RK. Physiological barriers to delivery of monoclonal antibodies and other macromolecules in tumors. *Cancer Res (Suppl).* 1990;50:814s–819s.
49. Netti PA, Hamberg LM, Babich JW, et al. Enhancement of fluid filtration across tumor vessels: implication for delivery of macromolecules. *Proc Natl Acad Sci USA.* 1999;96:3137–3142.

Concept of Systemic Therapy: Dose-Dense Chemotherapy

Tiffany A. Traina and Larry Norton

■ INTRODUCTION

Systemic chemotherapy and radiation are modalities of anticancer treatment that may initially appear quite different from one another. However, these two therapeutic approaches share fundamental similarities such as the delivery of toxic agents to achieve tumor cytoreduction while simultaneously preserving healthy host tissue. The concepts of tumor growth kinetics and the lessons learned through the use of mathematical models to predict optimal chemotherapy delivery may also be applicable to the delivery of radiation therapy.

Oftentimes, the choice of chemotherapy dose and schedule for clinical practice has been based on preclinical experiments and clinical trials that focus on toxicity as primary end points (1). However, the belief that dose escalation is proportional to benefit and that the chosen recommended dose is that which can be best tolerated has not been supported by the breast cancer literature (2–5). Additionally, the phenomenom of tachyphylaxis, whereby repeated dosing leads to waning effect, would caution against continued dosing to the point of maximum tolerability as more drug may not in fact be more effective. The trial-and-error approach to determining clinical dosing schedules is laborious and exhausts precious patient and financial resources. Therefore, improved methods for predicting optimal dosing schedules may lead to better regimens, which may also be more cost-efficient and expeditious.

Mathematical models are potentially useful tools whereby optimal drug schedule may be predicted. Experimental models have attempted to describe the fundamentals of tumor cell growth and kinetics. From these systems arose an improved understanding of tumor growth characteristics, a foundation for the key principles of chemotherapy and, eventually, recognition of the importance of dose scheduling. In this chapter, we review how mathematical models have led to a better understanding of tumor growth kinetics and have informed rational dosing schedules of chemotherapy that improved survival of patients with early-stage breast cancer. We also discuss the latest application of the Norton–Simon model—the creation of a method by which preclinical data may determine the optimal schedule and dose level of an anticancer drug or regimen. Similarities may be drawn between chemotherapy and the systemic delivery of radiation.

■ MATHEMATICAL MODELS OF TUMOR GROWTH KINETICS

Several mathematical models have been proposed to describe the fundamentals of tumor cell growth and kinetics (6–13). In one of the earliest models, Skipper and Schabel hypothesized that tumor growth is exponential and that growth rate is constant. Therefore, a dose of drug active against a uniformly sensitive population should always kill a constant fraction of cells, regardless of the size of the tumor at the start of treatment (the log-kill hypothesis) (14,15). This fixed, relative cytoreduction led to interest in postoperative adjuvant chemotherapy as small-volume micrometastases were predicted to be more easily eliminated. However, the log-kill model did not account for tumor regrowth between doses and could not completely explain tumor cytokinetics as evidenced by recurrences of breast cancer despite adjuvant chemotherapy. The next generation of mathematical models built upon these concepts was thus established.

The application of the Gompertzian equation, which describes population growth to tumor kinetics, improved our understanding of tumorigenesis (6). It is described as follows:

$$N(t) = N(0)\exp\{k[1-\exp(-bt)]\}$$

where $k = \log_e[N(\infty)/N(0)]$.

In this equation, N is the cell number, $N(0)$ is the starting size, t is the time of growth, and b is a constant. This equation has been noted to "best fit" clinical and experimental data and help design various clinical trials (16). Speer et al. (10) proposed a stochastic model by which tumor growth is largely Gompertzian. The main variation is that there are proposed spontaneous alterations in the parameters of b (decrease) and $N(\infty)$ (increase). This will result in growth "spurts" or random spontaneous changes in the growth rate of the tumor. The Speer model indicates that these events are independent of tumor size and, as a result, embraces a long-term maintenance chemotherapy program in the adjuvant setting. In this fashion, the random and continuous growth spurts of the tumor will be potentially exposed to cytotoxic agents. There are, however, insufficient data correlating the Speer model to clinical tumor growth. Interestingly, pure Gompertzian growth

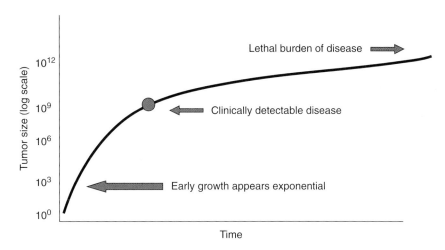

FIGURE 19.1 Gompertzian growth curve illustrating the nonconstant rate of population growth. The curve describes an early exponential phase of tumor growth, followed by a plateau phase.

appears to best correlate with animal and human tumor growth data (16).

Gompertzian growth is characterized by the nonconstant rate of cancer growth (Fig. 19.1). Tumor cell numbers increase over time; however, the relative rate of increase falls exponentially until the tumor reaches a plateau phase of very slow absolute growth (16–19). Although, all tumors seem to observe the characteristic Gompertzian curve, the plateau phase for a particular type of cancer may be theoretically greater than the lethal volume of tumor. Rapidly growing malignancies such as leukemia may appear to grow by nearly exponential growth because the host organism succumbs to the burden of disease well before the plateau phase is attained.

Norton and Simon refined the Skipper–Schabel log-kill model, taking into account the kinetic nature of population growth described by the Gompertzian equation. The underlying philosophy of the Norton–Simon hypothesis recognizes that a dynamic process such as tumor growth requires a treatment approach that considers the trajectory of cytokinetics. In this model, the rate of cytoreduction is proportional to the rate of tumor growth (9). In other words, log kill is not constant but rather is relative to the growth rate. This model predicts that small-volume tumors experience greater response to treatment because of their rapid growth rate in comparison to larger tumors with slower growth rates. Therefore, a kinetic advantage exists for treatment when tumor volume is small such as in the postoperative, adjuvant setting (20).

The Norton–Simon hypothesis acknowledged that without eradication of all cancer cells, rapid regrowth of micrometastases would occur as predicted by the Gompertzian curve. Investigators postulated that delivering chemotherapy at a greater rate (dose density) could optimize chemotherapy efficacy and that by minimizing the regrowth of cancer between doses of therapy, one could increase the cumulative cell kill and achieve greater clinical benefit (21). Preclinical data supported this hypothesis (22,23).

■ DELIVERY OF CYTOTOXIC THERAPY

▓ Dose density and validation of the Norton–Simon hypothesis

The superiority of dose density in chemotherapy scheduling was first supported in a multicenter, randomized, clinical trial in over 2000 patients with early-stage breast cancer receiving adjuvant therapy every 2 weeks rather than the conventional every-3-week schedule (doxorubicin and cyclophosphamide [AC] followed by paclitaxel [T]) (24). The design of this trial allowed for a true test of dose density as all patients received the same drugs, at the same individual and cumulative doses, in the same number of cycles for all arms of the trial. As predicted by the Norton–Simon mathematical model, the more dose-dense schedule (every 2 weeks rather than every 3 weeks) yielded a statistically significant 26% reduction in the average annual risk of recurrence and a significant 31% reduction in the average annual risk of death. The benefit of dose density was independent of other predictive factors such as the number of positive nodes, tumor size, and menopausal status. An updated analysis performed on November 30, 2005 and reflecting 6.5 years of follow-up from the date of last patient accrual was reported at the 2005 annual meeting of the American Society of Clinical Oncology and the 2005 annual San Antonio Breast Cancer Symposium (20,25). After 508 (26%) disease-free survival events and 370 (19%) overall survival events, a significant improvement in disease-free survival persisted for the dose-dense, every-2-week regimen (Hazard ratio 1.25, 95% CI 1.05 to 1.49, $p = 0.012$). An overall survival advantage was confirmed for the dose-dense (q2 week) schedule ($p < 0.05$).

Several trials have since supported the feasibility of dose-dense administration of chemotherapy (26–28). Additional trials have been consistent with the superiority of dose-dense treatment; however, trial designs must be critically examined (29,30). Too often, study arms confound results due to differing drugs and dose intensity between the experimental and control arms (31–33).

Recently, Sparano and colleagues reported the results of a large, randomized, multicenter trial that compared two taxanes (paclitaxel and docetaxel) administered in two schedules (every 3 weeks vs. weekly) following AC for the adjuvant treatment of women with early-stage breast cancer (34). The dose-dense regimen, weekly administration of paclitaxel was found to be superior in terms of both disease-free (OR 1.27 [1.03 to 1.57], $p = 0.006$) and overall survival (OR 1.32 [1.02 to 1.72], $p = 0.01$) when all treatment arms were compared to the less-dense regimen, paclitaxel every 3 weeks. The weekly schedule of paclitaxel also proved to be the best tolerated treatment arm with the lowest incidence of grade 3 or 4 adverse events, offering additional evidence that dose-dense chemotherapy schedules are not synonymous with greater toxicity.

■ APPLICATION OF THE NORTON–SIMON MODEL TO PREDICT OPTIMAL DOSING SCHEDULE

The practical application of the above model to intravenous bolus chemotherapy delivery concluded that maximization of effect can occur by (a) using effective drugs at optimal dose levels and (b) delivering drugs with as short a cycle length as feasible with the use of supportive measures to reduce toxicity. However, to date, the duration of our dosing schedule within a cycle has typically been determined by the limitation of intolerable toxicity. The need for a method of optimizing drug delivery schedules has been imperative as the possible iterations of dosing schedules are nearly limitless.

Norton and colleagues developed a method by which Gompertzian growth curves are fit to untreated and treated tumor models. From these data, a new curve can be generated that represents, at each point in time, the ratio of Gompertzian growth rates for treated tumor versus tumor in the control, untreated state. From this derivative, the magnitude of the impact of treatment at each point in time may be observed. It then logically follows that optimal drug delivery would proceed to the point of maximal perturbation of the curve or maximal therapeutic benefit (35). Continued treatment beyond the point of maximal drug effect may contribute to additional toxicity without significant incremental benefit.

This mathematical approach summarized here was applied to xenograft models treated with capecitabine (Xeloda, Roche), an orally administered prodrug of 5-fluorouracil.

■ Preclinical data

Capecitabine is an orally administered prodrug that has substantial antitumor activity against breast cancer (36–39). The drug is approved by the U.S. Food and Drug Administration (FDA) as monotherapy for treatment of patients with metastatic breast cancer resistant to anthracycline- and taxane-containing regimens, and also in combination with docetaxel for treatment of anthracycline-pretreated breast

cancer (40,41). After numerous dose finding trials in breast and other malignancies, the capecitabine dose and schedule of 2510 mg/m^2/day in two divided daily doses given for 14 days followed by a 7-day rest (14–7) was recommended as most suitable for phase III studies.

In practice, this dosing schedule has proven problematic. Capecitabine-associated toxicities of palmar–plantar erythrodysesthesia, diarrhea, and stomatitis have led to dose interruptions and reductions in approximately 34% to 65% of patients receiving capecitabine at the FDA-recommended dose level and schedule. As many as 12% to 16% of patients on clinical trials have discontinued capecitabine because of toxicity rather than disease progression (39,42). In clinical practice, physicians have empirically reduced dose levels of the drug or modified the 14–7 schedule to minimize intolerable toxicity (43). These adjustments to dosing schedule have been driven by toxicity and are chosen in the absence of theoretically motivated and experimentally determined guidelines.

When this mathematical method was applied to capecitabine in mice bearing MX-1 human breast cancer xenografts, the point of maximal drug effect was estimated to occur after approximately 7 days of treatment and was consistent across different dose levels tested (35). For treatment delivered beyond this point, the impact of capecitabine drug effect decreases consistently over the remaining days of a typical cycle. The model predicts that drug delivery beyond 7 days contributes to toxicity with diminishing anticancer benefit; therefore, the optimal cycle duration is predicted to be 7 days followed by a 7-day rest (7–7).

Preclinical experiments of the capecitabine 7–7 schedule in KPL-4 xenograft mouse models achieved a maximum tolerated dose (MTD) level of 1.75-fold higher than previously achieved with the conventional schedule (700 mg/kg/day vs. 400 mg/kg/day) (44). As predicted by the mathematical model, the capecitabine 7–7 dosing schedule achieved greater antitumor activity. This dosing schedule of capecitabine demonstrated statistically significant tumor regression and a survival benefit when compared with control (44).

■ Clinical validation of optimal dosing schedule

A phase I trial evaluated the tolerability and determined the MTD of capecitabine 7–7 in patients with breast cancer (45). Patients with measurable, histologically confirmed metastatic breast cancer with normal organ function were eligible for this trial. Any number of prior chemotherapy regimens were permitted. The MTD was defined as the highest dose for which the incidence of dose-limiting toxicity was less than 33%. A standard three-patient-per-cohort dose escalation schedule was used and patients in the started cohort received capecitabine 1500 mg flat dose orally twice daily for 7 days followed by a 7-day rest. There was no intrapatient dose escalation. Cohort dose levels increased by 500-mg increments. All patients within a cohort were monitored for 28 days prior to accrual to the next cohort. Radiographic response assessment was performed every 12 weeks using response evaluation criteria in solid tumors (RECIST) criteria. Treatment continued until disease progression, intolerable treatment-related toxicities, or withdrawal of consent.

Twenty-one patients were treated on study. The most frequently reported treatment-related, grade 2/3 adverse events were palmar–plantar erythrodysesthesia (29%), leukopenia/neutropenia (24%), and fatigue (19%). Grade 3 toxicity was transient and easily managed. Three patients experienced grade 3 palmar–plantar erythrodysesthesia; one of these patients also had grade 3 diarrhea. There were no grade 4 events.

This study concluded that capecitabine 7–7 is well tolerated at an MTD of 2000 mg twice daily. Comparisons across studies with differing patient populations and trial designs are wrought with confounding variables. However, the amount of capecitabine delivered at this dose and schedule appeared greater than that historically achieved in practice with the licensed recommended dose and schedule (2500 mg/m^2 for 14 days followed by a 7-day rest).

■ CONCLUSION AND FUTURE DIRECTIONS

Experience has established that mathematical modeling based on growth curve analysis can predict improved chemotherapy dosing schedules and thereby improve patient survival. The use of models is an intriguing approach for the systematic and rational design of treatment schedules. Application of this methodology to novel, systemic targeted therapies is ongoing. Similarly, the fundamentals learned from these models of tumor kinetics may be applied to the development of optimal systemic radiation delivery schedules. By using active therapies in the best possible schedules, as predicted by tumor cytokinetics and based on efficacy rather than toxicity, we can significantly improve the lives of patients with cancer.

■ REFERENCES

1. Chu E. Pharmacology of cancer chemotherapy: drug development. In: DeVita VT Jr, Hellman S, Rosenberg SA, eds. *Cancer: Principles and Practice of Oncology.* New York, NY: Lippincott Williams & Wilkins; 2005:307–317.
2. Fisher B, Anderson S, Wickerham DL, et al. Increased intensification and total dose of cyclophosphamide in a doxorubicin–cyclophosphamide regimen for the treatment of primary breast cancer: findings from National Surgical Adjuvant Breast and Bowel Project B-22. *J Clin Oncol.* 1997;15(5):1858–1869.
3. Henderson IC, Berry DA, Demetri GD, et al. Improved outcomes from adding sequential Paclitaxel but not from escalating Doxorubicin dose in an adjuvant chemotherapy regimen for patients with node-positive primary breast cancer. *J Clin Oncol.* 2003;21(6):976–983.
4. Winer EP, Berry DA, Woolf S, et al. Failure of higher-dose paclitaxel to improve outcome in patients with metastatic breast cancer: cancer and leukemia group B trial 9342. *J Clin Oncol.* 2004;22(11):2061–2068.
5. Peters WP, Dansey RD, Klein JL, et al. High-dose chemotherapy and peripheral blood progenitor cell transplantation in the treatment of breast cancer. *Oncologist.* 2000;5(1):1–13.
6. Norton L, Simon R, Brereton HD, et al. Predicting the course of Gompertzian growth. *Nature.* 1976;264:542–545.
7. Norton L, Simon R. The growth curve of an experimental solid tumor following radiotherapy. *J Natl Cancer Inst.* 1977;58:1735–1741.
8. Norton L, Simon R. Tumor size, sensitivity to therapy, and design of treatment schedules. *Cancer Treat Rep.* 1977;61(7):1307–1315.
9. Norton L, Simon R. The Norton–Simon hypothesis revisited. *Cancer Treat Rep.* 1986;70:163–169.
10. Speer J, Petrosky VE, Retsky MW, et al. A stochastic numerical model of breast cancer that simulates clinical data. *Cancer Res.* 1984;44:4124.
11. Spratt JA, von Fournier D, Spratt JS, et al. Mammographic assessment of human breast cancer growth and duration. *Cancer.* 1993;71(6):2020–2026.
12. Spratt JA, von Fournier D, Spratt JS, et al. Decelerating growth and human breast cancer. *Cancer.* 1993;71(6):2013–2019.
13. Koscielny S, Tubiana M, Valleron AJ. A simulation model of the natural history of human breast cancer. *Br J Cancer.* 1985;52(4):515–524.
14. Skipper H, Schabel FJ, Wilcox W. Experimental evaluation of potential anticancer agents XIII: on the criteria and kinetics associated with "curability" of experimental leukemia. *Cancer Chemother Rep.* 1964;35:1.
15. Skipper H. Laboratory models: some historical perspective. *Cancer Treat Rep.* 1986;70(1):3–7.
16. Norton L. A Gompertzian model of human breast cancer growth. *Cancer Res.* 1988;48:7067–7071.
17. Norton L. Evolving concepts in the systemic drug therapy of breast cancer. *Semin Oncol.* 1997;24(4 suppl 10):S10-3–S10-10.
18. Norton L. Theoretical concepts and the emerging role of taxanes in adjuvant therapy. *Oncologist.* 2001;6(suppl 3):30–35.
19. Piccart-Gebhart MJ. Mathematics and oncology: a match for life? *J Clin Oncol.* 2003;21(8):1425–1428.
20. Hudis C. Dose Dense Adjuvant Chemotherapy for Breast Cancer. Presented at the annual meeting of American Society of Clinical Oncology, Orlando, FL, 2005.
21. Norton L. Conceptual and practical implications of breast tissue geometry: toward a more effective, less toxic therapy. *Oncologist.* 2005;10(6):370–381.
22. Skipper HE. Kinetics of mammary tumor cell growth and implications for therapy. *Cancer.* 1971;28(6):1479–1499.
23. Skipper H. Analysis of multiarmed trials in which animals bearing different burdens of L1210 leukemia cells were treated with two, three, and four drug combinations delivered in different ways with varying dose intensities of each drug and varying average dose intensities. *Southern Res Inst Booklet 7.* 1986;420:87–92.
24. Citron ML, Berry DA, Cirrincione C, et al. Randomized trial of dose-dense versus conventionally scheduled and sequential versus concurrent combination chemotherapy as postoperative adjuvant treatment of node-positive primary breast cancer: first report of Intergroup Trial C9741/Cancer and Leukemia Group B Trial 9741. *J Clin Oncol.* 2003;21(8):1431–1439.
25. Hudis C, Citron ML, Berry D, et al. Five year follow-up of INT C9741: dose-dense (DD) chemotherapy (CRx) is safe and effective. *Breast Cancer Res Treat.* 2005;94.
26. Fornier MN, Seidman AD, Lake D, et al. Increased dose-density (DD) is feasible: a pilot study of epirubicin and cyclophosphamide (EC) followed by paclitaxel (T), at 10–11 day interval with filgrastim support, for women with early breast carcinoma (BC). In: *Proceedings of the American Society of Clinical Oncology.* 2005. Available at: http://meeting.ascopubs.org/cgi/content/abstract/23/16_suppl/616.
27. Dickler MN. A phase II study of bevacizumab with dose dense doxorubicin and cyclophosphamide (AC) followed by dose dense nanoparticle albumin bound paclitaxel for the treatment of early stage breast cancer. 2005.
28. Dang C, Smith K, Fornier M, et al. Mature cardiac safety results of dose-dense (DD) doxorubicin and cyclophosphamide (AC) followed by paclitaxel (T) with trastuzumab (H) in HER2/neu overexpressed/amplified breast cancer (BCA). In: *SABCS.* 2006.
29. Bonadonna G, Zambetti M, Valagussa P. Sequential or alternating doxorubicin and CMF regimens in breast cancer with more than three positive nodes. Ten-year results. *JAMA.* 1995;273(7):542–547.
30. Bonadonna G, Zambetti M, Moliterni A, et al. Clinical relevance of different sequencing of doxorubicin and cyclophosphamide, methotrexate, and Fluorouracil in operable breast cancer. *J Clin Oncol.* 2004;22(9):1614–1620.
31. Green MC, Buzdar AU, Smith T, et al. Weekly paclitaxel improves pathologic complete remission in operable breast cancer when compared with paclitaxel once every 3 weeks. *J Clin Oncol.* 2005;23(25):5983–5992.
32. Untch M, Konecny G, Ditsch N, et al. Dose-dense sequential epirubicin-paclitaxel as preoperative treatment of breast cancer: results of a randomised AGO study. In: *ASCO Annual Meeting.* 2002.
33. Therasse P, Mauriac L, Welnicka-Jaskiewicz M, et al. Final results of a randomized phase III trial comparing cyclophosphamide, epirubicin,

and fluorouracil with a dose-intensified epirubicin and cyclophosphamide + filgrastim as neoadjuvant treatment in locally advanced breast cancer: an EORTC-NCIC-SAKK multicenter study. *J Clin Oncol.* 2003;21(5):843–850.

34. Sparano JA, Wang M, Martino S, et al. Weekly paclitaxel in the adjuvant treatment of breast cancer. *N Engl J Med.* 2008;358(16):1663–1671.

35. Norton L, Dugan U, Young D, et al. Optimizing chemotherapeutic dose-schedule (CDS) by Norton–Simon modeling: capecitabine (Xeloda(®)). In: *Annual Meeting of American Association for Cancer Research.* Anaheim, CA; 2005.

36. Blum JL, Dieras V, Lo Russo PM, et al. Multicenter, phase II study of capecitabine in taxane-pretreated metastatic breast carcinoma patients. *Cancer.* 2001;92(7):1759–1768.

37. Blum JL, Jones SE, Buzdar AU, et al. Multicenter phase II study of capecitabine in paclitaxel-refractory metastatic breast cancer. *J Clin Oncol.* 1999;17(2):485–493.

38. Reichardt P, Von Minckwitz G, Thuss-Patience PC, et al. Multicenter phase II study of oral capecitabine (Xeloda(")) in patients with metastatic breast cancer relapsing after treatment with a taxane-containing therapy. *Ann Oncol.* 2003;14(8):1227–1233.

39. O'Shaughnessy JA, Blum J, Moiseyenko V, et al. Randomized, open-label, phase II trial of oral capecitabine (Xeloda) vs. a reference arm of intravenous CMF (cyclophosphamide, methotrexate and 5-fluorouracil) as first-line therapy for advanced/metastatic breast cancer. *Ann Oncol.* 2001;12(9):1247–1254.

40. Food and Drug Administration. *FDA Approves Xeloda for Breast Cancer.* Food and Drug Administration, ed. U.S. Department of Health and Human Services; 1998. Available at: http://timelines.com/1998/4/30/fda-approves-hoffmann-la-roches-xeloda.

41. Food and Drug Administration. *FDA Approves Xeloda in Combination with Taxotere for Advanced Breast Cancer.* Food and Drug Administration, ed. U.S. Department of Health and Human Services; 2001. Available at: http://www.highbeam.com/doc/1G1-79369986.htm.

42. Miller KD, Chap LI, Holmes FA, et al. Randomized phase III trial of capecitabine compared with bevacizumab plus capecitabine in patients with previously treated metastatic breast cancer. *J Clin Oncol.* 2005;23(4):792–799.

43. Hennessy BT, Gauthier AM, Michaud LB, et al. Lower dose capecitabine has a more favorable therapeutic index in metastatic breast cancer: retrospective analysis of patients treated at M. D. Anderson Cancer Center and a review of capecitabine toxicity in the literature. *Ann Oncol.* 2005;16(8):1289–1296.

44. Traina T, Theodoulou M, Higgins B, et al. In vivo activity of a novel regimen of capecitabine in a breast cancer xenograft model. *Breast Cancer Res Treat.* 2006;100(suppl 1):S279. (2006 San Antonio Breast Cancer Symposium Proceedings: Abstract 6071.)

45. Traina TA, Theodoulou M, Feigin K, et al. Phase I study of a novel capecitabine schedule based on the Norton–Simon mathematical model in patients with metastatic breast cancer. *J Clin Oncol.* 2008;26(11):1797–1802.

Modeling of the Systemic Cure with Targeted Radionuclide Therapy

Peter Bernhardt and Tod W. Speer

■ INTRODUCTION

Several new radiopharmaceuticals for targeted radionuclide therapy (TRT) of disseminated cancers are currently approaching routine use. In the following chapters, the clinical use of radiolabeled antibodies directed toward the CD20 antigen for treating non–Hodgkin lymphoma (NHL) is discussed. Further, the clinical approach of using smaller radiopharmaceuticals such as radiolabeled somatostatin analogs is reviewed. Currently, numerous preclinical and clinical trials using different radionuclides and targeting constructs are being investigated and are comprehensively described in this book.

One advantage of employing the concept of TRT is that it is a point-specific therapy, that is, the cytotoxic effect is mostly limited to the target site. This phenomenon is due to the fact that the emitted radiation, beta particles, low-energy electrons, and alpha particles ionize and cause lethal cell damage along a track length measured in nanometers to millimeters. The larger track length emissions may provide a benefit when the target site is distributed in a heterogenous fashion in the tumor tissue, or worse, the target site is lacking at some tissue locations. In these particular scenarios, a long particle range is of value, since the "cross-irradiation" will make the absorbed dose distribution more uniform than the distributions of available target sites. This is termed the cross-fire effect. However, too long of a path length of the emitted particles will be a potential drawback for the treatment of small tumor nests, in view of the fact that most of the energy will be deposited outside of the tumor.

Cancer that metastasizes will contain numerous tumors of different sizes. If the elusive "cure" is to be obtained, all of these tumors must be sterilized. But, due to the stochastic nature of cancer progression, it is difficult to predict that a patient will be cured after a given treatment. A more realistic method to help understand the potential for the systemic cure of cancer is to mathematically evaluate the probability of cure. In this chapter, we will describe how the metastatic cure probability (MCP) can be estimated by dynamic modeling. We will begin by describing the dosimetric properties of various therapeutic radionuclides. Then, the target-hit models for dose-response estimates as well as how the single-hit–single-target model is incorporated into the

modeling of tumor cure probability (TCP) will be described. Please note that we will not use the term tumor *control* probability, which is more commonly used in the literature. This is necessary to address the estimated probability for *cure* and not just the probability to control the disease. The TCP model is therefore integrated into the MCP model. For estimation of MCP, the metastatic distribution needs to be determined by dynamic modeling. By using the MCP model, it will be shown that the required absorbed tumor dose will differ for various radionuclides and for different metastatic distributions. In addition, multiple factors affecting MCP will be analyzed and discussed, and an example of the MCP estimate in a unique clinical case will be demonstrated.

■ DOSIMETRIC CHARACTERIZATION OF RADIONUCLIDES

Today, at least three electron-emitting radionuclides have proven to be useful in clinical applications: ^{90}Y, ^{177}Lu, and ^{131}I (1). Alpha-emitting radionuclides are just beginning to be used in the clinical setting. ^{223}Ra is approved in Europe for symptom relief of skeleton metastases and can perhaps even cause a prolongation of life in patients with severe dissemination of skeleton metastases (see Chapter 22). But the alpha emitter ^{211}At might be a more attractive radionuclide for targeted therapy. Several preclinical studies have shown its potential in the treatment of microscopic disease. Clinical studies have been performed with glioma, using an ^{211}At-labeled antitenascin antibody (see Chapter 27). Table 20.1 presents the physical properties of the four radionuclides: ^{90}Y, ^{177}Lu, ^{131}I, and ^{211}At, which will be used in this chapter for multiple analyses.

The decay mode of the three illustrated electron emitters is beta minus decay, with different mean energies of the emitted electrons. ^{90}Y emits electrons with very high energies, and the maximal range of the electrons is 11.3 mm. ^{177}Lu and ^{131}I emit electrons with mean energies of 133 and 182 keV, respectively. The maximal electron range for ^{177}Lu and ^{131}I is 1.8 and 3.3 mm, respectively. The maximal range for the alpha emitter ^{211}At is 93 μm, which is considerably shorter than the range for the electron emitters. This observation might seem to be a contradiction since the emitted energy is much higher (6300 keV). This phenomenon can

Table **20.1**	Physical properties of the radionuclides				
Radionuclide	Decay Mode	$T_{1/2}$	Energy (keV)	Range (mm)	p/e
^{90}Y	β^-	2.7 days	935	11.3	0
^{177}Lu	β^-	6.7 days	133	1.8	0.24
^{131}I	β^-	8.0 days	182	3.3	2.0
^{211}At	α	7.2 hours	6300	0.093	0

partly be explained by the fact that the alpha particle is approximately 8000 times heavier than an electron. This will result in a much slower speed for the alpha particle. This slow speed will increase the probability for an interaction with the biologic material, resulting in a dense ionization track. The linear energy transfer (LET) of the emitted alpha particles will be around 100 keV/μm; for electrons it will be less than 1 keV/μm.

The different ranges of the emitted charged particles will make the radionuclides more or less suitable for treatment of various-sized tumors (2,3). Figure 20.1 illustrates the dependence of the mean energy deposition in spherical tumors of different sizes (mass). In the figure, the smallest mass corresponds to a single cell with a mass of 1 ng. The cell diameter will be just above 12 μm. It is evident that only a very small fraction of the emitted energy from ^{90}Y will be deposited in single cells or small tumor nests. It is at tumor sizes larger than 1 g that almost all energy is effectively absorbed in the tumor tissue from ^{90}Y. In contrast, for the alpha emitter ^{211}At, all energy is effectively absorbed in a 1-μg tumor. For ^{177}Lu and ^{131}I, the corresponding tumor masses will be around 1 mg. Further, another important aspect in the judgment of radionuclides' suitability for targeted therapy is the emission of photons. The tumor–to–normal tissue mean absorbed dose ratio (TND) model was developed for analyzing the influence of charged particles and photons on the absorbed dose to tumor and normal tissue (4,5). In Figure 20.2, it can be observed that the

high photon abundance markedly reduces the TND for ^{131}I, which is not seen for the other radionuclides with a lower photon emission. ^{131}I has a photon to charged particle ratio (p/e) of 2 (Table 20.1), that is, most of the emitted energy is from photons. Too high of a photon abundance might cause severe normal tissue damage or toxicity, especially to the radiosensitive bone marrow (BM). However, a small fraction of emitted photons might be useful for quantification of uptake and dosimetric studies. The use of ^{177}Lu-labeled somatostatin analogues has enabled dosimetric evaluation of organ doses, which is especially important information for critical organs such as the kidneys. For ^{177}Lu-labeled somatostatin analogues, the estimated kidney dose is the factor that determines the total activity that will be administered to the patient, reducing the risk of late kidney failure. The very low abundance of photon emissions from ^{90}Y and ^{211}At makes it more difficult to quantify the activity distributions of these radionuclides. The most common approach for performing dosimetric evaluations of these radionuclides is to use a surrogate gamma-emitting radionuclide, such as ^{111}In, for the clinical evaluation. In another example, the radionuclide ^{86}Y has been used for positron emission tomography measurement, with resulting dosimetric calculations for ^{90}Y. The dosimetric evaluation is an important aspect in the understanding of tumor and normal tissue response; more precisely, the dose is incorporated into target-hit models for describing the response in tissues.

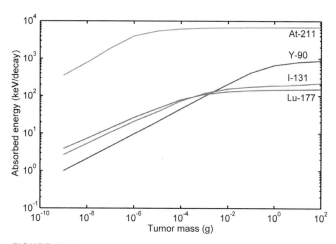

FIGURE 20.1 The absorbed energy per decay versus tumor mass with uniform activity distribution of At-211, Lu-177, I-131, and Y-90.

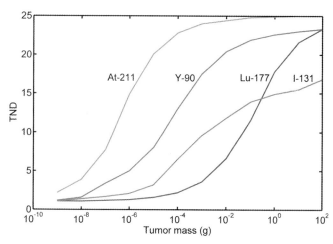

FIGURE 20.2 The tumor–to–normal tissue mean absorbed dose ratio (TND) versus tumor mass with uniform activity distribution.

■ TISSUE RESPONSE MODELS

Irradiation of tissue will induce DNA damage, which might be effectively repaired or result in permanent DNA damage. The permanent DNA damage will most likely result in cell death or potentially the late effect of cancer induction. The cellular response is a complex process that is driven by multiple signaling pathways and has been extensively studied in the field of radiobiology. Fortunately, in order to obtain a good model for describing tissue response to therapy, the molecular mechanism underlying this complex signaling does not have to be exactly known. By using target-hit models, the tissue response descriptions are simplified. In this example of modeling of an end point, that is, cell death, it is described as a function of the absorbed dose.

In the early era of radiation biology, cell survival studies revealed that cells responded almost exponentially to absorbed dose; when plotting the log of cell survival versus absorbed dose (see Chapters 6 and 27), the result is an observable shoulder on the cell survival curve (Fig. 20.3). With these results in mind, target-hit models were developed. In these models, the target in a cell can be regarded as any cellular structure leading to cell death when "hit." The "hit" is considered an ionization event that causes cell death when interacting with the target. All emitted particles will then create a number of potential hits along their track, where some of these hits might interact with the target and cause cell death. In this way the probability that a hit will cause cell death is achieved. The mathematical term, α, is a constant (for a given tumor or tissue) used to describe this probability for cell death. It represents the radiosensitivity of the cells (tissue) and can also be described as the initial slope of the cell survival curve. It is more convenient to have the radiosensitivity defined per absorbed dose instead of per track length; 1 Gy in a typical cell nucleus will have been created by approximately 1000 electron tracks.

The DNA in the cell nucleus appears to be the main target that results in cell death. The DNA damage that results in most cell deaths seems to be double-strand breaks (DSBs).

In spite of this, the constant, α, can be considered as the probability, per absorbed dose, of creating lethal DSBs. This process is regarded as the single-target–single-hit model, where the target is a lethal DSB, and the cell survival (S) versus absorbed dose will be a pure exponential function:

$$S = e^{-\alpha D}, \qquad (\text{Eq. 20.1})$$

where D is the mean absorbed dose.

The observed shoulder in many cell survival experiments can be largely explained by target-hit models, where multiple hits and/or multiple targets are used. The most common model is the linear-quadratic (LQ) model where the linear portion is explained by the single-hit model, described earlier, and the quadratic portion is a single-target–double-hit model. One way to describe the quadratic model is to consider single-strand break (SSB) induction. It is well known that multiple SSBs will be induced during irradiation, and that most of these SSBs will be repaired. However, if two SSBs are induced in close proximity before any repair can occur, these two SSBs will summate and induce a DSB. In this case, the DSBs have been induced by double hits. The constant β is used to describe this phenomenon. The value of β can be considered as the product of two probabilities of inducing SSB, that is, the cell survival will depend on β times the absorbed dose squared:

$$S = e^{-\beta D^2}. \qquad (\text{Eq. 20.2})$$

In the LQ model, the two models are combined:

$$S = e^{-\alpha D - \beta D^2}. \qquad (\text{Eq. 20.3})$$

The shoulder on the cell survival curve is often observed when high dose rates are employed, as with external beam irradiation where about 2 Gy/min is given. In radionuclide therapy, a nearly 1000-fold lower dose rate is delivered, and the quadratic portion of the LQ model will have less of an influence on the cell survival curve since many of the SSBs will be repaired; the probability that two SSBs will create a lethal DSB is reduced. In addition, when considering tumor responses to low dose, low dose rate radiotherapy (TRT), the quadratic term is often missing. As a result, there is either a "small" or "no" observable shoulder. So when estimating the surviving fraction for tumors after radionuclide therapy, the single-target–single-hit model is often used.

The value of the radiosensitivity of cells exposed to electrons and alpha particles is determined by the application of cell survival studies. For electrons, the radiosensitivity of a cell line may range from "radioresistant" with an α equal to 0.2 Gy^{-1} to "radiosensitive" with cells having an α equal to 0.5 Gy^{-1}. When analyzing cell survival curves, it can be concluded that the cytotoxicity of a given type of radiation is much higher for alpha particles (densely ionizing radiation) than for electrons (sparsely ionizing radiation). The estimation of the relative biologic effectiveness (RBE) between alpha particles and electrons can vary widely in studies, but in a recent discussion paper, an RBE of 5 was proposed (6). Also proposed was a new unit, the Barendsen (Bd), to be used as an equivalent absorbed dose unit. In this

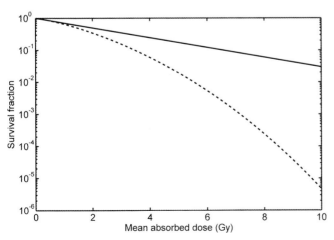

FIGURE 20.3 The survival curves for the linear *(solid line)* target-hit model ($S = e^{-\alpha D}$) and the linear quadric *(dashed line)* target-hit model ($S = e^{-\alpha D - \beta D^2}$).

chapter, the alpha dose factor will be given a weight of 5 and will still remain in the unit Gy. Accordingly, the doses used for the alpha emitter ^{211}At will be divided by 5 in order to obtain the physical parameter, "mean absorbed dose."

■ THE METASTATIC CURE PROBABILITY MODEL

In the previous section, it was shown that the cell survival fraction (S) changes with the absorbed dose. S will have a value between 0 and 1, and if we attempt to estimate the chance to sterilize a tumor cell we have to calculate the probability (p) for this single cell to be sterilized:

$$p = 1 - S. \qquad \text{(Eq. 20.4)}$$

Furthermore, in order to estimate the TCP, all of the probabilities for sterilization of the tumor must be multiplied:

$$\text{TCP} = p_1 p_2 p_3 \cdots p_n = \prod_{i=1}^{n} p_i. \qquad \text{(Eq. 20.5)}$$

Observe now that TCP depends on every single tumor cell probability to be sterilized, which in turn is dependent on the radiosensitivity and the absorbed dose (Equation 20.1). Consequently, having the absorbed dose to a single cell equal zero, or extremely low, the TCP will be equal to zero and the tumor cannot be regarded as cured. This can occur when the activity concentration is an extremely nonuniform distribution and short-range radiation is used. Further discussions on this topic will be undertaken later in this chapter, but for now, we assume that all tumor cells have the same radiosensitivity (α) and are exposed to an equal, uniform absorbed dose. In this case, the equation for TCP is simplified to:

$$\text{TCP} = (1 - e^{-\alpha D_T})^n. \qquad \text{(Eq. 20.6)}$$

The mean absorbed dose to the tumor (D_T) with uniform distributed activity concentration (C_T) will be:

$$D_T = \frac{C_T \times T_{\text{eff}} \times 1.6 \times 10^{-12} \times \sum_i E_i k_i \phi_{T,i}}{\ln 2}, \qquad \text{(Eq. 20.7)}$$

where T_{eff} is the effective half-life that will depend on the physical half-life (Table 20.1) and the biologic half-life of the

radiopharmaceutical. The parameter E_i is the energy (keV) of the charged particle or photon emitted per decay and k_i is the number of emitted charged particles or photons per decay; $\varphi_{T,i}$ is the absorbed energy fraction of the emitted charged particles or photons. The constant 1.6×10^{-13} converts the product to J/kg (Gy).

In Figure 20.4, the TCP for ^{211}At, ^{177}Lu, ^{131}I, and ^{90}Y versus tumor mass is illustrated. In this simulation, the spherical tumors contain identical activity concentrations; the activity concentration for each radionuclide is set so that the TCP for one of the studied tumors will be 0.9 or 0.99. In this fashion, it can be observed that the TCP is optimal at one specific tumor size. This optimal tumor size will be approximately 10^{-5}, 10^{-2}, 0.1, and 10 g for ^{211}At, ^{177}Lu, ^{131}I, and ^{90}Y, respectively (Fig. 20.4A). The shape of the TCP versus the logarithm of tumor mass is created by two phenomena: the change in the number of tumor cells and absorbed energy fraction. Initially only one cell needs to be sterilized and therefore very low doses (activities) are required. But, as the tumor mass increases, the relative cell numbers will increase accordingly. This effect will be considerable and TCP drops to almost zero. Figure 20.1 illustrates the concept that the absorbed energy fraction will increase exponentially as the tumor mass increases. At a certain tumor size (different for each radionuclide), all of the potential emitted energy will be absorbed by the tumor or tumor spheroid. This will result in an increased absorbed dose with increasing tumor size and the TCP will increase until the optimal tumor cure size is reached. Above this tumor size, the increase in absorbed energy will be minimal (plateau portion of curves in Fig. 20.1). Nevertheless, if the number of tumor cells continues to increase, the TCP will decrease due to a continued increase in tumor mass. For a tumor mass over 10 g, one other phenomenon can be observed for ^{131}I. This phenomenon is the absorption of a portion of the emitted photons by a larger tumor which will begin to influence the TCP and thereby increase the TCP once again (Fig. 20.4A). The p/e ratio is 2 for ^{131}I, whereas it is less than 0.2 for the other studied radionuclides; no observable photon attenuation effects are seen for ^{90}Y, ^{177}Lu, and ^{211}At.

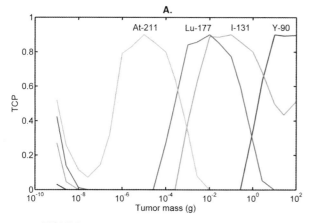
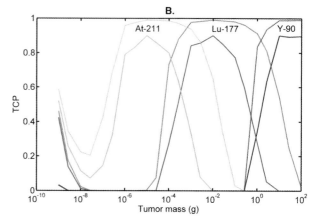

FIGURE 20.4 A: TCP = 0.9 versus tumor mass. The optimal tumor masses for ^{211}At, ^{177}Lu, ^{131}I, and ^{90}Y are about 10^{-5}, 10^{-2}, 0.1, and 10 g, respectively. B: TCP = 0.9 and 0.99 versus tumor mass. For improved clarity, of the figure, only three of the four studied radionuclides are presented.

The TCP model shows that different radionuclides will optimally target different sized tumors. This might lead to the conclusion that a "cocktail" of radionuclides is necessary to treat various sizes of tumors. However, a small increase in activity concentration will dramatically increase the TCP value at the optimal size; in Figure 20.4B, the TCP curves are plotted for TCP = 0.9 and 0.99 at the optimal TCP size. It can be seen that the curve will be broadened with increased activity concentration (dotted lines). If the activity concentration is further increased, high TCPs can be obtained for all tumor sizes. Such an analysis can provide useful information concerning the activity concentration required for obtaining high TCP values for all tumor sizes in metastatic disease. Of course, this would mean that the activity concentration and TCP would need to be estimated for all tumors of the metastatic process. Furthermore, the standard TCP model only describes the condition of isolated tumors; it does not include cross-irradiation from activity in the host organ. When the TCP model was translated into MCP estimates, it contained cross-irradiation and demonstrated that cross-irradiation could facilitate the elimination of some of the smallest tumor sizes (7,8). When we derive the formula where cross-irradiation is included, we also incorporate the tumor–to–normal tissue activity concentration (TNC) into the derivation of D_T:

$$TNC = \frac{C_T}{C_N},\qquad \text{(Eq. 20.8)}$$

where C_N is the activity concentration in the normal tissue that surrounds the tumor tissue. The D_T with inclusion of cross-irradiation will be

$$D_T = \frac{T_{eff} \times 1.6 \times 10^{-13}}{\ln 2} \times \frac{C_T}{TNC}$$

$$\left(\sum_i E_i k_i \phi_N + (TNC-1) \sum_i E_i k_i \phi_{T,i} \right). \quad \text{(Eq. 20.9)}$$

The MCP will be the product of all TCP and is equal to:

$$MCP = \prod_{j=1}^{m} TCP_j. \qquad \text{(Eq. 20.10)}$$

In addition to explaining the influence of cross-irradiation on the MCP, the MCP model has demonstrated efficacy as a tool for analyzing several other physical and biologic factors involved in predicting the therapeutic outcome. These factors are different radionuclide properties, variable activity concentration in tumors, tumor cell proliferation, and treatment start time (7–9). Before these factors are discussed in the following sections, it first must be demonstrated how metastatic distributions can be explained by dynamic modeling.

MODELS OF TUMOR GROWTH

There are several methods for describing tumor growth, but there are only a limited number of models that describe the dissemination of metastases in individual patients. A dynamic model for describing the dissemination of metastases has been proposed (10). We used this modeling approach to develop a method for simulating tumor disease and responses to radionuclide therapy, that is, the MCP. With simulation models, we will be able to handle complex tumor distributions (7,8). The model described by Iwata et al. was developed for analytical solutions and cannot handle more complex problems that require Monte Carlo (MC) simulations. With an MC model, it is easier to obtain stochastic variations of tumor number and size. The MC model will be used for the simulation of metastatic distributions.

One fundamental "input source" for the MC model is the description of tumor growth. In animal studies, tumor growth rates for several cell lines have been accurately determined. In contrast, in clinical studies, tumor growth rates have not been precisely determined. This is partly due to the fact that treatment is typically initiated shortly after the tumor has been diagnosed. Therefore, determinations of tumor growth rates are often based on only two tumor volume estimates. In preclinical and clinical studies, the tumor growth rate can be described by tumor volume doubling time (DT), or the time it takes a tumor to double its volume. Typical DT values are approximately 50 to 100 days. However, we recently demonstrated that DT is an incorrect parameter, when determined from only two volume estimates (11). This can be seen in the formula used in the determination of DT:

$$DT = \frac{t_2 - t_1}{\ln(V_2/V_1)}, \qquad \text{(Eq. 20.11)}$$

where V_1 and V_2 are the volumes determined in the two consecutive data sets and t_2-t_1 is the time difference between the data sets. It can be observed that DT is undefined when two subsequent tumor volume estimates are equal; the logarithm of $V_2/V_1 = 1$ is equal to zero, which makes Equation 20.11 undefined. Furthermore, the uncertainties in volume estimates, for example, those derived from computed tomography (CT), can result in two very similar tumor volume estimates, which leads to unrealistically large positive or negative DT values that must be excluded from the estimation of mean growth rate. This problem has been reported in some studies over many years, since Equation 20.11 was proposed by Collins et al. in 1956 (12), but no solution has been described. We resolved this problem by showing that specific growth rate (SGR), or the inverted DT, is defined for all growth rates:

$$SGR = \frac{\ln(V_2/V_1)}{t_2 - t_1}. \qquad \text{(Eq. 20.12)}$$

SGR also provides information about the fraction of tumor volume that grows every day (%/day), illustrating an improved description of the growth characteristics. When the DT and SGR were estimated for tumor measurements performed in several clinical studies, it could be concluded that the use of SGR resulted in a more rapid growth of tumors than previously determined with DT estimates (11). In this study, the mean SGR was determined for various tumor types: pancreatic carcinoma, primary lung cancer (adenocarcinoma, bronchioalveolar, squamous cell carcinoma, non–small cell lung cancer, and small cell lung cancer), metastatic lung cancer to bone and soft tissue, and hepatocellular carcinoma. The SGR ranged between 0.5 and 3%/day for these tumors. An SGR of 1%/day corresponds to a DT of 70 days. With a constant SGR the tumor will grow exponentially over time:

$$V = V_0\, e^{\text{SGR}\cdot t}, \qquad (\text{Eq. } 20.13)$$

where V_0 is the initial volume of one tumor cell.

In the tumor growth model described above, the SGR determination assumes exponential growth. However, several preclinical studies have demonstrated retardation of growth rate over time, termed Gompertzian or power-exponential growth. In clinical studies, this has not been clearly observed, most probably due to the limited data available and therapeutic intervention. In order to determine a decline in tumor growth rate, more than two data points are needed, which seldom are available. Iwata et al. analyzed data from four time points prior to therapy in a patient with hepatocellular carcinoma (10). From this data set, they observed a decline in growth rate over time and adopted the Gompertzian growth rate model, which appears to be the most accurate model to describe growth rate decline. Inclusion of the SGR into the Gompertzian model will generate the following formula for growth rate over time:

$$\frac{dV}{dt} = \text{SGR}_i V\, e^{-bt}, \qquad (\text{Eq. } 20.14)$$

where SGR_i is the initial growth rate of first tumor cell and b is the growth rate decline parameter. Several physiologic and biologic factors will influence the value of b, but a comprehensive review is beyond the scope of this chapter. However, as a tumor enlarges, some of these factors could potentially include an increased interstitial fluid pressure within the tumor, aberrant tumor vasculature, abnormal extracellular matrix, and necrosis; all potentially resulting in decreased available nutrients and increased hypoxia. From preclinical and clinical studies, the range of realistic b values can be determined. For example, assuming an SGR of 1%/day for a 10-g tumor and an $\text{SGR}_i = 35\%$ at inception of the tumor (in vitro studies of human cell lines seldom exhibit a cell rate proliferation higher than 35% [DT = 2 days]), the parameter b will be less than 0.0147. Observe that when $b = 0$ the growth retardation model will mirror the exponential model. Therefore we can merge the two models into one dynamic model of tumor growth: the general Gompertzian model.

In Figure 20.5, the general Gompertzian model is applied in order to simulate tumor volume versus time for a tumor having a volume of 10 g at the detection time (d) and an SGR_d (specific growth rate at the time of detection) of 1%/day. To demonstrate the growth characteristics of the Gompertzian model, the initial specific growth rates, SGR_i, were set to 1, 3, 10, or 35%/day. First it can be observed that when SGR_i is equal to SGR_d (1%/day), the growth curve will result in a pure exponential growth. The inception of the initial tumor cell, following the exponential growth

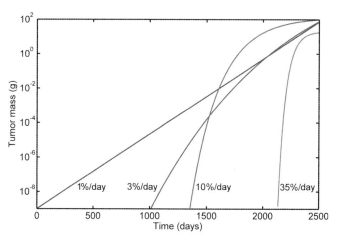

FIGURE 20.5 Simulation of the tumor growth with $\text{SGR}_d = 1\%$/day at the detection volume of 10 g. The growth curve for tumors with initial specific growth rates (SGR_i) of 1, 3, 10, and 35%/day, respectively, is demonstrated. With these initial specific growth rates, the inception times of the tumors will be 2313, 1265, 591, and 241 days before the detection of the 10-g tumor, respectively. Tumors having an initial specific growth rate of 35%/day will never reach the size of 100 g, following the Gompertzian growth model.

model, will be 2313 days before the detection day of the 10-g tumor; that is, the age of this 10-g tumor will be 6.3 years. If SGR_i was higher than 1%/day, the model will display the typical Gompertzian growth pattern and the inception time to the detection time will be decreased. For an SGR_i of 3, 10, or 35%/day, the inception time of the tumors will be 1265, 591, and 241 days before the detection time of the resulting 10-g tumor, respectively. If SGR_i is higher than 10%/day, the growth rate will decline to almost zero when the tumor has reached the size of 100 g; metastases with this type of growth characteristics will never become larger than 100 g. Tumors having initial SGRs of 35%/day will just be slightly larger than the detection size of 10 g.

In the current demonstration of dissemination modeling, we assume that the tumors follow Gompertzian growth with an SGR_i equal to 10%/day and that this tumor will have an SGR equal to 1%/day when reaching it reaches the size of 10 g. The growth characteristics of such a tumor are described by the 10%/day curve in Figure 20.5.

MODELS FOR METASTATIC FORMATION

Describing the progression of metastatic formation in patients is a process that involves many factors which are not easy to determine accurately. The equations derived for this complex system are not always possible to solve analytically. Therefore, limited models for metastatic formation have been created. Most developed models have been statistical or stochastic approaches for analyzing metastatic distributions. However, one dynamic model has been developed (10) where tumor growth, as the Gompertzian growth model, can be effectively incorporated. These authors tested the model on a patient with hepatocellular carcinoma and solved the equations analytically. This can be performed for such a case as hepatocellular carcinoma since it is reasonable to assume that the primary tumor and the metastases grow according to the same model. Typically, the metastases will remain confined to the liver for a significant period of time prior to dissemination. The resulting assumption, however, becomes more questionable when the tumors are systemically distributed and located in different host tissues; in this case, several different Gompertzian models may be needed that could make an analytical approach difficult. Therefore, we will use a simulation approach making the dynamic modeling more flexible.

The model of metastatic dissemination starts with the induction of the primary tumor. The primary tumor grows according to any growth description model; in our example, we use the Gompertzian model. The primary tumor will, at certain time points, exhibit the probability of producing new metastasis. The metastatic formation rate is described by

$$\frac{\mathrm{d}m}{\mathrm{d}t} = c \times V^f, \qquad \text{(Eq. 20.15)}$$

where c is the probability constant that a disseminated tumor cell will settle at a certain distance from the primary tumor and develop a metastatic lesion (Fig. 20.6). The value of c will range from 0 to a value that could result in death based on a large tumor burden. In the subsequent analyses, these values will be set to 1 kg, which might be a good approximation of a lethal tumor burden for most cancers.

The metastatic process will occur through hematogenous and/or lymphatic routes. The fractal dimension f can be assumed to correspond to the infiltration of vasculature and lymphatic channels (number of tumor cells that have access to possible routes of dispersion). When this value (f) is equal to 1, all cells in the tumor tissue are assumed to have the same probability of being capable of disseminating and forming new metastases. This physiologic condition would correspond to the tumor vasculature being uniformly distributed throughout the tumor. In the opposite direction, when f is equal to 0, this will reflect the clinical situation where only a single cell can potentially give rise to all metastases. A lower value for f may be relevant when considering cancer stem cell theory. Iwata et al. demonstrated that the fractal dimension f of blood vessels infiltrating the tumor (tumor vascularity tends to be superficial and lymphatic channels are lacking) was estimated to be close to 2/3, which can explain that the tumor cells closest to the tumor surface of the tumor have the highest probability of forming new metastases. Therefore, $f = 2/3$ will be used for dynamic modeling of metastatic formation and simulation of MCPs.

The newly created metastases will also be capable of forming new metastases with specific values of c and f. Of course, these values may differ depending on the tumor microenvironment and tissue location of the subsequent metastases. In this demonstration of the model, the values of c and f are equivalent to the primary tumor. In order to analyze the influence the metastatic formation rate (c) on the tumor distribution, it is assumed that all tumors grow with the same growth characteristic, that is, $SGR_i = 10\%/\text{day}$ and that a 10-g tumor has an $SGR_d = 1\%/\text{day}$. The simulation is performed by generating a random number at every time interval, which determines if a new metastatic lesion has been produced. This process is performed until a predetermined value of the size of the primary tumor, that is, 100 g in most of the simulations, has been achieved. Next, the simulation process is performed on all induced metastases. To obtain low uncertainties in the studies, more than 10,000 simulations should be performed. Depending on the complexity of the study, the simulations will take from seconds to hours on a standard computer.

Simulations of the influence of the metastatic formation rate constant (c) on the metastatic distribution are presented in Figure 20.7. Increasing the metastatic formation rate constant (0.01 to 10%/(day g)) will increase the frequency of metastases in the same order, but the shape of the curves

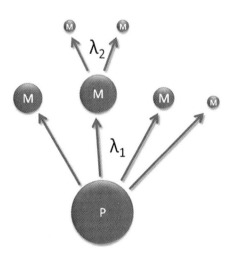

FIGURE 20.6 Illustration of the model of the metastatic process. P indicates the primary tumor that grows according to the Gompertzian model. From the primary tumor, metastases (M_i) are produced with a certain metastatic formation rate ($\lambda_1 = \mathrm{d}m/\mathrm{d}t$), growing at a certain distance from the primary tumor. The metastatic formation rate will depend on the size of the primary tumor. The created metastases can in turn produce new metastases with a new metastatic formation rate (λ_2) that will be specific for each metastasis.

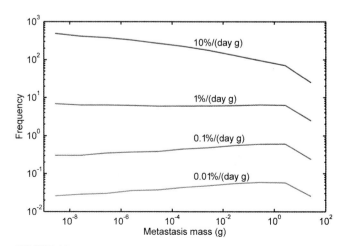

FIGURE 20.7 Simulation of metastatic distributions based on Gompertzian growth ($SGR_d = 1\%/\text{day}$, $SGR_i = 10\%/\text{day}$). The simulations are performed for four different metastatic rate constants, 0.01, 0.1, 1, and 10%/(day g).

will differ. For the lower c values, it is observed that the highest frequency of metastases occurs at 10 g. This is due to the lower probability of forming metastases and the induced metastases will grow according to the Gompertzian model; the growth is almost exponential in the beginning but slows during its progression. For $c = 1\%/(\text{day g})$, the frequency of metastases is almost equal for all metastatic volumes (mass) below 10 g. For the higher metastatic formation rate of $10\%/(\text{day g})$, the formation of new metastasis is so high that the highest frequency will result from the smallest volume of metastases. Such a high value of $10\%/(\text{day g})$ will give rise to a total tumor burden that most probably will be lethal for the patient (Table 20.2). With this value of c, multiple, grossly visible metastases will be observed. By defining the detection limit for tumors at 1 g, more than 100 metastases can be observed (Table 20.2). When c is less than $0.1\%/(\text{day g})$, the chance of detecting any metastasis is extremely low, and a cancer with a 100-g primary tumor might be considered to be free from metastases. Unfortunately, in this clinical scenario, there is still a high risk of undetectable metastases.

Simulation of MCP for different metastatic distributions

Even if the same growth characteristic was used in the previous section, the stochastic nature of the metastatic progression can be captured with the described simulation method. To determine the MCP, the activity concentration is adjusted so that the MCP is equal to 0.99. The absorbed dose required to sterilize the tumors will differ, depending on size or number of tumors. Therefore, the absorbed dose that will be generated in the largest tumor will be presented as the mean absorbed dose required for obtaining MCP = 0.99. Figure 20.8 presents the frequency distribution of the mean absorbed dose required to obtain MCP = 0.99 for ^{177}Lu, with an $SGR_d = 1\%/\text{day}$ (for a 10-g tumor) and an $SGR_i = 10\%/\text{day}$. In this case, the frequency distribution is almost a normal distribution and the highest required absorbed dose for a single simulation is 900 Gy and the lowest required absorbed dose is 600 Gy. The 90-percentile absorbed dose will be used to describe the mean absorbed dose required for cure; in this way, the MCP = 0.9 in a tumor population is obtained.

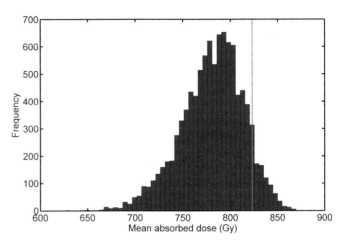

FIGURE 20.8 The ^{177}Lu mean absorbed dose distribution for MCP = 0.99 in a population of 10,000 individuals (10,000 simulations). The *vertical line* indicates the absorbed dose at the 90% percentile, which is the required absorbed (equivalent) dose for obtaining MCP equal to 0.9 ($MCP_{0.9}$).

Influence of metastatic formation rate on MCP

For cancers having the same general Gompertzian growth, the metastatic distribution will depend on the metastatic formation rate. In the previous section, the metastatic formation rate constant c was varied (0.01 to $10\%/(\text{day g})$) and this resulted in a powerful influence on the observed number of metastases (Table 20.2). If we now simulate the absorbed dose required for obtaining an MCP = 0.9 in a population using the four selected radionuclides (^{90}Y, ^{177}Lu, ^{131}I, and ^{211}At), it can be observed that the required absorbed dose will exhibit a large variance between the radionuclides and the different metastatic distributions (Table 20.3). The variation between the radionuclides is due to the different particle ranges of the radionuclides (Table 20.1). The long range of ^{90}Y will result in very low absorbed doses to micrometastases and consequently low TCP (Figs. 20.1 and 20.4). For obtaining a high TCP for micrometastases, the activity concentration needs to be increased considerably. The required absorbed dose to the primary tumor of 100 g will be as high as 28,000 Gy. Even when the metastatic formation rate constant is decreased to 0.01 and the tumor burden consists of very few micrometastases, a high absorbed dose is still required in order to obtain a cure (5200 Gy). This example demonstrates that a long-ranged particle emitter, such as ^{90}Y,

Table **20.2**	The simulated distributions of metastases for different metastatic formation rate constants (c)		
Metastatic Rate Constant (%/(day g))	**Detectable Metastases**	**Total Number of Metastases**	**Total Metastatic Mass (g)**
10	180	9000	1600
1	17	170	160
0.1	1.7	9.7	16
0.01	0.17	0.92	1.4

The number of detectable metastases is defined as all simulated metastasis over 1 g.

Table **20.3**	The mean equivalent doses required for different metastatic formation rate constants and different radionuclides; primary tumor mass equal to 100 g			
Metastatic Formation Rate (%/(day g))	**Mean Equivalent Dose (Gy)**			
	^{90}Y	**^{177}Lu**	**^{131}I**	**^{211}At**
10	28,000	1300	2800	660
1	17,000	820	1700	400
0.1	11,000	550	1100	260
0.01	5,200	290	550	100

is less suitable in adjuvant treatments, and perhaps also as a single radionuclide treatment of severe, widespread disseminated disease. However, the long particle range of ^{90}Y might be the best alternative when the activity distribution is nonuniformly distributed in larger tumors, and also when the TNC ratio is low; such as is the case with radioembolization of liver tumors. These two situations will be further discussed in the coming sections.

By choosing radionuclides with a short particle range, the required absorbed dose will be more appropriate and achievable. The lowest required absorbed dose (100 Gy) was obtained for ^{211}At, in the simulated adjuvant treatment setting. As previously mentioned, an equivalent dose was used for the simulations. Therefore, the physical mean absorbed dose will be less for ^{211}At, depending on the RBE. We choose not to set a weighting to the alpha particles since there is no consensus as to the actual RBE. Of note, an RBE of 5 has been proposed as an adequate value (6). Unfortunately, two physical factors might be a drawback for using ^{211}At for systemic therapy: the short physical half-life and the short range of the emitted particles. The physical half-life of ^{211}At is only 7.2 hours and will be a problem when using large macromolecules, such as antibodies, in systemic therapies; the slow kinetics of antibody penetration into tumors will result in nonspecific irradiation of normal tissue. This could be especially problematic regarding the radiosensitive BM. The other factor, the short range of the emitted alpha particle, will make it less suitable for heterogeneic activity distributions. The most extreme example of this might be in radioembolization of liver tumors where the distance between the loaded microspheres can be of the order of 1 mm. In such a situation, the maximal range of 93 μm will be useless in regard to obtaining a cure. The nonhomogenous distribution of antibodies can also be considerable in larger tumors making ^{211}At less suitable as monotherapy for treating bulky disease. It has been established that a fractional standard deviation of 20% (FSD = 0.2) will result in a 50% reduction of tumor cure with radionuclides (13), emphasizing the need to try and limit the influence of dose heterogeneity in TRT.

Both ^{177}Lu and ^{131}I might be more appropriate radionuclides for a single systemic treatment of metastatic disease, compared to ^{90}Y and ^{211}At. ^{131}I was introduced into the clinic more than 50 years ago for the treatment of thyroid cancers and benign disease (hyperthyroidism). In both situations very high activity concentrations can be obtained, resulting in successful outcomes. Due to the excellent clinical results, high availability, and relative low cost, ^{131}I is a very tempting radionuclide to embrace for use in TRT. However, the photon emission (p/e) is considerably high (Table 20.1). This will result in a more pronounced impact on the absorbed dose to normal tissues, as is the case with ^{131}I treatment of thyroid cancers (Fig. 20.2). The photons will be scattered throughout the body resulting in a uniform whole body dose. As a result, the radiosensitive BM will determine the maximum tolerated dose for the treatment. Recently, ^{177}Lu has become available as a therapeutic radionuclide. The physical properties of ^{177}Lu seem to be quite satisfying; it emits a lower level of photons (p/e = 0.24) that are useful for gamma camera measurements during therapy, but will result in a decreased total body exposure, compared to ^{131}I. ^{177}Lu emits electrons with a maximal range of 1.8 mm, making the required absorbed dose quite low for metastatic disease. The drawback for using ^{177}Lu seems to be the high accumulation in the kidneys. ^{177}Lu is attached to a targeting construct (e.g., peptide or antibody) by a chelate (DOTA), that is, as in the case with the ^{177}Lu-labeled somatostatin analogue, ^{177}Lu–DOTA–octreotate. This small molecular weight radiopeptide is processed through the kidneys by the mechanism of proximal tubular reabsorption that results in entrapment of ^{177}Lu in the renal interstitium (14). This entrapment can be reduced by infusing charged amino acids during treatment. The amino acids "block" the reabsorption of ^{177}Lu–DOTA–octreotate by approximately 50%. Regardless, the kidney is the major critical organ for radiopharmaceuticals of this size (conjugation to peptides; kidneys filtrate macromolecules ≤ 60 kDa) and therefore new treatment strategies for further reduction of the kidney uptake is warranted.

Influence of TNC on MCP

The previous section illustrated the influence of the metastatic rate constant on the simulated MCP for isolated tumors.

In these simulations with isolated tumors, it is understood that the surrounding normal tissue contains no activity. However, the realities of systemic therapy is that the activity will be distributed among the different tissues within the body and in this manner irradiate normal and target (tumor) tissue. Tumors infiltrate normal tissues and will therefore, more or less, receive cross-irradiation. The TNC for tissue where the tumors are embedded will determine the contribution of cross-irradiation. High TNC values tend to be in tissues such as bone and lymph nodes, whereas low TNC values are often observed in the liver. For ^{177}Lu–DOTA–octreotide, typical TNC values are 4 to 45 (15). For ^{90}Y-microspheres, delivery by the arterial system will dilute with venous blood in the normal liver and the TNC will be 4 to 6.

When performing the simulation for isolated tumors and with $c = 1\%$/(day g), the required equivalent doses were 17,000, 820, 1700, and 400 Gy for ^{90}Y, ^{177}Lu, ^{131}I, and ^{211}At, respectively (Table 20.3). When the tumors are embedded in normal tissue and exposed to cross-irradiation, the required absorbed dose will be decreased considerably (Fig. 20.9). With a TNC of 25 the required equivalent doses will be 870, 370, 490, and 250 Gy for ^{90}Y, ^{177}Lu, ^{131}I, and ^{211}At, respectively. Reasonable tumor doses might even be achieved for ^{90}Y when the TNC is further decreased; however, the normal tissue dose will of course be considerable. Having the TNC equal to 4, as is the fact with radioembolization, might result in the liver tissue being exposed to 100 Gy. The recommendation from the company that produces ^{90}Y resin microspheres is that the absorbed dose to the liver should be kept below 80 Gy. This value seems to

be high when compared with the dose limits derived from external beam radiation data. The higher tolerable liver dose with radioembolization might be due to the low dose rate situation (external beam radiation represents a high dose rate delivery) and the inhomogeneous distribution of microspheres. The possible sparing effect of inhomogeneous microsphere distribution must be compared with its distribution in the tumor tissue. Currently, clinical data on this subject is limited (see Chapters 23 and 24).

▇ Influence of treatment start time on MCP

An earlier treatment start time, when a more minimal disease state is present, should represent an advantage since the tumors will have less time to metastasize and grow. Additionally, large tumors (late treatment time) will have larger cell numbers (clonogens), poor perfusion, necrosis, and a heterogeneic targeting microenvironment. Table 20.4 shows the result of a simulation when the treatment starts at the size of either 100, 10, or 1 g of the primary tumor. In this simulation, it is seen that the required equivalent dose to the primary tumor will decrease from 370 to 230 Gy for ^{177}Lu, which must be regarded as a valuable decrease for the optimization of treatment protocols. Unfortunately, radionuclide therapy is not typically utilized as a first-line treatment. It is mostly administered to patients with advanced disease, those with a poor performance status, and as a second- or third-line therapy or greater. The one exception is the use of ibritumomab tiuxetan (Zevalin) as frontline consolidation for advanced follicular NHL (see Chapter 34). Since earlier treatment start times have a

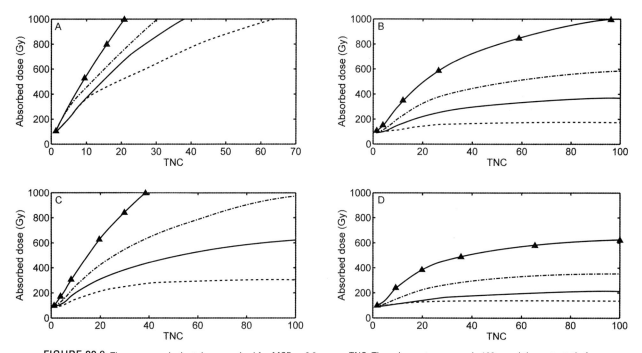

FIGURE 20.9 The mean equivalent dose required for MCP = 0.9 versus TNC. The primary tumor equals 100 g and the metastatic formation rate varies; 0.01 (*dashed lines*), 0.1 (*solid lines*), 1 (*dashed-dotted lines*), and 10%/(day g) (*triangles*). The results of the simulations are presented for the radionuclides: ^{90}Y (A), ^{177}Lu (B), ^{131}I (C), and ^{211}At (D).

Table **20.4**	The mean equivalent doses required for primary tumors with different sizes; TNC = 25, and c = 1%/(day g)			
	Mean Equivalent Dose (Gy)			
Primary Tumor (g)	**[90]Y**	**[177]Lu**	**[131]I**	**[211]At**
100	870	370	490	250
10	700	270	350	180
1	600	230	300	150

beneficial impact on a potential cure, it is hoped that TRT will be inserted earlier in the treatment schemata.

Influence of variable activity concentration and radiosensitivity on MCP

Gompertzian growth is characterized by an SGR that decreases with an increase in tumor size. This might be explained by a lower proportion of cells in a proliferative state as the tumor enlarges, perhaps due to a decrease in available nutrients. Regardless as a result the tumor may be less radiosensitive during progression. Furthermore, this reduced proliferation rate may also be caused by a decreased efficiency in the blood vessel system of large tumors, which will decrease oxygen support. Accordingly, the uptake of a radiopharmaceutical might be decreased due to this decreased perfusion. Recalling Equation 20.6, it can be seen that the same relative change in activity concentration (absorbed dose) and radiosensitivity will cause the same effect on TCP. A model (Norton–Simon hypothesis) (16,17) has been developed for the delivery of chemotherapy (18) during the more chemosensitive initial high proliferative state at the beginning of the Gompertzian growth curve (see Chapter 19). This model is similar to the Speer stochastic numerical model but the "assumption of uniform nascent growth is not supported" (17). However, the Norton–Simon hypothesis, and perhaps the Speer model, could be applied to TRT, where proliferating cells are more sensitive to radiation than dormant cells. This effect might be of the same magnitude as has been shown for increased activity concentration with a decreased tumor size (7,8).

Williams et al. developed a model that described uptake of radiopharmaceuticals as a function of time and demonstrated this validity in preclinical and clinical studies (19,20). In this model, it was assumed that the activity will follow an inverse power law function of tumor mass:

$$C_T(V) = C_T(V_0)V^{-d}, \qquad \text{(Eq. 20.16)}$$

where d is a fractal number of the activity distribution. It has been demonstrated that the network of blood vessels in tumors can be described by fractal geometries (21–24). The model developed by Williams et al. correlates the activity distribution to the fractal geometry of the blood vessels. In our previous work, we analyzed the impact of this phenomenon on the MCP. It was shown that even small values of the fractal dimension will have a great impact on MCP. A value of 0.1 and 0.2 will result in uptake, respectively, of approximately 10 and 100 times higher in the smallest tumors, compared to a primary tumor of 100 g. Simulations, using these values on the fractal parameter, will result in that the smallest tumors being less problematic, even when using [90]Y. As a result, very low equivalent doses would be required (Table 20.5). Further, the increased radiosensitivity of small tumors in accordance to the Gompertzian model dictum would predict for the increased possibility of sterilizing small tumors. However, since radionuclide therapy is a prolonged therapy over time (exponentially decreasing low dose, low dose rate), the more rapid proliferation of small tumors will potentially create an increasing number of new tumor cells (proliferation and repopulation) in comparison to larger tumors. This higher number of cells will require a higher equivalent dose for sterilization. For

Table **20.5**	The mean equivalent doses required for variable activity concentrations; TNC = 25, c = 1%/(day g), and primary tumor mass equal to 100 g			
	Mean Equivalent Dose (Gy)			
Fractal Dimension	**[90]Y**	**[177]Lu**	**[131]I**	**[211]At**
0	870	370	490	250
0.05	700	180	290	100
0.1	500	86	120	86
0.15	280	86	86	86

Table **20.6**	The mean equivalent doses required for different uniformity parameters; TNC = 25, c = 1%/(day g), primary tumor mass equal to 100 g, and d = 0			
	Mean Equivalent Dose (Gy)			
Uniformity Parameter	**[90]Y**	**[177]Lu**	**[131]I**	**[211]At**
0	870	370	490	250
0.25	870	450	540	430
0.5	870	530	590	710
1.0	870	700	700	1900

rapidly growing tumors with an SGR_i equal to 20%, a long physical half-life such as that for ^{177}Lu and ^{131}I may cause the required absorbed dose to be increased by 35%, but only 10% for [90]Y (7,8). The short half-life of [211]At will make it relatively ineffective for this proliferation effect.

A decreasing activity concentration relative to increasing tumor size might mean that the overall activity has decreased uniformly; however, it is more realistic that the decreased uptake (decreased activity concentration) will be the result of a more inhomogeneous distribution of the radiopharmaceutical. When the dose distribution inhomogeneity increases, it will negatively influence the MCP (25). Modeling of the absorbed dose distribution obtained for a given activity distribution is sparsely presented in the literature. Therefore, a very simplified version of the impact of dose distribution on the MCP will be performed. In this model, it is assumed that the activity concentration is distributed in such a way that the long-ranged radiation from ^{90}Y always will cause a uniform dose distribution:

$$D_{\text{eff}} \propto \left(\frac{R}{R^{90Y}} \right)^u, \qquad \text{(Eq. 20.17)}$$

where R is the range of the radionuclide in question (Table 20.1) and u is the relative uniformity parameter. With a value of zero for u, the dose distribution is uniform and no reduction in the effective dose (D_{eff}) will occur. An increased value of u will increase the dose distribution heterogeneity

(nonuniformity) so that the effective dose will decrease. This decrease is a function of the relative particle range. A better estimation might result from the use of point kernel data and a simulation of the situation of interest. However, this simplified model is adequate for addressing the important effect that the nonuniform activity concentration has on the MCP for the various radionuclides under investigation. Table 20.6 illustrates how an increase in nonuniform activity concentration will depend on the particle range. As can be seen, the efficacy of radionuclides with shorter path lengths is more significantly abrogated due to increasing dose nonuniformity (heterogeneity). Concerning ^{177}Lu and ^{131}I, there is a marked impact on the required equivalent dose. This effect, however, is much more pronounced for [211]At that appears to quickly become readily ineffective with increasing dose nonuniformity (large variations in activity concentration).

To overcome the problem created by nonuniform activity distributions in large tumors, external beam radiotherapy or radionuclides with long-ranged particle emissions might be useful to initially cytoreduce bulky tumors to a size that is more suitable for treatment with radionuclides that exhibit shorter path lengths, such as [177]Lu. Table 20.7 illustrates the result of such a simulation with u and d set to 0.5 and 0.1, respectively. The most optimal combination of radionuclides in this scenario seems to be a combination of ^{90}Y and [177]Lu. A low dose from [90]Y

Table **20.7**	Total mean equivalent doses for combination treatments with ^{90}Y; TNC = 25, c = 1%/(day g), primary tumor mass equal to 100 g, d = 0.1, and u = 0.5			
	Total Absorbed Dose (Gy)			
[90]Y Dose (Gy)	**[90]Y**	**[177]Lu**	**[131]I**	**[211]At**
0	500	200	200	680
10	500	160	210	480
20	500	170	220	330
40	500	190	240	280
80	500	345	290	340

would be used to cytoreduce the larger tumors and somewhat attenuate the negative impact of an initial nonuniform activity concentration. ^{177}Lu would then be administered for the remainder of the dose. As can be seen, the total mean absorbed dose that would be required for ^{90}Y or ^{177}Lu alone is lower than the necessary dose by using the paired radionuclide combination. This simulation indicates that it might be of value to combine multiple radionuclides and initiate clinical trials (26). However, an exact description and understanding of the influence that multiple radionuclide therapies will have on tumor growth, activity uptake, and its distribution in the tumor tissue is unknown. This, of course, makes a quantitative estimation of the impact of this therapeutic approach somewhat tenuous. Improved estimates of variables such as the fractal parameter d and the effective dose D_{eff} might be achieved by focusing on the modeling of the change in uptake of radionuclides during tumor growth and analyzing, for example, by autoradiography, the activity distributions in tumor tissues (27). The estimation of D_{eff} will be much improved by performing metastatic cure simulations of the dose distributions obtained from autoradiographs of human tumor tissue.

The MCP model applied to clinical data

Applying the MCP model to the evaluation of clinical trials might be a valuable tool for improving our understanding of the therapeutic effect of TRT. To date, the MCP model has been applied to (a) a theoretical comparative study of the potential of therapeutic radionuclides (7), (b) a preclinical study of ^{211}At radioimmunotherapy of ovarian cancer in nude mice (28), and (c) a hypothetical analysis of clinical data (8). The clinical data were obtained from a patient with hepatocellular carcinoma where four consecutive CT measurements of the primary tumor were performed (10). From this data set, the tumor growth was determined to follow Gompertzian growth; the SGR_d was approximately 0.55%/day for the largest measured tumor (25.4 g). From the Gompertzian model, it was determined that the "saturation size" of the tumors would be 73 g. In a series of three measurements or over time in a patient not receiving therapy, the number of metastases was 10, 28, and 48 tumors, respectively. This resulted in an estimation of a relatively rapid metastatic formation rate. The simulation of the required mean absorbed dose resulted in large values when the TNC values were greater than 10. However, if radioembolization with ^{90}Y-microspheres is applied, TNC values in the range of 2 to 10 are often obtained. For ^{90}Y, low TNC values are beneficial for sterilizing the small tumors. Table 20.8 shows the different TNC values and the required absorbed doses to the primary tumor (25.4 g) in order to obtain an MCP$_{90}$. TNC values, in radioembolization, of 8 or higher result in mean absorbed doses for sterilizing the tumor of greater than or equal to 340 Gy. With decreasing TNC, the required dose will be less; however, the mean absorbed dose to the liver will increase. In

Table **20.8**	The required mean absorbed dose to the tumor and the mean liver dose	
TNC	Tumor Dose (Gy)	Liver Dose (Gy)
2	110	55
4	200	50
6	270	45
8	340	42

radioembolization, these doses are achievable and the treatment is effective, but cure is seldom achieved. This effect might be explained by using doses that are too low due to the concern of inducing hepatic toxicity (radiation-induced liver disease). Other factors could include the possibility that the radiosensitivity is lower than the value of 0.35 used in the simulations, or that the microsphere distribution is inhomogeneous. In either scenario, it is important to have knowledge of the radiosensitivity as well as the perfusion distribution of the tumors. By using fractionated protocols it might be possible to select patients with a good response, caused by high radiosensitivity and/or well-perfused tumor tissue.

In this section it was possible to follow the tumor growth over four consecutive measurements. However, this is not possible in most clinical situations due to intervening therapy. In order to analyze the MCP for clinical data, we must utilize methods that process limited data in an optimal fashion. It has been shown that the growth rate can be determined by using the SGR method, where two data points are required before the initiation of treatment. If the SGR is obtained for multiple metastases in a patient, then correlating volumes and tumor sizes could be compared. If the SGR is decreasing as indicated by decreasing tumor size, growth deceleration is indicated (29). The SGR deceleration can also be studied in populations with similar cancers. From these population studies, it might be possible to determine the maximum tumor size of the cancer. This maximum size would indicate the tumor saturation level (Fig. 20.5). Accordingly, the parameters for Gompertzian growth could be determined. Continued investigations with the MCP model could be the analysis of clinical data and the subsequent evaluation of response rates of tumors to radionuclide therapy.

As a demonstration of how a TRT treatment will affect the metastatic distribution, an evaluation of tumor volume data from a patient with NHL was undertaken. The patient was a 58-year-old female, from Wisconsin, USA who was diagnosed with a stage-IV follicular NHL in February 2006. Interestingly, she presented with mostly osseous disease (CD20+ and BCL2+). She was initially treated with R-CHOP X 6. She experienced a 9-month remission. At the time of progression, she was treated with RICE X 2 in preparation for an autologous stem cell transplant. She underwent a stem cell harvest but was noted to again have disease

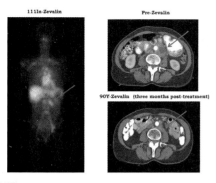

FIGURE 20.10 Patient treated with Zevalin (fourth-line therapy) for relapsed follicular non–Hodgkin lymphoma. The patient achieved a partial response of 10-month duration. Note the ^{111}In-Zevalin scan correlating to the pre-Zevalin CT scan.

Table 20.9	Tumor volumes estimated in the regrowth phase after treatment with ^{90}Y-Zevalin, and the corresponding SGR$_d$		
Tumor SGR$_d$	V_1	V_2	
1	1.08	10.6	0.77
2	2.01	10.7	0.56
3	0.22	0.94	0.48
4	2.25	129	1.36
5	34.2	257	0.68

progression after only experiencing a 2-month remission from the RICE chemotherapy. She was then treated with ifosamide, gemcitabine, vinorelbine, and prednisone X 2. She did not respond and was evaluated for treatment with Zevalin. She received 22 mCi (0.4 mCi/kg) of ^{90}Y-Zevalin and experienced a near-complete response as evaluated 3 months postinfusion (Fig. 20.10). Overall, she experienced a 10-month remission from therapy with Zevalin. At the time of progression, she was treated palliatively with two experimental drug regimens (on protocol) and then external beam radiotherapy, all of which resulted in no meaningful response. She eventually enrolled into hospice. Unfortunately, this case represents an all too common pattern in the treatment of follicular NHL. Patients are treated for a relapse with increasingly ineffective chemotherapy regimens before consideration is given to radioimmunotherapy (Zevalin or Bexxar). In this particular scenario, Zevalin was used as a fourth-line therapy and achieved a response that was equivalent to the initial R-CHOP regimen. This observation is particularly sanguine when one considers that it is well documented that sequential regimens for relapsed follicular NHL result in increased toxicity and shorter intervals of response (30). Realizing this, studies have been designed so that radioimmunotherapy for NHL is "moved" forward in the therapeutic schemata into a consolidative role. This, of course, translates into an earlier start time for the targeted radionuclide agent. In 2008, the "First-line Indolent Trial (FIT)" was published, and it documented a significant progression-free survival advantage for patients with stage III to IV low-grade NHL receiving Zevalin consolidation after induction with chemotherapy (31). The success of this trial has resulted in FDA approval for frontline therapy for Zevalin as well as an NCCN category I designation (see Chapter 34).

As noted earlier, the patient was treated with ^{90}Y-Zevalin and obtained an objective response to the treatment; however, the patient developed recurrent disease and the resulting metastatic rate was considerably high. In order to perform a simulated evaluation of the metastatic process, all visible sites of disease that were identified on a CT scan of the chest, abdomen, and pelvis were contoured using the radiation oncology treatment planning system, antibody-directed cellular cytotoxicity (ADCC) Pinnacle (Tod W. Speer, MD; University of Wisconsin School of Medicine, Department of Human Oncology). In this fashion, an attempt was made to establish an overall volume and a number of metastatic lesions over two separate observation points. These two points in time were at the partial response evaluation of Zevalin (3 months after treatment with Zevalin) until time of progression, 10 months later. Within these two points in time, representing 297 days, 6 observable metastases had become 80 metastases. The overall tumor burden had advanced from 58.7 g to 1458.4 g. With the obtained SGR values (Table 20.9), the Gompertzian model was applied with SGR$_i$ values ranging from the mean SGR$_d$ of 0.75%/day, that is, assuming exponential growth, to 5.5%/day. A value higher than 5.5%/day would result in a volume of disease greater than the largest tumor of 257 g, which was not identified in the patient (Fig. 20.5). Interestingly, the rapid appearance of metastases after the objective response could not be simulated with these parameters. However, the number of metastases and tumor volume does position reasonably well into Table 20.2, as long as a metastatic rate constant between 1 and 10%/(day g) can be assumed. The reason for this mathematical incongruence in a "treated" patient is most probably due to the fact that the ^{90}Y irradiation mainly cytoreduced the larger tumors, while the smaller metastases were less affected. This resulted in a "compression" of disease into a more limited range (Fig. 20.11). When recurring, the metastases presented as a more "massive attack" at a detectable level. Other potential problems with this model would include a disease process that is very resistant to therapy and harbors an elevated growth fraction due to multiple prior therapies (30). Also, during the contour phase, individual metastases were difficult to identify as lymph node regions tended to coalesce over time. This example, however, reveals the future direction of using MCP models for response evaluation of TRT.

■ Clinical correlation

Thus far, the presented data hve been derived meticulously on a microdosimetric scale. The following is an extrapolation

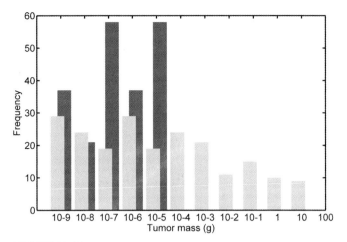

FIGURE 20.11 Simulation of the metastatic distribution before treatment *(gray bars)* and after treatment *(dark gray bars)* with ^{90}Y-Zevalin. The growth characteristics are based on the determination of SGR during the regrowth phase after treatment with ^{90}Y-Zevalin.

from known LQ models and clinical data (32). Fully human monoclonal antibodies (mAbs) are currently being designed for clinical use and fractionated treatments should be well tolerated (33). This can be contrasted to multiple administrations of murine or chimeric antibodies that typically result in high rates of seroconversion to human antiglobulin antibodies (HAGA) when used in TRT (34). Considering that radionuclides are more cytotoxic than common chemotherapy agents (35) and that response rates are significantly increased when anti-CD20 antibodies are radiolabeled (36,37), it should be compelling to initiate trials using TRT with fully human antibodies, such that fractionation schedules can be employed. Fractionation aside, the LQ formula can quantitate cell kill when using TRT. If a dose rate of 10 to 15 cGy/hr, an effective half-life of 4 days, half-time repair = 1.5 hours, $\alpha/\beta = 10$, and an absorbed tumor dose of 15 to 20 Gy are delivered by a single instillation, then a 2- to 3-log cell kill of malignant tissue should result. This scenario would sterilize 60% of clinically undetectable cell aggregates (10^3 cells), 30% of millimeter-size tumors (10^6 cells), or 20% of clinically apparent disease (10^9 cells) (38). Remarkably, responses of 60% to 80% are reported after single instillations of TRT when treating NHL. This most likely is due to the innate radiosensitivity of hematologic malignancies and due to the induced immune effector response (which typically is not present for solid tumors). If the current phase I and II trials using TRT as adjuvant therapy with chemotherapy for NHL are favorable, then the prototypical lymphoma model of TRT will be that of a single administration in the adjuvant setting. This is definitely a step in the right direction and certainly may be the maximum amount of radionuclide that can be tolerated in a combined modality setting by patients heavily pretreated with chemotherapy. Recognizing that tumor growth is governed by Gompertzian kinetics, multiple cycles of dose-dense chemotherapy are employed. Given subclinical tumor volumes of 10^3 to 10^5 cells, greater than or equal to 3 to 4 cycles of chemotherapy are prescribed to

exercise multilog cell kill. What, then, would be a reasonable fractionated schedule of TRT?

The current treatment regimens of TRT for NHL use single administrations resulting in dose rates of 1 to 10 cGy/hr and absorbed tumor doses in the range of 10 to 15 Gy (39). The typical administered activity ranges from 50 to 200 mCi for Bexxar and 20 to 30 mCi for Zevalin. This results in a total body (marrow) equivalent dose of 75 cGy and 47 to 69 cGy, respectively (40). Extrapolating from ^{131}I therapy for thyroid cancer, cumulative activities of greater than or equal to 1000 mCi may be given as long as dose-limiting BM is monitored and less than or equal to 3-Gy BM or less than or equal to 30-Gy lung is not reasonably breached (41). By all accounts, there does appear to be the potential for dose escalation and the safe delivery of multiple fractions of TRT. The time between fractions should be modeled after the effective half-life (interaction of the physical half-life of the radionuclide and the biologic clearance of the targeting construct). This is particularly sanguine when viewed in the context of our current ability to employ fully human antibodies, pretargeting, and BM support. Thus, it is not unreasonable to consider 3 to 6 cycles of "dose-dense" TRT, a treatment that could theoretically deliver greater than or equal to 60- to 100-Gy tumor dose and eradicate clinically detectable tumors (10^9 cells). The ability to deliver multiple fractions of TRT now exists with the advent of fully human mAbs. It is time to apply the principles of dose-dense chemotherapy delivery to TRT and investigate the feasibility and efficacy of multiple fractions (cycles) of these very promising agents. Whether considering radionuclides as an adjunct to delivery systems other than intact antibodies (42), the medical community must overcome current economic biases and work in unison (43). Continued computer analysis with the MCP remains front and center for the quest to cure metastatic epithelial carcinoma with a TRT approach.

■ REFERENCES

1. Uusijarvi H, Bernhardt P, Forssell-Aronsson E. Translation of dosimetric results of preclinical radionuclide therapy to clinical situations: influence of photon irradiation. *Cancer Biother Radiopharm.* 2007;22:268–274.
2. Goddu SM, Rao DV, Howell RW. Multicellular dosimetry for micrometastases: dependence of self-dose versus cross-dose to cell nuclei on type and energy of radiation and subcellular distribution of radionuclides. *J Nucl Med.* 1994;35:521–530.
3. Goddu SM, Howell RW, Rao DV. Cellular dosimetry: absorbed fractions for monoenergetic electron and alpha particle sources and S-values for radionuclides uniformly distributed in different cell compartments. *J Nucl Med.* 1993;35:303–316.
4. Bernhardt P, Benjegard SA, Kolby L, et al. Dosimetric comparison of radionuclides for therapy of somatostatin receptor-expressing tumors. *Int J Radiat Oncol Biol Phys.* 2001;51:514–524.
5. Bernhardt P, Forssell-Aronsson E, Jacobsson L, et al. Low-energy electron emitters for targeted radiotherapy of small tumours. *Acta Oncol.* 2001;40:602–608.
6. Sgouros G, Howell RW, Bolch WE, et al. MIRD commentary: proposed name for a dosimetric unit applicable to deterministic biological effects—the Barendsen (Bd). *J Nucl Med.* 2009;50:485–487.
7. Bernhardt P, Ahlman H, Forssell-Aronsson E, et al. Modelling of metastatic cure after radionuclide therapy: influence of tumor

distribution, cross-irradiation, and variable activity concentration. *Med Phys.* 2004;31:2628–2635.

8. Bernhardt P, Ahlman H, Forssell-Aronsson E, et al. Model of metastatic growth valuable for radionuclide therapy. *Med Phys.* 2003;30:3227–3232.

9. Bernhardt P, Forssell-Aronsson E. Estimation of metastatic cure after radionuclide therapy. *Q J Nucl Med Mol Imaging.* 2007;51:297–303.

10. Iwata K, Kawasaki K, Shigesada N. A dynamic model for the growth and size distribution of multiple metastatic tumors. *J Theor Biol.* 2000;203:177–186.

11. Mehrara E, Forssell-Aronsson E, Ahlman H, et al. Specific growth rate versus doubling time for quantitative characterization of tumor growth rate. *Cancer Res.* 2007;67:3970–3975.

12. Collins VP, Loeffler RK, Tivey H. Observations on growth rates of human tumors. *Am J Roentgenol Radium Ther Nucl Med.* 1956;76:988–1000.

13. O'Donoghue JA. Dosimetric principles of targeted radiotherapy. In: Abrams PG, Fritzberg AR, eds. *Radioimmunotherapy of Cancer.* New York, NY and Basel: Marcel Dekker, Inc.; 2000.

14. Bodei L, Cremonesi M, Ferrari M, et al. Long-term evaluation of renal toxicity after peptide receptor radionuclide therapy with 90Y-DOTA-TOC and 177Lu-DOTATATE: the role of associated risk factors. *Eur J Nucl Med Mol Imaging.* 2008;35:1847–1856.

15. Forrer F, Uusijarvi H, Waldherr C, et al. A comparison of ^{111}In-DOTA-TOC and ^{111}In-DOTATATE: biodistribution and dosimetry in the same patients with metastatic neuroendocrine tumors. *Eur J Nucl Med Mol Imaging.* 2004;31(9):1257–1262.

16. Norton L, Simon R, Brereton HD, et al. Predicting the time course of Gompertzian growth. *Nature.* 1976;264:542–545.

17. Norton L. A Gompertzian model of human breast cancer growth. *Cancer Res.* 1988;48:7067–7071.

18. Norton L. Evolving concepts in the systemic drug therapy of breast cancer. *Semin Oncol.* 1997;24(4 suppl 10):S10-3–S10-10.

19. Williams LE, Duda RB, Proffitt RT, et al. Tumor uptake as a function of tumor mass: a mathematic model. *J Nucl Med.* 1988;29:103–109.

20. Williams LE, Bares RB, Fass J, et al. Uptake of radiolabeled anti-CEA antibodies in human colorectal primary tumors as a function of tumor mass. *Eur J Nucl Med.* 1993;20:345–347.

21. Baish JW, Jain RK. Fractals and cancer. *Cancer Res.* 2000;60(14):3683–3688.

22. Baish JW, Jain RK. Cancer, angiogenesis and fractals. *Nat Med.* 1998;4(9):984.

23. Gazit Y, Baish JW, Safabakhsh N, et al. Fractal characteristics of tumor vascular architecture during tumor growth and regression. *Microcirculation.* 1997;4(4):395–402.

24. Jain RK. Normalizing tumor vasculature with anti-angiogenic therapy: a new paradigm for combination therapy. *Nat Med.* 2001;7:987–989.

25. O'Donoghue JA. Implications of nonuniform tumor doses for radioimmunotherapy. *J Nucl Med.* 1999;40:1337–1341.

26. Seregni E, Maccauro M, Coliva A, et al. Treatment with tandem [90Y]DOTA-TATE and [177Lu]DOTA-TATE of neuroendocrine tumors refractory to conventional therapy: preliminary results. *Q J Nucl Med Mol Imaging.* 2010;54:84–91.

27. Yokota T, Milenic DE, Whitlow M, et al. Microautoradiographic analysis of the normal organ distribution of radioiodinated single-chain Fv and other immunoglobulin forms. *Cancer Res.* 1993;53:3776–3783.

28. Elgquist J, Andersson H, Bernhardt P, et al. Administered activity and metastatic cure probability during radioimmunotherapy of ovarian cancer in nude mice with [211]At-MX35 F(ab')2. *Int J Radiat Oncol Biol Phys.* 2006;66(4):1228–1237.

29. Mehrara E, Forssell-Aronsson E, Ahlman H, et al. Quantitative analysis of tumor growth rate and changes in tumor marker level: specific growth rate versus doubling time. *Acta Oncol.* 2009;48:591–597.

30. Ansell SM, Schilder RJ, Pieslor PC, et al. Antilymphoma treatments given subsequent to Yttrium 90 Ibritumomab tiuxetan are feasible in patients with progressive non-Hodgkin's lymphoma: a review of the literature. *Clin Lymphoma.* 2004;5:202–204.

31. Morschhauser F, Radford J, Van Hoof A, et al. Phase III trial of consolidation therapy with Yttrium-90-ibritumomab tiuxetan compared with no additional therapy after first remission in advanced follicular lymphoma. *J Clin Oncol.* 2008;26:5156–5164.

32. Speer TW. Fully human monoclonal antibodies and targeted radionuclide therapy. *Blood.* 2009;112:2584–2585.

33. Hagenbeek A, Gadeberg O, Johnson P, et al. First clinical use of ofatumumab, a novel fully human anti-CD20 monoclonal antibody in relapsed or refractory follicular lymphoma: results of a phase 1/2 trial. *Blood.* 2008;111:5486–5495.

34. Wong JY. Basic immunology of antibody targeted radiotherapy. *Int J Radiat Oncol Biol Phys.* 2006;66:S8–S14.

35. Chen P, Mrkobrada M, Vallis KA, et al. Comparative antiproliferative effects of ^{111}In-DPTA-hEGF, chemotherapeutic agents and γ-radiation on EGFR-positive breast cancer cells. *Nucl Med Biol.* 2002;29:693–699.

36. Witzig TE, Gordon LI, Cabanillas F, et al. Randomized controlled trial of Yttrium-90-labeled ibritumomab tiuxetan radioimmunotherapy versus rituximab immunotherapy for patients with relapsed or refractory low-grade. Follicular or transformed B-cell non-Hodgkin's lymphoma. *J Clin Oncol.* 2002;20:2453–2463.

37. Davis TA, Kaminski MS, Leonard JP, et al. The radioisotope contributes significantly to the activity of radioimmunotherapy. *Clin Cancer Res.* 2004;10:7792–7798.

38. Fowler JF. Radiobiological aspects of low dose rates in radioimmunotherapy. *Int J Radiat Oncol Biol Phys.* 1990;18:1261–1269.

39. Macklis RM. Radioimmunotherapy as a therapeutic option for non-Hodgkin's lymphoma. *Semin Radiat Oncol.* 2007;17:176–183.

40. Wiseman GA, Kornmehl E, Leigh B, et al. Radiation dosimetry results and safety correlation from 90Y-ibritumomab tiuxetan radioimmunotherapy for relapsed or refractory non-Hodgkin's lymphoma: combined data from 4 clinical trials. *J Nucl Med.* 2003;44:465–474.

41. Dorn R, Kopp J, Vogt H, et al. Dosimetry-guided radioactive iodine treatment in patients with metastatic differentiated thyroid cancer: largest safe dose using a risk-adapted approach. *J Nucl Med.* 2003;44:451–456.

42. Speer TW. Proapoptotic receptor agonists, targeted radionuclide therapy, and the treatment of central nervous system malignancies: in regard to Fiveash et al. *Int J Radiat Oncol Biol Phys.* 2008;15:1273–1274.

43. Speer TW, Welsh JS. Will radioimmunotherapy survive? *Clin Adv Hematol Oncol.* 2008;6:233–237.

Unconjugated Therapy

131-I Ablation and Treatment of Well-Differentiated Thyroid Cancer

Kanchan Kulkarni, Douglas Van Nostrand, and Frank Atkins

■ INTRODUCTION

Thyroid cancer is one of the most commonly occurring cancers (1), and the National Cancer Institute estimates 37,200 new cases of thyroid cancer in the United States in 2009 (2). Well-differentiated thyroid cancer (WDTC), which includes papillary and follicular thyroid cancers, comprises the vast majority of thyroid cancers. Fortunately, WDTC cells are unique in their ability to concentrate iodine. As a result, for over 60 years, radioiodine has been an important part of the standard of care for the diagnosis and treatment of WDTC. Therefore, 131-I has been the primary radioisotope of choice for the ablation and treatment of WDTC (3,4). This chapter presents an overview of the use of 131-I in the ablation and treatment of WDTC, discussing the terminology, objectives, indications, side effects, and several guidelines for the selection of prescribed activity of radioiodine for ablation and treatment of WDTC.

■ TERMINOLOGY

▧ Ablation versus treatment

Although the terms "ablation" and "treatment" are frequently used interchangeably, some organizations believe it is useful to differentiate these terms based on objectives for the use of 131-I for therapy of WDTC. For example, the American Thyroid Association (ATA) guidelines state that the objective of ablation is "to eliminate the post surgical remnant in an effort to decrease the risk for loco-regional disease and to facilitate long term surveillance with whole body iodine scans and radioiodine and/or stimulated thyroglobulin measurements" (5). The European Consensus has defined ablation as "postsurgical administration of 131-I, whose aim is to destroy any thyroid tissue in the thyroid bed" (6). However, the use of the term "treatment" has been reserved for the administration of radioiodine for therapy of locoregional and/or distant metastases. For the purposes of this chapter, the terms "ablation" and "treatment" will be used as noted above.

▧ Dosage versus dose

The term "dose" is often used to refer to the quantity of activity of 131-I that is administered to a patient. Unfortunately, "dose" is also used to describe the amount of energy that is absorbed in the whole body, an organ, and/or a site of thyroid cancer from the radiation released during the radioactive decay of 131-I within the patient. To avoid this confusion in this chapter, we use the terms "dosage" and/or "prescribed activity" to refer to the quantity of 131-I administered to the patient and "dose" to refer to the amount of energy absorbed by the patient. Dosage or prescribed activity may be expressed either in the traditional units of *Curies* (Ci) or in the International System of Units (SI) as *Becquerels* (Bq). One Becquerel of any radioactive sample means that one of the atoms in the sample will disintegrate or decay per second, whereas one Curie represents 3.7×10^{10} disintegrations per second. "Dose" may also be expressed either in the traditional unit of absorbed dose, namely the *rad* (radiation *a*bsorbed *d*ose) or in the SI system as a *Gray* (Gy, where 1 gray is equal to 100 rad).

▧ Methods of selection of dosage of 131-I

The two principal methods used for selecting dosage of 131-I for either the ablation or treatments are "empiric" and "dosimetric," and an overview of these approaches is discussed in the following sections.

Empiric approach

The empiric method entails the administration of a fixed dosage of 131-I that has been recommended by various physicians and other medical organizations. Typically, an empiric regimen uses a standard fixed prescribed activity of 131-I, which may then be adjusted based on other factors such as (a) patient's height and weight, (b) the size of the primary tumor, (c) tumor histology, (d) age, (e) comorbid factors, (f) renal function, (g) convenience, (h) risk of potential side effects, and/or (i) institutional policies regarding hospitalization.

Selection of a dosage using an empiric approach has both advantages and disadvantages. The advantages include (a) ease of dosage selection, (b) a long history of use, and (c) well-documented information regarding the frequency and severity of side effects that have generally been considered acceptable. The disadvantage of empiric approach is that none of the empiric dosages is based on either one of the two fundamental principles of radiation therapy planning—namely, (a) determining and delivering radiation to the tumor for control while (b) determining and minimizing the radiation dose to the normal tissues.

Dosimetric approach

Dosimetry for the ablation or treatment of thyroid cancer patients has been used in the context of either (a) the calculation of maximum safe dosage that can be administered to a patient that would not exceed some limiting radiation absorbed dose to normal tissue and/or (b) the calculation of the radiation absorbed dose that would be delivered to thyroid tissue remnants and/or metastatic lesions. A few of the dosimetric approaches that have been used are outlined as follows.

Lesional dosimetry Lesional dosimetry for thyroid cancer refers to the calculation of the dosage of 131-I that will need to be administered to a specific patient to deliver a lethal or at least a "controlling" radiation dose to remnant thyroid tissue, recurrence, or metastases. Lesional dosimetry for thyroid cancer was first described by Maxon and colleagues (7,8), which was actually intended to establish the radiation absorbed dose that needed to be delivered to destroy lymph node metastasis. The advantages of the lesional dosimetry are (a) the potential of improving patient outcome by the selection and administration of dosages that have a greater chance of achieving a tumoricidal effect on the metastasis and (b) the identification of patients who will not benefit from 131-I ablation or treatment because a tumoricidal dose may not be delivered within constraints imposed on the maximum prescribed activity that can be administered to the patient. However, lesional dosimetry has significant disadvantages. The calculation of a tumoricidal dose to a lesion requires information such as the volume, the uptake, and the residence time of 131-I of each lesion, which can all be difficult to measure accurately. Additional disadvantages include increased cost, patient inconvenience because measurements must typically be made daily over a period of 5 to 7 days, and limited availability of this technique.

Whole body dosimetry Whole body dosimetry is used to calculate a safe prescribed activity that can be administered that will not exceed a generally accepted radiation absorbed dose to a critical organ, which for 131-I is typically the hematopoietic system. Several models have been proposed to calculate this activity and some of these approaches have been modified over time. One of the original approaches was first published in 1948 by Marinelli et al. (9) and was later refined by Lovinger in 1956 (10). Since then, the Medical Internal Radiation Dose (MIRD) Committee was established by the Society of Nuclear Medicine whose function was, and continues to be, to provide a more sophisticated alternate approach to calculating the radiation absorbed dose to various organs from internally deposited radionuclides (11). Based on this early formalism, whole body dosimetry was first described by Benua and colleagues (12,13), which calculated the maximum tolerated activity (MTA) that could be administered to a given patient without exceeding a maximum tolerable dose (MTD) of 200 rad to the patient's blood. Using MIRD calculations and selecting a somewhat higher limiting dose of 300 rad to the bone marrow, a prescribed activity as high as 1040 mCi (38.5 GBq) has been adminis-

tered (14). Whole body dosimetry likewise has several benefits and limitations. One major advantage is that the approach could identify those patients who would have received 200 rad or more to their blood, had the standard, empiric dosage been administered. This situation occurs in as many as 11% to 19% of patients (15,16). Conversely, the whole body dosimetric technique potentially allows the safe administration of a prescribed activity of 131-I larger than an empiric fixed prescribed activity for patients with metastatic disease, thereby delivering a higher radiation absorbed dose to their metastases. Furthermore, whole body dosimetry has a long history of use and safety—as long as and in many cases longer than the experience with the various empiric fixed dosages. However, whole body dosimetry is not without limitations. First, it does not calculate the radiation absorbed dose to the metastasis and therefore cannot be used to predict the tumoricidal effect of the calculated dosage. Consequently, even though the MTA may be administered, a therapeutic effect still may not be achieved. In addition, while whole body dosimetry calculates a safe dose to the blood as a surrogate for the bone marrow, it does not evaluate any other organs such as the salivary glands. However, research is under way to better assess and reduce the radiation absorbed dose to the salivary glands. Some other limitations of the whole body dosimetric approach include increased inconvenience to the patient, increased costs, and a lack of resources to support this technique at most facilities. Finally, outcome studies have not been performed to evaluate the various empiric fixed-dosage approaches or dosimetric approaches.

Percent 48-hour whole body retention As noted earlier, many facilities do not perform whole body dosimetry because it is a complex and time-consuming procedure (12,17). For this reason, some investigators have suggested alternative approaches aimed at simplifying the dosimetric procedure. For example, Thomas et al. (18) have proposed using sequential whole body external counting as a predictor of the blood concentration and clearance, thereby eliminating the need for blood samples. Sisson and Carey (19) proposed using only the measurement of the relative whole body retention of 131-I at a single time point, namely at 48 hours after administration of the diagnostic prescribed activity, to subsequently adjust the empiric prescribed activity of 131-I. Sisson (20) later proposed several criteria based on the fractional 48-hour retention as a guide for increasing and decreasing the empiric activity of 131-I. The following general, but still ill-defined, recommendations were made based on the percent retention at 48 hours: (a) if less than 9%, then increase the activity of 131-I; (b) if less than 5%, then increase the activity of 131-I by 50% to 100%; (c) if more than 24.8%, then decrease the activity of 131-I; and (d) if more than 40%, then substantially decrease the activity of 131-I. Only limited data are available about the use of this approach in the selection of a prescribed activity, and it is consequently not routinely used in clinical practice.

However, this concept was expanded by Van Nostrand and colleagues (21), in which the MTA as determined by whole body dosimetry was compared with the percent

48-hour whole body retention in a group of 142 patients. Based on this comparison, a biexponential regression model was determined and proposed as an easier, more quantitative single measurement to identify those patients whose empiric fixed dosages should be reduced or could be increased without exceeding 200 rad to the blood. Van Nostrand and colleagues (22) subsequently evaluated the application of this simplified dosimetry model and have demonstrated that it could be used as an alternative method of estimating the maximum activity for a patient's treatment for metastatic WDTC. The benefits of the percent 48-hour whole body retention include (a) no additional patient visits, (b) minimal expense, (c) could easily be performed in most nuclear medicine facilities, and (d) an approach that would identify those patients whose empiric fixed dosages should be reduced and those whose dosage could be increased.

ABLATION

Objectives of radioiodine ablation

The objectives of radioiodine ablation are variable and multiple. As already discussed earlier, the ATA guidelines state that the goal of ablation is "... to eliminate the post surgical remnant in an effort to decrease the risk for loco-regional disease and to facilitate long term surveillance with whole body iodine scans and radioiodine/or stimulated thyroglobulin measurements" (5). The objectives as defined in the European Consensus are as follows: " (1) 131-I treatment of residual postoperative microscopic tumor foci may decrease the recurrence rate and possibly mortality rate, (2) 131-I ablation of residual normal thyroid tissue facilitates the early detection of recurrence based on serum thyroglobulin measurement and eventually on 131-I whole body scan (WBS), and (3) a high activity of 131-I permits sensitive post-therapy WBS, 2–5 days post administration and may reveal previously undiagnosed tumors" (6).

Indications of radioiodine ablation

Several organizations and medical societies have proposed a list of indications for radioiodine ablation. The ATA recommendations are noted in Table 21.1 (5). These recommendations are based on the American Joint Commission of Cancer TNM staging (Table 21.2) (23), and their recommendations are graded based on available evidence (Table 21.3). The European Consensus recommendations are based on the risk of recurrence and cancer-specific mortality (Table 21.4) (6), and the British Thyroid Association recommendations were developed based on retrospective studies and recent consensus statements (Table 21.5) (24).

In summary, 131-I ablation is indicated in most patients except those who (a) are post–total thyroidectomy and younger than 45 years and (b) have tumor diameter less than 1 cm, no positive lymph nodes, no invasion beyond the capsule, no aggressive histology, and no metastases. In all other patients, 131-I ablation is almost universally recommended; however, multiple other factors such as patient's health status and iodine avidity should be considered. Pregnancy is an absolute contraindication for ablation, and breast-feeding must be discontinued. In addition, it is

Table 21.1	American Thyroid Association recommendations for indications of ablation	
Stage	**Patient and Tumor Characteristics**	**Recommendations**
Stage I	■ For patients <45 years old, any T, any N, M0 ■ For patients ≥45 years old, T1, any N0, M0	Ablation is recommended in selected patients who have stage I disease, especially who have multifocal disease, nodal metastases, extrathyroidal or vascular invasive, or more aggressive histology—*Recommendation B*
Stage II	■ For patients <45 years old, any T, any N, M1 ■ For patients ≥45 years old, T2, any N0, M0	Ablation is recommended for all patients who have stage II disease <45 years old and most patients ≥45 years old—*Recommendation B*
Stage III	■ For patients ≥45 years old, T3: any N0, M0; T1: N1a, M0; T2: N1a, M0; T3: N1a, M0	Ablation is recommended for all patients—*Recommendation B*
Stage IV	■ For patients ≥45 years old, T4a: any N0, M0; T4a: N1a, M0; T1: N1b, M0; T3: N1b, M0; T2: N1b, M0; T4a: N1b, M0; T4b: any N, M0; Any T: any N, M1	Ablation is recommended for all patients—*Recommendation B*

Data from Cooper DS, Doherty GM, Haugen BR, et al. Management guidelines for patients with thyroid nodules and differentiated thyroid cancer. *Thyroid.* 2006;16(2):109–142.

Table **21.2**		**TNM classification of differentiated thyroid cancer**	
Tumor size	■ Tx	Primary tumor cannot be assessed but without extrathyroidal invasion	
	■ T0	No evidence of primary tumor	
	■ T1	Tumor 2 cm or less in greatest dimension limited to the thyroid	
	■ T2	Tumor >2 cm but <4 cm in greatest dimension and limited to the thyroid	
	■ T3	Tumor 4 cm in greatest dimension or tumor of any size extending to tissue around the thyroid	
	■ T4a	Tumor of any size extending beyond the thyroid capsule and invading local soft tissues, larynx, trachea, esophagus, or recurrent laryngeal nerve	
	■ T4b	Tumor invading prevertebral fascia or encases carotid artery or mediastinal vessels	
Nodes	■ Nx	Regional nodes not assessed by surgery	
	■ N0	No metastases to regional nodes	
	■ N1	Metastases to regional nodes are present	
	■ N1a	Metastases to level VI nodes	
	■ N1b	Metastases to unilateral, bilateral, contralateral cervical, or superior mediastinal node metastases	
Metastases	■ MX	Presence of distant metastases cannot be assessed	
	■ M0	No distant metastases	
	■ M1	Distant metastases are present	

Stage	**Younger Than 45 Years**	**45 Years or Older**
Stage I	Any T, any N, M0	T1, N0, M0
Stage II	Any T, any N, M1	T2, N0, M0
Stage III	Not applicable	T3, N0, M0, or any T, N1A, M0
Stage IV A	Not applicable	T4a, N0, M0 T4a, N1a, M0 T1, N1b, M0 T2, N1b, M0 T3, N1b, M0 T4a, N1b, M0
Stage IV B	Not applicable	T4b, any N, M0
Stage IV C	Not applicable	Any T, any N, M1

Data from Greene F, Page D, Fleming I, et al. *AJCC Cancer Staging Manual.* 6th ed. 2002. http://www.amazon.com/AJCC-Cancer-Staging-Manual-6th/dp/0387952713

our recommendation that any patient who has recently stopped breast-feeding should be imaged with 123-I to assess uptake in the breast prior to ablation. With significant uptake of 123-I in the breast, the breast may receive a significant radiation absorbed dose from the 131-I for ablation.

Selection of dosage

Empiric dosage recommendations range from 30 to 200 mCi (1.1 to 7.4 GBq) of 131-I for ablation, which is summarized in Table 21.6 for the ATA, European Consensus, and British Thyroid Association (5,6,24). In general, an empiric regimen is used for ablation of residual thyroid tissue. Dosimetry is generally reserved for patients with locoregional and/or distant metastatic thyroid cancers and is discussed in detail later in this chapter.

■ TREATMENT OF METASTATIC WDTC

Objectives of radioiodine treatment

The objectives of 131-I treatment in WDTC can be (a) curative, (b) adjuvant, or (c) palliative purposes. For palliative therapy, the objective is typically to reduce pain and/or increase function for the patient. For adjuvant therapy combined with other interventions such as surgery, the objectives are to reduce the likelihood of recurrence and increase survival.

Indications for radioiodine treatment

The ATA, European, and British Consensus guidelines for the indications of 131-I treatment are summarized in Table 21.7 (5,6,24). In brief, indications for 131-I treatment

Table **21.3**	American Thyroid Association (ATA): definitions of recommendations
Recommendation A	**Strongly recommends.** Based on good evidence that the service or intervention can improve important health outcomes. Evidence includes consistent results from well-designed, well-conducted studies in representative populations that directly assess effects on health outcomes.
Recommendation B	**Recommends.** Based on fair evidence that the service or intervention can improve important health outcomes. The evidence is sufficient to determine effects on health outcomes, but the strength of evidence is limited by number, quality, or consistency of individual studies; generalizability to routine practice; or indirect nature of evidence based on health outcomes.
Recommendation C	**Recommends.** Based on expert opinion.
Recommendation D	**Recommends against.** Based on expert opinion.
Recommendation E	**Recommends against.** Based on fair evidence that the service or intervention does not improve important health outcomes or that harms outweigh benefits.
Recommendation F	**Strongly recommends against.** Based on good evidence that the service or intervention does not improve important health outcomes or that harms outweigh benefits.
Recommendation I	**Recommends neither for nor against.** The evidence is insufficient for or against providing the service or intervention because evidence is lacking that the service or intervention improves health outcomes, the evidence is poor quality, or the evidence is conflicting. As a result, balance of benefits or harms cannot be determined.

Data from Cooper DS, Doherty GM, Haugen BR, et al. Management guidelines for patients with thyroid nodules and differentiated thyroid cancer. *Thyroid.* 2006;16:109–142.

include locoregional metastases, as well as pulmonary metastasis with the potential of being curative in patients with iodine-avid diffuse pulmonary metastases and negative radiographs (i.e., x-ray and computed tomography [CT]) (25). 131-I treatment may be used as an adjuvant therapy when combined with other treatments such as surgery, radiofrequency ablation, and/or external beam radiotherapy (EBRT). In the case of brain metastases, 131-I treatment should only be considered after other options such as surgery, EBRT, or stereotactic radiosurgery have been

Table **21.4**	European Consensus (EC) recommendations for indications of ablation	
Patient and Tumor Characteristics		**Recommendations**
■ Complete surgery;		No indication for ablation
■ Favorable histology;		
■ Unifocal, T ≤1 cm, N0, M0; and		
■ No extra thyroid extension		
■ Distant metastases or		Definite indication
■ Incomplete tumor resection, and/or		
■ Complete tumor resection but high risk for recurrence or mortality: tumor extension beyond thyroid capsule (T3 or T4) or lymph node involvement		
■ Less than total thyroidectomy or		Probable indication
■ No lymph node dissection or		
■ Age <18 years or		
■ T1 >1 cm and T2, N0, M0, and/or		
■ Unfavorable histology		

Data from Pacini F, Schlumberger M, Dralle H, et al. European Thyroid Cancer Taskforce. European Consensus for the management of patients with differentiated thyroid carcinoma of the follicular epithelium. *Eur J Endocrinol.* 2006;154(6):787–803.

Table **21.5**	British Consensus (BC) recommendations for indications of ablation

Patient and Tumor Characteristics	Recommendations
Patients should satisfy all the criteria for 131-I ablation to be omitted:	
■ Complete surgery	No indication for ablation
■ Favorable histology	
■ Tumor unifocal ≦1 cm in diameter, N0, M0, or minimally invasive FTCs, without vascular invasion <2 cm in diameter	
■ No extension beyond the thyroid capsule	
■ Distant metastasis	Definite indication
■ Incomplete tumor resection	
■ Complete tumor resection but high risk of recurrence or mortality (tumor extension beyond thyroid capsule or more than 10 involved lymph nodes and more than 3 lymph nodes with extracapsular spread)	
■ Less than total thyroidectomy (inferred from operation nodes or pathology reports, or when ultrasound or isotope scan shows significant postoperative thyroid remnant)	Probable indication
■ Status of lymph node not assessed by surgery	
■ Tumor size >1 cm and <4 cm in diameter	
■ Tumors <1 cm in diameter with unfavorable histology	
■ Multifocal tumors <1 cm	

FTC, follicular thyroid cancer.
Data from Perros P, Clarke SEM, Franklin J, et al. *Guidelines for the Management of Thyroid Cancer. British Thyroid Association, Royal College of Physicians of London.* Suffolk, England: Lavenham Press; 2007:18.

excluded. Again, more detail is available within the designated tables.

Selection of dosage

The optimal treatment dosage for patients with metastatic WDTC is even more controversial, especially with the lack of adequate studies evaluating the outcomes of the many different empiric fixed-dosage or dosimetric approaches.

The ATA guidelines and the European and British Consensus guidelines for selection of prescribed activity are summarized in Table 21.8. Empirically prescribed activities for metastatic thyroid cancer are typically in the range of 150 to 300 mCi (5.5 to 11.1 GBq). Beierwaltes (26) proposed dosages in the range of 150 mCi (5.55 GBq) to 175 mCi (6.48 GBq) for cervical lymph node metastases, 175 mCi (6.48 GBq) to 200 mCi (7.4 GBq) for pulmonary metastases, and 200 mCi (7.4 GBq) for bone metastases. However, there are many

Table **21.6**	American Thyroid Association (ATA), European, and British Consensus recommendations for selection of dosage of 131-I for ablation

Association	Recommendations
ATA	■ "The minimum activity of 30–100 mCi (1.1–3.7 GBq) necessary to achieve successful remnant ablation should be chosen, particularly for low-risk patients." —*Recommendation B* ■ "If residual microscopic disease is suspected or documented, or if there is a more aggressive tumor histology (e.g. tall cell, insular, columnar cell carcinoma), then higher activities, 100–200 mCi (3.7–7.4 GBq) may be appropriate." —*Recommendation C*
European Consensus	■ "Definite indication of ablation: High activity ≧100 mCi (3.7 GBq) after thyroid hormone withdrawal." ■ "Probable Indication: High or low activity: 100 or 30 mCi (3.7 or 1.1 GBq)"
British Consensus	■ The current recommendation for remnant ablation is 100 mCi (3.7 GBq)

Table 21.7   ATA, European, and British Consensus guidelines for indications for 131-I treatment of locoregional and distant metastases

ATA	European Consensus	British Consensus
Regional nodes		
"For regional nodal metastases discovered on DxWBS, radioiodine is usually used, although surgery is typically used in the presence of bulky disease or disease amenable to surgery found on anatomic imaging such as ultrasound, CT scanning, or MRI. Radioiodine is also used adjunctively after surgery for regional nodal disease or aerodigestive invasion if residual disease is present or suspected." —*Recommendation I*	■ "Treatment is based on the combination of surgery and 131-I, in those with 131-I uptake. ■ When complete surgical excision is not possible, external beam radiotherapy (EBRT) may be indicated if there is no significant 131-I uptake within the tumor."	■ "Surgical re-exploration is the preferred method of management, usually followed by 131-I therapy."
Pulmonary metastases		
■ "Pulmonary micrometastasis should be treated with radioiodine therapy, repeated every 6–12 months as long as the disease continues to respond . . ."—*Recommendation A* ■ "Radioiodine-avid macronodular metastases should be treated with radioiodine, and treatment repeated when objective benefit is demonstrated (decrease in the size of the lesions, decreasing thyroglobulin) but complete remission is not common and survival remains poor."—*Recommendation B*	■ "In the case of 131-I uptake, treatment consists of 131-I administration following prolonged withdrawal."	■ "These sites of metastases are usually not amenable to surgery should be treated with 131-I therapy." ■ "In tumors with radioiodine uptake, the preferred treatment is repeated doses of radioiodine."
Bone metastases		
■ "Complete surgical resection of isolated symptomatic metastases has been associated with improved survival and should be considered, especially in patients less than 45 years old" and "Radioiodine therapy of iodine-avid bone metastases has been associated with improved survival and should be used."—*Recommendation B*	"Bone metastases should be treated by a combination of surgery whenever possible, 131-I treatment if uptake is present in the metastases, and external beam radiotherapy either as resolute treatment or as pain control . . ."	■ "Extensive bony metastases are generally not curable by 131-I therapy alone. For solitary or limited number of bony metastases that are not cured by 131-I therapy, EBRT with/without resection and/or embolization should be considered in selected cases."
Central nervous system (CNS) metastases		
"Complete surgical resection of central nervous system metastases should be considered regardless of radioiodine avidity, as it is associated with significantly longer survival."—*Recommendation B.* ■ "CNS lesions that are not amenable to surgery should be considered for external beam irradiation. Often, targeted approaches (such as radiosurgery) are employed to limit the radiation exposure of the surrounding brain tissue . . ."—*Recommendation C* "If CNS metastases do concentrate radioiodine, then radioiodine could be considered. If radioiodine is being considered, prior external beam radiotherapy and concomitant glucocorticoid therapy are strongly recommended to minimize the effects of a potential TSH-induced increase in tumor size and the subsequent inflammatory effects of the radioiodine."—*Recommendation C*	■ "Whenever possible they should be resected; if not resectable and non-iodine-avid, external beam radiation may provide palliation. Usually they carry a poor prognosis."	■ "EBRT has an important palliative role in management along with surgery if possible."

DxWBS, diagnostic whole body scan.

Table **21.8**	American Thyroid Association (ATA), European, and British Consensus recommendations for selection of dosage of 131-I for treatment of metastatic disease
Pulmonary	
ATA	"The selection of radioiodine activity to administer for pulmonary micrometastases can be made empirically [100–300 mCi (3.7–11.1 GBq)] or estimated by dosimetry to limit whole body retention to 80 mCi (2.96 GBq) at 48 hours and 200 cGy (rad) to the red bone marrow."—*Recommendation B*
European Consensus	"An activity ranging between 100 and 200 mCi (3.7 and 7.4 GBq) [or higher] is administered every 4–8 months during the first 2 years and thereafter at longer intervals . . ." "There is no maximum limit for the cumulative 131-I activity that can be given to patients with persistent disease."
British Consensus	"131-I activities ranging from 100–275 mCi (3.7–10.1 GBq) at 3–9 month intervals have been employed, the usual being 150 mCi (5.5 GBq) given every 4–6 months until 131-I uptake is no longer evident." "There is no maximum limit to the cumulative 131-I dose that can be given to patients with persistent disease."
Bone	
ATA	"The radioiodine activity administered can be given empirically [150–300 mCi (5.5–11.1 GBq) or estimated by dosimetry."—*Recommendation B*
European Consensus	No recommendations given
British Consensus	No recommendations given
Brain	
No specific recommendations given	

other empiric fixed-dosage approaches (Fig. 21.1). Schlumberger et al. (27) use an initial dose of 100 mCi (3.7 GBq) to treat lung and bone metastases, which may be repeated every 3 to 6 months. Menzel et al. (28) adopted a more aggressive approach of using 300 mCi (11.1 GBq) of empiric fixed dosage at short intervals of 3 months with a maximum administered activity of 1200 mCi (44.4 GBq) during 1 year.

Although an empiric dosage is a convenient approach, a significant number of patients may be "undertreated" or "overtreated" depending on the activity selected (15,16). In this context, "over" and "under" treatment refers to whether a given empiric dosage of 131-I would have potentially delivered more than or less than the MTD of 200 rad (cGy) to the blood as determined by the Benua and Leeper approach (12,13).

Dosimetrically determined dosages have been reported to range from 50 mCi or less to over 1000 mCi (1.85 to 37 GBq) (14,16). The actual prescribed activity is often less than the maximal dosimetrically determined activity. Additional guidance regarding the whole body retention at 48 hours is that (a) it should not exceed 120 mCi (4.44 GBq) if no pulmonary metastases are present and (b) it should not exceed 80 mCi (2.96 GBq) if diffuse pulmonary metastases are present. The treatment dosage determined by dosimetry

may be modified based on other considerations including tumor histology, burden of metastatic disease, radioiodine avidity, patient's health status, pulmonary function tests, total cumulative 131-I activity, absolute neutrophil count, absolute platelet count, side effects from previous treatments, and radiation safety considerations and restrictions.

Until data become available that demonstrate whether empiric dosages or dosimetrically determined dosages are superior for the treatment of locoregional and/or distant metastases or for that matter whether one empiric, fixed-dosage regimen is better than another, we believe that the rational choice for selecting a dosage of 131-I for treatment is to adopt an approach that is based on at least one of the two fundamentals of radiation therapy planning, namely assessing and limiting radiation absorbed dose to normal tissue.

Success of treatment

Discussing the success of 131-I therapy is complicated for many multiple reasons: numerous prognostic factors, variability in the objectives of therapy, and lack of controlled studies. Several retrospective studies (27,29–32) assessing the outcome of patients with distant metastases are available with variable amounts and frequency of iodine used

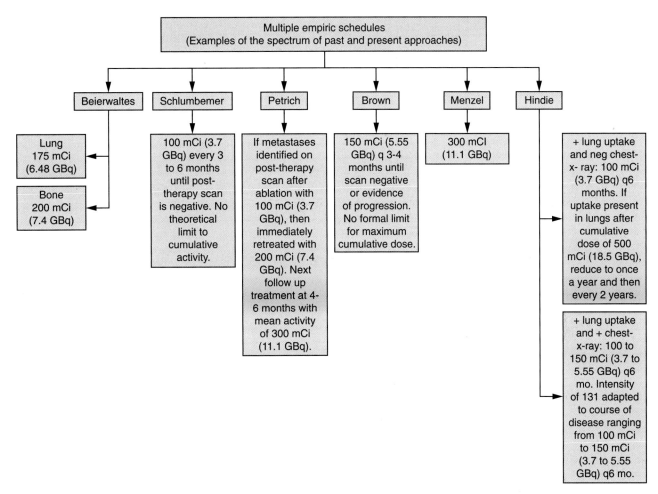

FIGURE 21.1 Emperic dose schedules for matastatic WDTC. Redrawn with permission from Wartofsky L, Van Nostrand D, eds. *Thyroid Cancer: A Comprehensive Guide to Clinical Management.* 2nd ed. Totowa, NJ: Humana Press; 2006:419.

for treatment, variability in patient population, metastatic sites, and lengths of follow-up.

Pulmonary metastases

Numerous factors including patient's age (33,34), radioiodine avidity (35,36), pattern on CT (37,38), and uptake on fluorodeoxyglucose positron emission tomography scans (39,40) have all been shown to influence the prognosis in patients with pulmonary metastases from WDTC (41,42). The data on some reported patterns of metastatic disease and response to 131-I treatment in some of the representative publications are presented (Table 21.9).

Bone metastases

The overall prognosis of patients with bone metastases is poor. Some factors reported to influence outcome in these patients are age, time of diagnosis, and radioiodine avidity (33,34,41,43–46). The outcome of these patients reported by some investigators is presented (Table 21.10).

Miscellaneous

Other metastases such as renal, muscle, mediastinum, brain, liver, kidney, skin, and pancreas are less common. No exten-

sive data are available on the success of radioiodine treatments in these patients.

■ SIDE EFFECTS

Patients often experience early- and/or late-onset side effects from the radioiodine ablation or treatment, which are summarized in Table 21.11. It is not our intent to do an exhaustive review of side effects when excellent reports are available by multiple authors (7,42,48–61). However, we would like to focus on just one potential side effect, namely the risk and incidence of second primary malignancies (SPMs) as a consequence of radioiodine treatment.

SPMs within the digestive tract, bladder, breast, bone and soft tissues, and hematologic malignancies are reported to occur more frequently in patients receiving 131-I than in patients not receiving 131-I (62–67). Data from some large studies are summarized in Table 21.12. In our opinion, the risk of SPM is overall low. The risk may be influenced by multiple factors such as patients' inherent risk, the cumulative administered activity, and frequency of administration of 131-I.

Table **21.9**   **Patient outcome in pulmonary metastases from WDTC**

Pattern of Disease	Investigator	Number of Patients	10-Year Survival	Complete Remission
Normal chest x-ray, positive 131-I scan	Casara et al. (41)	42	96%	78%
	Hindie et al. (42)	11	90%	73%
Abnormal chest x-ray, positive 131-I scan	Casara et al. (41)	54	36%	3.7%
	Hindie et al. (42)	9	78%	22%
Abnormal chest x-ray, negative 131-I scan	Casara et al. (41)	38	11%	None
		9 (negative 131-I scan)	0%	
Micronodular pattern	Massin et al. (37)	11	77% at 8 years	9/11 patients
	Nemec et al. (38) (fine pattern)	25	59%	
Macronodular pattern	Massin et al. (37)	13		3/13 patients
	Nemec et al. (38) (coarse pattern)	33	14%	

WDTC, well-differentiated thyroid cancer.

Table **21.10**   **Patient outcome in bone metastases from WDTC**

Author	Number of Patients	5-Year Survival (%)	10-Year Survival (%)	Complete Remission (%)
Brown et al. (44)	21	7	0	0
Schlumberger et al. (27)	108		21	10
Bernier et al. (47)	109	15		
Pittas et al. (45)	146	25	13	
Zettinig et al. (46)	41	59	39	

WDTC, well-differentiated thyroid cancer.

Table **21.11**   **Side effects of 131-I**

A. Early side effects

1. Ageusia

2. Abnormalities in smell

3. Nausea

4. Acute sialoadenitis

5. Epistaxis

6. Thyroiditis

7. Cystitis

8. Gastritis

9. Bleeding or edema in metastatic deposits

10. Acute pneumonitis

11. Transient ovarian or testicular failure

12. Transient effects such as hair loss

13. Fatigue due to hypothyroidism

B. Late side effects

1. Chronic sialoadenitis and resultant xerostomia or salivary duct obstruction

2. Chronic or recurrent conjunctivitis

Table **21.11**	Side effects of 131-I *(Continued)*
3. Lacrimal gland inflammation and resultant xerophthalmia	
4. Epistaxis	
5. Nasolacrimal duct obstruction	
6. Radiation fibrosis	
7. Hematologic toxicity and bone marrow depression	
8. Second primary malignancies (SPMs)	

Table **21.12**	Risk of second primary malignancies following RAI
Author	**Findings**
Sawka et al. (62)	■ Data from 16,502 individuals: 8473 received RAI
	■ The relative risk (RR) of SPMs in thyroid cancer survivors treated with RAI showed a slight but statistically significant increase at 1.19 (95% confidence interval [CI] 1.04, 1.36, $p = 0.010$), relative to thyroid cancer survivors not treated with RAI using a minimum latency period of 2–3 years after thyroid cancer diagnosis
	■ The RR of leukemia was small but statistically significant in thyroid cancer survivors treated with RAI, with an RR of 2.5 (95% CI 1.13, 5.53, $p = 0.024$)
	■ Did not observe a significantly increased risk of the following cancers related to prior RAI treatment: bladder, breast, central nervous system, colon and rectum, digestive tract, stomach, pancreas, kidney (and renal pelvis), lung, or melanoma of skin
Rubino et al. (63)	■ European cohort: 6841 patients
	■ Overall significantly increased risk of 27% (95% CI: 15–40)
	■ An increased risk of both solid tumors and leukemia with increasing cumulative activity, with an excess absolute risk of 14.4 solid cancers and 0.8 leukemias per Becquerel of 131-I
	■ Positive relationship between 131-I administration and occurrence of bone and soft tissue, colorectal, and salivary gland cancers
Brown et al. (64)	■ 30,278 patients
	■ 2158 patients who developed a total of 2338 nonthyroid malignancies
	■ The overall risk of second primary malignancies is slightly increased for thyroid cancer survivors over that of the general U.S. population
Bhattacharyya and Chien (65)	■ 18,882 cases of DTC treated without RAI and 10,349 cases treated with RAI were identified
	■ 6.7% of patients without RAI vs. 4.8% with RAI developed SPM
	■ Breast or prostate followed by colon or lung cancers were most common sites for both groups
	■ Use of RAI does not elevate the risk of SPM
Verkooijen et al. (66)	■ 282 patients
	■ The standardized incidence rate (SIR) for all cancers after the diagnosis of DTC in this study population was not increased (1.13; CI: 0.68–1.69). However, they found an increased SIR of 2.26 (CI: 1.60–3.03) for all cancers either following or preceding DTC, which is mainly caused by an SIR of 3.95 (CI: 2.06–6.45) for breast cancer
	■ Patients with DTC have an overall increased SIR for SPM but not for second primary tumors following I-131 therapy. These findings suggest a common etiologic and/or genetic mechanism instead of a causal relation
Subramanian et al. (67)	■ 70,844 thyroid cancer survivors from 13 full text papers
	■ The incidence of SPMs in thyroid cancer survivors was increased with an SIR of 1.20 (95% CI: 1.17, 1.24) based on pooled data from six studies)
	■ The SIR of the following SPMs was significantly increased: salivary gland, stomach, colon/colorectal, breast, prostate, kidney, brain/central nervous system, soft tissue sarcoma, non–Hodgkin lymphoma, multiple myeloma, leukemia, bone/joints, and adrenal
	■ A significantly reduced risk of lung and cervical cancers was observed
	■ Thyroid cancer survivors are at increased risk of SPMs, which may be related to disease-specific treatments or genetic predisposition

DTC, differentiated thyroid cancer; RAI, radioactive iodine; SPMs, second primary malignancies.

■ SUMMARY

131-I therapy continues to be an important tool in the management of WDTC. As more studies are published, our understanding and methods of selecting the appropriate dosages for ablation and treatment of WDTCs will likewise improve.

■ REFERENCES

1. Niccoli P, Wion-Barbot N, Caron P, et al. Interest of routine measurement of serum calcitonin: study in a large series of thyroidectomized patients. The French Medullary Study Group. *J Clin Endo and Metab.* 1997;82:338–341.
2. Available at: http://www.cancer.gov/cancertopics/types/thyroid. Accessed October 10, 2009.
3. Seidlin SM, Marinelli LD, Oshry E. Radioactive iodine therapy: effect of functioning metastases of adenocarcinoma of the thyroid. *JAMA.* 1946;132:838–847.
4. Siegel E. The beginnings of radioiodine therapy of metastatic thyroid carcinoma: a memoir of Samuel M. Seidlin, M. D. (1895–1955) and his celebrated patient. *Cancer Biother Radiopharm.* 1999;14:71–79.
5. Cooper DS, Doherty GM, Haugen BR, et al. Management guidelines for patients with thyroid nodules and differentiated thyroid cancer. *Thyroid.* 2006;16:109–142.
6. Pacini F, Schlumberger M, Dralle H, et al. European consensus for the management of patients with differentiated thyroid carcinoma of the follicular epithelium. *Eur J Endocrinol.* 2006;154:787–803.
7. Maxon HR, Thomas SR, Hertzbert VS, et al. Relation between effective radiation dose and outcome of radioiodine therapy for thyroid cancer. *N Engl J Med.* 1983;309:937–941.
8. Thomas SR, Maxon HR, Kereiakes JG. In vivo quantitation of lesion radioactivity using external counting methods. *Med Phys.* 1976; 3:253–255.
9. Marinelli LD, Quimby EH, Hine GJ. Dosage determination with radioactive isotopes: practical considerations in therapy and protection. *Am J Roentgenol Radium Ther.* 1948;59:260–281.
10. Lovinger R, Holt JG, Hine JG. Internally administered radioisotopes. In: Attix F, Roesch W, Tolin E, eds. *Radiation Dosimetry.* New York, NY: Academic Press; 1956:803–875.
11. Snyder WS, Ford MR, Warner GG, et al. "S" absorbed dose per unit cumulated activity for selected radionuclides and organs. In: *MIRD Pamphlet No.11.* Reston, VA: Society of Nuclear Medicine; 1975.
12. Benua RS, Cicale NR, Sonenberg M, et al. The relation of radioiodine dosimetry to results and complications in the treatment of metastatic thyroid cancer. *Am J Roentgenol Radium Ther Nucl Med.* 1962; 87:171–182.
13. Leeper RD, Shimaoka K. Treatment of metastatic thyroid cancer. *Clin Endocrinol Metab.* 1980;9:383–404.
14. Dorn R, Kopp J, Vogt H, et al. Dosimetry guided radioactive iodine treatment in patients with metastatic differentiated thyroid cancer: largest safe dose using a risk-adapted approach. *J Nucl Med.* 2003; 44:451–456.
15. Tuttle RM, Pentlow K, Qualey R, et al. Empiric Radioactive Iodine (RAI) Dosing Regimens Frequently Exceed Maximum Tolerated Activity Levels in Elderly Patients with Metastatic Thyroid Cancer. Presented at the 74th annual meeting, American Thyroid Association, Los Angeles, CA; October 2002:198. Abstract.
16. Kulkarni K, Van Nostrand D, Atkins F, et al. The relative frequency in which empiric dosages of radioiodine would potentially over-treat or under-treat patients who have metastatic well-differentiated thyroid cancer. *Thyroid.* 2006;16:1019–1023.
17. Van Nostrand D, Atkins F, Yeganeh F, et al. Dosimetrically determined doses of radioiodine for the treatment of metastatic thyroid carcinoma. *Thyroid.* 2002;12:121–134.
18. Thomas SR, Samaratunga RS, Sperling M, et al. Predictive estimate of blood dose from external counting data preceding radioiodine therapy for thyroid cancer. *Nucl Med Biol.* 1993;20:157–162.
19. Sisson JC, Carey JE. Thyroid carcinoma with high levels of function: treatment with 131-I. *J Nucl Med.* 2001;42:975–983.
20. Sisson JC. Practical dosimetry of 131I in patients with thyroid carcinoma. *Cancer Biother Radiopharm.* 2002;17:101–105.
21. Van Nostrand D, Atkins F, Kulkarni K, et al. The utility of percent 48-hour whole body retention for modifying empiric amounts of I-131 for the treatment of thyroid carcinoma [abstract]. *J Nucl Med.* 2006; 47(1):324P.
22. Van Nostrand D, Atkins F, Moreau S, et al. Utility of the radioiodine whole-body retention at 48 hours for modifying empiric activity of 131-iodine for the treatment of metastatic well-differentiated thyroid carcinoma. *Thyroid.* 2009;19:1093–1098.
23. Greene F, Page D, Fleming I, et al. *AJCC Cancer Staging Manual.* 6th ed. 2002.
24. Perros P, Clarke SEM, Franklin J, et al. *Guidelines for the Management of Thyroid Cancer. British Thyroid Association, Royal College of Physicians of London.* Suffolk, England: Lavenham Press; 2007:18.
25. Van Nostrand D. Radioiodine treatment of distant metastases. In: Wartofsky L, Van Nostrand D, eds. *Thyroid Cancer: A Comprehensive Guide to Clinical Management.* Totowa, NJ: Humana Press; 2006:433–446.
26. Beierwaltes WH. The treatment of thyroid carcinoma with radioactive iodine. *Semin Nucl Med.* 1978;8:79–94.
27. Schlumberger M, Challeton C, De Vathaire F. Radioactive iodine treatment and external radiotherapy for lung and bone metastases from thyroid carcinoma. *J Nucl Med.* 1996;37:598–605.
28. Menzel C, Grunwald F, Schomburg A, et al. "High-dose" radioiodine therapy in advanced differentiated thyroid carcinoma. *J Nucl Med.* 1996;37:1496–1503.
29. Haq M, Harmer C. Differentiated thyroid carcinoma with distant metastases at presentation: prognostic factors and outcome. *Clin Endocrinol (Oxf).* 2005;63(1):87–93.
30. Sampson E, Brierley JD, Le LW, et al. Clinical management and outcome of papillary and follicular (differentiated) thyroid cancer presenting with distant metastasis at diagnosis. *Cancer.* 2007;110(7): 1451–1456.
31. Sugitani I, Fujimoto Y, Yamamoto N. Papillary thyroid carcinoma with distant metastases: survival predictors and the importance of local control. *Surgery.* 2008;143(1):35–42.
32. Showalter TN, Siegel BA, Moley JF, et al. Prognostic factors in patients with well-differentiated thyroid cancer presenting with pulmonary metastasis. *Cancer Biother Radiopharm.* 2008;23(5):655–659.
33. Ruegemmer JJ, Hay ID, Bergstralh E, et al. Distant metastases in differentiated thyroid carcinoma: a multivariate analysis of prognostic variables. *J Clin Endocrinol Metab.* 1988;67:501–508.
34. Dinneen SF, Valimali MJ, Bergstralh EJ, et al. Distant metastases in differentiated thyroid carcinoma: 100 cases observed at one institution during 5 decades. *J Clin Endocrinol Metab.* 1995;80:2041–2045.
35. Samaan NA, Schultz PN, Haynie TP, et al. Pulmonary metastases of differentiated thyroid carcinoma: treatment results in 101 patients. *J Clin Endocrinol Metab.* 1985;60:376–380.
36. Ronga G, Filesi M, Montaseno T, et al. Lung metastases from differentiated thyroid carcinoma. A 40 years' experience. *Q J Nucl Med Mol Imaging.* 2004;48:12–19.
37. Massin JP, Savoie JC, Garnier H, et al. Pulmonary metastases in differentiated thyroid carcinoma. Study of 58 cases with implications for the primary tumor treatment. *Cancer.* 1984;53:982–992.
38. Nemec J, Zamrazil V, Pohunkova D, et al. Radioiodide treatment of pulmonary metastases of differentiated thyroid cancer. Results and prognostic factors. *Nuklearmedizin.* 1979;18:86–90.
39. Wang W, Larson SM, Fazzari M, et al. Prognostic value of [18F] fluorodeoxyglucose positron emission tomographic scanning in patients with thyroid cancer. *J Clin Endocrinol Metab.* 2000;85:1107–1113.
40. Robbins RJ, Wan Q, Grewal RK, et al. Real-time prognosis for metastatic thyroid carcinoma based on 2-[18F]fluoro-2-deoxy-D-glucose-positron emission tomography scanning. *J Clin Endocrinol Metab.* 2006;91(2):498–505.
41. Casara D, Rubello D, Saladini G, et al. Different features of pulmonary metastases in differentiated thyroid cancer: natural history and multivariate statistical analysis of prognostic variables. *J Nucl Med.* 1993;34:1626–1631.
42. Hindie E, Melliere D, Lange F, et al. Functioning pulmonary metastases of thyroid cancer: does radioiodine influence the prognosis? *Eur J Nucl Med Mol Imaging.* 2003;30:974–981.
43. Petrich T, Widjaja A, Musholt TJ, et al. Outcome after radioiodine therapy in 107 patients with differentiated thyroid carcinoma and initial bone metastases: side-effects and influence of age. *Eur J Nucl Med.* 2001;28:203–208.
44. Brown AP, Greening WP, McCready VR, et al. Radioiodine treatment of metastatic thyroid carcinoma: the Royal Marsden Hospital experience: *Br J Radiol.* 1884;57:323–327.

45. Pittas AG, Adler M, Fazzari M, et al. Bone metastases from thyroid carcinoma: clinical characteristics and prognostic variables in one hundred forty-six patients. *Thyroid.* 2000;10:261–268.

46. Zettinig G, Fueger B, Passier C, et al. Long-term follow-up of patients with bone metastases from differentiated thyroid carcinoma-surgery or conventional therapy? *Clin Endocrinol.* 2002;56:377–382.

47. Bernier MO, Leenhardt L, Hoang C, et al. Survival and therapeutic modalities in patients with bone metastases of differentiated thyroid carcinomas. *J Clin Endocrinol Metab.* 2001;86:1568–1573.

48. Van Nostrand D, Freitas J. Side effects of 131-I for ablation and treatment of well-differentiated thyroid carcinoma. In: Wartofsky L, Van Nostrand D, eds. *Thyroid Cancer: A Comprehensive Guide to Clinical Management.* Totowa, NJ: Humana Press; 2006:459–484.

49. Smith MB, Xue H, Takahashi H, et al. Iodine 131 thyroid ablation in female children and adolescents: long-term risk of infertility and birth defects. *Ann Surg Oncol.* 1994;1(2):1228–1231.

50. Hyer S, Vini L, O'Connell M, et al. Testicular dose and fertility in men following I(131) therapy for thyroid cancer. *Clin Endocrinol (Oxf).* 2002;56(6):755–758.

51. Dottorini ME, Lomuscio G, Mazzucchelli L, et al. Assessment of female fertility and carcinogenesis after iodine-131 therapy for differentiated thyroid carcinoma. *J Nucl Med.* 1995;36(1):21–27.

52. Mazzaferri EL, Jhiang SM. Long-term impact of initial surgical and medical therapy on papillary and follicular thyroid cancer. *Am J Med.* 1994;97(5):418–428. Erratum in: *Am J Med.* 1995;98(2):215.

53. Hyer S, Kong A, Pratt B, et al. Salivary gland toxicity after radioiodine therapy for thyroid cancer. *Clin Oncol (R Coll Radiol).* 2007;19(1):83–86.

54. Solans R, Bosch JA, Galofré P, et al. Salivary and lacrimal gland dysfunction (sicca syndrome) after radioiodine therapy. *J Nucl Med.* 2001;42(5):738–743.

55. Schlumberger M, De Vathaire F. 131 iodine: medical use. Carcinogenic and genetic effects [in French]. *Ann Endocrinol (Paris).* 1996;57(3):166–176.

56. De Vathaire F, Schlumberger M, Delisle MJ, et al. Leukemias and cancers following iodine-131 administration for thyroid cancer. *Br J Cancer.* 1997;75(5):734–739.

57. Pacini F, Cetani F, Miccoli P, et al. Outcome of 309 patients with metastatic differentiated thyroid carcinoma treated with radioiodine. *World J Surg.* 1994;18(4):600–604.

58. Günter HH, Schober O, Schwarzrock R, et al. Long-term hematologic changes caused by radioiodine treatment of thyroid cancer. II. Bone marrow changes including leukemia [in German]. *Strahlenther Onkol.* 1987;163(7):475–485.

59. Raza H, Khan AU, Hameed A, et al. Quantitative evaluation of salivary gland dysfunction after radioiodine therapy using salivary gland scintigraphy. *Nucl Med Commun.* 2006;27(6):495–499.

60. Lin WY, Shen YY, Wang SJ. Short-term hazards of low-dose radioiodine ablation therapy in postsurgical thyroid cancer patients. *Clin Nucl Med.* 1996;21(10):780–782.

61. Ceccarelli C, Canale D, Vitti P. Radioactive iodine (131I) effects on male fertility. *Curr Opin Urol.* 2008;18(6):598–601.

62. Sawka AM, Thabane L, Parlea L, et al. Second primary malignancy risk after radioactive iodine treatment for thyroid cancer: a systematic review and meta-analysis. *Thyroid.* 2009;19(5):451–457.

63. Rubino C, de Vathaire F, Dottorini ME, et al. Second primary malignancies in thyroid cancer patients. *Br J Cancer.* 2003;89:1638–1644.

64. Brown AP, Chen J, Hitchcock YJ, et al. The risk of second primary malignancies up to three decades after the treatment of differentiated thyroid cancer. *J Clin Endocrinol Metab.* 2008;93(2):504–515.

65. Bhattacharyya N, Chien W. Risk of second primary malignancy after radioactive iodine treatment for differentiated thyroid carcinoma. *Ann Otol Rhinol Laryngol.* 2006;115(8):607–610.

66. Verkooijen RB, Smit JW, Romijn JA, et al. The incidence of second primary tumors in thyroid cancer patients is increased, but not related to treatment of thyroid cancer. *Eur J Endocrinol.* 2006; 155(6):801–806.

67. Subramanian S, Goldstein DP, Parlea L, et al. Second primary malignancy risk in thyroid cancer survivors: a systematic review and meta-analysis. *Thyroid.* 2007;17:1277–1288.

22

Unconjugated Radiopharmaceuticals

Paul E. Wallner

■ INTRODUCTION

Although far from being scientifically precise or universally accepted, the term "unconjugated" radiopharmaceutical has been generally defined as referring to those radioactive isotopes that target specific disease sites by virtue of chemical, biologic, or physical affinity, rather than by virtue of carrier agents to which they are tagged. Because of the untagged nature of their use, the class of agents has occasionally been referred to in the literature as "naked" radiopharmaceuticals (1). The approval for testing and use of these agents is under the authority of the US Food and Drug Administration (FDA), Center for Drug Evaluation and Research, and Office of Oncology Drug Products (2). Transport, handling, safety, educational credentials, and user approval is under the regulatory mandate of the US Nuclear Regulatory Commission (NRC) that refers to the agents as "unsealed" radioisotopes. NRC responsibility is at the national level and for 17 states and territories. Thirty-three state regulatory agencies operate independently in oversight of the agents by agreement with the NRC. The NRC is provided advice regarding the agents by the Advisory Committee for the Medical Use of Isotopes. The operative regulations related to unconjugated radioisotopes reside in Title 10 of the Code of Federal Regulations, Part 35 (10 CFR 35) (3).

By common usage, the class of unconjugated agents has also included those agents such as Samarium-153 and Rhenium-186 and -188, which are typically administered bound to various chemical chelating agents (4). Particular localization properties of individual agents and the clinical circumstances involved will determine routes of administration, but individual agents have been delivered via intravenous, intra-arterial, intracavitary, intra-articular, and direct intralesional approaches. This variability of site and administration has been especially true for phosphorous-32 that has uniquely been studied using oral administration (5).

Pecher first reported the use of a beta-emitting radioisotope for management of intractable metastatic bone pain in 1942 (6). Because the family of unconjugated radionuclides has demonstrated a chemical affinity for bone, the predominant thrust of investigation and clinical utility has been for primary and secondary malignancies of bone and bone marrow, but other target sites have been considered. In some instances, these alternative uses have remained a part of the therapeutic armamentarium, but for many alternative indications, the availability, presumed safety profile, and ease of handling of nonradioactive agents such as corticosteroids and systemic chemotherapy have reduced interest and enthusiasm regarding the agents. The relative difficulty of access to innovative candidate radionuclides, diminished levels of investigation, and absence of use from many training curricula have further exacerbated the problem (1).

The radionuclides currently recognized as having effectiveness in the management of painful bone metastases, especially in circumstances of increased osteoblastic activity such as primary prostate, breast, and lung cancer, exhibit their proclivity for bone targeting because of a chemical similarity to calcium and relationship to that element on the periodic table. The agents may directly substitute for stable analogs in hydroxyapatite or may be chemisorbed on the hydroxyapatite surface of the phosphate moiety of phosphonate chelates (4).

Agents with decay profiles that include a gamma emission component may be utilized for scanning purposes to document uptake and the disseminated nature of bone pathology. Prior to utilization of pure beta emitters, scanning with ^{99m}Tc is appropriate to verify disseminated osseous disease. The intensity of uptake on pretherapeutic injection scanning does not necessarily coincide with therapeutic efficacy, and widely disseminated disease may actually produce dilution of dose and potentially reduced effectiveness (4).

Regardless of the precise method of chemical or physical affinity, all of the agents studied for palliation of osseous metastatic bone pain have fared better than placebos in randomized trials, but there is little evidence that the response or morbidity profile of the various agents varies significantly among the agents themselves. In addition, there is little evidence that dose escalation either in individual or cumulative doses will improve effectiveness. Sequenced administration has been investigated, but if an initial intervention has not produced a significant level or duration of response, there is little evidence that additional administrations will increase effectiveness but will predictably increase morbidity (4).

Rapid and significant localization in bone by all agents will generally limit potential morbidity to myelosuppression, which, in patients with adequate marrow reserve, will usually be mild, and manifested initially within 1 week postadministration with evidence of thrombocytopenia. Leukopenia may develop somewhat later, but all sequelae typically reverse without intervention within 8 to 10 weeks. Circulating isotope not immediately incorporated into bone is typically excreted in urine, so patients with reduced renal function may not be ideal candidates for the agents and, if used, should have blood counts monitored carefully. Administration is routinely on an outpatient basis, so radiation protection measures for low-level radiation in urine should be practiced (3). Palliative effects may be observed within 3 to 5 days but usually peak at approximately 7 to 10 days and the beneficial effects may last for months. At this point, subsequent administrations can be considered. When used for management of bone pain, all of the agents in this class can exhibit a flare in pain within 24 to 72 hours postinjection that may last for 5 to 7 days. Appropriate analgesic management must be provided during this period. In the treatment of metastatic prostate cancer, prostate specific antigen (PSA) levels may begin to decline within several days, but the rapidity of decline, nadir of the PSA level, and duration of PSA response are not satisfactory predictors of improved outcomes (4). The bone-seeking agents have been and continue to be used primarily in metastatic prostate cancer, and evidence of effectiveness in breast and lung cancer is limited with responses noted in primarily osteoblastic metastases. Plain radiographs of symptomatic metastatic sites should be obtained prior to use of systemic agents for palliation of bone pain. If there is evidence of possible impending fracture, stabilization and/or external beam radiation should be initiated prior to systemic radionuclide therapy. If painful vertebral metastasis is apparent clinically, computed tomography or magnetic resonance imaging of the painful vertebral segments should be obtained prior to administration of isotope to ensure that no epidural disease is present. If this pathology is discovered, external beam radiation or surgery should be carried out prior to systemic isotope therapy.

Intravenous administration of all agents should be given slowly over 1 to 5 minutes, through indwelling catheters with clear and unobstructed flow clearly validated, adequate hydration, and careful radiation precautions for patients and staff.

■ AGENTS

▓ Phosphorus-32

Physical properties

$t_{1/2}$—14.3 days

Radiation decay: β (1.71 MeV maximum and 0.69 MeV mean)

γ—none

Clinical utility

Phosphorus-32 (^{32}P) represents one of the earliest agents in this class and perhaps the most frequently studied for a wide variety of indications and routes of administration. In its aqueous form (Na_2PO_3), the agent was employed for the systemic therapy of chronic myelogenous leukemia and polycythemia vera. Orthopedic surgeons and rheumatologists have evaluated the agent for intra-articular management of persistent synovial effusions and hemarthroses secondary to hemophilia and leukemia (7,8). In addition, the agent has been placed into indwelling catheters to treat central nervous system lesions.

The colloidal form of the agent (as chromic phosphate) became a standard modality for the management of malignant pleural and peritoneal effusions in the 1960s and 1970s, driving numerous clinical investigations. Anecdotal reports suggesting significant activity were infrequently corroborated in randomized clinical trials. Following drainage of abdominal ascites or pleural effusions, up to 5 mCi of the agent was instilled and patients were placed in various positions to enhance distribution. The nature of the disease processes and prior therapy often predisposed patients to preinstillation adhesions with bowel or lung immobility and a uniform distribution of the agent proved difficult. This indication has largely been replaced by instillations of various antibiotic or chemotherapeutic compounds (9–11).

Following identification of a subset of early-stage, high-risk ovarian cancer patients (FIGO stage Ia or Ib (grade 3), or stage 1c or II (any grade), or any stage I/II patient with clear-cell histology, the Gynecologic Oncology Group, North Central Cancer Treatment Group, and Southwest Oncology Group undertook a randomized trail assigning patients to either a single dose of 15 mCi of intraperitoneal ^{32}P or cyclophosphamide 1 g/m^2 and cisplatin 100 mg/m^2 every 21 days for three cycles. Prior to instillation of the radioactive material through multiperforated indwelling peritoneal dialysis catheters, ^{99m}Tc was instilled to ensure free flow and even distribution of the therapeutic agent. Intraperitoneal ^{32}P was administered within 10 days but not more than 6 weeks following laparotomy. Ten-year follow-up of the study population suggested a modest reduction in intra-abdominal recurrence rate for the chemotherapy population but only a small and nonsignificant improvement in survival. These findings were corroborated by other reports (12).

In the 1990s, Order et al. reported a series of patients treated with direct intralesional infusions of ^{32}P colloidal chromic phosphate for unresectable tumors of the liver, central nervous system, pancreas, and head and neck. The observation of extralesional extravasation of isotope was apparently overcome by preinstillation of macroaggregated albumin to induce capillary and arteriole blockade prior to isotope infusion. Intense activity and doses were documented, but improvements in local control and survival were inconclusive (13,14).

^{32}P localization in bone created interest in use of the orthophosphate form of the isotope for painful skeletal metastases with 85% of the administered dose ultimately incorporated into bone. Priming regimens including androgenic agents, prior to isotope administration, were prolonged, beneficial results were modest, and myelotoxicity was significant. The use of this agent for this indication has largely been abandoned.

Strontium-89 chloride (Metastron, GE Healthcare, Chalfont St. Giles, UK)

Physical properties

$t_{1/2}$—50.5 days
Radiation decay: β (1.463 MeV maximum and 0.583 MeV mean)
γ—none

The calcium analog strontium-89 (^{89}Sr) chloride is administered as an intravenous injection at doses of 4 mCi, given slowly.

Clinical utility

Porter and coworkers (15), in a Trans-Canada study, compared ^{89}Sr with bisphosphonates in the prophylactic setting in an attempt to reduce subsequent development of additional osseous metastasis. Results were comparable in both arms with a reduced cost of therapy in the ^{89}Sr arm. Low-grade hematologic toxicity in the radiation arm did not require intervention. In an attempt to build upon currently established palliative results, a randomized phase III trial is under way to investigate the use of weekly doxorubicin (20 mg/m^2) with ^{89}Sr after response to induction chemotherapy (16).

Samarium-153 EDTMP (lexidronam: Sm-153-ethylenediaminetetramethylenephosphonate) (Quadramet, Cytogen, Princeton, NJ)

Physical properties

$t_{1/2}$—46.3 hours
Radiation decay: β (0.81 MeV maximum and 0.23 MeV mean)
γ (103 keV maximum)

Clinical utility

Samarium-153 EDTMP (^{153}Sm) is a bone-seeking agent consisting of radioactive samarium and a telephosphonate chelator, ethylenediaminetetramethylenephosphonate. The recommended therapeutic dose is 1.0 mCi/kg, administered intravenously over a period of 1 minute through a secure indwelling catheter and followed by a saline flush.

Extensive preclinical and clinical investigations have demonstrated the safety and effectiveness profile of ^{153}Sm-EDTMP (17). Although primarily used alone, there is increasing interest in consideration of combination therapy with the bisphosphonates and taxane-based chemotherapeutics.

The use of ^{153}Sm-EDTMP has been evaluated in osseous metastases for primary osteosarcomas (18). Anderson and coworkers investigated the use of gemcitabine as a radiosensitizer to increase ^{153}Sm-EDTMP effectiveness. Using 30 mCi/kg (average of 1640 mCi), they found acceptable toxicity and objective response in 8 of 14 patients investigated.

Radium-223 chloride

Physical properties

$t_{1/2}$—11.4 days
Radiation decay: α (6 MeV maximum)
γ (270 keV maximum)

Clinical utility

Although not available for commercial distribution in the United States, there has been interest in ^{223}Ra in the treatment of metastatic hormone-refractory prostate cancer involving multiple bone sites. Nilsson et al. at the Karolinska Hospital and Institute in Stockholm reported initial findings in 2005, comparing the safety and effectiveness of ^{223}Ra with ^{89}Sr (19). The group had carried out preclinical studies prior to this phase I investigation. They concluded that at relevant dose levels, the agent was well tolerated and justified extension into phase II and III studies. Following focal external beam radiation to selected sites, patients were randomly assigned to treatment with ^{223}Ra or placebo in a double-blinded manner. One primary end point, bone alkaline phosphatase levels, was significantly decreased in the treatment arm and the time to PSA increase was significantly lengthened. Hematologic toxicity in both groups was equivalent. The time to first skeletal-related event was significantly increased in the ^{223}Ra cohort and can be considered as a measure of quality of life, taking into account increase in pain or analgesic requirements; new neurologic symptoms or fractures; or additional surgical, radiologic, or systemic therapy. In this limited report, survival in the treated group was significantly extended. Subsequent reports have confirmed these findings and a commercially prepared formulation of the agent (Alpharadin, Algeta ASA, Oslo, Norway) was granted an investigational new drug application approval by the FDA in February 2008 for phase I trials in the United States (20).

Rhenium-186 HEDP (etidronate—hydroxyethylidene diphosphate)

Physical properties

$t_{1/2}$—3.8 days
Radiation decay: β (1.07 MeV maximum and 0.336 mean)
γ (0.137 MeV maximum)

Although not commercially available in the United States, ^{186}Rh-HEDP has been studied in phase I trials in Europe in association with autologous peripheral blood stem cell rescue in the management of hormone-refractory prostate cancer metastatic to bone (21). Promising results have led to initiation of phase II trials.

Rhenium-188 HEDP (etidronate—hydroxyethylidene diphosphate)

Physical properties

$t_{1/2}$—16.9 hours
Radiation decay: β (2.1 MeV maximum and 0.779 mean)
γ (0.155 MeV maximum and 0.061 mean)

Clinical utility

Although not commercially available in the United States, [188]Re-HEDP has been studied in Europe for some time. The agent is produced by a generator similar to that used to produce ^{99m}Tc, enabling wide availability at relatively low cost. Liepe et al. (22) reported treatment of 46 patients with multiple bone metastases from breast and prostate cancer with pain. Thirty-one received [188]Re-HEDP (3300 MBq) and 25 received [153]Sm-EDTMP (37 MBq/kg of body weight). All patients had a single injection of isotope. Patients with prostate cancer received hormone therapy for 6 months before isotope therapy and during the postisotope observation period. Thirty-nine patients received bisphosphonates for 6 months prior to study treatment with discontinuance of the agents 1 month prior to isotope administration. In posttherapy evaluation, only the [188]Re-HEDP group had a statistically significant improvement in Karnofsky performance score. Pain relief within 2 weeks of treatment was noted in 77% of the [188]Re-HEDP group and 73% of the [153]Sm-EDTMP group. These results were not statistically significant and there was no significant difference between responses in the patients with prostate or breast cancer. A brief flare reaction was noted in 17% of patients in both groups within 14 days of therapy, and the majority of patients demonstrated a maximum of grade I anemia within 12 weeks of therapy based on the 1979 WHO criteria. Grade I thrombocytopenia was noted in two patients with each isotope, and one patient in the [188]Re-HEDP group experienced grade II thrombocytopenia. Grade I leucopenia was noted in one patient in each group. All cases of thrombocytopenia and leucopenia reversed within 12 weeks after therapy. Similar findings have been reported by other investigators (23,24).

REFERENCES

1. Wallner PE. "Naked" radiopharmaceuticals. *Int J Radiat Oncol Biol Phys.* 2006;6(2 suppl):S60–S61.
2. U.S. Food and Drug Administration; Office of Oncology Drug Products: Division of Medical Imaging and Hematologic Products (DMIHP) or Division of Biologic Oncology Products (DBOP). Available at: http://www.fda.gov/cder/Offices/OODP/DMIHP_products2.htm http://www.fda.gov/cder/Offices/OODP/DBOP_products.htm. Accessed December 5, 2009.
3. U.S. NRC. Part 35—Medical use of byproduct material. Available at: http://www.nrc.gov/reading-rm/doc-collections/cfr/part035/. Accessed December 5, 2009.
4. Silberstein EB. Teletherapy and radiopharmaceutical therapy of painful bone metastases. *Semin Nucl Med.* 2005;35:152–158.
5. Nair N. Relative efficacy of ^{32}P and ^{89}Sr in palliation of skeletal metastases. *J Nucl Med.* 1999;40:256–261.
6. Pecher P. Biological investigation with radioactive calcium and strontium: preliminary report on the use of radioactive strontium in the treatment of metastatic bone cancer. *Univ Calif Publ Pharmacol.* 1942;11:117–149.
7. Siegel HJ, Luck JV Jr, Siegel ME, et al. Advances in radionuclide therapeutics in orthopaedics. *J Am Acad Orthop Surg.* 2004;12:55–64.
8. Soroa VE, del Huerto Velazquez Espeche M, Giannone C, et al. Effects of radiosynovectomy with p-32 colloid therapy in hemophilia and rheumatoid arthritis. *Cancer Biotherm Radiopharm.* 2005;20:344–348.
9. Potter ME, Partridge EE, Shingleton HM, et al. Intraperitoneal chromic phosphate in ovarian cancer: risks and benefits. *Gynecol Oncol.* 1989;32:314–318.
10. Soper JT, Berchuk A, Dodge R, et al. Adjuvant therapy with intraperitoneal chromic phosphate (32P) in women with early ovarian carcinoma after comprehensive surgical staging. *Obstet Gynecol.* 1992;79:993–997.
11. Spanos WJ Jr, Day T Jr, Jose B, et al. Use of P-32 in stage III epithelial carcinoma of the ovary. *Gynecol Oncol.* 1994;54:35–39.
12. Young RC, Brody MF, Nieberg RK, et al. Adjuvant treatment for early ovarian cancer: a randomized phase III trial of intraperitoneal ^{32}P or intravenous cyclophosphamide and cisplatin—a Gynecologic Oncology Group study. *J Clin Oncol.* 2003;21(23)4350–4355.
13. Order SE, Siegel JA, Lustig RA, et al. A new method of delivering radioactive cytotoxic agents in solid cancers. *Int J Radiat Oncol Biol Phys.* 1994;30:715–720.
14. Firusian N, Dempke W. An early phase II study of intratumoral P-32 chromic phosphate injection therapy for patients with refractory solid tumors and solitary metastases. *Cancer.* 1999;85;980–987.
15. Porter AT, McEwan AJ, Powe JE, et al. Results of a randomized phase-III trial to evaluate the efficacy of strontium-89 adjuvant to local field external beam irradiation in the management of endocrine resistant metastatic prostate cancer. *Int J Radiat Oncol Biol Phys.* 1993;25: 805–813.
16. Tu SM, Lin SH. Current trials using bone-targeting agents in prostate cancer. *Cancer J.* 2008;14(1):35–39.
17. Sartor O. Overview of samarium Sm 153 lexidronam in the treatment of painful metastatic bone disease. *Rev Urol.* 2004;6(S 10):S3–S12.
18. Anderson PM, Wiseman GA, Erlandson L, et al. Gemcitabine radiosensitization after high-dose samarium for osteoblastic osteosarcoma. *Clin Cancer Res.* 2005;11(19):6895–6900.
19. Nilsson S, Larsen RH, Fossa SD, et al. First clinical experience with α-emitting radium-223 in the treatment of skeletal metastases. *Clin Cancer Res.* 2005;11(12):4451–4459.
20. Nilsson S, Franzen L, Parker C, et al. Bone-targeted radium-223 in symptomatic, hormone-refractory prostate cancer: randomised, multicentre, placebo-controlled phase II study. *Lancet Oncol.* 2007;8: 587–594.
21. O'Sullivan JM, McCready VR, Flux G, et al. High activity rhenium-186 HEDP with autologous peripheral blood stem cell rescue: a phase I study in progressive hormone refractory prostate cancer metastatic to bone. *Br J Cancer.* 2002;86:1715–1720.
22. Liepe K, Runge R, Kotzerke, J. The benefit of bone-seeking radiopharmaceuticals in the treatment of metastatic bone pain. *J Cancer Res Clin Oncol.* 2005;131:60–66.
23. Li S, Liu J, Zhang H, et al. Rhenium-188 HEDP to treat painful bone metastases. *Clin Nucl Med.* 2001;26(11):919–922.
24. Zhang H, Tian M, Li S, et al. Rhenium-188-HEDP therapy for the palliation of pain due to osseous metastases in lung cancer patients. *Cancer Biother Radiopharm.* 2003;18:719–726.

Yttrium-90 Radioembolization for the Therapy of Primary and Metastatic Liver Malignancies

Ahsun Riaz, Robert J. Lewandowski, Laura Kulik, and Riad Salem

■ INTRODUCTION

The past decade has seen an increase in the incidence of primary liver tumors (1). Due to limited role of surgical and systemic therapies, locoregional therapies are establishing their role in the management of liver tumors. The minimization of systemic toxicity and a favorable outcome make its use very promising. This chapter presents an overview of the general concepts associated with yttrium-90 and its specific use in different primary and secondary malignancies of the liver.

▧ Vascular anatomy of the liver and its tumors

The portal vein is the predominant source of blood supply to the parenchyma of the liver. This vascularization allows for the hepatocytes to carry out their metabolic functions. It also makes the liver a common organ for the development of metastatic disease.

The arterial supply is summarized as follows. The celiac trunk gives off the common hepatic artery that continues to become the proper hepatic artery. The proper hepatic artery branches into the right and left hepatic arteries that supply the corresponding lobes of the liver. The cystic artery supplies the gall bladder and usually arises from the right hepatic artery. The right and left hepatic arteries give rise to the segmental branches. These eventually branch into the small vessels found in the portal triads. Hepatic tumors are hypervascular structures that are predominantly supplied by branches of the hepatic artery (2). Their blood supply may often arise from parasitization from extrahepatic sites. Thus, hepatic tumors in one segment of the liver may become vascularized from vessels of adjacent segments or adjacent structures.

▧ History of radioembolization

The use of external radiation for liver tumors traditionally has had limited value due to the sensitivity of the normal parenchyma to the tumoricidal radiation dose (3,4). A mean liver dose greater than 35 Gray (Gy) often leads to the development of a radiation-induced liver disease (RILD), a clinical syndrome of ascites, anicteric hepatomegaly, and elevation of liver enzymes. Conformal beam therapy, which uses a three-dimensional approach rather than broad axial plane techniques, has been shown to minimize the toxicity to normal hepatic parenchyma (5). However, even when using conformal beam therapy, radiation is delivered to normal hepatic parenchyma adjacent to the tumor, which limits the maximum dose that can be delivered to the tumor without compromising safety.

Figure 23.1 illustrates the treatment catheter positioned in the right hepatic artery, perfusing multiple hypervascularized hepatic metastases. Thus, given the vasculature of tumors, radioembolization provides a mode of delivering localized radiotherapy to the tumor. A radiation dose of up to 150 Gy can be administered minimizing the complications of external radiation. Radioembolization has been shown to have promising outcomes in primary and secondary hepatic malignancies by numerous investigators.

Nolan and Grady first used yttrium^{90} oxide (^{90}Y$_2$O$_3$) contained in a metal particle (50 to 100 μm) and injected it intra-arterially (6). The study had a small number of patients but showed a favorable response, observed by the reduction in size of palpable masses. The next study using ^{90}Y was published in 1982. Mantravadi et al. studied the effect and distribution of ^{90}Y after whole liver delivery via the hepatic artery. This study concluded that patients with hypervascular tumors are much more likely to benefit from this treatment (7). An animal study concluded that portal fibrosis was seen after the use of radioactive microspheres (8). A dose-escalation study performed on animals formed the basis of the phase I dose-escalation evaluations in humans (9). Shepherd et al. conducted a phase I dose-escalation study using ^{90}Y-microspheres in 10 patients. Extrahepatic shunting was assessed using technetium-99m–labeled macroaggregated albumin (^{99m}Tc-MAA). None of the patients in this study experienced hematologic toxicity in contrast to earlier studies. This study stressed the value of assessing angiographic findings and extrahepatic shunting before treatment (10). The technical aspects of dosimetry, radioassays, safety, and efficacy were discussed by many studies that followed (11,12). Lau et al.

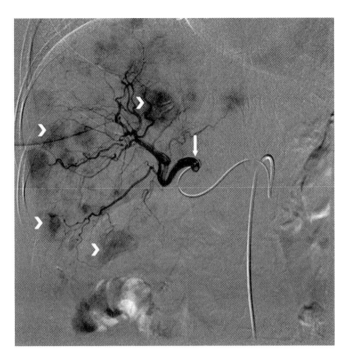

FIGURE 23.1 An angiogram of a patient with neuroendocrine (carcinoid) metastases to the liver. The contrast is being injected in the right hepatic artery *(arrow)* showing multiple hypervascular tumors *(arrowheads* on some examples*)* within the right lobe of the liver.

showed that tumor response was proportional to the dose delivered with improved survival in patients receiving greater than 120 Gy (13). Geschwind et al. published their landmark comprehensive analysis on using ^{90}Y for hepatocellular carcinoma (HCC), which showed improved survival in Okuda I when compared with Okuda II (4) (Okuda classification uses tumor- and liver-related parameters for staging).

■ YTTRIUM-90 MICROSPHERES

The radioactive isotope that is most commonly used for radioembolization is yttrium-90 (^{90}Y). It is a pure beta emitter with maximum beta energy of 2.28 MeV and average beta energy of 934 keV per disintegration. ^{90}Y has a half-life of 64.2 hours. It decays into the stable element Zirconium-90. The range of tissue penetration of the emissions is 2.5 to 11 mm.

■ Pretreatment evaluation

The imaging diagnosis of the hepatic tumors is beyond the scope of this chapter. Laboratory workup is essential to determine the pretreatment functional status of the liver. Clinical evaluation is required to stratify the patients according to the Eastern Cooperation Oncology Group (ECOG) performance status. Patients with an ECOG performance status of greater than two are not considered ideal candidates for this treatment.

Pretreatment angiography

The aortogram assesses the tortuosity and the presence of atherosclerosis in the aorta. The superior mesenteric angiogram

and celiac trunk angiogram allows the interventional radiologist with an opportunity to study the vascular anatomy of the liver in detail. The patency of the portal vein and the presence of arterioportal shunting are assessed. The inadvertent spread of the microspheres is prevented by a meticulous study of the vascular anatomy of the liver and collateral nontarget flow (14).

Prophylactic embolization of the gastroduodenal artery and right gastric artery is thus recommended as a safe and efficacious mode of minimizing the risks of hepatoenteric flow, particularly if using resin microspheres (15–17). Other vessels that may need to be embolized are the falciform, inferior esophageal, left inferior phrenic, accessory left gastric, supraduodenal, and retroduodenal arteries.

^{99m}Tc-MAA is used to assess splanchnic and pulmonary shunting. The proximity of the duodenum and stomach to the liver may make it difficult to assess shunting to these portions of the gastrointestinal tract by using nuclear medicine scans. Thus, it is important to correlate the findings of angiography to the findings of the ^{99m}Tc-MAA scan. Lung shunt fraction (LSF) is used to calculate the dose delivered to the lungs, and appropriate adjustment for this parameter minimizes the risk of radiation pneumonitis.

Diagnostic mesenteric angiography is necessary to ensure that the blood supply to the lesions has been adequately identified. Incomplete assessment of the blood supply to the tumor may lead to incomplete targeting and treatment.

Available devices

TheraSphere (MDS Nordion, Ottawa, Canada) consists of nonbiodegradable glass microspheres with diameters ranging between 20 and 30 μm (^{90}Y is an integral component of the glass). It has been approved by the Food and Drug Administration (FDA) in 1999 for unresectable HCC, potentially leading to resection or transplantation. Further, it has recently been approved for use in HCC patients with partial or branch portal vein thrombosis (PVT). Vials of six different activities are available: 3, 5, 7, 10, 15, and 20 gigabecquerel (GBq). The only difference in the vials is the number of spheres; for example, 1.2 million microspheres are present in a vial with an activity of 3 GBq. At the time of calibration, each microsphere has an activity of 2500 Bq. The activity of the vial varies inversely with the time elapsed after calibration.

SIR-Spheres consist of biodegradable resin microspheres. These spheres have a slightly larger diameter and lower specific activity per microsphere than TheraSphere and hence may be associated with an increased embolic effect. The use of SIR-Spheres was approved by the FDA for metastatic colorectal cancer (CRC) to the liver in 2002. These two devices are compared in Table 23.1. The use of ^{90}Y-microspheres as a transcatheter therapy is termed "radioembolization" but is also known as "selective internal radiation therapy." The small particle size allows deep penetration into the tumor and hence increased efficacy with minimal toxicity due to embolic effects.

Table **23.1**	Available yttrium-90 microspheres	
Parameter	**TheraSphere**	**SIR-Spheres**
Radionuclide	Yttrium-90	Yttrium-90
Half-life (hours)	64.2	64.2
Maximum beta emission (MeV)	2.28	2.28
Maximum gamma emission (keV)	0	0
Material	Glass microsphere	Resin microsphere
Size of particle (μm)	20–30	20–60
Embolic effect	Mild	Moderate
Activity	3–20 GBq	3 GBq
Number of particles per treatment	1.2–8 million	30–60 million
Images of particles		

Dose calculation for TheraSphere

Three-dimensional reconstruction of the target site allows the calculation of the volume of the liver to be infused. Volume of target site in cubic centimeters is then used to calculate the mass in grams by multiplying it by a factor of 1.03. The activity (A) in gigabecquerel administered to the target area of the liver, assuming uniform distribution of microspheres, is calculated using the following formula:

$$A = \frac{D \times M}{50},$$

where D is the dose administered in Gray and M is the mass in kilograms. Using this formula, it can be said that a dose of 50 Gy will be administered to 1 kg of tissue, if 1 GBq of ^{90}Y is given.

The dose given to the treated mass also depends on the percent residual activity (R) in the vial after treatment and the LSF that is calculated beforehand. These factors are accounted for in the following formula:

$$D = \frac{A \times 50 \times (1-\text{LSF}) \times (1-R)}{M}.$$

Dose calculation for SIR-Spheres

The model of dosimetry for SIR-Spheres is based on whole liver infusion. The calculated gigabecquerel of the whole liver is multiplied by the percentage of the target site as a proportion of the whole liver. There are three methods for dosimetry of SIR-Spheres recommended by the manufacturers. The partition method is seldom used, as it is applicable only in special circumstances. The empiric method is outlined in Table 23.2.

The most widely used body surface area (BSA) method is as follows:

$$A = \text{BSA} - 0.2 + (\% \text{ tumar burden}/100),$$

where A is the activity in gigabecquerel, BSA is the body surface area in meters squared (m^2), and % tumor burden is the percentage of the liver that is involved by tumor.

Transcatheter ^{90}Y radioembolization

The tumor is approached using its arterial supply and the vial is injected into the vessel feeding the tumor. The distribution of the tumor is the factor that allows the treatment to be selective, that is, to one lobe, or superselective, that is, to one segment. The apparatus for the administration of ^{90}Y is designed to minimize the radiation exposure to the persons involved in the procedure. The presence of a physicist throughout the case ensures that proper protocols are followed to minimize accidental radiation exposure. This is an outpatient procedure and the patient is discharged on the same day (18).

Table **23.2** The Empiric Method	
Percent Tumor Involvement of Liver (%)	**Recommended Yttrium-90 Activity for Treatment (GBq)**
<25	2
25–50	2.5
>50	3

Posttreatment assessment

The response to treatment has to be monitored both clinically and radiologically. The regular follow-up laboratory work analysis includes the hepatic panel and tumor markers such as alpha-fetoprotein in the case of HCC, to monitor any potential toxicity due to treatment or clinical improvement in the patient. Cross-sectional imaging is performed at 1 month posttreatment and then the patients are followed with scans every 3 months to assess response to treatment or progression of disease. World Health Organization size criteria and the European Association for the Study of the Liver necrosis criteria are used to assess response in the target lesions (19). The conventional anatomic imaging studies are not able to assess tumor response until 6 weeks have elapsed after treatment, and functional magnetic resonance imaging may have a role in earlier detection of tumor response (20).

■ PRIMARY LIVER TUMORS

Radioembolization has been extensively studied as a treatment option of the most common primary malignant tumor, HCC. Its use in the management of intrahepatic cholangiocarcinoma (ICC) has also been studied and will be discussed briefly.

Radioembolization for hepatocellular carcinoma

Patient selection

The management of HCC is a multidisciplinary task. The patients should be selected for radioembolization after a consensus of the team consisting of hepatologists, oncologists, transplant surgeons, and interventional radiologists. As discussed later, the role of radioembolization is not limited by the stage of the disease.

Indications and efficacy

Patients within Transplant Criteria Patients within Milan criteria, that is, single lesion less than 5 cm or three or less lesions all less than 3 cm, are eligible for transplantation. Resection is possible only if liver cirrhosis is well compensated. The use of surgical options is the gold standard of treatment for these patients. Orthotopic liver transplantation (OLT) has a limited role due to the limited availability of donor organs and the dropout of patients due to tumor progression. Radioembolization has been shown to limit progression of HCC. This allows the patient more time to wait for donor organs and thus increases their chance of undergoing OLT. Thus, it has a role of bridging the patient to OLT (21).

Patients Beyond Transplant Criteria Patients who are outside transplant criteria but do not have malignant PVT or metastatic HCC are also candidates for radioembolization. Radioembolization in these patients has been shown to downstage the disease to that within transplant criteria.

This allows patients who were initially outside Milan criteria to be eligible for transplant. There is an increase in overall survival in these patients as well (21).

Patients with Advanced Disease Patients with PVT have been shown to have a good response to treatment after radioembolization. The presence of PVT excludes these patients from the transplant criteria. Systemic therapy with sorafenib has been shown to have a significant improvement in survival in patients with advanced disease. A survival benefit has been shown with the use of radioembolization in patients with malignant vascular involvement (22). The presence of distant metastases, that is, lung and adrenals, is a contraindication to this treatment, as a survival benefit has not been shown for this subset of patients.

Radioembolization has been shown to be a safe and effective tool in the management of HCC. The response rate and improvement in survival have established its role in many centers around the world for the management of HCC.

Radioembolization for intrahepatic cholangiocarcinoma

Resection of ICC is an option in patients who have resectable disease. Surgical resection has been shown to modestly improve survival. The use of transarterial chemoembolization for cholangiocarcinoma has been studied and a trend for improvement in survival has been shown, but toxicity remains high. Radioembolization has been shown to be effective in the treatment of HCC, but its role in the management of ICC has not been extensively studied. A pilot study analyzing the use of ^{90}Y in 24 patients with biopsy-proven ICC has shown a favorable response to treatment and favorable survival outcomes (23). The patients with a better performance status according to the ECOG had a significantly better survival in this study.

■ SECONDARY LIVER TUMORS

Metastatic disease to the liver is common due to its unique anatomy. Extrahepatic metastasis and comorbidities limit the role of surgical resection in these patients (24). The use of radioembolization alone and as a conjunct to systemic chemotherapy has been well published.

Radioembolization for metastatic colorectal carcinoma

Resection is the only curative option available for CRC that has metastasized to the liver, but only less than 10% patients have disease that is resectable (24). Some commonly used chemotherapeutic agents are Fluorouracil (5-FU), Oxaliplatin, Irinotecan (CPT-11), Bevacizumab, Cetuximab, and Capecitabine. The favorable role of radioembolization in treatment of metastatic CRC to the liver has been published.

Patient selection

Patients who have unresectable liver metastases and are on systemic chemotherapy or have failed to respond to first- or second-line chemotherapeutic agents are considered as candidates for internal radiation. Carcinoembryonic antigen is measured and radiologic studies are performed before and after treatment to assess response to treatment. Fluorodeoxyglucose positron emission tomography shown to have increased sensitivity over computed tomography in assessing tumor response to radioembolization in the treatment of metastatic CRC.

Efficacy of radioembolization

The combination of systemic therapy and radioembolization in a randomized control trial has been shown to have a significantly better tumor response, a longer time to progression, survival benefit, and an acceptable safety profile than systemic chemotherapy alone (25). Dose-escalation studies have shown increased tumor response with increasing doses (26).

Radioembolization for metastatic neuroendocrine tumors

Liver metastases from neuroendocrine tumors (NETs) are common. Carcinoid, VIPomas, gastrinomas, and somatostatinomas are some examples. Systemic chemotherapy and ablative procedures have been shown to have a modest benefit in these patients. Patients with unresectable disease are candidates for radioembolization. Clinical improvement, chromogranin A, and imaging studies before and after treatment are used to assess response to treatment. Radioembolization of metastatic disease to the liver from a primary neuroendocrine neoplasia has been shown to be safe and effective. Prolonged response to treatment of greater than 2 years has also been seen (27,28).

Radioembolization for metastatic mixed neoplasia

Hepatic metastases from primary neoplasia other than CRC and NET are referred to as mixed neoplasia. Radioembolization for breast cancer metastases to the liver (29) has been described. Although there is significant radiologic response after treatment, the survival benefit of this treatment in these patients has not been established (30). Radioembolization has also been used to treat secondary liver tumors from various primary sources. This mode of treatment is an effective alternative to patients who have failed chemotherapy or have become chemorefractory (31).

■ COMPLICATIONS OF RADIOEMBOLIZATION

Postradioembolization syndrome

The following mild clinical complications may be seen after radioembolization: fatigue, nausea, vomiting, anorexia, fever, abdominal discomfort, and cachexia (32–34). These are usually not severe enough to require hospitalization. Some serious adverse events related to radioembolization are explained below.

Hepatobiliary toxicity

Hepatic dysfunction

Hepatic toxicity is measured by a change in liver enzymes and metabolites, that is, alanine aminotransferase, aspartate aminotransferase, alkaline phosphatase, albumin, and bilirubin. It is difficult to assess if liver toxicity is due to worsening of hepatic cirrhosis or is due to radioembolization in patients with HCC (35). Toxicity rates following radioembolization have been between 15% and 20% (35,36). Ascites and jaundice may be seen clinically. The histologic hallmark of veno-occlusive disease may be seen in severe cases. Hepatic toxicity may be severe and lead to significant morbidity and mortality (36). The presence of various factors such as a deranged hepatic function at baseline, age, and activity delivered may predispose patients to the hepatotoxic effects of radioembolization. Kennedy et al. observed RILD in 4% of patients after radioembolization with resin microspheres (37).

Biliary injury

Several authors have evaluated biliary complications (21,22). It has been shown that radiation cholecystitis and grade 3 bilirubin toxicity are rare. Kulik et al. treated 108 patients with HCC. Patients with and without PVT received a cumulative dose of 139.7 and 131.9 Gy, respectively. Ibrahim et al. treated 24 patients diagnosed with cholangiocarcinoma with 48 ^{90}Y treatments. The overall median dose to the liver was 105.1 Gy and the accumulated median dose to the lung was 8.4 Gy. No patients developed a symptomatic radiation pneumonitis. One patient (4%) developed a gastroduodenal ulcer that necessitated surgical intervention.

Portal hypertension

Postradioembolization fibrosis leads to a decrease in the volume of the treated lobe. The time for development of portal hypertension is variable (38). It is more often associated with bilobar treatment and its incidence is increased in patients who have chemotherapy-associated steatohepatitis. Despite imaging findings suggestive of portal hypertension, clinically significant occurrence of portal hypertension is low (38).

Radiation pneumonitis

Radiation pneumonitis has been seen when the LSF is greater than 13% (39). Radiation pneumonitis is a restrictive pulmonary dysfunction. The LSF is used to calculate the dose that would be administered to the lung, and an absolute contraindication to radioembolization is the predicted administration of a dose greater than or equal to 30 Gy to the lungs in a single treatment or greater than 50 Gy as a cumulative dose after multiple treatments (40). Radiation pneumonitis can be diagnosed clinically and on finding consolidation on chest x-rays.

Gastrointestinal complications

The inadvertent spread of microspheres to the gastrointestinal tract is responsible for complications such as ulceration (41,42). This complication is severe and may require surgical intervention. Meticulous mapping of the blood vessels to look for aberrant vasculature arising from branches of the hepatic artery that supply the gastrointestinal tract can prevent the occurrence of ulceration. Nevertheless, prophylactic use of proton pump inhibitors is recommended.

Vascular injury

Transcatheter ^{90}Y radioembolization is an invasive procedure. The incidence of vascular injury is very low and mostly has been seen in patients who were already on systemic chemotherapy (43). Systemic chemotherapy might cause weakening of the vessel wall leading to an increased susceptibility to injury.

■ CONCLUSIONS

Radioembolization represents an innovative treatment approach that has gained increased awareness and clinical use during the past 15 years. Patients are able to resume normal activities shortly following treatment with minimal side effects. Treatment planning requires important steps including (a) visceral angiography to map out tumor-perfusing vessels and to embolize collaterals; (b) assessment of LSF; (c) determination of the optimal therapeutic dose; (d) radiation monitoring and safety procedures; (e) calculation of residual activity and efficiency of radiation delivery.

Selection of patients with adequate hepatic reserve and good functional status will maximize the beneficial therapeutic effect of this therapy with minimal risk to normal liver parenchyma. This treatment has also shown to be beneficial for patients presenting with metastatic disease who have intrahepatic progression despite standard of care chemotherapy. The potential to increase survival and improve quality of life makes radioembolization an important treatment modality in the management of liver tumors. The occurrence of adverse events can be minimized by careful assessment of angiographic findings before treatment; these occur rarely and can usually be managed conservatively.

■ REFERENCES

1. El-Serag HB. Hepatocellular carcinoma and hepatitis C in the United States. *Hepatology.* 2002;36:S74–S83.
2. Gyves JW, Ziessman HA, Ensminger WD, et al. Definition of hepatic tumor microcirculation by single photon emission computerized tomography (SPECT). *J Nucl Med.* 1984;25:972–977.
3. Ingold JA, Reed GB, Kaplan HS, et al. Radiation hepatitis. *Am J Roentgenol Radium Ther Nucl Med.* 1965;93:200–208.
4. Geschwind JF, Salem R, Carr BI, et al. Yttrium-90 microspheres for the treatment of hepatocellular carcinoma. *Gastroenterology.* 2004;127: S194–S205.
5. Dawson LA, McGinn NJ, Ensminger WD. Preliminary results of escalated focal liver radiation and hepatic artery floxuridine for unresectable liver malignancies. *Am Soc Clin Oncol.* 1999;18:86.
6. Nolan TR, Grady ED. Intravascular particulate radioisotope therapy: clinical observations of 76 patients with advanced cancer treated with 90-yttrium particles. *Am Surg.* 1969;35:181–188.
7. Mantravadi RV, Spigos DG, Tan WS, et al. Intraarterial yttrium 90 in the treatment of hepatic malignancy. *Radiology.* 1982;142:783–786.
8. Wollner I, Knutsen C, Smith P, et al. Effects of hepatic arterial yttrium 90 glass microspheres in dogs. *Cancer.* 1988;61:1336–1344.
9. Wollner IS, Knutsen CA, Ullrich KA, et al. Effects of hepatic arterial yttrium-90 microsphere administration alone and combined with regional bromodeoxyuridine infusion in dogs. *Cancer Res.* 1987;47: 3285–3290.
10. Shepherd FA, Rotstein LE, Houle S, et al. A phase I dose escalation trial of yttrium-90 microspheres in the treatment of primary hepatocellular carcinoma. *Cancer.* 1992;70:2250–2254.
11. Yan ZP, Lin G, Zhao HY, et al. An experimental study and clinical pilot trials on yttrium-90 glass microspheres through the hepatic artery for treatment of primary liver cancer. *Cancer.* 1993;72:3210–3215.
12. Andrews JC, Walker SC, Ackermann RJ, et al. Hepatic radioembolization with yttrium-90 containing glass microspheres: preliminary results and clinical follow-up. *J Nucl Med.* 1994;35:1637–1644.
13. Lau WY, Leung WT, Ho S, et al. Treatment of inoperable hepatocellular carcinoma with intrahepatic arterial yttrium-90 microspheres: a phase I and II study. *Br J Cancer.* 1994;70:994–999.
14. Covey AM, Brody LA, Maluccio MA, et al. Variant hepatic arterial anatomy revisited: digital subtraction angiography performed in 600 patients. *Radiology.* 2002;224:542–547.
15. Liu DM, Salem R, Bui JT, et al. Angiographic considerations in patients undergoing liver-directed therapy. *J Vasc Interv Radiol.* 2005;16:911–935.
16. Murthy R, Nunez R, Szklaruk J, et al. Yttrium-90 microsphere therapy for hepatic malignancy: devices, indications, technical considerations, and potential complications. *Radiographics.* 2005;25(suppl 1):S41–S55.
17. Cosin O, Bilbao JI, Alvarez S, et al. Right gastric artery embolization prior to treatment with yttrium-90 microspheres. *Cardiovasc Intervent Radiol.* 2007;30:98–103.
18. Salem R, Thurston KG, Carr BI, et al. Yttrium-90 microspheres: radiation therapy for unresectable liver cancer. *J Vasc Interv Radiol.* 2002;13:S223–S229.
19. Riaz A, Kulik L, Lewandowski RJ, et al. Radiologic-pathologic correlation of hepatocellular carcinoma treated with internal radiation using yttrium-90 microspheres. *Hepatology.* 2009;49:1185–1193.
20. Rhee TK, Naik NK, Deng J, et al. Tumor response after yttrium-90 radioembolization for hepatocellular carcinoma: comparison of diffusion-weighted functional MR imaging with anatomic MR imaging. *J Vasc Interv Radiol.* 2008;19:1180–1186.
21. Kulik LM, Atassi B, van Holsbeeck L, et al. Yttrium-90 microspheres (TheraSphere) treatment of unresectable hepatocellular carcinoma: downstaging to resection, RFA and bridge to transplantation. *J Surg Oncol.* 2006;94:572–586.
22. Kulik LM, Carr BI, Mulcahy MF, et al. Safety and efficacy of (90)Y radiotherapy for hepatocellular carcinoma with and without portal vein thrombosis. *Hepatology.* 2008;47:71–81.
23. Ibrahim SM, Mulcahy MF, Lewandowski RJ, et al. Treatment of unresectable cholangiocarcinoma using yttrium-90 microspheres: results from a pilot study. *Cancer.* 2008;113:2119–2128.
24. Welsh JS, Kennedy AS, Thomadsen B. Selective internal radiation therapy (SIRT) for liver metastases secondary to colorectal adenocarcinoma. *Int J Radiat Oncol Biol Phys.* 2006;66:S62–S73.
25. Gray B, Van Hazel G, Hope M, et al. Randomised trial of SIR-Spheres plus chemotherapy vs. chemotherapy alone for treating patients with liver metastases from primary large bowel cancer. *Ann Oncol.* 2001; 12:1711–1720.
26. Goin JE, Dancey JE, Hermann GA, et al. Treatment of unresectable metastatic colorectal carcinoma to the liver with intrahepatic Y-90 microspheres: a dose-ranging study. *World J Nucl Med.* 2003;2:216–225.
27. Rhee TK, Lewandowski RJ, Liu DM, et al. ^{90}Y Radioembolization for metastatic neuroendocrine liver tumors: preliminary results from a multi-institutional experience. *Ann Surg.* 2008;247:1029–1035.
28. Kennedy AS, Dezarn WA, McNeillie P, et al. Radioembolization for unresectable neuroendocrine hepatic metastases using resin 90Y-microspheres: early results in 148 patients. *Am J Clin Oncol.* 2008; 31:271–279.
29. Coldwell D, Nutting C, Kennedy AK. Treatment of Hepatic Metastases from Breast Cancer with Yttrium-90 SIR-Spheres Radioembolization.

Presented at the annual meeting of the Society of Interventional Radiology, New Orleans, LA, 2005.

30. Jakobs TF, Hoffmann RT, Fischer T, et al. Radioembolization in patients with hepatic metastases from breast cancer. *J Vasc Interv Radiol.* 2008;19:683–690.
31. Sato KT, Lewandowski RJ, Mulcahy MF, et al. Unresectable chemorefractory liver metastases: radioembolization with ^{90}Y microspheres—safety, efficacy, and survival. *Radiology.* 2008;247:507–515.
32. Kennedy AS, Coldwell D, Nutting C, et al. Resin ^{90}Y-microsphere brachytherapy for unresectable colorectal liver metastases: modern USA experience. *Int J Radiat Oncol Biol Phys.* 2006;65:412–425.
33. Salem R, Lewandowski RJ, Atassi B, et al. Treatment of unresectable hepatocellular carcinoma with use of 90Y microspheres (TheraSphere): safety, tumor response, and survival. *J Vasc Interv Radiol.* 2005;16:1627–1639.
34. Murthy R, Xiong H, Nunez R, et al. Yttrium 90 resin microspheres for the treatment of unresectable colorectal hepatic metastases after failure of multiple chemotherapy regimens: preliminary results. *J Vasc Interv Radiol.* 2005;16:937–945.
35. Young JY, Rhee TK, Atassi B, et al. Radiation dose limits and liver toxicities resulting from multiple yttrium-90 radioembolization treatments for hepatocellular carcinoma. *J Vasc Interv Radiol.* 2007;18:1375–1382.
36. Sangro B, Gil-Alzugaray B, Rodriguez J, et al. Liver disease induced by radioembolization of liver tumors: description and possible risk factors. *Cancer.* 2008;112:1538–1546.
37. Kennedy AS, McNeillie P, Dezarn WA, et al. Treatment parameters and outcome in 680 treatments of internal radiation with resin 90Y-microspheres for unresectable hepatic tumors. *Int J Radiat Oncol Biol Phys.* 2009;74(5):1494–1500.
38. Jakobs TF, Saleem S, Atassi B, et al. Fibrosis, portal hypertension, and hepatic volume changes induced by intra-arterial radiotherapy with 90yttrium microspheres. *Dig Dis Sci.* 2008;53:2556–2563.
39. Leung TW, Lau WY, Ho SK, et al. Radiation pneumonitis after selective internal radiation treatment with intraarterial 90yttrium-microspheres for inoperable hepatic tumors. *Int J Radiat Oncol Biol Phys.* 1995;33:919–924.
40. TheraSphere Yttrium-90 microspheres [package insert]. Kanata, Canada: MDS Nordion; 2004.
41. Murthy R, Brown DB, Salem R, et al. Gastrointestinal complications associated with hepatic arterial Yttrium-90 microsphere therapy. *J Vasc Interv Radiol.* 2007;18:553–561; quiz 562.
42. Carretero C, Munoz-Navas M, Betes M, et al. Gastroduodenal injury after radioembolization of hepatic tumors. *Am J Gastroenterol.* 2007;102:1216–1220.
43. Murthy R, Eng C, Krishnan S, et al. Hepatic yttrium-90 radioembolotherapy in metastatic colorectal cancer treated with cetuximab or bevacizumab. *J Vasc Interv Radiol.* 2007;18:1588–1591.

Radioembolization with Yttrium-90 Microspheres for Primary and Metastatic Hepatic Cancer

Andrew Kennedy and James Welsh

■ INTRODUCTION

Radioembolization (RE) is defined as the intra-arterial delivery of micron-sized radioisotope-tagged particles that preferentially and permanently embed in tumor as opposed to normal tissue. The technique is specified through fluoroscopic guidance of intravascular catheters with endpoints of adequate coverage of tumor by implanted microspheres inferred by changes in tumor vascular flow. Radiation dose planning, administration and delivery of radiation, is modified on the basis of tumor and hepatic volumes which are essential considerations for the safety and efficacy of the procedure. This treatment modality delivers effective doses of radiation to primary or metastatic liver lesions via infusions directly into the hepatic arterial circulation. In the United States, the technique is Food and Drug Administration approved for liver metastases secondary to colorectal carcinoma and is under investigation for treatment of other liver malignancies, including hepatocellular carcinoma (HCC) and neuroendocrine tumors (NET). In older literature the terms "selective internal radiation therapy" and "Y-90 microsphere brachytherapy" were used to describe this treatment; a multidisciplinary panel of experts recommended the term "radioembolization" as a more accurate description. This is now the accepted term (1).

RE selectively targets a high radiation dose of yttrium-90 (^{90}Y), a beta emitter, to all tumors within the liver, regardless of their cell of origin or location, while at the same time limiting to within tolerable levels the dose to normal liver parenchyma (2–5). Preferential deposition of microspheres embedded with ^{90}Y within the tumor capillary bed causes a tumoricidal dose (Fig. 24.1) of radiation (100 to 1000+ Gray [Gy]) to be absorbed over a limited range (mean tissue penetration 2.5 mm; maximum 11 mm) for a limited time (2); ^{90}Y decays to stable zirconium-90 with an average half-life of 2.67 days (64.2 hours).

The expanding literature reports good and encouraging results in both retrospective and prospective reports as demonstrated by low acute or late toxicity and high response rates. Use of this treatment modality has led to improved time to liver progression and extended overall patient survival. The main side effects include fatigue, pain, and nausea/vomiting. Although phase III trials of RE as first-line treatment of patients with metastatic colorectal cancer are ongoing, sufficient phase II and retrospective clinical data support the use of RE in salvage therapy for most patients in this setting. Patients with HCC, NET, as well as cancer in other primary sites, including breast and lung, have also shown promising response and survival.

Worldwide approximately 20,000 patients will have received this revolutionary treatment by the end of 2009. The main body of evidence from prospective studies, and particularly from randomized controlled trials, is with ^{90}Y resin microspheres (SIR-Spheres® microspheres; Sirtex Medical, Sydney, Australia) in colorectal and other liver metastases (6–18), but several single-arm studies have reported the results of using ^{90}Y glass microspheres (TheraSphere®; MDS Nordion, Ottawa, Canada) in HCC (19–22).

■ ELIGIBILITY

A Consensus Panel Report by the Radioembolization Brachytherapy Oncology Consortium provides detailed guidelines for RE eligibility and patient selection (23). The multidisciplinary team carefully assesses which patients are most likely to benefit from this treatment modality. Eligible patients include those with unresectable hepatic primary or metastatic cancer and liver-dominant tumor burden. Because a small amount of normal liver tissue immediately adjacent to the tumor will be destroyed by radiation, sufficient liver reserve is required. The appropriateness of RE is governed in each patient by the number of well-established and accepted parameters for liver reserve and vascular access. The important indicators of adequate liver tolerance for RE include a lack of ascites, normal synthetic liver function (e.g., albumin greater than 3 g/dL), and normal total bilirubin of less than 2.0 mg/dL (less than 34 µmol/L).

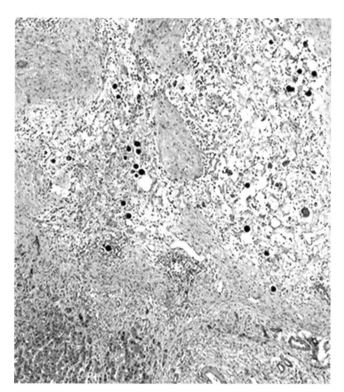

FIGURE 24.1 Photomicrograph of hematoxylin and eosin stained hepatic tissue showing microspheres (black spheres) embedded in tissue that was formally metastatic colon cancer but is now only fibrosis. Original magnification 100×.

■ CLINICAL INDICATIONS

Because the nature of primary and secondary hepatic malignancies differs, therapy should be tailored to the disease. Patients considered for RE therapy would include those with (a) unresectable hepatic primary or metastatic cancer, (b) liver-dominant tumor burden, and (c) a life expectancy of at least 3 months. Good candidates for referral are also those patients with an Eastern Cooperative Oncology Group (ECOG) performance status of 0 to 2, particularly for certain tumor types where RE can be safely combined with systemic chemotherapy.

It is notable that the responses seen with newer combination chemotherapy regimens sometimes convert patients with unresectable liver metastases to resectable status. The integration of combination therapy with irinotecan, oxaliplatin, and bevacizumab has improved response rates and survival of patients with metastatic colorectal cancer, as demonstrated in large randomized trials (24–26). In metastatic colorectal cancer, RE therapy is given (a) alone after failure of first-line chemotherapy, (b) with FUDR during first-line therapy, or (c) during first- or second-line chemotherapy on a clinical trial, and (d) in salvage therapy combined with 5FU, leucovorin, oxaliplatin, or irinotecan. Similarly, patients with hepatic metastases from other primary sites should be offered standard systemic treatment options with known survival benefit before ^{90}Y treatment. In the case of primary liver tumors, patients should undergo hepatology and transplant evaluations to determine the optimal treatment strategy. Earlier integration of RE into the treatment paradigm can provide the added options of using systemic chemotherapy synergistically as a radiosensitizer and/or to control extrahepatic metastases; permitting a reduction in hepatic disease, thereby improving the potential for ablation, resection, and transplantation; and conserving remaining liver function, thus allowing for the possibility of improved patient survival and quality of life.

Contraindications to RE therapy may include (a) pretreatment ^{99m}Tc macroaggregated albumin (MAA) scan demonstrating the potential of ≥30 Gy to the lung or any flow to the gastrointestinal tract (Fig. 24.2) resulting in extrahepatic deposition of ^{99m}Tc-MAA that cannot be corrected

FIGURE 24.2 A: ^{99m}Tc-MAA scan (coronal view) showing a normal liver to lung shunt of 6% and an abnormal shunt. B: An abnormal ^{99m}Tc-MAA scan with both stomach uptake and an excessive shunting of microparticles (45%) to the lungs.

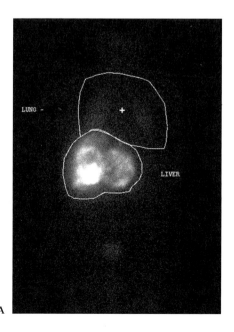

A

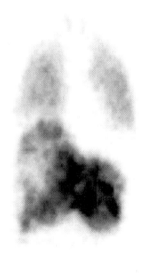

B

Table **24.1**	Most common acute (0–30 days) and delayed (31+ days) grade 2–3 toxicities (CTCae 3.0) (27)			
	Incidence Grade			
Side Effect	**2**	**3**	**Clinical Presentation**	**Prevention/Treatment**
Constitutional total	43%	1%		
Weight loss	3%	0%	Days 0–7 posttreatment	Antiemetics, low-dose steroids for 7 days
Fatigue	37%	1%	Days 0–14 posttreatment	Low-dose steroids for 7 days
Fever	2%	0%	Days 0–3 posttreatment	Pan-cultures not necessary, acetaminophen in low doses safe for 3–7 days
Gastrointestinal total	25%	5%		
Nausea	9	1	Days 0–3 posttreatment	Antiemetics, low-dose steroids for 7 days
Emesis	6	1	Days 0–3 posttreatment	Antiemetics, low-dose steroids for 7 days
Pain	11	2	Days 0–14 posttreatment	Analgesics prn
Ulceration	5% (median) (0–20%)		Nausea, pain beyond day #14 posttreatment	Prophylactic embolization of GDA, gastric arteries
Radiation Cholecystitis	<1%		Persistent abdominal pain	Avoid cystic artery
Hepatic Abscess	<1%		Abdominal pain, septic symptoms	Prophylactic antibiotics in patients with violated ampulla or prior Whipple
Biochemical	16%	2%	Steady rise first 6 weeks posttreatment, return to baseline by 12 weeks posttreatment	Appropriate radiation dose selection
Radiation pancreatitis	<1%		Abdominal pain, elevated enzymes typical for pancreatitis	Supportive care
Radiation-induced liver disease (RILD)	<1% (median) (0–4%)		Progressive ascites and elevation of alkaline phosphatase, AST, ALT, and ± total bilirubin, ammonia levels	Steroids, supportive care
Radiation pneumonitis	<1%		Can be asymptomatic, but serious cases present with pleural effusion and can progress to ARDS	Steroids, supportive care

AST, aspartate aminotransferase; ALT, alanine aminotransferase; ARDS, acute respiratory distress syndrome; and GDA, gastroduodenal artery.

by catheter embolization techniques, (b) excessive tumor burden with limited hepatic reserve, (c) elevated total bilirubin level (greater than 2.0 mg/dL) in the absence of a reversible cause, and (d) compromised portal vein, unless selective or superselective RE can be performed. Patients with prior radiotherapy involving the liver should be carefully reviewed on a case-by-case basis (23). Microsphere RE is conducted using a multidisciplinary team approach. The well-integrated team involves representatives from interventional radiology, radiation oncology, nuclear medicine, medical oncology, surgical oncology, and medical physics.

Toxicity

The typical side-effect profile for RE is generally of lower intensity than the profiles of transarterial embolization or transarterial chemoembolization (TACE) with virtually no cases of true postembolization syndrome. Most current reports in the literature use the Common Toxicity Criteria of Adverse Events (CTCae) 3.0, although a large part of the literature uses CTCae 2.0 and World Health Organization (WHO) criteria. The most common side effects, their clinical

presentations, and treatments are summarized in Table 24.1 (27). Special cases to consider are patients with neuroendocrine primary tumors with typical symptoms of ongoing carcinoid syndrome prior to liver treatment. As is the case with embolic therapy to the liver in these tumor types, release of active peptides from abrupt tumor lysis can lead to severe symptoms. Although rare, respiratory distress and/or dangerous hypertension can result even while the patient is receiving microsphere therapy in the interventional suite. Emergent supportive care including escalating doses of Sandostatin (octreotide) is used to reverse the acute effects and stabilize the patient.

Radiation details

The U.S. Nuclear Regulatory Commission (NRC) guidelines for the approved use of radioactive microspheres as a brachytherapy procedure follow the Code of Federal Register 35, under 10, part 35.1000, and are very similar in most respects to conventional brachytherapy procedures (http://www.nrc.gov/materials/miau/med-use-toolkit/microsphere.html). This treatment may be prescribed only by authorized users that satisfy the training and experience requirements for this type of brachytherapy. The NRC Licensing Guidance for ^{90}Y microspheres states that the written directive (prescription) should be made in terms of absorbed radiation dose or equivalent dose (i.e., rad, Gy, rem, or Sv) to the primary target and should specify a maximum allowed dose to sites outside the target. Although both commercial manufacturers describe procedures for dose calculation in their product material, the calculations often have little relation to the true dose delivered. Only certain activities can be ordered, and the treatment time is then determined so the calculated activity will be delivered.

Recognizing the extreme difficulty (to impossibility) of determining the actual absorbed dose to tumors in most clinical settings, the NRC has allowed prescription of treatment for SIR-Spheres® to be based on a model that was used in earlier clinical trials. In this fashion, three factors determine the prescribed activity: (a) the extent of disease (i.e., fraction of liver involved with tumor), (b) fractional shunting to the lung, and (c) the amount of the liver to be treated (i.e., right, left, or both lobes).

Dosimetry

To better understand the following activity calculations (Equations 24.1 to 24.4 below) for ^{90}Y microspheres, let us review the schema developed by the Medical Internal Radiation Dose (MIRD) Committee of the Society of Nuclear Medicine.

In this formalism, the dose rate ($\dot{D}$) can be written as

$$\dot{D} = k\frac{A}{m}|E|, \qquad \text{(Eq. 24.1)}$$

where k is a constant to yield the dose rate in desired units, A the source activity, m the mass of tissue that the radiation is absorbed within, and $\langle E \rangle$ the average energy emitted per nuclear transition. Since we are dealing with a source undergoing nuclear decay, the activity of the source is not constant in time. Also the source is permanently implanted in the patient with no biologic excretion. Thus, the activity as a function of time is described by the radioactive decay equation

$$A(t) = A_0 e^{-\ln(2)t/T}, \qquad \text{(Eq. 24.2)}$$

where A_0 is the calibrated activity, t the time from calibration, and T the half-life of the radioactive source. The absorbed dose, calculated by integrating overall time, is then given by the following

$$D = \frac{k\langle E \rangle A_0}{m}\int_0^\infty e^{-\ln(2)t/T}dt = k\frac{A_0}{m}\langle E \rangle\frac{T}{\ln(2)} \qquad \text{(Eq. 24.3)}$$

From the published decay data in MIRD format, the average energy released in the β-decay of ^{90}Y is 0.9337 MeV (Bq s)$^{-1}$ or 0.5385 Gy kg (GBq h)$^{-1}$, assuming that all of the energy of the β-decay is absorbed in tissue (20). Using the

half-life $T = 64.2$ hours, the total radiation-absorbed dose after the complete β-decay of ^{90}Y is given by

$$D[\text{Gy}] = 49.9\frac{A_0[\text{GBq}]}{m[\text{kg}]} \qquad \text{(Eq. 24.4)}$$

The difference between the 49.9 constant given here and the 49,670 constant used in the partition model method for ^{90}Y resin microspheres is explained by taking the mass in kilograms instead of grams and using current values for the average energy released in the decay process.

Selection of ^{90}Y activity with resin microspheres

All patients undergo computed tomography (CT) treatment planning with reconstruction of the liver volumes (whole liver, and right and left lobes). The selection of activity for treatment is individualized according to histologic tumor type; vascularity of the tumor; uptake characteristics as seen on the angiogram, CT, and MAA scan; performance status of the patient; and whether concurrent chemotherapy will be given. Activity to be infused is calculated prospectively by one of two methods described in the manufacturer's User's Manual and Package Insert:

(I) Body surface area (BSA) method;
(II) Partition model method.

The following description will apply to the BSA method.

BSA method

The BSA method varies the prescribed activity of ^{90}Y according to the size of the patient and the proportion of tumor involvement within the liver. This is the most widely used method for determining the prescribed activity of ^{90}Y resin microspheres.

The patient's BSA is normally derived from a weight/height chart but can also be calculated using the following equation

$$\text{BSA}[\text{m}^2] = 0.20247 \times (\text{height}[\text{m}])^{0.725} \times (\text{weight}[\text{kg}])^{0.425} \qquad \text{(Eq. 24.5)}$$

The prescribed activity is then calculated using the BSA together with the volume of tumor (V_T) and overall volume of liver including tumor ($V_T + V_L$) (calculated from the CT or magnetic resonance imaging [MRI] scan), by the following equation

$$A[\text{GBq}] = (\text{BSA} - 0.2) + \frac{V_T}{V_T + V_L}, \qquad \text{(Eq. 24.6)}$$

where A = activity (GBq)
V_T = volume of tumor (cm^3) from CT/MRI scan
V_L = volume of liver (cm^3) from CT/MRI scan

Prescribed activity calculations for lobar treatments

In the case of lobar treatments, for example, a single lobar treatment for disease in only one lobe, or for sequential lobar treatments for disease in both lobes, the BSA formula should be modified as follows:

$$A_{lobe}[GBq] = \left(BSA - 0.2 + \left\{\frac{V_{Tumor\ lobe}}{V_{Total\ lobe}}\right\}\right) \cdot \left(\frac{V_{Total\ lobe}}{V_{Total\ Liver}}\right),$$

where A_{lobe} = activity in the lobe (GBq)
$V_{Tumor\ lobe}$ = volume of tumor (cm^3) in the lobe
$V_{Total\ lobe}$ = volume of lobe including tumor (cm^3)
$V_{Total\ Liver}$ = volume of whole liver including tumor (cm^3)

Required activity reductions

The prescribed activity of ^{90}Y resin microspheres may need to be reduced depending on specific factors including excessive (greater than 10%) shunting to the lung or if hepatic function is compromised.

Excessive lung shunting

The ^{99m}Tc-MAA study is conducted during the work-up procedure in order to determine the proportion of ^{90}Y resin microspheres and therefore radiation that may reach the lungs through arteriovenous shunting. Excessive lung shunting may be defined in either of two ways: (a) as a degree of liver to lung shunting that will lead to a cumulative lung dose of 30 Gy or more and (b) more simplistically, as liver to lung shunting of greater than 10%.

It is recommended by a consensus panel that the cumulative lung dose be less than 30 Gy, although the manufacturer of the ^{90}Y resin microspheres recommends less than 25 Gy and preferably less than 20 Gy (7).

The activity that may potentially reach the lung can be calculated by the following formula

$$A_{lung}[GBq] = A_{total} \times \frac{L}{100},$$

where A_{lung} = lung activity (GBq)
A_{total} = total prescribed activity (GBq)
L = lung shunt (%)

The resulting lung dose, given a certain amount of activity shunting from the liver to the lung, can be calculated by the following formula

$$D_{lung}(Gy) = \frac{49670 \times A_{lung}}{M_{lung}},$$

where D_{lung} = lung dose (Gy)
A_{lung} = lung activity (GBq)
M_{lung} = mass of the lung (g)

As the lung is largely filled with air, CT/MRI scans cannot be used to measure the volume of the lung parenchyma and hence an estimation of 1000 mL is made. For the purpose of calculating tissue mass, all tissue densities are estimated at 1 g/mL.

A more simplistic definition of excessive lung shunting has been employed by the manufacturer of ^{90}Y resin microspheres. This definition recommends reducing the prescribed activity of ^{90}Y resin microspheres if the lung shunting is greater than 10%.

RADIATION SAFETY

Because the ^{90}Y used in RE is a pure beta emitter with a half-life of just 64.2 hours, radiation safety issues are typically not problematic. The manufacturer-provided Lucite shielding effectively blocks the beta radiation and, thanks to its low average atomic number, does not generate significant bremsstrahlung gamma radiation. Under ordinary circumstances, the dose to personnel from fluoroscopy approximates the dose from the microspheres during the procedure. The area in which particular care should be exerted is in the prevention and rapid cleanup of any spills. Unlike unsealed radiopharmaceuticals in solution that dry in place after a spill, the microspheres, once dry, can roll about and move with the air current, presenting a hazard. The microspheres can also wedge themselves into tiny crevices on tabletops or equipment, becoming practically impossible to remove. Appropriate planning and care reduces this risk and contamination of interventional radiology suites is extremely rare. Radiation precaution should follow guidelines of the consensus panel (23).

LIVER ANATOMY, VASCULATURE, TUMOR VASCULATURE

Because metastatic lesions in the liver preferentially receive their blood supply from the hepatic artery whereas normal liver parenchyma is fed primarily through the hepatic portal vein (28,29), this provides a natural means of selectively delivering radiation via infused radioactive microspheres. In 1970 Lien and Ackerman (30) described silicone rubber casts of tumor vessels forming a ring around the periphery of the tumor in a plexus, such that tumors larger than 0.03 g received about three quarters of their blood supply from the hepatic artery. This estimate has been confirmed in experimental investigations of microspheres of varying sizes (31). The metastatic tumor vasculature tends to differ in other ways, including increased capillary diameter and length, greater intercapillary distances, higher endothelial proliferation rates, arterial-venous fistulas, and loss of the typical vascular hierarchy of arterioles, capillaries, venules, and then veins (32).

In addition to the anatomic differences between tumor and normal liver vasculature, there is a differential physiologic response to vasoconstrictors (33). For example, animal experiments demonstrated that normal hepatic arterioles constrict in response to a 50-μg bolus injection of angiotensin II, whereas tumor vasculature exhibits a diminished reaction (34). Therefore, an injection of such a vasoconstrictor will selectively shunt blood toward tumor tissue. This difference can, in principle, be exploited clinically to further improve the selective targeting of tumors over normal liver when using RE. Given the relative radioresistance of hypoxic cells compared to well-oxygenated cells, the aim of microsphere therapy is to maximize trapping of spheres where there is little hypoxia or necrosis—that is, in the tumor periphery rather than the core.

The recommended microsphere size (25 to 35 μm) has been suggested by several investigations (32,35) to balance the objectives of depositing the microspheres within the tumor but not allowing passage through to the venous circulation. Despite the size difference between glass (25 μm) and resin (35 μm) microspheres, Kennedy et al. (2) did not observe any obvious difference in the embolic location of the microspheres on a detailed pathologic examination of liver tissues from treated patients; both microsphere types preferentially localized in the periphery of the tumors. The differences between the microsphere types regarding average sphere size, specific gravity (3.2 g/mL glass vs. 1.6 g/mL resin), and number of particles infused (2 million vs. 50 million, respectively) also made no difference in the particle distribution. Thus, the available data suggest that despite the differences between them, both of the commercially available microsphere products are effective and equivalent in their targeting aims (27).

■ PATIENT EVALUATION, WORKUP, TESTING PRETREATMENT

Treatment with ^{90}Y microspheres is a two-stage process involving an extensive work-up procedure to assess the appropriateness of the patient for treatment and to prepare the liver for radiation and the treatment procedure itself (23). During the workup, three-phase contrast CT and/or gadolinium-enhanced MRI of the liver should be conducted for assessment of tumor and nontumor volume, portal vein patency, and extent of extrahepatic disease. The liver vasculature is then meticulously mapped by a trans-femoral hepatic angiogram to identify any vessels that could carry microspheres away from the liver to the stomach, duodenum, or gallbladder, and to plan the subsequent administration of ^{90}Y microspheres. The gastroduodenal, right gastric, and other extrahepatic arteries are then embolized in order to isolate the hepatic circulation.

To evaluate hepatopulmonary shunting, a simulation of the actual treatment is then performed with technetium-99m labeled macroaggregated albumin (^{99m}Tc-MAA) particles that approximate the size of the microspheres. The ^{99m}Tc-MAA allows for planar and/or single photon emission computed tomography (SPECT) gamma-camera imaging, which can identify the proportion of the microparticles that have passed through to the lungs or can alert the treatment team to any deposition in the gastrointestinal tract. Approximately 20% of patients with HCC and less than 5% of those with liver metastases may have a lung-shunt fraction of greater than 20% and consequently could be unsuitable for treatment if the ^{99m}Tc-MAA simulation suggests they will receive more than 30 Gy exposure to the lungs. One to 3 weeks later, prior to the injection of ^{90}Y microspheres, occlusion is reassessed.

■ TREATMENT PROCEDURE

The RE procedure has been described elsewhere in detail (1,23,36). Treatment comprises two phases: as described, the performance of a hepatic angiogram the week before treatment as well as simulation of microsphere delivery using albumin particles through the hepatic artery. Then, after the procedure, SPECT gamma imaging is used to detect shunting of albumin particles into the gastrointestinal or pulmonary vasculature.

■ CLINICAL RESULTS

Clinical studies have demonstrated that RE using ^{90}Y microspheres has the potential to provide substantial clinical benefits through increased progression-free periods and length of survival, as well as through improved response rates (Fig. 24.3). Studies conducted so far have been small in size, although at least 30 prospective trials have been reported to date. A number of larger randomized controlled trials are examining the role of ^{90}Y resin microspheres in combination with chemotherapy for the treatment of colorectal hepatic metastases. Other trials under way are assessing ^{90}Y microspheres either in combination with chemotherapy or as monotherapy in noncolorectal metastases and in primary liver tumors. The results of these studies, which will take several years to complete, will help to further define the role of RE as a cancer treatment.

The following sections discuss a few of the largest and most current studies for hepatic metastases from colorectal, hepatocellular, neuroendocrine, and breast cancers, as well as miscellaneous tumor types.

■ COLORECTAL CANCER

Localized high-dose tumor-directed radiation is an effective treatment for reducing the burden of colorectal liver metastases (mCRC) (6–11,22,24,26,37–45) (Table 24.2). A single treatment with RE induces profound cytoreduction of mCRC in the liver and significantly prolongs time to progression (TTP), progression-free survival (PFS), and overall survival (OS) even among patients with highly chemorefractive disease. For the first-line treatment of patients with or without extrahepatic metastases, RE augments the treatment response of systemic chemotherapy in patients with advanced unresectable liver metastases, with a PFS and OS as well as response rates that compare favorably with phase II/III data for modern chemotherapy regimens with or without biologics. Moreover, the addition of ^{90}Y resin microspheres to 5FU/LV chemotherapy has been associated with a significant improvement in health-related quality of life (46).

The results of prospective clinical trials suggest that patients could derive increased benefit from earlier access to RE, most notably in combination with chemotherapy and at an early line of therapy (7,10,11,40). Several prospective

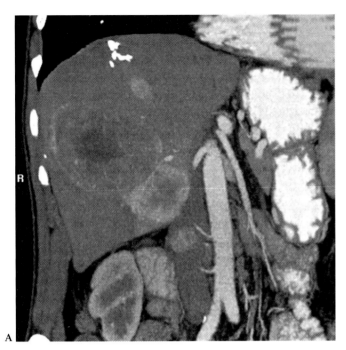
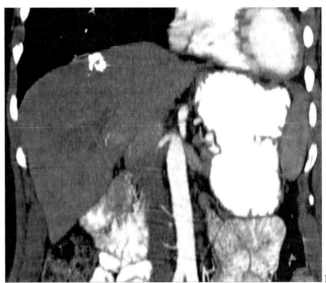

FIGURE 24.3 A: Pretreatment CT scan image of a patient 1 week prior to a single treatment with ^{90}Y resin microspheres. B: Same patient with CT (RECIST) complete response at 5 months postradiation.

studies have provided efficacy and safety data on RE alone or combined with a radiosensitizing chemotherapy regimen as salvage therapy in patients with mCRC that is refractory to standard-of-care chemotherapy options (11,38,40,45, 47–49). The increased response rate with RE plus first-line chemotherapy may also improve the likelihood for potentially curative resection or ablation (50), or induce stabilization of hepatic disease through a radiation lobectomy (11,45,51,52).

The results of clinical trials combining RE with second- or third-line chemotherapy indicate that an objective response may be seen in 30% to 48% of patients (8,10,47). Furthermore, studies in chemorefractory patients have reported that disease progression is delayed following RE and that survival is prolonged compared to either randomized, matched-pair, or historical controls (11,38,40, 45,47–48).

■ HEPATOCELLULAR CANCER

Over the last 10 years, significant data have emerged regarding the role of RE in hepatocellular carcinoma (HCC) (Table 24.3) (22,37,42–44,53). RE may be an option for patients who are not candidates for transplant or resection, and for whom conventional therapies may have limited efficacy and have an urgent need for bridging procedures to enable surgery, ablation, or transplantation. A number of recent reports have supported the effectiveness of ^{90}Y labeled microspheres to treat intermediate to advanced disease in patients with good overall functional performance and liver reserve, and in a

limited role to treat unresectable early-stage disease and patients with portal vein involvement (21–22,42–44, 53–61). By using stringent selection criteria and conservative models for calculating delivered radiation activity, RE can be performed safely in cirrhotic patients without causing significant postembolization syndrome or radiation-induced liver disease, even with multiple treatments (21–22,54). RE compares favorably with TACE in terms of efficacy and tolerability and can be used in a broader group of patients than TACE, including those with more advanced disease, with or without portal vein thrombosis (22,62).

Salem et al., in a prospective longitudinal study of clinical outcomes in a large single-center cohort of HCC patients, recently reported evaluations of those patients who had the greatest potential for successful outcomes with RE treatment (44). In 526 treatments given to 291 patients, where the 30-day mortality rate was 3%, factors predictive of survival included baseline age; sex; performance status; presence of portal hypertension; tumor distribution; levels of bilirubin, albumin, and alpha-fetoprotein; and WHO/EASL response rate.

Sangro and coinvestigators, reporting preliminary results from a multicenter European study, showed tumor nodularity as well as extent of disease at treatment were strong predictors of survival following RE (60). In 250 patients treated with ^{90}Y resin microspheres between 2003 and 2009 at eight European centers, CLIP score, extrahepatic disease, total bilirubin above median, and the number of nodules was retrospectively identified as significant independent predictors of OS.

Table 24.2 Representative summary of clinical outcomes from prospective clinical trials and key retrospective studies of radioembolization using ^{90}Y microspheres for the treatment of colorectal cancer liver metastases

Lead Author, Year	n	Treatment	ORR	SD	Median TTP[a] or PFS[b]		Median Survival	
First-line								
Sharma 2007 (9)	20	^{90}Y resin microspheres + FOLFOX-4	90%	10%	9.3 months[b]		nr	
					14.2 months[b]	In liver only		
Tan 2008[c] (87)	16	^{90}Y resin microspheres + (FOLFOX or 5FU/LV)	82%		9.2 months[b]		>21.9 months	
Second- or third-line								
van Hazel 2009 (10)	25	^{90}Y resin microspheres + irinotecan	48%	39%	6.0 months[b]		12.2 months	
Mixed setting: first-line through to salvage therapy of treatment-refractory disease								
Mulcahy 2009 (47)	72	^{90}Y glass microspheres	40.3%	44.5%	15.4 months		14.5 months	$p < 0.0001$
		ECOG 0					23.5 months	
		ECOG 1					6.7 months	
		ECOG 2					4.0 months	
		Responders (WHO criteria or by PET)					23.5 months	$p < 0.0001$
		Nonresponders					8.5 months	
Salvage therapy of treatment-refractory disease								
Seidensticker 2009 (49)	58	^{90}Y resin microspheres	nr	nr	5.5 months[b]	$p < 0.001$	8.3 months	$p < 0.001$
		Best supportive care	nr	nr	2.1 months[b]		3.5 months	
Cosimelli 2008 (11)	50	^{90}Y resin microspheres	24%	24%	4.0 months[b]		13.0 months	$p = 0.0006$
		Responders (CR + PR + SD)					16.0 months	
		Nonresponders (PD)					8.0 months	
Jakobs 2008 (38)[c]	41	^{90}Y resin microspheres	17%	61%	5.9 months[a]		10.5 months	$p = 0.0001$
		Responders (PR)					29.3 months	
		Responders (SD)					10.9 months	
							4.3 months	
Kennedy 2006 (39–40)[c]	208	^{90}Y resin microspheres	35.5%	55%	7.2 months[a]			
		Responders					10.5 months	$p = 0.0001$
		Nonresponders and historical controls					4.5 months	

[a]TTP: time to progression.
[b]PFS: progression-free survival.
[c]Retrospective study.
ORR, objective response rate (complete response + partial response); SD, stable disease; and nr, not reported.

Table 24.3 **Representative summary of clinical outcomes from prospective clinical trials and retrospective studies of radioembolization using ^{90}Y microspheres for the treatment of hepatocellular carcinoma**

Lead Author, Year	Design	n	Second Line	Treatment/Prognostic Group	ORR	SD	Median TTP	Median Survival	
Salem 2009 (44)	Retrospective cohort	291[a]	13%	^{90}Y glass microspheres	42%	nr	7.9 months	nr	
				BCLC A	21%	nr	25.1 months	26.9 months	nr
				BCLC B	42%	nr	13.3 months	17.2 months	
				BCLC C, no EHD	40%	nr	6.0 months	7.3 months	
				BCLC C, with EHD	11%	nr	3.1 months	5.4 months	
Sangro 2009 (53)	Retrospective cohort	250	18%	^{90}Y resin microspheres	nr	nr	nr	14.1 months	$p < 0.001$
				BCLC A	nr	nr	nr	22.1 months	
				BCLC B	nr	nr	nr	19.4 months	
				BCLC C	nr	nr	nr	10.0 months	
Riaz 2009 (43)	Retrospective cohorts	104	nr	^{90}Y glass microspheres	77%	nr	nr	27.3 months	ns $p = 0.72$
	Nonrandomized	100	nr	TACE	71%	nr	nr	26.0 months	
Iñarrairaegui 2009 (37)	Retrospective cohort	72	40%	^{90}Y resin microspheres	nr	nr	nr	12 months	$p = 0.001$
				≤5 nodules				22 months	
				>5 nodules				8 months	
Minocha 2008 (42)	Retrospective cohort	205	nr	^{90}Y glass microspheres					
				Child A	nr	nr	nr	14.9 months	ns $p = 0.21$
				Child B	nr	nr	nr	6 months	
Kulik 2008 (22)	Prospective phase II	71	nr	^{90}Y glass microspheres					
				No PVT	nr	nr	nr	15.4 months	$p = 0.0052$
	First- or second-line, advanced disease with PVT	25		Branch PVT	nr	nr	nr	10.0 months	
		12		Main PVT	nr	nr	nr	4.4 months	

[a]Includes patients with extrahepatic disease.

ORR, objective response rate (complete response + partial response); SD, stable disease; TTP, time to progression; nr, not reported; ns, not statistically significant; PVT, portal vein thrombosis.

Table **24.4** Representative summary of outcomes from prospective clinical trials and retrospective studies of radioembolization using ^{90}Y microspheres for the treatment of neuroendocrine tumor (NET) liver metastases

Lead Author, Year	n	Treatment	ORR	SD	Symptomatic Response	Median TTP	Median Survival	
Kalinowski 2009 (14)	9	^{90}Y resin microspheres	66%	33%	Improved HRQoL	11 months	57% alive at 36 months	
Kennedy 2008 (64)[a]	148	^{90}Y resin microspheres	63.2%	22.7%	nr	nr	70 months	
King 2008 (12)	34	^{90}Y resin microspheres + 5FU	50%	14.7%	55%	nr	59% alive at 35.2 months	
Rhee 2008 (63)	42							
	20	^{90}Y resin microspheres	50%	44%	nr	nr	28 months	ns ($p = 0.82$)
	22	^{90}Y glass microspheres	53.8%	38.5%	nr	nr	22 months	

[a]Retrospective study.
ORR, objective response rate (complete response + partial response); SD, stable disease; TTP, time to progression; HRQoL, health-related quality of life; nr, not reported; and ns, not statistically significant.

Thus, for unresectable HCC patients presenting with portal vein occlusion/thrombosis, the published clinical experience presented independently by a number of centers demonstrates a favorable risk/benefit ratio for ^{90}Y microsphere therapy, with minimal toxicity compared to more embolic therapies such as TACE.

▪ NEUROENDOCRINE CANCERS

RE has been used to treat tumors from a range of primary neuroendocrine sites, including carcinoid and islet cell carcinomas as well as nonfunctional, asymptomatic tumors.

Initial clinical studies and retrospective studies on a large cohort of patients with metastatic neuroendocrine tumors (mNETs) indicate that RE is well tolerated and highly effective in achieving a durable hepatic tumor response and ameliorating symptoms (Table 24.4) (12–14,63,64). The benefits of RE appear to extend from use in early lines of treatment through to salvage of refractory disease (13,14,41,65,66).

In a retrospective review conducted across 10 clinical centers, 148 patients with unresectable liver metastases from mNET were treated with ^{90}Y resin microspheres (64). The acute and delayed toxicity was very low and quality-of-life

Table **24.5** Summary of clinical outcomes from clinical trials and studies of radioembolization for the treatment of breast cancer liver metastases

Lead Author, Year	n	Treatment	ORR	SD	Median TTP	Median Survival	
Treatment hiatus or chemorefractory disease							
Coldwell 2007 (67)[a]	44	^{90}Y resin microspheres	47%[b]	47%[b]	nr	86% alive at 14 months	
Chemorefractory disease							
Jakobs 2008 (15)	30	^{90}Y resin microspheres	61%[b]	35%[b]	nr	11.7 months	$p = 0.005$
		Responders (PR)				23.6 months	
		Nonresponders (SD or PD)				5.7 months	
		No EHD				16 months	$p = 0.077$
		EHD				9.6 months	
Bangash 2007 (68)	27	^{90}Y glass microspheres	39%[c]	52%[c]	nr	nr	
		ECOG 0				6.8 months	ns ($p = 0.24$)
		ECOG 1–3				2.6 months	
		<25% liver involvement				9.4 months	$p = 0.0001$
		>25% liver involvement				2.0 months	

[a]Retrospective study.
[b]By RECIST.
[c]By WHO criteria.
ORR, objective response rate (complete response + partial response); SD, stable disease; TTP, time to progression; nr, not reported; ns, not statistically significant; and EHD, extrahepatic disease.

measures obtained prospectively before and after RE compared favorably to other loco-regional therapies. The effective disease control and effect on quality of life following RE merits its consideration as an option for both functional and nonfunctional mNETs.

BREAST CANCER

For patients with a metastatic disease burden larger than 3 cm, RE has been reported to provide clinical benefits in patients failing initial lines of chemotherapy or who are chemotherapy-refractory (15,67,68). Three published studies describe RE for breast cancer liver metastases, either during a hiatus between lines of chemotherapy or in patients who are refractory to standard-of-care chemotherapy (Table 24.5) (15,67,68). To date, there are no published data on the use of RE in combination with any chemotherapy regimens in this setting.

MISCELLANEOUS CANCERS

RE has been used worldwide in other cancer settings including, as a partial listing, the following: cholangiocarcinoma (69–76), gastric (69,72,73,75–77), gastrointestinal stromal tumor (69,72,73,78–80), duodenum (76), head and neck (69), mouth (78), pancreas (51,64,69,72,76–82), squamous cell (including that of anus, of oral cavity) (75,76, 78–80,83), unknown primary origin (51,72–74,76,78,83), melanoma (cutaneous, ocular, choroidal) (51,69,72,73,75, 76,79,82,84–86), thymus (69,79,82), sarcoma (51,69,83), thyroid (51,69,76,79), endometrial (72,79,80,83), lung (69,72,76, 79,83), renal (69,79,80), gallbladder (69,72,76), small bowel, adrenal gland (76), esophagus (69,72,76,77,83), ovary (69,72,76,83), cervix (76), prostate (73,74,80), hepatic angiosarcoma (73,76), bone (69), bladder (69,76), lymphoma (76), and parotid gland (76).

CONCLUSIONS

RE using ^{90}Y microspheres has demonstrated acceptable toxicity and impressive efficacy in formal clinical trials and single-institution experience for unresectable primary and metastatic hepatic tumors. Studies have investigated the use of RE alone and in combination with chemotherapy (9,10,87). Effective implementation of this treatment requires a well-integrated multidisciplinary team approach, careful patient selection, and imaging for evaluation and as pretreatment simulation. Radiation safety issues should not be problematic if appropriate precautions are taken. Several innovative investigations of RE for other hepatic malignancies and in combination with newer chemotherapy agents and targeted biologic therapies are under way or in planning.

REFERENCES

1. Salem R, Thurston KG. Radioembolization with 90Yttrium microspheres: a state-of-the-art brachytherapy treatment for primary and secondary liver malignancies. Part 1: technical and methodologic considerations. *J Vasc Interv Radiol*. 2006;17:1251–1278.
2. Kennedy AS, Nutting C, Coldwell D, et al. Pathologic response and microdosimetry of (90)Y microspheres in man: review of four explanted whole livers. *Int J Radiat Oncol Biol Phys*. 2004;60:1552–1563.
3. Burton MA, Gray BN, Kelleher DK, et al. Selective internal radiation therapy: validation of intraoperative dosimetry. *Radiology*. 1990;175:253–255.
4. Burton MA, Gray BN, Klemp PF, et al. Selective internal radiation therapy: distribution of radiation in the liver. *Eur J Cancer Clin Oncol*. 1989;25:1487–1491.
5. Gray BN, Burton MA, Kelleher DK, et al. Selective internal radiation (SIR) therapy for treatment of liver metastases: measurement of response rate. *J Surg Oncol*. 1989;42:192–196.
6. Gray B, Van Hazel G, Hope M, et al. Randomised trial of SIR-Spheres plus chemotherapy vs. chemotherapy alone for treating patients with liver metastases from primary large bowel cancer. *Ann Oncol*. 2001;12:1711–1720.
7. Van Hazel G, Blackwell A, Anderson J, et al. Randomised phase II trial of SIR-Spheres plus flrorouracil/leucovrin chemotherapy versus fluororacil/leucovorin chemotherapy alone in advanced colorectal cancer. *J Surg Oncol*. 2004;88:78–85.
8. Lim L, Gibbs P, Yip D, et al. A prospective evaluation of treatment with Selective Internal Radiation Therapy (SIR-Spheres) in patients with unresectable liver metastases from colorectal cancer previously treated with 5-FU based chemotherapy. *BMC Cancer*. 2005;5:132.
9. Sharma RA, Van Hazel GA, Morgan B, et al. Radioembolization of liver metastases from colorectal cancer using yttrium-90 microspheres with concomitant systemic oxaliplatin, fluorouracil, and leucovorin chemotherapy. *J Clin Oncol*. 2007;25:1099–1106.
10. van Hazel GA, Pavlakis N, Goldstein D, et al. Treatment of fluorouracil-refractory patients with liver metastases from colorectal cancer by using yttrium-90 resin microspheres plus concomitant systemic irinotecan chemotherapy. *J Clin Oncol*. 2009;27:4089–4095.
11. Cosimelli M, Mancini R, Carpanese L, et al. Clinical safety and efficacy of 90yttrium resin microspheres alone in unresectable, heavily pre-treated colorectal liver metastases: results of a phase II trial. ASCO Annual Meeting Proceedings. *J Clin Oncol*. 2008;26:Abstract 4078.
12. King J, Quinn R, Glenn DM, et al. Radioembolization with selective internal radiation microspheres for neuroendocrine liver metastases. *Cancer*. 2008;113:921–929.
13. Meranze SG, Bream PR, Grzeszczak E, et al. Phase II clinical trial of yttrium-90 resin microspheres for the treatment of metastatic neuroendocrine tumor. *Soc Interv Radiol*. 2007:Abstract 422.
14. Kalinowski M, Dressler M, Konig A, et al. Selective internal radiotherapy with yttrium-90 microspheres for hepatic metastatic neuroendocrine tumors: a prospective single center study. *Digestion*. 2009;79:137–142.
15. Jakobs TF, Hoffmann RT, Fischer T, et al. Radioembolization in patients with hepatic metastases from breast cancer. *J Vasc Interv Radiol*. 2008;19:683–690.
16. Sangro B, Bilbao JI, Boan J, et al. Radioembolization using 90Y-resin microspheres for patients with advanced hepatocellular carcinoma. *Int J Radiat Oncol Biol Phys*. 2006;66:792–800.
17. Lau WY, Ho S, Leung TW, et al. Selective internal radiation therapy for nonresectable hepatocellular carcinoma with intraarterial infusion of 90yttrium microspheres. *Int J Radiat Oncol Biol Phys*. 1998;40:583–592.
18. Lau WY, Leung WT, Ho S, et al. Treatment of inoperable hepatocellular carcinoma with intrahepatic arterial yttrium-90 microspheres: a phase I and II study. *Br J Cancer*. 1994;70:994–999.
19. Dancey JE, Shepherd FA, Paul K, et al. Treatment of nonresectable hepatocellular carcinoma with intrahepatic 90Y-microspheres. *J Nucl Med*. 2000;41:1673–1681.
20. Steel J, Baum A, Carr B. Quality of life in patients diagnosed with primary hepatocellular carcinoma: hepatic arterial infusion of cisplatin versus 90-yttrium microspheres (TheraSphere). *Psychooncology*. 2004;13:73–79.
21. Salem R, Lewandowski R, Roberts C, et al. Use of yttrium-90 glass microspheres (TheraSphere) for the treatment of unresectable hepatocellular carcinoma in patients with portal vein thrombosis. *J Vasc Interv Radiol*. 2004;15:335–345.
22. Kulik LM, Carr BI, Mulcahy MF, et al. Safety and efficacy of 90Y radiotherapy for hepatocellular carcinoma with and without portal vein thrombosis. *Hepatology*. 2008;47:71–81.
23. Kennedy A, Nag S, Salem R, et al. Recommendations for radioembolization of hepatic malignancies using yttrium-90 microsphere brachytherapy: a consensus panel report from the radioembolization

brachytherapy oncology consortium. *Int J Radiat Oncol Biol Phys.* 2007;68:13–23.

24. Goldberg RM, Sargent DJ, Morton RF, et al. A randomized controlled trial of fluorouracil plus leucovorin, irinotecan, and oxaliplatin combinations in patients with previously untreated metastatic colorectal cancer. *J Clin Oncol.* 2004;22:23–30.

25. Grothey A, Sargent D, Goldberg RM, et al. Survival of patients with advanced colorectal cancer improves with the availability of fluorouracil-leucovorin, irinotecan, and oxaliplatin in the course of treatment. *J Clin Oncol.* 2004;22:1209–1214.

26. Hurwitz H, Fehrenbacher L, Novotny W, et al. Bevacizumab plus irinotecan, fluorouracil, and leucovorin for metastatic colorectal cancer. *N Engl J Med.* 2004;350:2335–2342.

27. Kennedy AS, Salem R. Comparison of two 90Yttrium microsphere agents for hepatic artery brachytherapy. In: *Proceedings of the 14th International Congress on Anti-Cancer Treatment.* 2003;1:156.

28. Breedis C, Young G. The blood supply of neoplasms in the liver. *Am J Pathol.* 1954;30:969–984.

29. Ackerman NB, Lien WM, Kondi ES, et al. The blood supply of experimental liver metastases I: the distribution of hepatic artery and portal vein blood to "small" and "large" tumors. *Surgery.* 1970;66:1067–1072.

30. Lien WM, Ackerman NB. The blood supply of experimental liver metastases II: a microcirculatory study of the normal and tumor vessels of the liver with the use of perfused silicone rubber. *Surgery.* 1970;68:334–340.

31. Meade VM, Burton MA, Gray BN, et al. Distribution of different sized microspheres in experimental hepatic tumours. *Eur J Cancer Clin Oncol.* 1987;23:37–41.

32. Hirst DG. Blood flow and its modulation in malignant tumors. In: Willmott N, Daly JM, eds. *Microspheres and Regional Cancer Therapy.* 1st ed. Boca Raton, FL: CRC Press; 1994:31–56.

33. Willmott N, Goldberg J, Anderson J, et al. Abnormal vasculature of solid tumours: significance for microsphere-based targeting strategies. *Int J Radiat Biol.* 1991;60:195–199.

34. Burton MA, Gray BN, Coletti A. Effect of angiotensin II on blood flow in the transplanted sheep squamous cell carcinoma. *Eur J Cancer Clin Oncol.* 1988;24:1373–1376.

35. Jirtle R, Clifton KH, Rankin JH. Measurement of mammary tumor blood flow in unanesthetized rats. *J Natl Cancer Inst.* 1978;60:811.

36. Lewandowski RJ, Sato KT, Atassi B, et al. Radioembolization with 90Y microspheres: angiographic and technical considerations. *Cardiovasc Intervent Radiol.* 2007;30:571–592.

37. Iñarrairaegui M, D'Avola D, Rodriguez M, et al. Prognostic factors among patients with hepatocellular carcinoma (HCC) treated by Y90-radioembolization (Y90-RE). 44th Annual Meeting of the European Association for the Study of the Liver (EASL). *J Hepatol.* 2009; 20:S291. Abstract 795.

38. Jakobs TF, Hoffmann RT, Dehm K, et al. Hepatic yttrium-90 radioembolization of chemotherapy-refractory colorectal cancer liver metastases. *J Vasc Interv Radiol.* 2008;19:1187–1195.

39. Kennedy A. 90Y-microsphere brachytherapy in unresectable colorectal liver metastases. *Am J Hemat Oncol Rev.* 2006;5:1–5.

40. Kennedy AS, Coldwell D, Nutting C, et al. Resin 90Y-microsphere brachytherapy for unresectable colorectal liver metastases: modern USA experience. *Int J Radiat Oncol Biol Phys.* 2006;65:412–425.

41. Kennedy AS, Dezarn WA, McNeillie P, et al. Fractionation, dose selection, and response of hepatic metastases of neuroendocrine tumors after 90 Y-microsphere brachytherapy. *Brachytherapy.* 2006;5:103–104.

42. Minocha J, Kulik L, Ibrahim SM, et al. Prognostic value of lung shunting fraction in patients undergoing yttrium-90 radioembolization for HCC. *Second International Liver Cancer Association meeting;* September 2008:Abstract P-115.

43. Riaz A, Lewandowski RJ, Ryu RK, et al. Chemoembolization vs radioembolization: comparison of toxicity, imaging response and long-term outcomes in 100 TACE vs. 104 Y90 patients. Abstract presentation at Society of Interventional Radiology (SIR) 34th Annual Scientific Meeting. *J Vasc Interv Radiol.* 2009;26:Abstract 215.

44. Salem R, Lewandowski RJ, Mulcahy MF, et al. Radioembolization for hepatocellular carcinoma using yttrium-90 microspheres: a comprehensive report of long-term outcomes. *Gastroenterology.* 2010;138:52–64.

45. Van den Eynde M, Hendlisz A, Peeters M, et al. Prospective randomized study comparing intra-arterial injection of yttrium-90 resin microspheres with protracted IV 5FU continuous infusion versus IV 5FU continuous infusion alone for patients with liver-limited metastatic colorectal cancer refractory to standard chemotherapy.

Poster presentation at the American Association of Clinical Oncology (ASCO) Annual Meeting. *J Clin Oncol.* 2009;27:Abstract 4096.

46. van Hazel G, Turner D, Gebski V. Impact of 90Y resin microspheres on health-related quality of life (HRQoL) in patients with colorectal cancer (CRC) liver metastases receiving first-line chemotherapy. *American Society of Clinical Oncology (ASCO) Gastrointestinal Cancers Symposium.* 2009:Abstract 419.

47. Mulcahy MF, Lewandowski RJ, Ibrahim SM, et al. Radioembolization of colorectal hepatic metastases using yttrium-90 microspheres. *Cancer.* 2009;115:1849–1858.

48. Ricke J, Rühl R, Seidensticker M, et al. Extensive liver-dominant colorectal (CRC) metastases failing multiple lines of systemic chemotherapy treated by 90Y radioembolisation: a matched-pair analysis. Poster presentation, 11th World Congress of Gastrointestinal Cancer. *Ann Oncol.* 2009;20:Abstract PD-002.

49. Seidensticker M, Rühl R, Kraus P, et al. Radioembolization with yttrium-90 resin microspheres as a salvage treatment for refractory liver-dominant colorectal metastases: a matched-pair analysis. Presented as a poster at ECCO 15/34th ESMO. *Eur J Cancer Suppl.* 2009; 7:343. Abstract 6071.

50. Folprecht G, Grothey A, Alberts S, et al. Neoadjuvant treatment of unresectable colorectal liver metastases: correlation between tumour response and resection rates. *Ann Oncol.* 2005;16:1311–1319.

51. Hoffmann RT, Jakobs TF, Kubisch CH, et al. Radiofrequency ablation after selective internal radiation therapy with yttrium90 microspheres in metastatic liver disease—is it feasible? *Eur J Radiol.* 2010;74:199–205.

52. Van den Eynde M, Flamen P, El Nakadi I, et al. Inducing resectability of chemotherapy refractory colorectal liver metastasis by radioembolization with yttrium-90 microspheres. *Clin Nucl Med.* 2008;33:697–699.

53. Sangro B, Cianni R, Ezziddin S, et al. Predictors of survival following radioembolization using 90Y-labeled resin microspheres in unresectable hepatocellular carcinoma (HCC): results from a European multi-center evaluation. Poster presentation at the American Association for the Study of the Liver; 2009:Abstract 1712.

54. Iñarrairaegui M, Thurston KG, Martinez-Cuesta A. Radioembolization of hepatocellular carcinoma in patients presenting with portal vein occlusion: a safety analysis. *2nd International Liver Cancer Association meeting;* 2008:Abstract P-140.

55. Goin JE, Dancey JE, Roberts CA, et al. Comparison of post-embolization syndrome in the treatment of patients with unresectable hepatocellular carcinoma: trans-catheter arterial chemo-embolization versus yttrium-90 glass microspheres. *World J Nucl Med.* 2004;3:49–56.

56. Goin JE, Salem R, Carr BI, et al. Treatment of unresectable hepatocellular carcinoma with intrahepatic yttrium 90 microspheres: factors associated with liver toxicities. *J Vasc Interv Radiol.* 2005;16:205–213.

57. Goin JE, Salem R, Carr BI, et al. Treatment of unresectable hepatocellular carcinoma with intrahepatic yttrium 90 microspheres: a risk-stratification analysis. *J Vasc Interv Radiol.* 2005;16:195–203.

58. Riaz A, Kulik L, Lewandowski RJ, et al. Radiologic–pathologic correlation of hepatocellular carcinoma treated with internal radiation using yttrium-90 microspheres. *Hepatology.* 2009;49:1185–1193.

59. Young JY, Rhee TK, Atassi B, et al. Radiation dose limits and liver toxicities resulting from multiple yttrium-90 radioembolization treatments for hepatocellular carcinoma. *J Vasc Interv Radiol.* 2007;18: 1375–1382.

60. Sangro B, Carpanese L, Ezziddin S, et al. Nodularity is a strong predictor of survival following treatment with radioembolisation using 90Y-labelled resin microspheres in unresectable hepatocellular carcinoma: preliminary results from a European multi-centre evaluation. *Presented at the 3rd International Liver Cancer Association 2009 Annual Conference.* Milan, Italy; September 4–6, 2009. Abstract P-129 2009.

61. Lewandowski RJ, Kulik LM, Riaz A, et al. A comparative analysis of transarterial downstaging for hepatocellular carcinoma: chemoembolization versus radioembolization. *Am J Transplant.* 2009;9: 1920–1928.

62. Okuda K, Ohnishi K, Kimura K, et al. Incidence of portal vein thrombosis in liver cirrhosis: an angiographic study in 708 patients. *Gastroenterology.* 1985;89:279–286.

63. Rhee TK, Lewandowski RJ, Liu DM, et al. 90Y radioembolization for metastatic neuroendocrine liver tumors: preliminary results from a multi-institutional experience. *Ann Surg.* 2008;247:1029–1035.

64. Kennedy AS, Dezarn WA, McNeillie P, et al. Radioembolization for unresectable neuroendocrine hepatic metastases using resin 90Y-microspheres: early results in 148 patients. *Am J Clin Oncol.* 2008;31:271–279.

65. Murthy R, Kamat P, Nunez R, et al. Yttrium-90 microsphere radioembolotherapy of hepatic metastatic neuroendocrine carcinomas after hepatic arterial embolization. *J Vasc Interv Radiol.* 2008;19:145–151.

66. McGrath S, Kennedy A, Dezarn W. Resin 90Y-microsphere radioembolisation is effective in controlling hepatic metastases from neuroendocrine primary cancers. Emerging trends in radioembolization using microspheres: *3rd Annual Clinical Symposium.* May 4–5, 2007.

67. Coldwell DM, Kennedy AS, Nutting CW. Use of yttrium-90 microspheres in the treatment of unresectable hepatic metastases from breast cancer. *Int J Radiat Oncol Biol Phys.* 2007;69:800–804.

68. Bangash AK, Atassi B, Kaklamani V, et al. 90Y radioembolization of metastatic breast cancer to the liver: toxicity, imaging response, survival. *J Vasc Interv Radiol.* 2007;18:621–628.

69. Kennedy AS, McNeillie P, Dezarn WA, et al. Treatment parameters and outcome in 680 treatments of internal radiation with resin 90Y-microspheres for unresectable hepatic tumors. *Int J Radiat Oncol Biol Phys.* 2009;74:1494–1500.

70. Coldwell D. Treatment of unresectable nodular cholangiocarcinoma with yttrium-90 microspheres. *Ann Oncol.* 2006;17:vi56. Abstract P-102.

71. Ibrahim SM, Mulcahy MF, Lewandowski RJ, et al. Treatment of unresectable cholangiocarcinoma using yttrium-90 microspheres: results from a pilot study. *Cancer.* 2008;113:2119–2128.

72. Gulec SA, Mesoloras G, Dezarn WA, et al. Safety and efficacy of Y-90 microsphere treatment in patients with primary and metastatic liver cancer: the tumor selectivity of the treatment as a function of tumor to liver flow ratio. *J Transl Med.* 2007;5:15.

73. Lim L, Gibbs P, Yip D, et al. Prospective study of treatment with selective internal radiation therapy spheres in patients with unresectable primary or secondary hepatic malignancies. *Intern Med J.* 2005;35:222–227.

74. Bailey W, Little A, Lim L, et al. Ytrium-90 microsphere hepatic artery embolization in the treatment of nonresectable hepatic malignancy. Australasian Radiology Conference 2003. *Australasian Radiol.* 2004;48:A4–A5.

75. Rowe BP, Weiner R, Foster J, et al. 90Yttrium microspheres for nonresectable liver cancer: the University of Connecticut Health Center experience. *Conn Med.* 2007;71:523–528.

76. Sato KT, Lewandowski RJ, Mulcahy MF, et al. Unresectable chemorefractory liver metastases: radioembolization with 90Y microspheres—safety, efficacy, and survival. *Radiology.* 2008;247:507–515.

77. Cianni R, Satarelli A, Notarianni E, et al. Radioembolism (yttrium-90) of hepatic liver metastases. A preliminary experience. *Cardiovasc Interv Radiol.* 2006:Abstract 49.1.9.

78. Khodjibekova M, Szyszko T, Khan S, et al. Selective internal radiation therapy with yttrium-90 for unresectable liver tumours. *Rev Recent Clin Trials.* 2007;2:212–216.

79. Jakobs TF, Hoffmann RT, Yu M, et al. Yttrium-90 (SIR-Spheres®) treatment for metastatic cancer to the liver: midterm result. *World Conference on Interventional Oncology.* 2006;Session L1.

80. Wong CY, Qing F, Savin M, et al. Reduction of metastatic load to liver after intraarterial hepatic yttrium-90 radioembolization as evaluated by [18F]fluorodeoxyglucose positron emission tomographic imaging. *J Vasc Interv Radiol.* 2005;16:1101–1106.

81. Stubbs R, Wickremesekera S. Selective internal radiation therapy (SIRT): a new modality for treating patients with colorectal liver metastases. *HPB (Oxford).* 2004;6:133–139.

82. Pöpperl G, Helmberger T, Münzing W, et al. Selective internal radiation therapy with SIR-Spheres in patients with nonresectable liver tumors. *Cancer Biother Radiopharm.* 2005;20:200–208.

83. Stuart JE, Tan B, Myerson RJ, et al. Salvage radioembolization of liver-dominant metastases with a resin-based microsphere: initial outcomes. *J Vasc Interv Radiol.* 2008;19:1427–1433.

84. Kennedy AS, Nutting C, Jakobs T, et al. A first report of radioembolization for hepatic metastases from ocular melanoma. *Cancer Invest.* 2009;27:682–690.

85. Dhanasekaran R, Khanna V, Lawson D, et al. Survival benefits of yttrium-90 radioembolization (SIR-Spheres) for hepatic metastasis from melanoma: preliminary study. Society of Interventional Radiology (SIR) 34th Annual Scientific Meeting. *J Vasc Interv Radiol.* 2009;26:S65. Abstract 167.

86. Gonsalves C, Eschelman DJ, Sullivan KL, et al. Selective internal radiation therapy (SIRT) as salvage therapy for uveal melanoma (UM) hepatic metastases. ASCO Annual Meeting Proceedings. *J Clin Oncol.* 2009;27:Abstract 9066.

87. Tan TH, Kosmider S, Yip D, et al. Clinical experience of selective internal radiation therapy in combination with systemic chemotherapy as first-line therapy in patients with unresectable hepatic metastases from colorectal cancer. ASCO Annual Meeting Proceedings. *J Clin Oncol.* 2008;26:Abstract 15080.

Conjugated Therapy

Radioimmunotherapy of Colorectal Cancer

Jeffrey Y.C. Wong, Lawrence E. Williams, and Paul J. Yazaki

■ INTRODUCTION

Colorectal cancer is the third most common form of cancer in the United States and represents approximately 10% of all cancer cases. There were an estimated 112,340 new cases of colon cancer and 41,420 new cases of rectal cancer, with an estimated 52,180 deaths from this disease in the United States in 2007. Primary therapy for localized rectal cancer is surgery. Radiation therapy, either in the neoadjuvant or adjuvant setting, plays an important role particularly for rectal cancer. Postoperative radiation therapy and chemotherapy is recommended after surgery for pT3 and/or N1-2 disease. Preoperative combined radiation therapy and chemotherapy is also utilized for uT3-4 and/or node-positive disease followed by surgery and postoperative chemotherapy. This approach can be successful in preserving anal sphincter function for distal lesions. For locally advanced disease that is initially unresectable, preoperative chemotherapy and radiation therapy can often reduce the size of the primary tumor, allowing for successful surgical resection. Intraoperative radiation therapy can also be used to decrease local recurrence for difficult to resect, advanced, or recurrent tumors. Radiation therapy is also effective in palliating disease that often causes pain or bleeding.

Given the important role radiotherapy has in this disease, utilizing antibodies directed against tumor-associated antigens as a method to deliver targeted systemic radiotherapy or radioimmunotherapy (RIT) is appealing. The concept of a "magic bullet" that would target therapy specifically to tumor while avoiding normal tissues was initially proposed almost a century ago by Paul Ehrlich. One of the earliest efforts using antibodies to target radiotherapy was by Beierwaltes et al. who reported in 1951 a complete clinical response in 14 advanced melanoma patients treated with ^{131}I-labeled rabbit polyclonal antibodies (1). Since then, dozens of clinical trials have evaluated radiolabeled polyclonal, monoclonal, and genetically engineered antibodies for therapy. Much of this effort has been in patients with colorectal cancer, since many of the monoclonal antibodies (MAbs) initially evaluated were directed to pancarcinoma tumor–associated antigens, such as carcinoembryonic antigen (CEA) and tumor-associated glycoprotein (TAG-72) that are expressed in a high percentage of colorectal cancers. Through this experience there is now a clearer understanding of the factors, including antibody-, antigen-, tumor-, and host-related factors, that influence this form of targeted therapy.

RIT demonstrated significant promise in laboratory models, and has been translated to the clinic for the radiosensitive hematologic malignancies, with overall response rates ranging from 30% to 85% (2–10). The recent FDA approval of two radiolabeled anti-CD20 MAbs for clinical use highlights the potential for antibody-guided systemic radiotherapy (11,12). Clinical results in colorectal cancer and other solid tumors have been more modest but remain encouraging, and clinical trials continue. Current interest is focused on using RIT in a minimum tumor burden setting either as monotherapy or in combination with other systemic therapies. Clinical trials are also evaluating novel antibody-based pretargeting strategies that have the potential to increase radiation dose to tumor relative to normal organs.

This chapter reviews the clinical experience of RIT in colorectal cancer, the factors that influence the efficacy and toxicity of RIT, and the strategies that have been and are currently being pursued in the clinic to further optimize this form of targeted therapy.

■ FACTORS TO CONSIDER IN DELIVERY OF RIT

Antibody factors

Over the last several decades, there have been continued refinements in the production and design of antibodies used for antibody-targeted radiation therapy. Initial efforts utilized polyclonal antibodies, which were produced by collection of antiserum after immunization of a given species, such as rabbit, to a specific antigen. Polyclonal antibodies were heterogeneous in specificity and affinity and recognized a number of different sites (epitopes) on the antigen. Initial trials at Johns Hopkins and then by Radiation Therapy Oncology Group (RTOG) evaluated ^{131}I-labeled polyclonal antiferritin produced in a variety of species in combination with external beam radiation, doxorubicin, and 5-fluoruracil (5-FU) in patients with hepatoma, and reported a 7% complete response and 41% partial response rate (13). Polyclonal ^{131}I-anti-CEA antibodies were also evaluated in clinical trials by the same group at Johns Hopkins (14).

In 1975, Kohler and Milstein (15) developed the hybridoma technique that allowed for the production of MAbs. This involved the immunization of mice against a target antigen and then immortalization of the antibody-producing B-cells from that mouse by fusion with myeloma cells to produce a hybridoma. The selected hybridoma could produce large quantities of a specific MAb with high specificity. This allowed for the rapid expansion of clinical trials evaluating radiolabeled MAbs to a variety of tumor-associated antigens.

More recently, large immunized, naive or synthetic antibody libraries displayed on bacterial phage have been developed. Briefly, these phage display libraries express a diverse repertoire of antibody-binding domains on the surface of the phage coat, allowing the selection of binders against the antigen of choice. The DNA encoding the antibody can be sequenced, subcloned, and expressed for further evaluation. Using this technology, libraries on the order of 10^{10} independent members can be rapidly screened for the identification of new candidates or for affinity maturation or humanization of existing hybridomas. Human antibodies have also been produced recently through the use of transgenic mice that have the murine immunoglobulin loci "knocked out" and replaced with human immunoglobulin genes. Transgenic mice are immunized with the target antigen, and human antibodies are then produced through the hybridoma technique.

Immunoglobulins have a molecular weight of approximately 150 kDa and are composed of two pairs of light and heavy polypeptide chains, which are linked by disulfide bridges. Specifically, the IgG_1 light chain consists of the variable light (V_L) and constant light chains (C_L), and the heavy chain consists of the variable heavy (V_H), constant heavy C_H1 domain, hinge, and constant C_H2 and C_H3 domains (Fig. 25.1). The antigen-binding region of the antibody consists of the V_L, V_H, C_L, and C_H1 domains, also known as the Fab portion of the antibody. The Fc portion consists of the C_H2 and the C_H3 domains and contains receptor-binding sites that are involved in a number of immune response effector functions. Effector functions that have been associated with the Fc portion include complement-dependent mediated cytotoxicity and antibody-dependent cellular cytotoxicity. An IgG_1 antibody is bivalent, having two antigen-binding sites, one on each "arm" of the Y-shaped molecule.

Antibody molecular size

Antibody molecular size can influence the rate of antibody clearance from the circulation and penetration of the antibody into the tumor. Whole immunoglobulins with a molecular weight of 150 kDa tend to clear slowly from circulation. Prolonged circulation of a radiolabeled antibody can contribute to an increased dose to marrow and increased hematologic toxicity. In addition, given the size of whole immunoglobulins, the diffusion distances from blood vessels are reduced compared to smaller molecules, limiting penetration and uptake into tumor. To further improve antibody-guided radiation therapy, many investigators have evaluated a variety of different antibody fragments or recombinant constructs.

Initial efforts generated enzymatically produced antibody fragments. The whole immunoglobulin can be digested by the

FIGURE 25.1 Antibody fragments produced from whole immunoglobulin by enzyme digestion or genetic engineering.

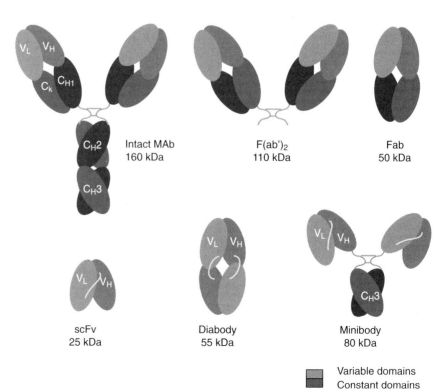

Intact MAb
160 kDa

F(ab')₂
110 kDa

Fab
50 kDa

scFv
25 kDa

Diabody
55 kDa

Minibody
80 kDa

Variable domains
Constant domains

enzymes pepsin or papain, resulting in bivalent F(ab')$_2$ of 120 kDa in size or monovalent Fab of 28 kDa in size, respectively (Fig. 25.1). These smaller fragments demonstrate superior tumor penetration and clear rapidly from the circulation. However, clearance that is too rapid can sometimes reduce the total amount of antibody uptake in tumor compared to intact antibodies. In addition, some of the F(ab')$_2$ fragments are unstable and degrade in circulation, necessitating chemically linking or stabilizing the two arms of the F(ab')$_2$.

Recently, genetic engineering has allowed synthesis of antibody constructs of various molecular size and valency (Fig. 25.1). Fvs represent the smallest antibody fragment that still retains antigen-binding specificity and consists of the V_H and V_L chains joined by a short polypeptide linker to form a single-chain Fv (scFv) that is monovalent. Diabodies can be created by shortening this linker and forcing cross-pair dimerization of scFvs, resulting in an antibody construct that has two antigen-recognition sites or is bivalent. Slightly larger antibody constructs have been synthesized without the C_H1 domain and/or C_H2 domain, such as the anti-CEA minibody that is 80 kDa and bivalent (Fig. 25.1). Monovalent fragments or constructs have been chemically linked to produce divalent, trivalent, and multivalent species. Table 25.1 lists some of these engineered constructs that have been produced and evaluated mostly in preclinical studies.

Affinity and avidity

Affinity relates to the binding interaction between the antigen and antibody and reflects the ratio of the association versus dissociation rate constants. The overall tendency of antibody binding to antigen is dependent on not only affinity but also the number of binding sites and is termed "avidity." The optimum antibody-binding affinity for therapy is yet to be clearly defined. Some studies have reported a correlation between affinity and tumor uptake while others have not (31). High-affinity antibodies may have a disadvantage by having a greater tendency to bind to circulating antigen before reaching the tumor site or binding in the immediate perivascular region that limits its diffusion into all areas of the tumor (32).

Antibody immunogenicity

Antibody immunogenicity can potentially limit tumor targeting or the ability to deliver repeat therapy administrations. Early clinical trials with murine MAbs produced through hybridoma technology had the disadvantage of being recognized as foreign by the patient's immune system. This led to the formation of human anti-mouse antibodies (HAMA) in 50% to 100% of patients after single administration (33–36). The formation of HAMA can hasten blood clearance and also compromise the therapeutic efficacy of subsequently administered antibody (35,37). Using recombinant DNA technology, antibody immunogenicity can be reduced by modification of the antibody molecule, replacing murine with human antibody domains to varying degrees. Chimeric antibodies retain the murine variable domains fused to a human Fc. Humanized antibodies have only the murine complementarity-determining

Table **25.1**	Select engineered or chemically cross-linked antibody fragments evaluated in experimental tumor systems			
Study (First Author)	Construct	Valency	MW (kDa)	Antigen
Colcher (16)	scFv B6.2	Monovalent	25	NCA
Wu (17)	scFv 212, scFvC28	Monovalent	28	CEA
Adams (18)	scFvC6.5 diabody	Bivalent	50	her2/neu
Rossi (19)	Diabody of hMN14	Bivalent	54	CEA
Wu (20)	GS8 T84.66 diabody	Bivalent	55	CEA
Goel (21)	[sc(Fv)$_2$]$_2$	Tetravalent	58	TAG-72
Pavlinkova (22)	(scFv)$_2$ CC49 diabody	Bivalent	60	TAG-72
Rossi (23)	Triabody hMN14	Trivalent	80	CEA
Yazaki (24)	GS18 Flex T84.66 minibody	Bivalent	80	CEA
Iliades (25)	Triabody of scFv 11-1G10	Trivalent	85	N9 neuraminidase
King (26)	DFM (di-Fab)	Bivalent	95	TAG-72
Rossi (23)	Tetrabody of hMN-14	Tetravalent	120	CEA
Shu (27)	SCAΔCLCH1	Bivalent	120	TAG-72
Slavin-Chiorini (28)	cB72.3ΔCH2	Bivalent	120	TAG-72
King (26)	TFM (tri-Fab)	Trivalent	150	TAG-72
Slavin-Chiorini (29)	huCC49ΔCH2	Bivalent	153	TAG-72
Santos (30)	SCIgHuCC49db	Tetravalent	160	TAG-72

regions or binding loops retained. Chimeric or humanized antibodies potentially allow for multiple administrations without alteration of clearance rate, biodistribution, or tumor targeting. Recently, human antibodies have been produced for clinical evaluation. Other methods to reduce the immunogenicity of murine antibodies include the use of smaller antibody fragments, veneering that modifies the murine residues on the surface of the antibody molecule, and the use of immunosuppressive agents such as cyclosporin A (38–40).

Both chimeric and humanized antibodies have been evaluated in the clinic. Table 25.2 compares the immunogenicity of some of the murine, chimeric, and humanized radiolabeled MAbs that have been evaluated in clinical trials. Chimerization and humanization have decreased immunogenicity of most antibody constructs (52,55–59). Not all humanized MAbs have low immunogenicity. A 47% immune response rate was seen with hMN-14 (53) and a 63% immune response rate with humanized MAb A33 (60). However, this is still substantially lower than the 100% rate observed for their murine counterparts (43,47).

Challenges still remain regarding immunogenicity of antibodies since recent efforts have attempted to add additional components or to modify the antibody molecule to improve it as a delivery vehicle for radiotherapy. For example, macrocyclic chelates with improved stability and binding capability for the radionuclide, when conjugated to the immunoglobulin, have been shown in some cases to result in increased immunogenicity (61). Multistep pretargeted radioimmunotherapy approaches that fuse or conjugate avidin or streptavidin to the antibody have been shown to increase immunogenicity of the protein (62).

Antigen factors

There are over 100 tumor-associated antigens that have been identified, but only a limited number are used as targets for radioimmunotherapy (Table 25.3). Candidate target molecules include overexpressed oncogene products and their receptors, members of the epidermal growth factor receptor (EGFR) family, vascular endothelial growth factor receptors, development-related epitopes such as neural cell adhesion molecule (NCAM), extracellular epitopes with an extracellular matrix location (tenascin), CEA, prostate-specific membrane antigen (PSMA), and high-molecular weight glycoprotein mucins. The ideal target tumor antigen would be one that is highly expressed on the surface of all cells within the tumor with minimal expression in normal tissues and with little shedding into the vascular system. Most target antigens in RIT trials are preferentially expressed by tumor compared to normal tissue. Antigens such as CEA are expressed on the luminal side of the gastrointestinal (GI) mucosa, and are not readily available to anti-CEA antibodies delivered systemically. Shed antigens can complex circulating antibody and hasten antibody clearance, potentially reducing antibody targeting to tumor.

In general, antigen expression is heterogeneous within the tumor. One advantage of using radiolabeled antibodies involves the cross-fire effect that occurs when ionizing radiation still reaches a non–antigen-expressing cell if neighboring antigen-expressing cells bind the radiolabeled antibody. In addition, some surface target antigens internalize after binding to antibody, which may become problematic since this can result in metabolism and dehalogenation, resulting in loss of the radiolabel from the antibody (63). Esteban et al.

Table **25.2**	**Antibody immunogenicity following a single administration (select solid tumor RIT trials)**			
Study (First Author)	**Antibody**	**Type**	**No. of Patients**	**Percent Anti-Antibody Response**
Breitz (41)	[186]Re-NR-LU-10	Murine	15	100
Meredith (42)	^{131}I-CC49	Murine	15	100
Welt (43)	^{131}I-MAb A33	Murine	23	100
Mulligan (44)	^{177}Lu-CC49	Murine	9	100
Yu (45)	^{131}I-COL-1	Murine	18	83 prevented add'n RIT in 2
Behr (46)	^{131}I-NP-4	Murine	32	94
Juweid (47)	^{131}I-MN-14	Murine	14	100
Meredith (48)	^{131}I-cB72.3	Chimeric	12	58
Weiden (49)	[186]Re-NR-LU-13	Chimeric	8	75
Meredith (50)	[125]I-17-1A	Chimeric	15	13
Wong (51)	^{90}Y-cT84.66	Chimeric	21	52 prevented add'n RIT in 8
Kramer (52)	^{111}In-huBrE3	Humanized	7	14
Hajjar (53)	^{131}I-hMN-14	Humanized	15	47
Goldsmith (54)	^{90}Y-huJ591	Humanized	19	0
Borjesson (55)	[186]Re-BIWA 4	Humanized	20	10

Table **25.3**	Select monoclonal antibodies evaluated for RIT	
Malignancy	**Antigen**	**Antibody**
Colorectal cancer	CEA	cT84.66, hMN-14, A5B7
	TAG-72	B72.3, CC49
	A33	Anti-A33
	Ep-CAM	NR-LU-10, NR-LU-13
	DNA histone H1	chTNT-1/B
Breast cancer	MUC1	huBrE-3, m170
	L6	chL6
	TAG-72	CC49
	CEA	cT84.66
Ovarian cancer	MUC1	HMFG1
	Folate receptor	cMov18
	TAG-72	B72.3, CC49
Prostate cancer	PSMA	huJ591
	TAG-72	CC49
Lung cancer	DNA histone H1	chTNT-1/B
	TAG72	CC49
Head and neck cancer	CD44v6	U36, BIWA4
Gliomas	EGFR	425
	Tenascin	816C, BC4
Melanoma	p97	96.5
Renal cancer	G250 glycoprotein	cG250
Medullary thyroid	CEA	cT84.66, hMN-14, NP-4
Neuroblastoma	Ganglioside G_{D2}	3F8
	NCAM	UJ13A, ERIC-1

demonstrated down-modulation of antigen expression after antibody binding, which limited targeting of a second cycle of administered antibody (64).

■ Radionuclides

A number of factors are considered when selecting appropriate radionuclides for RIT, including emission characteristics, physical half-life, cost, availability, and linkage chemistry. Table 25.4 lists some of the radionuclides that have been used in clinical RIT trials. Radionuclides usually used for therapy produce intermediate and long-range beta emissions, which have a range of several millimeters to a centimeter in tissue, making them suitable for therapy of macroscopic disease. In addition, the range in tissue of these beta emissions allows for a potential cross-fire effect, where despite heterogeneous targeting of the radiolabeled antibody, radiation can reach not only the antibody-targeted cell but also neighboring nontargeted cells. Some radionuclides, such as iodine-131 (^{131}I), lutetium-177 (^{177}Lu), and copper-67 (^{67}Cu), also have a gamma emission that may be useful for imaging and tracking of the radiolabeled agent.

However, gamma emissions have no significant role in therapy and have the disadvantage of contributing to radiation dose to normal organs and to personnel, especially with ^{131}I, which has a relatively energetic and abundant gamma emission.

The physical half-life of the radionuclide should be comparable to the biologic half-life of the antibody and the time needed for the antibody to target to tumor. For most intact antibodies this is at least 24 hours. Antibodies labeled with shorter-lived radionuclides, such as rhenium-188 (^{188}Re), bismuth-212 (^{212}Bi), and astatine-211 (^{211}At), will have suffered significant decay of activity prior to maximum uptake in the tumor. Radionuclides with shorter half-lives may be more suitable for low molecular weight and faster targeting antibody constructs and fragments.

Initially ^{131}I was used in clinical RIT trials since it was readily available and labeling methods were well established, with iodine usually covalently linked to the antibody through tyrosine residues. However, with radioiodinated antibodies the iodine can be enzymatically dehalogenated after administration, leading to loss of some of the radioactivity from the antibody before it can reach the tumor. In

Table **25.4** **Select radionuclides for clinical use**

Radionuclide	Decay Mode	Physical Half-Life	Max. Particulate Energy (%)	Max. Range in Tissue (mm)	Gamma Energy (%)	Potential Advantages	Potential Disadvantages
Iodine-131 (^{131}I)	Beta	8.0 d	807 keV (1)	2.4	364 keV (81)	Available	Dehalogenation
	Gamma		606 keV (86)			Inexpensive	γ emission (organ exposure and radiation safety issues)
			336 keV (13)				
Yttrium-90 (^{90}Y)	Beta	64 h	2.29 MeV (100)	11.9	None	Metal chemistry	Bone seeker
						No γ exposure	Does not image
Rhenium-186 (^{186}Re)	Beta	91 h	1.07 MeV (77)	5.0	137 keV (9)	^{99m}Tc chemistry	Scarce
	Gamma		934 keV (23)				
	Electron capture						
Rhenium-188 (^{188}Re)	Beta	16.9 h	2.12 MeV (80)	10.6	155 keV (15)	^{99m}Tc chemistry	Scarce
	Gamma		1.96 MeV (20)				Short half-life
Lutetium-177 (^{177}Lu)	Beta	6.7 d	500 keV (86)	1.6	206 keV (11)	γ for imaging	Bone seeker
	Gamma						Scarce
Iodine-125 (^{125}I)	Electron capture	60 d	35 keV (100)	0.0002	None	Short range	Long half-life
							Does not image
							Requires internalization
Copper-67 (^{67}Cu)	Beta	62 h	577 keV (20)	2.2	184 keV (47)	Metal chemistry	Scarce
	Gamma		484 keV (35)		92 keV (24)	γ for imaging	
			395 keV (45)				
Bismuth-212 (^{212}Bi)	Alpha	1 h	6.05 MeV α (25)	0.09	None	High RBE	Scarce
	Beta		2.27 MeV β (40)				Short half-life
							Unstable daughter
Astatine-211 (^{211}At)							
	Alpha	7 h	5.87 MeV α (100)	0.09	None	High RBE	Scarce
							Short half-life

RBE, relative biologic effectiveness.

addition, if bound to tumor antigen and internalized into the cell, as in some tumor systems, further dehalogenation is possible (63). Free iodine can deposit in the thyroid, kidneys, bladder, salivary glands, and the stomach, although thyroid uptake can be mitigated through the use of blocking agents such as SSKI that are initiated prior to and continued until clearance of radiolabeled antibody has occurred.

Yttrium-90 (^{90}Y) and other radioactive metals, such as ^{186}Re, ^{188}Re, ^{177}Lu, and ^{67}Cu, are not covalently linked to the

antibody but are linked through an intermediary chelate. Unlike iodine, more of the radionuclide remains linked to the antibody after administration. As a result more activity and radiation dose can be delivered to organs such as liver and kidney, as antibody is cleared by these organs. Free ^{90}Y and ^{177}Lu will target to cortical bone, potentially adding to marrow dose and hematological toxicity. The radiometals, ^{186}Re, ^{188}Re, ^{177}Lu and ^{67}Cu, have suitable beta emissions for therapy, but at this time are not as readily available, limiting their widespread use in clinical trials.

A few studies have utilized ^{125}I that decays by electron capture and requires internalization of the radiolabeled antibody into the tumor cell and subsequent intranuclear localization of the radionuclide to realize cytotoxic effects. In colorectal cancer ^{125}I-labeled antibodies have been delivered systemically with only modest hematopoietic toxicities, despite the relatively long half-life of the radionuclide (65,66).

Alpha particle–emitting radionuclides are also being investigated for RIT and may potentially be better suited for the treatment of microscopic disease, given their very short range. Other advantages include their high LET (linear energy transfer) and high RBE (relative biologic effectiveness) characteristics. Disadvantages include a very short half-life on the order of hours for some radionuclides and limited availability. Clinical experience thus far has been limited, with no clinical trials reported in colorectal cancer (67,68). An in vivo study reported using a ^{212}Bi-labeled B72.3, an anti-TAG72 antibody, in LS174T colon cancer intraperitoneal (IP) tumor–bearing mouse model. Mice receiving single or multiple doses of IP ^{212}Bi-labeled B72.3 had significant tumor reduction compared to controls treated with either unlabeled B72.3 or ^{212}Bi-labeled nonspecific antibody (69).

Tumor factors

Tumor physiology is complex. Tumors rapidly develop, often outgrowing their blood supply. This results in spatial heterogeneity of tumor vascularization. Some areas are well vascularized, oxygenated, and rapidly growing, while other areas are poorly perfused, necrotic or hypoxic, and slower growing. Blood flow within tumor is often erratic and slow in many portions. Tumor vasculature is also leaky, leading to increased interstitial pressure in regions of the tumor. Interstitial pressure tends to be higher in poorly perfused regions. These physiologic factors work to impede macromolecule uptake, resulting in reduced antibody uptake, limited penetration of the antibody into tumor, and spatial heterogeneity of antibody deposition, resulting in radioactivity primarily deposited in the well-vascularized areas with lower interstitial pressure (70).

As tumor size increases, these physiologic barriers to antibody uptake exponentially increase, significantly limiting tumor uptake and radiation dose. For example, Williams et al., in a review of in vivo studies utilizing tumor-bearing mouse models with subcutaneous xenografts, observed an inverse power–law relationship between radiolabeled MAb uptake and tumor volume for both solid tumors and lymphomas (71). It should be noted that there have been inverse correlations demonstrated between tumor uptake u (%ID/g) and tumor mass m (g) in both human tumor xenografts (71) and clinical colorectal cancer cases (72). In the former, using the LS174T human colorectal tumor model in nude mice, the correlations were of the following form:

$$u(\%ID/g) = Bm^A$$

where A and B were determined via least-square fitting at a given time point. In both intravenous (IV) and IP injections, values varied between -0.39 and -0.46 for B72.3 and cT84.66 intact antibodies. The B parameter was much more variable due to implantation site and antibody factors. A clinical study on colorectal primary tumors reported by Williams et al. (72) had a slope value of -0.362 with a 2% confidence level ($n = 19$ consecutive colorectal patients). For colon tumors exhibiting such variation, one may expect that RIT will be more effective for smaller lesions. A decrease of one order of magnitude in lesion size can result in increased uptake (and hence dose) by approximately a factor of 2.4 in the clinical situation. Such an analysis implies that adjuvant RIT for minimal or microscopic disease may be an optimal application of targeting radiolabeled antibodies.

Host factors

The radiation dose to tumor is determined by how much of the administered radiolabeled antibody reaches, accumulates, and is retained at the tumor site. Radiolabeled antibody uptake to normal organs, the rate of clearance from circulation, and the rate of metabolism all impact on the amount of radiolabeled antibody available to target the tumor compartment. Clearance and biodistribution of the agent can vary depending on the antibody, antigen, chelate linker, radionuclide, overall tumor burden, and clearance organ function. Radiolabeled antibodies that are cleared too rapidly from circulation may have limited access to antigen sites at the tumor. Antibody fragments and constructs of molecular weight of less than approximately 50 kDa tend to clear rapidly through the kidney and, depending on its isoelectric charge, may actually be retained within the renal parenchyma, leading to additional dose to kidneys.

Variability of clearance kinetics and biodistribution from patient to patient further adds to the challenge of delivering therapy to tumor and to the complexity of estimating organ and tumor doses for a given patient. Some groups have developed pharmacokinetic models for a given radioimmunotherapeutic to help with dose estimation in addition to the standard use of serial images (73).

The amount of antibody protein administered with the radiolabeled dose can have a significant impact on activity localizing to the tumor. With some antibodies, increasing the milligrams of antibody protein administered will reduce liver and/or spleen uptake, keeping more in circulation and resulting in an increase in tumor uptake of the antibody. This has been observed in both animal models and patients (74,75).

CLINICAL RESULTS IN COLORECTAL CANCER

Much of the preclinical and clinical work evaluating radiolabeled antibodies for imaging and therapy of solid tumors is in colorectal cancer, and continues to be an active area of clinical investigation.

Tables 25.5 and 25.6 summarize results of clinical RIT trials to date that have treated patients with colorectal cancer.

Table 25.5 Anti-CEA radioimmunotherapy trials in colorectal cancer

Radiolabeled Antibody	Antibody Type	Trial Type	No. Treated (No. CRC)	Objective Responses (%)	Minor/Mixed Response or Stable Disease (%)	Comments
^{131}I-NP-4 (46)	Murine IgG$_1$	I/II	57 (29)	1/57 (2)	4/57 (7)	
^{131}I- NP4 F(ab')$_2$ (76)	Murine IgG$_1$ F(ab')$_2$	I	13 (8)		4/13 (31)	Small-volume disease
^{131}I-NP4 (77)	Murine IgG$_1$	I/II	6 (6)	1/6 (13%)	5/6 (88) CEA ↓	Liver Metastases, RIT combined with hyperthermia
^{186}Re-MN-14 (78)	Murine IgG$_1$	I	11 (10)			30–80 mCi/m^2 in 2–3 divided doses every 3–4 days
^{131}I-hMN-14 (53)	Humanized IgG$_1$	I	17 (14)			
^{131}I-hMN-14 (79)	Humanized IgG$_1$	I	12 (2)	2/11 (16)	5/11 (45)	Small-volume lesions ≤ 2.5 cm
^{131}I-hMN-14 (80)	Humanized IgG$_1$	II	21 (21)	3/19 (16)	8/19 (42)	Small-volume lesions ≤ 3.0 cm
^{131}I-hMN-14 (80)	Humanized IgG$_1$	II	9 (9)	7/9 NED 24–36 + months		Adjuvant RIT after R0 resection Liver Metastases
^{131}I-hMN-14 (81)	Humanized IgG$_1$	II	23 (23)	DFS 18 months		Adjuvant RIT after R0 resection Liver Metastases
				OS 68 months		Median F/U 64 months
				5 yr survival 51.3%		
^{131}I-hMN-14 (82)	Humanized IgG$_1$	II	23 (23)	DFS 18 months		Adjuvant RIT after R0 resection Liver Metastases
				OS 59 months		Median F/U 91 months
				5 yr survival 42.1%		
^{131}I-hMN-14 (83)	Humanized IgG$_1$	II	32 (32)	DFS 18 mo adjuvant RIT vs. 6 mo nonadjuvant RIT		Resection Liver Metastases/24 patients 2 cycles
						16 no gross residual (adjuvant RIT)
						16 gross residual (nonadjuvant RIT)
Bispecific anti-CEA hMN-14 – anti-DTPA-indium + ^{131}I-di-DTPA-indium hapten (84)	Coupling of Fab' from hMN-14 and murine m734	I	22 (9)		9/20 (45)	Pretargeting approach
^{90}Y-cT84.66 (51)	Chimeric IgG$_1$	I	22 (18)		12/22 (54)	DTPA infusion post-RIT
					7/22 >50% ↓ CEA (33)	
^{90}Y-cT84.66 (85)	Chimeric IgG$_1$	I	13 (7)		5/13 (38)	DOTA-conjugated antibody
						DTPA infusion after RIT
^{90}Y-cT84.66 (86)	Chimeric IgG$_1$	I	21 (21)		12/21 (57)	RIT 16.6 mCi/m^2
						5-FU 5 day CI 700–1000 mg/m^2
						DTPA infusion after RIT

Table **25.5** *(Continued)*

Radiolabeled Antibody	Antibody Type	Trial Type	No. Treated (No. CRC)	Objective Responses (%)	Minor/Mixed Response or Stable Disease (%)	Comments
^{90}Y-cT84.66 (87)	Chimeric IgG$_1$	I	32 (19)	1/32 (3)	10/32 (31)	RIT 16 .6 mCi/m^2
						Gemcitabine 30– 165 mg/m^2 days 1, 3
^{90}Y-cT84.66 (unpublished)	Chimeric IgG$_1$	I	15 (8)		8/15 (53)	IP RIT
						DTPA infusion after RIT
^{90}Y-cT84.66 (unpublished)	Chimeric IgG$_1$	I	7 (2)		4/7 (57)	IP RIT 19 mCi/m^2
						IP gemcitabine 40– 80 mg/m^2 days 1, 4, 8
^{90}Y-cT84.66 (unpublished)	Chimeric IgG$_1$	I	13 (13)	5 no progression (4–37 months)		RIT 16.6 mCi/m^2 day 9
						Hepatic arterial FUdR 0.1–0.2 μg/kg/d × 14 d
						Systemic gemcitabine 105 mg/m^2 days 9, 11
						Liver Metastases resection
^{186}Re-NR-CO-2 F(ab′)$_2$ (41)	Murine IgG$_1$ F(ab′)$_2$	I	31 (27)	1/31 (3)	11/31 (35)	Hepatic arterial infusion in five patients
^{131}I-A5B7 (88)	Murine IgG$_1$ / F(ab′)$_2$	I/II	19 (17)	2/19 (11)		
^{131}I-A5B7 (89)	Murine IgG$_1$	I/II·	12 (11)		1/10 (10)	RIT combined with CA4P
^{131}I-COL-1 (45)	Murine IgG$_{2a}$	I	18 (16)		4/18 (22)	
^{131}I-F6 F(ab′)$_2$ (90)	Murine IgG$_1$ F(ab′)$_2$	I/II	10 (10)	1/9 (11)	3/9 (33)	Autologous marrow cells reinfused in five patients
^{131}I-F6 F(ab′)$_2$ (91)	Murine IgG$_1$	II	13 (13)	DFS 12 months		Adjuvant RIT after R0 resection of Liver Metastases
				OS 50 months		Median F/U 127 months
^{131}I-MAb 35, MAb B7, MAb B93 F(ab′)$_2$ (92)	Murine IgG$_1$ F(ab′)$_2$	Pilot	6 (6)		4/6 (67)	Limited Liver Metastases
					5/6 ↓ CEA (88)	External beam RT

NED, no evidence of disease; DFS, disease-free survival; OS, overall survival; IP, intraperitoneal; RT, external beam radiotherapy; CA4P, combretastatin-A-4-phosphate.

Early trials utilized ^{131}I as the radionuclide due to availability and ease of labeling, with subsequent trials using radiometals such as ^{90}Y, ^{186}Re, and ^{177}Lu. Although different MAbs and radionuclides have been evaluated, comparable results have been observed in most trials. The majority have been phase I trials reporting on a relatively limited number of patients. Most of the antibodies studied have been administered at low protein doses (~5 to 50 mg), have not demonstrated clinical immunomodulatory or antitumor properties, and have therefore served primarily as a delivery vehicle for radiation. Most patients received a single therapy infusion, with only a subset receiving a limited number of additional infusion cycles. Dose-limiting toxicity has been hematologic, primarily thrombocytopenia and leukopenia. As is typical of phase I trials, patients who were entered often had advanced, bulky, chemotherapy refractory disease, progressing into therapy.

Table **25.6**   **Radioimmunotherapy trials directed against antigens other than CEA in colorectal cancer**

Radiolabeled Antibody	Antibody Type	Trial Type	No. Treated (No. CRC)	Objective Responses (%)	Minor/Mixed Response or Stable Disease (%)	Comments
TAG-72						
^{131}I-cB72.3 (93)	Chimeric IgG$_4$	I	12 (12)		4/12 (33)	
^{131}I-cB72.3 (48)	Chimeric IgG$_4$	I	12 (12)		4/12 (33)	12–18 mCi/m^2 weekly × 2–3
^{131}I-CC49 (94)	Murine IgG$_1$	I	24 (24)		6/24 (25)	
^{131}I-CC49 (95)	Murine IgG$_1$	II	15 (15)		3/14 (21)	
^{131}I-CC49 (96)	Murine IgG$_1$	II	15 (15)		5/15 (33)	IL-1 to reduce hematologic toxicity
^{131}I-CC49 (97)	Murine IgG$_1$	I	6 (6)			15 mCi/m^2 biweekly × 4
^{177}Lu-CC49 (44)	Murine IgG$_1$	I	9 (3)		2/9 (22)	
^{131}I-CC49 (98)	Murine IgG$_1$	I	14 (11)			Autologous stem cells reinfused
^{90}Y-CC49 (99)	Murine IgG$_1$	I	12 (5)		2/12 (17)	Autologous stem cells reinfused
CC49 scFv –SA ^{90}Y-DOTA-biotin (100)	Tetrameric CC49 scFv fusion construct	Pilot	6 (6)		2/6 (33)	Pretargeting approach
TAG-72+ CEA						
^{131}I-COL-1 and ^{131}I-CC49 (101)	Murine IgG$_1$	II	14 (14)		4/14 (29)	Alpha-interferon to ↑ antigen expression
^{131}I-F023C5, BW494/32, B72.3, AUA1 (102)	Murine IgG$_1$	II	16 (16)	4/15 (27) (2 CR)	9/15 (60)	IP in all patients (also IV in 3)
A33						
^{131}I-A33 (43)	Murine IgG$_{2a}$	I/II	23 (23)		3/20 (15)	
^{125}I-A33 (66)	Murine IgG$_{2a}$	I/II	21 (21)		14/20 (70)	
^{131}I-huA33 (103)	Humanized IgG$_1$	I	15 (15)		4/15 (27)	
Ep-CAM						
^{125}I-CO 17-1A (65)	Murine IgG$_{2a}$	I	53 (25)	1/53 (2)	11/53 (21)	Liver RT 15 Gy in 46 patients
^{125}I-17-1A (50)	Chimeric IgG$_1$	I	28 (28)		10/28 (36)	
^{186}Re-NR-LU-10 (41)	Murine IgG$_{2a}$	I	15 (10)			
^{186}Re-NR-LU-13 (49)	Chimeric IgG$_1$	I	9 (4)		2/9 (22)	
NR-LU-10-SA + ^{90}Y-DOTA-biotin (104)	Murine IgG$_{2a}$	I	40 (10)	2/40 (5)	4/40 (10)	Pretargeting approach
NR-LU-10-SA + ^{90}Y-DOTA-biotin (105)	Murine IgG$_{2a}$	II	25 (25)	2/25 (8)	4/25 (16)	Pretargeting approach
DNA Histone H1						
^{131}I-chTNT-1/B (106)	Chimeric IgG$_1$	I	21 (21)		5/21	
^{131}I-chTNT-1/B (107)	Chimeric IgG$_1$	Pilot	6 (2)	NS	NS	Adjuvant RIT after RFA of Liver Metastases
						Feasibility study

CR, complete response; IP, intraperitoneal; IL-1, interleukin-1; RT, external beam radiotherapy; RFA, radiofrequency ablation; NS, not stated.

In this patient population, studies have reported primarily stable disease and serologic, mixed, or minor responses (43,50,51,53,94), with objective responses being infrequent (41,46,47,79,88,90,108–111). On the basis of the clinical experience thus far, there appears to be no clear advantage to a particular radionuclide–antibody combination.

CEA trials

The majority of RIT trials in colorectal cancer have evaluated antibodies directed against CEA. CEA was first characterized by Gold and Freedman (112) and is expressed by approximately 95% of colorectal cancers, with limited expression by other normal tissues, making it an attractive target for RIT. One of the first therapy trials was reported by Lane et al. (88) who administered ^{131}I-A5B7 anti-CEA murine MAb to 19 patients (17 colorectal cancers) in a phase I/II study: ten received intact IgG$_1$ and nine the F(ab')$_2$. One partial response and one complete response of 4 weeks duration were observed. Although clearance, organ biodistribution, organ dosimetry, and toxicity were similar between the intact and F(ab')$_2$, the F(ab')$_2$ localized more rapidly to tumor, supporting the hypothesis that smaller antibody fragments penetrate tumor more rapidly.

The Goldenberg group also described much of the early efforts. Behr et al. (46) reported on 57 patients treated in a phase I/II trial treated with ^{131}I-NP-4. Twenty patients received up to four cycles of therapy. One patient with a partial remission, four with minor/mixed responses, and seven with stabilization of disease were observed. An inverse correlation with antibody uptake versus tumor size was seen. Faster blood clearance rates were observed in the 29 patients with colorectal cancer, especially those with large tumor burden in liver, or in patients who developed a HAMA response to the agent. The authors suggested that because of interpatient variability of clearance rates, administered activity should be individualized on the basis of dosimetry.

Carrying forth on these principles, the same group evaluated the F(ab')$_2$ of NP-4 labeled with ^{131}I in a phase I trial of 13 patients (eight with colorectal cancer) with small-volume disease ($\leq$3 cm diameter). Administered activity was determined using individual patient dosimetry to deliver a given dose to bone marrow. Mixed responses were seen in two patients and stable disease in four patients of 3.5 to 7 months duration (76).

MN-14, a murine MAb with 10-fold higher affinity to CEA (1×10^{-9} L/mol) than NP-4, was subsequently evaluated in 11 patients (10 with colorectal cancer) in a phase I trial labeled with ^{188}Re (78). ^{188}Re was felt to be attractive for therapy since it decays through a beta emission with maximum energy comparable to ^{90}Y, but it also emits a low abundance of (15%) 155 keV gamma emission that can be used for imaging and tracking the radiopharmaceutical. Given the short half-life of the radionuclide (17 hours), the therapy was delivered in two to three divided doses with 3 to 4 days between infusions. Hepatic and renal uptakes were higher than with ^{131}I-labeled anti-CEA antibodies, although dose-limiting toxicity was still hematologic. No therapeutic effects were observed. The authors concluded that high administered activities were possible on an outpatient basis with this agent, but given the short half-life, ^{188}Re may be a more suitable in scenarios of rapid tumor uptake of the antibody, such as with low-molecular-weight antibody fragments or constructs, smaller volume tumors, or regional administration.

More recently, hMN-14, a humanized version of MN-14, has been evaluated and radiolabeled with ^{131}I in patients primarily with colorectal cancer with small-volume disease or as adjuvant therapy postsurgery. These trials are described in more detail in the section "Strategies to Optimize RIT in Colorectal Cancer: Minimal Tumor Burden Setting."

The anti-CEA antibody, T84.66, has been extensively evaluated at City of Hope. Murine T84.66 is an IgG$_1$ MAb with high specificity and affinity ($\sim$1.16 $\times$ 10^{11} M^{-1}) for CEA (113,114). It recognizes the A3 domain of the CEA molecule and has little cross-reactivity with normal tissues. Using ^{111}In-labeled murine T84.66, Beatty et al. (115) demonstrated successful targeting and imaging of colon cancer with this antibody.

A less immunogenic, high-affinity human–mouse chimeric T84.66 was then developed (IgG$_1$ isotype) for therapy (113). Chimeric T84.66 (cT84.66) was radiolabeled with ^{111}In and evaluated in two pilot imaging/biodistribution trials in patients with CEA-producing malignancies (116,117). These trials demonstrated that ^{111}In-cT84.66 targeted CEA-producing tumors with results comparable to other ^{111}In-labeled intact anti-CEA antibodies, immunogenicity was less after single administration of up to 105 mg of antibody protein compared to intact murine MAbs, the antibody was well tolerated, and potentially therapeutic radiation doses could be delivered to some tumors and regional metastatic lymph nodes.

A phase I therapy trial was then initiated administering ^{90}Y-DTPA-cT84.66 (51). Of 22 patients treated, 12 had colorectal cancer. All patients were heavily pretreated and had progressive disease prior to entry on this trial. Ca-DTPA (diethylenetriaminepentaacetic acid) chelate was infused for 72 hours after therapy infusion to bind the small percentage of ^{90}Y that disassociates from the antibody and to help hasten its excretion through the urinary system, thereby preventing its potential deposition in bone and contribution to marrow dose. Maximum tolerated dose (MTD) was reached at 22 mCi/m^2. Twelve patients demonstrated stable disease or a mixed response and seven demonstrated greater than or equal to 50% decrease in serum CEA levels.

A separate phase I trial with DOTA (1,4,7,10-tetraazacyclododecane-N,N0,N00,N000-tetraacetic acid)-conjugated cT84.66 radiolabeled with ^{90}Y was also carried out in 13 patients (seven with colorectal cancer) with chemotherapy refractory progressive disease (85). Five patients demonstrated stable disease after therapy. Mean tumor dose was 2355 cGy after single-cycle therapy with higher doses estimated for smaller lesions, particularly nodal areas, suggesting that therapy may be best suited for the minimal tumor burden setting. The MTD was defined at 13.4 mCi/m^2. Ca-DTPA infusion post-RIT was needed to reduce hematopoietic toxicity and allow dose escalation beyond 8 mCi/m^2. There appeared to be no clear advantage to DOTA-conjugated versus DTPA-conjugated ^{90}Y-cT84.66.

Subsequent trials at City of Hope with ^{90}Y-cT84.66 have used DTPA-conjugated antibody and have evaluated IP regional administration or RIT in combination with various chemotherapy agents in advanced disease and in the minimal tumor burden setting. These trials are described in more detail in the section "Strategies to Optimize RIT in Colorectal Cancer."

Finally, a phase I therapy trial of a humanized version of T84.66 labeled with ^{90}Y is currently under way. Immunogenicity appears to be further reduced with only 1 of 10 patients developing a human antihuman antibody (HAHA) response (unpublished data), compared to 11 of 21 after single administration of ^{90}Y-DTPA-cT84.66 (51).

Other anti-CEA MAbs have been studied in clinical trials on a more limited basis. The high-affinity anti-CEA murine MAb COL-1 was evaluated by Yu et al. labeled with ^{131}I in a phase I trial (45). Four of 18 patients (16 with colorectal cancer) demonstrated stable disease of 1.5 to 4 months duration. Faster clearance rates of the antibody were observed in patients with large tumor burden or high serum CEA levels, an observation reported in other studies (46).

Ychou et al. reported on 10 patients with unresectable liver metastases from colorectal cancer treated with ^{131}I-F6 F(ab')$_2$ (90). Autologous bone marrow was harvested in all patients. Administered activity ranged from 87 to 300 mCi. Five of six patients treated at 300 mCi had reinfusion of marrow. One partial response and two patients with stable disease were observed.

Breitz et al. (41) evaluated the anti-CEA F(ab')$_2$ fragment of NR-CO-02 in 31 patients (27 with colorectal cancer) in a phase I trial. The antibody was labeled with ^{186}Re, which is attractive for therapy since it has a half-life of 3.7 days, comparable with the tumor localization kinetics of intact antibodies, emits primarily a beta particle with maximum energy of 1.07 MeV, and has a low-abundance gamma emission (137 keV) suitable for antibody imaging and tracking. One partial response was seen. Eleven other patients demonstrated stable disease. Five patients received the agent through hepatic arterial infusion and demonstrated comparable pharmacokinetics to patients receiving the agent intravenously. Marrow toxicity was dose limiting. Although renal uptake and dose was greater than that seen with other ^{131}I- or ^{90}Y-labeled antibodies, no significant nephrotoxicity was observed. In 17 patients with minimal prior therapy, the MTD was not reached at 200 mCi/m^2.

▓ TAG-72 trials

Tumor-associated glycoprotein (TAG-72) has been an antigen target for RIT trials in patients with adenocarcinomas, including colorectal cancer. TAG-72 was first identified as the target antigen for the MAb B72.3, which had been generated from the membrane fraction of breast adenocarcinomas (118). TAG-72 is expressed by approximately 80% of colorectal cancers with very little expression in normal tissues (119).

Radiolabeled murine MAb B72.3 was initially evaluated in imaging trials (120–122). A chimeric version of B72.3 was then developed and evaluated labeled with ^{131}I in a phase I therapy trial by Meredith et al. (93). Of 12 patients with colorectal cancer, four demonstrated stable disease and received a second cycle of therapy. Seven patients developed a HAMA response. An MTD of 36 mCi/m^2 was defined with dose-limiting toxicity being hematopoietic. The MTD was reduced compared to other ^{131}I-labeled intact murine MAbs. The added toxicity was felt to be secondary to its prolonged plasma half-life of 242 hours (56), which resulted in increased total body and marrow doses. The authors concluded that ^{131}I-B72.3 had limited potential as a radioimmunotherapeutic agent due to its unexpectedly high immunogenicity that prevented multiple administrations and its long plasma half-life that increased hematopoietic toxicity.

Subsequent RIT trials evaluated CC49, a murine MAb with higher affinity for TAG-72 (1.62 × 10^{10} L/mol) than B72.3, and demonstrated better relative tumor uptake compared to B72.3 in clinical trials (123). An initial phase I trial reported by Divgi et al. (94) entered 24 patients with colorectal cancer. Escalating doses of 15 to 90 mCi/m^2 ^{131}I-CC49 were administered with an MTD defined by hematopoietic toxicity at 75 mCi/m^2. Six patients demonstrated stable disease after first cycle and subsequently received a second cycle, resulting in a mixed response in one of these patients. This was followed by a phase II trial reported by Murray et al. (95) who treated 15 patients with colorectal cancer at the previously defined MTD of 75 mCi/m^2. Of 14 evaluable patients, no objective responses were seen and three patients demonstrated stable disease after one cycle but went on to progress after second cycle.

Mulligan et al. (44) evaluated CC49 labeled with ^{177}Lu in nine patients (three with colorectal cancer). ^{177}Lu has a lower energy, less abundant gamma emission compared to ^{131}I and, compared to ^{90}Y, a lower energy beta emission and less myelosuppression in animal models (124). An MTD of 15 mCi/m^2 was defined. No antitumor effects were observed. Although hematopoietic toxicity was acceptable, the authors concluded that the prolonged uptake of activity in the marrow and reticuloendothelial system limited the amount of activity that could be administered.

Subsequent trials with radiolabeled CC49 using strategies to reduce hematopoietic toxicity and fractionate administration of activity to improve efficacy have also been performed, and are reported in more detail in the section "Strategies to Optimize RIT in Colorectal Cancer."

▓ A33 trials

A33 is an attractive target antigen for RIT. It is a 43-kDa transmembrane glycoprotein that is highly expressed by colonic cells. Unlike CEA, it is not shed into circulation. MAb once bound to A33 antigen will internalize, resulting in the rapid tumor localization and increased retention and uptake at the tumor site. Welt and colleagues first evaluated MAb A33 labeled with ^{131}I in a phase I/II trial of 23 patients with progressive colorectal cancer (43). An MTD of 75 mCi/m^2 was reached with 13 patients treated at dose levels from 78 to 94 mCi/m^2. Three patients demonstrated a mixed response and an additional two patients had a 22% and 30% decrease in CEA. Variable uptake was seen in normal bowel but GI symptoms were mild.

^{125}I-MAb A33 was also evaluated in a subsequent phase I/II trial (66). Twenty-one patients with chemotherapy refractory colorectal cancer received a dose of 50 to 350 mCi/m^2 (97 to 728 mCi). No dose-limiting toxicity was observed up to 350 mCi/m^2. Transient grade 3 thrombocytopenia was seen in one patient. No GI toxicity was documented. One patient had a mixed response and three patients had a decrease in serum CEA levels.

Recently, Chong et al. (103) evaluated ^{131}I-huA33, a humanized version of MAb A33, in a phase I trial. Fifteen patients with colorectal cancer were treated at 20 to 50 mCi/m^2 and an MTD was established at 40 mCi/m^2 with hematopoietic toxicity as dose limiting. Four patients developed a HAHA response. Tumor dose estimates ranged from 12 to 33 Gy and four patients with smaller volume disease demonstrated stable disease.

Ep-CAM trials

Epithelial cellular adhesion molecule (Ep-CAM), also known as 17-1A antigen, is a 40-kDa transmembrane glycoprotein. It is expressed by GI epithelium and some epithelial cancers, including colorectal cancer (125). It is not shed into the circulation.

Initial trials evaluated the murine IgG$_{2a}$ MAb, 17-1A. The antibody was labeled with ^{125}I, taking advantage of the fact that 17-1A is internalized after binding with surface antigen. Markoe et al. (65) reported on 53 patients (25 with colorectal cancer) treated as part of a phase I study. Most received approximately three cycles of therapy (range 1 to 17) at 3 to 25 mCi per infusion cycle. One patient with partial response of 3 months duration, 1 mixed response of 12 months duration, and 10 patients with stable disease of 3 to 8 months duration were observed. How much of the observed antitumor effect can be attributed to the RIT is somewhat difficult to determine since most of the 46 patients with hepatic metastases also received 15 Gy (1.5 Gy × 10) whole-liver external beam radiotherapy in an attempt to increase RIT uptake to hepatic lesions. No significant hepatotoxicity was reported with this combination.

Meredith et al. (50) subsequently evaluated in a phase I study a chimeric version of 17-1A also labeled with ^{125}I. Twenty-eight patients with colorectal cancer received a singe cycle of therapy ranging from 20 to 250 mCi. For activities above 150 mCi, the activity was administered as separate 50 to 100 mCi infusions every 4 days. Ten patients were

noted to have stable disease when assessed at 6 weeks post therapy. No significant bone marrow suppression or other dose-limiting toxicities were reported.

^{186}Re-NR-LU10 is a murine IgG$_{2a}$, which was evaluated in 15 patients (10 with colorectal cancer) as part of a phase I study (41). An MTD of 90 mCi/m^2 was defined on the basis of hematologic dose-limiting toxicity. Estimated mean radiation dose to marrow was 0.6, liver 2.9, lung 1.4, and kidney 5.7 cGy/mCi. Serum half-life ($T_{1/2}$) β was 26.3 hours. All patients developed a HAMA response. No objective response or other antitumor effects were reported.

The chimeric version of the antibody NR-LU13 labeled with ^{186}Re was evaluated in nine patients (four with colorectal cancer) by Weiden et al. (49). Patients received 25 or 60 mCi/m^2 administered as a single infusion. Estimated mean radiation dose to marrow was 1.3, liver 3.6, lung 3.3, and kidney 12.6 cGy/mCi. As with the murine version of the antibody, kidney uptake was higher than seen with other intact radiolabeled antibodies. Serum $T_{1/2}$ β was slower compared to the murine antibody at 36.5 hours. Immunogenicity was reduced compared to the murine antibody, with six of eight patients developing a human antichimeric antibody (HACA) response. Two patients demonstrated stable disease when reassessed at 6 weeks. Pretargeting approaches using the NR-LU10 antibody have also been evaluated, and are described in more detail in the section "Strategies to Optimize RIT in Colorectal Cancer."

Colon-specific antigen-p trials

Colon-specific antigen-p is a tumor-associated antigen expressed by approximately 60% of colorectal cancers. It is also found in normal colonic mucosa, primarily in the mucin-secreting goblet cells. Sharkey et al. (126) evaluated ^{131}I-Mu-9 in 25 patients (21 with colorectal cancer) as part of a phase I trial. In tumor-bearing animal models, ^{131}I-Mu-9 demonstrated higher tumor uptake, longer tumor retention, and greater antitumor effects than RIT with anti-CEA antibodies. Thirteen patients were treated with intact ^{131}I-Mu-9 and 12 patients were treated with the ^{131}I-Mu-9 F(ab')$_2$. Administered activity was determined on the basis of the amount needed to achieve 450 cGy to marrow. The mean blood half-life for the intact antibody and the F(ab')$_2$ was 41 and 19 hours, respectively. Compared to the intact antibody, the smaller F(ab')$_2$ construct cleared faster, resulting in not only lower marrow doses but also lower tumor uptake, resulting in comparable tumor-to-marrow dose ratios. No antitumor effects were reported.

DNA histone trials

Recently, RIT directed against intracellular antigens have been explored. ^{131}I-chimeric (ch)-TNT-1/B targets areas of tumor necrosis by targeting a complex of double-stranded DNA and histone H1 antigens. Encouraging results were initially seen with intratumoral injections of this radiolabeled antibody in gliomas and lung cancers (127). Street et al. (106) recently reported the first results of systemic administration of ^{131}I-ch TNT-1/B in a phase I trial of 21 patients with advanced colorectal cancer. The antibody was biotinylated for this study to increase tumor uptake. Administered activities ranged from 0.35 to 1.79 mCi/kg (30.3 to 157.6 mCi), with an MTD defined at 1.79 mCi/kg. Tumor doses ranged from 365 to 4560 cGy (mean 2534 cGy). Five of 21 patients demonstrated stable disease.

STRATEGIES TO OPTIMIZE RIT IN COLORECTAL CANCER

RIT demonstrated promise in animal models with dozens of studies in tumor-bearing animal models documenting significant tumor growth delay and cures in a wide variety of solid tumor types (128–131). Tumor doses often exceeded 10 to 15 Gy after a single infusion (132,133). In some preclinical studies RIT achieved comparable tumor growth delays as equivalent doses of single fraction or conventionally fractionated external beam radiation therapy (132–138) or equitoxic doses of chemotherapy (139). Initial clinical trials evaluating biodistribution and pharmacokinetics confirmed tumor targeting and demonstrated that therapeutic doses of radiation to tumor were potentially achievable (117,140–144).

However in the clinic, RIT in colorectal cancer and other solid tumors has not realized the gains as hoped for from preclinical results. As summarized earlier (Tables 25.5 and 25.6), objective responses have been infrequent with most antitumor effects reported as stable disease, serologic, minor, and mixed responses of approximately 3 to 9 months duration. This is in contrast to the clinical results observed in hematologic malignancies with objective responses ranging from 30% to 85% (2–10).

A number of factors have been put forth to explain the limited responses seen. With hematologic malignancies, much of the observed response rates can be attributed to the immunologic effects of the antibody itself (145), which is not the case for most radiolabeled antibodies directed against solid tumors. With regards to colorectal cancer, many of the preclinical studies utilized the colon cancer cell line LS174T, which is one of the most radiosensitive and one of the highest expressors of tumor-associated antigens such as CEA and TAG-72 among colorectal cancer lines (132,146). Therefore, the level of RIT targeting and tumor response observed in animal models may not have reflected values normally encountered in the clinic.

Other factors involve those that restrict antibody targeting and uptake to the tumor more so for solid tumors than lymphomas. These include differences in tumor physiology, tumor vascularity, antigen accessibility, and heterogeneity of antigen expression (147,148). However, these factors probably play a minor role since the clinical literature demonstrates no significant differences in estimated RIT dose to tumor between solid tumors and hematologic malignancies. This suggests that the difference in radiosensitivity is the major factor in explaining differences in response rates between solid tumors and hematologic malignancies.

Table 25.7 compares tumor doses achieved after single administration of nonmyeloablative activities of RIT for solid tumors and lymphomas and demonstrates that tumor doses are comparable for most antibodies evaluated in the clinic. Median and mean doses are approximately 10 to 20 Gy, with select tumors occasionally achieving doses of 20 to 70 Gy or greater. In our experience with ^{90}Y-cT84.66 anti-CEA RIT, approximately 25% of tumors achieve tumor doses greater than 15 to 20 Gy after single infusion. These data support the hypothesis that the differences in response rates between solid tumors and hematologic malignancies are largely due to differences in radiosensitivity, not due to differences in tumor antibody uptake. This is even after accounting for effects of unlabeled antilymphoma antibodies, since clinical trials have demonstrated no significant response rates with unlabeled antibodies such as Lym-1 (156,157), or, as in the case of ^{90}Y-ibritumomab, a 24% increase in response rate was observed with the addition of radiolabeled antibody compared to unlabeled antibody alone in a recent randomized trial (145).

Although tumor doses with RIT are a fraction of what can be delivered by teletherapy or brachytherapy, doses currently achievable are at levels that can potentially result in clinically important antitumor effects in solid tumors, particularly in subclinical or microscopic disease settings. With conventionally fractionated external beam radiotherapy, Withers et al. (158) reviewed the clinical literature evaluating adjuvant radiation for solid tumors and noted an inverse linear relationship between radiation dose and tumor recurrence rate with doses ranging from 2000 to 5000 cGy. More importantly, there was no threshold effect and doses in the range of 2000 cGy had measurable effects in the adjuvant setting. Clinical trials have also demonstrated important antitumor effects in rectal cancer with doses in the range of 3000 cGy (159,160). Finally, doses as low as 3000 cGy conventionally fractionated have been combined with chemotherapy in esophageal and anal cancer, resulting in pathologic complete responses (161–163). Therefore, the dose delivered to a tumor, achievable through RIT, may have more clinical importance in low tumor burden situations and/or as an additional agent added to a multiagent systemic therapy approach.

Further improving RIT clinical outcomes in solid tumors would require increasing radiation dose to tumor or increasing the biologic effect of that targeted dose. Strategies to achieve this goal include (a) improving the antibody delivery system to either increase antibody targeting to tumor or decrease uptake to critical organs; (b) decreasing dose-limiting toxicity (usually marrow toxicity), which would allow for escalation of administered activity; (c) altering the tumor environment to enhance radiolabeled macromolecule targeting; and (d) increasing the tumoricidal effect of the targeted radiation dose through combined modality approaches.

Optimization strategies that have been specifically explored include reduction of hematologic toxicity through hematopoietic stem cell support, the use of agents to upregulate antigen expression, engineered immunoconstructs,

Table **25.7**	Tumor doses and objective response rates from select solid tumor and lymphoma RIT trials				
Study (First Author)	**Radionuclide-Antibody**	**Tumor Type**	**No. of Tumors Analyzed**	**Tumor Dose (cGy/Cycle)**	**Objective Response Rate (%)**
Meredith (42)	^{131}I-CC49	Prostate	4	208–1083	0
Juweid (76)	^{131}I-NP4 F(ab')$_2$	Colorectal, lung, pancreas, thyroid	4	511–6476	0
DeNardo (108)	^{131}I-chL6	Breast	7	120–3700 (~1300 mean)	40
Van Zanten-Pryzbysz (149)	^{131}I-cMOv18	Ovary	3	600–3800	0
Breitz (41)	^{186}Re-NR-CO-2 F(ab')$_2$	Lung, colorectal, breast, ovary, renal	5	500–2100	4
Postema (55,150)	^{186}Re-hu BIWA 4	Head and neck	16	380–7610 (1240 median)	0
DeNardo (151)	^{90}Y-BrE-3	Breast	16	442–1887	0
Wong (86)	^{90}Y-cT84.66	Colorectal	31	46–6400 (mean 1320)	0
Chong (103)	^{131}I-huA33	Colorectal		1173–3273 (mean 2119 at 50 mCi/m^2)	0
Street (106)	^{131}I-cTNT-1/B	Colorectal		365–4560 (mean 2534 at 1.79 mCi/kg)	0
Wiseman (152)	^{90}Y-ibritumomab	Non-Hodgkin lymphoma	18	580–6700 (1700 median)	67
Kaminski (153)	^{131}I-tositumomab	Non-Hodgkin lymphoma	NS	141–2584 (925 mean)	79
Lamborn (154)	^{131}I-Lym-1	Non-Hodgkin lymphoma	45	16–1485 (241 median)	54
Vose (155)	^{131}I-LL2	Non-Hodgkin lymphoma	NS	166–861	33

NS, not stated.

regional administration, combined modality approaches, and therapy in the minimal tumor burden or adjuvant setting. Antibody-based, pretargeting delivery strategies that seek to amplify the differences between tumor and normal organ uptake also continue to be actively explored and are promising.

Reducing dose-limiting hematopoietic toxicity

Since hematologic toxicity is often dose limiting, groups have explored dose intensification strategies using stem cell or bone marrow reinfusion after myeloablative doses of radiolabeled MAbs. Most have been phase I studies treating a limited number of patients with breast (164–168), medullary thyroid (169), or GI malignancies (90,98,99). Tempero and colleagues (99) in a phase I study administered ^{131}I-CC49 to 14 patients (12 with colorectal cancer) as a single infusion at administered activities of 50 to 300 mCi/m^2 followed by hematopoietic stem cell reinfusion. Although no extrahematopoietic dose-limiting toxicities were observed, the study was stopped due to limited tumor doses achieved (630 to 3000 cGy) and an absence of any antitumor effects. The same group

evaluated ^{90}Y-CC49 in 12 patients with advanced GI malignancies (five with colorectal cancer) with administered activities ranging from 0.3 to 0.5 mCi/kg followed by hematopoietic stem cell reinfusion. As in the previous study, no extrahematopoietic dose-limiting toxicities were observed. Tumor doses ranged from 180 to 3000 cGy. Although no objective responses were observed, two patients demonstrated stable disease of 2 and 4 months duration. In summary, hematopoietic stem cell and marrow reinfusion has permitted higher myeloablative activities to be administered, but it appears that dose intensification alone will not result in the level of objective response rates initially hoped for, and may need to be combined with other optimization strategies.

Other approaches include those by Wheeler et al. (96) who administered interleukin-1 (IL-1) after RIT in an attempt to reduce hematopoietic toxicity. Twelve patients with metastatic colorectal cancer received 0.4 μg/kg IL-1 on days −5 to −1 prior to a dose of 75 mCi/m^2 ^{131}I-CC49. When compared to historical controls receiving the same dose of ^{131}I-CC49 alone, the authors concluded that IL-1 did not significantly reduce hematopoietic toxicity and did not permit administration of higher activities.

Fractionation of administered activity

In most published animal and clinical studies, RIT is delivered as a single infusion or, if repeated, administered approximately 4 to 6 weeks later after recovery of blood counts, similar to many chemotherapy schedules. Fractionated RIT usually involves administration of the total activity through divided infusions spaced days to a week apart instead of as a single infusion and takes advantage of the differences in uptake and clearance kinetics of activity between tumor and normal tissues, such that with the appropriate fractionation schedule, the ratio between tumor dose and marrow dose can be amplified. The optimum schedule therefore may be dependent on a complex interplay of multiple factors including uptake and clearance kinetics of the antibody construct, decay kinetics of the radionuclide, tumor size, change in tumor size with each administration, radiosensitivity of tumor and organs, and clearance kinetics of the individual patient. Factors such as tumor reoxygenation, repopulation, and cell cycle redistribution may also theoretically play a role, but have not been studied extensively in experimental models. A number of groups have reported in animal models less hematopoietic toxicity and greater antitumor effects if the administered activity is delivered in smaller divided doses every few days, weekly, or biweekly, rather than as a single infusion (21,170–172). Others have seen not only reduced toxicity but also reduced tumor growth suppression (173).

Meredith et al. (48) used a fractionated RIT schedule with ^{131}I-chimeric B72.3. Patients with colorectal cancer received 28 or 36 mCi/m^2 in 2 to 3 weekly fractions of 12 to 18 mCi/m^2. There was a modest but statistically significant ($p = 0.04$) decrease in hematopoietic toxicity adjusted for whole-body dose when compared to a similar population treated on an earlier trial (93) who received similar doses of ^{131}I-chimeric B72.3 but as a single infusion. Of the 12 patients treated, 1 experienced a minor response of 17+ months duration and 3 had stable disease after the first cycle of therapy but subsequently progressed after the second cycle.

Divgi et al. (97) also evaluated a fractionated schedule with the anti-TAG-72 antibody CC49 radiolabeled with ^{131}I. Six patients with colorectal cancer received 15 mCi/m^2 biweekly up to a maximum of four infusions. The immunomodulating agent deoxyspergualin was administered after each infusion to reduce the likelihood of a HAMA response. This schedule was well tolerated with no dose-limiting toxicities observed. No major antitumor effects were observed.

Modifying tumor environment

Upregulation of tumor antigen expression as a means of increasing antibody targeting and radiation dose to tumor has been explored. Alpha- and gamma-interferon have been shown to increase tumor-associated antigen expression, including CEA and TAG-72, in vitro (174,175) and in vivo (176,177). The effects of interferon on CEA expression were greatest in colorectal cell lines that were low-to-moderate CEA producers. In animal models this translated into increased therapeutic efficacy of RIT (178,179). Kuhn et al. (180) demonstrated in colon cancer–bearing animal models greater tumor growth suppression with gamma-interferon combined with anti-CEA ^{90}Y-ZCE025 RIT, compared to ^{90}Y-ZCE025 alone or radiolabeled nonspecific antibody with interferon. In addition, gamma-interferon increased tumor CEA expression and treatment efficacy when combined with a second cycle of anti-CEA ^{90}Y-ZCE025 RIT (181).

Increased CEA and TAG-72 expression has also been documented in patients receiving interferon (182–185). In patients with colorectal cancer, Meredith et al. (101) administered alpha-interferon at 3×10^6 IU per day on days −5 to +3 to increase CEA and TAG-72 expression and antibody uptake to tumor. On day 0 ^{131}I-COL-1 anti-CEA and ^{131}I-CC49 anti-TAG-72 were administered for a total administered activity of 75 mCi/m^2. This second optimization strategy of using a "cocktail" of anti-TAG-72 and anti-CEA antibodies was based on preclinical studies that demonstrated increased tumor antibody uptake (186) and increased therapeutic effect (187) with a combination of radiolabeled MAbs recognizing two distinct epitopes instead of one. An increase in estimated radiation dose to tumors was noted when compared to tumor doses from a previous study (95) that administered 75 mCi/m^2 ^{131}I-CC49 without interferon in patients with colorectal cancer. For extrahepatic tumors, radiation doses ranged from 393 to 1327 cGy with and 592 to 745 cGy without interferon.

Strategies to modify the tumor vasculature to increase blood flow or vascular leakage, using vasoactive agents, vasoactive immunoconjugates, radiation therapy, or hyperthermia, have been explored primarily in experimental models (188). Interest has been on an emerging class of agents directed against the tumor neovasculature. Jain et al. (189,190) and others have proposed using antiangiogenic agents, such as anti-VEGF (vascular endothelial growth factor) antibodies, to "prune" or normalize the tumor vasculature, decrease tumor interstitial pressure, and increase tumor perfusion, which should result in increased macromolecule delivery. In some experimental models tumor oxygenation is also increased (190), which can add to potential effects of RIT.

In a similar strategy Burke et al. have looked at using cyclic RGD peptide, which recognizes the $\alpha v \beta 3$ integrin receptor on tumor neovasculature. In a tumor-bearing breast cancer mouse model, the combination of RGD peptide and ^{90}Y-chimeric L6 RIT resulted in higher tumor uptake of antibody, and a greater percentage of mice cured than either therapy alone (191,192). In colorectal cancer tumor-bearing mice, Kinuya et al. (193) combined the antiangiogenic agent 2-methoxyestradiol with ^{131}I-A7 RIT and demonstrated prolonged survival with the combination, compared to either agent alone. Recently, Bodet-Milin et al. (194) combined ^{131}I-F6 anti-CEA RIT and bevacizumab (anti-VEGF) in medullary thyroid cancer–bearing mice and reported an increase in tumor growth delay with the combination compared to either agent alone.

The vascular disrupting agent combretastatin-A-4-phosphate (CA4P) has been shown to increase tumor retention of ^{131}I-AB7 anti-CEA antibody, resulting in increased radiation dose (195) and significant increase in tumor growth suppression compared to ^{131}I-AB7 RIT alone (196). On the basis of these encouraging preclinical results, a phase I/II trial was initiated and preliminary results recently reported (89). Twelve patients (11 with colorectal cancer) received ^{131}I-A5B7 anti-CEA MAb given on day 1 and CA4P on days 2 and 3. Dynamic contrast-enhancing MRI demonstrated reduction in tumor vascular kinetics in 9 of 12 patients. Dose-limiting hematopoietic toxicity was observed at ^{131}I-A5B7 administered activities of 1600 MBq/m^2 (43.2 mCi/m^2) and CA4P of 54 mg/m^2. Of 10 evaluable patients, 1 had stable disease.

Regional administration

Regional administration to optimize uptake at the tumor site relative to dose-limiting normal organs has also been explored. Preclinical (197,198) and clinical (199) studies indicate that IP administration has pharmacologic advantages over IV administration for cancers confined to the peritoneal cavity, due to increased antibody uptake in tumor, particularly for small-volume disease (198–201).

Only a limited number of IP RIT trials have been performed in patients with colorectal cancer. Riva et al. (102) conducted a phase II study of IP RIT in 18 patients with metastatic colorectal cancer. A second optimization strategy using a mixture of four different ^{131}I radiolabeled antibodies directed against three different epitopes was used. Three patients also received IV RIT. Administered activities ranged from 21 to 150 mCi, resulting in tumor doses of 768 to 4628 cGy. Multiple cycles of therapy were administered to most patients. Results were encouraging. Of 15 evaluable patients, 2 achieved a complete response of 6+ and 12+ months duration, and 2 patients had a partial response of 3 and 16 months duration. An additional 3 patients demonstrated stable disease from 3 to 11 months duration. Of 10 patients with elevated serum CEA, 6 showed a decrease in CEA by an average of 84%.

At City of Hope, a phase I trial of IP-administered anti-CEA ^{90}Y-cT84.66 was recently completed in patients with CEA-expressing malignancies, with disease primarily confined to the peritoneal cavity (Table 25.5). Fifteen patients (eight with colorectal cancer) received 5, 7, 10.5, 14, or 19 mCi/m^2. Nine patients received one cycle, four patients two cycles, and one patient three cycles. Toxicities as expected were primarily hematopoietic although not dose limiting even at the highest administered activity of 19 mCi/m^2. Eight patients demonstrated antitumor effects. One patient had a mixed response with resolution of malignant ascites. Seven patients demonstrated stable disease of 3 to 7 months duration, of which one patient demonstrated a reduction in malignant ascites and another patient demonstrated resolution of pelvic fascial thickening and pelvic pain. The highest dose level on this trial (19 mCi/m^2)

resulted in less than or equal to grade 2 toxicity. The therapeutic index appeared to be improved with IP compared to IV administration of ^{90}Y-cT84.66 (51), since the MTD reached with IV-administered antibody was lower at 16.6 mCi/m^2.

New constructs

Recombinant antibodies can be designed with improved biodistribution and pharmacokinetic properties to optimize their use for therapy. Recombinant DNA methodology has enabled antibodies to be engineered for the selection of molecular size, affinity, valency, effector functions, site-specific conjugation, and humanization.

A limiting factor of intact antibodies is their relatively slow blood clearance. Serum half-lives can extend from days to weeks, resulting in higher doses to marrow and hematopoietic toxicity. Antibody fragments and other low-molecular-weight antibody constructs may ultimately prove superior for therapy due to their faster clearance, greater tumor penetration (70), more uniform distribution in tumor (202), higher initial dose rate in tumor (203), decreased immunogenicity (204), and higher tumor-to-background ratios. These factors offer the potential for higher administered activities and increased tumor doses for the same level of toxicity.

Initial efforts evaluated Fab and F(ab')$_2$ fragments generated by enzymatic digestion. In vivo studies demonstrated superior tumor-to-blood dose ratios over the intact antibody (131,205,206). Radiolabeled F(ab')$_2$ and Fab' fragments have also been evaluated as radioimmunotherapeutics in the clinic with some success (Tables 25.5 and 25.6) (41,76,88,90,92). However, the observed antitumor effects with F(ab')$_2$ and Fab' fragments appear to be no better than their intact antibody counterparts. This is probably due to the fact that although blood clearance may be more rapid with fragments, retention time in tumor is also reduced, resulting in no significant improvement in centigray dose to tumor over the intact antibody for equitoxic administered activities.

More recent efforts have used recombinant DNA technology to genetically engineer antibody constructs with properties to improve tumor-to-normal organ biodistribution, enhance in vivo stability, reduce immunogenicity, aid in conjugation and radiolabeling, and increase clearance kinetics. Constructs have ranged from approximately 25 to 160 kDa in size. The genes encoding the antibody's variable light (V$_L$) and variable heavy (V$_H$) domains can be cloned and linked by a contiguously encoded peptide into a single-chain (sc) Fv construct. This small monovalent scFv, 28 kDa, clears rapidly from the circulation, increasing the tumor-to-blood ratio, thus making them attractive as potential imaging agents (207,208). However, the absolute peak uptake and retention time in tumors are often reduced, limiting their effective use as therapy agents (207–210). In addition, low-molecular-weight constructs can filter through the renal glomeruli, resulting in increased kidney uptake and radiation dose compared to higher molecular weight constructs.

A more suitable construct for therapy would perhaps be bivalent and of intermediate molecular weight to exhibit uptake and retention in tumor comparable to intact antibodies, but with faster clearance times, resulting in an improved therapeutic ratio. Multivalent, intermediate-molecular-weight constructs have been produced through covalent linking of monovalent fragments (20,21,24–26,28,30,209, 211–213). Alternatively, single-chain monomers can be engineered with properties that promote spontaneous formation of dimeric and trimeric species. For example, Wu and colleagues at the City of Hope (214) engineered a series of recombinant fragments derived from the intact anti-CEA T84.66 MAb (Fig. 25.1). This cognate family of anti-CEA constructs was radioiodinated and compared to each other in a mice bearing human colorectal cancer xenografts. The scFv gave low peak tumor uptake of 2% to 3% injected dose per gram (%ID/g). The diabody (55 kDa), which is formed by the cross-pair dimerization of two scFv monomers, gave improved peak tumor uptake of 10 to 15 %ID/g with longer retention time in tumor than the scFv monomer. The minibody (80 kDa), formed by the self-association of two scFv-C_H3 single-chain monomers, gave peak tumor uptakes of over 20% to 30% ID/g, which exceeded that of the diabody and F(ab')$_2$ and approached that of the intact antibody. When evaluated in tumor-bearing animal models, radioiodinated cT84.66 minibody demonstrated a tumor-to-blood dose ratio of 5.5 compared to 3.4 for the intact antibody and 3.9 for the F(ab')$_2$ fragment. This translated into the potential for higher administered activities with the minibody while maintaining the same toxicity profile and predicted for up to a 60% increase in radiation dose to tumor at maximum administered activities (215).

Wong et al. recently completed a pilot imaging trial (216) evaluating the biodistribution and tumor targeting properties of the cT84.66 minibody labeled with ^{123}I in patients with colorectal cancer. Ten patients received an imaging dose of 5 to 10 mCi (1 mg) of ^{123}I-minibody prior to planned surgery. Tumor imaging was observed in seven of the eight patients who had gross disease found at surgery. The blood clearance was faster than intact cT84.66 with a $T_{1/2}\beta$ of 29.8 hours compared to the intact cT84.66 antibody (98.3 hours) seen in an earlier study (217). Results were comparable to an earlier trial at City of Hope evaluating a ^{123}I-F(ab')$_2$ fragment of cT84.66 in 19 patients with colorectal cancer planned for surgery. In this trial 13 patients demonstrated imaging of at least one known site and serum $T_{1/2}\beta$ was 29 hours (unpublished data).

To further evaluate its potential as a therapy agent, a similar study was performed at City of Hope evaluating ^{111}In-DOTA-cT84.66 minibody. Five patients received the agent, with four of five demonstrating tumor imaging. In one patient, targeting was seen in pelvic soft tissue areas. Later, after resection of this area, micrometastatic disease was discovered, suggesting that this targeting construct can identify small-volume disease. The serum $T_{1/2}$ was 52.1 hours, which was longer than that for ^{123}I-minibody, probably reflecting the longer half-life on [111]I and dehalogenation,

which occurs with radioiodinated MAbs. Mean radiation dose to liver was 19.6, kidney 33.3, lung 1.5, and marrow 2.2 cGy/mCi [90]Y. Renal doses were higher than predicted from animal studies (24). There was no evidence of minibody degradation on serum high-performance liquid chromatography after administration that would potentially explain this level of renal uptake. Mean tumor dose based on four lesions was 12.4 (6.8 to 25.1) cGy/mCi [90]Y. Tumor-to-marrow ratio was 5.6, comparable to that seen in murine models. However, this was less than the ratio of 10.5 seen for intact ^{90}Y-DTPA-cT84.66 (51) and the ratio of 11.6 for ^{90}Y-DOTA-cT84.66 (85) seen in previous phase I trials (51,85). On this basis, it was concluded that the therapeutic ratio of the minibody was not clearly superior when compared to the intact cT84.66 MAb.

Other groups have investigated similar strategies (210,218–222). Forero and colleagues recently reported on a 153-kDa ^{131}I-labeled humanized C_H2 domain-deleted construct (HuCC49ΔCH$_2$) derived from CC49 anti-TAG72 (223). Blood clearance $T_{1/2}$ was 20 hours, comparable to cT84.66 minibody. This was faster than that seen for ^{131}I-labeled intact murine CC49, which was 50 hours. All four patients demonstrated targeting to tumor with a mean tumor-to-marrow dose ratio of 7.3, predicting that over a threefold increase of administered activity was possible compared to ^{131}I-intact murine CC49. A phase I dose escalation therapy trial in metastatic colorectal cancer was initiated, and preliminary results indicate reduced hematologic toxicity compared to intact murinen ^{131}I-CC49. At the initial dose level of 75 mCi/m^2, only 25% of patients (one of four) developed greater than grade 3 hematopoietic toxicity, compared to greater than 60% of patients with ^{131}I-murine CC49 in a previous trial (224).

▪ Pretargeting delivery systems

Pretargeting or a multistep approach may overcome the limitations of direct-radiolabeled antibody therapy. Pretargeting separates the antibody's slow pharmacokinetics from the rapid delivery of a therapeutic radionuclide ligand. This strategy is described in more detail elsewhere (Chapter 14) and as such will only be discussed here as it applies to colorectal cancer therapy.

The basic steps of pretargeting include the following: (a) a modified unlabeled antitumor antibody is administered and allowed to localize to the tumor; (b) a clearing agent is added, which binds the unbound antibody in the circulation, forming complexes that are rapidly cleared out through the hepatobiliary system; (c) a hapten, consisting of a radionuclide linked to a low-molecular-weight ligand, is administered, which rapidly targets to the antibody bound on tumor, with fast clearance of the unbound fraction from blood by the kidneys. The end result is an increase in the therapeutic ratio primarily through a decrease in radiation dose to marrow and normal tissue, allowing for increased administered activities.

Pioneering work utilized the high-binding affinity streptavidin– or avidin–biotin system in which an antibody–

streptavidin conjugate or a biotinylated antibody is coupled to a reciprocal ligand bearing the therapeutic radionuclide (62,225,226). Results using pretargeted approaches have been promising in animal models (227,228) and are now being actively studied in the clinic (105,229–235). However, immunogenicity to the bacteria-derived reagents, such as streptavidin, has limited the ability to deliver multiple administrations.

Bispecific antibodies provide an attractive alternative for pretargeting by fusing antitumor targeting to the capture of the low-molecular-weight hapten (236). Bispecific antibodies have one arm of the antibody recognizing the tumor antigen and the other recognizing the radiolabeled ligand. The unlabeled bispecific antibody is first administered and allowed to localize to the tumor site. This is followed by infusion of a radiolabeled ligand, which then targets to the tumor by binding to the second arm of the antibody. While initial studies used chemically conjugated (237) or quadroma fusions (238), recombinant DNA technology has enabled the production of human or humanized molecules to lower the potential for immunogenicity.

The antihapten antibody can be highly specific for the radiometal–chelate complex, exhibiting vastly reduced binding affinity if a different metal is used to coordinate the complex (239). To circumvent this metal specificity, Goldenberg and colleagues at the Garden State Cancer Center have generated antibodies against the hapten peptide, histamine-succinyl-glycine (HSG), which is independent of the radionuclide or chelate (240). This provides a platform technology that enables multivalency and multifunctionality, where for example two antitumor Fabs can self-assemble with an anti-HSG Fab (241).

To date, there have been a number of RIT trials in colorectal cancer using pretargeting strategies. A phase I trial was performed using a streptavidin-conjugated NR-LU-10 murine MAb (NR-LU-10-SA) directed against Ep-CAM (104,242). Forty patients with refractory adenocarcinomas (10 with colorectal cancer) were treated. Patients first received NR-LU-10-SA, followed 48 hours later by a clearing agent (human serum albumin-galactose-biotin) to clear any unbound NR-LU-10-SA from circulation. This was then followed by administration of 10 to 140 mCi/m^2 ^{90}Y-DOTA-biotin. GI toxicity (diarrhea) was dose limiting at 140 mCi/m^2 due to antibody targeting to normal gut. Hematopoietic toxicity was not dose limiting. Mean radiation dose estimates to kidney were 11.5, bowel 10.6, and marrow 0.15 cGy/mCi. Two partial and four minor responses were observed.

This was followed by a phase II trial using the same pretargeting antibody system in patients with metastatic colorectal cancer (105). Twenty-five patients received 110 mCi/m^2 ^{90}Y-DOTA-biotin. GI toxicity was the most frequent toxicity observed with 16% of patients experiencing grade 4 toxicity and 16% experiencing grade 3 toxicity. Grade 3 and 4 hematopoietic toxicities were less frequent. In addition, two patients developed a significant elevation in serum creatinine 7 to 8 months after therapy, which could

not be explained by other factors or disease. Dose estimates were performed in three patients with mean doses of 2102, 2864, and 33 cGy to small intestine, kidneys, and marrow, respectively. All patients developed an immune response to the antibody, streptavidin, and radiolabeled conjugate. Two partial responses of 16 weeks duration were observed. Four patients had stable disease of 10 to 20 weeks duration. In summary, although objective responses were seen in both the phase I and II studies of NR-LU-10-SA pretargeting RIT, uptake of antibody to normal intestine and kidney, and the resulting GI toxicity and possible nephrotoxicity, potentially limits the use of this particular agent.

Forero-Torres et al. (100) reported their initial experience using a similar three-step pretargeted RIT approach that utilized an antibody fusion construct directed against TAG-72. Nine patients with metastatic colorectal cancer first received CC49 fusion protein, a tetrameric scFv fusion construct conjugated to streptavidin. This was followed 48 hours later by a synthetic monobiotinylated poly-N-acetyl galactosoamine compound clearing agent. Twenty-four hours later all patients received ^{111}In-DOTA-biotin for pharmacokinetics and dosimetry purposes, with the latter six patients also receiving ^{90}Y-DOTA-biotin at 10 mCi/m^2. The mean plasma $T_{1/2}$ was 23 hours. Greater than 95% of the CC49 fusion protein was cleared within 6 hours after administration of the clearing agent. Mean tumor dose was 29.3 (7.9 to 121.6) cGy/mCi. Estimated mean radiation doses to kidney, liver, whole body, and marrow were 3.7, 7.04, 0.52, and 0.21 cGy/mCi, respectively. Two of six demonstrated stable disease of 12 weeks and 6 months duration. No significant hematopoietic, renal, hepatic, or infusion-related toxicities were observed in this initial cohort. All patients developed an immune response to the agent. Estimated mean tumor dose to marrow radiation dose was 139:1 and tumor dose to whole-body dose 56:1. The authors predicted for the ability to deliver greater radiation dose to tumor with this fusion construct compared to a radiolabeled intact antibody.

Recently, Kraeber-Bodere et al. (84) described a two-step pretargeted RIT approach, utilizing a chimeric bispecific anti-CEA/anti-DTPA-indium antibody. The bispecific antibody was formed by coupling Fab' fragments of hMN14 anti-CEA and murine m734 anti-DTPA-indium. Twenty-two patients (nine with colorectal cancer) were treated on this phase I trial. Patients received bispecific antibody at 75 mg/m^2 (11 patients) or 40 mg/m^2 (11 patients), followed 5 days later by escalating administered activities of ^{131}I-di-DTPA-indium bivalent hapten (1.9 to 5.5 GBq/m^2). The primary toxicity was hematopoietic, which was more frequent at the 75 mg/m^2 level. At the 40 mg/m^2 level, the MTD of ^{131}I-di-DTPA-indium bivalent hapten was 3 GBq (81.1 mCi). At the 40 mg/m^2 level, the mean radiation dose to tumor, kidney, liver, and whole body was 18.5, 2.4, 1.9, and 0.38 Gy, respectively. Of 20 evaluable patients, 9 demonstrated stable disease of 3 months to greater than 12 months duration. A HAMA response was seen in one patient and HAHA response in four patients.

Combined modality approaches

RIT and chemotherapy

Multiple preclinical studies have documented additive or supra-additive antitumor effects when RIT is combined with radiation-enhancing chemotherapy or other systemic agents, including gemcitabine (243–245), taxanes (246,247), cisplatin (248), 5-FU (249–251), doxorubicin (252), halogenated pyrimidines (253), topoisomerase inhibitors (249,254,255), tirapazamine (256,257), EGFR tyrosine kinase inhibitors (258), and anti-EGFR MAbs (259). A growing number of clinical trials are evaluating the feasibility and potential improved efficacy of concomitant chemotherapy and RIT, either by adding chemotherapy to MTDs of RIT or adding RIT as additional therapy to established chemotherapy regimens. RIT and chemotherapy trials have been performed in a number of different solid tumor types including ovarian, breast, prostate, medullary thyroid, and colorectal cancer (260–264). In some studies, the strategy of chemotherapy and RIT has often been combined with other strategies, including regional delivery, interferon, and hematopoietic stem cell support. These trials demonstrate the feasibility of combined modality systemic therapy incorporating RIT.

Wong et al. at City of Hope (86) reported the results of a phase I trial combining systemic ^{90}Y-cT84.66 anti-CEA RIT and a 5-day continuous infusion of 5-FU in patients with metastatic colorectal cancer. ^{90}Y-cT84.66 administered activity ranged from 16.6 to 20.6 mCi/m^2 and 5-FU dose levels were escalated from 700 to 1000 mg/m^2. Thirteen patients received one cycle and eight patients received two cycles of combined therapy. The MTD was 16.6 mCi/m^2 of ^{90}Y-cT84.66 and 1000 mg/m^2/day of 5-FU, comparable to that expected for each agent alone, demonstrating the feasibility of this combination. Of 21 patients treated, 1 mixed response and 11 with stable disease of 3 to 8 months duration were observed. Mean tumor dose was 1320 cGy (46 to 6400 cGy). 5-FU did not appear to alter the pharmacokinetics and biodistribution of cT84.66. Of 19 evaluable patients, 5 developed a HACA response that was less frequent than that observed with ^{90}Y-cT84.66 alone where 13 of 21 developed a HACA response (51), suggesting that the 5-FU may have played a role in reducing immune response to the chimeric antibody.

As with external beam radiotherapy, gemcitabine may also act as a radiosensitizer when combined with RIT. Our group observed a significant increase in tumor growth delay with gemcitabine and ^{90}Y-cT84.66 in LS174T colon cancer–bearing nude mice without significant additional toxicity (unpublished data). Several other preclinical in vivo studies have demonstrated a synergistic antitumor effect with the combination of RIT and gemcitabine in a number of GI malignancy models, including colorectal cancer (244,245,265–269). A phase I study evaluating concomitant ^{90}Y-cT84.66 anti-CEA RIT and gemcitabine has recently been completed at City of Hope (Table 25.5) (87). Thirty-two patients with CEA-expressing advanced

carcinomas (18 with colorectal cancer) refractory to standard therapies were treated. Each received 16.6 mCi/m^2 ^{90}Y-cT84.66 (day 1) and gemcitabine at escalating doses (days 1 and 3). Gemcitabine doses ranged from an initial dose level of 30 mg/m^2 to 165 mg/m^2, at which point dose-limiting toxicity was reached with grade 3 rash and grade 4 neutropenia. The MTD was determined to be 150 mg/m^2. For tumors greater than 9 cc estimated mean tumor dose was 13.9 Gy (2 to 35 Gy). For smaller lesions 0.3 to 5 cc in size, mean tumor dose was 33.9 Gy (14.1 to 192 Gy), suggesting that higher dose may be achievable with very small lesions, as predicted from preclinical models. One patient experienced a partial response, one a mixed response, and nine stable disease. Twelve of 32 developed a HACA response that was less frequent than that with ^{90}Y-cT84.66 alone (51), suggesting that, as with 5-FU, the addition of gemcitabine may have reduced the incidence of HACA.

Also recently completed at City of Hope is a pilot study of IP-administered ^{90}Y-cT4.66 anti-CEA RIT and IP gemcitabine in patients with CEA-expressing cancers with disease primarily confined to the peritoneal cavity. Seven patients (two with colorectal cancers) received 19 mCi/m^2 ^{90}Y-cT84.66 and gemcitabine at escalating doses on days 1, 4, and 8. Six patients received 40 mg/m^2/d and one patient 80 mg/m^2/d gemcitabine. The combination was well tolerated with no dose-limiting toxicities observed. Results were encouraging with four of seven patients demonstrating antitumor effects (one with mixed response and three with stable disease of 2 to over 15 months duration). One had complete resolution of malignant ascites, while another had greater than 50% reduction of ascites, no longer requiring frequent abdominal paracenteses.

In summary, combining RIT with single-agent chemotherapy 5-FU or gemcitabine appears to be feasible with acceptable toxicity and has resulted in antitumor activity in heavily pretreated patients. Similar efforts should continue in the appropriate patient populations and should consider combining RIT with established chemotherapy regimens possibly in less heavily pretreated patients.

RIT and external beam radiotherapy

Combined modality approaches should also evaluate the combination of RIT and external beam radiation therapy for a number of reasons (270). The two modalities combined may deliver a higher cumulative radiation dose to the tumor than either modality alone. If external beam radiotherapy precedes RIT, radiolabeled macromolecule uptake can potentially be increased through reduction in tumor size (271), increase in vascular permeability (272,273), or increase in antigen expression (274–276). If RIT precedes external beam radiation, low-dose-rate RIT irradiation has been shown to potentiate tumoricidal effects of subsequent external beam radiotherapy in vitro through mechanisms that involve a G2 block, which puts cells in a more sensitive phase of the cell cycle (277), or through a phenomenon termed "protracted exposure radiosensitization" as described by Williams et al. (278).

Clinical trials combining local regional external beam radiotherapy with RIT have been completed with acceptable toxicity in patients with hepatobiliary cancers (13,14,65,279) and high-grade gliomas (280–282). Combining total body irradiation (TBI) as a form of systemic external beam radiotherapy with RIT in a myeloablative transplant setting has also been performed in patients with breast, prostate (283), and hematologic malignancies (6,284–286) with cumulative marrow doses up to approximately 40 Gy reported (284).

Only a limited number of external beam radiotherapy and RIT-combined therapy efforts have been reported for colorectal cancer. Markoe et al. (65) treated 53 patients (25 with colorectal cancer) with ^{125}I-17-1A anti-Ep-CAM antibody in a phase I study. Forty-six patients with liver metastases also received 1500 cGy whole-liver radiotherapy in 10 daily fractions to increase RIT uptake to hepatic lesions. No significant hepatotoxicity was reported with this combination. One partial response of 3 months duration, 1 mixed response of 12 months duration, and 10 patients with stable disease of 3 to 8 months duration were observed.

Buchegger et al. (92) also combined RIT with liver radiotherapy in six patients with metastatic colorectal cancer. RIT consisted 127 to 227 mCi of ^{131}I-anti-CEA F(ab')$_2$ derived from three different murine MAbs. RIT was administered after a dose of 20 Gy (2 Gy per fraction) to the liver in three patients. In the other three patients, 10 Gy at 2.5 Gy per fraction was delivered first, followed by RIT, and then an additional 10 Gy. Hematopoietic toxicity was the primary toxicity. Grade 1 to 3 transient elevations in liver transaminases and alkaline phosphatase were observed. One minor response, three patients with stable disease, and five patients with a decrease in CEA were reported.

Although the experience is limited, combining RIT with external beam radiotherapy appears to be feasible and is associated with acceptable toxicity. Efforts evaluating RIT as an adjunct to external beam radiotherapy should continue to be evaluated in clinical trials in colorectal cancer as well as in other solid tumors.

RIT and hyperthermia

Hyperthermia has demonstrated promise in experimental models as a means of enhancing the efficacy of RIT through a number of possible mechanisms, which include increasing tumor antigen expression (287,288), increasing tumor blood flow and/or vascular permeability, decreasing tumor interstitial pressure, radiosensitization by inhibition of sublethal damage and potentially lethal damage repair (289–291), and direct cytotoxic effects on tumor. Wong et al. (287) heated LS174T colon cancer cells in vitro at 42°C/1 hour, 43°C/1 hour, and 45°C/30 minutes and observed a decrease in CEA membrane expression in the initial 24 hours followed by a two- to threefold increase, and a peaking at 3 days and

returning toward baseline by the fifth to sixth day. The magnitude of effect was directly related to the magnitude of cell kill by each heating schedule.

Multiple in vivo studies have demonstrated an increase in antibody uptake to tumor with hyperthermia (292–298). The sequencing schedule appears to be important. For example, Kinuya et al. (297) administered ^{131}I-A7 anticolorectal RIT in LS180 colon cancer–bearing mice. Hyperthermia to 43°C/1 hour was administered either 2 days before, 2 days after, or immediately after RIT. Increased tumor uptake and a 2.4-fold increase in radiation dose to tumor were observed if hyperthermia was delivered immediately after RIT. This translated into greater tumor growth delay compared to RIT alone, hyperthermia alone, and untreated controls. In contrast, hyperthermia 2 days prior to RIT resulted in a 30% decrease in radiation dose to tumor.

Mittal et al. (298) treated LS174T colon cancer–bearing mice with ^{131}I-anti-CEA C110, followed 2 days later with 42.5°C/45 minutes hyperthermia. Greater tumor growth delay was seen when hyperthermia was added to RIT. The same group then performed a phase I/II combined therapy trial of ^{131}I-NP4 anti-CEA RIT combined with hyperthermia. Results from six patients, all with liver metastases, were reported. RIT (30 or 60 mCi/m^2) was administered IV followed 24 hours later by 42°C interstitial hyperthermia to the liver lesions. One partial response was observed and two of three patients had resolution of abdominal pain after therapy.

RIT and immunotherapy

Using radiotherapy as a means to synergize immunotherapy has received recent attention (299,300). Radiotherapy can potentially enhance the efficacy of immunotherapy through a number of potential mechanisms. Tumor cell death after irradiation can release antigens that can then activate or potentiate an immune response against tumor (300). Radiation therapy can alter the tumor cell phenotype, by increasing expression of tumor-associated antigens, such as CEA, upregulate tumor chemokines and adhesion molecules (301), and upregulate Fas and major histocompatability complex (MHC) molecules (302) expression that can work in concert to enhance immune recognition. Low-dose TBI in murine models can enhance effects of subsequent adoptive transfer of tumor-specific T-cells by selectively depleting cell populations that compete for needed cytokines (303).

The combination of RIT and immunotherapy is therefore intriguing. Recently, Chakraborty et al. (304) evaluated the combination of anti-CEA RIT (^{90}Y-COL-1) and vaccine therapy in a colon cancer–bearing transgenic mouse model for human CEA. The combination resulted in a significant increase in survival compared to either therapy alone. RIT resulted in an upregulation of Fas by tumor cells and an increase in infiltrating CEA-specific CD8$^+$ T-cells in tumor. The investigators concluded the combination of RIT and vaccine therapy promotes a more effective antitumor response, and should be considered in future trial designs.

RIT directed against new target antigens

MAbs directed against new target antigens show promise as RIT agents. Fibroblast activation protein (FAP) is a cell surface glycoprotein expressed by reactive stromal cells in epithelial tumors, including a high percentage of colorectal cancers. Welt et al. (305) administered an imaging dose of ^{131}I-MAbF19 anti-FAP just prior to planned surgery to 17 patients with hepatic metastases from colorectal cancer. Selective targeting of tumor was observed in 15 of 17 patients. Tumor-to-liver ratios as high as 21:1 and tumor-to-serum ratios as high as 9:1 were reported. Recently, ^{131}I-labeled sibrotuzumab, the humanized version of MAbF19, was administered to 26 patients (20 with colorectal cancer) (306). ^{131}I-sibrotuzumab showed no uptake to normal organs on nuclear scans and tumor targeting at 24 to 48 hours postadministration. Therapy trials are reportedly ongoing.

MAbs, such as cetuximab and bevacizumab, have recently been FDA approved and now play an important role in therapy for a variety of solid tumors, including colorectal cancer. These antibodies are also being evaluated to deliver RIT. This concept is attractive since these antibodies have known antitumor effects that can add to the antitumor effects of RIT and also can potentially enhance the effects of the targeted radiation.

Cetuximab, an MAb directed against EGFR, is now used in the treatment of colorectal cancer in combination with standard chemotherapy regimens in patients with metastatic disease and is currently being evaluated in the adjuvant setting with FOLFOX4 and FOLFOX6 (307). The antitumor effects of the antibody may also enhance the efficacy of radiotherapy (308,309) although the exact mechanism is unclear. In a recent phase III randomized trial in head and neck cancer, the combination of cetuximab and radiotherapy significantly improved median overall survival, progression-free survival, and median duration of locoregional control compared to radiotherapy alone (310). Preclinical in vivo studies have also reported increased efficacy with EGFR-inhibiting agents and RIT (258,311), including a recent preclinical study combining ^{177}Lu-CHX-A"-DTPA-huA33 and cetuximab in colorectal cancer (312).

Radiolabeled anti-EGFR MAbs have been evaluated in animal models and in a limited number of clinical trials to assess biodistribution, tumor targeting, and its potential as a radioimmunoimaging and radioimmunotherapy agent. Goldenberg et al. (313) evaluated biodistribution and tumor localization of ^{111}In-labeled murine 225 anti-EGFR in mice bearing high-EGFR–expressing vulvar squamous cell cancer tumors. At 3 days postadministration, tumor uptake was 28 %ID/g, with mean tumor-to-blood uptake ratio of 4.5 and mean tumor-to-liver uptake ratio of 6.7.

This was followed by an imaging and biodistribution trial with ^{111}In-MAb 225 in 19 patients with squamous cell lung cancer (75). The antibody protein was increased for each cohort from 1 to 300 mg. All tumors imaged if 20 g or more were administered. With increasing antibody protein, there was a decrease in liver uptake and increase in tumor uptake. At the 300-mg level, mean percentage injected dose of tumor was 3.1%, liver 21.6%, heart 4.3%, and bowel 24.5%. The low tumor uptake and low tumor-to-organ uptake ratios appear to limit the potential of MAb 225 as a radioimmunotherapy agent.

Recently, Milenic et al. (314) evaluated ^{111}In-cetuximab in mice bearing a variety of tumor xenografts. For the human colon cancer line LS174T, tumor uptake at 72 hours was high at 52 %ID/g, with blood uptake of 10.6 %ID/g and liver uptake of 7.9 %ID/g. The authors conclude that ^{111}In-cetuximab may be a useful radioimmunoconjugate for imaging and therapy.

Bevacizumab, an anti-VEGF MAb, has recently been introduced as part of standard systemic therapy regimens for metastatic colorectal cancer. An initial randomized trial demonstrated significant improvement in survival, progression-free survival, and duration of response with the addition of bevacizumab to IFL (irinotecan, 5-flurouracil, and leucovorin) compared to IFL alone (315). Bevacizumab is currently being evaluated in combination with other chemotherapy regimens in colorectal cancer as first-line therapy for metastatic disease and in the adjuvant setting (307). Preclinical models also report that bevacizumab combined with RIT can potentially increase antitumor effects compared to RIT alone (194).

Evaluation of bevacizumab as a possible radioimmunoconjugate for imaging and therapy are in the preclinical stages. Stollman et al. (316) recently performed imaging and biodistribution studies in LS174T colon cancer–bearing mice administered ^{111}In-labeled or ^{125}I-labeled bevacizumab. At 3 days postadministration mean tumor uptake of ^{111}In-bevacizumab was 19.4 %ID/g, which is comparable to the levels observed for ^{111}In-anti-CEA antibodies evaluated in the same tumor-bearing mouse model. Tumor uptake was highest (20 to 25 %ID/g) when unlabeled antibody protein doses were kept low, suggesting that with higher antibody protein levels, tumor-binding sites become less available for targeting by the radiolabeled antibody. Tumor uptake was lower for ^{125}I-bevacizumab (mean 9.6% ID/g at 3 days). Bevacizumab labeled with [89]Zr or alpha particle–emitting radionuclides (317,318) have also been evaluated in vivo and have demonstrated targeting to tumor and successful tumor imaging.

Minimal tumor burden setting

Tumor size plays a dominant role in influencing antibody uptake and, as a result, clinically important outcomes are predicted if systemic RIT is applied in the subclinical or microscopic disease setting. Jain et al. (70,319) have identified key physiologic factors that limit uptake of macromolecules. These factors include spatial heterogeneity of tumor vascularity, increased interstitial pressure in poorly vascularized areas, and limited diffusion distances of macromolecules, which work to significantly limit the ability of the antibody to reach all sites within the tumor. These factors are amplified as the tumor grows, resulting in an exponential decrease in tumor antibody uptake, which has been demonstrated in vivo (320–323) and in clinical trials (324,325). Given this inverse exponential relationship, a very modest reduction in tumor size will result in a substantial increase in antibody uptake.

RIT should therefore have its greatest impact in the adjuvant setting and in the treatment of minimal or microscopic disease. For example, an improvement of survival and the prevention of liver metastases have been shown in animal models when RIT is delivered with adjuvant intent (142,326). Subsequent clinical trials evaluated this strategy in patients with small-volume disease. Behr et al. (79) reported initial phase I trial results in 12 colorectal cancer patients with metastatic lesions less than or equal to 2.5 cm. Patients received a single administration of 50 to 70 mCi/m^2 ^{131}I-hMN14 anti-CEA RIT. An MTD of 60 mCi/m^2 was established. Of 11 evaluable patients, two partial responses and five minor/mixed responses of up to 12 months duration were observed.

This study was followed by a phase II study of 30 patients with colorectal cancer and liver metastases who received a single administration of ^{131}I-hMN14 anti-CEA RIT (60 mCi/m^2) (80). Of 19 evaluable patients who had small-volume disease of less than or equal to 3.0 cm, three experienced a partial response of 3 to 15 months duration and eight patients had a minor response of 3 to 14 months duration. Five patients received a second cycle at time of progression at 8 to 16 months, which resulted in partial responses in two of those five patients. In addition, nine patients receive RIT after an R0 resection of hepatic metastases, and therefore received RIT for microscopic disease similar to an adjuvant setting. Seven of nine patients remained disease free at more than 24 to 36 months, which compared favorably to historical controls at the same institution receiving 5-FU-based regimens posthepatic resection.

These initial encouraging observations led to a phase II adjuvant RIT trial of ^{131}I-hMN14 administered after resection of colorectal cancer liver metastases (Table 25.5) (82,327). In the most recent report, 23 patients who underwent R0 resection for liver metastases from colorectal cancer received a single administration of 40 to 60 mCi/m^2 of ^{131}I-hMN14 anti-CEA (82). Results were compared to a contemporaneous control group of 19 patients from the same institution treated postresection with 5-FU-based chemotherapy regimens. Median follow-up for the RIT group was 91 months and for the control group 51 months. A statistically significant improvement in median overall survival with the RIT group (58 versus 31 months) was reported. Median disease-free survival was greater for the RIT group (18 versus 12 months) but the difference did not reach statistical significance. The investigators concluded that a prospective randomized trial to evaluate ^{131}I-hMN14

as adjuvant therapy in this patient population was warranted given the suggestion of a survival advantage.

This same group recently reported preclinical results of an ongoing trial evaluating the feasibility of administering two courses of RIT after resection of liver metastases in patients with colorectal cancer (83). Thirty-two patients received a dose of 40 to 50 mCi/m^2 ^{131}I-hMN14 anti-CEA, with 24 receiving a second RIT administration. Toxicity after the first RIT cycle was comparable with the toxicity from the second RIT cycle. Sixteen patients had no residual disease detectable after surgery and comprised the group that received adjuvant RIT. With follow-up of 21 months, disease-free survival was 18 months for the adjuvant group and 6 months for the nonadjuvant group. The authors concluded that a second cycle of RIT is feasible with acceptable toxicity. A future randomized trial is planned that will compare two cycles of RIT versus RIT and chemotherapy as adjuvant therapy in the same population.

An adjuvant RIT trial in colorectal cancer was recently carried out by Ychou et al. (91) who administered a preoperative "diagnostic" dose of ^{131}I-F6 F(ab')$_2$ anti-CEA (8 to 10 mCi) prior to planned surgery. A total of 22 patients were entered on trial and all of them had 1 to 4 liver metastases. After R0 resection, 13 patients, including 10 who had tumor-to-liver uptake ratios of greater than 5, received 180 to 200 mCi of ^{131}I-F6 F(ab')$_2$ anti-CEA RIT. With a median follow-up of 127 months, median disease-free survival was 12 months and median overall survival was 50 months. One patient remained disease free at 93 months. The investigators concluded that RIT is feasible after surgery in this poor prognostic group and that RIT, possibly combined with chemotherapy, should be further evaluated in this clinical setting.

At the City of Hope, an ongoing phase I trial has been designed to evaluate the feasibility and toxicities of ^{90}Y-cT84.66 anti-CEA RIT combined with hepatic arterial fluorodeoxyuridine (FUdR) and systemic gemcitabine in colorectal cancer patients after resection and/or radiofrequency ablation of liver metastases. No dose-limiting toxicities have been observed to date in 13 patients with FUdR of 0.1 to 0.2 µg/kg/d × 14 days, gemcitabine 105 mg/kg, and RIT 16 .6 mCi/m^2. Four patients remain progression free at over 4 to 37 months (Table 25.5).

In summary, preclinical studies predict that RIT should have its greatest impact in the minimum tumor burden or adjuvant setting. Initial clinical trials are promising and demonstrate feasibility of RIT alone or in combination with chemotherapy in the posthepatic resection setting. Further trials are warranted to better define the potential benefits of this approach.

■ SUMMARY

The fields of Radiation Oncology and Nuclear Medicine are entering an exciting era with therapies being delivered in a more targeted fashion through an increasing number of novel approaches. The targeting of external beam radiotherapy now integrates functional and anatomic tumor imaging to guide delivery of conformal radiation to tumors. There are a growing number of biologically targeted radiation therapy agents that include not only radiolabeled immunoconstructs, but also radiolabeled peptides, radiolabeled liposomes (328,329), radiolabeled nanoparticles (330), and agents such as strontium-89 and samarium-153 that selectively target bone metastases.

RIT adds an important new dimension to therapies available to the radiation oncologist. As one of the first forms of biologically targeted radiation therapy, RIT is now a standard therapy for some non-Hodgkin lymphomas. The role of RIT for colorectal cancer and other solid tumors is yet to be clearly defined, but clinical results remain promising and warrant further investigation. The limitations and challenges of RIT are now better appreciated. Optimization strategies will further improve the efficacy of RIT by improving antibody-based delivery systems, modifying the tumor microenvironment to increase targeted dose, and maximizing dose effect. Although a number of strategies to increase tumor uptake and antitumor effects of these agents have proven encouraging, it is likely that no one strategy will be sufficient and that multiple strategies will be needed to realize clinically important results in colorectal cancer. As with other emerging targeted therapies, the greatest potential for RIT will not be as monotherapy, but as therapy integrated into established multimodality regimens, used as adjuvant or consolidative therapy in patients with minimal or micrometastatic disease.

REFERENCES

1. Beierwaltes WH. Radioiodine-labeled compounds previously or currently used for tumour localization. In: Agency IAE, ed. *Proceedings of an Advisory Group Meeting on Tumour Localization with Radioactive Agents, Panel Proceedings Series*. Vienna, Austria: International Atomic Energy Agency; 1974;47–56.
2. Press OW, Eary JF, Appelbaum FR, et al. Radiolabeled-antibody therapy of B-cell lymphoma with autologous bone marrow support [see comments]. *N Engl J Med*. 1993;329:1219–1224.
3. Kaminski MS, Zasadny KR, Francis IR, et al. Radioimmunotherapy of B-cell lymphoma with ^{131}I-anti-B1 (anti-CD20) antibody. *N Engl J Med*. 1993;329:459–465.
4. Knox SJ, Goris ML, Trisler K, et al. Yttrium-90-labeled anti-CD20 monoclonal antibody therapy of recurrent B-cell lymphoma. *Clin Cancer Res*. 1996;2:457–470.
5. DeNardo GL, Lewis JP, DeNardo SJ, et al. Effect of Lym-1 radioimmunoconjugate on refractory chronic lymphocytic leukemia. *Cancer*. 1994;73:1425–1432.
6. Appelbaum FR, Matthews DC, Eary JF, et al. Use of radiolabeled anti-CD33 antibody to augment marrow irradiation prior to marrow transplantation for acute myelogenous leukemia. *Transplantation*. 1992;54:829–833.
7. Matthews DC, Appelbaum FR, Eary JF, et al. Development of a marrow transplant regimen for acute leukemia using targeted hematopoietic irradiation delivered by ^{131}I-labeled anti-CD45 antibody, combined with cyclophosphamide and total body irradiation. *Blood*. 1995;85:1122–1131.
8. Jurcic JG, Caron PC, Nikula TK, , et al. Radiolabeled anti-CD33 monoclonal antibody M195 for myeloid leukemias. *Cancer Res*. 1995;55:5908s–5910s.
9. Juweid M, Sharkey RM, Markowitz A, et al. Treatment of non-Hodgkin's lymphoma with radiolabeled murine, chimeric, or humanized LL2, an anti-CD22 monoclonal antibody. *Cancer Res*. 1995;55:5899s–5907s.
10. Vriesendorp HM, Herpst JM, Germack JL, et al. Phase I-II studies of yttrium-labeled antiferritin treatment for end-stage Hodgkin's disease, including radiation therapy oncology group 87-01. *J Clin Oncol*. 1991;9:918–928.
11. Gordon LI, Witzig TE, Wiseman GA, et al. Yttrium-90 ibritumomab tiuxetan radioimmunotherapy for relapsed or refractory low-grade non-Hodgkin's lymphoma. *Semin Oncol*. 2002;29:87–92.
12. Zelenetz AD. A clinical and scientific overview of tositumomab and iodine I-131 tositumomab. *Semin Oncol*. 2003;30:22–30.
13. Order SE, Stillwagon GB, Klein JL, et al. Iodine-131 anti-ferritin, a new treatment modality in hepatoma: a Radiation Therapy Oncology Group study. *J Clin Oncol*. 1985;3:1573–1582.
14. Stillwagon GB, Order SE, Klein JL, et al. Multi-modality treatment of primary nonresectable intrahepatic cholangiocarcinoma with ^{131}I-anti-CEA: a Radiation Therapy Oncology Group study. *Int J Radiat Oncol Biol Phys*. 1987;5:687–695.
15. Kohler G, Milstein C. Continuous cultures of fused cells secreting antibody of predefined specificity. *Nature*. 1975;256:495–497.
16. Colcher D, Bird R, Roselli M, et al. In vivo tumor targeting of a recombinant single-chain antigen binding protein. *J Natl Cancer Inst*. 1990;82:1191–1197.
17. Wu AM, Chen W, Raubitschek AA, et al. Tumor localization of anti-CEA single-chain Fvs: improved targeting by non-covalent dimers. *Immunotechnology*. 1996;2:21–36.
18. Adams GP, Schier R, McCall AM, et al. Prolonged in vivo tumour retention of a human diabody targeting the extracellular domain of human HER2/neu. *Br J Cancer*. 1998;77:1405–1412.
19. Rossi EA, Chang CH, McBride W, et al. Development of bispecific diabodies for tumor therapy by pretargeting methodology. *Proc Am Assoc Cancer Res*. 2002;43:1015.
20. Wu AM, Williams LE, Zieran L, et al. Anti-carcinoembryonic antigen (CEA) diabody for rapid tumor targeting and imaging. *Tumor Target*. 1999;4:47–58.
21. Goel A, Augustine S, Baranowska-Kortylewicz J, et al. Single-dose versus fractionated radioimmunotherapy of human colon carcinoma xenografts using ^{131}I-labeled multivalent CC49 single-chain FVs. *Clin Cancer Res*. 2001;7:175–184.
22. Pavlinkova G, Booth BJ, Batra SK, et al. Radioimmunotherapy of human colon cancer xenografts using a dimeric single-chain Fv antibody construct. *Clin Cancer Res*. 1999;5:2613–2619.
23. Rossi EA, Chang CH, Karacay H, et al. Tumor targeting with humanized anti-CEA diabodies, triabodies, and tetrabodies. *Proc Am Assoc Cancer Res*. 2002;43;911.
24. Yazaki PJ, Wu AM, Tsai SW, et al. Tumor targeting of radiometal labeled anti-CEA recombinant T84.66 diabody and T84.66 minibody: comparison to radioiodinated fragments. *Bioconjug Chem*. 2001;12:220–228.
25. Iliades P, Kortt AA, Hudson PJ. Triabodies: single chain Fv fragments without a linker form trivalent trimers. *FEBS Lett*. 1997;409:437–441.
26. King DJ, Turner A, Farnsworth AP, et al. Improved tumor targeting with chemically cross-linked recombinant antibody fragments. *Cancer Res*. 1994;54:6176–6185.
27. Shu L, Qi CF, Schlom J, et al. Secretion of a single-gene-encoded immunoglobulin from myeloma cells. *Proc Natl Acad Sci U S A*. 1993;90:7995–7999.
28. Slavin-Chiorini DC, Horan Hand PH, Kashmiri SV, et al. Biologic properties of a CH2 domain-deleted recombinant immunoglobulin. *Int J Cancer*. 1993;53:97–103.
29. Slavin-Chiorini DC, Kashmiri SVS, Lee H-S, et al. A CDR-grafted (humanized) domain-deleted antitumor antibody. *Cancer Biother Radiopharm*. 1997;12:305–316.
30. Santos AD, Kashmiri SV, Hand PH, et al. Generation and characterization of a single gene-encoded single-chain tetravalent antitumor antibody. *Clin Cancer Res*. 1999;5:3118s–3123s.
31. Langmuir VK, Mendonca HL, Woo DV. Comparisons between two monoclonal antibodies that bind to the same antigen but have differing affinities: uptake kinetics and ^{131}I-antibody therapy efficacy in multicell spheroids. *Cancer Res*. 1992;52:4728–4734.
32. Jain RK. Barriers to drug delivery in solid tumors. *Sci Am*. 1994;271(1):58–65.
33. Schroff RW, Foon KA, Beatty SM, et al. Human anti-murine immunoglobulin responses in patients receiving monoclonal antibody therapy. *Cancer Res*. 1985;45:879–885.
34. Courtenay-Luck NS, Epenetos AA, Moore R, et al. Development of primary and secondary immune responses to mouse monoclonal antibodies used in the diagnosis and therapy of malignant neoplasms. *Cancer Res*. 1986;46:6489–6493.

35. Leichner PK, Order SE, Klein JL. Y-90 antiferritin dosimetry in hepatoma. *Int J Radiat Oncol Biol Phys.* 1989;17:241.

36. Goldman-Leikin RE, Kaplan EH, Zimmer AM, et al. Long-term persistence of human anti-murine antibody responses following radioimmunodetection and radioimmunotherapy of cutaneous T- cell lymphoma patients using ^{131}I-T101. *Exp Hematol.* 1988;16:861–864.

37. Pimm MV, Perkins AC, Armitage NC, et al. The characteristics of blood-borne radiolabeled antibodies and the effect of anti-mouse IgG antibodies on localization of radiolabeled monoclonal antibody in cancer patients. *J Nucl Med.* 1985;26:1011–1023.

38. Weiden PL, Wolf SB, Breitz HB, et al. Human anti-mouse antibody suppression with cyclosporin A. *Cancer.* 1994;73:1093–1097.

39. Ledermann JA, Begent RH, Bagshawe KD, et al. Repeated antitumour antibody therapy in man with suppression of the host response by cyclosporin A. *Br J Cancer.* 1988;58:654–657.

40. Richman CM, DeNardo SJ, O'Grady LF, et al. Radioimmunotherapy for breast cancer using escalating fractionated doses of [131]I -labeled chimeric L6 antibody with peripheral blood progenitor cell transfusions. *Cancer Res.* 1995;55:5916s–5920s.

41. Breitz HB, Weiden PL, Vanderheyden J-L, et al. Clinical experience with rhenium-186-labeled monoclonal antibodies for radioimmunotherapy: results of phase I trials. *J Nucl Med.* 1992;33:1099–1109.

42. Meredith RF, Bueschen AJ, Khazaeli MB, et al. Treatment of metastatic prostate carcinoma with radiolabeled antibody CC49. *J Nucl Med.* 1994;35:1017–1022.

43. Welt S, Divgi CR, Kemeny N, et al. Phase I/II study of iodine-131-labeled monoclonal antibody A33 in patients with advanced colon cancer. *J Clin Oncol.* 1994;12:1561–1571.

44. Mulligan T, Carrasquillo JA, Chung Y, et al. Phase I study of intravenous Lu-labeled CC49 murine monoclonal antibody in patients with advanced adenocarcinoma. *Clin Cancer Res.* 1995;1:1447–1454.

45. Yu B, Carrasquilo J, Milenic D, et al. Phase I trial of iodine-131-labeled COL-1 in patients with gastrointestinal malignancies: influence of serum carcinoembryonic antigen and tumor bulk on pharmacokinetics. *J Clin Oncol.* 1996;6:1798–1809.

46. Behr TM, Sharkey RM, Juweid ME, et al. Phase I/II clinical radioimmunotherapy with an iodine-131-labeled anti-carcinoembryonic antigen murine monoclonal antibody IgG. *J Nucl Med.* 1997;38:858–870.

47. Juweid M, Swayne LC, Sharkey RM, et al. Prospects of radioimmunotherapy in epithelial ovarian cancer: results with iodine-131-labeled murine and humanized MN-14 anti-carcinoembryonic antigen monoclonal antibodies. *Gynecol Oncol.* 1997;67:259–271.

48. Meredith RF, Khazaeli MB, Liu T, et al. Dose fractionation of radiolabeled antibodies in patients with metastatic colon cancer. *J Nucl Med.* 1992;33:1648–1653.

49. Weiden PL, Breitz HB, Seiler CA, et al. Rhenium-186-labeled chimeric antibody NR-LU-13: pharmacokinetics, biodistribution and immunogenicity relative to murine analog NR-LU-10. *J Nucl Med.* 1993; 34:2111–2119.

50. Meredith RF, Khazaeli MB, Plott WE, et al. Initial clinical evaluation of iodine-125-labeled chimeric 17-1A for metastatic colon cancer. *J Nucl Med.* 1995;36:2229–2233.

51. Wong JYC, Chu DZ, Yamauchi DM, et al. Phase I radioimmunotherapy trials evaluating Y-90 labeled anti-CEA chimeric T84.66 in patients with metastatic CEA-producing malignancies. *Clin Cancer Res.* 2000;6:3855–3863.

52. Kramer EL, Liebes L, Wasserheit C, et al. Initial clinical evaluation of radiolabeled MX-DTPA humanized BrE-3 antibody in patients with advanced breast cancer. *Clin Cancer Res.* 1998;4:1679–1688.

53. Hajjar G, Sharkey RM, Burton J, et al. Phase I radioimmunotherapy trial with iodine-131-labeled humanized MN-14 anti-carcinoembryonic antigen monoclonal antibody in patients with metastatic gastrointestinal and colorectal cancer. *Clin Colorectal Cancer.* 2002; 2:31–42.

54. Goldsmith SJ, Vallabhajosula S, Kostakoglu L, et al. ^{90}Y-DOTA-huJ591: radiolabeled anti-PSMA humanized monoclonal antibody for the treatment of prostate cancer: phase I dose escalation studies. *J Nucl Med.* 2002;43(5):158P.

55. Borjesson PKE, Postema EJ, Roos JC, et al. Phase I therapy study with Re-186-labeled humanized monoclonal antibody BIWA 4 (bivatuzumab) in patients with head and neck squamous cell carcinoma. *Clin Cancer Res.* 2003;9:3961s–3972s.

56. Khazaeli MB, Saleh MN, Liu TP, et al. Pharmacokinetics and immune response of ^{131}I-chimeric mouse/human B72.3 (human g4) monoclonal antibody in humans. *Cancer Res.* 1991;51:5461–5466.

57. LoBuglio AF, Wheeler RH, Trang J, et al. Mouse/human chimeric monoclonal antibody in man: kinetics and immune response. *Proc Natl Acad Sci U S A.* 1989;86:4220–4224.

58. Goodman GE, Hellstrom I, Yelton DE, et al. Phase I trial of chimeric (human–mouse) monoclonal antibody L6 in patients with non-small-cell lung, colon, and breast cancer. *Cancer Immunol Immunother.* 1993;36:267–273.

59. Khazaeli MB, Wheeler R, Rogers K, et al. Initial evaluation of a human monoclonal antibody (HA-1A) in man. *J Biol Response Mod.* 1990;9: 178–184.

60. Ritter G, Cohen LS, Williams C, et al. Serological analysis of human anti-human antibody responses in colon cancer patients treated with repeated doses of humanized monoclonal antibody A33. *Cancer Res.* 2001;61:6851–6859.

61. Khazaeli MB, Conry RM, LoBuglio AF. Human immune response to monoclonal antibodies. *J Immunother.* 1994;15:42–52.

62. Meredith RF, Buchsbaum DJ. Pretargeted radioimmunotherapy. *Int J Radiat Oncol Biol Phys.* 2006;66:S57–S59.

63. Press OW, Shan D, Howell-Clark J, et al. Comparative metabolism and retention of iodine-125, yttrium-90, and indium-111 radioimmunoconjugates by cancer cells. *Cancer Res.* 1996;56:2123–2129.

64. Esteban JM, Kuhn JA, Felder B, et al. Carcinoembryonic antigen expression of resurgent human colon carcinoma after treatment with therapeutic doses of ^{90}Y-alpha-carcinoembryonic antigen monoclonal antibody. *Cancer Res.* 1991;51:3802–3806.

65. Markoe AM, Brady LW, Woo D, et al. Treatment of gastrointestinal cancer using monoclonal antibodies. *Front Radiat Ther Oncol.* 1990;24:214–224.

66. Welt S, Scott AM, Divgi CR, et al. Phase I/II study of iodine-125-labeled monoclonal antibody A33 in patients with advanced colon cancer. *J Clin Oncol.* 1996;14:1787–1797.

67. Jurcic JG, McDevitt MR, Sgouros G, et al. Phase I trial of targeted alpha-particle therapy for myeloid leukemias with bismuth-213-HuM 195 (ANTI-CD33). *Proc ASCO.* 1999;18:79.

68. Jurcic JG, Larson SM, Sgouros G, et al. Targeted α particle immunotherapy for myeloid leukemia. *Blood.* 2002;100:1233–1239.

69. Simonson RB, Ultee ME, Hauler JA, et al. Radioimmunotherapy of peritoneal human colon cancer xenografts with site-specifically modified [212]Bi-labeled antibody. *Cancer Res.* 1990;50:985s–988s.

70. Jain RK. Physiological barriers to delivery of monoclonal antibodies and other macromolecules in tumors. *Cancer Res (Suppl).* 1990;50: 814s–819s.

71. Williams LE, Duda RB, Proffitt RT, et al. Tumor uptake as a function of tumor mass: a mathematic model. *J Nucl Med.* 1988;29:103–109.

72. Williams LE, Bares RB, Fass J, et al. Uptake of radiolabeled anti-CEA antibodies in human colorectal primary tumors as a function of tumor mass. *Eur J Nucl Med.* 1993;20:345–347.

73. Odom-Maryon TL, Williams LE, Chai A, et al. Pharmacokinetics modeling and absorbed dose estimation for a chimeric anti-CEA antibody (cT84.66) in humans. *J Nucl Med.* 1997;38:1959–1966.

74. Beatty BG, Beatty JD, Williams LE, et al. Effect of specific antibody pretreatment on liver uptake of ^{111}In-labeled anticarcinoembryonic antigen monoclonal antibody in nude mice bearing human colon cancer xenografts. *Cancer Res.* 1989;49:1587–1594.

75. Divgi CR, Welt S, Kris M, et al. Phase I and imaging trial of indium-111-labeled anti-epidermal growth factor receptor monoclonal antibody 225 in patients with squamous cell lung carcinoma. *J Natl Cancer Inst.* 1991;83:97–104.

76. Juweid ME, Sharkey RM, Behr T, et al. Radioimmunotherapy of patients with small-volume tumors using iodine-131-labeled anti-CEA monoclonal antibody NP-4 F(ab')₂. *J Nucl Med.* 1996;37:1504–1510.

77. Mittal BB, Zimmer MA, Sathiaseelan V, et al. Phase I/II trial of combined ^{131}I anti-CEA monoclonal antibody and hyperthermia in patients with advanced colorectal adenocarcinoma. *Cancer.* 1996;78: 1861–1870.

78. Juweid M, Sharkey RM, Swayne LC, et al. Pharmacokinetics, dosimetry and toxicity of rhenium-188-labeled anti-carcinoembryonic antigen monoclonal antibody, MN-14, in gastrointestinal cancer [see comments]. *J Nucl Med.* 1998;39:34–42.

79. Behr TM, Salib AL, Liersch T, et al. Radioimmunotherapy of small volume disease of colorectal cancer metastatic to the liver: preclinical evaluation in comparison to standard chemotherapy and initial results of a phase I clinical study. *Clin Cancer Res.* 1999;5:3232s–3242s.

80. Behr TM, Liersch T, Greiner-Bechert L, et al. Radioimmunotherapy of small-volume disease of metastatic colorectal cancer. Results of a

phase II trial with the Iodine-131-labeled humanized anti-carcinoembryonic antigen antibody hMN-14. *Cancer*. 2002;94:1373–1381.

81. Liersch T, Meller J, Kulle B, et al. Phase II trial of carcinoembryonic antigen radioimmunotherapy with ^{131}I-labetuzumab after salvage resection of colorectal metastases in the liver: five-year safety and efficacy results. *J Clin Oncol*. 2005;23:6763–6770.

82. Liersch T, Meller J, Bittrich M, et al. Update of carcinoembryonic antigen radioimmunotherapy with ^{131}I-labetuzumab after salvage resection of colorectal liver metastases: comparison of outcome to a contemporaneous control group. *Ann Surg Oncol*. 2007;14:2577–2590.

83. Liersch T, Meller J, Sahlmann C, et al. Repeated anti-CEA-radioimmunotherapy (RAIT) with 131-iodine-labetuzumab (phase II study) versus single dose RAIT after salvage resection of colorectal liver metastases (CRC-LM) [Abstract]. *J Clin Oncol*. 2008;26(15S pt 1):198s.

84. Kraeber-Bodere F, Rousseau C, Bodet-Milin C, et al. Targeting, toxicity, and efficacy of 2-step, pretargeting radioimmunotherapy using a chimeric bispecific antibody and ^{131}I-labeled bivalent hapten in a phase I optimization clinical trial. *J Nucl Med*. 2006;47:247–255.

85. Wong JYC, Chu DZ, Williams LE, et al. A phase I trial of ^{90}Y-DOTA-anti-CEA chimeric T84.66 (cT84.66) radioimmunotherapy in patients with metastatic CEA-producing malignancies. *Cancer Biother Radiopharm*. 2006;21:88–100.

86. Wong JYC, Shibata S, Williams LE, et al. A phase I trial of Y-90-anti-carcinoembryonic antigen chimeric T84.66 radioimmunotherapy with 5-fluorouracil in patients with metastatic colorectal cancer. *Clin Cancer Res*. 2003;9:5842–5852.

87. Shibata S, Raubitschek A, Leong L, et al. A phase I study of a combination of yttrium-90 labeled anti-CEA antibody and gemcitabine in patients with CEA producing advanced malignancies. *Clin Cancer Res*. 2009;15:2935–2941.

88. Lane DM, Eagle KF, Begent RH, et al. Radioimmunotherapy of metastatic colorectal tumours with iodine-131-labelled antibody to carcinoembryonic antigen: phase I/II study with comparative biodistribution of intact and F(ab')₂ antibodies. *Br J Cancer*. 1994;70:521–525.

89. Gaya AM, Violet J, Dancey G, et al. A phase I/II trial of radioimmunotherapy with 131-iodine-labelled A5B7 anti-CEA antibody (^{131}I-A5B7) in combination with combretastatin A4-phosphate (CA4P) in advanced gastrointestinal carcinomas. *J Clin Oncol*. 2008;26:629s.

90. Ychou M, Pelegrin A, Faurous P, et al. Phase-I/II radio-immunotherapy study with iodine-131-labeled anti-CEA monoclonal antibody F6 F(ab')₂ in patients with non-resectable liver metastases from colorectal cancer. *Int J Cancer*. 1998;75:615–619.

91. Ychou M, Azria D, Menkarios C, et al. Adjuvant radioimmunotherapy trial with iodine-131-labeled anti-carcinoembryonic antigen monoclonal antibody F6 F(ab')₂ after resection of liver metastases from colorectal cancer. *Clin Cancer Res*. 2008;14:3487–3493.

92. Buchegger F, Allal AS, Roth A, et al. Combined radioimmunotherapy and radiotherapy of liver metastases from colorectal cancer: a feasibility study. *Anticancer Res*. 2000;20:1889–1896.

93. Meredith RF, Khazaeli MB, Plott WE, et al. Phase I trial of iodine-131-chimeric B72.3 (human IgG4) in metastatic colorectal cancer. *J Nucl Med*. 1992;33:23–29.

94. Divgi CR, Scott AM, Dantis L, et al. Phase I radioimmunotherapy trial with iodine-131-CC49 in metastatic colon carcinoma. *J Nucl Med*. 1995;36:586–592.

95. Murray JL, Macey DJ, Kasi LP, et al. Phase II radioimmunotherapy trial with ^{131}I-CC49 in colorectal cancer. *Cancer*. 1994;73:1057–1066.

96. Wheeler RH, Meredith RF, Saleh MN, et al. A phase II trial of IL-1 + radioimmunotherapy (RIT) in patients (pts) with metastatic colon cancer [Meeting abstract]. *Proc Annu Meet Am Soc Clin Oncol*. 1994;13:295.

97. Divgi CR, Scott AM, Gulec S, et al. Pilot radioimmunotherapy trial with ^{131}I-labeled murine monoclonal antibody CC49 and deoxyspergualin in metastatic colon carcinoma. *Clin Cancer Res*. 1995;1503–1510.

98. Tempero M, Leichner P, Dalrymple G, et al. High-dose therapy with iodine-131-labeled monoclonal antibody CC49 in patients with gastrointestinal cancers: a phase I trial. *J Clin Oncol*. 1997;15:1518–1528.

99. Tempero M, Leichner P, Baranowska-Kortylewicz J, et al. High-dose therapy with 90-yttrium-labeled monoclonal antibody CC49: a phase I trial. *Clin Cancer Res*. 2000;6:3095–3102.

100. Forero-Torres A, Shen S, Breitz H, et al. Pretargeted radioimmunotherapy (RIT) with a novel anti-TAG-72 fusion protein. *Cancer Biother Radiopharm*. 2005;20:379–390.

101. Meredith RF, Khazaeli MB, Plott WE, et al. Phase II study of dual ^{131}I-labeled monoclonal antibody therapy with interferon in patients with metastatic colorectal cancer. *Clin Cancer Res*. 1996;2:1811–1818.

102. Riva P, Marangolo M, Tison V, et al. Treatment of metastatic colorectal cancer by means of specific monoclonal antibodies conjugated with iodine-131: a phase II study. *Nucl Med Biol*. 1991;18:109–119.

103. Chong G, Lee FT, Hopkins W, et al. Phase I trial of ^{131}I-huA33 in patients with advanced colorectal carcinoma. *Clin Cancer Res*. 2005;11:4818–4826.

104. Breitz H, Knox S, Weiden P, et al. Pretargeted radioimmunotherapy with antibody-streptavidin and Y-90 DOTA-biotin (avidin): result of a dose escalation study. *J Nucl Med*. 1998;39(5):71P.

105. Knox SJ, Goris ML, Tempero M, et al. Phase II trial of yttrium-90-DOTA-biotin pretargeted by NR-LU-10 antibody/streptavidin in patients with metastatic colon cancer. *Clin Cancer Res*. 2000;6:406–414.

106. Street HH, Goris ML, Fisher GA, et al. Phase I study of ^{131}I-chimeric (ch) TNT-1/B monoclonal antibody for the treatment of advanced colon cancer. *Cancer Bull*. 2006;21:243–256.

107. Anderson PM, Wiseman GA, Lewis BD, et al. A phase I safety and imaging study using radiofrequency ablation (RFA) followed by ^{131}I-chTNT-1/B radioimmunotherapy adjuvant treatment of hepatic metastases. *Cancer Ther*. 2003;1:283–291.

108. DeNardo SJ, O'Grady LF, Richman CM, et al. Radioimmunotherapy for advanced breast cancer using I-131-ChL6 antibody. *Anticancer Res*. 1997;17:1745–1751.

109. Juweid ME, Hajjar G, Swayne LC, et al. Phase I/II trial of ^{131}I-MN-14F(ab)₂ anti-carcinoembryonic antigen monoclonal antibody in the treatment of patients with metastatic medullary thyroid carcinoma. *Cancer*. 1999;85:1828–1842.

110. Steffens MG, Boerman OC, de Mulder PH, et al. Phase I radioimmunotherapy of metastatic renal cell carcinoma with ^{131}I-labeled chimeric monoclonal antibody G250. *Clin Cancer Res*. 1999;5:3268s–3274s.

111. Lashford L, Jones D, Pritchard J, et al. Therapeutic application of radiolabeled monoclonal antibody UJ13A in children with disseminated neuroblastoma. *NCI Monogr*. 1987;53–57.

112. Gold P, Freedman SO. Demonstration of tumor-specific antigens in human colonic carcinoma by immunological tolerance and absorption techniques. *J Exp Med*. 1965;121:439.

113. Neumaier M, Shively L, Chen FS, et al. Cloning of the genes for T84.66, an antibody that has a high specificity and affinity for carcinoembryonic antigen, and expression of chimeric human/mouse T84.66 genes in myeloma and Chinese hamster ovary cells. *Cancer Res*. 1990;50:2128–2134.

114. Neumaier M, Zimmermann W, Shively L, et al. Characterization of a cDNA clone for the nonspecific cross-reacting antigen (NCA) and a comparison of NCA and carcinoembryonic antigen. *J Biol Chem*. 1988;263:3202–3207.

115. Beatty JD, Duda RB, Williams LE, et al. Pre-operative imaging of colorectal carcinoma with 111-In-labeled anti-carcinoembryonic antigen monoclonal antibody. *Cancer Res*. 1986;46:6494–6502.

116. Wong JY, Chu DZ, Yamauchi D, et al. Dose escalation imaging trial evaluating indium-111-labeled anti-CEA chimeric monoclonal antibody (cT84.66) in presurgical colorectal cancer patients. *J Nucl Med*. 1998;39:2097–2104.

117. Wong JY, Thomas GE, Yamauchi D, et al. Clinical evaluation of indium-111-labeled chimeric anti-CEA monoclonal antibody. *J Nucl Med*. 1997;38:1951–1959.

118. Johnson VG, Schlom J, Paterson AJ, et al. Analysis of a human tumor-associated glycoprotein (TAG-72) identified by monoclonal antibody B72.3. *Cancer Res*. 1986;46:850–857.

119. Molinolo A, Simpson JF, Thor A, et al. Enhanced tumor binding using immunohistochemical analyses by second generation anti-tumor-associated glycoprotein 72 monoclonal antibodies versus monoclonal antibody B72.3 in human tissue. *Cancer Res*. 1990;50:1291–1298.

120. Cohen AM, Martin EW Jr, Lavery I, et al. Radioimmunoguided surgery using iodine-125 B72.3 in patients with colorectal cancer. *Arch Surg*. 1991;126:349–352.

121. Carrasquillo JA, Sugarbaker P, Colcher D, et al. Peritoneal carcinomatosis: imaging with intraperitoneal injection of I-131-labeled B72.3 monoclonal antibody. *Radiology*. 1988;167:35–40.

122. Colcher D, Carrasquillo JA, Esteban JM, et al. Radiolabeled monoclonal antibody B72.3 localization in metastatic lesions of colorectal cancer patients. *Int J Rad Appl Instrum B*. 1987;14:251–262.

123. Divgi CR, Scott AM, McDermott K, et al. Clinical comparison of radiolocalization of two monoclonal antibodies (mAbs) against the TAG-72 antigen. *Nucl Med Biol.* 1994;21:9–15.

124. Schlom J, Siler K, Milenic DE, et al. Monoclonal antibody-based therapy of a human tumor xenograft with a 177-lutetium-labeled immunoconjugate. *Cancer Res.* 1991;51:2889–2896.

125. Gottlinger HG, Funke I, Johnson JP, et al. The epithelial cell surface antigen 17-1A, a target for antibody-mediated tumor therapy: its biochemical nature, tissue distribution and recognition by different monoclonal antibodies. *Int J Cancer.* 1986;38:47–53.

126. Sharkey RM, Goldenberg DM, Vagg R, et al. Phase I clinical evaluation of a new murine monoclonal antibody (Mu-9) against colon-specific antigen-p for targeting gastrointestinal carcinomas. *Cancer.* 1994;73:864–877.

127. Yu L, Ju D-W, Chen W-C, et al. ^{131}I-chTNT radioimmunotherapy of 43 patients with advanced lung cancer. *Cancer Biother Radiopharm.* 2006;21:5–14.

128. Buchsbaum DJ. Experimental radioimmunotherapy. *Semin Radiat Oncol.* 2000;10:156–167.

129. Knox SJ. Overview of studies on experimental radioimmunotherapy. *Cancer Res.* 1995;55:5832s–5836s.

130. Buras RR, Beatty BG, Williams LE, et al. Radioimmunotherapy of human colon cancer in nude mice. *Arch Surg.* 1990;125:660–664.

131. Pedley RB, Boden JA, Boden R, et al. Comparative radioimmunotherapy using intact or F(ab')₂ fragments of ^{131}I anti-CEA antibody in a colonic xenograft model. *Br J Cancer.* 1993;68:69–73.

132. Buras RR, Wong JYC, Kuhn JA, et al. Comparison of radioimmunotherapy and external beam radiotherapy in colon cancer xenografts. *Int J Radiat Oncol Biol Phys.* 1993;25:473–479.

133. Buchsbaum DJ, Ten Haken RK, Heidorn DB, et al. A comparison of ^{131}I-labeled monoclonal antibody 17-1A treatment to external beam irradiation on the growth of LS174T human colon carcinoma xenografts. *Int J Radiat Oncol Biol Phys.* 1990;18:1033–1041.

134. Wessels BW, Vessella RL, Palme DF, et al. Radiobiological comparison of external beam irradiation and radioimmunotherapy in renal cell carcinoma xenografts. *Int J Radiat Oncol Biol Phys.* 1989;17:1257–1263.

135. Knox SJ, Goris ML, Wessels BW. Overview of animal studies comparing radioimmunotherapy with dose equivalent external beam irradiation [see comments]. *Radiother Oncol.* 1992;23:111–117.

136. Langmuir VK, Fowler JF, Knox SJ, et al. Radiobiology of radiolabeled antibodies as applied to tumor dosimetry. AAPM Report 40. *Med Phys.* 1993;20:601–610.

137. Wong JYC, Buras RR, Kuhn JA, et al. Strategies to improve the efficacy of radioimmunotherapy: radiobiologic and dosimetric considerations. In: Dewey WC, Edington M, Fry RJM, et al., eds. *Radiation Research: A Twentieth Century Perspective.* San Diego, CA: Academic Press; 1992:647–652.

138. Fowler JF. Radiobiological aspects of low dose rates in radioimmunotherapy. *Int J Radiat Oncol Biol Phys.* 1990;18:1261–1269.

139. Blumenthal RD, Sharkey RM, Natale AM, et al. Comparison of equitoxic radioimmunotherapy and chemotherapy in the treatment of human colonic cancer xenografts. *Cancer Res.* 1994;54:142–151.

140. de Bree R, Roos JC, Plaizier MABD, et al. Selection of monoclonal antibody E48 IgG or U36 IgG for adjuvant radioimmunotherapy in head and neck cancer patients. *Br J Cancer.* 1997;75:1049–1060.

141. Breitz HB, Fisher DR, Weiden PL, et al. Dosimetry of rhenium-186-labeled monoclonal antibodies: methods, prediction from technetium-99m-labeled antibodies and results of phase I trials [see comments]. *J Nucl Med.* 1993;34:908–917.

142. Colnot DR, Roos JC, de Bree R, et al. Safety, biodistribution, pharmacokinetics, and immunogenicity of [99]m-Tc-labeled humanized monoclonal antibody BIWA 4 (bivatuzumab) in patients with squamous cell carcinoma of the head and neck. *Cancer Immunol Immunother.* 2003;52:576–582.

143. Nanus DM, Milowsky MI, Kostakoglu L, et al. Clinical use of monoclonal antibody HuJ591 therapy: targeting prostate specific membrane antigen. *J Urol.* 2003;170:S84–S89.

144. Larson SM, Carrasquillo JA, Krohn KA, et al. Localization of ^{131}I-labeled p97-specific Fab fragments in human melanoma as a basis for radiotherapy. *J Clin Invest.* 1983;72:2101–2114.

145. Witzig T, Gordon LI, Cabanillas F, et al. Randomized controlled trial of yttrium-90-labeled ibritumomab tiuxetan radioimmunotherapy versus rituximab immunotherapy for patients with relapsed or refractory low-grade, follicular, or transformed B-cell non-Hodgkin's lymphoma. *J Clin Oncol.* 2002;20:2453–2463.

146. Wong JY, Williams LE, Demidecki AJ, et al. Radiobiologic studies comparing yttrium-90 irradiation and external beam irradiation in vitro. *Int J Radiat Oncol Biol Phys.* 1991;20:715–722.

147. Bertagnolli MM. Radioimmunotherapy for colorectal cancer. *Clin Cancer Res.* 2005;11:4637–4638.

148. Divgi C. What ails solid tumor radioimmunotherapy? *Cancer Biother Radiopharm.* 2006;21:81–84.

149. van Zanten-Przybysz I, Molthoff C, Roos JC, et al. Radioimmunotherapy with intravenously administered ^{131}I-labeled chimeric monoclonal antibody MOv18 in patients with ovarian cancer. *J Nucl Med.* 2000;41:1168–1176.

150. Postema EJ, Borjesson PK, Buijs WC, et al. Dosimetric analysis of radioimmunotherapy with [186]Re-labeled bivatuzumab in patients with head and neck cancer. *J Nucl Med.* 2003;44:1690–1699.

151. DeNardo SJ, Kramer EL, O'Donnell RT, et al. Radioimmunotherapy for breast cancer using indium-111/yttrium-90 BrE-3: results of a phase I clinical trial. *J Nucl Med.* 1997;38:1180–1185.

152. Wiseman GA, White CA, Stabin M, et al. Phase I/II ^{90}Y-zevalin (yttrium-90 ibritumomab tiuxetan, IDEC-Y2B8) radioimmunotherapy dosimetry results in relapsed or refractory non-Hodgkin's lymphoma. *Eur J Nucl Med.* 2000;27:766–777.

153. Kaminski MS, Zasadny KR, Francis IR, et al. Iodine-131-anti-B1 radioimmunotherapy for B-cell lymphoma. *J Clin Oncol.* 1996;14:1974–1981.

154. Lamborn KR, DeNardo GL, DeNardo SJ, et al. Treatment-related parameters predicting efficacy of Lym-1 radioimmunotherapy in patients with B-lymphocytic malignancies. *Clin Cancer Res.* 1997;3:1253–1260.

155. Vose JM, Colcher D, Gobar L, et al. Phase I/II trial of multiple dose ^{131}I-MAb LL2(CD22) in patients with recurrent non-Hodgkin's lymphoma. *Leuk Lymphoma.* 2000;38:91–101.

156. Hu E, Epstein AL, Naeve GS, et al. A phase 1a clinical trial of LYM-1 monoclonal antibody serotherapy in patients with refractory B cell malignancies. *Hematol Oncol.* 1989;7:155–166.

157. Hu P, Hornick JL, Glasky M, et al. A chimeric lym-1/interleukin 2 fusion protein for increasing tumor vascular permeability and enhancing antibody uptake. *Cancer Res.* 1996;56:4998–5004.

158. Withers HR, Peters LJ, Taylor JMG. Dose–response relationship for radiation therapy of subclinical disease. *Int J Radiat Oncol Biol Phys.* 1995;31:353–359.

159. Dahl O, Horn A, Morild I, et al. Low-dose preoperative radiation postpones recurrences in operable rectal cancer: results of a randomized multicenter trial in western Norway. *Cancer.* 1990;66:2286–2294.

160. Gerard A, Buyse M, Nordlinger B, et al. Preoperative radiotherapy as adjuvant treatment in rectal cancer. Final results of a randomized study of the European Organization for Research and Treatment of Cancer (EORTC). *Ann Surg.* 1988;208:606–614.

161. Franklin R, Steiger Z, Vaishampayan G, et al. Combined modality therapy for esophageal squamous cell carcinoma. *Cancer.* 1983;51:1062–1071.

162. Nigro ND, Seydel HG, Considine B, et al. Combined preoperative radiation and chemotherapy for squamous cell carcinoma of the anal canal. *Cancer.* 1983;51:1826–1829.

163. Roth JA, Putnam JB, Lichter AS, et al. Cancer of the esophagus. In: DeVita VT, Hellman S, Rosenberg SA, eds. *Cancer: Principles and Practice of Oncology.* 4th ed. Philadelphia, PA: Lippincott Williams & Wilkins; 1993:776–817.

164. Schrier DM, Stemmer SM, Johnson T, et al. High-dose [90]Y Mx-diethylenetriaminepentaacetic acid (DTPA)-BrE-3 and autologous hematopoietic stem cell support (AHSCS) for the treatment of advanced breast cancer: a phase I trial. *Cancer Res.* 1995;55:5921s–5924s.

165. Cagnoni PJ, Ceriani RL, Cole W, et al. High-dose radioimmunotherapy with ^{90}Y-hu-BrE-3 followed by autologous hematopoietic stem cell support (AHSCS) in patients with metastatic breast cancer. *Cancer Biother Radiopharm.* 1999;14(4):318.

166. Richman CM, DeNardo SJ, O'Donnell RT, et al. Dosimetry-based therapy in metastatic breast cancer patients using ^{90}Y monoclonal antibody 170H.82 with autologous stem cell support and cyclosporin A. *Clin Cancer Res.* 1999;5:3243s–3248s.

167. Richman CM, DeNardo SJ, O'Grady LF, et al. Radioimmunotherapy for breast cancer using escalating fractionated doses of ^{131}I-labeled chimeric L6 antibody with peripheral blood progenitor cell transfusions. *Cancer Res.* 1995;55:5916s–5920s.

168. Wong JYC, Somlo G, Odom-Maryon T, et al. Initial results of a phase I trial evaluating yttrium-90 (^{90}Y) chimeric T84.66 (cT.84.66) anti-CEA

antibody and autologous stem cell support in CEA-producing metastatic breast cancer. *Clin Cancer Res.* 1999;5:3224s–3231s.

169. Juweid ME, Hajjar G, Stein R, et al. Initial experience with high-dose radioimmunotherapy of metastatic medullary thyroid cancer using ^{131}I-MN-14 F(ab)$_2$ anti-carcinoembryonic antigen MAb and AHSCR [see comments]. *J Nucl Med.* 2000;41:93–103.

170. Buchsbaum D, Khazaeli MB, Liu T, et al. Fractionated radioimmunotherapy of human colon carcinoma xenografts with ^{131}I-labeled monoclonal antibody CC49. *Cancer Res.* 1995;55:5881s–5887s.

171. DeNardo GL, Schlom J, Buchsbaum DJ, et al. Rationales, evidence, and design considerations for fractionated radioimmunotherapy. *Cancer.* 2002;94:1332–1348.

172. Vogel CA, Galmiche MC, Buchegger F. Radioimmunotherapy and fractionated radiotherapy of human colon cancer liver metastases in nude mice. *Cancer Res.* 1997;57:447–453.

173. Violet JA, Dearling JLJ, Green AJ, et al. Fractionated ^{131}I anti-CEA radioimmunotherapy: effects on xenograft tumour growth and haematological toxicity in mice. *Br J Cancer.* 2008;99:632–638.

174. Greiner JW, Guadagni F, Hand PH, et al. Augmentation of tumor antigen expression by recombinant human interferons: enhanced targeting of monoclonal antibodies to carcinomas. *Cancer Treat Res.* 1990;51:413–432.

175. Yan X, Wong JYC, Esteban JM, et al. Effects of recombinant human gamma-interferon on carcinoembryonic antigen expression of human colon cancer cells. *J Immunother.* 1992;11:72–84.

176. Greiner JW, Guadagni F, Noguchi P, et al. Recombinant interferon enhances monoclonal antibody-targeting of carcinoma lesions in vivo [published erratum appears in *Science.* 1987 May 8;236(4802):657]. *Science.* 1987;235:895–898.

177. Guadagni F, Roselli M, Schlom J, et al. In vitro and in vivo regulation of human tumor antigen expression by human recombinant interferons: a review. *Int J Biol Markers.* 1994;9:53–60.

178. Greiner JW, Guadagni F, Roselli M, et al. Improved experimental radioimmunotherapy of colon xenografts by combining ^{131}I-CC49 and interferon-gamma. *Dis Colon Rectum.* 1994;37:S100–S105.

179. Kuhn JA, Wong JYC, Beatty BG, et al. Interferon enhancement of radioimmunotherapy for colon carcinoma in vivo. *J Nucl Med.* 31(5):850.

180. Kuhn JA, Beatty BG, Wong JY, et al. Interferon enhancement of radioimmunotherapy for colon carcinoma. *Cancer Res.* 1991;51:2335–2339.

181. Kuhn JA, Wong JYC, Beatty BG, et al. Gamma interferon enhancement of a multiple treatment regimen for radioimmunotherapy. *Antibody Immunoconjug Radiopharm.* 1992;4:837–845.

182. Greiner JW, Guadagni F, Goldstein D, et al. Evidence for the elevation of serum carcinoembryonic antigen and tumor-associated glycoprotein-72 levels in patients administered interferons. *Cancer Res.* 1991;51:4155–4163.

183. Greiner JW, Guadagni F, Goldstein D, et al. Intraperitoneal administration of interferon-gamma to carcinoma patients enhances expression of tumor-associated glycoprotein-72 and carcinoembryonic antigen on malignant ascites cells. *J Clin Oncol.* 1992;10:735–746.

184. Macey DJ, Grant EJ, Kasi L, et al. Effect of recombinant α-interferon pharmacokinetics, biodistribution, toxicity, and efficacy of ^{131}I-labeled monoclonal antibody CC49 in breast cancer: a phase II trial. *Clin Cancer Res.* 1997;3:1547–1555.

185. Slovin SF, Scher HI, Divgi CR, et al. Interferon-γ and monoclonal antibody ^{131}I-labeled CC49: outcomes in patients with androgen-independent prostate cancer. *Clin Cancer Res.* 1998;4:643–651.

186. Simpson JF, Primus FJ, Schlom J. Complementation of expression of carcinoembryonic antigen and tumor associated glycoprotein-72 (TAG-72) in human colon adenocarcinomas. *Int J Biol Markers.* 1991;6:83–90.

187. Blumenthal RD, Kashi R, Stephens R, et al. Improved radioimmunotherapy of colorectal cancer xenografts using antibody mixtures against carcinoembryonic antigen and colon-specific antigen-p. *Cancer Immunol Immunother.* 1991;32:303–310.

188. Buchsbaum DJ. Experimental tumor targeting with radiolabeled ligands. *Cancer.* 1997;80:2371–2377.

189. Jain RK. Normalizing tumor vasculature with anti-angiogenic therapy: a new paradigm for combination therapy. *Nat Med.* 2001;7:987–989.

190. Lee CG, Heijn M, di Tomaso E, et al. Anti-vascular endothelial growth factor treatment augments tumor radiation response under normoxic or hypoxic conditions. *Cancer Res.* 2000;60:5565–5570.

191. Burke PA, DeNardo SJ, Miers LA, et al. Cilengitide targeting of αvβ3 integrin receptor synergizes with radioimmunotherapy to increase efficacy and apoptosis in breast cancer xenografts. *Cancer Res.* 2002;62:4263–4272.

192. DeNardo SJ, Burke PA, Leigh BR, et al. Neovascular targeting with cyclic RGD peptide (cRGDf-ACHA) to enhance delivery of radioimmunotherapy. *Cancer Biother Radiopharm.* 2000;15:71–79.

193. Kinuya S, Yokoyama K, Koshida K, et al. Improved survival of mice bearing liver metastases of colon cancer cells treated with a combination of radioimmunotherapy and antiangiogenic therapy. *Eur J Nucl Med Mol Imaging.* 2004;31:981–985.

194. Bodel-Milin C, Salaun P-Y, Paris F, et al. Toxicity and efficacy of combined radioimmunotherapy and bevacizumab (avastin) in mouse model of medullary thyroid carcinoma. *Cancer Biother Radiopharm.* 2008;23(4):517.

195. Lankester KL, Maxwell RJ, Pedley RB, et al. Combretastatin A-4-phosphate effectively increases tumor retention of the therapeutic antibody, ^{131}I-A5B7, even at doses that are sub-optimal for vascular shut-down. *Int J Oncol.* 2007;30:453–460.

196. Pedley RB, Hill SA, Boxer GM, et al. Eradication of colorectal xenografts by combined radioimmunotherapy and combretastatin a-4 3-O-phosphate. *Cancer Res.* 2001;61:4716–4722.

197. Rowlinson G, Snook D, Busza A, et al. Antibody-guided localization of intraperitoneal tumors following intraperitoneal or intravenous antibody administration. *Cancer Res.* 1987;47:6528–6531.

198. Koppe MJ, Soede AC, Pels W, et al. Experimental radioimmunotherapy of small peritoneal metastases of colorectal origin. *Int J Cancer.* 2003;106:965–972.

199. Colcher D, Esteban J, Carrasquillo JA, et al. Complementation of intracavitary and intravenous administration of a monoclonal antibody (B72.3) in patients with carcinoma. *Cancer Res.* 1987;47:4218–4224.

200. Ward BG, Mather SJ, Hawkins LR, et al. Localization of radioiodine conjugated to the monoclonal antibody HMFG2 in human ovarian carcinoma: assessment of intravenous and intraperitoneal routes of administration. *Cancer Res.* 1987;47:4719–4723.

201. Chatal JF, Saccavini JC, Gestin JF, et al. Biodistribution of indium-111-labeled OC 125 monoclonal antibody intraperitoneally injected into patients operated on for ovarian carcinomas. *Cancer Res.* 1989;49:3087–3094.

202. Behr TM, Blumenthal RD, Memtsoudis S, et al. Cure of metastatic human colonic cancer in mice with radiolabeled monoclonal antibody fragments. *Clin Cancer Res.* 2000;6:4900–4907.

203. Dale RG. Radiobiological assessment of permanent implants using tumour repopulation factors in the linear quadratic model. *Br J Radiol.* 1989;62:241–244.

204. Juweid M, Sharkey RM, Behr T, et al. Targeting and initial radioimmunotherapy of medullary thyroid carcinoma with ^{131}I-labeled monoclonal antibodies to carcinoembryonic antigen. *Cancer Res.* 1995;55:5946s–5951s.

205. Buchegger F, Mach JP, Folli S, et al. Higher efficiency of ^{131}I-labeled anti-carcinoembryonic antigen monoclonal antibody F(ab')$_2$ as compared to intact antibodies in radioimmunotherapy of established human colon carcinoma grafted in nude mice. *Recent Results Cancer Res.* 1996;141:19–35.

206. Buchegger F, Pelgrin A, Delaloye B, et al. Iodine-131-labeled MAb F(ab')$_2$ fragments are more efficient and less toxic than intact anti-CEA antibodies in radioimmunotherapy of large human colon carcinoma grafted in nude mice. *J Nucl Med.* 1990;31:1035–1044.

207. Begent RH, Verhaar MJ, Chester KA, et al. Clinical evidence of efficient tumor targeting based on single-chain Fv antibody selected from a combinatorial library. *Nat Med.* 1996;2:979–984.

208. Larson SM, El Shirbiny AM, Divgi CR, et al. Single chain antigen binding protein (sFv CC49): first human studies in colorectal carcinoma metastatic to liver. *Cancer.* 1997;80:2458–2468.

209. Milenic DE, Yokota T, Filpula DR, et al. Construction, binding properties, metabolism, and tumor targeting of a singly-chain Fv derived from the pancarcinoma monoclonal antibody CC49. *Cancer Res.* 1991;51:6363–6371.

210. Adams GP, McCartney JE, Tai M-S, et al. Highly specific in vivo tumor targeting by monovalent and divalent forms of 741F8 anti-c-erbB-2 single-chain Fv. *Cancer Res.* 1993;53:4026–4034.

211. Beresford G, Pavlinkova G, Booth BJ, et al. Binding characteristics and tumor targeting of a covalently linked divalent CC49 single-chain antibody. *Int J Cancer.* 1999;81:911–917.

212. Storto G, Buchegger F, Waibel R, et al. Biokinetics of a F(ab')$_3$ iodine-131 labeled antigen binding construct (MAb 35) directed against CEA in patients with colorectal carcinoma. *Cancer Biother Radiopharm.* 2001;16:371–379.

213. Casey JL, Napier MP, King DJ, et al. Tumour targeting of humanised cross-linked divalent-Fab' antibody fragments: a clinical phase I/II study. *Br J Cancer.* 2002;86:1401–1410.

214. Wu AM, Williams LE, Bebb GG, et al. Selection of engineered antibody fragments for targeting and imaging applications. In: Hori W, ed. *Antibody Engineering: New Technologies, Applications, and Commercialization.* Vol 2. Southborough: IBC BioMedical Library; 1997: 163–183.

215. Williams LE, Wu AM, Yazaki PJ, et al. Numerical selection of optimal tumor imaging agents with application to engineered antibodies. *Cancer Biother Radiopharm.* 2001;16:25–35.

216. Wong JYC, Chu DZ, Williams LE, et al. Pilot trial evaluating a I-123 labeled 80-kilodalton engineered anticarcinoembryonic antigen antibody fragment (cT84.66 minibody) in patients with colorectal cancer. *Clin Cancer Res.* 2004;10:5014–5021.

217. Wong JYC, Thomas GE, Yamauchi D, et al. Clinical evaluation of an Indium-111-labeled chimeric anti-CEA monoclonal antibody. *J Nucl Med.* 1997;38:1951–1959.

218. Whitlow M, Bell BA, Feng SL, et al. An improved linker for single-chain Fv with reduced aggregation and enhanced proteolytic stability. *Protein Eng.* 1993;6:989–995.

219. Cumber AJ, Ward ES, Winter G, et al. Comparative stabilities in vitro and in vivo of a recombinant mouse antibody FvCys fragment and a bisFvCys conjugate. *J Immunol.* 1992;149:120–126.

220. Pack P, Pluckthun A. Miniantibodies: use of amphipathic helices to produce functional, flexibly linked dimeric Fv fragments with avidity in *Escherichia coli. Biochemistry.* 1992;31:1579–1584.

221. Holliger P, Prospero T, Winter G. "Diabodies": small bivalent and dispecific antibody fragments. *Proc Natl Acad Sci U S A.* 1993;90:6444–6448.

222. Kostelny SA, Cole MS, Tso JY. Formation of a bispecific antibody by the use of leucine zippers. *J Immunol.* 1992;148:1547–1553.

223. Forero A, Meredith RF, Khazaeli MB, et al. A novel monoclonal antibody design for radioimmunotherapy. *Cancer Biother Radiopharm.* 2003;18:751–759.

224. Meredith RF, Forero A, Khazaeli M, et al. Radioimmunotherapy of colon cancer with an improved humanized monoclonal antibody design. *Int J Radiat Oncol Biol Phys.* 2002;54(suppl 2):98.

225. Reilly RM. Radioimmunotherapy of solid tumors: the promise of pretargeting strategies using bispecific antibodies and radiolabeled haptens. *J Nucl Med.* 2006;47:196–199.

226. Barbet J, Kraeber-Bodere F, Chatal JF. What can be expected from nuclear medicine tomorrow? *Cancer Biother Radiopharm.* 2008;23: 483–503.

227. Boerman OC, van Schaijk FG, Oyen WJ, et al. Pretargeted radioimmunotherapy of cancer: progress step by step. *J Nucl Med.* 2003; 44:400–411.

228. Press OW, Corcoran MC, Subbiah K, et al. A comparative evaluation of conventional and pretargeted radioimmunotherapy of CD20-expressing lymphoma xenografts. *Blood.* 2001;98:2535–2543.

229. Kraeber-Bodere F, Bardet S, Hoefnagel CA, et al. Radioimmunotherapy in medullary thyroid cancer using bispecific antibody and iodine-131-labeled bivalent hapten: preliminary results of a phase I/II clinical trial. *Clin Cancer Res.* 1999;5:3190s–3198s.

230. Vuillez JP, Kraeber-Bodere F, Moro D, et al. Radioimmunotherapy of small cell lung carcinoma with the two-step method using a bispecific anti-carcinoembryonic antigen/anti-diethylenetriaminepentaacetic acid (DTPA) antibody and iodine-131 Di-DTPA hapten: results of a phase I/II trial. *Clin Cancer Res.* 1999;5:3259s–3267s.

231. Grana C, Chinol M, Robertson C, et al. Pretargeted adjuvant radioimmunotherapy with yttrium-90-biotin in malignant glioms patients: a pilot study. *Br J Cancer.* 2002;86:207–212.

232. Paganelli G, Bartolomei M, Ferrari M, et al. Pre-targeted locoregional radioimmunotherapy with ^{90}Y-biotin in glioma patients: phase I study and preliminary therapeutic results. *Cancer Biother Radiopharm.* 2001;16:227–235.

233. Grana C, Bartolomei M, Handkiewicz D, et al. Radioimmunotherapy in advanced ovarian cancer: is there a role for pre-targeting with ^{90}Y-biotin? *Gynecol Oncol.* 2004;93:691–698.

234. Weiden PL, Breitz HB. Pretargeted radioimmunotherapy (PRIT) for treatment of non-Hodgkin's lymphoma (NHL). *Crit Rev Oncol/Hematol.* 2001;40:37–51.

235. Forero A, Weiden PL, Vose JM, et al. Phase I trial of a novel anti-CD20 fusion protein in pretargeted radioimmunotherapy for B-cell non-Hodgkin lymphoma. *Blood.* 2004;104:227–236.

236. Goldenberg DM, Chatal JF, Barbet J, et al. Cancer imaging and therapy with bispecific antibody pretargeting. *Update Cancer Ther.* 2007;2:19–23.

237. Stickney DR, Anderson LD, Slater JB, et al. Bifunctional antibody: a binary radiopharmaceutical delivery system for imaging colorectal carcinoma. *Cancer Res.* 1991;51:6650–6655.

238. Allard WJ, Moran CA, Nagel E, et al. Antigen binding properties of highly purified bispecific antibodies. *Mol Immunol.* 1992;29: 1219–1227.

239. Reardan DT, Meares CF, Goodwin DA, et al. Antibodies against metal chelates. *Nature.* 1985;316:265–268.

240. Rossi EA, Chang CH, Losman MJ, et al. Pretargeting of carcinoembryonic antigen-expressing cancers with a trivalent bispecific fusion protein produced in myeloma cells. *Clin Cancer Res.* 2005; 11:7122s–7129s.

241. Rossi EA, Goldenberg DM, Cardillo TM, et al. Stably tethered multifunctional structures of defined composition made by the dock and lock method for use in cancer targeting. *Proc Natl Acad Sci U S A.* 2006;103:6841–6846.

242. Murtha A, Weiden P, Knox S, et al. Phase I dose escalation trial of pretargeted radioimmunotherapy (PRIT) with yttrium-90. *Proc Am Soc Clin Oncol.* 1998;17:438a.

243. Gold DV, Schutsky K, Modrak D, et al. Low-dose radioimmunotherapy (^{90}Y-PAM4) combined with gemcitabine for the treatment of experimental pancreatic cancer. *Clin Cancer Res.* 2003;9:3929s–3937s.

244. Karacay H, Sharkey RM, Gold DV, et al. Pretargeted radioimmunotherapy of pancreatic cancer xenografts: TF10-^{90}Y-IMP-288 alone and combined with gemcitabine. *J Nucl Med.* 2009;50:2008–2016.

245. Okazaki S, Tempero MA, Colcher D. Combination radioimmunotherapy and chemotherapy using ^{131}I-B72.3 and gemcitabine. *Proc Am Assoc Cancer Res.* 1998;39:310.

246. DeNardo SJ, Kukis DL, Kroger LA, et al. Synergy of Taxol and radioimmunotherapy with yttrium-90-labeled chimeric L6 antibody: efficacy and toxicity in breast cancer xenografts. *Proc Natl Acad Sci U S A.* 1997;94:4000–4004.

247. O'Donnell RT, DeNardo SJ, Miers LA, et al. Combined modality radioimmunotherapy with Taxol and ^{90}Y-Lym-1 for Raji lymphoma xenografts. *Cancer Biother Radiopharm.* 1998;13:351–361.

248. Kievit E, Pinedo HM, Schluper HMM, et al. Addition of cisplatin improves efficacy of I-131-labeled monoclonal antibody 323/A3 in experimental human ovarian cancer. *Int J Radiat Oncol Biol Phys.* 1997;38:419–428.

249. Blumenthal RD, Osorio L, Leon E, et al. Multimodal preclinical radioimmunotherapy (RAIT) in combination with chemotherapy of human colonic tumors: selection between 5-fluorouracil (5-FU) and irinotecan (CPT-11). *Proc Am Assoc Cancer Res.* 2002;43:479.

250. Kinuya S, Yokoyama K, Tega H, et al. Efficacy, toxicity and mode of interaction of combination radioimmunotherapy with 5-fluorouracil in colon cancer xenografts. *J Cancer Res Clin Oncol.* 1999;125:630–636.

251. Remmenga SW, Colcher D, Gansow O, et al. Continuous infusion chemotherapy as a radiation-enhancing agent for yttrium-90-radiolabeled monoclonal antibody therapy of a human tumor xenograft. *Gynecol Oncol.* 1994;55:115–122.

252. Behr TM, Wulst E, Radetzky S, et al. Improved treatment of medullary thyroid cancer in a nude mouse model by combined radioimmunotherapy: doxorubicin potentiates the therapeutic efficacy of radiolabeled antibodies in a radioresistant tumor type. *Cancer Res.* 1997;57:5309–5319.

253. Buchsbaum DJ, Khazaeli MB, Davis MA, et al. Sensitization of radiolabeled monoclonal antibody therapy using bromodeoxyuridine. *Cancer.* 1994;73:999–1005.

254. Roffler SR, Chan J, Yeh MY. Potentiation of radioimmunotherapy by inhibition of topoisomerase I. *Cancer Res.* 1994;54:1276–1285.

255. Ng B, Liebes L, Kramer E, et al. Synergistic activity of radioimmunotherapy with prolonged topotecan infusion in human breast cancer xenograft. *Proc Annu Meet Am Assoc Cancer Res.* 1997;38:a1659.

256. Blumenthal RD, Taylor A, Osorio L, et al. Optimizing the use of combined radioimmunotherapy and hypoxic cytotoxin therapy as a function of tumor hypoxia. *Int J Cancer.* 2001;94:564–571.

257. Langmuir VK, Mendonca HL. The combined use of ^{131}I-labeled antibody and the hypoxic cytotoxin SR 4233 in vitro and in vivo. *Radiat Res.* 1992;132:351–358.

258. Lee FT, Mountain AJ, Kelly MP, et al. Enhanced efficacy of radioim-munotherapy with ^{90}Y-CHA-A''-DTPA-hu3S193 by inhibition of epidermal growth factor receptor (EGFR) signaling with EGFR tyrosine kinase inhibitor AG1478. *Clin Cancer Res.* 2005;11(suppl 19):7086s.

259. van Gog FB, Brakenhoff RH, Stigter-van Walsum M, et al. Perspectives of combined radioimmunotherapy and anti-EGFR antibody therapy for the treatment of residual head and neck cancer. *Int J Cancer.* 1998;77:13–18.

260. Meredith RF, Alvarez RD, Partridge EE, et al. Intraperitoneal radioim-munochemotherapy of ovarian cancer: a phase I study. *Cancer Biother Radiopharm.* 2001;16:305–315.

261. Alvaraz RD, Huh WK, Khazaeli MB, et al. A phase I study of combined modality 90-yttrium-CC49 intraperitoneal radioimmunotherapy for ovarian cancer. *Clin Cancer Res.* 2002;8:2806–2811.

262. Richman CM, DeNardo SJ, O'Donnell RT, et al. Combined modality radioimmunotherapy (RIT) in metastatic prostate (PC) and breast cancer (BC) using paclitaxel (PT) and a MUC-1 monoclonal antibody m170, linked to yttrium-90 (Y-90): a phase I trial. In: *Annual Meeting ASCO.* 2004;23:176.

263. Sharkey RM, Hajjar G, Yeldell D, et al. A phase I trial combining high-dose Y-90-labeled humanized anti-CEA monoclonal antibody with Doxorubicin and peripheral blood stem cell rescue in advanced medullary thyroid cancer. *J Nucl Med.* 2005;46:620–633.

264. Wong JYC. Systemic targeted radionuclide therapy: potential new areas. *Int J Radiat Oncol Biol Phys.* 2006;66:S74–S82.

265. Gold DV, Modrak DE, Schutsky K, et al. Combined 90-yttrium-DOTA-labeled PAM4 antibody radioimmunotherapy and gemcita-bine radiosensitization for the treatment of a human pancreatic cancer xenograft. *Int J Cancer.* 2004;109:618–626.

266. Graves SS, Dearstyne E, Lin Y, et al. Combination therapy with pre-target CC49 radioimmunotherapy and gemcitabine prolongs tumor doubling time in a murine xenograft model of colon cancer more effectively than either monotherapy. *Clin Cancer Res.* 2003;9: 3712–3721.

267. Koppe MJ, Oyen WJG, Bleichrodt RP, et al. Combination therapy using gemcitabine and radioimmunotherapy in nude mice with small peritoneal metastases of colonic origin. *Cancer Biother Radiopharm.* 2006;21:506–514.

268. Gold P, Schutsky K, Cardillo TM. Successful treatment of pancreatic cancer by combined gemcitabine and low dose radioimmunothe-rapy with ^{90}Y-labeled PAM4 antibody. *Proc Am Assoc Cancer Res.* 2002;43:395.

269. Cardillo TM, Blumenthal R, Ying Z, et al. Combined gemcitabine and radioimmunotherapy for the treatment of pancreatic cancer. *Int J Cancer.* 2002;97:386–392.

270. Raben D, Buchsbaum DJ. Combined external beam radiotherapy and radioimmunography. In: Syrigos KN, Harrington KJ, eds. *Targeted Therapy for Cancer.* Oxford: Oxford University Press; 2003:76–91.

271. Wong JY, Williams LE, Hill LR, et al. The effects of tumor mass, tumor age, and external beam radiation on tumor-specific antibody uptake. *Int J Radiat Oncol Biol Phys.* 1989;16:715–720.

272. Msirikale JS, Klein JL, Schroeder J, et al. Radiation enhancement of radiolabelled antibody deposition in tumors. *Int J Radiat Oncol Biol Phys.* 1987;13:1839–1844.

273. Kalofonos H, Rowlinson G, Epenetos AA. Enhancement of monoclonal antibody uptake in human colon tumor xenografts following irradiation. *Cancer Res.* 1990;50:159–163.

274. Kunala S, Macklis RM. Ionizing radiation induces CD-20 surface expression on human B cells. *Int J Cancer (Radiat Oncol Invest).* 2001;96:178–181.

275. Peter RU, Beetz A, Ried C, et al. Increased expression of the epidermal growth factor receptor in human epidermal keratinocytes after exposure to ionizing radiation. *Radiat Res.* 1993;136:65–70.

276. Hareyama M, Imai K, Kubo K, et al. Effect of radiation on the expression of carcinoembryonic antigen of human gastric adenocarcinoma cells. *Cancer.* 1991;67:2269–2274.

277. Knox SJ, Sutherland W, Goris ML. Correlation of tumor sensitivity to low-dose-rate irradiation with G2/M-phase block and other radiobiological parameters. *Radiat Res.* 1993;135:24–31.

278. Williams JA, Williams JR, Yuan X, et al. Protracted exposure radiosensitization of experimental human malignant glioma. *Radiat Oncol Investig.* 1999;6:255–263.

279. Order SE, Klein JL, Leichner PK, et al. 90-Yttrium antiferritin—a new therapeutic radiolabeled antibody. *Int J Radiat Oncol Biol Phys.* 1986; 12:277–281.

280. Emrich JG, Brady LW, Quang TS, et al. Radioiodinated (I-125) monoclonal antibody 425 in the treatment of high grade glioma patients. *Am J Clin Oncol.* 2002;25:541–546.

281. Reardon DA, Akabani G, Coleman RE, et al. Phase II trial of murine ^{131}I -labeled antitenascin monoclonal antibody 81C6 administered into surgically created resection cavities of patients with newly diagnosed malignant gliomas. *J Clin Oncol.* 2002;20(5):1389–1397.

282. Goetz C, Rachinger W, Poepperl G, et al. Intralesional radioimmuno-therapy in the treatment of malignant glioma: clinical and experimental findings. *Acta Neurochir.* 2003;88:69–75.

283. Carabasi M, Khazaeli MB, Tilden AB, et al. Autologous stem cell transplantation for breast and prostate cancer after combined modality therapy with radioimmunotherapy plus external beam radiation. *Blood.* 94(10 suppl 1):333a.

284. Bunjes D, Buchmann I, Duncker C, et al. Rhenium-188-labeled anti-CD66 monoclonal antibody to intensify the conditioning regimen prior to stem cell transplantation for patients with high-risk acute myeloid leukemia or myelodysplastic syndrome: results of a phase I-II study. *Blood.* 2001;98:565–572.

285. Rottinger EM, Bartkowiak D, Bunjes D, et al. Enhanced renal toxicity of total body irradiation combined with radioimmunotherapy. *Stra-hlenther Onkol.* 2003;179:702–707.

286. Matthews DC, Appelbaum FR, Eary JF, et al. Phase I study of ^{131}I-anti-CD45 antibody plus cyclophosphamide and total body irradiation for advanced acute leukemia and myelodysplastic syndrome. *Blood.* 1999;94:1237–1247.

287. Wong JY, Mivechi NF, Paxton RJ, et al. The effects of hyperthermia on tumor carcinoembryonic antigen expression. *Int J Radiat Oncol Biol Phys.* 1989;17:803–808.

288. Davies Cde L, Rofstad EK, Lindmo T. Hyperthermia-induced changes in antigen expression on human FME melanoma cells. *Cancer Res.* 1985;45:4109–4114.

289. Spiro IJ, McPherson S, Cook J, et al. Sensitization of low-dose-rate irradiation by non-lethal hyperthermia. *Radiat Res.* 1991;127: 111–114.

290. Raaphorst GP, Heller DP, Bussey AM, et al. Thermal radiosensitiza-tion by 41 degrees celsius hyperthermia during low-dose-rate irradiation in human normal and tumor cell lines. *Int J Hyperthermia.* 1991;10:263–270.

291. Sakurai H, Mitsuhashi N, Takahashi T, et al. Enhanced cytotoxicity in combination of low dose-rate irradiation with hyperthermia in vitro. *Int J Hyperthermia.* 1996;12:355–366.

292. Hauck ML, Zalutsky M. Enhanced tumour uptake of radiolabelled antibodies by hyperthermia. Part II: application of the thermal equi-valency equation. *Int J Hyperthermia.* 2005;21:13–27.

293. Hauck ML, Zalutsky MR. Enhanced tumour uptake of radiolabelled antibodies by hyperthermia. Part I: timing of injection relative to hyperthermia. *Int J Hyperthermia.* 2005;21:1–11.

294. Hosono MN, Hosono M, Endo K, et al. Effect of hyperthermia on tumor uptake of radiolabeled anti-neural cell adhesion molecule antibody in small-cell lung cancer xenografts. *J Nucl Med.* 1994;35: 504–509.

295. Kinuya S, Yokoyama K, Hiramatsu T, et al. Combination radioimmu-notherapy with local hyperthermia: increased delivery of radioim-munoconjugate by vascular effect and its retention by increased antigen expression in colon cancer xenografts. *Cancer Lett.* 1999; 140:209–218.

296. Stickney DR, Gridley DS, Kirk GA, et al. Enhancement of monoclonal antibody binding to melanoma with single dose radiation or hyper-thermia. *NCI Monogr.* 1987;3:47–52.

297. Kinuya S, Yokoyama K, Michigishi T, et al. Optimization of radioim-munotherapy interactions with hyperthermia. *Int J Hyperthermia.* 2004;20:190–200.

298. Mittal BB, Zimmer AM, Sathiaseelan V, et al. Effects of hyperthermia and iodine-131-labeled anticarcinoembryonic antigen monoclonal antibody on human tumor xenografts in nude mice. *Cancer.* 1992;70:2785–2791.

299. Hodge JW, Guha C, Neefjes J, et al. Synergizing radiation therapy and immunotherapy for curing incurable cancers: opportunities and challenges. *Oncology.* 2008;22:1064–1070.

300. DeMaria S, Bhardwaj N, McBride WH, et al. Combining radiotherapy and immunotherapy: a revived partnership. *Int J Radiat Oncol Biol Phys.* 2005;63:655–666.

301. Baluna RG, Eng TY, Thomas CR. Adhesion molecules in radiotherapy. *Radiat Res.* 2006;166:819–831.

302. Garnett CT, Palena C, Chakraborty M. Sublethal irradiation of human tumor cells modulates phenotype resulting in enhanced killing by cytoxic T lymphocytes. *Cancer Res.* 2004;64:7985–7994.

303. Gattinoni L, Finkelstein SE, Klebanoff CA. Removal of homeostatic cytokine sinks by lymphodepletion enhances the efficacy of adoptively transferred tumor-specific CD8+ T cells. *J Exp Med.* 2005;202: 907–912.

304. Chakraborty M, Gelbard A, Carrasquillo JA, et al. Use of radiolabeled monoclonal antibody to enhance vaccine-mediated antitumor effects. *Cancer Immunol Immunother.* 2008;58:1173–1183.

305. Welt S, Divgi CR, Scott AM, et al. Antibody targeting in metastatic colon cancer: a phase I study of monoclonal antibody F19 against a cell-surface protein of reactive tumor stromal fibroblasts. *J Clin Oncol.* 1994;12:1193–1203.

306. Scott AM, Wiseman G, Welt S, et al. A phase I dose-escalation study of Sibrotuzumab in patients with advanced or metastatic fibroblast activation. *Clin Cancer Res.* 2003;9:1639–1647.

307. de Gramont A, Tournigand C, Andre T, et al. Targeted agents for adjuvant therapy of colon cancer. *Semin Oncol.* 2006;33:S42–S45.

308. Bonner JA, Raisch KP, Trummell HQ, et al. Enhanced apoptosis with combination C225/radiation treatment serves as the impetus for clinical investigation in head and neck cancers. *J Clin Oncol.* 2000;18 (suppl):47s–53s.

309. Zips D, Krause M, Yaromina A, et al. Epidermal growth factor receptor inhibitors for radiotherapy: biological rationale and preclinical results. *J Pharm Pharmacol.* 2008;60:1019–1028.

310. Bonner JA, Harari PM, Giralt J, et al. Radiotherapy plus cetuximab for squamous-cell carcinoma of the head and neck. *N Engl J Med.* 2006;354:567–578.

311. Kelly MP, Lee ST, Lee FT, et al. Therapeutic efficacy of ^{177}Lu-CHX-A″-DTPA-hu3S193 radioimmunotherapy in prostate cancer is enhanced by EGFR inhibition or docetaxel chemotherapy. *Prostate.* 2009;69: 92–104.

312. Lee FT, Yuen A, Osborn A, et al. Combined modality ^{177}Lu-CHX-A″-DTPA HUA33 radioimmunotherapy of colorectal cancer xenografts. *Cancer Biother Radiopharm.* 2008;23(4):518.

313. Goldenberg A, Masui H, Divgi C, et al. Imaging of human tumor xenografts with an indium-111-labeled anti-epidermal growth factor receptor monoclonal antibody. *J Natl Cancer Inst.* 1989;81:1616–1625.

314. Milenic DE, Wong KJ, Baidoo KE, et al. Cetuximab: preclinical evaluation of a monoclonal antibody targeting EGFR for radioimmunodiagnostic and radioimmunotherapeutic applications. *Cancer Biother Radiopharm.* 2008;23:619–631.

315. Hurwitz H, Fehrenbacher L, Novotny W, et al. Bevacizumab plus irinotecan, fluorouracil, and leucovorin for metastatic colorectal cancer. *N Engl J Med.* 2004;350:2335–2342.

316. Stollman TH, Scheer MGW, Leenders WPJ, et al. Specific Imaging of VEGF-A expression with radiolabeled anti-VEGF monoclonal antibody. *Int J Cancer.* 2008;122:2310–2314.

317. Nagengast WB, De Vries EGE, Hospers GA, et al. In vivo VEGF imaging with radiolabeled bevacizumab in a human ovarian tumor xenograft. *J Nucl Med.* 2007;48:1313–1319.

318. Abbas-Rizvi SM, YanJun Song E, Raja C, et al. Preparation and testing of bevacizumab radioimmunoconjugates with bismuth-213 and bismuth-205/bismuth-206. *Cancer Biol Ther.* 2008;7:1547–1554.

319. Jain RK. Haemodynamic and transport barriers to the treatment of solid tumours. *Int J Radiat Biol.* 1991;60:85–100.

320. Buras R, Williams LE, Beatty BG, et al. A method including edge effects for the estimation of radioimmunotherapy absorbed doses in the tumor xenograft model. *Med Phys.* 1994;21:287–292.

321. Wong JYC, Williams LE, Demidecki AJ, et al. Radiobiologic studies comparing yttrium-90 irradiation and external beam irradiation in vitro. *Int J Radiat Oncol Biol Phys.* 1991;20:715–722.

322. Philben VJ, Jakowatz JG, Beatty BG, et al. The effect of tumor CEA content and tumor size on tissue uptake of indium-111-labeled anti-CEA monoclonal antibody. *Cancer.* 1986;57:571–576.

323. O'Donoghue JA, Bardies M, Wheldon TE. Relationships between tumor size and curability for uniformly targeted therapy with beta-emitting radionuclides [see comments]. *J Nucl Med.* 1995;36:1902–1909.

324. Behr TM, Sharkey RM, Juweid ME, et al. Variables influencing tumor dosimetry in radioimmunotherapy of CEA-expressing cancers with anti-CEA and antimucin monoclonal antibodies. *J Nucl Med.* 1997;38: 409–418.

325. de Bree R, Kuik DJ, Quak JJ, et al. The impact of tumour volume and other characteristics on uptake of radiolabelled monoclonal antibodies in tumour tissue of head and neck cancer patients. *Eur J Nucl Med.* 1998;25:1562–1565.

326. Behr TM, Salib AL, Liersch T, et al. Radioimmunotherapy of small volume disease of colorectal cancer metastatic to the liver: preclinical evaluation in comparison to standard chemotherapy and initial results of a phase I clinical study. *Clin Cancer Res.* 1999;5:3232s–3242s.

327. Zelefsky MJ. Prostate cancer. In: Perez CA, Brady LW, Halperin EC, et al., eds. *Principles and Practice of Radiation Oncology.* 4th ed. Philadelphia, PA: Lippincott Williams & Wilkins; 2004:1692–1762.

328. Sofou S, Thomas JL, Lin HY, et al. Engineered liposomes for potential α-particle therapy of metastatic cancer. *J Nucl Med.* 2004;45:253–260.

329. Harrington KJ, Mohammadtaghi S, Uster PS, et al. Effective targeting of solid tumors in patients with locally advanced cancers by radiolabeled pegylated liposomes. *Clin Cancer Res.* 2001;7:243–254.

330. Li L, Wartchow CA, Shen Z, et al. Y-90 labeled anti-Flk-1 antibody (anti-Flk-1-NP-Y90): a novel anti-angiogenesis therapy using nanoparticles. *Proc Am Assoc Cancer Res.* 2002;43:1006.

Radioimmunotherapy of Unresectable Hepatocellular Carcinoma

Stanley Order

Hepatocellular carcinoma (HCC) is a significant cancer worldwide (1). It is increasing in incidence in the United States (2). When it cannot be surgically removed (unresectable) the prognosis is very poor (3). Its frequency is highest in Africa and Asia. It has been estimated to cause greater than 1.2 million deaths annually (4). In addition to resection, orthotopic liver transplantation (OLT) is the only potentially curative treatment (5). My extensive experience with unresectable HCC evolved to the concept of three classifications: (a) tumors producing alpha-fetoprotein (AFP+), usually of viral etiology, rapidly dividing, and an extremely poor prognosis (4,6,7); (b) tumors not producing alpha-fetoprotein (AFP−), often associated with chemical or hormonal factors, slower growing, often massive, and clinically producing symptoms later than AFP+ tumors; and (c) fibrolamellar carcinoma, a unique subtype of HCC, representing about 5% of cases in North America (8). The etiology is unknown and the mean age at presentation is 23 to 26 years. It is not associated with cirrhosis and it has a better overall prognosis than the other types of HCC (6,7,9).

The etiology of HCC can be viral, metabolic (i.e., hemochromatosis or alcoholic cirrhosis), toxin (aflatoxin), hormonal, or chemical (oil industry). The development of HCC is often preceded by cirrhosis. The relationship between hepatitis and HCC is well documented and has been addressed by hepatitis vaccination in Taiwan, resulting in a subsequent reduction in HCC incidence (6).

■ CLINICAL PRESENTATION AND EVALUATION

The unresectable tumors tend to present with late symptoms. Patients typically experience abdominal fullness, weight loss, fatigue, pain, fever, gynecomastia, and jaundice as presenting symptoms. Further confusion is added by the presentation of fibrolamellar hepatoma (9–12). Tumors related to AIDS also exhibit younger presenting age distributions.

Aside from the physical examination, a computed tomography (CT) scan or magnetic resonance imaging, AFP, liver chemistries, ferritin, blood urea nitrogen, creatinine, and complete blood count are obtained. A needle biopsy will help confirm the diagnosis of HCC. An evaluation of tumor size and the potential for resection is undertaken. Comparative studies can be accomplished by using CT tumor volumetrics (13,14) (Figs. 26.1 and 26.2).

▒ Radioimmunotherapy of HCC

HCC is known to synthesize and secrete ferritin, most often in the form of apoferritin (lacking iron) (15). At the time of the initial radioimmunotherapy (RIT) studies, authorities were convinced that tumors would have specific tumor antigens that would be unique. This has not been true and useful antigens are tumor "associated" or are normal tissue antigens exaggerated or amplified by the cancer. It was therefore inferred that ferritin, being a ubiquitous normal tissue element (spleen, marrow), would also be targeted by antiferritin radioimmunoglobulin (16,17). Antiferritin immunoglobulin was synthesized by immunizing rabbits, pigs, horses, and monkeys with ferritin derived from patients diagnosed with Hodgkin disease (derived from the spleen). Early data using electrophoresis in polyacrylamide gels, however, indicated that ferritin was quite different between tumors and normal tissue (14,15). It was shown that radiolabeled, tumor-associated antiferritin antibody preparations preferentially targeted malignant tissue over normal tissue in both experimental and clinical studies (16–19). For example, a 2.9-fold greater dose deposition was found in animal tumors treated with /sup 131/I-antiferritin compared to tumors treated with /sup 131/I-normal immunoglobulin G (IgG). The deposition was equivalent for the primary tumor and for metastases of similar size (17).

In our clinical studies, in order to calculate tumor dose, the tumor volume had to be determined along with the radionuclide deposition (13,14,19,20). The initial dosimetric analysis involved 22 patients diagnosed with HCC who were administered ^{131}I-labeled antiferritin IgG. The antibodies were polyclonal and were affinity-column purified. Tumor and normal liver volume computations were performed using a computerized axial tomographic scan analysis (13,14,20). The activity deposition was determined for tumor and normal liver tissue as well as the effective half-life of the radionuclide in tumor, normal liver, and total body. The administered activity of ^{131}I-labeled antiferritin IgG ranged from 32 to 157 mCi. The tumor volumes at the time of the administration of the radiolabeled antibody ranged from 220 to 3020 cm^3 and the normal liver volumes ranged from 900 to 4620 cm^3. For smaller tumors (220 to 1700 cm^3), the mean tumor-to-liver specific activity was 4.8:1. For larger tumors (2290 to 3020 cm^3), there was reduced uptake of the radiolabeled antibody and the mean

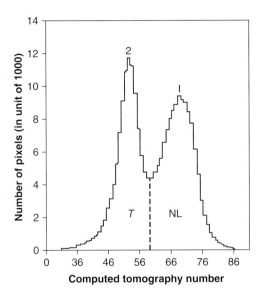

FIGURE 26.1 **Global histogram used to calculate tumor (T) and normal liver (NL) volume.** It was produced by reconstructing the entire liver and summating a histogram from each CT slice. Gaussian fitting functions were used to generate various peaks based upon pixel analysis. In this example, peak 1 represents NL and peak 2 represents T. The *dashed line* represents the CT threshold density between T and NL.

tumor-to-liver specific activity was 1.6:1. Although administered activities of 50 mCi were well tolerated, there was no additional tumor saturation benefit above 30 mCi. Coupled with tumor effective half-life information and toxicity data, the treatment regimen of administering 30 mCi of radiolabeled antibody on day 0 and 20 mCi on day 5 was derived (20).

These principles were further developed and integrated into multiple Radiation Therapy Oncology Group (RTOG) studies (19). A total of 105 patients with HCC were treated on three sequential phase I to II RTOG trials. In all trials, therapy began with external beam radiotherapy (EBRT) combined with chemotherapy (doxorubicin and 5-fluorouricil [5-FU]).

The ^{131}I-antiferritin was delivered as 30 mCi and 20 mCi on day 0 and day 5. Toxicity was hematologic, largely caused by thrombocytopenia. Cyclic therapy was then initiated with antibodies from different species of animals: rabbit, pig, monkey, and bovine. The next step was to successfully integrate chemotherapy (15-mg doxorubicin and 500-mg 5-FU) with the ^{131}I-antiferritin. The EBRT and chemotherapy produced a 22% partial remission rate. Further treatment with ^{131}I-antiferritin and chemotherapy resulted in a further response of 48% (7% complete response; 41% partial response). Patients who were AFP+ and AFP− had median survivals of 5 months and 10.5 months, respectively. The longest complete response duration was 3.5 years and the longest partial response duration was 5.7 years (19).

A phase III trial was initiated (21). A total of 98 patients with unresectable HCC were randomized. All patients received induction therapy consisting of 21-Gy EBRT delivered in seven fractions to the whole liver. The EBRT was delivered concurrently with 15-mg doxorubicin and 500-mg 5-FU. The chemotherapy only arm contained 50 patients and the radioimmunotherapy (RIT; ^{131}I-antiferritin) plus low-dose chemotherapy (15-mg doxorubicin and 500-mg 5-FU) arm contained 48 patients. The chemotherapy arm received chemotherapy at a dose of 60-mg/m^2 doxorubicin and 500-mg/m^2 5-FU every 3 weeks. The RIT arm received 30- and 20-mCi ^{131}I-antiferritin on day 0 and day 5 every 8 weeks. Each administration of RIT was delivered with low-dose chemotherapy, as stated above. Crossover was allowed for disease progression. The partial remission rates and survival analysis yielded no significant differences between the two arms. It was noted that 7 out of 11 (64%) AFP− patients who failed chemotherapy achieved a remission when crossing over to the RIT arm. None of the patients receiving chemotherapy would be converted to surgically resectable. In another analysis, the 11 patients who crossed over from the chemotherapy arm to the RIT arm were further analyzed and found to have converted to a resectable state (22). Three were resected for cure (Fig. 26.3). Another important observation was that

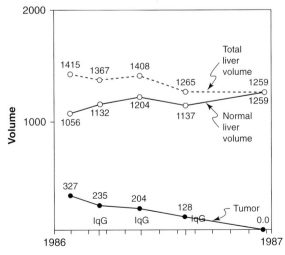

FIGURE 26.2 Characteristic changes in total liver, normal liver, and tumor volumes following therapy with ^{131}I-antiferritin IgG. The patient was a 22-year-old female diagnosed with an unresectable, nodular HCC (AFP−).

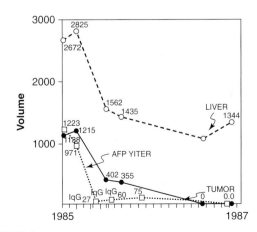

FIGURE 26.3 Changes in volume of normal liver and tumor, following therapy with ^{131}I-antiferritin IgG. The patient had an AFP+ tumor and was converted to a resectable state. Following resection, she was a long-term survivor at the time of the initial report.

the patients on the west coast, managed by Dr Stephen Leibel, had an elevated AFP titer (AFP+). They tended to be Asian, had cirrhosis and a shortened median survival in comparison to the patients from the east coast. The patients from the east coast tended to lack an AFP titer (AFP−) and had a median survival of 10 months, compared to 5 months for AFP+ patients (21,22). Careful analysis revealed that the tumor volumetrics of AFP+ patients exhibited an initial tumor reduction following treatment with RIT and then an expansion of tumor prior to the next cycle of treatment. Thus, it would appear that tumor cell division (proliferation) was more rapid in these patients with an elevated AFP titer. This realization seems to indicate that the effective time of therapy used in the protocol was surpassed by the rather quick proliferation rate of AFP+ tumors. Therefore, the 8-week therapeutic window of ^{131}I-antiferritin was potentially too long. What was the ultimate goal of radioimmunoglobulin therapy? It was the conversion of unresectable HCC to a resectable state (22). Clearly, downstaging of HCC prior to resection improves the prognosis of this disease (23). Of course, the most promising role of radiolabeled antibody therapy is in the treatment of microscopic disease.

The safety and pharmacokinetics of Licartin (^{131}I metuximab) were investigated in phase I/II trials (24). Licartin is an antibody fragment, F(ab')$_2$, that targets HAb18G/CD147, an HCC-associated antigen. In a phase I trial, 28 patients received 9.25 to 37.0 MBq/kg (0.25 to 1.0 mCi/kg) via hepatic artery infusion. In a subsequent phase II multicenter trial, 106 patients were administered 27.75 MBq/kg (0.75 mCi/kg) on day 1 of a 28-day cycle. Life-threatening toxicities did not occur. The maximum tolerated dose was 27.75 MBq/kg (0.75 mCi/kg). The serum clearance was biphasic with a half-life of 90.56 to 63.93 hours. In the phase II trials, tumor was adequately targeted. In 73 patients (completing two cycles), 6 (8.22%) had a partial response, 14 (19.18%) had a minor response, and 43 (58.9%) exhibited stable disease. The 21-month survival rate was 44.54%. Progression-free patients had a significantly higher survival rate ($p < 0.0001$). It was concluded that Licartin was safe and active in patients diagnosed with HCC.

Realizing that radiolabeled monoclonal antibodies or antibody fragments are most effective in treating small-volume disease, Licartin was tested as an adjuvant therapy for patients with HCC undergoing OLT (25). A total of 60 post-OLT patients with HCC (three fourth of which were outside of the Milan criteria) (5) were randomized to 15.4 MBq/kg (0.42 mCi/kg) of Licartin, three fractions at 28-day intervals versus placebo. At 1 year of follow-up, the recurrence rate was significantly decreased by 30.4% ($p = 0.0174$) and the survival rate was significantly increased by 20.6% ($p = 0.0289$) in the Licartin group. No significant toxicities were observed (25).

Currently, there are two trials using Licartin that are ongoing, but not recruiting participants. In the first trial (NCT00819650), patients with HCC receiving a curative R0 resection are randomized to postoperative Licartin or no further treatment. Licartin is administered in three doses at 28-day intervals, beginning at week 4 after liver resection. In the second trial (NCT00829465), patients with unresectable HCC are randomized to transcatheter arterial chemoembolization (TACE) or Licartin combined with TACE.

▓ Frontiers of nonresectable hepatoma

Prevention of HCC can be accomplished by avoiding aflatoxin and using appropriate immunizations against hepatitis B and C. That being said, several new and intriguing approaches warrant mentioning.

One such approach to radioimmunoglobulin therapy is a consideration of targeting viral antigens as novel tumor targets in virus-associated cancer, such as hepatitis B and C virus–associated HCC, human papilloma virus–associated cervical cancer, and Epstein–Barr virus–associated lymphomas. Unlike the tumor-associated antigens that are present in some normal tissues but are amplified in cancer, the antigens from virus-associated cancer would presumably not be related to normal tissues (12,26,27). This approach is different than other approaches in RIT and potentially will increase specificity and minimize toxicity (26,27).

Another approach is the use of radioactive cisplatin. Patients with HCC who had failed a variety of therapeutic approaches but still had a reasonable performance status and could receive further treatment were given intra-arterial cisplatin, 50 mg/m^2. This was in contrast to the more conventional intravenous dose of 150 mg/m^2 (28). Remissions were achieved with this reduced dose. Therefore, radioactive cisplatin was synthesized by making platinum itself radioactive, ^{195m}Pt-cisplatin (low-energy electron emitter). Our initial study was limited to 1 mCi in order to demonstrate the uptake of cisplatin at the 50-mg/m^2 intra-arterial dose (28–30). Realizing that auger electrons were being emitted, it was accepted that the radiobiologic effect or relative biological effectiveness (RBE) was equal to 4.8 (forming DNA adducts). Animal studies substantiated that radioactive cisplatin could be an effective antitumor drug (31). The energy of these low-energy electrons ranges from 23 to 183 keV per decay (28,29,31,32). A phase II trial was poised to be initiated in unresectable HCC using radioactive cisplatin. Although the trial was approved by the FDA, the author's health and the lack of sufficient funds to support this study resulted in its withdrawal. Thus, as more biologic information is gathered on HCC, a sophisticated radiation delivery system should be possible by radioimmunoglobulin and by radiopharmaceuticals.

■ REFERENCES

1. Cook CG. Hepatocellular carcinoma: one of the world's most common malignancies. *Q J Med*. 1985;57:705–798.
2. El-Serag HB, Mason AC. Rising incidence of hepatocellular carcinoma in the United States. *N Engl J Med*. 1999;340:745–750.

3. McDermott WV, Cady B, Georgi B, et al. Primary cancer of the liver. Evaluation, treatment, and prognosis. *Arch Surg*. 1989;124: 552–554.

4. Knop R, Berg CD, Ihde D. Primary liver cancer in the adult. In: Moosa AR, Robson MC, Schimpff, eds. *Comprehensive Textbook of Oncology*. Baltimore, MD: Williams & Wilkins; 1956:1087–1096.

5. Koschny R, Schmidt J, Ganten TM, et al. Beyond Milan criteria—chances and risks of expanding transplantation criteria for HCC patients with liver cirrhosis. *Clin Transplant*. 2009;23:49–60.

6. Linsell A. Primary liver cancers: epidemiology and etiology. In: Wanebo AJ, ed. *Hepatic and Biliary Cancer*. New York, NY: Marcell Dekker; 1987:3–15.

7. Chang MH, Chen CJ, Lai MS, et al. Universal hepatitis B vaccination in Taiwan and the incidence of hepatocellular carcinoma in children. Taiwan Childhood Hepatoma Study Group. *N Engl J Med*. 1997;336: 1855–1859.

8. Nzeako UC, Goodman ZD, Ishak KG. Comparison of tumor pathology with duration of survival of North American patients with hepatocellular carcinoma. *Cancer*. 1995;76:579–588.

9. Berman MM, Libbey NP, Foster JH. Hepatocellular carcinoma. Polygonal cell type with fibrous stroma—an atypical variant with a favorable prognosis. *Cancer*. 1980;46:1448–1455.

10. Craig JR, Peters RL, Edmonson HA, et al. Fibrolamellar carcinoma of the liver: a tumor of adolescents and young adults with distinctive clinico-pathologic features. *Cancer*. 1980;46:372–379.

11. Epstein BE, Pajak TF, Haulk TL, et al. Metastatic nonresectable fibrolamellar hepatoma: prognostic features and natural history. *Am J Clin Oncol*. 1999;22:22–28.

12. Chen DS, Hoger BH, Nelson J, et al. Detection and properties of hepatitis B viral DNA in liver tissues from patients with hepatocellular carcinoma. *Hepatology*. 1982;2:S42–S46.

13. Yang NC, Leichner PK, Fishman EK, et al. CT volumetrics of primary liver cancers. *J Compt Asst Tomgr*. 1986;10:621–628.

14. Ettinger DS, Leichner PK, Siegelman SS, et al. Computer tomography assisted volumetric analysis of primary liver tumor as a measure of response to therapy. *Am J Clin Oncol*. 1985;8:413–418.

15. Richter GW. Comparison of ferritins from neoplastic and non-neoplastic human cells. *Nature*. 1965;207:616–618.

16. Ettinger DS, Dragon LH, Klein J. et al. Isotopic immunoglobulin in an integrated multimodal treatment program for a primary liver cancer: a case report. *Cancer Treat Rep*. 1979;63:131–134.

17. Rostock RA, Klein JL, Leichner PK, et al. Selective tumor localization in experimental hepatoma by radiolabeled antiferritin antibody. *Int J Radiat Oncol Biol Phys*. 1983;9:1345–1350.

18. Rostock RA, Klein JL, Leichner PK, et al. Distribution of and physiologic factors that affect/sup 131/I-antiferritin tumor localization in experimental hepatoma. *Int J Radiat Oncol Biol Phys*. 1984;10:1135–1141.

19. Order SE, Stillwagon GB, Klein JL, et al. Iodine 131 antiferritin, a new treatment modality in hepatoma: a Radiation Therapy Oncology Group Study. *J Clin Oncol*. 1985;3:1573–1582.

20. Leichner PK, Klein JL, Siegelman SS, et al. Dosimetry of 131I-labeled antiferritin in hepatoma: specific activities in the tumor and liver. *Cancer Treat Rep*. 1983;67:647–658.

21. Order SE, Pajak T, Leibel S, et al. A randomized prospective trial comparing full dose chemotherapy to 131I antiferritin: an RTOG study. *Int J Rad Oncol Biol Phys*. 1989;20:953–963.

22. Sitzmann JV, Order SE, Klein JL, et al. Conversion by new treatment modalities of nonresectable to resectable hepatocellular cancer. *J Clin Oncol*. 1987;5:1566–1573.

23. Tang Z-Y, Zhou X-D, Ma Z-C, et al. Downstaging followed by resection plays a role in improving prognosis of unresectable hepatocellular carcinoma. *Hepatobiliary Pancreat Dis Int*. 2004;3:495–498.

24. Chen Z-N, Mi L, Xu J, et al. Targeting radioimmunotherapy of hepatocellular carcinoma with iodine (^{131}I) metuximab injection: clinical phase I/II trials. *Int J Radiat Oncol Bio Phys*. 2006;65:435–444.

25. Xu J, Shen Z-Y, Chen X-G, et al. A randomized controlled trial of Licartin for preventing hepatoma recurrence after liver transplantation. *Hepatology*. 2007;45:269–276.

26. Wang XG, Revskaya E, Bryan RA, et al. Treating cancer as an infectious disease—viral antigens as novel targets for treatment and potential prevention of tumors of viral etiology. *PLoS One*. 2007;2:e1114.

27. Dadachova E, Wang X-G, Casadevall. Targeting the virus with radioimmunotherapy in virus-associated cancers. *Cancer Biother Radiopharm*. 2007;22:303–308.

28. Court WS, Order SE, Siegel JA, et al. Remission and survival following monthly intra-arterial cisplatinum in nonresectable hepatoma. *Cancer Invest*. 2002;20:613–625.

29. Melia WM, Westaby D, Williams R. Diamminochloride platinum (cis-platinum) in the treatment of hepatocellular carcinoma. *Clin Oncol*. 1981;7:275–280.

30. Howell RW, Kassis AI, Adelstein SJ, et al. Radiotoxicity of platinum-195m-labeled tans-platinum (II) in mammalian cells. *Radiat Res*. 1994;140:55–62.

31. Areberg J, Wennerberg J, Johnsson A, et al. Antitumor effect of radioactive cisplatinum (191 pt) on nude mice. *Int J Radiat Oncol Biol Phys*. 2001;49:827–832.

32. Areberg J, Norrgren K, Mattsson S. Absorbed doses to patients from ^{191}Pt-, ^{193m}Pt- and ^{195m}Pt-cisplatin. *Appl Radiat Isot*. 1999;51:581–586.

Evolution of Radiotherapy Toward a More Targeted Approach for CNS Malignancies

Tod W. Speer, Jeffrey P. Limmer, Dawn Henrich, Jennifer Buskerud,
Betty Vogds, Denise VanderKooy, and Darryl Barton

◼ INTRODUCTION

It has been over a century since the discovery of x-rays by Conrad Roentgen. Almost immediately, the potential of radiation for treating malignancies was recognized. Although the mainstay for treating central nervous system (CNS) tumors is surgery, radiotherapy has been established as the most effective adjuvant therapy in this setting. Unfortunately, with the exception of adjuvant temozolomide chemotherapy (1), little progress has been made over the past 20 years when treating gliomas (2). Approximately one half of the 18,000 newly diagnosed CNS neoplasms in the United States are glioblastoma multiforme (GBM) (3) and the majority will die from the disease in less than 2 years. This dismal outcome greatly underscores the need for new and effective therapies.

Benign ependymomas aside, all glial tumors exhibit anatomic and pathologic correlates of invasion (4). Despite more than 60 years of intense study, this particular characteristic remains poorly defined. Undoubtedly, it is a complex interplay between the tumor growth fraction, proliferative rate, lineage of cell origin, as well as host cellular and extracellular barriers (5). Regardless, complete surgical extirpation of the tumor remains elusive. Therefore, the utilization of radiotherapy, whether by external beam techniques, brachytherapy, or a more targeted approach, remains a vital adjunct to surgery in the management of CNS malignancies.

Fortunately, the Department of Energy has continued to increase its financial commitment for "science," for the years 2008 to 2010. This will lead to progressive research and identification of potential radionuclides for imaging and therapy. Most likely, the next-generation "breakthrough therapy" will consist of a culmination of improved imaging, surgery, radiation delivery technique, radiation sensitization, chemotherapy, targeting agents, and the understanding and utilization of molecular profiling (6). If one considers the failure of recent dose-escalation attempts utilizing external beam radiotherapy (EBRT) when treating glioma, perhaps a targeted radionuclide therapy (TRT) approach will be of considerable merit. TRT potentially allows for the most conformal, intensity modulated, and guided radiation therapy known. The potential for

dose escalation, with this form of therapy, is promising. Phase I and II studies are currently being explored.

If the cure for CNS malignancies were brought to fruition in the immediate future, quality-of-life issues would certainly remain as portions of the destructive process from the malignancy and therapies cannot be reversed. The field of stem cell research may ultimately help allay or even reverse some of the current neurologic deficits that are so debilitating.

On a less sanguine note, one must be ever diligent with regards to the promising phase I and II data that have often shown considerable merit. History is replete with phase III trial failures based on early successes (7) when treating glioma. Quite obviously, level I data are scant and patient selection will often determine the outcome of nonrandomized trials. The objective of this chapter is to provide an overview of the radiation physics, radiobiology, and the various radiation delivery mechanisms, leading to the development of TRT, for CNS tumors.

◼ RADIOBIOLOGY

There are three general methods to deliver therapeutic radiation to patients with a malignant disease. The first method consists of local/regional therapy from an external source, such as the radiation generated from kilovoltage units, teletherapy γ-ray units (cobalt-60), linear accelerators, nuclear reactors (neutrons), or cyclotrons (protons). The second method consists of the local implantation (permanent or temporary) of sealed sources, termed brachytherapy. The third method is the local, compartmental, or systemic delivery of unsealed sources. The unsealed sources may be unconjugated ("naked" radionuclide, i.e., ^{153}Sm, ^{131}I) or conjugated (radionuclide bound to a targeting construct, i.e., ibritumomab tiuxetan, Zevalin, tositumomab, Bexxar).

Radiobiology may be simply defined as the interaction between ionizing radiation and biologic systems. In reality, the field of radiobiology is anything but simple. It is exceedingly complex. Its complexity is embodied in the writings, over many decades, of such leaders as Fowler, Hall, Withers, Orton, and Elking. For a comprehensive review of radiobiology, the reader is referred to such writings. The purpose of this section is to supply a brief overview of important radiobiology concepts.

William Conrad Roentgen discovered "x-rays" in 1895. The first radiograph was performed in 1896. During the same year, Henri Becquerel discovered "natural radioactivity" (8). In 1898 Pierre and Marie Curie postulated the existence of polonium and radium in pitchblende (uraninite), and they eventually isolated radium in 1902. Due to its lack of abundance (100 µg/ton of ore) and short half-life (138 days), it was virtually impossible to isolate polonium in the late 1800s with the existing techniques. Polonium was eventually isolated in 1944 (Dayton, Ohio). Becquerel performed the first "self-imposed" radiobiology experiment by accidentally leaving a vial, containing 200 mg of radium, in his breast pocket for 6 hours. As a result, he described the development of skin erythema and ulceration that required many weeks to heal (9). Later, Pierre Curie produced a similar skin reaction on his forearm using a similar radium exposure. Within a few short years, researchers in Germany and France reported on the radiation sensitivity of mitotically active cells in testes. Unfortunately, much of the early radiobiology data documented in the German literature, prior to WWII, are not well known (10). However, the groundwork of Reisner, Miescher, and Strandqvist in the 1930s to the 1950s subsequently gave rise to the "Golden Age of Radiobiology" (11), as some refer to it today.

An x-ray or photon is a form of electromagnetic radiation that is produced extranuclearly, typically by accelerating electrons into a high atomic mass material, such as tungsten. This process will produce x-rays as the electrons rapidly decelerate, in a process called "bremsstrahlung" or "braking radiation" (12). This is the basic premise by which modern accelerators operate. A γ-ray is electromagnetic radiation that is emitted from a radioactive isotope. Both forms of radiation can be described by wave and particle theory.

When radiation interacts with biologic material, excitation or ionization may occur. If the imparted energy does not exceed a certain threshold, an electron in the material will only be raised to a higher energy state and not ejected. This is termed excitation. Ionization occurs when the imparted energy is great enough to cause ejection of one or more orbital electrons from an atom or molecule in the material. The energy released in an ionization event is 33 eV (13). The radiation causing the ionization is hence termed ionizing radiation. Ionizing radiation can be either electromagnetic (photons or γ-rays) or particulate (electrons, α-particles, neutrons, protons, heavy charged particles). The particulate radiation is generally considered directly ionizing and electromagnetic radiation is generally considered indirectly ionizing. Directly ionizing radiation interacts with and "directly" alters the molecular structure of the biologically important molecule or target, such as an α-particle causing a DNA double-strand break. Indirectly ionizing radiation interacts with the target molecule through intermediary products, such as a photon producing

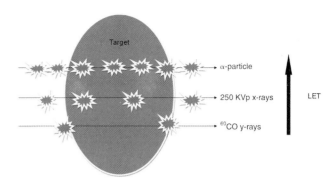

FIGURE 27.1 Schematic representation of ionization tracks produced by different types of radiation with increasing linear energy transfer (LET). Closely spaced ionization events represent densely ionizing radiation (as opposed to sparsely ionizing radiation). In general, radiation with a higher LET will have a higher relative biologic effectiveness (RBE). The ionization tracks, from top to bottom, represent α-particles, 250 kVp x-rays, and ^{60}Co γ-rays.

free radicals that will subsequently interact with DNA. As ionizing radiation interacts with biologic material, the resulting ionizing events are distributed along the path of the incident photon or particulate radiation. If the ionizing events are separated by relatively large distances in space, the radiation is termed "sparsely ionizing." If the ionizing radiation is geometrically very close, the radiation is termed "densely ionizing" (Fig. 27.1). The amount of energy that is deposited per unit length is termed the linear energy transfer (LET), and is usually defined by kiloelectron volt per micrometer. Typical LET values for various forms of radiation are shown in Table 27.1. Because these different types of radiation cause different biologic effects, a means for comparison was developed and called the relative biologic effectiveness (RBE). Classically, the RBE is defined as the ratio of the dose of a known, standard radiation (250 kVp x-rays) to the dose of a "test" radiation, which results in the same biologic end point.

Many targets have been proposed as the recipient cause of the biologic impact of radiation. These include DNA, lipids and proteins, cell membrane (14), mitochondria (15), and microvasculature (16). It is largely asserted that it is

Table **27.1**	The linear energy transfer (LET) values of various types of radiation.
Type of Radiation	**LET (keV/µm)**[a]
^{60}Co γ-rays	0.2–0.3
250 kVp x-rays	2.0
Protons[b]	0.5–5.0
Neutrons[b]	12–150
α-Particles[b]	100–150
Heavy charged ions[b]	100–2500

[a]As defined by the International Commission of Radiological Units: LET = L = dE/dl (dE is the average energy locally delivered to the biologic medium by the radiation, when traversing the distance, dl).
[b]Range of energies.

the interaction of ionizing radiation with the cell DNA that leads to a lethal event. Using a polonium-tipped microneedle, α-particle radiation (range, 25 to 35 μm from needle tip) was directed to different regions of a cell. When doses as high as 100,000 cGy were directed at large portions of the cytoplasm only (and within 2 to 3 μm of the nucleus), there was no negative impact on subsequent cell proliferation. However, with an α-particle fluence of 0.3 to 3.0 particles/μm², penetrating only 1 to 2 μm into the nucleus, 92% of the cells either died or had a significantly diminished reproductive integrity. The conclusion determined it only takes a few α-particles to traverse several cubic micrometers into the nucleus (location of the DNA) for the negative impact on cell survival to occur (17). In general, the consequences of this interaction of radiation with the cell nucleus or DNA may result in the cell undergoing quiescence, apoptosis, mitotic catastrophe, replicative senescence, accelerated senescence, treatment-induced senescence, terminal differentiation, terminal growth arrest, or necrosis (18–21).

If the log surviving fraction of cells is plotted against the dose of radiation delivered in a single fraction, a cell survival curve is generated. Because radiation will kill an equal proportion or percentage of cells per dose (not equal number), a component of the cell survival/dose relation is logarithmic. As a result, the following becomes evident. If 3 Gy will inactivate 50% of the cells, then increasing the dose to 6, 9, and 12 Gy will result in a 25%, 12.5%, and 6.25% surviving fraction, respectively. For prokaryotic systems, such as bacteria, the log surviving fraction versus dose (albeit much greater than that required for mammalian cells) results in a straight line (Fig. 27.2). Quite simply, this represents an exponential cell kill with a linear increase in dose, signifying a response to single hits. Eukaryotic (mammalian cells) systems differ from bacteria cells in that there is a "shoulder" on the initial cell survival curve, at lower doses. This represents a region of reduced efficiency in cell killing. Another important concept, all parameters being equal, is that larger tumors simply require larger doses of radiation for tumor control probability. Figure 27.3 demonstrates tumor control probability versus tumor volume for a given

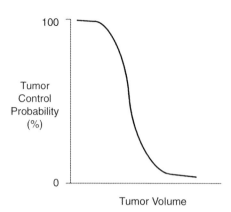

FIGURE 27.3 Relation between tumor control and volume of tumor (number of clonogens), for a given dose of radiation.

dose or regimen of radiotherapy. If one considers a large tumor with 10,000 clonogens (cells capable of continued replication) versus a smaller tumor with 100 clonogens and applies the above logarithmic cell-kill concept, it takes more radiation to reach a less than one surviving clonogen number in the larger tumor as opposed to the smaller tumor. Less than one surviving clonogen should translate into 100% tumor control probability.

For mammalian cells, when dose (Gy) is plotted on the abscissa for single fractions of radiation and log surviving fraction is plotted on the ordinate, the resulting cell survival curve appears different than the typical straight line of prokaryotic systems (Fig. 27.4). Qualitatively, the curve can be described as having a shoulder in the low-dose region. At higher doses, the curve changes into a straight line; however, there are data to support that some cell survival curves continue to curve or bend "downward," even in the range of high doses per fraction.

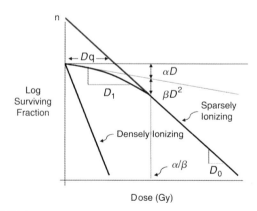

FIGURE 27.4 Mammalian cell survival curve; the shape of the curve represents the single-hit, multitarget model (initial shoulder and then straight line). The continuously bending linear-quadratic (LQ) cell survival curve is not shown for simplification. For illustrative purposes, the parameters α, β, and α/β are included (representing the LQ model); n, D_q, D_1, and D_0 are included (representing the single-hit, multitarget model). D_q and n define the width of the shoulder region. D_1 is the initial slope where cell killing is proportional to dose (αD). D_0 represents the final slope where cell killing is proportional to the dose squared (βD_2). The α/β ratio for the cell population is defined as the dose when the linear (αD) component of cell killing is equal to the quadratic (βD_2) component.

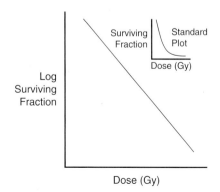

FIGURE 27.2 Cell survival curve for prokaryotic system representing an exponential cell kill with a linear increase in dose (kilogray). The inset represents a standard plot of the same data.

It is less than a perfect world when one tries to account for the actual molecular mechanisms involved in the appearance of the actual cell survival curves. Several models have been developed to explain the observed findings of the response of eukaryotic cells to radiation. Almost all models and theory can account for the actual shape of the curve, but it is exceedingly difficult to actually ascertain which model truly represents the biologic and molecular mechanisms of the interaction of radiation and cells in vivo. Therefore, a few brief comments, about two prevailing radiobiology models used to try and explain mammalian cell survival curves, are warranted.

The single-hit, multitarget model (Fig. 27.4) assumes that the radiation damage must accumulate before the resulting effect becomes evident. This dose–response relation can be mathematically described by $S = e^{-D/D_0}$, where S is the surviving fraction of cells after a given dose (D) and D_0 represents the dose that reduces the cell population to 0.37 ($1/e$) of a value on the exponential (straight) portion of the cell survival curve. The initial slope, D_1, results from single-event cell kill and the final slope, D_0, results from multi-event cell kill. The extrapolation number, n, and the quasithreshold, D_q, measure the width of the shoulder of the curve. If n is large, the shoulder is broad and the cells tend to be more resistant to radiation in this dose range. Hence, more radiation is required to result in the same proportion of cells killed as would result on the straight portion of the curve (compare slopes of D_1 and D_0). The quasithreshold represents a dose range below which there is no impact on cell survival. Since there truly is no such threshold, it is termed "quasi" or an "almost" threshold (22). The terms D_q, D_0, and n can be described by $\log_e n = D_q/D_0$. For densely ionizing radiation the cell survival curve is a straight line.

The linear-quadratic (LQ) model was developed to try and better explain a continuously bending (not depicted in Fig. 27.4) cell survival curve, rather than an initial shoulder and final slope (straight line) which is applicable only to the multitarget model. A problem with the multitarget model is that it predicts an initial cell-kill slope of zero (no cell kill) at very low doses and this is simply not the case, as typified in experiments using increased fractionation or low dose rate treatment approaches (23). The accumulation of damage or "sublesions" in cells (24), often referred to as sublethal damage, was proposed to account for some of these observations. The LQ model assumes that there are two components to cell kill; the first component (α) is proportional to dose (initial slope; linear cell kill described by a single-hit process), and the second component (β) is proportional to the square of the dose (final slope; quadratic cell kill described by a two-hit process). They can be mathematically expressed as $S = e^{-\alpha D - \beta D^2}$ (22). These coefficients are felt to represent nonrepairable (α) and repairable (β) components of cell damage (11). In this expression, S is the fraction of surviving cells after dose, D, whereas α and β are constants for a given cell line. These two different components of cell killing are equal if

$D = \alpha/\beta$, or, stated differently, the linear and quadratic components of cell killing are equal when the dose is equal to the ratio of α to β. At a dose where α/β is greater than 1 or less than 1, the α or β component to cell killing predominates, respectively. As previously mentioned, the LQ model describes a continually bending cell survival curve. The LQ model has largely replaced the single-hit, multitarget model.

The goal of radiation oncology is to maximize dose to the tumor while sparing as much normal tissue as possible. In order to fully utilize radiation as an effective treatment modality, an understanding of early- and late-responding tissues is necessary. Early-responding tissues typically exhibit high cell propagation rates. Relevant examples would include skin, hair follicles, and mucosa. Radiation damage will become apparent in these tissues within weeks after the initial radiation exposure. Late-responding tissues exhibit low or no cell propagation rates. Relevant examples would include brain, spinal cord, kidneys, and peripheral nerves. Radiation damage will become apparent in these tissues only after months or years after the initial radiation exposure. In general, there is not a direct relationship between acute side effects induced in early-responding tissues and the subsequent development of complications in late-responding tissues. Additionally, acute radiation reactions tend to respond to therapeutic interventions, whereas late complications tend to be more difficult to manage and often will not respond significantly to current therapies. Therefore, a greater chance for tumor control and a lower chance for complications results in a larger therapeutic ratio or gain. Concerning the delivery of radiation, the therapeutic ratio can be maximized by (a) decreasing the dose to normal tissues (conformal techniques, IMRT, proton therapy, four-dimensional planning), (b) combined modality approaches (combining surgery, chemotherapy, biologics, targeting agents, and radiopharmaceuticals with radiation), and (c) modification of the delivery of radiation in order to exploit radiobiology properties (fractionation, duration of treatment, dose rate, and type of radiation [photons, protons, charged particles, neutrons]). The following portion of this section will focus on the modification of the delivery of radiation, namely fractionation, treatment time considerations, and dose rate.

Standard fractionation, in the United States, can be characterized as delivering 1.8- to 2.0-Gy fractions, 5 days/week. For potentially curative clinical situations, such as head and neck squamous cell carcinoma, this would translate into delivering between 66 and 72 Gy over 6.5 to 7.5 weeks. Fractionation evolved early in the history of radiobiology with the understanding that there was a sparing of late-responding tissues relative to the tumor, compared to high-dose single-fraction regimens. Because the shoulder region of the cell survival curve is repeated with each fraction, the overall dose must be increased to help offset this "less effective" radiation (a dose region where it is less likely that sublethal damage will accumulate). A deviation from the standard fractionation schedule is termed "altered fractionation." The three most common altered fractionation schedules are hyperfractionation, accelerated fractionation, and hypofractionation. These schedules attempt to increase tumor control by delivering higher biologically effective doses. Hyperfractionation consists of using more than one fraction per day. The dose used for each fraction is less than that used in standard fractionation (i.e., 1.1 to 1.6 Gy, twice daily). This results in a total daily dose of 2.2 to 3.2 Gy. The overall final treatment schedule dose is higher than conventional doses. An example would be 76.8 Gy, 64 fractions, twice daily, for an overall treatment time of 32 days. In contrast, a standard fractionation regimen would consist of 70.0 Gy, 35 fractions, once daily, for an overall treatment time of 35 days. Hyperfractionation exploits the differences between early- and late-responding tissues. Accelerated fractionation shortens the overall treatment time (5 to 6 weeks vs. 7 weeks), using standard daily doses (1.8 to 2.0 Gy), and keeping the overall treatment schedule dose similar to standard fractionation schedules. This can be accomplished, for example, by treating 6 days/week (instead of 5 days) or by using a concomitant boost technique. Accelerated fractionation attempts to address the problem of accelerated repopulation of tumor clonogens. Hypofractionation is the delivery of daily doses larger than 2 Gy, shorter overall treatment times, and lower overall doses. Hypofractionation regimens take advantage of "treating off the shoulder region" (greater cell kill per fraction) of the cell survival curve and combat accelerated repopulation of tumor tissue. A concern about using a hypofractionation regimen, in a curative fashion, would be the potential of greater, late, and normal tissue complications.

There appears to be a reproducible difference in how early- and late-responding tissues respond to fractionated radiation. Early-responding tissue has less of an ability to recover between fractions of radiation, compared to late-responding tissue. As a result, fractionation tends to diminish potential complications in late-responding tissue while remaining relatively effective against tumors and early-responding tissue. The relation of the impact of fractionated radiation on early- and late-responding tissue may also be described in terms of the α/β ratio. This is, in fact, the ratio of the linear to the quadratic component of the cell survival curve for each respective tissue. In general, early-responding tissues (and tumor) are assigned high values for the α/β ratio, usually in the 7- to 20-Gy range, with 10 Gy being a typical value. Late-responding tissue typically has an α/β ratio of 1 to 5 Gy (25). Thus, the α/β ratio may be used to quantify the effects of different fractionation regimens on early- and late-responding tissues. Of course, if tumors and late-responding tissues exist as representing a spectrum of α/β ratios, then local control and toxicity data may be rather variable. It may simply be too difficult to apply specific α/β ratios to tissues when other factors such as tumor hypoxia, tumor volume, repopulation, and patient-specific variables may prevail. In fact, there is some evidence that prostate cancer may have an α/β ratio similar to late-responding tissue (26).

Another radiobiology principle that is intimately related to overall treatment time and fractionation is the concept of repopulation. Repopulation represents the proliferation of clonogens within the tumor (or stem cells within normal tissue) during fractionated radiotherapy. This process will diminish the effectiveness of radiotherapy by eventually increasing the number of clonogens that need sterilizing during the radiation therapy course. The initiation of repopulation appears to be stimulated by a cytotoxic event (injury) and represents a complex relation between growth fraction and cell cycle kinetics. In general, repopulation is not felt to begin immediately but after a several-week delay from the beginning of radiotherapy (27,28). Repopulation becomes "accelerated" when the tumor doubling time is shorter during therapy than the doubling time prior to the initiation of therapy. In fact, it has been estimated that 0.6 Gy/day is lost due to repopulation in head and neck squamous cell carcinoma (27). Due to accelerated repopulation, treatment breaks or protraction of a radiation course can have a significant negative impact on tumor control. Altered fractionation programs, therefore, have been designed to ultimately shorten the overall treatment time with an attempt to abrogate the negative impact of accelerated repopulation. (*Note*: Hyperfractionation uses an overall similar treatment time, compared to standard fractionation regimens, but the final dose is increased, thus ultimately resulting in a shorter treatment time for the larger end dose.)

Dose rate is another important determinant of the biologic response to irradiation. When the dose rate is lowered, the impact on cell kill is lessened. The dose rate effect seems to result from the repair of sublethal damage. As the dose rate is lowered, the ability of a cell to repair the damage increases. The resulting cell survival curve becomes "shallower" or, in other terms, D_0 decreases; the curves also tend to "lose" the shoulder region. Low dose rate radiation tends to spare normal tissue (low α/β ratio) to a greater degree compared to malignant tissue (high α/β ratio). The dose-rate effect is most pronounced between 1 and 100 cGy/min (22). At these low dose rates, some cell lines will actually exhibit an increase in cell kill compared to higher dose rates. This is felt to be secondary to the cells being "blocked" in G2, a more radiosensitive portion of the cell cycle. This phenomenon is termed the inverse dose-rate effect.

It has been known for many decades that molecular oxygen is one of the most powerful agents for enhancing the effects of ionizing radiation. Early studies revealed that 150 to 200 μm was the maximum range that oxygen would diffuse from a blood vessel and into tissue. These distances were confirmed by histopathologic analysis of tumors (29). Thus, it was inferred that tumor cells ranged from fully anoxic (greater distances from blood vessels in areas of necrosis) to fully oxic (close proximity to blood vessels). Intermediate regions could potentially harbor hypoxic and radioresistant clonogenic cells. Subsequently, it has been extensively confirmed by in vitro and in vivo studies that hypoxic cells are more radioresistant than well-oxygenated cells (30–32). In an effort to measure the benefit of oxygen as a dose-modifying agent, the oxygen enhancement ratio (OER) has been developed. The OER is defined as the ratio of the dose required to achieve the same end point (i.e., cell survival) under hypoxic conditions to that under oxic or aerobic conditions. Typical values are 2.5 to 3.0 for large fractions of sparsely ionizing radiation and 1.0 for high-LET irradiation (23).

Due to the benefit of oxygenation, a single fraction of radiation will preferentially spare hypoxic regions of the tumor. As a result, multiple fractions of radiation should slowly increase the hypoxic cell fraction within a tumor, rendering it relatively incurable with a large number of hypoxic and radioresistant cells remaining at the end of therapy. It has been shown, however, that this is not the case and that the hypoxic fraction of cells within a tumor is the same at the beginning as at the end of therapy (33). This occurs because of the process of reoxygenation, which returns the proportion of hypoxic cells back to the level that existed prior to each fraction. If the time between fractions is sufficient to allow for reoxygenation, then tumor hypoxia should potentially have a minimal impact on tumor control probability.

■ BRACHYTHERAPY

External beam radiation remains the most effective adjuvant therapy for treating CNS malignancies. The Brain Tumor Study Group confirmed a survival benefit of EBRT, following surgery for patients with malignant glioma, in the landmark 1978 publication (34). The radiotherapy arm of this study revealed a significant improvement in median survival, from 14 weeks (surgery only) to 36 weeks (surgery and radiotherapy; $p = 0.001$). During the following decades, there was considerable interest in utilizing radiotherapy in an effort to improve survival when treating this extremely resilient disease. It is quite clear that dose escalation with EBRT in excess of 60 Gy has no significant impact on survival (35,36) and often exceeds normal tissue tolerance. In fact, it has been shown that there is typically no incidence of CNS necrosis with external beam doses less than 57 Gy compared to 18% incidence of CNS necrosis with external beam doses greater than 64.8 Gy (37). Considering that most recurrences of high-grade gliomas are local (38,39), there has been a recent emphasis on more localized and focal radiation techniques such as radiosurgery and brachytherapy. The obvious goal is to safely escalate the dose of radiation to the high-risk portion of the CNS and minimize normal tissue exposure, hence increasing the therapeutic ratio. However, due to the infiltrating nature of these tumors, local targeting with a more focal radiation technique appears to be a formidable task.

Brachytherapy for CNS tumors has a long history. The first brachytherapy treatment of glioma was reported in 1914 (40). This somewhat cumbersome, free-hand treatment technique was soon surpassed by the less-invasive delivery of radiotherapy using "teletherapy machines." During this time period, there was also the concurrent development of stereotactic localization devices (frame-based and frameless). This, coupled with the improved availability and an increase in choice of radioisotopes, resulted in a resurgence of interest in CNS brachytherapy throughout the 1970s and 1980s. Encouraging initial single institution experiences seemed to indicate a survival advantage for selected patients treated with stereotactic-guided brachytherapy (41,42). However, due to the invasive nature of the procedure, the potential for hemorrhage, infection, necrosis, and frequent need for reoperation, there was reasonable concern for restraint. Criticism, claiming "patient selection" as the cause for the initial favorable results, was often levied (43). Obviously, there was considerable pressure for level I data via prospective randomized studies. The answer came from two phase III trials (44,45) published in 1998 and 2002. Although different in design, each study used a combination of EBRT and a stereotactic-guided temporary ^{125}I implant. The conclusion of each study was that there was no statistically significant survival benefit for the patients receiving the brachytherapy (see below). As a result, there has been a rather marked decrease in the utilization of brachytherapy for primary and recurrent CNS malignancies over the ensuing years (46). This is not to say, however, that brachytherapy is no longer a viable option for certain clinical situations involving brain tumors (47). Today, more than ever, radiotherapy remains one of the most effective standalone or adjuvant therapies for this type of disease. There appears to be a strong potential for a dose–effect relationship when reviewing external beam (48) and brachytherapy (49) data. When this concept is taken in context with improved imaging modalities, the potential therapeutic ratio enhancement of brachytherapy due to improved radiobiology, the fact that radioisotopes are more cytotoxic than commonly used chemotherapy agents (50), and that there are new and intriguing radionuclide delivery techniques, further preclinical and clinical investigation is certainly warranted.

The intrigue of utilizing brachytherapy in CNS malignancies is largely due to the potential normal tissue sparing from low dose rate irradiation and the inverse-square law. Commonly used radioisotopes for CNS brachytherapy are shown in Table 27.2. Selection of the isotope often depends on availability, half-life, activity, energy, dose rate, and shielding requirements that potentially impact exposure risk to health care personnel. A select group of patients with cystic lesions or craniopharyngiomas may benefit from the direct instillation of colloidal ^{32}P, ^{90}Y, or ^{198}Au (51–55). Typically this technique will deliver between 20,000 and 40,000 cGy to the cyst wall, assuming a uniform dispersion of the radionuclide within the cystic structure. It has been estimated that the dose will often be less than the actual calculated dose due to the phenomenon of "plating" (56). Plating represents a nonuniform distribution of the radiocolloid. A review of the CNS brachytherapy literature reveals that ^{125}I is the most commonly used encapsulated or sealed

Table **27.2** Commonly used isotopes for CNS brachytherapy.					
Isotope	Half-Life	Typical Dose Rate (cGy/h)	Energy (MeV)	Decay/Product	Exposure Rate Constant (Γ)
^{60}Co	5.263 years	>1000	1.25	$\beta \rightarrow \beta, \gamma$	13.07
^{252}Cf	2.645 years	>350	2.3	$\alpha \rightarrow n$	
^{125}I[a]	60.2 days	3–8 (permanent)			
		40–70 (temporary)	0.027–0.035	EC $\rightarrow$ x	1.46
^{192}Ir	74.2 days	80–100 (LDR)			
		120–360 (HDR)	0.38	EC, $\beta \rightarrow \beta, \gamma$	4.69
^{198}Au[b]	2.7 days	–	0.412	$\beta \rightarrow \beta, \gamma$	2.38
^{32}P[c]	14.28 days	–	1.7	$\beta \rightarrow \beta$	–
^{90}Y[c]	2.67 days	–	2.3	$\beta \rightarrow \beta$	–

[a]Seeds or organically bound aqueous solution.
[b]Seeds and colloidal preparation (for cystic lesions).
[c]Colloidal preparation (for cystic lesions).
$\Gamma = R \times cm^2 \times mCi^{-1} \times h^{-1}$; β, beta particle; γ, gamma irradiation; n, neutron; EC, electron capture; x, characteristic x-rays.
LDR, low dose rate; HDR, high dose rate.

source isotope. This is mainly due to its availability, low half-value layer, and low exposure rate constant. Personnel near the patient can actually acquire shielding from a standard lead apron (47). ^{125}I decays by electron capture (EC), which results in an excited state of ^{125}Te. ^{125}Te will then spontaneously decay to a stable ground state, emitting a 35.5-keV photon. Also, due to EC and internal conversion, characteristic x-rays are produced with energies between 27 and 35 keV. All electron emissions and photons (with energies less than 5 keV) are filtered by the titanium capsule (57). Typically, permanent ^{125}I implants are planned with dose rates in the range of 3 to 8 cGy/h while temporary ^{125}I implants are planned with dose rates in the range of 40 to 70 cGy/h (47). Some have concluded that the preferred stereotactic implant is a temporary procedure, utilizing ^{125}I at a dose rate of 10 cGy/h, and prescribing a reference dose of 60 Gy to the margin of the tumor. With this approach, "toxic vasogenic edema" has virtually been eliminated in these series of patients (58,59). With the advent of remote afterloading technology, different isotopes, such as ^{192}Ir (60–64), ^{252}Cf (65), and ^{60}Co (66), have been employed.

Patient selection for brachytherapy is critical. Although there are slight variations between institutions, it is generally accepted that patients should have solitary, well-demarcated lesions that are typically less than 6 cm in maximum dimension. There should not be involvement of the leptomeninges, corpus callosum, or evidence of subependymal spread (41,44,45,59). A high performance status (KPS ≥ 70) is desirable and some institutions exclude patients with involvement of their speech center due to "quality-of-life" issues (42). As a result of this selective triage for brachytherapy candidates, only 10% to 30% of all patients with high-grade gliomas will be eligible for the procedure (43,67).

The typical CNS brachytherapy program consists of an attempt at maximum surgical debulking of the tumor, implantation of radioactive sources or delivery device

(catheters or balloon), and EBRT (68,69). The EBRT is variably sequenced (44,45); some institutions have incorporated hyperthermia (70,71) and most will utilize chemotherapy at some point in the treatment process (44,45,72). Interstitial CNS brachytherapy can be broadly classified as either "open" (craniotomy and source placement) or "closed" (stereotactic source placement). The open technique involves layering of permanent, titanium-encapsulated radioactive seeds, connected with suture, into the resection cavity. Alternatively, the seeds can be placed directly into the adjacent tissue of the resection cavity. In all cases, the seeds are fixed in place with an application of fibrin glue, cyanoacrylate, or a tissue adhesive (73–75). A permutation of the open technique involves placement of a balloon catheter (Gliasite, Cytyc Surgical Products) into the resection cavity that is then afterloaded via a subcutaneous port (76–79). The balloon is instilled with an organically bound aqueous solution of ^{125}I (Iotrex). The closed technique involves the placement of temporary or permanent radioactive sources using computed tomography (CT)- or magnetic resonance imaging (MRI)-guided stereotactic localization (42,59). Often, a template is attached to the stereotactic frame to aid with catheter spacing. The initial, outer catheters are secured to the scalp. After appropriate dosimetric calculations, a smaller caliber catheter, containing the radioactive sources, is placed within the larger initial catheter. This array is left in place so that the calculated dose is delivered to the tumor volume. Most implants are adequately performed by using 2 to 10 catheters, each containing two to six seeds (47). When the treatment is complete, all catheters are removed en block in the operating room or at bedside.

Most CNS brachytherapy studies are retrospective or are of phase I and II design. Of course, all of these studies are subject to the possibility of selection bias (80). It has been shown that patients with GBM, eligible for brachytherapy, exhibit improved median survivals compared to those that are ineligible (13.9 months vs. 5.8 months, $p = 0.0001$), when they are treated in the same manner, with surgery, EBRT, and chemotherapy (43). Conversely, using the Radiation Therapy Oncology Group (RTOG) recursive partitioning analysis, it has been shown that patients with malignant glioma experience a survival benefit from a ^{125}I implant that is not purely based on selection bias (81).

In general, the median survival for patients receiving either a temporary or permanent ^{125}I brachytherapy implant as part of their initial therapy is 6 to 23 months (42,44, 45,58,59,69,73,82) for GBM and 31 to 39.3 months (59,73,82) for anaplastic astrocytoma (AA). For recurrent lesions, the median survivals are 11.7 to 16 months (59,74,75) for GBM and 13 to 17 months (59,75) for AA. When the data are combined (GBM and AA), the median survival is 6 to 11.5 months (42,72,83–85). The results for high dose rate afterloading techniques with ^{192}Ir, ^{252}Cf, and ^{60}Co are disappointingly similar with median survivals of 6 to 17 months for GBM and AA (63,65,66).

There have been two prospective randomized clinical trials using CNS brachytherapy as a portion of the initial management of CNS glioma. The first study was performed by Princess Margaret Hospital (PMH) and the University of Toronto and was published in 1998 (44). The second study, performed by the Brain Tumor Cooperative Group (BTCG; NIH trial 87-01), was published in 2002 (45).

The PMH study accrued patients from 1986 to 1996. A temporary stereotactic ^{125}I implant was utilized after EBRT. A total of 140 patients, diagnosed with a supratentorial malignant astrocytoma (gliosarcoma in 2 patients), were randomized to either EBRT (50 Gy/25 fractions; 69 patients) or EBRT (50 Gy/25 fractions; 71 patients) followed by the brachytherapy procedure (60 Gy minimum peripheral tumor dose at 70 cGy/h). Patients were selected with a Karnofsky Performance Status (KPS) ≥70 and maximum tumor size ≤6 cm. There could be no involvement of the corpus callosum. Of note, one patient in the EBRT arm actually received an implant and eight patients in the EBRT plus implant arm did not receive an implant (five disease progression, two myocardial infarction, one pulmonary emboli; 11% of treatment arm). The study was analyzed on an "intention-to-treat" basis and the median survival for the EBRT versus EBRT plus implant arm was 13.2 months versus 13.8 months ($p = 0.49$). If only the patients who received the implant as part of their therapy were analyzed (63 patients), their median survival was 15.7 months. In all fairness, however, patients should also be excluded from the analysis of the EBRT arm, during the same time period due to progression of disease or death from various comorbidities. Although this particular information was not reported in the study, the survival in this group of patients would also most likely improve. Regardless, this represents a subset analysis and was not an intended end point. There was a 15% (15/63) significant complication rate attributed to the implant. Overall, 26% of the patients received chemotherapy at the time of relapse (all received oral CCNU, two patients received intravenous carmustine, and two patients

received PCV). A partial or subtotal excision was accomplished as the initial surgery in 86% of the patients and reoperation was aggressively performed in 32% of the patients. Both of these surgical events were equally distributed between both treatment arms. Analysis of the pattern of failure revealed a 93% failure at the original site in the EBRT arm versus 82% in the implant arm.

The BTCG accrued patients from 1987 to 1994 and also used a temporary stereotactic ^{125}I implant (60 Gy total implant dose, at 40 cGy/h, prescribed to enclose the enhancing tumor). In this study, the EBRT (60.2 Gy/35 fractions) was delivered after the implant. The randomization was to implant plus EBRT plus BCNU (133 patients) versus EBRT plus BCNU (137 patients). The patients were equally stratified by age, KPS (≥50), gender, histology (85% GBM, 10% AA, 3% anaplastic oligodendroglioma, 2% malignant mixed glioma), and date of operation. Anatomic exclusion criteria included a tumor that crossed midline, multicentric tumors, and lack of contrast enhancement (target) following initial surgery. Because the implant was performed prior to the EBRT, all patients received the intended brachytherapy procedure. The median survival in the EBRT plus implant plus BCNU versus EBRT plus BCNU arm was 17.02 months versus 14.7 months ($p = 0.101$).

In spite of the valiant efforts of multiple institutions over the last several decades, there does not appear to be a clear survival advantage of the use of CNS brachytherapy when compared to surgical resection and EBRT, with or without chemotherapy. What appears quite obvious is that the greatest influence on survival continues to be patient selection parameters such as performance status, histology, age, size of the incipient lesion, the amount of tumor removed at initial operation, and the use of reoperation. However, on close scrutiny of the brachytherapy data there does appear to be a dose–effect response. Although not significantly impacting on survival, brachytherapy does seem to alter the recurrence pattern in some studies (44,86), although this is not a uniform finding (59,87). Considering that radiotherapy remains the most effective adjuvant treatment, it is not unreasonable to consider further dose escalation, and perhaps a favorable alteration of the therapeutic ratio, by employing an approach such as TRT. But first, let us explore the history and potential of another form of targeted therapy, neutron capture therapy.

■ NEUTRON CAPTURE THERAPY

Neutron capture therapy (NCT) is defined as the activation of a stable nuclide, by neutrons, resulting in the subsequent release of ionizing radiation. Tumor cells are initially loaded with the stable nuclide. When the nuclide has cleared from the blood and normal tissues (assuming preferential uptake in malignant tissue), neutrons from an external source are used to activate the nuclide and produce a targeted cytotoxic event in the tumor. At least in theory, this form of treatment represents a true form of "binary therapy." A binary system typically consists of two nontoxic components. Each component by itself is harmless.

When combined, however, cell death will ensue (88). NCT has been proposed for ^{10}B, ^{157}Gd (89), and ^{235}U (90). Neutron sources are typically external and produced by nuclear reactors (91) in the form of thermal neutrons (E_n less than 0.5 eV), epithermal neutrons (E_n less than 10 keV), or mixed thermal and epithermal neutron beams (92). Epithermal neutron beams are attractive because the neutrons lose energy and fall into the thermal range as they traverse tissue. This allows for greater depth of penetration when compared to nearly pure thermal neutron beams. In fact, a standard epithermal reactor beam will result in peak thermalization of the neutrons at approximately 2 cm below the skull surface (93). Regardless, beam contamination with photons and fast neutrons continues to be a problem. Accelerator-based neutron sources are being developed (94). These systems produce the neutron beam by accelerating protons into a ^{7}Li target. Internal neutron sources, using ^{252}Cf brachytherapy, have been suggested for boron neutron capture therapy (BNCT) (95). This form of NCT, however, has not reached the clinical setting for CNS malignancies. Currently, all clinical data have been generated using boron as the capture agent. Natural boron consists of 80% ^{11}B and 20% ^{10}B (96). ^{10}B is the nuclide with the large neutron capture cross-section. It is generally accepted that the intracellular ^{10}B concentration must be $\geq$20 μg/g tumor (97) or approximately 10^9 ^{10}B atoms/cell (98). This concentration must be achieved in $\geq$90% of the tumor cells (99) in order for NCT to be successful. It has been calculated that a thermal neutron fluence of 10^{12} to 10^{13} n/cm^2 is necessary in order to sustain the boron neutron capture (BNC) reaction (100).

BNCT involves the nuclear reaction ^{10}B + ^{1}n → ^{7}Li + ^{4}He. The concept was first proposed in 1936 (101). The reaction is based on the ability of ^{10}B to react with thermal neutrons (0.025 eV). It occurs with a high probability and has a nuclear cross-section of 3838 barns (102). The characteristics of common NCT agents are listed in Table 27.3. A barn is defined as 10^{-24} cm^2. The larger the barn number, the greater the probability of a reaction or capture event. In general, the probability for neutron capture is high for low-energy (thermal) neutrons and low for high-energy (fast) neutrons, for a given nucleus. The cross-section of ^{10}B can be contrasted to the fission reaction of ^{235}U that has a cross-section of 583 barns and fission

product release energy of 200.0 MeV (90). Interestingly, ^{157}Gd has a cross-section of 255,000 barns but the reaction must be located in the nucleus, due to the short range (0 to 150 nm) of the Auger and Coster–Kronig electrons, in order for cellular damage to occur. BNC liberates an α-particle and a recoiling lithium nucleus with an energy of 2.79 MeV (6% probability) or an α-particle and lithium nucleus with an energy of 2.31 MeV (94% probability) plus a lithium nucleus and γ with an energy of 0.48 MeV (97). The α-particle and Li nucleus are of high LET and are responsible for the cytotoxic effect. The resulting γ radiation has minimal local biologic impact but may contribute to the whole body dose. Additionally, the γ radiation may serve as a means to measure dose, as the γ emission will be concentrated in a region of local ^{10}B concentration, in a neutron activated treatment area. The path length of the high-LET particles is between 5 and 9 μm, approximately one cell diameter (97). The obvious goal of BNC therapy is to supply a selective cytotoxic treatment to the malignancy, while sparing normal tissues. Weighted doses between 60 and 70 Gy can be reasonably delivered with BNC therapy in approximately 1 hour as opposed to 6 to 7 weeks with standard external beam photon therapy (103).

Initial studies using BNCT to treat GBM were performed at the Brookhaven National Laboratory (BNL) in 1951 (104), using isotopically enriched borax (105). Another series of patients ($n = 17$) were treated at BNL (105–107) between 1959 and 1961 and ($n = 18$) at the Massachusetts Institute of Technology (MIT) (105,107–109) between 1959 and 1961 (96). These trials concluded in 1961 and the results have been analyzed (110). The disappointing results seemed to be primarily due to lack of specificity of the boron agents for the tumor (tumor:blood ratio less than 1), high blood boron concentrations (leading to vascular injury), and the inability of thermal neutrons to reach deep-seated (greater than 6 cm depth) tumors. These problems often resulted in severe skin reactions and damage to normal tissues. BNCT was thus discontinued in the United States at this time. In the late 1960s, it was initiated in Japan (111,112) under the guidance of Dr Hatanaka, who performed a prior 2-year fellowship at MIT with Dr Sweet (97,113). It was during this fellowship that Dr Hatanaka learned of the pioneering procedure to lessen scalp and bone dose by reflecting these

Nuclide	Cross-Section (Barns)	Reaction	Path Length	Energy (MeV)
^{1}H	0.33	^{1}H + n → ^{2}H + γ[a]	–	2.22
^{14}N	1.75	^{14}N + n → ^{14}C + ^{1}H	10–11 μm	0.626
^{10}B	3838	^{10}B + n → ^{7}Li + ^{4}He	5–9 μm	2.79
^{157}Gd	255,000	^{157}Gd + n → ^{158}Gd + γ[b]	0–150 nm	7.94
^{235}U	583	^{235}U + n → ^{86}Kr + ^{136}Xe[c]	11–18 μm	200.00

Table 27.3 Neutron capture of various nuclides

[a]Radiative capture.
[b]Auger cascade.
[c]Many possible fission products.

structures at the time of neutron treatment. The Japanese approach, therefore, was to use sodium mercaptoundecahydrododecaborate, $Na_2B_{12}H_{11}SH$ (BSH), as the neutron capture agent (113). Of note, BSH is generally not felt to cross the blood–brain barrier (BBB), although a CNS malignancy will cause BBB disruption due to local invasion (96), hence allowing some accumulation of BSH. BSH can be contrasted to p-boronophenylalanine (BPA), another commonly used neutron capture agent, which does cross the BBB (96). In the Japanese series, BSH was initially given intra-arterially and eventually intravenously. The tumors were maximally surgically debulked. During the actual neutron treatment, a skin and bone flap was raised to avoid excessive radiation damage, as reported in the early BNL and MIT experiences. As the technique evolved, a silastic sphere was placed into the resection cavity in an attempt to further improve upon the depth of penetration of the thermal neutron beam. Eventually, BNCT trials resumed in the United States and Europe and epithermal neutron beams were used in order to increase neutron depth of penetration and decrease the dose to the scalp, thus abrogating the need for a skin and bone flap. More recent trials in Japan have initiated BNCT with epithermal beams (114). Favorable initial reports with long-term survivors (112,115) led to a renewed interest of BNCT in many countries. However, an analysis of patients from the United States, treated in these Japanese series, was performed (116). Between 1987 and 1994, 14 patients were identified. Two patients were excluded, one deceased and the next of kin could not be contacted for permission to review the medical information; the second patient actually had a primary CNS lymphoma. A matched cohort of patients with high-grade glioma, treated by conventional therapy, was compared to the 12 remaining patients treated by BNCT in Japan. There was no significant difference in survival between the two groups.

The results from more recent BNCT trials performed in the United States, Japan, Finland, Sweden, the Netherlands, and the Czech Republic have been extensively reviewed (97,103,117). In general, the results appear to support a baseline level of efficacy comparable to standard therapy (Table 27.4) (93,97,104,105,115,118–124). It appears that further research is warranted. Clinical investigations continue in the United States, Japan, Europe, and Argentina. Areas of active research include improved neutron sources (accelerator-based neutron production and reliable collimation), more targeted boron delivery agents, new neutron capture agents,

Table **27.4**	**BNC for malignant glioma and other brain tumors**				
Facility (Year)	**Beam/Fraction/Number of Fields/Dose**	**Neutron Capture Agent**	**Patients (n)**	**Median Survival (Months)**	**References**
Japan; multiple[a] (1968–1995)	Thermal neutrons[b]/1/1/ 10.4–11.3 Gy	BSH (60–80 mg/kg)	n = 149; GBMF = 64; AA = 39	GBMF = 21.33 AA = 60.36	115
The Netherlands; Petten Irradiation Facility (1997–2002)	Epithermal neutrons/4/ 1–2/8.6–11.4 Gv	BSH (100 mg/kg)	n = 26; GBMF = 26	No data; phase I dose searching	97,118,119
Finland; FiR1 (1999–2001 P-01; 2001 P-03)	Epithermal neutrons/1/ 2/25–29 Gy (W)[c]	BPA (290–400 mg/kg P-01; 290 mg/kg P-03)	n = 21; GBMF = 18, P-01; GBMF = 3, P-03	61% 1 year OAS	120
Sweden; Studsvik Medical AB (2001–2002)	Epithermal neutrons/1/ 2/8.0–15.5 Gy (W)[d]	BPA (900 mg/kg)[e]	n = 17; GBMF = 17	GBMF = 18[f]	97,121
Czech Republic; LVR-15 (2001)	Thermal neutrons/1/ 1/<14.2 Gy (W)	BSH (100 mg/kg)	n = 5; GBMF = 5	Less than conventional therapy	97,122
USA, Harvard-MIT; MITR-II, M67 (1996–1999)[g]	Epithermal neutrons/ 1–2/1–3/8.8–14.2 Gy[h]	BPA (250–350 mg/kg)	n = 22; GBMF = 20[i]	All patients = 13	97,105, 123,124
USA, BNL, BMRR (1994–1999)	Epithermal neutrons/1/ 1–3/8.9–15.9 Gy-Eq	BPA (250–330 mg/kg)	n = 53; GBMF = 53	1 field = 14.8 2 fields = 12.1 3 fields = 11.9	93,104

[a]Hitachi training (HTR), Japan Atomic Research Institute (JJR-3), Musashi Institute of Technology (MuITR), Kyoto University (KUR), and Japan Atomic Research Institute (JRR-2).
[b]Skin and bone flap removed during the irradiation process; silastic-covered sphere or tube placed in resection cavity.
[c]Weighted dose.
[d]Estimated peak normal brain dose.
[e]Infusion of BPA performed over 6 hours.
[f]No prior therapy other than surgery.
[g]Only US facility treating with BNCT.
[h]RBE-Gy (sum of the physical dose for each component in the neutron beam, weighted by its RBE).
[i]Two patients with melanoma.
BSH, mercaptoundecahydrododecaborate; BPA, p-boronophenylalanine; GBMF, glioblastoma multiforme; AA, anaplastic astrocytoma; BNL, Brookhaven National Laboratory; OAS, overall survival.

Table **27.5**	Commonly used radionuclides for TRT				
Radionuclide	Physical Half-Life	E_{max} (MeV)	Maximum Range in Tissue	LET (keV/μm)	Approximate Cell Diameters
β-Emitters		*β-Particle*		*0.2*	
^{90}Y	2.7 days	2.30	12.0 mm		400–1100
^{131}I	8.0 days	0.81	2.0 mm		10–230
^{177}Lu	6.7 days	0.50	1.5 mm		4–180
^{186}Re	3.8 days	1.10	3.6 mm		
^{188}Re	17.0 hours	2.10	11.0 mm		200–1000
^{67}Cu	2.6 days	0.60	2.8 mm		5–210
α-Emitters		*α-Particle*		*80*	
^{213}Bi	45.7 minutes	5.87	70–100 μm		7–10
^{211}At	7.2 hours	5.87	55–60 μm		5–6
Low-Energy Electron Emitters		*Low-Energy Electron*		*4–26*	
^{125}I	60.1 days	0.35	2–500 nm		1
^{67}Ga	3.3 days	0.18	2–500 nm		1
^{111}In	2.83 days	0.04–0.2	2–500 nm		1

better dosimetry, improved dose components (lowering of fast neutron and photon contamination of the primary beam as well as lessening of the proton and gamma dose to normal tissue from the interaction of neutrons with hydrogen and nitrogen), combined modality approaches (photons and neutrons), fractionation of the neutron beam, and the overwhelming need for randomized trials. If BNCT can become more targeted, the delivery of neutron irradiation moved from the realm of "unfriendly" nuclear reactors to hospital environments, and favorable randomized results reported, perhaps this form of therapy has a chance to survive.

■ TARGETED RADIONUCLIDE THERAPY

Currently, the most cytotoxic agents known are α, β, and the low-energy (Auger) electron-emitting radionuclides. It has been estimated that 1 g of unconjugated ^{210}Po, an intense α-emitter, would be lethal to as many as 10 million humans (http://en.wikipedia.org/wiki/polonium_210#isotopes). On a molar basis, ^{111}In is 85, 200, and 300 times more cytotoxic than the commonly used chemotherapy agents, paclitaxol, methotrexate, and Adriamycin (125). The properties of commonly employed radionuclides for TRT are shown in Table 27.5 (126–129). TRT is a treatment modality that employs the conjugation or bonding of a radionuclide to a delivery construct that has a high avidity for the specific tumor cell or target. Based on the path length, the LET, and the decay properties, it is generally accepted that Auger or low-energy electron emitters are best suited to sterilize single cells, α-emitters for cell clusters or preangiogenic micrometastases, and β-emitters for bulkier lesions. Cell-kill modeling indicates that the ideal location for Auger electron

emitters is in the cell nucleus in close proximity to the DNA and α-emitters on the cell surface or in the cytoplasm. β-Emitters generally exert their toxicity through the "crossfire" effect (130), but there is certainly some variation depending on the ultimate energy of the emitted electron.

Typically, the delivery construct (see Part I; Chapters 2 to 5) consists of an intact antibody, an antibody fragment, peptide, or some type of affinity ligand (Table 27.6). The size of the construct has significant ramifications concerning biodistribution, excretion, and tumor penetration (131). Ultimately, the larger antibodies will remain bound to solid tumors to a greater extent than antibody fragments. Unfortunately, the longer biologic half-life of intact antibodies will lead to increased dose to normal tissues, most notably, the bone marrow. Even though modern medicine is capable of manufacturing fully human mAbs the intact antibodies are often

Table **27.6**	The size of different targeting constructs
Targeting Construct	Size (kDa)
IgG	150
CH2-deletion	125
Minibody	100
F(ab')$_2$	100
Fab'	50
scFv	25
Affibodies	6–7
Peptides	1–2

kept in a murine form in order to facilitate their clearance in an attempt to limit marrow toxicity (i.e., Zevalin/Bexxar). The route of delivery for such constructs, as applied to CNS malignancies, can be systemic, intracavitary, intracompartmental, or intratumor. Additionally, there appears to be several ways by which the therapeutic ratio of TRT can be enhanced. These include fractionation, pretargeting, protection of normal tissues, and a combined modality approach. Although TRT has been utilized for treating neuroblastoma, brain metastasis, and meningeal disease, this section will refer to its specific clinical application as it applies to treating grade III and IV astrocytoma.

The perfect antigenic target would be highly expressed on the tumor cell (tumor specific) and neither expressed within normal tissue nor secreted or "shed" systemically. If internalization occurs, then an α- or low-energy electron emitter should be considered as the therapeutic radionuclide. In reality, the best targets tend to be excessively expressed in the malignant tissue and expressed to a lesser degree in benign tissue. To date, the most commonly identified antigenic targets for CNS malignancies are the epidermal growth factor receptor (EGFR), neural cell adhesion molecule (NCAM), tenascin, placental alkaline phosphatase (PLAP), and phosphatidyl inositide. The EGFR is variably amplified in malignant tissue and is also present in benign tissue. NCAM is present in both benign and malignant glioma cells and tenascin is an extracellular glycoprotein ubiquitously expressed in glioma. A comprehensive review of clinical trials using TRT to treat CNS malignancies is listed in Table 27.7 (132–155).

Most of the trials to date are of "dose-searching pilot" or phase I design. The evolution of these trials has seen the delivery route move from systemic (intra-arterial or intravenous) to local instillation of the TRT agent into a surgically created resection cavity (SCRC). Even though the BBB is often partially disrupted by a rapidly growing CNS malignancy, this phenomenon is not well defined and 150-kDa antibodies would still not likely cross to a significant degree, although there does appear to be an element of nonspecific uptake from a systemic delivery (133). As a result, studies using the systemic approach often deliver EBRT in conjunction with TRT. It has been well documented that EBRT will cause an increase in the permeability of the BBB and increase vascular leakage (156–158). Regardless, it has been disappointingly estimated that only 0.001% to 0.01% of the systemically delivered antibody will penetrate each gram of solid tumor (135). Furthermore, biopsy data have revealed that a single systemic injection of radiolabeled anti-EGFR antibody will deliver only 0.02% of the injected activity per gram of tumor, resulting in a dose of only 100 to 200 cGy (133).

Direct instillation of the TRT agent into the SCRC is an attractive alternative to the systemic approach. Unlike other malignant sites where the potential for systemic spread mandates a systemic approach, this is not the case for malignant gliomas. The local approach is accomplished by injecting or instilling the TRT agent directly into the SCRC via an Ommaya or Rickham catheter. Preliminary dosimetry is performed to ensure localization within the surgical bed and

that no direct communication with the ventricular system has occurred. Institutions using this technique have utilized murine, chimeric, or humanized monoclonal antibodies attached to ^{131}I, ^{90}Y, ^{188}Re, and ^{211}At. Other important treatment variances include fractionation, pretargeting, and a combined modality approach using EBRT and chemotherapy. The success of this therapy will depend on meaningful penetration of the TRT agent into the local brain parenchyma such that the monoclonal antibodies (or targeting construct) can bind to areas of microscopic extension of malignant cells at some distance from the SCRC margin. It is still unknown as to what impact the healing process/inflammation at the surgical margin has on the success of antibody penetration. Also, it is well known that binding site barrier phenomena, interstitial tumor pressure, aberrant tumor vasculature, and a recusant extracellular tumor matrix will significantly impede antibody penetration.

Hopkins et al. (159) obtained biopsy data from three patients with glioma who received two to three cycles of either ^{131}I or ^{90}Y-ERIC-1 (anti-NCAM antibody), directly instilled into a SCRC. Relevant assumptions were that the SCRCs were spherical, the radionuclide was spread evenly around the resection margin, 100% of the TRT agent was bound to its target, and diffusion into the resection margin was uniform. It was shown that "modest" diffusion occurred and the process was exponential. The peak dose occurred between 0.16 and 0.18 cm beyond the resection margin and 4.4% to 5.8% of the peak dose was delivered to a depth of 2 cm. Of note, NCAM is expressed on benign and malignant cells and perhaps a more tumor-specific antigen would allow for greater depth of penetration. Certainly, smaller targeting constructs have been shown to penetrate to a greater depth in brain parenchyma, compared to intact antibodies (149). Using the same antibody, radiolabeled with ^{131}I and instilled into a SCRC, Papanastassiou (135) showed that diffusion occurred from 0.5 to 1.0 cm (SPECT). The range of antibody binding to the target was 8% to 80%. Dosimetry revealed tumor doses between 110 and 3768 Gy in four analyzed patients. Because the R_{95} (thickness of tissue where 95% of the β energy is deposited) for ^{131}I is only 0.992 mm, it was concluded that a more optimal radionuclide would potentially be ^{90}Y with an R_{95} of 5.94 mm (135). Assuming a 2-cm SCRC and 100% binding, as much as 351 Gy could be delivered to the tumor with a single instillation of 18.2 mCi of ^{90}Y-ERIC-1. This calculation resulted in an impressive minimum tumor/whole brain dose ratio of 140:1 (136).

Using ^{131}I-81C6 (antitenascin monoclonal antibody), dose-limiting toxicity (DLT) was reached with a single injection (fraction) of 80 mCi for leptomeningeal disease (intrathecal delivery), 100 mCi for heavily pretreated and recurrent glioma (into SCRC), and 120 mCi for de novo glioma (into SCRC), also receiving EBRT and chemotherapy (145). Using a standard, fixed, mCi dose, a wide range of absorbed doses (18 to 186 Gy) will be delivered to a depth of 2 cm beyond the SCRC margin (150). On further analysis, an optimal dose of 44 Gy to 2 cm beyond SCRC was identified. Doses less than 44 Gy resulted in increased recurrence rates and doses greater

Table **27.7** Clinical trials of TRT for treating CNS malignancies.

Study/Institute/ Publish Date (Reference)	Design/ Cohort Years	Nuclide- Antibody/ Type	Antigen or Target/ Antigen Tested on Tumor	Tumor Type = No. of Patients/ Presentation/KPS	Route	Activity Per Fraction/No. of Fractions
Epenetos/London/ 1985 (132)	Case report/ 1984	^{131}I-9A/murine	EGFR/yes	GBM = 1/R/not stated	IA	45 mCi/1
Kalofonos/London/ 1989 (133)	Phase I/ no data	^{131}I-EGFR1, ^{131}I-H17E2/ murine	EGFR, PLAP/yes	GBM = 5 AA = 3 BSG = 2/R/not stated	IA (n = 5) IV (n = 5)	40–140 mCi/1
Brady/Philadelphia/ 1990 (134)	Phase I–II/ no data	^{125}I-425/murine	EGFR/no	GBM = 4 AA = 6 LGG = 3 ACA = 1 Unknown = 1/R/ not stated	IA (1)	8–75 mCi/≥2 11/15 patients
Papanastassiou/UK/ 1993 (135)	Pilot study/ no data	^{131}I-ERIC-1/murine	NCAM/no	Glioma = 7/R = 6, DN = 1/not stated	SCRC or intracystic via O/R	36–59 mCi/1
Hopkins/UK/1995 (136)	Pilot study/ 1992–1993	^{90}Y-ERIC-1/murine	NCAM/no	GBM = 10 AA = 4 LGG = 1/R/not stated	SCRC or intratumor via O/R	11–25 mCi/1–3
Bigner/Duke/1998 (137)	Phase I/ 1992–1996	^{131}I-81C6/murine	Tenascin/yes	GBM = 26 AA = 3 AO = 2 Epen = 1 MM = 2/R/KPS ≥ 50	SCRC via O/R	20–120 mCi/1
Riva/Cesena/1999 (138)	Phase I and II/ 1990–1997	^{131}I-BC2, BC4/murine	Tenascin/yes	GBM = 91 AA = 10 LGG = 2 AO = 7, O = 1/R and DN/KPS ≥ 60	SCRC via O/R	5–75 mCi/3–6 (2)
Cokgor/Duke/2000 (139)	Phase I/ 1993–1998	^{131}I-81C6/murine	Tenascin/yes	GBM = 32 AA = 3 AO = 5 O = 2/DN/KPS ≥ 50	SCRC via O/R	20–180 mCi/1
Pagnelli/Milan/ 2001 (140)	Phase I/ no data	^{90}Y-BC4/murine	Tenascin/no data	GBM = 16 AA = 8/R/KPS ≥ 60	SCRC via O/R	15–30 mCi/2 (4)
Pöpperl/Munich/ 2002 (141)	Phase I/ no data	^{131}I-BC4/murine	Tenascin/no data	GBM = 8 AA = 4/DN/KPS > 70	SCRC via O/R	30 mCi (6)/1–5
Emrich/Drexel/2002 (142)	Phase II/ 1987–1997	^{125}I-425/murine (7)	EGFR/no data	GBM = 118 AA = 55/DN/KPS = 80	IV or IA	140 mCi (8)/3 (9)
Grana/EIO/2002 (143)	Phase II/ 1994–1997	^{90}Y-BC4/murine	Tenascin/yes	GBM = 20 AA = 17 (12)/DN/ KPS > 70	IV (13)	59 mCi/m^2/1
Wygoda/Poland/ 2002 (144)	Phase III/ no data	^{125}I-425/murine	EGFR/no	GBM = 8 AA = 4 (16)/DN/ not stated	IV (17)	50 mCi/3

Other Therapies	MTD/DLT	BBB Disruption via EBRT	Type of Surgery/ Residual	Pretargeting/ HAMA	RFN	POF	Median Survival (Months)
Prior S and EBRT (70 Gy)	ND/none	No	None/ enlarging mass	No/no data	0%	No data	Improved symptoms and partial response via CT
Prior S (80%), EBRT (100%), C (10%)	ND/none	No	Not stated/no data	No/1/10 (10%)	No data	No data	40% clinical and 30% CT improvement
Prior S (100%), EBRT (100%)	50 mCi/ neurologic	No	Not stated/no data	No/no data	1/15 (7%)	No data	GBM and AA = 5.5 (relapse-free interval)
Prior S (100%)	59 mCi/ neurologic	No	Gross total resection/ no data	No/no data	1/7 (14%)	No data	No data
Prior S (100%), EBRT (100%)	ND/none	No	Gross total resection/no excessive tumor	No/no data	No data	No data	All = 6
Prior S (100%), EBRT (73%), C (55%)	100 mCi/ neurologic	No	SCRC/tumor ≤1 cm from SCRC margin	No/17/30 (57%)	0%	34% non contiguous; 91% ≤2 cm of SCRC	GBM = 14 All = 15
S (100%), EBRT (100%), C (54%)	70 mCi/CNS edema at ≥ MTD	No	Maximum debulking/ 52 < 2 cm³, 39 > 3 cm³	No/(59%) (3)	3/111 (2.7%)	83.5% local, 16.4% distant	GBM = 19 AA ≥ 46 A0 = 23 0 = 31
S (100%), EBRT 1 month after ¹³¹I-81C6	120 mCi/ neurologic	No	Gross total resection/ ≤1 cm tumor	N0/34/38 (89%)	1/42 (2.4%)	No data	GBM = 17.3 All = 19.8
Prior S (100%), EBRT (100%)	30 mCi/ neurologic (5)	No	Surgical debulking/ no data	Yes/no data	0%	No data	GBM = 20 AA = 52
S (100%), EBRT (100%)	ND/none	Yes	Surgical debulking/ no data	No/8/12 (67%)	No data	No data	All = 18.5
S (100%), EBRT (100%), C (32%)	50 mCi/none	Yes	Surgical debulking (10)/no data	No/no HAMA (11)	No data	No data	GB = 13.4 AA = 50.9
S (100%), EBRT (100%), C (24%)	ND/none	Yes	Absence of gross disease after surgery/ no data	Yes/(20%) (14)	0%	No data	Control GBM = 8 AA = 33 Treatment GBM = 35.5 AA = NR (15)
S (100%), EBRT (100%), C (0%)	None/none	Yes	Macroscopic radical surgery/ no data	No/no data	0%	No data	Control All = 3/4 Treatment All = 5/7 (18)

(Continued)

Table 27.7 *(Continued)*

Study/Institute/ Publish Date (Reference)	Design/ Cohort Years	Nuclide- Antibody/ Type	Antigen or Target/ Antigen Tested on tumor	Tumor Type = No. of Patients/ Presentation/KPS	Route	Activity Per Fraction/No. of Fractions
Reardon/Duke/2002 (145)	Phase II/ 1996–2000	^{131}I-81C6/murine	Tenascin/yes	GBM = 27 AA = 4 AO = 2/DN/KPS ≥ 70	SCRC via O/R	120 mCi/1
Goetz/Munich and Cesena/2003 (146)	Phase I/1995 publication	^{90}Y and ^{131}I-BC4/murine	Tenascin/yes	GBM = 24 AA = 13/DN/KPS ≥ 70	SCRC via O/R	30 mCi/2.96 (19)
Bartolomei/Milan/ 2004 (147)	Phase II/ no data	^{90}Y-BC4/murine	Tenascin/no data	GBM = 73/R/KPS ≥ 70 Group A = 38 Group B = 35 (23)	SCRC via O/R	10–25 mCi/2–7
Boiardi/Milan/2005 (148)	Phase I/ 1999–2001	^{90}Y-BC4/murine	Tenascin/no data	GBM = 25/R/KPS > 60	SCRC via O/R	5–25 mCi/2 (26)
Mamelak/Los Angeles/ 2006 (149)	Phase I/ no data	^{131}I-TM-601 (28)/ synthetic peptide	Phosphatidyl inositide	GBM = 17 AA = 1/R/KPS ≥ 60	SCRC via O/R	10 mCi/1
Reardon/Duke/2006 (150)	Phase II/ 1996–2003	^{131}I-81C6/murine	Tenascin/no data	GBM = 33 AA = 6 AO = 2 GS = 1 M = 1/R/KPS ≥ 60	SCRC via O/R	100 mCi (29)/1
Reardon/Duke/2006 (151)	Phase I/ 1999–2002	^{131}I-81C6/chimeric	Tenascin/yes	GBM = 38 AA = 7 AO = 2/R and DN/KPS > 60	SCRC via O/R	<80–120 mCi/1
Wygoda/Poland/ 2006 (152)	Phase III/ no data	^{125}I-425/murine	EGFR/no	GBM = 12 AA = 6/DN/Zubrod 0–2	IV	52 mCi/3
Casaco/Cuba/2007 (153)	Phase I/ no data	^{188}Re-h-R3/ humanized	EGFR/no data	GBM = 8 AA = 3/R/not stated	Intratumor	10–15 mCi/1
Reardon/Duke/2008 (154)	Phase II/ 2002–2004	^{131}I-81C6/murine	Tenascin/yes	GBM = 15 AA = 6/DN/ KPS ≥ 60 (34)	SCRC via O/R	25–150 mCi (35)/1
Zalutsky/Duke/2008 (155)	Phase I/ 1998–2001	^{211}At-81C6/ chimeric	Tenascin/yes	GBM = 14 AA = 1 AO = 3/R/KPS > 70	SCRC via O/R	1.9–9.2 mCi/1

(1) Antibody delivered via internal carotid or vertebral artery system after cannulation of femoral artery.
(2) Patients had multiple cycles (every 30–60 days) for three cycles, and then repeated after 4–6 months (three cycles, *n* = 24; four cycles, *n* = 18; five cycles, *n* = 10; six cycles, *n* = 6).
(3) Largest HAMA titer in those receiving ≥3 cycles.
(4) Each fraction 8–10 weeks apart.
(5) Three patients infected at catheter site.
(6) Average dose.
(7) Internalizing antibody.
(8) Mean cumulative dose.
(9) Once per week × 3; 50 mCi/dose, IV or IA.
(10) 30/55 (55%) debulking for AA; 93/118 (79%) debulking for GBMF.
(11) No HAMA with ≤3 doses of targeted radionuclide.

Other Therapies	MTD/DLT	BBB Disruption Via EBRT	Type of Surgery/ Residual	Pretargeting/ HAMA	RFN	POF	Median Survival (Months)
S (100%), EBRT 1 month after [131]I-81C6	Previously done/ neurologic	No	Gross total resection/ ≤1-cm tumor	No/27/30 (90%)	1/33 (3%)	No data	GBM = 19.9 All = 21.7
S (100%), EBRT (100%), C (0%)	ND/none (20)	Yes	Surgical debulking/ minimal (21)	No/8/12 (67%)	0%	No data	GBM = 17 AA = NR (22)
Prior S (100%), EBRT (100%). C (41%)	ND/none	No	Surgical debulking/ no data	Yes/no data	3/73 (4%) (24)	No data	Group A 17.5 Group B 25.0 (25)
Prior S (100%), EBRT (100%), C (100%)	None/none (27)	No	Partial resection/75% had tumor >2 cm	Yes/no data	0%	No data	18 months OAS = 42%
Prior S (100%), EBRT (100%), C (100%)	ND/none	No	Surgical debulking/ no data	No/not tested	0%	No data	All = 6.75
Prior S (100%), EBRT (93%), C (53%)	100 mCi/ none (30)	No	Maximum debulking/ ≤1-cm tumor	No/27/34 (79%)	0% (31)	2/43 (5%) failed in opposite hemisphere	GBM/GS = 16.0 AA/AO = 24.75
(32)	80 mCi/ hematologic and neurologic	No	SCRC/little or no residual	No/19/41 (46%)	0%	14/47 (30%) distant failure	Stratum A and B GBM = 21.5 AA = 57.6 Stratum C GBM = 12.2 AA = NR
(33)	None/none	Yes	Maximum debulking/ <2 mL or no residual	No/no data	0%	Treatment 8/8 (100%) local Standard 9/9 (100%) local	Treatment All = 14 Standard All = 13 p = 0.23
Not stated	10 mCi/ neurologic	Not stated	No data/no data	No/no data	No data	No data	No data
S (100%), EBRT (95%), C (95%) (36)	Previously done/mild and limited	Yes (3/20 patients)	Gross total resection/ ≤1-cm tumor	No/17/17 (100%)	1/20 (5%)	1/20 (5%) distant, 19/20 (95%) local	GBM = 22.6 AA = NR
Prior S (100%), EBRT (100%), C (44%)	None/none	No	Gross total resection/ ≤1-cm tumor	No/5/15 (33%)	0%	Local in all but one case	GBM = 13.5 AA = 13.0 AO = 29

(12) Control group, $n = 18$, S + EBRT ± C, only; treatment group, $n = 19$, S + EBRT + ^{90}Y-BC4 ± C.

(13) Targeted radionuclide delivered 1 month after EBRT.

(14) 90% antistreptavidin antibodies; 70% antiavidin antibodies.

(15) Significant survival advantage for treatment versus control group for GBMF ($p = 0.014$) and AA ($p = 0.002$).

(16) GBMF: EBRT + [125]I-425, $n = 5$, EBRT only, $n = 3$. AA: EBRT + [125]I-425, $n = 2$, EBRT only, $n = 2$.

(17) Targeted radionuclide therapy initiated during fourth week of EBRT and repeated at 1-week intervals for three fractions.

(18) Crude survival.

(19) Patients at Cesena received ^{90}Y-BC4 and ^{131}I-BC4 in unspecified dose schedule; 30 mCi/fraction ^{131}I-BC4 used in Munich; mean number of fractions 2.96/patient, maximum of 8, given every 6–8 weeks.

(20) Two patients developed skin necrosis, at injection site on scalp, requiring surgical closure.

(21) No or "small" enhancement on MRI.

(22) AA 5-year survival = 85%.

Table **27.7**   *(Continued)*

(23) Group A = ^{90}Y-BC4 alone; group B = ^{90}Y-BC4 + Temodar.

(24) All three patients still had viable tumor with necrosis.

(25) Significant survival advantage for group B versus group A ($p < 0.01$).

(26) All patients were treated with ^{90}Y-BC4 (two cycles, 10 weeks apart), PCV chemotherapy, and mitoxantrone via O/R at 4 mg every 20 days.

(27) No toxicity from targeted radionuclide therapy; 44% of patients experienced grade 3–4 hematologic toxicity secondary to PCV chemotherapy; five cases had O/R removed secondary to local decubitus or aseptic osteitis.

(28) TM-601 is a synthetic 36 amino acid peptide (chlorotoxin), derived from scorpion venom. TM-601 binds to phosphatidyl inositide on the lamellipodia of tumor cells.

(29) Average dose to 2-cm rim of tissue of SCRC = 46 Gy; range = 18–186 Gy; 58% of the patients received chemotherapy after ^{131}I-81C6.

(30) One patient experienced irreversible neurotoxicity (grade 2 hemiparesis worsened to grade 3); 23% developed reversible acute hematologic toxicity.

(31) 6/43 (14%) had a stereotactic biopsy showing gliosis and necrosis.

(32) Patients divided onto stratum A (newly diagnosed and intreated; SCRC and catheter → ^{131}I-81C6 → EBRT → chemotherapy for 1 year), stratum B (newly diagnosed and prior EBRT; initial S → EBRT → SCRC and catheter → ^{131}I-81C6 → chemotherapy for 1 year), stratum C (recurrent disease; SCRC and catheter → ^{131}I-81C6 → chemotherapy for 1 year); the dose to a 2-cm margin of the SCRC was A = 32 Gy, B = 45 Gy, and C = 40 Gy.

(33) Treatment group (S + EBRT + 125I-425; $n = 8$); standard therapy group (S + EBRT; $n = 10$).

(34) One patient excluded from study due to subgaleal leak (therefore, $n = 20$).

(35) Injected activity, into the SCRC, ranged from 25 to 150 mCi. This was done in order to deliver a uniform dose of 44 Gy ± 10% to a 2-cm rim of the SCRC. This was achieved in 20/21 (95%) patients.

(36) 17/20 patients were treated with S + ^{131}I-81C6 → EBRT + C; 3/20 patients were treated with S + EBRT → ^{131}I-81C6 + C.

MTD, maximum tolerated dose; DLT, dose-limiting toxicity; BBB, blood–brain barrier; HAMA, human antimouse antibody; RFN, reoperation for necrosis; POF, pattern of failure; EGFR, epidermal growth factor receptor; NCAM, neural cell adhesion molecule; GBM, glioblastoma multiforme; ACA, metastatic adenocarcinoma; IA, intra-arterial; IV, intravenous; AA, anaplastic astrocytoma; AO, anaplastic oligodendroglioma; Epen, ependymoma; MM, malignant melanoma; LGG, low-grade glioma; O, oligodendroglioma; R, recurrent presentation; DN, de novo at presentation; SCRC, surgically created resection cavity; O/R, Ommaya or Rickham catheter; S, surgery; EBRT, external beam radiotherapy; C, chemotherapy; ND, not determined; NR, median survival not reached; EIO, European Institute of Oncology; PLAP, placental alkaline phosphatase; BSG, brain stem glioma; GS, gliosarcoma; M, metastatic lesion; OAS, overall survival.

than 44 Gy resulted in a higher rate of necrosis. A trend toward significant improvement in median survival was shown for patients receiving 40 to 48 Gy versus less than 40 Gy (160). Refining the technique further, it was shown that 20/21 patients could be successfully dosed to 44 Gy by varying the initial injection activity and considering the volume of the SCRC (154). Zalutsky et al. showed that a high-LET, α-emitting radioconjugate (^{211}At-81C6) could be safely delivered in a small cohort of glioma patients (155). Interestingly, histopathology appears to correlate with prognosis. Biopsy data from patients with a suspected recurrence, after receiving ^{131}I-labeled antitenascin 81C6 antibody, were analyzed. Three types of histologic patterns were evident: "proliferative glioma," "quiescent glioma," and "negative for neoplasm." The median survival for each histopathologic pattern was 3.5, 15.0, and 27.5 months, respectively ($p < 0.0001$). Considering total dose (external beam radiation plus radiolabeled antibody), patients receiving less than 86 Gy or greater than 86 Gy had median survivals of 7 and 19 months, respectively ($p < 0.002$) (161).

Table 27.7 indicates that the range of maximum tolerated dose (MTDs), of the studies reviewed, was between 10 and 120 mCi. There were many variables that could potentially account for the noted range. In general, by performing dosimetry for a given radionuclide delivery construct, a specific absorbed dose can be calculated to a predetermined depth from the SCRC margin. It has been shown that ^{131}I-antitenascin 81C6 can deliver 2000, 90, and 34 Gy to the cavity interface, at 1- and 2-cm depth, respectively (160,161). The median survival (Table 27.7) for TRT in treating glioma appears extremely favorable when compared to other treatment approaches. For de novo lesions, the median survival range is 50.9 to 57.6 months (three studies not reaching

median survival at the time of the report) for AA and 13.4 to 35.5 months for GB. For recurrent lesions, the median survival range is 13.0 to 52.0 months (one study not reaching median survival at the time of the report) for AA and 14.0 to 25.0 months for GB.

Building upon the data generated by Duke University, Bradmer Pharmaceuticals has developed two clinical trials using the ^{131}I-antitenascin antibody (Neuradiab) for treating glioblastoma (WHO grade IV astrocytoma). The first trial (Glass-Art) is a phase III study that randomizes patients with untreated glioblastoma to standard therapy (surgery, radiotherapy, and temozolomide) versus standard therapy plus Neuradiab. In the experimental arm, dosimetry is performed and a calculated dose of radiolabeled antibody is delivered via a Rickham catheter. The Neuradiab therapeutic dose is given after surgery and prior to the initiation of radiotherapy and temozolomide. The second trial is a phase II study designed to treat patients with recurrent glioblastoma with surgery, Neuradiab, and bevacizumab. This trial is not yet open for patient recruitment. The Glass-Art trial began enrolling patients in 2008. Although "ongoing," the trial is currently not recruiting participants. Bradmer Pharmaceuticals continues to seek development partners and has submitted multiple grants for potential funding. On March 3, 2010, the company released a proposal for private placement.

Further improvements can be expected as this field matures and phase II and III data are generated. Unlike sealed source brachytherapy, there appears to be a very low rate of CNS toxicity and subsequent need for surgical intervention to remove necrotic regions. Areas of active research include variable sized targeting agents (162,163), utilization of humanized (153,164) or fully human (165) constructs, engineering antibodies (166), clinically appropriate radionuclides

(130,167), antibody and radionuclide "cocktails" (168,169), alteration of the affinity of the targeting agent (170), selection of more promising targets (171), high-LET radionuclides (172–174), pretargeting (128,175), improved neutron capture techniques (176), combined modality approaches (177,178), fractionation (179–181), BBB disruption (182–185), extracorporeal technology (186–190), and an improved understanding of the tumor microenvironment (191) and growth kinetics (192).

■ REFERENCES

1. Stupp R, Mason WP, van den Bent MJ, et al. Radiotherapy plus concomitant and adjuvant temozolomide for glioblastoma. *N Engl J Med.* 2005;352:987–996.
2. Deorah S, Lynch CF, Sibenaller ZA, et al. Trends in brain cancer incidence and survival in the United States: surveillance, epidemiology, and end results program, 1973 to 2001. *Neurosurg Focus.* 2006;20:E1.
3. Robins HI, Chang S, Butowski N, et al. Therapeutic advances for glioblastoma multiforme: current status and future prospects. *Curr Oncol Rep.* 2007;9:66–70.
4. Giese A, Westphal M. Glioma invasion in the central nervous system. *Neurosurgery.* 1996;39:235–250.
5. Annabi B, Bouzeghrane M, Moumdjian R, et al. Probing the infiltrating character of brain tumors: inhibition of RhoA/ROK-mediated CD44 cell surface shedding from glioma cells by green tea catechin EGCg. *J Neurochem.* 2005;94:906–916.
6. Chakravarti A, Tyndall E, Palanichamy K, et al. Impact of molecular profiling on clinical trial design for glioblastoma. *Curr Oncol Rep.* 2007;9:71–79.
7. Perry JR. Bias, benefit, or both: evaluating new glioma therapies. *Neurosurg Focus.* 1998;4:e9.
8. Bedford JS, Dewey WC. Radiation Research Society 1952–2002. Historical and current highlights in radiation biology: has anything important been learned by irradiating cells? *Radiat Res.* 2002;158:251–291.
9. Hall EJ, Astor M, Bedford, et al. Basic radiobiology. *Am J Clin Oncol.* 1988;11:220–252.
10. Willers H, Beck-Bornholdt HP. Origins of radiotherapy and radiobiology: separation of the influence of dose per fraction and overall treatment time on normal tissue damage by Reisner and Miescher in the 1930s. *Radiother Oncol.* 1996;38:171–173.
11. Fowler JF. Development of radiobiology for oncology—a personal view. *Phys Med Biol.* 2006;51:R263–R286.
12. Khan FM. *The Physics of Radiation Therapy.* Baltimore, MD: Williams and Wilkins; 1984:41.
13. Hall EJ. *Radiobiology for the Radiologist.* 3rd ed. Philadelphia, PA: J.B. Lippincott Co.; 1988:3.
14. Kolesnick R, Fuks Z. Radiation and ceramide-induced apoptosis. *Oncogene.* 2003;22(37):5897–5906.
15. Taneja N, Tjalkens R, Philbert M, et al. Irradiation of mitochondria initiates apoptosis in a cell free system. *Oncogene.* 2001;20(2):167–177.
16. Garcia-Barros M, Paris F, Cordon-Cardo C, et al. Tumor response to radiotherapy regulated by endothelial cell apoptosis. *Science.* 2003; 300(5622):1155–1159.
17. Munro TR. The relative radiosensitivity of the nucleus and cytoplasm of Chinese hamster fibroblasts. *Radiat Res.* 1970;42:451–470.
18. Rainaldi G, Romano R, Indovina P, et al. Metabolomics using ¹H-NMR of apoptosis and necrosis in HL60 leukemia cells: differences between the two types of cell death and independence from the stimulus of apoptosis used. *Radiat Res.* 2008;169:170–180.
19. Janicke RU, Engels IH, Dunkern T, et al. Ionizing radiation but not anticancer drugs causes cell cycle arrest and failure to activate the mitochondrial death pathway in MCF-7 breast carcinoma cells. *Oncogene.* 2001;20:5043–5053.
20. Roninson IB. Tumor cell senescence in cancer treatment. *Cancer Res.* 2003;63:2705–2715.
21. Chang B, Broude EV, Dokmanovic M, et al. A senescence-like phenotype distinguishes tumor cells that undergo terminal proliferation arrest after exposure to anticancer agents. *Cancer Res.* 1999;59:3761–3767.
22. Hall EJ. *Radiobiology for the Radiologist.* 5th ed. Philadelphia, PA: Lippincott Williams and Wilkins; 2000.

23. Zeman EM. Biologic basis of radiation oncology. In: Gunderson LL, Tepper JE, eds. *Clinical Radiation Oncology.* 2nd ed. Philadelphia, PA: Churchill Livingstone; 2007.
24. Kellerer AM, Rossi HH. A generalized formulation of dual radiation action. *Radiat Res.* 1978;75:471–488.
25. Willers H, Held, KD. Introduction to clinical radiation biology. *Hematol Oncol Clin N Am.* 2006;20:1–24.
26. Fowler J, Chappell R, Ritter M. Is alpha/beta for prostate tumors really low? *Int J Radiat Oncol Biol Phys.* 2001;50(4):1021–1031.
27. Withers H, Taylor J, Maciejewski B. The hazard of accelerated tumor clonogen repopulation during radiotherapy. *Acta Oncol.* 1988;27:131–146.
28. Fowler JF. Non-standard fractionation in radiotherapy. *Int J Radiat Oncol Biol Phys.* 1984;10:755–759.
29. Thomlinson RH, Gray LH. The histologic structure of some human lung cancers and the possible implications for radiotherapy. *Br J Cancer.* 1955;9:539–549.
30. Powers WE, Tolmach LJ. Demonstration of an anoxic component in a mouse tumor-cell population by in vivo assay of survival following irradiation. *Radiology.* 1964;83:328–336.
31. Moulder JE, Rockwell S. Hypoxic fractions of solid tumors: experimental techniques, methods of analysis, and a survey of existing data. *Int J Radiat Oncol Biol Phys.* 1984;10(5):695–712.
32. Carlson DJ, Stewart RD, Semenenko VA, et al. Effects of oxygen on intrinsic radiation sensitivity: a test of the relationship between aerobic and hypoxic linear-quadratic (LQ) model parameters. *Med Phys.* 2006;33(9):3105–3115.
33. Van Putten LM, Kallman RF. Oxygenation status of a transplantable tumor during fractionated radiation therapy. *J Natl Cancer Inst.* 1968;40(3):441–451.
34. Walker MD, Alexander E Jr, Hunt WE, et al. Evaluation of BCNU and/or radiotherapy in the treatment of anaplastic gliomas. A cooperative clinical trial. *J Neurosurg.* 1978;49:333–343.
35. Walker MD, Green SB, Byar DP, et al. Randomized comparisons of radiotherapy and nitrosoureas for the treatment of malignant glioma after surgery. *N Engl J Med.* 1980;303:1323–1329.
36. Bleehen NM, Stenning SP. A medical research council trial of two radiotherapy doses in the treatment of grades 3 and 4 astrocytoma. The Medical Research Council Brain Tumour Working Party. *Br J Cancer.* 1991;64:769–774.
37. Marks JE, Wong J. The risk of cerebral radionecrosis in relation to dose, time and fractionation. A follow up study. *Prog Exp Tumor Res.* 1985;29:210–218.
38. Hochberg FH, Pruitt A. Assumptions in the radiotherapy of glioblastoma. *Neurology.* 1980;30:907–911.
39. Wallner KE, Galicich JH, Krol G, et al. Patterns of failure following treatment for glioblastoma multiforme and anaplastic astrocytoma. *Int J Radiat Oncol Biol Phys.* 1989;17:1129–1139.
40. Frazier C. The effects of radium emanations upon brain tumors. *Surg Gynecol Obstet.* 1920;31:236–239.
41. Gutin PH, Phillips TL, Wara WM, et al. Brachytherapy of recurrent malignant brain tumors with removable high-activity iodine-125 sources. *J Neurosurg.* 1984;60:61–81.
42. Malkin MG. Interstitial brachytherapy of malignant gliomas: the Memorial Sloan-Kettering Cancer Center experience. *Recent Results Cancer Res.* 1994;135:117–125.
43. Florell RC, Macdonald DR, Irish WD, et al. Selection bias, survival, and brachytherapy for glioma. *J Neurosurg.* 1992;76:179–183.
44. Laperriere NJ, Leung PM, McKenzie S, et al. Randomized study of brachytherapy in the initial management of patients with malignant astrocytoma. *Int J Radiat Oncol Biol Phys.* 1998;41:1005–1011.
45. Selker RG, Shapiro WR, Burger P, et al. The Brain Tumor Cooperative Group NIH trial 87-01: a randomized comparison of surgery, external radiotherapy, and carmustine vs. surgery, interstitial radiotherapy boost, external radiotherapy, and carmustine. *Neurosurgery.* 2002;51: 343–355.
46. McDermott MW, Berger MS, Kunwar AT, et al. Stereotactic radiosurgery and interstitial brachytherapy for glial neoplasms. *J Neurooncol.* 2004;69:83–100.
47. Vitaz TW, Warnke PC, Tabar V, et al. Brachytherapy for brain tumors. *J Neurooncol.* 2005;73:71–86.
48. Walker MD, Strike TA, Sheline GE, et al. An analysis of dose–effect relationship in the radiotherapy of malignant gliomas. *Int J Radiat Oncol Biol Phys.* 1979;5:1725–1731.
49. Sneed PK, Lamborn KR, Larson DA, et al. Demonstration of brachytherapy boost dose–response relationships in glioblastoma multiforme. *Int J Radiat Oncol Biol Phys.* 1996;35:37–44.

50. Bailey KE, Costantini DL, Cai Z, et al. Epidermal growth factor inhibition modulates the nuclear localization and cytotoxicity of Auger electron-emitting radiopharmaceutical ^{111}In-DTPA–human epidermal growth factor. *J Nucl Med.* 2007;48:1562–1570.

51. Hood TW, Shapiro B, Taren JA, et al. Treatment of cystic astrocytomas with intracavitary phosphorus 32. *Acta Neurochir (Wien).* 1987;39:34–37.

52. Lunsford LD, Gumerman L, Levine G. Stereotactic intracavitary irradiation of cystic neoplasms of the brain. *Appl Neurophysiol.* 1985;48:46–150.

53. Zeng T, Zong-hui L, Gui-quan K, et al. CT-guided stereotactic injection of radionuclide in treatment of brain tumors. *Chin Med J.* 1992;105:987–991.

54. Kobayashi T, Kageyama N, Ohara K, et al. Internal irradiation for cystic craniopharyngioma. *J Neurosurg.* 1981;55:896–903.

55. Zengmin T, Zonghui L, Yungan W, et al. Stereotactic intratumoral irradiation of huge craniopharyngioma. *Chin J Oncol.* 1996;18:234–236.

56. Fig LM, Shapiro B, Taren J, et al. Distribution of [^{32}P]-chromic phosphate colloid in cystic brain tumors. In: *Proceedings of the Meeting of the American Society for Stereotactic and Functional Neurosurgery*; 1992; 59:166–168.

57. Khan FM. *The Physics of Radiation Therapy*. Baltimore, MD: Williams and Wilkins; 1984:360.

58. Ostertag CB. Interstitial implant radiosurgery of brain tumors: radiobiology, indications, and results. *Recent Results Cancer Res.* 1994;135:105–116.

59. Scharfen CO, Sneed PK, Wara WM, et al. High activity iodine-125 interstitial implant for gliomas. *Int J Radiat Oncol Biol Phys.* 1992;24:583–591.

60. Johannesen TB, Watne K, Lote K, et al. Intracavitary fractionated balloon brachytherapy in glioblastoma. *Acta Neurochir.* 1999;141(2):127–133.

61. Micheletti E, La Face B, Feroldi P, et al. High-dose-rate brachytherapy for poor-prognosis, high-grade glioma: (phase II) preliminary results. *Tumori.* 1996;82:339–344.

62. Matsumoto K, Nakagawa M, Higashi H, et al. Preliminary results of interstitial ^{192}Ir brachytherapy for malignant gliomas. *Neurol Med Chir (Tokyo).* 1992;32:739–746.

63. Chun M, McKeough P, Wu A, et al. Interstitial iridium-192 implantation for malignant brain tumors. Part II: clinical experience. *Br J Radiol.* 2002;62:158–162.

64. Kolotas C, Birn G, Baltas D, et al. CT guided interstitial high dose rate brachytherapy for recurrent malignant gliomas. *Br J Radiol.* 1999;72:805–808.

65. Patchell RA, Yaes RJ, Beach L, et al. A phase I trial of neutron brachytherapy for the treatment of malignant gliomas. *Br J Radiol.* 1997;70:1162–1168.

66. Kumar PP, Good RR, Jones EO, et al. Survival of patients with glioblastoma multiforme treated by intraoperative high-activity cobalt 60 endocurietherapy. *Cancer.* 1989;64:1409–1413.

67. Bernstein M, Laperriere N. Indications for brachytherapy for brain tumors. *Acta Neurochir.* 1995;63:25–28.

68. Chin HW, Lefkowitz DM, Eisenberg MD, et al. Treatment options in high-grade brain tumors: brain brachytherapy. *Radiographics.* 1992;12:721–729.

69. Videtic GMM, Gaspar LE, Eisenberg MD, et al. Implant volume as a prognostic variable in brachytherapy decision-making for malignant gliomas stratified by the RTOG recursive partitioning analysis. *Int J Radiat Oncol Biol Phys.* 2001;51(4):963–968.

70. Stea B, Kittelson L, Cassady JR, et al. Treatment of malignant gliomas with interstitial irradiation and hyperthermia. *Int J Radiat Oncol Biol Phys.* 1992;24:657–667.

71. Sneed PK, Stauffer PR, Gutin PH, et al. Interstitial irradiation and hyperthermia for treatment of recurrent malignant brain tumors. *Neurosurgery.* 2002;28:206–215.

72. Chamberlain MC, Barba D, Kormanik P, et al. Concurrent cisplatin therapy and iodine 125 brachytherapy for recurrent malignant brain tumors. *Arch Neurol.* 1995;52:162–167.

73. Fernandez PM, Zamorano L, Yakar D, et al. Permanent iodine-125 implants in up-front treatment of malignant gliomas. *Neurosurgery.* 1995;36(3):467–473.

74. Patel S, Breneman J, Warnick RE, et al. Permanent iodine-125 interstitial implants for the treatment of recurrent glioblastoma multiforme. *Neurosurgery.* 2000;46(5):1123–1130.

75. Halligan JB, Stelzer KJ, Rostomily RC, et al. Operation and permanent low activity ^{125}I brachytherapy for recurrent high-grade astrocytomas. *Int J Radiat Oncol Biol Phys.* 1996;35(3):541–547.

76. Dempsey JF, Williams JA, Stubbs JB, et al. Dosimetric properties of a novel brachytherapy balloon applicator for the treatment of malignant brain-tumor resection-cavity margins. *Int J Radiat Oncol Biol Phys.* 1998;42:421–429.

77. Johannesen TB, Watne K, Lote K, et al. Intracavity fractionated balloon brachytherapy in glioblastoma. *Acta Neurochir.* 1999;141:127–133.

78. Chan TA, Weingart JD, Parisi M, et al. Treatment of recurrent glioblastoma multiforme with gliasite brachytherapy. *Int J Radiat Oncol Biol Phys.* 2005;62(4):1133–1139.

79. Gabayan AJ, Green SB, Sanan A, et al. Gliasite brachytherapy for treatment of recurrent malignant gliomas: a retrospective multi-institutional analysis. *Neurosurgery.* 2006;58(4):701–708.

80. Haines SJ. Moving targets and ghosts of the past: outcome measurement in brain tumour therapy. *J Clin Neurosci.* 2002;9:109–112.

81. Videtic GM, Gaspar LE, Shamsa F, et al. Use of the RTOG recursive partitioning analysis to validate the benefit of iodine-125 implants in the primary treatment of malignant gliomas. *Int J Radiat Oncol Biol Phys.* 1999;45:687–692.

82. Kitchen ND, Hughes SW, Taub NA, et al. Survival following interstitial brachytherapy for recurrent malignant glioma. *J Neurooncol.* 1994;18:33–39.

83. Bernstein M, Laperriere N, Glen J, et al. Brachytherapy for recurrent malignant astrocytoma. *Int J Radiat Oncol Biol Phys.* 1994;30:1213–1217.

84. Gutin PH, Prados MD, Phillips TL, et al. External irradiation followed by an interstitial high activity iodine-125 "boost" in the initial treatment of malignant gliomas: NCOG study 6G-82-2. *Int J Radiat Oncol Biol Phys.* 1991;21:601–606.

85. Ryken TC, Hitchon PW, VanGilder JC, et al. Interstitial brachytherapy versus cytoreductive surgery in recurrent malignant glioma. *Stereotact Funct Neurosurg.* 1994;63:241–245.

86. Wen PY, Alexander E III, Black PM, et al. Long term results of the stereotactic brachytherapy used in the initial treatment of patients with glioblastoma. *Cancer.* 1994;73(12):3029–3036.

87. Agbi CB, Bernstein M, Laperriere N, et al. Patterns of recurrence of malignant astrocytoma following stereotactic interstitial brachytherapy with iodine-125 implants. *Int J Radiat Oncol Biol Phys.* 1992;23:321–326.

88. Crossley EL, Ziolkowski EJ, Coderre JA, et al. Boronated DNA-binding compounds as potential agents for boron neutron capture therapy. *Mini Rev Med Chem.* 2007;7:303–313.

89. De Stasio G, Rajesh D, Casalbore P, et al. Are gadolinium contrast agents suitable for gadolinium neutron capture therapy? *Neurol Res.* 2005;27:387–398.

90. Hainfeld JF. Uranium-loaded apoferritin with antibodies attached: molecular design for uranium neutron-capture therapy. *Proc Natl Acad Sci U S A.* 1992;89:11064–11068.

91. Harling O, Riley K. Fission reactor neutron sources for neutron capture therapy—a critical review. *J Neurooncol.* 2003;2:7–17.

92. Kageji T, Nagahiro S, Matsuzaki K, et al. Boron neutron capture therapy using mixed epithermal and thermal neutron beams in patients with malignant glioma-correlation between radiation dose and radiation injury and clinical outcome. *Int J Radiat Oncol Biol Phys.* 2006;65(5):1446–1455.

93. Diaz AZ, Coderre JA, Chanana AD, et al. Boron neutron capture therapy for malignant gliomas. *Ann Med.* 2000;32:81–85.

94. Blue TE, Yanch JC. Accelerator-based epithermal neutron sources for boron neutron capture therapy of brain tumors. *J Neurooncol.* 2003;62:19–31.

95. Rivard MJ, Zamenhof RG. Moderated ^{252}Cf neutron energy spectra in brain tissue and calculated boron neutron capture dose. *Appl Radiat Isot.* 2004;61:753–757.

96. Carlsson J, Forssell-Aronsson E, Glimelius B, et al. Radiation therapy through activation of stable nuclides. *Acta Oncol.* 2002;41:629–634.

97. Barth RF, Coderre JA, Vincente MGH, et al. Boron neutron capture therapy of cancer: current status and future prospects. *Clin Cancer Res.* 2005;11(11):3987–4002.

98. Tolphin EI, Wellum GR, Dohan FC, et al. Boron neutron capture therapy of cerebral gliomas: II. Utilization of the blood–brain barrier and tumor-specific antigens for selective concentrations of boron in gliomas. *Oncology.* 1975;32:223–246.

99. Fowler JF, Kinsella TJ. The limiting radiosensitisation of tumours by S-phase sensitizers. *Br J Cancer.* 1996;74(suppl XXVII):S294–S296.

100. Barth RF, Soloway AH, Fairchild RG, et al. Boron neutron capture therapy for cancer. *Cancer.* 1992;70(12):2995–3007.

101. Locher GL. Biological effects and therapeutic possibilities of neutrons. *Am J Roentgenol Radium Ther.* 1936;36:1–13.

102. Beddoe AH. Boron neutron capture therapy. *Br J Radiol*. 1997;70: 665–667.

103. Barth RF, Joensuu H. Boron neutron capture therapy for the treatment of glioblastomas and extracranial tumors: as effective, more effective or less effective than photon irradiation? *Radiother Oncol*. 2007;82: 119–122.

104. Diaz AZ. Assessment of the results from the phase I/II boron neutron capture therapy trials at the Brookhaven National Laboratory from a clinician's point of view. *J Neurooncol*. 2003;62:101–109.

105. Palmer MR, Goorley JT, Kiger WS, et al. Treatment planning and dosimetry for the Harvard-MIT phase I clinical trial of cranial neutron capture therapy. *Int J Radiat Oncol Biol Phys*. 2002;53(5):1361–1379.

106. Farr LE, Sweet WH, Robertson JS, et al. Neutron capture therapy with boron in the treatment of glioblastoma multiforme. *Am J Roentgenol*. 1954;71:279–291.

107. Goodwin JT, Farr LE, Sweet WH, et al. Pathological study of eight patients with glioblastoma multiforme treated by neutron-capture therapy using boron 10. *Cancer*. 1955;8:601–615.

108. Asbury AK, Ojemann MD, Nielson SL, et al. Neuropathologic study of fourteen cases of malignant brain tumor treated by boron-10 slow neutron capture therapy. *J Neuropathol Exp Neurol*. 1972;31:278–303.

109. Sweet WH. Practical problems in the past in the use of boron-neutron capture therapy in the treatment of glioblastoma multiforme. In: *Proceedings of the First International Symposium on Neutron Capture Therapy. Brookhaven National Laboratory Reports 51730*; October 12–14, 1983: 376–378.

110. Slatkin DN. A history of boron neutron capture therapy of brain tumours. Postulation of a brain radiation dose tolerance limit. *Brain*. 1991;114:1609–1629.

111. Hatanaka H. Boron neutron capture therapy for brain tumors. In: Karin ABMF, Laws E, eds. *Glioma*. Berlin: Springer-Verlag; 1991:233–249.

112. Hatanaka H, Nakagawa Y. Clinical results of long-surviving brain tumor patients who underwent boron neutron capture therapy. *Int J Radiat Oncol Biol Phys*. 1994;28(5):1061–1066.

113. Soloway AH, Hatanaka H, Davis MA. Penetration of brain and brain tumor. VII. Tumor-binding sulfhydryl boron compounds. *J Med Chem*. 1967;10:714.

114. Miyatake S-I, Kajimoto Y, Kawabata S, et al. Clinical results of modified BNCT for malignant glioma using two boron. In: *Abstracts of the 11th World Congress on Neutron Capture Therapy*. Boston, MA; October 11–15, 2004:61.

115. Nakagawa Y, Hatanaka H. Boron neutron capture therapy. Clinical brain tumor studies. *J Neurooncol*. 1997;33(1–2):105–115.

116. Laramore GE, Spence AM. Boron neutron capture therapy (BNCT) for high-grade gliomas of the brain: a cautionary note. *Int J Radiat Oncol Biol Phys*. 1996;36(1):241–246.

117. van Rij CM, Wilhelm AJ, Sauerwein WAG, et al. Boron neutron capture therapy for glioblastoma multiforme. *Pharm World Sci*. 2005; 27:92–95.

118. Vos MJ, Turowski B, Zanella FE, et al. Radiologic findings in patients treated with boron neutron capture therapy for glioblastoma multiforme within EORTC trial 11961. *Int J Radiat Oncol Biol Phys*. 2005; 61(2):392–399.

119. Wittig A, HideghetynK, Paquis P, et al. Current clinical results of the EORTC-study 11961. In: Sauerwein W, Moss R, Wittig A, eds. *Research and Development in Neutron Capture Therapy*. Bologna: Monduzzi Editore; 2002:1117–1122.

120. Joensuu H, Kankaanranta L, Seppala L, et al. Boron neutron capture therapy of brain tumors: clinical trials at the Finnish facility using boronophenylalanine. *J Neurooncol*. 2003;62:123–134.

121. Capala J, Stenstam BH, Skold K, et al. Boron neutron capture therapy for glioblastoma multiforme: clinical studies in Sweden. *J Neurooncol*. 2003;62(1–2):135–144.

122. Honova H, Safanda M, Petruzelka L, et al. Neutron capture therapy in the treatment of glioblastoma multiforme. Initial experience in the Czech Republic. *Cas Lek Cesk*. 2004;143(1):44–47.

123. Busse PM, Harling OK, Palmer MR, et al. A phase-I clinical trial for cranial BNCT at Harvard-MIT. In: *Program and Abstracts, Ninth International Symposium on Neutron Capture Therapy for Cancer*. Osaka, Japan; 2000:27–28.

124. Busse PM, Harling OK, Palmer MR, et al. A critical examination of the results from the Harvard-MIT program phase I clinical trial of neutron capture therapy for intracranial disease. *J Neurooncol*. 2003;62(1–2):111–121.

125. Chen P, Mrkobrada M, Vallis KA, et al. Comparative antiproliferative effects of (111)In-DTPA-hEGFR, chemotherapeutic agents and

gamma-radiation on EGFR-positive breast cancer cells. *Nucl Med Biol*. 2002;29(6):693–699.

126. Ercan MT, Caglar M. Therapeutic radiopharmaceuticals. *Curr Pharm Des*. 2000;6(11):1085–1121.

127. Kassis AI, Adelstein SJ. Radiobiologic principles in radionuclide therapy. *J Nucl Med*. 2005;46(suppl 1):4S–12S.

128. Goldenberg DM, Sharkey RM, Paganelli G, et al. Antibody pretargeting advances cancer radioimmunodetection and radioimmunotherapy. *J Clin Oncol*. 2006;24(5):823–834.

129. Sharkey RM, Goldenberg DM. Targeted therapy of cancer: new prospects for antibodies and immunoconjugates. *CA Cancer J Clin*. 2006;56;226–243.

130. Karagiannis TC. Comparison of different classes of radionuclides for potential use in radioimmunotherapy. *Hell J Nucl Med*. 2007;10(2): 82–88.

131. Wong JYC. Basic immunology of antibody targeted radiotherapy. *Int J Radiat Oncol Biol Phys*. 2006;66(suppl 2):s8–s14.

132. Epenetos AA, Courtenay-Luck N, Pickering D, et al. Antibody guided irradiation of brain glioma by arterial infusion of radioactive monoclonal antibody against epidermal growth factor receptor and blood group A antigen. *Br Med J*. 1985;290(May):1463–1466.

133. Kalofonos HP, Pawlikowska TR, Hemingway A, et al. Antibody guided diagnosis and therapy of brain gliomas using radiolabeled monoclonal antibodies against epidermal growth factor receptor and placental alkaline phosphatase. *J Nucl Med*. 1989;30:1636–1645.

134. Brady LW, Markoe AM, Woo DV, et al. Iodine-125-labeled anti-epidermal growth factor receptor-425 in the treatment of glioblastoma multiforme. *Front Radiat Ther Oncol*. 1990;24:151–160 [discussion 161–165].

135. Papanastassiou V, Pizer BL, Coalham HB, et al. Treatment of recurrent and cystic malignant gliomas by a single intracavity injection of ^{131}I monoclonal antibody: feasibility pharmacokinetics and dosimetry. *Br J Cancer*. 1993;67:144–151.

136. Hopkins K, Chandler C, Bullimore J, et al. A pilot study of the treatment with recurrent malignant glioma with intratumoral yttrium-90 radioimmunoconjugates. *Radiother Oncol*. 1995;34:121–131.

137. Bigner DD, Brown MT, Friedman AH, et al. Iodine-131-labled antitenascin monoclonal antibody 81C6 treatment of patients with recurrent malignant gliomas: phase I trial results. *J Clin Oncol*. 1998;16: 2202–2212.

138. Riva P, Franceschi G, Frattarelli M, et al. [131]I radioconjugated antibodies for the locoregional radioimmunotherapy of high-grade malignant glioma. *Acta Oncol*. 1999;38(3):351–359.

139. Cokgor I, Akabani G, Kuan CT, et al. Phase I trial results of iodine-131-labeled antitenascin monoclonal antibody 81C6 treatment of patients with newly diagnosed malignant gliomas. *J Clin Oncol*. 2000; 18:3862–3872.

140. Paganelli G, Bartolomei M, Ferrari M, et al. Pre-targeted locoregional radioimmunotherapy with ^{90}Y-biotin in glioma patients: phase I study and preliminary therapeutic results. *Cancer Biother Radiopharm*. 2001;16(3):227–235.

141. Pöpperl G, Götz C, Gildehaus FJ, et al. Initial experience with locoregional radioimmunotherapy using 131I-labelled monoclonal antibodies against tenascin (BC-4) for treatment of glioma (WHO III and IV). *Nuklearmedizin*. 2002;41(3):120–128.

142. Emrich JG, Brady LW, Quang TS, et al. Radioiodinated (I-125) monoclonal antibody 425 in the treatment of high grade glioma patients. *Am J Clin Oncol*. 2002;25(6):541–546.

143. Grana C, Chinol M, Robertson C, et al. Pretargeted adjuvant radioimmunotherapy with yttrium-90-biotin in malignant glioma patients: a pilot study. *Br J Cancer*. 2002;86:207–212.

144. Wygoda Z, Tarnawski R, Brady L, et al. Simultaneous radiotherapy and radioimmunotherapy of malignant gliomas with anti-EGFR antibody labeled with iodine 125. Preliminary results. *Nucl Med Rev*. 2002;5(1):29–33.

145. Reardon DA, Akabani G, Coleman RE, et al. Phase II trial of murine ^{131}I-labeled antitenascin monoclonal antibody 81C6 administered into surgically created resection cavities of patients with newly diagnosed malignant gliomas. *J Clin Oncol*. 2002;20:1389–1397.

146. Goetz C, Riva P, Poepperl G, et al. Locoregional radioimmunotherapy in selected patients with malignant glioma: experiences, side effects and survival times. *J Neurooncol*. 2003;62:321–328.

147. Bartolomei M, Mazzetta C, Handkiewicz-Junak D, et al. Combined treatment of glioblastoma patients with locoregional pre-targeted 90Y-biotin radioimmunotherapy and temozolomide. *Q J Nucl Med*. 2004;48:220–228.

148. Boiardi A, Bartolomei M, Silvani A, et al. Intratumoral delivery of mitoxantrone in association with 90-Y radioimmunotherapy (RIT) in recurrent glioblastoma. *J Neurooncol.* 2005;72:125–131.

149. Mamelak AN, Rosenfeld S, Bucholz R, et al. Phase I single-dose study of intracavitary-administered iodine-131-TM-601 in adults with recurrent high-grade glioma. *J Clin Oncol.* 2006;24:3644–3650.

150. Reardon DA, Akabani G, Coleman RE, et al. Salvage radioimmunotherapy with murine iodine-131-labeled antitenascin monoclonal antibody 81C6 for patients with recurrent primary and metastatic malignant brain tumors: phase II study results. *J Clin Oncol.* 2006;24:115–122.

151. Reardon DA, Quinn JA, Akabani G, et al. Novel human IgG2b/murine chimeric antitenascin monoclonal antibody construct radiolabeled with 131I and administered into the surgically created resection cavity of patients with malignant glioma: phase I trial results. *J Nucl Med.* 2006;47(6):912–918.

152. Wygoda Z, Kula D, Bierzynska-Macyszyn G, et al. Use of monoclonal anti-EGFR antibody in the radioimmunotherapy of malignant gliomas in the context of EGFR expression in grade III and IV tumors. *Hybridoma.* 2006;25(3):125–132.

153. Casaco A, Lopez G, Garcia I, et al. Phase I single-dose study of intracavitary-administered nimotuzumab labeled with 188-Re in adult recurrent high-grade glioma. *Cancer Biol Ther.* 2007;7(3):333–339.

154. Reardon DA, Zalutsky MR, Akabani G, et al. A pilot study: 131I-antitenascin monoclonal antibody 81C6 to deliver a 44-Gy resection cavity boost. *Neuro-oncol.* 2008;10(April):182–189.

155. Zalutsky MR, Reardon DA, Akabani G, et al. Clinical experience with α-particle-emitting 211At: treatment of recurrent brain tumor patients with 211At-labeled chimeric antitenascin monoclonal antibody 81C6. *J Nucl Med.* 2008;49(1):30–38.

156. Qin DX, Zheng R, Tang J, et al. Influence of radiation on the blood–brain barrier and optimum time of chemotherapy. *Int J Radiat Oncol Biol Phys.* 1990;19:1507–1510.

157. Quang TS, Brady LW. Radioimmunotherapy as a novel treatment regimen: 125I-labeled monoclonal antibody 425 in the treatment of high-grade brain gliomas. *Int J Radiat Oncol Biol Phys.* 2004;58:972–975.

158. Cao Y, Tsien CI, Shen Z, et al. Use of magnetic resonance imaging to assess blood–brain/blood–glioma barrier opening during conformal radiotherapy. *J Clin Oncol.* 2005;23(18):4127–4136.

159. Hopkins K, Chandler C, Eatough J, et al. Direct injection of 90Y MoAbs into glioma tumor resection cavities leads to limited diffusion of the radioimmunoconjugates into normal brain parenchyma: a model to estimate absorbed radiation dose. *Int J Radiation Oncol Biol Phys.* 1998;40(4):835–844.

160. Akabani G, Reardon DA, Coleman RE, et al. Dosimetry and radiographic analysis of 131I-labeled anti-tenascin 81C6 murine monoclonal antibody in newly diagnosed patients with malignant gliomas: a phase II study. *J Nucl Med.* 2005;46:1042–1051.

161. McLendon RE, Akabani G, Friedman HS, et al. Tumor resection cavity administered iodine-131-labeled antitenascin 81C6 radioimmunotherapy in patients with malignant glioma: neuropathology aspects. *Nucl Med Biol.* 2007;34:405–413.

162. Schumacher T, Hofer S, Eichhorn K, et al. Local injection of the 90Y-labelled peptidic vector DOTATOC to control gliomas of WHO grades II and III: an extended pilot study. *Eur J Nucl Med.* 2002;29:468–493.

163. Kneifel S, Bernhardt P, Uusijarvi H, et al. Individual voxelwise dosimetry of targeted 90Y-labelled substance P radiotherapy for malignant gliomas. *Eur J Nucl Med Mol Imaging.* 2007;34:1388–1395.

164. Torres LA, Coca MA, Batista JF, et al. Biodistribution and internal dosimetry of the 188Re-labelled humanized monoclonal antibody anti-epidermal growth factor receptor, nimotuzumab, in the locoregional treatment of malignant gliomas. *Nucl Med Commun.* 2008;29:66–75.

165. Speer TW. Fully human monoclonal antibodies and targeted radionuclide therapy. *Blood.* 2008;112:2584–2585.

166. Liu XY, Pop LM, Vitetta ES. Engineering therapeutic monoclonal antibodies. *Immunol Rev.* 2008;222:9–27.

167. Kassis AI. Therapeutic radionuclides: biophysical and radiologic principles. *Semin Nucl Med.* 2008;38:358–366.

168. Logtenberg T. Antibody cocktails: next-generation biopharmaceuticals with improved potency. *Trends Biotechnol.* 2007;25:390–394.

169. Wheldon TE, O'Donoghue JA, Barrett A, et al. The curability of tumours of differing size by targeted radiotherapy using 131I or 90Y. *Radiother Oncol.* 1991;21:91–99.

170. Adams GP, Schier R, Marshall K, et al. Increased affinity leads to improved selective tumor delivery of single-chain Fv antibodies. *Cancer Res.* 1998;58:485–490.

171. Carlsson J, Ren ZP, Wester K, et al. Planning for intracavitary anti-EGFR radionuclide therapy of gliomas. Literature review and data on EGFR expression. *J Neurooncol.* 2006;77:33–45.

172. O'Donoghue JA, Wheldon TE. Targeted radiotherapy using Auger electron emitters. *Phys Med Biol.* 1996;41:1973–1992.

173. Mulford DA, Scheinberg DA, Jurcic FG. The promise of targeted α-particle therapy. *J Nucl Med.* 2005;46:199S–204S.

174. Cordier D, Forrer F, Bruchertseifer F, et al. Targeted alpha-radionuclide therapy of functionally critically located gliomas with 213Bi-DOTA-[Thi8,Met(O2)11]-substance P: a pilot trial. *Eur J Nucl Med Mol Imaging.* 2010;37:1335–1344.

175. Urbano N, Papi S, Ginanneschi M, et al. Evaluation of a new biotin–DOTA conjugate for pretargeted antibody-guided radioimmunotherapy (PAGRIT®). *Eur J Nucl Med.* 2007;34:68–77.

176. Barth RF. Boron neutron capture therapy at the crossroads: challenges and opportunities. *Appl Radiat Isot.* 2009;67:S3–S6.

177. Speer TW. Proapoptotic receptor agonists, targeted radionuclide therapy, and the treatment of central nervous system malignancies: in regard to Fiveash et al. *Int J Radiat Oncol Biol Phys.* 2008;71:507–516.

178. Al-Ejeh F, Darby JM, Brown MP. Chemotherapy synergizes with radioimmunotherapy targeting La autoantigen in tumors. *PLoS One.* 2009;4:e4630.

179. Shen S, Duan J, Meredith RF, et al. Model prediction of treatment planning for dose-fractionated radioimmunotherapy. *Cancer.* 2002;94:1264–1269.

180. DeNardo GL, Scholm J, Buchsbaum DJ, et al. Rationales, evidence, and design considerations for fractionated radioimmunotherapy. *Cancer.* 2002;94:1332–1348.

181. DeNardo G, DeNardo S. Dose intensified molecular targeted radiotherapy for cancer-lymphoma as a paradigm. *Semin Nucl Med.* 2010;40:136–144.

182. Hynynen K. Macromolecular delivery across the blood–brain barrier. *Methods Mol Biol.* 2009;480:175–185.

183. Stamatovic SM, Keep RF, Andjelkovic AV. Brain endothelial cell–cell junctions: how to "open" the blood brain barrier. *Curr Neuropharmacol.* 2008;6:179–192.

184. Cruickshank GS, Ngoga D, Detta A, et al. A cancer research UK pharmacokinetic study of BPA–mannitol in patients with high grade glioma to optimize uptake parameters for clinical trial of BNCT. *Appl Radiat Isot.* 2009;67:S31–S33.

185. Van Vulpen M, Kal HB, Taphoorn MJ, et al. Changes in blood–brain barrier permeability induced by radiotherapy: implications for timing of chemotherapy? [Review]. *Oncol Rep.* 2002;9:683–688.

186. Strand SE, Jonsson BA, Ljungberg M, et al. Radioimmunotherapy dosimetry—a review. *Acta Oncol.* 1993;32:807–817.

187. Strand SE, Ljungberg M, Tennvall J, et al. Radio-immunotherapy dosimetry with special emphasis on SPECT quantification and extracorporeal immuno-adsorption. *Med Biol Eng Comput.* 1994;32:551–561.

188. Martensson L, Nilsson R, Ohlsson T, et al. Improved tumor targeting and decreased normal tissue accumulation through extracorporeal affinity adsorption in a two-step pretargeting strategy. *Clin Cancer Res.* 2007;13:5572s–5576s.

189. Martensson L, Nilsson R, Ohlsson T, et al. High-dose radioimmunotherapy combined with extracorporeal depletion in a syngeneic rat tumor model—evaluation of toxicity, therapeutic effect and tumor model. *Cancer Biother Radiopharm.* 2008;23:517. (Abstract 14, *Twelfth Conference on Cancer Therapy with Antibodies and Immunoconjugates,* Parsippany, NJ, October 16–18, 2008.)

190. Nemecek ER, Green DJ, Fisher DR, et al. Extracorporeal adsorption therapy: a method to improve targeted radiation delivered by radiometal-labeled monoclonal antibodies. *Cancer Biother Radiopharm.* 2008;23:181–191.

191. Jain RK. Normalization of tumor vasculature: an emerging concept in antiangiogenic therapy. *Science.* 2005;307:58–62.

192. Khaitan D, Chandna S, Arya MB, et al. Establishment and characterization of multicellular spheroids from a human glioma cell line; implications for tumor therapy. *J Transl Med.* 2006;4:1–13.

Targeted Radionuclide Therapy for Medullary Thyroid Cancer

Aurore Oudoux, Pierre-Yves Salaun, Jean-François Chatal,
Jacques Barbet, David M. Goldenberg, and Françoise Kraeber-Bodéré

■ INTRODUCTION

Medullary thyroid cancer (MTC) is a neoplasm of the C cells and accounts for less than 8% of thyroid cancers. C cells secrete calcitonin (Ct), other polypeptides and glycoproteins, such as carcinoembryonic antigen (CEA) and somatostatin. The primary treatment of sporadic or hereditary MTC is total thyroidectomy with dissection of ipsilateral and central lymph nodes, extended in some cases to contralateral dissection. Many patients are cured by this surgical intervention. However, a number of patients show persistent disease after primary surgery, as documented by measurable serum Ct (1). Patients with localized residual disease and/or distant metastases may survive for several years or progress rapidly. Thus, highly reliable prognostic factors are needed for an early distinction between high-risk patients who need to be treated and low-risk patients who warrant a "watch-and-wait" behavior. For systemic treatment of patients with rapidly progressing metastatic MTC, chemotherapy is not considered a valid therapeutic option (2,3). It is too early to evaluate the potential effectiveness of tyrosine kinase inhibitors, multikinase inhibitors, and VEGFR inhibitors, even if phase II studies have shown a transient stabilization in 30% to 50% of patients (4–6). Targeted radiotherapy, in particular pretargeted radioimmunotherapy (PRAIT), has been another innovative treatment modality.

■ PRETHERAPEUTIC EVALUATION: PROGNOSTIC INDICATORS AND IMAGING

Among the various prognostic parameters that could identify high- and low-risk groups, advanced age, advanced stage of the disease, and associated multiple endocrine neoplasia (MEN) 2B are commonly accepted factors of poor prognosis (7). Recently, the presence of node metastasis was confirmed as the most significant factor affecting the outcome of the disease (8). Kebebew et al. (9) concluded that the EORTC prognostic scoring system, which takes into account age, gender, nature, and stage of the disease for all thyroid cancers, had the highest predictive value. Moreover, the presence of a somatic mutation in the RET oncogene and a high Ki67 expression are considered as risk factors (10,11).

Measuring Ct and CEA doubling-times (DT) is another way of looking at tumor progression rate. Ct DT is an independent predictor of survival, with a high predictive value, in a population of patients who have not normalized their Ct, even after repeated surgery (12).

Several imaging methods should be proposed for a patient with an abnormal residual Ct level persisting after complete surgery: ultrasonography and computed tomography (CT) for neck exploration, and CT for chest, abdomen, and pelvis. Magnetic resonance imaging (MRI) appears to be a sensitive imaging technique for detecting spread to bone/bone marrow and liver (13,14). Whole-body FDG-PET also appears of interest in progressive MTC patients with 83% sensitivity for neck, 85% for mediastinum, 75% for lung, 60% for liver, and 67% for bone metastases (15). Moreover, maximum SUV correlates with Ct DT with possible prognostication value (15).

■ PRETARGETED RADIOIMMUNOTHERAPY

For radioresistant solid tumors such as MTC, pretargeting strategies have been proposed to increase the therapeutic index when compared with directly labeled mAb and to improve the tumor absorbed doses (16). The Affinity Enhancement System (AES) is a pretargeting technique that uses a bispecific monoclonal antibody (BsmAb) and a radiolabeled bivalent hapten. In this system, the affinity of the hapten for the BsmAb is limited (Kd = 10^{-8} mol/L), but the bivalent hapten binds avidly to the immunoconjugate bound to the surface of target cells, whereas hapten–BsmAb complexes in the circulation, dissociates, and excess hapten are cleared, at least in part, through the kidneys. AES radioimmunotherapy (RIT) using anti-CEA × anti-DTPA murine BsmAb (F6-734) and di-DTPA-^{131}I hapten has been evaluated in CEA-expressing MTC (TT cells) xenografted mice (17–22). Increased tumor-to-normal tissue ratios, which may be further improved by adding a chase step, have been demonstrated (17,18). PRAIT was as efficient as the directly labeled antibody and was markedly less toxic (19). Repeated treatments with AES agents increased efficacy without increasing toxicity (20). Moreover, PRAIT efficacy was improved by using chemotherapy such as paclitaxel and pretreatment by antiangiogenic agents (21).

The first feasibility study assessed the murine F6-734 BsmAb and the di-DTPA-^{131}I hapten in five patients with recurrence of MTC (22). Dosimetric results showed that small lesions received potentially tumoricidal irradiation (up to 4.7 cGy/MBq), a dose comparable with that delivered by iodine-131 therapy to neck metastases from differentiated thyroid carcinoma (1.2 to 3.8 cGy/MBq for lesions of 8 to 40 g) (23). A phase I/II clinical trial was performed with the same reagents in 26 MTC patients (24). Immunoscintigraphy showed good tumor targeting. Tumor doses ranged from 0.1 to 5.0 cGy/MBq. Dose-limiting toxicity was hematologic and maximum tolerated activity was estimated at 1.8 GBq/m^2 in the group of patients with suspected bone marrow involvement. Preliminary data analysis showed a significant analgesic effect in five cases, five minor tumor responses, and four biologic responses. The therapeutic responses were observed mainly in patients with a small tumor burden and after repeated courses of RIT.

Because hematologic toxicity was relatively high and immune responses frequent, further optimization of the treatment, including the development of chimeric or humanized BsmAb, was considered necessary. A phase I optimization study was designed to determine the safety, antitumor efficacy, and targeting ability of the chimeric anti-CEA hMN-14 (humanized CEA antibody) × m734 (murine antihapten–chelate antibody) BsmAb administered at two different doses, escalating ^{131}I-di-DTPA-indium hapten activity injected 5 days later, optimizing the pretargeting interval in 22 patients with CEA-expressing tumors (non-MTC: 13 patients, MTC: 9 patients) (25,26). The overall rate of detection of lesions was 70% of 19 evaluable patients (49 anatomic sites). The main lesions that were not imaged well were lung (32% false negative) and liver (54% false negative). These lesions, however, were typically less than 1 cm. Dosimetry for patients receiving 75 mg/m^2 BsmAb was as follows: mean tumor absorbed dose was 10.7 Gy (range, 1.7 to 53.5 Gy), whole-body dose was 0.38 Gy (range, 0.14 to 0.57 Gy), liver dose was 1.9 Gy (range, 0.7 to 3.5 Gy), and kidney dose was 2.4 Gy (range, 1.5 to 3.9 Gy). The respective tumor-to-normal tissue mean ratios were 25 Gy (range, 3.0 to 102 Gy), 6.2 Gy (range, 0.5 to 31 Gy), and 7.0 Gy (range, 0.8 to 33 Gy). For patients receiving 40 mg/m^2 BsmAb, the dosimetry was as follows: mean tumor absorbed dose was 18.5 Gy (range, 2.4 to 49.3 Gy), whole-body dose was 0.33 Gy (range, 0.25 to 0.41 Gy), liver dose was 1.4 Gy (range, 0.7 to 2.3 Gy), and kidney dose was 2.1 Gy (range, 1.5 to 4.1 Gy). The respective tumor-to-normal tissue mean ratios were 55 Gy (range, 7.1 to 150 Gy), 14 Gy (range, 1.5 to 73 Gy), and 8.5 Gy (range, 1.4 to 22 Gy). The rate of tumor stabilization was 45% in the 1-year assessment. HAMA (human antimouse antibody) elevation was observed in 8% of patients and HAHA (human antihuman antibody) in 33%. The conclusion of the study was that disease stabilization occurred mostly at an antibody dose of 75 mg/m^2, but hematologic toxicity was reduced with the 40 mg/m^2 dose. It was also shown that severe hematologic toxicity occurred in patients with MTC as opposed to those with other CEA-expressing tumors. This may be related to the high incidence of bone involvement with MTC. It appeared that the maximum activity that could be administered to MTC patients was 1.8 GBq (48.6 mCi)/m^2.

Six years after the first PRAIT phase I/II trial, a retrospective study was conducted to compare the survival of 29 MTC patients given pretargeted RIT with that of 39 contemporaneous untreated patients for whom data were collected by the French Endocrine Tumor Study Group (GTE) (27). Long-term disease stabilization was observed in 53% of the MTC patients, as documented by morphologic imaging (CT, MRI) and serial Ct and CEA serum measurements. Overall survival (OS) was significantly longer in high-risk (Ct DT < 2 years) treated patients than in high-risk untreated patients (median OS, 110 vs. 61 months; p < 0.030). Forty-seven percent of patients, defined as biologic responders (by at least a more than 100% increase in Ct DT), experienced significantly longer survival than nonresponders (median OS, 159 vs. 109 months; p < 0.035) or untreated patients (median OS, 159 vs. 61 months; p < 0.010). Treated patients with bone/bone-marrow disease had a longer survival than patients without such involvement (10-year OS of 83% vs. 14%; p < 0.023). Toxicity was mainly hematologic and related to bone/bone-marrow tumor spread.

Following the encouraging results obtained in the phase I/II studies, a phase II PRAIT study has been developed in progressive MTC patients with Ct DT shorter than 5 years. Forty-five patients have been treated, receiving 40 mg/m^2 of hMN-14xm734 BsmAb and 1.8 GBq (48.6 mCi)/m^2 ^{131}I-di-DTPA 4 to 6 days apart. Six patients were retreated. A preliminary analysis was performed (September 2008) in 33 evaluable patients who received 35 treatments, with 15 months follow-up (6 to 36 months). A patient was considered unresponsive if progression according to Response Evaluation Criteria in Solid Tumors (RECIST), FDG-PET, or biomarker serum concentration was observed at 3 months post-RIT, or no effect on CEA or Ct DT (at least 100% CEA or Ct DT variation) was obtained. Tumor targeting was visualized in all cases. The sensitivity of immunoscintigraphy was 92%. Allergic reactions were observed during two BsmAb infusions, grade 1 liver toxicity after 3 out of 35 (8.5%) injections, and grade 3/4 hematologic toxicity after 19 out of 35 (54%) injections. Efficacy was observed after 18 out of 35 (51%) injections, with a time-to-progression of 18 months (6 to 36) for RECIST and 15 months (6 to 36) for PET and biomarker levels. Efficacy was found in 62% of patients in the low-risk group, 53% in the intermediate-risk group, and 50% in the high-risk group.

■ OTHER RADIONUCLIDE THERAPIES

MIBG-^{131}I therapy, which can be performed in about 35% of patients with a moderate to high tumor uptake, is generally limited to a symptomatic progression (28). ^{90}Y–DOTA–TOC is another radiopharmaceutical agent that has been used successfully for the treatment of endocrine gastroenteropancreatic tumors and has been extended to patients with MTC. In a phase II clinical trial, 31 progressive metastatic MTC patients were injected with a median cumulative activity of 12.6 GBq (340.5 mCi) [^{90}Y–DOTA]–TOC (29). Interestingly, a posttherapeutic prolongation of Ct DT of at least 100% (12) was found in 58% of patients, and a significantly longer survival was observed in responders as compared to nonresponders. Unfortunately, it is difficult to draw any valid conclusions with regard to a potential survival benefit because of the lack of pretherapeutic selection of patients based on validated prognostic factors, such as Ct DT (12). Indeed, patients with progressive disease but long Ct DT, beyond 2 to 5 years, can benefit from very long periods of survival in the absence of treatment. Moreover, it is important to highlight that only 60% to 70% of MTC express somatostatin receptors, whereas more than 90% of MTC express CEA.

CONCLUSIONS

Currently there is no approved drug for the systemic treatment of metastatic MTC. No real survival benefit has been convincingly documented with chemotherapy and it is too early to evaluate the potential effectiveness of multikinase inhibitors or radiolabeled somatostatin analogs. PRAIT is another innovative treatment modality that has convincingly shown a survival benefit in patients with rapidly progressing metastatic disease. A randomized phase III clinical trial is warranted to confirm these results, but due to the low frequency of MTC, it would take many years to accrue a sufficient number of patients, especially if only patients with short Ct DT are included. Additional years would be necessary for the survival analysis.

REFERENCES

1. Machens A, Schneyer U, Holzhausen HJ, et al. Prospects of remission in medullary thyroid carcinoma according to basal calcitonin level. *J Clin Endocrinol Metab*. 2005;90:2029–2034.
2. Schlumberger M, Abdelmouene N, Delisle MJ, et al. Treatment of advanced medullary thyroid cancer with an alternating combination of 5 FU-streptozocin and 5 FU-dacarbazine, The Groupe d'Etude des Tumeurs à Calcitonine (GETC). *Br J Cancer*. 1995;71:363–365.
3. Wu LT, Averbuch SD, Ball DW, et al. Treatment of advanced medullary thyroid carcinoma with a combination of cyclophosphamide, vincristine, and dacarbazine. *Cancer*. 1994;73:432–436.
4. De Groot JWB, Zonnenberg BA, Quarles van Ufford-Mannesse P, et al. A phase II trial of imatinib therapy for metastatic medullary thyroid carcinoma. *J Clin Endocrinol Metab*. 2007;92:3466–3469.
5. Frank-Raue K, Fabel M, Delorme S, et al. Efficacy of imatinib mesylate in advanced medullary thyroid carcinoma. *Eur J Endocrinol*. 2007; 157:215–220.
6. Cohen EE, Rosen LS, Vokes EE, et al. Axitinib is an active treatment for all histologic subtypes of advanced thyroid cancer: results from a phase II study. *J Clin Oncol*. 2008;26:4708–4713.
7. Modigliani E, Cohen R, Campos JM, et al. Prognostic factors for survival and for biochemical cure in medullary thyroid carcinoma: results in 899 patients. *Clin Endocrinol*. 1998;48:265–273.
8. Miccoli P, Minuto MN, Ugolini C, et al. Clinically unpredictable prognostic factors in the outcome of medullary thyroid cancer. *Endocr Relat Cancer*. 2007;14:1099–1105.
9. Kebebew E, Ituarte PH, Siperstein AE, et al. Medullary thyroid carcinoma. Clinical characteristics, treatment, prognostic factors, and a comparison of staging systems. *Cancer*. 2000;88:1139–1148.
10. Elisei R, Cosci B, Romei C, et al. Prognostic significance of somatic RET oncogene mutations in sporadic medullary thyroid cancer: a 10-year follow-up study. *J Clin Endocrinol Metab*. 2008;93:682–687.
11. Tisell LE, Oden A, Muth A, et al. The Ki67 index a prognostic marker in medullary thyroid carcinoma. *Br J Cancer*. 2003;89:2093–2097.
12. Barbet J, Campion L, Kraeber-Bodéré F, et al. Prognostic impact of serum calcitonin and carcinoembryonic antigen doubling-times in patients with medullary thyroid carcinoma. *J Clin Endocrinol Metab*. 2005;90:6077–6084.
13. Dromain C, de Baere T, Lumbroso J, et al. Detection of liver metastases from endocrine tumors: a prospective comparison of somatostatin receptor scintigraphy, computed tomography, and magnetic resonance imaging. *J Clin Oncol*. 2005;23:70–78.
14. Mirallié E, Vuillez JP, Bardet S, et al. High frequency of bone/bone marrow involvement in advanced medullary thyroid cancer. *J Clin Endocrinol Metab*. 2005;90:779–788.
15. Oudoux A, Salaun PY, Bournaud C, et al. Sensitivity and prognostic value of positron emission tomography with F-18-fluorodeoxyglucose and sensitivity of immunoscintigraphy in patients with medullary thyroid carcinoma treated with anticarcinoembryonic antigen-targeted radioimmunotherapy. *J Clin Endocrinol Metab*. 2007;92:4590–4597.
16. Barbet J, Kraeber-Bodéré F, Vuillez JP, et al. Pretargeting with the affinity enhancement system for radioimmunotherapy. *Cancer Biother Radiopharm*. 1999;14:153–166.
17. Hosono M, Hosono M, Kraeber-Bodéré F, et al. Biodistribution and dosimetry study in medullary thyroid cancer xenograft using bispecific antibody and iodine-125-labeled bivalent hapten. *J Nucl Med*. 1998;39:1608–1613.
18. Mirallié E, Sai-Maurel C, Faivre-Chauvet A, et al. Improved pretargeted delivery of radiolabelled hapten to human tumour xenograft in mice by avidin chase of circulating bispecific antibody. *Eur J Nucl Med Mol Imaging*. 2005;32:901–909.
19. Kraeber-Bodere F, Faivre-Chauvet A, Sai-Maurel C, et al. Bispecific antibody and bivalent hapten radioimmunotherapy in CEA-producing medullary thyroid cancer xenograft. *J Nucl Med*. 1999;40: 198–204.
20. Kraeber-Bodere F, Faivre-Chauvet A, Sai-Maurel C, et al. Toxicity and fficacy of radioimmunotherapy in carcinoembryonic antigen-producing medullary thyroid cancer xenograft: comparison of iodine ^{131}I-labeled F(ab')$_2$ and pretargeted bivalent hapten and evaluation of repeated injections. *Clin Cancer Res*. 1999;5:3183s–3189s.
21. Kraeber-Bodéré F, Saï-Maurel C, Campion L, et al. Enhanced antitumor activity of combined pretargeted radioimmunotherapy and paclitaxel in medullary thyroid cancer xenograft. *Mol Cancer Ther*. 2002;1:267–274.
22. Bardies M, Bardet S, Faivre-Chauvet A, et al. Bispecific antibody and iodine-131-labeled bivalent hapten dosimetry in patients with medullary thyroid or small-cell lung cancer, *J Nucl Med*. 1996;37: 1853–1859.
23. Thomas SR, Maxon MR, Kereiakes JG, et al. Quantitative external counting techniques enabling improved diagnostic and therapy decisions in patients with well-differentiated thyroid cancer. *Radiology*. 1977;122:731–737.
24. Kraeber-Bodere F, Bardet S, Hoefnagel CA, et al. Radioimmunotherapy in medullary thyroid cancer using bispecific antibody and iodine 131-labeled bivalent hapten: preliminary results of a phase I/II clinical trial. *Clin Cancer Res*. 1999;5:3190–3198.
25. Kraeber-Bodere F, Faivre-Chauvet A, Ferrer L, et al. Pharmacokinetics and dosimetry studies for optimisation of carcinoembryonic antigen x anti-hapten bispecific antibody mediated pretargeting of iodine-131-labeled hapten in a phase I radioimmunotherapy trial. *Clin Cancer Res*. 2003;9:3973–3981.
26. Kraeber-Bodere F, Rousseau C, Bodet-Milin C, et al. Targeting, toxicity and efficacy of 2-step, pretargeted radioimmunotherapy using a chimeric bispecific antibody and 131-I-labeled bivalent hapten in a phase I optimisation clinical trial. *J Nucl Med*. 2006;47:247–255.
27. Chatal JF, Campion L, Kraeber-Bodéré F, et al. Survival improvement in patients with medullary thyroid carcinoma who undergo pretargeted anti-carcinoembryonic-antigen radioimmunotherapy: a collaborative study with the French Endocrine Tumor Group. *J Clin Oncol*. 2006;24:1705–1711.
28. Hoefnagel CA. Metaiodobenzylguanidine and somatostatin in oncology: role in management of neural crest tumours. *Eur J Nucl Med*. 1994;21:561–581.
29. Iten F, Müller B, Schindler C, et al. Response to [90Yttrium-DOTA]-TOC treatment is associated with long-term survival benefit in metastasized medullary thyroid cancer: a phase II clinical trial. *Clin Cancer Res*. 2007;13:6696–6702.

Ovarian Cancer: Background and Clinical Perspectives

Jörgen Elgqvist, Ragnar Hultborn, Sture Lindegren, and Stig Palm

◾ INTRODUCTION

◾ Epidemiology

Ovarian carcinoma is most frequently of epithelial origin and is the fifth most common cause of cancer deaths among females in the United States and Europe. The median age is approximately 65 years. Approximately 22,000 patients are diagnosed yearly and 15,000 of them succumb to the disease in the United States (1). In Sweden, the 10-year relative survival is 37%. The lifetime risk of developing an epithelial ovarian cancer (EOC) is 1 out of 70, but individuals with heredity (5% to 10% of all cancers, among them BRCA1 and BRCA2 mutations) carry a much higher risk, up to 44%. The incidence of EOC differs between countries (2) and has decreased, especially in the United States and northern Europe (1.2% annually), probably as a consequence of the increasing use of oral contraceptives. However, the mortality rate has not correspondingly decreased in spite of intensified treatment.

◾ Pathogenesis

The most common EOC, serous cystadenocarcinoma, arises from the epithelial surface lining derived from the coelomic epithelium of the primitive mesoderm. Cancer development is probably related to regeneration and proliferation of the epithelium occurring at each ovulation, frequently also leaving inclusion epithelial cysts beneath the surface of the ovaries. Epidemiologically, the risk of developing EOC seems to be related to the number of incessant ovulations, and to some degree, it is also related to the use of oral contraceptives and parity. Progestins may decrease the risk by inducing epithelial apoptosis. BRCA1 and BRCA2 mutations and mismatch repair deficiency potentiate the risk of developing this malignancy.

In addition to serous EOC, there are other morphologic subtypes, such as, mucinous, endometrioid, clear cell, Brenner-type, mixed, and undifferentiated cancers. The morphology of the most common type, serous cystadenocarcinoma, resembles the epithelium of the fallopian tube but may be very heterogeneous with high-grade atypia and frequent mitotic figures. The molecular pathways leading to EOC have been suggested to be either a continuous progression from early borderline tumors to invasive cancers (type I) or a rapid de novo emergence of an aggressive cancer (type II) (3).

◾ Stage

Like other malignancies, prognosis and treatment of EOC is dependent on the topographic spread of the tumor. Stage I is defined as a tumor confined to the ovary/ovaries. In stage II, the tumor extends to other pelvic structures. Stage III, the most common stage at diagnosis, is defined as a malignancy extending to the peritoneal cavity beyond the confines of the pelvis and/or invasion of retroperitoneal, iliac, or inguinal lymph nodes. Stage IV is defined as a spread to distant organs.

◾ Symptoms and diagnoses

Unfortunately, early-stage tumors present few signs and symptoms. Nonspecific abdominal complaints often lead to a delay in diagnosis, resulting in wide spread intraperitoneal (i.p.) dissemination at presentation for a majority of patients (stage III) as well as distant metastases (stage IV). The diagnosis is established by gynecologic examination including vaginal ultrasonography as well as computed tomography (CT) together with the serum marker protein CA-125. Unfortunately, screening programs for early diagnosis have not been uniformly successful due to lack of specificity and sensitivity of available tests.

◾ Treatment

Surgery is the mainstay of therapy for EOC. It includes bilateral salpingo-oophorectomy and total abdominal hysterectomy, omentectomy, nodal sampling, and peritoneal cytology. Surgery may be the sole curative treatment for early-stage cancers (stage I). However, the vast majorities of cases are diagnosed in more advanced stages and are treated by cytoreductive surgery to remove as much as possible the macroscopic disease from the peritoneal surfaces. Regional lymphadenectomies will frequently identify spread to iliac and retroperitoneal lymph nodes (4).

In stage II and higher, surgery is not curative by itself but has to be supported by intravenous (i.v.) cytotoxic therapy and sometimes i.p. chemotherapy. There is also a history of whole abdominal or moving-strip external beam radiotherapy for such stages of ovarian carcinoma (5). Also, i.p. radiotherapy using colloid preparations of ^{198}Au or ^{32}P (6,7) has been applied. Despite extensive cytoreductive surgery and modern chemotherapy, with complete remissions (CRs) at second-look laparotomy (SLL) and normalization of the serum marker cancer antigen 125 (CA-125), most patients in stage III recur and succumb to their disease. The clinical feature of recurrence is the development of ascites derived from progression of remaining viable peritoneal microscopic deposits of cancer cells after primary therapy. The clinical progression of this incurable situation is dominated by the accumulation of ascites, intestinal adhesions, and obstructions. This progression may be temporarily palliated by chemotherapy or, in some circumstances, local external beam radiotherapy.

Since these types of complications predominate, efforts have been directed to develop more effective treatments by using i.p. chemotherapy or radioimmunotherapy (RIT). Intraperitoneal chemotherapy has demonstrated the importance of i.p. treatment shown as a reduction in recurrences and a decrease in mortality but at a cost of increased toxicity (8). The use of ^{90}Y, conjugated to a monoclonal antibody (mAb) and studied in a large prospective randomized controlled study, unfortunately did not demonstrate a survival benefit (9,10). This trial will be discussed later in the clinical studies section.

■ TARGETING CONSTRUCTS

Much effort has gone into developing treatment strategies against ovarian cancer based on the concept of targeted radionuclide therapy (TRT). Below is a list of the main targeting constructs that have been used for bringing the radionuclide to the target, in preclinical and clinical studies.

HMFG1. This murine mAb is directed to an epitope of the MUC1 gene product. MUC1 is a large, heavily glycosylated mucin (more than 400 kDa) expressed on the apical surface of the majority of secretory epithelial cells (11). MUC1 is overexpressed in 90% of adenocarcinomas, including cancers of the ovary (12). The extracellular portion of the MUC1 protein mainly consists of a variable number of highly conserved 20 amino acid repeats (9). HMFG1 has been used in clinical studies (9,13).

HMFG2. This murine mAb is directed to a large mucin-like molecule normally produced by the lactating breast. The mAbs react with similar components expressed by the majority (more than 90%) of ovarian, breast, and other carcinomas (14). The HMFG2 epitope is generally expressed at a higher level in tumors (15). HMFG2 has been used in one clinical study (13).

AUA1. This murine immunoglobulin G1 (IgG1) mAb detects an antigen expressed by a wide range of adenocarcinoma, including the majority (more than 90%) of carcinomas of the ovary. The antigen is a 40-kDa glycoprotein (16). AUA1 has been used in one clinical study (13).

H17E2. This murine IgG1 mAb is directed to placental and placental-like alkaline phosphatase (PLAP) (17). This enzyme is expressed as a surface membrane antigen (~67 kDa) of many neoplasms, including 60% to 85% of ovarian carcinomas (18,19). H17E2 has been used in one clinical study (13).

Hu2PLAP. This is a human IgG1 κ mAb that has the same specificity as the murine H17E2 mAb described earlier. Hu2PLAP has been used in one clinical study (20).

H317. This is a murine IgG mAb developed after immunization with syncytiotrophoblast microvilli preparations from term placenta. It is specific for the L-phenylalanine inhibitable PLAP. H317 has been used in one clinical study (20).

Trastuzumab. Trastuzumab (Herceptin; Genentech, South San Francisco, CA) is a humanized IgG1 mAb that recognizes the extracellular domain of the HER-2/neu oncoprotein (21). Trastuzumab has been used in one animal study (22).

Pertuzumab. This human mAb binds to the dimerization domain II of HER-2. Pertuzumab is based on the human IgG1 κ framework sequences and is produced in Chinese hamster ovary cells. It has been used in one animal study (23).

B72.3. This murine mAb has been shown to be immunoreactive with the glycoprotein complex TAG-72 (more than 200 kDa) with the characteristics of a mucin (24–26). TAG-72 expression has been shown in the majority of ovarian carcinomas tested (27). B72.3 has been used in clinical studies (28,29).

CC49. This murine mAb is a high-affinity murine product that reacts with the tumor-associated glycoprotein 72 (TAG-72), which is expressed by the majority of common epithelial tumors (30). CC49 has been used in one animal study (31) and in clinical studies (32–36).

OC125. This murine mAb is directed against the tumor marker CA-125 and has been used in clinical studies (37–39).

MOv18. This murine mAb recognizes and reacts with a surface antigen, which is a membrane folate–binding glycoprotein of 38 kDa expressed on approximately 90% of all human ovarian carcinomas (40–42). MOv18 (murine and in some cases chimeric) has been used in animal studies (43–46) and in clinical studies (47–52).

MX35. This murine IgG1 mAb is directed toward a cell-surface glycoprotein of approximately 95 kDa on OVCAR-3 cells (53) and is expressed strongly and homogeneously on approximately 90% of human EOCs (54). The antigen recognized by MX35 is characterized as the sodium–dependent phosphate transport protein 2b (NaPi2b) (55). MX35 F(ab')2 has been used in animal studies (56–61) and in one clinical study (62).

NR-LU-10. This IgG2b murine mAb is reactive with a glycoprotein (~40 kDa) expressed on most carcinomas of epithelial origin (63,64). NR-LU-10 has been used in clinical studies (65,66).

A5B7. This is an anti-CEA IgG1 mAb that has been used in one large animal model (sheep) study (67).

17-1A. This chimeric mAb is directed to an approximately 39-kDa membrane-associated pancarcinoma glycoprotein (68,69). It has been used in one animal study (70).

323/A3. This murine mAb is directed to an approximately 39-kDa membrane–associated pancarcinoma glycoprotein (same as 17-1A) (68,69). It has been used in one animal study (70).

hCTMO1. This antibody was constructed by taking the short hypervariable regions of the murine mAb CTMO1 and grafting them into a human IgG4, and is directed to a glycoprotein expressed on malignant cells of epithelial origin (71,72). hCTMO1 has been used in one clinical study (73).

OV-TL3. This is a murine IgG1 mAb that recognizes a cell-surface antigen highly expressed on more than 90% of ovarian carcinomas (74). It has been used in one clinical study (75).

139H2. This is a IgG1 mAb that binds to a protein determinant of episialin (76). 139H2 has been used in one animal study (77).

P-P4D. This targeting construct is a pseudosymmetrical covalent dimer of the monomeric peptide P-P4. It has been used in one animal study (78).

PAI2. This targeting construct is a plasminogen activator inhibitor type 2 and is a member of the serine protease inhibitor (Serpin) superfamily and forms SDS-stable 1:1 complexes with urokinase plasminogen activator (uPA) (79). It has been used in one animal study (79).

Affibody. Affibody molecules are composed of alpha helices and lack disulfide bridges. Two such molecular constructs, $(Z_{HER2:4})_2$ and $(Z_{HER2:342})_2$ (~15 kDa), have been used in animal studies (80–82).

■ RADIONUCLIDES

In TRT, the cytotoxic effect is mediated by a radionuclide, brought to the target by the targeting construct. Below is a list of the radionuclides used in both animal and clinical studies. The list includes a presentation of their physical characters and in which studies they have been used.

Actinium-225 (^{225}Ac). This alpha (α)-particle emitter decays with a half-life of 10 days in which four α-particles are emitted. The source of ^{225}Ac is mainly ^{225}Ra which is extracted from ^{229}Th. ^{229}Th has its origin in the development of nuclear weapons based on ^{233}U. The α-particle emitted from ^{225}Ac has an energy of 5.8 MeV (mean linear energy transfer [LET] ≈ 120 keV/μm) and the daughters are ^{221}Fr ($t\frac{1}{2}$ = 4.8 min, E = 6.3 MeV, mean LET ≈ 118 keV/μm), ^{217}At ($t\frac{1}{2}$ = 32.3 ms, E = 7.1 MeV, mean LET ≈ 109 keV/μm), and ^{213}Bi ($t\frac{1}{2}$ = 45.6 min, E = 8.4 MeV, mean LET ≈ 99 keV/μm). The decays are accompanied by gamma (γ)-radiation, enabling scintigraphy and dosimetry. ^{225}Ac is produced by the natural decay of ^{233}U, and also by accelerator-based techniques. ^{225}Ac has been used in one animal study (22).

Astatine-211 (^{211}At). This α-particle emitter is cyclotron produced by the bombardment of a bismuth target with 28 MeV helium nuclei via the nuclear reaction ^{207}Bi(α,2n)^{211}At. ^{211}At decays with a half-life of 7.2 hours in two ways: (a) via emission of an α-particle (E = 5.9 MeV) to ^{207}Bi or (b) via an electron capture process to ^{211}Po. ^{207}Bi decays with a half-life of 31.6 years to ^{207}Pb (stable). ^{211}Po decays with a half-life of 0.5 seconds to ^{207}Pb via α-particle emission (E = 7.4 MeV). The 5.9- and 7.4-MeV α-particles have a mean LET of approximately 122 and 106 keV/μm and a particle range in tissue of approximately 48 and 70 μm, respectively. The decays are accompanied by γ-radiation, enabling scintigraphy and

dosimetry. ^{211}At has been used in animal studies (43–46, 56–61,81,83,84) and in one clinical study (62).

Bismuth-213 (^{213}Bi). Due to its relatively long-lived parent radionuclide ^{225}Ac, this α-particle emitter is available via a generator-based technology. ^{213}Bi decays with a half-life of 45.6 minutes to ^{209}Bi (stable) during which it emits an α-particle of 8.4 MeV (mean LET and particle range in tissue: ~99 keV/μm and 89 μm, respectively. The α-particle emission is accompanied by γ-radiation, enabling scintigraphy and dosimetry. ^{213}Bi has been used in animal studies (78,79).

Yttrium-90 (^{90}Y). This radionuclide is chemically similar to the lanthanoids and decays with a half-life of 64 hours by the emission of electrons (β⁻) with a maximum energy of approximately 2.2 MeV (E_{mean} = 933 keV). The emitted electrons have a maximum range in tissue of approximately 12 mm (mean range ≈ 4 mm) and a mean LET of ≈ 0.2 keV/μm. Due to the emission of *bremsstrahlung*, scintigraphy with a γ-camera is feasible. ^{90}Y has been used in one animal study (31) and in clinical studies (9,10,28,32,38,85–89).

Lutetium-177 (^{177}Lu). This radionuclide has a half-life of 6.7 days and decays by the emission of β⁻-particles with a maximum energy of 497 keV (E_{mean} = 133 keV), which have a maximum range in tissue of approximately 2 mm (mean range ≈ 0.2 mm), and a mean LET of less than 0.1 keV/μm. It also emits γ-radiation (208 keV) enabling scintigraphy and dosimetry. ^{177}Lu can be produced in large scale owing to the high thermal neutron capture cross section of ^{176}Lu (2100 barn) using moderate flux reactors. ^{177}Lu has been used in animal studies (23,31,36,82) and in clinical studies (13,33,34,90).

Iodine-131 (^{131}I). This radionuclide has a half-life of 8 days and decays by the emission of β⁻-particles with a maximum energy of 807 keV (E_{mean} = 182 keV, mean LET ≈ 0.1 keV/μm), which have a maximum range in tissue of approximately 3.6 mm (mean range ≈ 0.4 mm). It emits γ-radiation (364 keV) enabling scintigraphy and dosimetry. ^{131}I has been used in animal studies (67,70,77) and in clinical studies (13,29,36,37,39,47–52,91–93).

Rhenium-186 (^{186}Re) and Rhenium-188 (^{188}Re). ^{186}Re has a half-life of 3.7 days and decays by β⁻-particle emission with maximum energy of 1.07 MeV (mean LET ≈ 0.1 keV/μm), 90% of it delivered within approximately 1.8 mm. The γ-radiation enables scintigraphy and dosimetry. ^{186}Re has been used in clinical studies (65,66). ^{188}Re has a half-life of 17 hours and decays by β⁻-particle emission with maximum energy of 795 keV (mean LET ≈ 0.1 keV/μm). The γ-radiation enables scintigraphy and dosimetry. ^{188}Re has been used in one clinical study (35).

■ LABELING CHEMISTRY OF α-PARTICLE EMITTERS

Alpha-particle emitters are attractive due to their physical and chemical characteristics. In contrast to β⁻-particles, α-particles have high LET and relatively short particle ranges, approximately 75 μm, and the halogen ^{211}At and the metal

[213]Bi have been recognized as promising candidates for RIT of ovarian cancer. As mentioned earlier, [213]Bi is obtained from the decay of [225]Ac in a generator resin column system (94). The chemistry of coupling [213]Bi to substances, for example, proteins and peptides, is well established and in labeling the reaction times can be kept short with generally good radiochemical yields (95). The short half-life (45.6 minutes) could be favorable for i.p. administration but perhaps problematic if the treatment is given systemically. The advantage with [211]At over [213]Bi is the longer half-life (7.2 hours), allowing time for radiopharmaceuticals and time to reach the tumor once injected. The halogen characteristics of [211]At allow coupling to a number of substances (96). A common approach has been the use of tumor-specific mAbs as carriers in which promising preclinical results have been obtained (46,58). The preclinical work with [211]At has resulted in two phase I studies: one study for the treatment of malignant glioma at Duke University Medical Center, Durham, NC, USA (97), and another study for the treatment of ovarian carcinoma, at Sahlgrenska University Hospital, Gothenburg, Sweden (62).

Despite the fact that preclinical [211]At-RIT research has been translated into two clinical phase I studies, there are still factors hampering clinical progress. The major obstacle is the radionuclide availability (98). Until recently, it has also been very difficult to obtain clinical amounts of labeled mAbs due to suboptimal chemical procedures (99). [211]At is the heaviest member of the halogen family and early on it was expected that it would resemble the electrophilic substitution chemistry of iodine when coupled to proteins. However, direct electrophilic astatination of proteins produced very unstable products. A mechanism for the direct interaction of [211]At with proteins has been proposed by Visser et al., indicating that unlike iodine, which mainly binds to tyrosyl residues, [211]At undergoes an electrophilic reaction with unsubstituted thiols on the protein (100). Since then, several different reagents have been developed for the synthesis of [211]At intermediates, involving the formation of stable [211]At–carbon bonds. The common feature of these reagents is *N*-succinimidyl-aryl-alkyl-tin (activated tin ester, ATE) for [211]At destannylation and *N*-acylation of the amino groups on the protein (101).

The conventional route for astatination of proteins using these reagents involves two radiochemical steps: labeling of a bifunctional reagent and conjugation of the labeled reagent to the protein. At high radioactivity concentrations, problems with this procedure have been recognized due to radiolytic effects in the reaction solvent affecting the redox chemistry of the nuclide, destroying the reagent, and affecting the immunoreactivity of the final product (102). This being the case, high concentration of mAbs is required in the conjugation reaction for good radiochemical yields. This has hampered the synthesis of a product with high specific radioactivity and radioactivity amounts required for clinical applications.

Similar to metal labeling for metals, in which a bifunctional chelate is conjugated to the protein prior to labeling, the ATE reagent can be conjugated to the protein prior to astatination. This direct astatination of immunoconjugates generally results in high yields and high specific radioactivity, even at conditions with high radioactivity concentration (103). A similar approach is used by Wilbur et al., with a different type of reagent. Their reagent is based on boron cage chemistry in which [211]At is attached forming a stable [211]At–boron bond (104). It has been shown that the bond strength of the [211]At–boron is higher than that of the [211]At–carbon bond (105). This is important, especially when labeling compounds are smaller than IgG and F(ab')2, for example, F(ab), scFv, or minibodies. The smaller fragments are mainly catabolized in the kidneys and are released and reabsorbed in normal tissue to a higher degree if labeled via the ATE reagent than if labeled by the boron cage reagents.

■ ANIMAL STUDIES

A number of animal studies have been performed during the past 20 years, investigating the pharmacokinetics, toxicity, and therapeutic efficacy using TRT. Presented below is a selection of these studies using different radionuclides as well as different targeting constructs. The studies are paragraphed based on the radionuclide used, that is, [225]Ac, [211]At, [213]Bi, ^{90}Y, ^{177}Lu, or [131]I.

▧ Animal study using the α-particle emitter [225]Ac

An interesting study was performed using [225]Ac-trastuzumab, which was tested for immunoreactivity, internalization, and cytotoxicity using SKOV-3 cells (22). [225]Ac-trastuzumab retained immunoreactivity (50% to 90%) and rapidly internalized into cells (50% at 2 hours). Different therapies were assessed, using unlabeled trastuzumab and 8.1, 12.2, and 16.6 kBq of [225]Ac-trastuzumab or [225]Ac-labeled control antibody. The therapies were initiated 9 days after tumor seeding. Groups of control mice and mice administered unlabeled trastuzumab had median survivals of 33, 37, or 44 days, respectively. Median survival was 52 to 126 days with [225]Ac-trastuzumab and 48 to 64 days for [225]Ac-control mAb. Deaths from toxicity occurred at the highest activity levels. The study showed that i.p. administration of [225]Ac-trastuzumab extended survival significantly in mice at levels that produce no apparent toxicity. The advantage of [225]Ac is that it emits a cascade of α-particles, as described earlier, implying a very high cytotoxic effect if all the α-particle emissions occur in close vicinity to the target volume, that is, the tumor cell nuclei. The disadvantage is that when [225]Ac decays, the atom will be separated from its targeting construct, making the remaining α-particle cascade an unspecific irradiation, potentially leading to both toxicity and dosimetry problems. Therefore, [225]Ac should be used with caution in situations other than during intracavitary treatments or when the radioimmunocomplex is rapidly internalized into the tumor cell nuclei.

■ Animal studies using the α-particle emitter [211]At

Astatine ([211]At) is a promising radionuclide in RIT due to its suitable half-life (7.2 hours) and relatively short particle range (~70 μm). The current drawback is its limited availability due to the fact that it is cyclotron produced. The potential problem with unspecific irradiation (as described in the preceding section for [225]Ac) is negligible due to the fact that the α-particle emanating from the second decay route (from [211]Po to [207]Pb) occurs with a very short half-life (0.5 seconds), that is, in close vicinity to the target volume (106). Andersson et al. have performed studies investigating the pharmacokinetics and therapeutic efficacy of [211]At-labeled mAbs (43–46). In one of those studies, the purpose was to compare the therapeutic efficacy of [211]At-MOv18 and ^{131}I-MOv18 (46). The study used OVCAR-3 cells growing i.p. in mice. Two weeks after the i.p. inoculation of 1×10^7 tumor cells, 20 mice were treated i.p. with MOv18 labeled with either [211]At (310 to 400 kBq) or [131]I (5.1 to 6.2 MBq). The pharmacokinetics of the labeled antibody in tumor-free animals was studied and the resulting absorbed dose to bone marrow was estimated. When the mice were treated with [211]At-MOv18, nine out of ten mice were free of macro- and microscopic tumors compared with three out of ten when ^{131}I-MOv18 was used. The equivalent dose to bone marrow was 2.4 to 3.1 Sv from [211]At-MOv18 and 3.4 to 4.1 Sv from ^{131}I-MOv18. The study showed that the therapeutic efficacy of [211]At-MOv18 was high, and superior to that using ^{131}I-MOv18.

Several other investigations using [211]At-mAbs have been completed (56–61,83,84). In one such study in mice, the purpose was to estimate the efficacy of RIT using [211]At-MX35 F(ab')2 or [211]At-rituximab F(ab')2 (nonspecific) against differently sized ovarian cancer deposits on the peritoneum, and to calculate absorbed dose to tumors and critical organs (56). At 1 to 7 weeks after inoculation, animals were i.p. treated with approximately 400 kBq [211]At-MX35 F(ab')2, approximately 400 kBq [211]At-rituximab F(ab')2, or unlabeled rituximab F(ab')2. Eight weeks after each treatment, the mice were sacrificed and the presence of tumors and ascites was determined. When given treatment 1, 3, 4, 5, or 7 weeks after cell inoculation, the tumor-free fraction (TFF) was 0.95, 0.68, 0.58, 0.47, and 0.26 or 1.00, 0.80, 0.20, 0.20, and 0.0 when treated with [211]At-MX35 F(ab')2 or [211]At-rituximab F(ab')2, respectively. The conclusion of the study was that treatment with [211]At-MX35 F(ab')2 or [211]At-rituximab F(ab')2 resulted in a TFF of 0.95 to 1.00 when the tumor radius was 30 μm or less. The TFF was decreased (TFF ≤ 0.20) for the nonspecific [211]At-rituximab F(ab')2 when the tumor radius exceeded the range of the α-particles. The tumor-specific mAb resulted in a significantly better TFF, for different tumor sizes, explained by a high mean absorbed dose (more than 22 Gy) from the activity bound to the tumor surface, probably in addition to some contribution from penetrating activity.

Bäck et al. evaluated the relative biologic effectiveness (RBE) of [211]At-mAb (61). The endpoint was growth inhibition (GI) of subcutaneous OVCAR-3 xenografts. The animals received an i.v. injection of [211]At-MX35 F(ab')2 (0.33, 0.65, and 0.90 MBq). External irradiation of the tumors was performed with [60]Co. To compare the biologic effects of the two radiation qualities, the mean value for GI was plotted for each tumor as a function of its corresponding absorbed dose. From exponential fits of these curves, the absorbed doses required for a GI of 0.37 (D_{37}) were derived, and the RBE of [211]At was calculated. The absorbed doses in tumors were 1.35, 2.65, and 3.70 Gy. The value for D_{37} was 1.59 ± 0.08 Gy (mean ± SEM). Tumor growth after ^{60}Co irradiation resulted in a D_{37} of 7.65 ± 1.0 Gy. The RBE of [211]At irradiation was calculated to be 4.8 ± 0.7 Gy.

In another study, different HER-2 binding affibody molecules were labeled with [211]At, using both the N-succinimidyl-para-astatobenzoate (PAB) and a decaborate-based linker, and the biodistribution in tumor bearing mice was investigated (81). The influence of L-lysine and Na-thiocyanate on the [211]At uptake in normal tissues was also studied. Compared with a previous biodistribution with ^{125}I, the [211]At biodistribution using the PAB linker showed higher uptake in lungs, stomach, thyroid, and salivary glands, indicating release of free [211]At. When the decaborate-based linker was used, the uptake in those organs was decreased, but instead, high uptake in kidneys and liver was found. The uptake, when using the PAB linker, could be significantly reduced in some organs by the use of L-lysine and/or Na-thiocyanate. The conclusion of the study was that affibody molecules have suitable blood kinetics for TRT with [211]At; the labeling chemistry, however, affects the distribution in normal organs to a high degree and needs to be improved to allow clinical use.

■ Animal studies using the α-particle emitter [213]Bi

This radionuclide, with its well-established chemistry and generator-based availability, has recently achieved more attention. Still, one drawback is its relatively short half-life (45.6 minutes), which necessitates a rapid specificity, once injected. Using [213]Bi in intracavitary or i.p. applications, or using pretargeting techniques, could, however, overcome this potential problem. One study utilizing [213]Bi was performed by Knör et al. who developed peptidic radioligands, targeting tumor cell–associated urokinase receptors (uPAR, CD87) (78). DOTA-conjugated, uPAR-directed ligands were synthesized on solid phase. The biodistribution of [213]Bi-P-P4D was analyzed in mice 28 days after i.p. inoculation of OV-MZ-6 ovarian tumor cells in the absence or presence of the plasma expander gelofusine. Specific binding of [213]Bi-P-P4D to monocytoid U937 and OV-MZ-6 cells was demonstrated using the natural ligand of uPAR, pro-uPA, or a soluble form of uPAR, suPAR, as competitors. The [213]Bi-P-P4D displayed superior binding to OV-MZ-6 cells in vitro, and accumulation of [213]Bi-P-P4D in tumor tissue was demonstrated by biodistribution analysis in mice bearing i.p. OV-MZ-6–derived tumors. Gelofusine reduced kidney uptake of [213]Bi-P-P4D by half. The conclusion of the study was that ovarian tumor cells overexpressing uPAR were specifically targeted in vitro and in vivo by [213]Bi-P-P4D, and the kidney uptake of [213]Bi-P-P4D was distinctly reduced by using gelofusine.

Another study that used [213]Bi was performed by Song et al. who investigated the pharmacokinetics, toxicity, and in vivo stability of [213]Bi-PAI2, and determined whether a prior injection of a metal chelator (Ca-DTPA) or lysine could reduce toxicity by decreasing renal uptake (79). Two chelators (CHX-A″-DTPA and cDTPA) were used for preparation of the [213]Bi-PAI2 conjugate, for i.p. administration in mice and ear vein injection in rabbits. Neither mice nor rabbits showed any short-term toxicity over 13 weeks at 1420 and 120 MBq/kg [213]Bi-PAI2, respectively. The kidney uptake was decreased threefold by blocking with lysine. Radiation nephropathy was observed at 20 to 30 weeks in mice, whereas severe renal tubular necrosis was observed at 13 weeks in rabbits. The conclusion was that nephropathy was the dose-limiting toxicity, and that lysine was effective in reducing the kidney uptake. The maximum tolerated doses (MTDs) were 350 and 120 MBq/kg for mice and rabbits, respectively. The research group had earlier demonstrated the in vitro cytotoxicity and in vivo inhibition of tumor growth in breast, prostate, pancreatic, and ovarian cancer (107–111).

■ Animal study using the β⁻-particle emitter ^{90}Y

Owing to efforts at developing strategies for RIT against ovarian cancer (32), the same research group also investigated pretargeted RIT in an i.p. tumor model (LS174T) using four CC49 anti-TAG-72 single-chain antibodies linked to streptavidin as a fusion protein (CC49 fusion protein) (31). A synthetic clearing agent was administered i.v. 1 day later to produce hepatic clearance of unbound CC49. A low-molecular-weight radiolabeled reagent composed of biotin conjugated to the chelating agent 7,10-tetra-azacyclododecane-N,N',N'',N'''-tetraacetic acid (DOTA) complexed with ^{111}In, ^{90}Y, or ^{177}Lu was injected 4 hours later. The radiolocalization to tumor sites was superior with i.p. administration of radiolabeled DOTA-biotin as compared with i.v. administration. Imaging and biodistribution studies showed good tumor localization with ^{111}In- or ^{177}Lu-DOTA-biotin. Tumor localization of ^{111}In-DOTA-biotin was 43% ID/g (percentage of injected dose per gram) and 44% ID/g at 4 and 24 hours with the highest normal tissue localization in the kidney with 6% ID/g at 48 and 72 hours. ^{90}Y-DOTA-biotin at doses of 14.8 to 22.2 MBq or ^{90}Lu-DOTA-biotin at doses of 22.2 to 29.6 MBq produced significant prolongation of survival compared with controls ($p = 0.03$ and $p < 0.01$). The conclusion of the study was that pretargeted RIT using regional administration of CC49 fusion protein and i.p. ^{90}Y- or ^{177}Lu-DOTA-biotin is a therapeutic strategy in the LS174T i.p. tumor model and that this strategy may be applicable to humans. LS174T is a human colon cancer cell line, but as it was used in an i.p. setting in this study together with CC49 (which reacts with the TAG-72, expressed by the majority of common epithelial tumors), we think it is relevant to present the results.

■ Animal studies using the β⁻-particle emitter ^{177}Lu

In the first study presented, ^{177}Lu-pertuzumab was used against disseminated HER-2-positive micrometastases (23) and showed good targeting properties in mice bearing HER-2-overexpressing xenografts. The absorbed dose in tumors was more than five and seven times higher than that in blood and in any other normal organ, respectively. ^{177}Lu-pertuzumab delayed tumor progression compared with controls (no treatment, $p < 0.0001$; pertuzumab, $p < 0.0001$; and ^{177}Lu-labeled irrelevant mAb, $p < 0.01$). No adverse side effects of the treatment could be detected. The conclusion of the study was that the results could support clinical studies using ^{177}Lu-pertuzumab.

In another fairly recent study, Tolmachev et al. utilized a ^{177}Lu-labeled anti-HER-2 affibody molecule ($Z_{HER2:342}$) targeting xenografts (82). The small size (~7 kDa) resulted in rapid glomerular filtration and high renal accumulation of radiometals. Reversible binding to albumin reduced the renal excretion and uptake. The dimeric affibody molecule $(Z_{HER2:342})_2$ was fused with an albumin-binding domain (ABD) conjugated with the isothiocyanate derivative of CHX-A″-DTPA and labeled with ^{177}Lu. Fusion with ABD enabled a 25-fold reduction of renal uptake in comparison with the nonfused dimer molecule $(Z_{HER2:342})_2$, and the biodistribution showed high specific uptake of the conjugate in HER-2-expressing tumors. Treatment of SKOV-3 microxenografts (high HER-2 expression) with 17 or 22 MBq ^{177}Lu-CHX-A″-DTPA-ABD-$(Z_{HER2:342})_2$ completely prevented formation of tumors. In LS174T xenografts (low HER-2 expression), this treatment resulted in a small but significant increase of survival. The conclusion of the study was that fusion with ABD improved the in vivo biodistribution and highlighted ^{177}Lu-CHX-A-DTPA-ABD-$(Z_{HER2:342})_2$ as a candidate for treatment of disseminated tumors with high HER-2 expression.

■ Animal study using the β⁻-particle emitter ^{131}I

Turner et al. (67) reported a large animal study of human tumors in cyclosporin-immunosuppressed sheep to evaluate and measure tumor uptake of ^{131}I-mAbs. Human tumor cells were orthotopically inoculated (~10^7 cells): SKMEL melanoma subcutaneously; LS174T and HT29 colon carcinoma into bowel, peritoneum, and liver; and JAM ovarian carcinoma into ovary and peritoneum. Tumor xenografts grew within 3 weeks and generally maintained their histologic appearance, although a few tumor deposits showed a variable degree of dedifferentiation. Regional lymph node metastases were demonstrated for xenografts of melanoma and ovarian carcinoma. The anti-CEA mAb A5B7 labeled with ^{131}I was i.v. administered. Peak uptake at 5 days in orthotopic tumors in gut was 0.027% and 0.034% ID/g in hepatic metastases with tumor to blood ratios of 2 to 2.5. Nonspecific tumor uptake in melanoma was 0.003% ID/g. The conclusion was that the uptake of labeled mAb in human tumors in sheep was comparable with the uptake observed in patients, and this sheep model may be more realistic than mice xenografts for prediction of efficacy of RIT.

CLINICAL STUDIES

During the past 20 years, several clinical studies have been performed. The studies presented below comprise a selection of different radionuclides as well as different targeting constructs, and are organized by paragraph based on the radionuclide used, that is, [211]At, ^{90}Y, ^{177}Lu, ^{131}I, or [186]Re.

Clinical study using the α-particle emitter [211]At

So far, only one clinical study has utilized [211]At for treating ovarian cancer. It was performed by Andersson et al. (62) who investigated the pharmacokinetics and toxicity in a phase I study of α-RIT using [211]At-MX35 F(ab')2. Nine patients underwent laparoscopy 2 to 5 days before therapy, and the abdominal cavity was inspected to exclude presence of macroscopic tumor growth or adhesions. Patients were infused with 20.1 to 101 MBq (0.54 to 2.73 mCi)/L [211]At-MX35 F(ab')2 via a peritoneal catheter. Gamma-camera scans were acquired at three to five occasions and a SPECT scan at 6 hours after infusion (Fig. 29.1). Samples of blood, urine, and peritoneal fluid were collected at 1 to 48 hours (Fig. 29.2). Hematology, together with renal and thyroid functions, was followed for a median of 23 months. Pharmacokinetics and dosimetric results were related to the initial activity concentration (IC) of the infusion. The decay-corrected activity concentration decreased with time

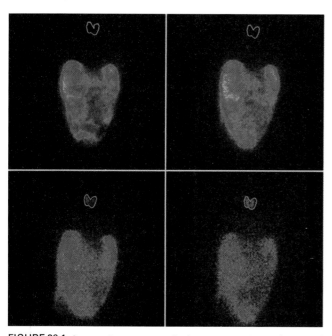

FIGURE 29.1 Consecutive anteroposterior decay-corrected scans (γ-camera) of the abdominal and thoracic area of a patient in the study by Andersson et al. (62). The thyroid uptake, which is indicated by a region of interest in each panel, was not blocked in this patient. Images were acquired at 1.5 (top left), 5 (top right), 11.5 (bottom left), and 19.5 (bottom right) hours after infusion of [211]At-MX35 F(ab')₂. The figure is reprinted by permission of the Society of Nuclear Medicine. (Please see Color Insert).

in the peritoneal fluid to 50% IC at 24 hours, increased in serum to 6% IC at 45 hours, and increased in the thyroid to less than 20% IC with blocking (potassium perchlorate/iodide). The cumulative urinary excretion was 40 kBq/(MBq/L) at 24 hours. The estimated absorbed dose to different structures was: peritoneum, 15.6 ± 1.0 mGy/(MBq/L); red bone marrow, 0.14 ± 0.04 mGy/(MBq/L); urinary bladder wall, 0.77 ± 0.19 mGy/(MBq/L); unblocked thyroid, 24.7 ± 11.1 mGy/(MBq/L); blocked thyroid, 1.4 ± 1.6 mGy/(MBq/L) (mean ± 1 SD). No adverse effects were observed. The study indicated that by i.p. [211]At-MX35 F(ab')2, it is possible to achieve therapeutic absorbed doses in microscopic tumors without significant toxicity. A multicenter, phase II study is currently being planned, intended as an upfront adjuvant treatment for a patient population that has received cytoreductive surgery and chemotherapy.

Clinical studies using the β⁻-particle emitter [90]Y

An important study was performed by Verheijen et al. (9). This multinational (74 centers; 17 countries; recruiting patients between 1998 and 2003) open-label, randomized phase III study compared ^{90}Y-HMFG1 (against the MUC 1 antigen) plus standard treatment versus standard treatment alone in patients with EOC who had attained a complete clinical remission after cytoreductive surgery and platinum-based chemotherapy. Eight hundred forty-four stage Ic to IV patients were screened, of whom 447 with a negative SLL were randomly assigned to receive either a single dose of ^{90}Y-HMFG1 plus standard treatment (224 patients) or standard treatment alone (223 patients). Patients in the active treatment (TRT) arm received an i.p. dose of 25 mg ^{90}Y-HMFG1 to provide 666 MBq (18 mCi)/m². After a median follow-up of 3.5 years, 70 patients had died in the active treatment arm compared with 61 in the control arm. Cox proportional hazards analysis of survival demonstrated no difference between treatment arms. In the TRT arm, 104 patients experienced relapse compared with 98 patients in the standard treatment arm. No difference in time to relapse was observed between the two study arms. The conclusion was that a single i.p. administration of ^{90}Y-HMFG1 to patients with EOC, who had a negative SLL after primary therapy, did not extend survival or time to relapse. The reason for the failure of the treatment could perhaps be explained by the choice of radionuclide. When treating microscopic disease with high-energy β⁻-particles emitted from ^{90}Y, the electron will have too long a range in order to deliver high enough energy to the tumor cell nuclei. It has been extensively modeled that high-energy β⁻-particle emissions will not deposit large amounts of energy (absorbed energy) into tumor spheroids below a certain size. However, there are other concerns about this study that warrant comment: (a) entry was allowed onto the study even if dispersal of the TRT agent (^{90}Y-HMFG1) could not occur in an entire quadrant of the abdomen due to adhesions. The adhesions were assessed by laparoscopy, CT scan,

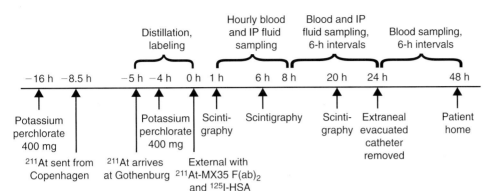

FIGURE 29.2 Schematic overview of the logistics of the therapeutic procedures in the phase I study by Andersson et al. (62). i.p., intraperitoneal. The figure is reprinted by permission of the Society of Nuclear Medicine.

or isotope diffusion scan. Although it is rather intuitive that a diffusion scan will allow a reasonable assessment of adhesions, it is less obvious that laparoscopy or a CT scan will discern between one or two quadrants of adhesions. This allowance could potentially result in a significant underdosing of 25% or less of the abdominal cavity. Importantly, there was no mention of how these patients (no adhesions vs. one quadrant with adhesions) were stratified between each treatment arm. (b) The TRT arm contained 3% more stage III and IV patients. (c) The TRT arm had a higher mean CA-125 level after laparoscopy (never explained). (d) The TRT arm had 8 percentage points more patients with residual disease after initial surgery (44.2% vs. 35.9%). (e) Seven percentage points (19.7% vs. 12.5%) more patients in the standard arm received consolidation chemotherapy. (f) The overall antibody mass (25 mg) may have been insufficient to help provide a concentration gradient to help "push" the radiolabeled antibody into the tumors (Chapter 12). This can be contrasted to the 250 mg/m^2 of cold antibody used with Zevalin or the 450 mg total antibody dose used with Bexxar. (g) Twenty percent of the injected dose can enter the systemic circulation. (h) The radiolabeling process was performed by each institution and not centralized. Although a radiolabeling efficiency of 95% was confirmed with thin-layer chromatography, there was no mention of immunoreactivity quality assurance (potential loss of affinity of the antibody for the antigen, as a result of the radiolabeling process). (i) During the accrual time period, single institution experiences tended to report higher conversion rates to an open laparotomy (from a SLL) than was reported in the current study (59% vs. 5%) (9). (j) Eighteen percent of the patients in the TRT arm had 60% or less MUC1 staining (unknown impact). (k) There was no pattern of failure analysis (i.p. vs. distant).

The pattern of failure analysis eventually came to fruition (10). Case report forms of all patients with disease recurrence were reviewed to determine site and date of recurrent disease. The 447 patients were included with a median follow-up of 3.5 years. Relapse was seen in 104 out of 224 patients in the TRT arm and 98 out of 223 patients in the control arm. Significantly fewer i.p. ($p < 0.05$) and more extraperitoneal ($p < 0.05$) relapses occurred in the TRT arm. Time to i.p. recurrence was significantly longer ($p = 0.0019$) and time to extraperitoneal recurrence was significantly shorter for the TRT arm ($p < 0.001$). In a subset analysis, the impact of i.p.

TRT on i.p. relapse-free survival was even greater and could only be seen in a subgroup of patients with residual disease after primary surgery. Although there was no survival benefit for ^{90}Y-HMFG1 i.p. instillation as consolidation treatment for EOC, an improved control of i.p. disease was found, which appeared to be offset by increased extraperitoneal recurrences. It was proposed that the transient myelosuppression (alteration of the immune system) induced by therapy with ^{90}Y-HMFG1 indirectly caused the greater number of extraperitoneal metastases. Most likely, this observation is simply the result of an alteration in the failure pattern due to a greater number of patients in the treatment arm benefiting from a greater i.p. control, since distant metastases will not be observed due to overwhelming local symptoms. Also, for reasons mentioned earlier, it is possible that the treatment arm was skewed with more advanced disease. Stewart et al. (85) and Hird et al. (88) previously published studies with ^{90}Y-HMFG1 in 1990 showing manifest myelotoxicity and poor therapeutic efficacy. Maraveyas et al. (89) reported in 1994, using ^{90}Y-CITC-DTPA-HMFG1, that bone marrow toxicity was the dose-limiting factor and recommended an activity level of 684.5 MBq (18.5 mCi)/m^2 for subsequent treatments.

Since ^{90}Y has been used on a rather wide scale, we would also like to present some studies performed earlier. Nicholson et al. reported on survival of patients who received single-dose i.p. RIT after achieving a CR with standard management (112). Twenty-five patients with EOC, stages Ic to IV, received i.p. RIT following completion of chemotherapy. Upon achieving a CR, they received a single dose of 25 mg of ^{90}Y-HMFG1, 666 MBq (18 mCi)/m^2. In addition, using a database of 84 North Thames Ovary Group (NTOG) patients known to be disease free at the end of chemotherapy, estimated survival curves were constructed. Close matches were found for 20 of the 25 patients. Median survival had not been reached at a median follow-up of 59 months for the RIT cases and 27 months for controls (NTOG). Survival at 5 years was 80% for the RIT cases and 55% for controls ($p = 0.0035$). The Cox model estimated long-term (10-year) survival of 70% for patients who received RIT, compared with 32% for those who did not ($p = 0.003$). All patients developed serologic evidence of human anti-mouse antibodies (HAMAs). The conclusion of this study was a likely survival benefit for patients with ovarian cancer who receive i.p. RIT in an adjuvant setting.

In another study, Epenetos et al. investigated the long-term survival of patients with advanced ovarian cancer treated with RIT following cytoreductive surgery and platinum-based chemotherapy (87). Eligibility criteria included patients with histologic evidence of ovarian cancer stages Ic to IV. Fifty-two patients entered the study, 31 had residual disease following standard chemotherapy and 21 patients had achieved CR. The treatment consisted of a single i.p. administration of 25 mg HMFG1 labeled with 666 MBq (18 mCi)/m^2 of ^{90}Y, survival being the primary endpoint. In the group of 21 patients who had achieved CR following surgery, conventional chemotherapy, and i.p. RIT, the median survival had not been reached with a maximum follow-up of 12 years. Survival at greater than 10 years was 78%. The conclusion of this study was that a substantial proportion of patients who achieve a CR with conventional therapy can achieve a long-term survival benefit if treated with i.p. ^{90}Y-HMFG1.

In 1999, Rosenblum et al. performed a dose-escalating, multiarm phase I study of ^{90}Y-B72.3 i.p. administration (28). The first arm (three patients/dose level) received i.p. infusion of either 2 or 10 mg B72.3 labeled with 37, 370, 555, or 925 MBq ^{90}Y. Pharmacokinetic studies showed that ^{90}Y-B72.3 persisted in peritoneal fluid with a half-life of more than 24 hours after i.p. administration. Biopsy specimens of bone and marrow obtained at 72 hours after administration showed significant content of the label in bone (0.015% ID/g) with relatively little in marrow (0.005% ID/g). The MTD was 370 MBq (10 mCi), mainly due to hematologic toxicity and platelet suppression. In an effort to suppress the bone uptake, patients were treated with a continuous i.v. infusion of ethylenediaminetetraacetic acid (EDTA) immediately before i.p. administration of ^{90}Y-B72.3. The second arm was treated with 370, 555, 740, 925, 1110, 1295, 1480, or 1665 MBq ^{90}Y-B72.3 for a total of 38 patients. Dose-limiting toxicities were thrombocytopenia and neutropenia. Analysis of biopsy demonstrated that the bone and marrow content of the ^{90}Y was 15-fold lower (less than 0.001% ID/g) than a group without EDTA. Four responses were noted in patients who received 555 to 1110 MBq ^{90}Y-B72.3, with response durations of 1 to 12 months. The conclusion of this study was that EDTA has a myeloprotective effect, which allows safe i.p. administration of higher doses of ^{90}Y-B72.3.

An interesting study was performed that investigated pretargeted RIT based on the avidin–biotin system, where the therapeutic efficacy and toxicity was evaluated in 38 advanced ovarian cancer patients (86). The therapy was performed according to the following three-step protocol: biotinylated mAbs and avidin were i.p. injected (first and second step) and 12 to 18 hours later, ^{90}Y-biotin (either i.v. or i.p.) was injected as the third step. Sixteen out of 38 patients were treated by i.p. injection only, whereas the other 22 patients received the combined treatment (i.v. + i.p.), the dose ranging from 370 to 3700 MBq of ^{90}Y-biotin. Both therapeutic regimens were well tolerated, but two patients showed temporary grade III to IV hematologic toxicity. Considering therapeutic efficacy, in the i.p. group, 6%

of the patients had an objective tumor reduction, 31% had stabilization of disease, and progression was seen in 50%. In the group of combined treatment, 9% of the patients achieved objective responses, 32% showed stable disease, and 41% had a progression. The conclusion of this study was excellent tolerability and a good potential therapeutic role of pretargeted RIT in advanced ovarian cancer and that the patients with minimal residual disease would probably be the best served by pretargeted RIT using ^{90}Y-biotin.

Alvarez et al. determined the feasibility and MTD of ^{90}Y-CC49 as the RIT component of an i.p. combined modality treatment for recurrent ovarian cancer (32). A phase I study of ^{90}Y-CC49 RIT was conducted in ovarian cancer patients who had persistent or recurrent intra-abdominal disease, had failed one or two prior chemotherapy regimens, and demonstrated TAG-72 expression. Patients were treated with a previously established combined modality treatment protocol of subcutaneous interferon (IFN) α2b, i.p. paclitaxel, and increasing dosages of i.p. ^{90}Y-CC49. The patients were monitored for toxicity, generation of HAMA response, and clinical efficacy. Twenty eligible patients were treated per study specifications, all previously treated with debulking and paclitaxel/carboplatin-based chemotherapy. The patients included were 11 women with persistent disease at the time of SLL and 9 women with delayed recurrence. RIT treatment was primarily associated with hematologic toxicity. The MTD of i.p. ^{90}Y-CC49 was established at 895.4 MBq/m^2. Of 9 patients with measurable disease, 2 had partial responses lasting 2 and 4 months. Of 11 patients with nonmeasurable disease, the median time to progression was 6 months in 7 patients who recurred. The conclusion of this study was that ^{90}Y-CC49 RIT in combination with IFN α2b and i.p. paclitaxel is feasible and well tolerated at a dose of less than or equal to 895.4 MBq/m^2.

■ Clinical studies using the β$^-$-particle emitter ^{177}Lu

Considering the much shorter range of the emitted β$^-$-particles from ^{177}Lu (mean range ≈ 0.2 mm) compared with those emitted from ^{90}Y (mean range ≈ 4 mm), ^{177}Lu theoretically has a higher therapeutic index than ^{90}Y for a microscopic disease, due to its ability to more specifically irradiate the tumor cells while sparing healthy tissue. Meredith et al. enrolled 12 ovarian cancer patients who failed chemotherapy in a phase I study of i.p. ^{177}Lu-CC49 treatment (33). The patients had disease confined to the abdominal cavity ± retroperitoneal lymph nodes, adequate organ function, and no previous radiation. Side effects included mild marrow suppression (marrow doses of 0.11 to 0.54 Gy). The MTD had not been reached with levels of 370, 666, 925, and 1110 MBq/m^2. Scintigraphy revealed localization consistent with tumor in 11 of 12 patients. One of eight patients with gross disease had more than 50% tumor reduction after therapy, while six progressed and one went off study with stable disease. In the group of patients with microscopic or occult disease, one relapsed at 10 months and three remained without evidence of disease after 18 months. The conclusion of this study was that i.p. ^{177}Lu-CC49-RIT was well tolerated and appeared to have some antitumor effect against chemotherapy-resistant ovarian cancer in the peritoneal cavity.

Meredith et al. also performed a phase I study to examine the feasibility of combining IFN and paclitaxel with i.p. ^{177}Lu-CC49-RIT (90). Patients with recurrent or persistent ovarian cancer confined to the abdominal cavity after first-line therapy were enrolled. Human recombinant alpha IFN was administered as four subcutaneous injections of 3×10^6 U on alternate days beginning 5 days before RIT to increase the expression of the tumor-associated antigen, TAG-72. The addition of IFN increased hematologic toxicity such that the MTD of the combination was 1.5 GBq/m^2 compared with ^{177}Lu-CC49 alone (1.7 GBq/m^2). Taxol (Paclitaxel) was given i.p. 48 hours before RIT. It was initiated at 25 mg/m^2 and escalated at 25 mg/m^2 increments to 100 mg/m^2. Subsequent groups of patients were treated with IFN + 100 mg/m^2 taxol + escalating doses of ^{177}Lu-CC49. Three or more patients were treated in each dose group and 34 patients were treated with the three-agent combination. The therapy was well tolerated with the expected reversible hematologic toxicity. The MTD for ^{177}Lu-CC49 was 1.5 GBq/m^2 when given with IFN + 100 mg/m^2 taxol. Four of 17 patients with CT measurable disease had a partial response and 4 of 27 with nonmeasurable disease had progression-free intervals of 18+, 21+, 21+, and 37+ months. The conclusion of this study was that the combination of i.p. taxol chemotherapy (100 mg/m^2) with RIT ^{177}Lu-CC49 and IFN was well tolerated, with bone marrow suppression as the dose-limiting toxicity.

In 1997, Alvarez et al. enrolled 27 ovarian cancer patients, who failed prior chemotherapy, into a phase I/II study of i.p. ^{177}Lu-CC49 treatment (34). The patients had disease confined to the abdominal cavity ± retroperitoneal lymph nodes. The most common side effects from the treatment were delayed, transient arthralgia (10/27) and marrow suppression with 1.7 GBq/m^2, which was the MTD. One of 13 patients with gross disease had more than 50% tumor reduction after therapy, whereas most others with gross disease progressed. Seven of nine patients with less than 1-cm nodules progressed in 21 months or less, and two of nine remained without evidence of disease at 4 to 5 months. Of the five patients with microscopic or occult disease, one relapsed at 10 months and four remained without evidence of disease at more than 6 to 35 months. Marrow suppression was dose limiting during i.p. RIT ^{177}Lu-CC49. The conclusion of this study was that an antitumor effect against chemotherapy-resistant ovarian cancer existed, resulting in prolonged disease-free survival of most patients with microscopic disease.

Clinical studies using the β⁻-particle emitter ^{131}I

This radionuclide has been used in several studies, some of which are presented below. Partly due to its long half-life (8 days), problems with bone marrow suppression have been evident. The long half-life and gamma emission are also a concern regarding the unintentional irradiation of

staff, relatives, and other patients. An explanation as to why some patients have not benefited from this form of therapy with ^{131}I is that the disease has been "macroscopic" at the time of treatment. As a result, the shorter path length of the emitted electron will not adequately penetrate larger tumors. In 1987, Epenetos et al. evaluated 24 patients with persistent EOC after treatment with chemotherapy (with or without external beam irradiation). These patients were treated with i.p. ^{131}I-mAbs, HMFG1, HMFG2, AUA1, and H17E2 (13). Acute side effects were mild abdominal pain, pyrexia, diarrhea, and moderate reversible pancytopenia. Eight patients with large volume disease, that is, tumor diameter greater than 2 cm, did not respond to antibody-guided irradiation and died of progressive disease within 9 months of treatment. Sixteen patients had small volume (less than 2 cm) disease at the time of treatment with radio-labeled mAbs. Seven patients failed to respond, and of nine initial responders, four patients remained alive and free from disease 6 months to 3 years after treatment. Doses greater than 5.2 GBq were more effective than lower doses. The conclusion of this study was that the i.p. administration of 5.2 GBq (140.5 mCi) or more of ^{131}I-mAbs represents a potentially effective form of therapy for patients with small volume stage III ovarian cancer.

Two years later, Stewart et al. enrolled 28 patients with assessable residual ovarian cancer after cytoreductive surgery and chemotherapy, to receive i.p. ^{131}I-mAbs (HMFG1, HMFG2, AUA1, or H17E2) (91). There was no response in eight patients with tumor diameters greater than 2 cm, a partial response in two of the fifteen patients with tumor diameters less than 2 cm, and a complete response in three of the other five patients. Six additional patients received ^{90}Y-mAbs for residual ovarian cancer, leading to no response in one patient with nodules more than 2 cm, and a partial response in one of the other five patients with tumor nodules less than 2 cm. The absorbed dose received by the peritoneal serosa was less than 5 Gy which was insufficient to account for the observed tumor response. Significant bone marrow suppression was observed with ^{131}I activities more than 4.44 GBq (120 mCi) and with ^{90}Y activities more than 481 MBq (13 mCi). The authors concluded that the hematopoietic bone marrow was the dose-limiting organ.

The same research group also treated 36 patients with ovarian cancer with i.p. ^{131}I-mAbs (HMFG1, HMFG2, AUA1, H17E2) (93). The activity was increased from 740 to 5846 MBq (20 to 158 mCi), and pharmacokinetics and toxicity were evaluated. Five patients who had developed HAMA were re-treated, and the pharmacokinetics and toxicity of the first and second treatment were compared. Patients receiving their first therapeutic instillation (HAMA negative) had a maximum of 25% (range 19.8% to 39.8%) of the injected activity identified in their circulation. This was accompanied by severe marrow suppression at ^{131}I activities more than 4.44 GBq (120 mCi). The five HAMA-positive patients had only 5% injected activity in the systemic circulation (range 3.8% to 6%), with rapid urinary excretion and negligible marrow suppression. In 31 patients with assessable disease, there were no responses in 8 patients with gross disease (tumors greater than 2 cm), partial responses in 2 out of 15 patients with tumors less than 2 cm, and complete responses in 3 out of 6 patients with microscopic disease.

Crippa et al. performed a study in which 16 of 19 enrolled patients with minimal residual disease of ovarian cancer (macroscopic disease less than 5 mm or positive blind biopsies and/or positive peritoneal washing), demonstrated by surgical second look, underwent i.p. RIT with ^{131}I-MOv18 (mean dose 14 mg of MOv18 with 3.7 GBq [100 mCi] of ^{131}I) 30 to 40 days after the second-look procedure (92). Clinical follow-up and/or third-look evaluation performed 90 days after RIT showed CR in five patients, no change (NC) in six patients, and progressive disease in five patients. A follow-up study showed long-term maintained CR in one patient (34 months) and relapses in the other four patients after a mean disease-free period of 10.5 months. The five NC patients showed clinical or instrumental progression after a mean disease-free period of 13 months. The toxicity of RIT was negligible, with only one patient showing mild and transient bone marrow suppression. HAMA production was demonstrated in 94% of patients. The conclusion of this study was that RIT appeared to be a promising therapeutic approach to treat minimal residual disease of ovarian cancer.

A phase II study published in 1999 investigated the efficacy of i.p. RIT in patients with minimal residual ovarian adenocarcinoma after primary treatment with surgery and chemotherapy (37). Six patients with residual macroscopic (less than 5 mm) or microscopic disease, as shown by laparotomy and biopsies, received i.p. RIT. All had initial stage III epithelial carcinoma and were treated with debulking surgery and one line (four patients) or two lines (two patients) of chemotherapy. RIT was performed with 60 mg of OC125 F(ab')2 mAb labeled with 4.44 GBq (120 mCi) of ^{131}I injected 5 to 10 days after the surgical procedure. Systematic laparoscopy or laparotomy with biopsies performed 3 months after the RIT in five patients (clinical progression was seen in one patient) showed NC in three patients and progression in two patients. The toxicity was mainly hematologic and HAMA production was demonstrated in all six patients. The conclusion of this study was that little therapeutic benefit could be shown from i.p. RIT in patients with residual ovarian carcinoma.

Finally, van Zanten-Przybysz et al. investigated the safety and pharmacokinetics of ^{131}I-MOv18 in patients with ovarian cancer and estimated the absorbed dose to cancer-free organs and tumors (47). They administered patients an i.v. and i.p. instillation of MOv18 IgG, labeled with different radionuclides (48). To study the kinetics of MOv18 in the latter study, patients were divided into two groups. Fifteen patients received MOv18 labeled with ^{131}I, ^{125}I, and ^{123}I (for imaging). Seven patients underwent surgery 2 days, seven patients 6 days, and one patient 3 days postinjection. Radioactivity was measured in blood, ascites, and biopsies of tumor and of several normal tissues. No anti-MOv18 responses were observed. At 2 days postinjection, a significant difference in tumor uptake was found in favor of the

i.v. route of administration (4.9% and 2.4% ID/kg for i.v. and i.p., respectively; $p < 0.0001$). Uptake in solid tumor tissue in ovarian cancer patients undergoing surgery 6 days postinjection was not significantly different ($p = 0.79$) for both routes (3.8% and 3.9% ID/kg for i.v. and i.p., respectively). The conclusion of this study was that no advantage could be demonstrated for the i.p. route with respect to tumor uptake. The i.p. route could, however, be advantageous with respect to bone marrow toxicity.

Clinical studies using the β⁻-particle emitters ^{186}Re or ^{188}Re

Very few studies have been published using these radionuclides. However, Jacobs et al. performed a phase I study to determine the MTD, toxicity, and response of persistent and recurrent ovarian carcinoma to i.p. injection of ^{186}Re-NR-LU-10 (66). A single dose of 25 mg/m^2 of mAb conjugated with 925 to 5550 MBq (25 to 150 mCi)/m^2 ^{186}Re was administered i.p. to 17 patients. Severe myelosuppression was observed at 5.55 GBq (150 mCi)/m^2 of ^{186}Re in two patients. Other toxicities included low-grade fever and transient skin rash. Hepatic enzyme elevation was seen in 12 of 17 patients but was not clinically significant. Decreased tumor size was demonstrated in 4 of 7 patients with disease measuring less than 1 cm at the time of treatment (4 of 17 total). Responders had serum CA-125 levels of 35 U/mL or less at the time of treatment and received one regimen of chemotherapy. The conclusion of this study was that the immunoconjugate could be administered i.p. with acceptable toxicity and produce objective responses after a single dose in patients with minimal disease. The problem with this radionuclide is that in order to increase the therapeutic efficacy, a higher absorbed dose must be delivered to the tumor. This could potentially be achieved by injecting larger amounts of activity and increasing the specificity of the treatment. However, considering the long half-life of ^{186}Re (3.7 days), this could cause toxicity problems, especially regarding the bone marrow.

This concept was partly investigated in a study by Macey et al. in which the design was to compare different β⁻-particle emitters and determine whether a shorter half-life could reduce red marrow (RM) toxicity for i.p. RIT (35). The radionuclides ^{188}Re, ^{166}Ho, ^{177}Lu, ^{186}Re, ^{131}I, and ^{90}Y were labeled to CC49. Blood and whole body retention biokinetic information acquired from 26 patients who received i.p. RIT with ^{177}Lu-CC49 were used as input data. The residence time and RM absorbed doses were calculated. In this model, ^{188}Re was found to deliver the lowest RM absorbed dose, primarily because it had the shortest half-life, whereas ^{90}Y delivered the highest RM dose (high energy, long path length). Based on limiting the RM absorbed dose to 2 Gy, the maximum administered activity of each radionuclide was as follows: ^{188}Re: 6.2 GBq (167.6 mCi), ^{166}Ho: 4.1 GBq (110.8 mCi), ^{177}Lu: 3.9 GBq (105.4 mCi), ^{186}Re: 2.6 GBq (70.2 mCi), ^{131}I: 2.2 GBq (59.5 mCi), and ^{90}Y: 1.3 GBq (35.1 mCi). Table 29.1 lists the various preclinical and clinical studies used to investigate EOC.

Table 29.1 References in which the different targeting constructs and radionuclides have been used

	α-Particle Emitters				β⁻-Particle Emitters			
	^{225}Ac	^{211}At	^{213}Bi	^{90}Y	^{177}Lu	^{131}I	^{186}Re/^{188}Re	—[a]
HMFG1	—	—	—	*9, 10, 85, 87–89*	13	*91, 93*	—	*20*
HMFG2	—	—	—	—	13	*91, 93*	—	*20*
AUA1	—	—	—	—	13	*91, 93*	—	—
H17E2	—	—	—	—	13	*91, 93*	—	*20*
Hu2PLAP	—	—	—	—	—	—	—	*20*
H317	—	—	—	—	—	—	—	*20*
Trastuzumab[b]	22	—	—	—	—	—	—	—
Pertuzumab[b]	—	—	—	—	23	—	—	—
B72.3	—	—	—	*28, 86*	—	29	—	—
CC49	—	—	—	*31, 32*	*31, 33, 34, 90*	36	35	—
OC125	—	—	—	*38*	—	*37, 39*	—	—
(c)MOv18[c]	—	*43–46*	—	*86*	—	*47–52, 92*	—	75
MX35	—	*56–61, 62, 83, 84*	—	—	—	—	—	—
NR-LU-10	—	—	—	—	—	—	*65, 66*	—
A5B7	—	—	—	—	—	67	—	—
17-A1	—	—	—	—	—	70	—	—
323/A3	—	—	—	—	—	70	—	—
hCTM01	—	—	—	—	—	—	—	***73***
OV-TL 3	—	—	—	—	—	—	—	***75***
139H2	—	—	—	—	—	77	—	—
P-P4D	—	—	78	—	—	—	—	—
PAI2	—	—	79	—	—	—	—	—
Affibody[b]	—	81	—	—	82	—	—	—

[a]The study was performed without therapeutic radionuclides for investigating pharmacokinetics, antigen expression, and tumor uptake.
[b]Trasuzumab, pertuzumab, and affibody are the only commercially available constructs.
[c]Some studies were performed with a chimeric version of MOv18.
Notes: Italic text indicates a clinical study. Bold text indicates human/humanized antibody.

■ RADIATION DOSIMETRY

In the management of ovarian cancer patients, radionuclide therapy will normally only be considered for targeting small cell clusters that cannot be visually identified and removed by surgical means. In practice, the presence of tumor cells can only be assumed based on previous clinical experience of recurrent disease in similar patients. The situation of delivering radiation to target single cells or small cell clusters, whose number and size are not known, requires special attention to the dosimetry. Also, under these circumstances, the radiation must be optimized in order to deliver a high radiation dose to tumor cells and a correspondingly low dose to healthy tissue.

Without direct physical detection of the targets, some qualified assumptions can be made to support the dosimetric calculations. The first is that as the targets were not identified and removed in conjunction with laparoscopic examination, their size can be estimated to have a length/diameter of a few millimeters or less. The other assumption is that the targets are either floating in the peritoneal fluid or are attached to its lining. Both assumptions form the basis for i.p. radionuclide therapy, but dosimetry can further guide the design of a more detailed therapeutic regimen.

In radionuclide therapy, it is the activity concentration and the absorbed fraction of the released energy in the tumors that determine the outcome. This suggests that for targets larger than approximately 1 mm, β^--emitters, such as ^{90}Y, ^{177}Lu, and ^{131}I with electron ranges up to approximately 10 mm, are acceptable. Smaller residual tumor cell clusters (i.e., less than a few hundred micrometers) would be considerably more effectively irradiated by α-particles, with a range of approximately 75 μm. Different dosimetry methods, some involving microdosimetry, can be applied to verify these general statements (113).

Based on assumptions regarding the tumor size and distribution, the estimated absorbed dose to tumor cells and tumor cell clusters in patients can be based on measuring the infused activity; imaging its distribution with, for example, a γ-camera; sampling the peritoneal fluid; and measuring the transport of radioactive substance to tissues outside the peritoneum. The absorbed dose to tumor cells could also be estimated based on the knowledge of the binding kinetics of the mAbs (84). Without detailed microdosimetric techniques, a first approximation on absorbed dose to single cells can be to estimate the dose to the peritoneal fluid. This is determined by the concentration of radioactivity in the fluid over time. This means that the absorbed dose to the peritoneum, as well as single cells and small microscopic tumors situated there, is computed as half the equilibrium absorbed dose of relevant activity concentration in the abdominal cavity. However, if the targeting molecule successfully reaches its target, then this first approximation is a gross underestimation of the actual absorbed dose to the cells. On the other hand, if the target clusters are larger than the range of the emitted radiation, some inner cells may not receive any absorbed radiation dose at all, assuming non-vascularized tumors during i.p. treatment. Attempts have been made in animal models to determine the actual absorbed radiation dose to cell clusters on the peritoneal lining in mice receiving i.p. RIT (56). These controlled experiments have involved retrospective electron-scanning imaging and elaborate microdosimetric calculations. These technologies have, however, not matured for clinical use, so it is reasonable to use the other approach for dosimetry, that is, adjust the therapies to a level that is below the tolerance for the critical organs. One must also remember that only a very small fraction (typically less than 1%) of the radiation energy released in the therapies discussed here will be deposited in tumor cells.

For most radionuclide therapies, even for i.p. administration, the bone marrow is the critical organ limiting the administered activity. The bone marrow dosimetry can be based on serum activity concentration data, since the activity concentration in red bone marrow is directly proportional to the serum activity concentration via the RM extracellular fluid fraction (114). However, for i.p. α-RIT, using the relatively short-lived ^{211}At, it was shown that the bone marrow dose was low and well below any tolerance dose for the infused radioactivity in a clinical phase I study (62). Instead, focus was placed on dose to the thyroid, and

when a thyroid-blocking agent was introduced, dose to the peritoneal lining. This illustrates the various assumptions that must be made for dosimetry in i.p. radionuclide therapy, and also suggests how dosimetry can assist in the design and evaluation of a clinical study.

SUMMARY AND FUTURE PROSPECTS

Despite a decline in incidence and an intensification of treatment, the mortality of EOC has not decreased during the past decades. Most patients are diagnosed at an advanced stage and the majority will succumb, suffering from abdominal complications. With present diagnostics, screening for early-stage ovarian cancer has not been successful, but efforts in finding proteins in serum indicating early ovarian cancer is a vision for future improvements in ovarian cancer survival. Other approaches are the development of targeted techniques, with higher efficacy and less toxicity than present day treatments, some of which have been presented in this chapter. Such targeted therapies may include ligands, substrate analogs, or antibodies, resulting in upregulation of receptors or surface antigens. The antibodies may exhibit efficiency on its own or as a conjugate to toxins or radionuclides. Since the clinical pattern is dominated by abdominal spread and complications, such therapeutic measures are primarily directed intraperitoneally. Although a successful i.p. therapy may eradicate abdominal disease and complications, extraperitoneal metastases may ultimately become "unmasked." Most likely, a combination of abdominal and systemic modalities is required.

Since the current available standard treatments frequently fail to cure micrometastatic disease, RIT using short-ranged high efficiency α-particle emitters, for example, ^{211}At or ^{213}Bi, depositing the energy in the immediate vicinity of targeted cells, is an attractive approach, possibly in combination with β^--particle emitters aimed at larger tumor cell clusters. This procedure may be added as a "boost" after cytoreductive surgery and systemic chemotherapy, primarily intraperitoneally but possibly also intravenously by pretargeted approaches, based, for example, on the avidin/streptavidin–biotin system. This systemic adjunctive approach may be particularly relevant if the disease includes, for example, retroperitoneal vascularized metastases to the lymph nodes (31,115,116). Another important concept that could potentially improve the therapeutic index would be the use of fractionated RIT, as applied to external beam radiation therapy, resulting in decreased toxicity while retaining the therapeutic efficacy (60). Auger emitters might also offer an interesting alternative to the above-mentioned radionuclides, because emitted electrons have low energy (mostly << 1 keV), and therefore a short path length in tissue. However, to effectively damage the DNA, the Auger emitter has to be incorporated into the DNA, which is a biologic challenge.

Potential disadvantages with an i.p. treatment are that the i.p. catheter could cause pain and discomfort for the patient, it could leak (possibly lowering the therapeutic efficacy and causing radiation protection problems for the staff), and it could cause infection and risk of peritonitis. Also, for the i.p. treatments to be successful, especially when using radionuclides that emit short-range particles, loculation and/or adhesions are undesirable and could hamper the therapeutic outcome. The potential problem of toxicity (e.g., bone marrow, renal, and peritoneum) and HAMA response always needs to be addressed. A number of review articles have been published, regarding RIT in general and RIT against i.p. ovarian cancer in particular, discussing advantages and disadvantages (117–134).

Several parameters can influence the i.p. therapeutic outcome, for example: specificity of targeting construct, antigen expression (135), loss of immunoreactivity of targeting construct, amount of unlabeled antibody, diffusion barriers for penetration of the targeting construct into tumor cell clusters, choice of radionuclide (half-life and particle range), low specific radioactivity, and tumors located extraperitoneally. When treating microscopic disease, the choice of β^--particle emitters could be problematic due to the inability of the β^--particles to deliver high enough energy to the target volume, that is, the tumor cell nuclei. This is presumably the reason why the clinical studies performed hitherto using β^--particle emitters have failed when trying to treat microscopic disease.

A proof of concept with an i.p. treatment advantage has been shown in a phase III study by the Gynecologic Oncology Group that included women undergoing initial therapy for advanced ovarian cancer (136), and the advantage of i.p. compared with i.v. administration for the localization of radiolabeled mAbs to microscopic peritoneal disease has been shown both in animal models and in human studies (125,137,138). Finally, in order to be able to properly compare and evaluate different treatment strategies, the need to conduct controlled, randomized, multicenter clinical trials with sufficient patient numbers, enabling statistical significance to occur, must be emphasized.

■ ACKNOWLEDGMENTS

Tod Speer (MD at the Department of Human Oncology, School of Medicine and Public Health, University of Wisconsin) and Lars Jacobsson (Professor at the Department of Radiation Physics, Sahlgrenska Academy, University of Gothenburg) are acknowledged for wise additional contributions to the chapter. Sofia Frost (PhD student at the Department of Radiation Physics, Sahlgrenska Academy, University of Gothenburg) is acknowledged for meticulous proofreading.

■ REFERENCES

1. Choi M, Fuller CD, Thomas CR, et al. Conditional survival in ovarian cancer: results from the SEER dataset 1988-2001. *Gynecol Oncol.* 2008; 109:203–209.
2. Sant M, Allermani C, Santaquilani M, et al. Eurocare 4. Survival of cancer patients diagnosed in 1995–1999. *Eur J Cancer.* 2009;45:931–991.
3. Shih M, Kurman RJ. Ovarian tumorigenesis: a proposed model based on morphological and molecular genetic analysis. *Am J Surg Path.* 2004;164:1511–1518.
4. Panici PB, Maggioni A, Hacker N, et al. Systemic aortic and pelvic lymphadenectomy versus resection of bulky nodes only in optimally debulked advanced ovarian cancer: a randomized clinical trial. *J Nat Cancer Inst.* 2005;97:560–566.
5. Einhorn N, Tropé C, Ridderheim M, et al. A systematic overview of radiation therapy effects in ovarian cancer. *Acta Oncol.* 2003;42:562–566.
6. Varia MA, Stehman FB, Bundy BN, et al. Intraperitoneal radioactive phosphorus (^{32}P) versus observation after negative second-look laparotomy for stage III ovarian carcinoma: a randomized trial of the Gynecologic Oncology Group. *J Clin Oncol.* 2003;21:2849–2855.
7. Rosenhein NB, Leichner PK, Vogelsang G. Radiocolloids in the treatment of ovarian cancer. *Obstet Gynecol Surv.* 1979;34:708–720.
8. Jaaback K, Johnson N. Intraperitoneal chemotherapy for the initial management of primary epithelial ovarian cancer [review]. *The Cochrane Library.* 2009;4:1–34.
9. Verheijen RH, Massuger LF, Benigno BB, et al. Phase III trial of intraperitoneal therapy with yttrium-90-labeled HMFG1 murine monoclonal antibody in patients with epithelial ovarian cancer after a surgically defined complete remission. *J Clin Oncol.* 2006;24:571–578.
10. Oei AL, Verheijen RH, Seiden MV, et al. Decreased intraperitoneal disease recurrence in epithelial ovarian cancer patients receiving intraperitoneal consolidation treatment with yttrium-90-labeled murine HMFG1 without improvement in overall survival. *Int J Cancer.* 2007;120:2710–2714.
11. Gendler SJ. MUC1, the renaissance molecule. *J Mammary Gland Biol Neoplasia.* 2001;6:339–353.
12. Mukherjee P, Madsen CS, Ginardi AR. Mucin 1-specific immunotherapy in a mouse model of spontaneous breast cancer. *J Immunother.* 2003;26:47–62.
13. Epenetos AA, Munro AJ, Stewart S, et al. Antibody-guided irradiation of advanced ovarian cancer with intraperitoneally administered radiolabeled monoclonal antibodies. *J Clin Oncol.* 1987;512:1890–1899.
14. Arklie J, Taylor-Papadimitriou J, Bodmer WF, et al. Differentiation antigens expressed by epithelial cells in the lactating breast are also detectable in breast cancers. *Int J Cancer.* 1981;28:23–29.
15. Burchell J, Durbin H, Taylor-Papadimitriou J. Complexity of expression of antigenic determinants recognised by monoclonal antibodies HMFG1 and HMFG2 in normal and malignant human mammary epithelial cells. *J Immunol.* 1983;131:508–513.
16. Epenetos AA, Nimmon CC, Arklie J, et al. Radioimmunodiagnosis of human cancer in an animal model using labeled tumor associated monoclonal antibodies. *Br J Cancer.* 1982;46:1–8.
17. Travers P, Bodmer WF. Preparation and characterisation of monoclonal antibodies against placental alkaline phosphatase and other human trophoblast-associated determinants. *Int J Cancer.* 1984;33: 633–641.
18. Benham FJ, Povey MS, Harris H. Placental-like alkaline phosphatase in malignant and benign ovarian tumours. *Clin Chim Acta.* 1978; 86:201–215.
19. Sunderland CA, Davis JO, Stirrat GM. Immunohistology of normal and ovarian cancer tissue with monoclonal antibody to placental alkaline phosphatase. *Cancer Res.* 1984;44:4496–4502.
20. Kosmas C, Kalofonos HP, Hird V, et al. Monoclonal antibody targeting of ovarian carcinoma. *Oncology.* 1998;55:435–446.
21. Carter P, Presta L, Gorman CM, et al. Humanization of an anti-p185^{HER2} antibody for human cancer therapy. *Proc Natl Acad Sci.* 1992;89: 4285–4289.
22. Borchardt PE, Yuan RR, Miederer M, et al. Targeted Actinium-225 in vivo generators for therapy of ovarian cancer. *Cancer Res.* 2003;63: 5084–5090.
23. Persson M, Gedda L, Lundqvist H, et al. ^{177}Lu-pertuzumab: experimental therapy of HER-2-expressing xenografts. *Cancer Res.* 2007;67: 326–331.
24. Thor A, Gorstein F, Ohuchi N, et al. Tumor-associated glycoprotein (TAG-72) in ovarian carcinomas defined by monoclonal antibody B72.3. *J Natl Cancer Inst.* 1986;76:995–1006.
25. Wolf BC, D'Emilia JC, Salem RR, et al. Detection of the tumor associated glycoprotein antigen (TAG-72) in premalignant lesions of the colon. *J Natl Cancer Inst.* 1989;81:1913–1917.
26. Johnson VG, Schlom J, Paterson AJ, et al. Analysis of a human tumor-associated glycoprotein (TAG-72) identified by monoclonal antibody B72.3. *Cancer Res.* 1986;46:850–857.
27. Nuti M, Teramoto YA, Mariani-Costantini R, et al. A monoclonal (B72.3) defines patterns of distribution of a novel tumor-associated antigen in human mammary carcinoma cell populations. *Int J Cancer.* 1982;29:539–545.

28. Rosenblum MG, Verschraegen CF, Murray JL, et al. Phase I study of ^{90}Y-labeled B72.3 intraperitoneal administration in patients with ovarian cancer: effect of dose and EDTA coadministration on pharmacokinetics and toxicity. *Clin Cancer Res.* 1999;5:953–961.

29. Colcher D, Esteban J, Carrasquillo JA, et al. Complementation of intracavitary and intravenous administration of a monoclonal antibody (B72.3) in patients with carcinoma. *Cancer Res.* 1987;47:4218–4224.

30. Schlom J, Colcher D, Suer K, et al. Tumor targeting with monoclonal antibody B72.3: experimental and clinical results. In: Goldenberg D, ed. *Cancer Imaging with Radiolabeled Antibodies.* Boston, MA: Kluwer Academic; 1990.

31. Buchsbaum DJ, Khazaeli MB, Axworthy DB, et al. Intraperitoneal pretarget radioimmunotherapy with CC49 fusion protein. *Clin Cancer Res.* 2005;11:8180–8185.

32. Alvarez RD, Huh WK, Khazaeli MB, et al. A phase I study of combined modality ^{90}Y-CC49 intraperitoneal radioimmunotherapy for ovarian cancer. *Clin Cancer Res.* 2002;8:2806–2811.

33. Meredith RF, Partridge EE, Alvarez RD, et al. Intraperitoneal radioimmunotherapy of ovarian cancer with lutetium-177-CC49. *J Nucl Med.* 1996;37:1491–1496.

34. Alvarez RD, Partridge EE, Khazaeli MB, et al. Intraperitoneal radioimmunotherapy of ovarian cancer with ^{177}Lu-CC49: a phase I/II study. *Gynecol Oncol.* 1997;65:94–101.

35. Macey DJ, Meredith RF. A strategy to reduce red marrow dose for intraperitoneal radioimmunotherapy. *Clin Cancer Res.* 1999;5:3044–3047.

36. Buchsbaum DJ, Rogers BE, Khazaeli MB, et al. Targeting strategies for cancer radiotherapy. *Clin Cancer Res.* 1999;5:3048–3055.

37. Mahé MA, Fumoleau P, Fabbro M, et al. A phase II study of intraperitoneal radioimmunotherapy with iodine-131-labeled monoclonal antibody OC-125 in patients with residual ovarian carcinoma. *Clin Cancer Res.* 1999;5:3249–3253.

38. Hnatowich DJ, Chinol M, Siebecker DA, et al. Patient distribution of intraperitoneally administered yttrium-90-labeled antibody. *J Nucl Med.* 1988;29:1428–1434.

39. Muto MG, Finkler NJ, Kassis AI, et al. Intraperitoneal radioimmunotherapy of refractory ovarian carcinoma utilizing Iodine-131-labeled monoclonal antibody OC125. *Gynaecol Oncol.* 1992;45:265–272.

40. Boerman OC, van Niekerk CC, Makkink K, et al. Comparative immunohistochemical study of four monoclonal antibodies directed against ovarian carcinoma-associated antigens. *Int J Gyn Path.* 1991;10:15–25.

41. Miotti S, Canevari S, Mènard S, et al. Characterization of human ovarian carcinoma-associated antigens defined by novel monoclonal antibodies with tumor-restricted specificity. *Int J Cancer.* 1987;39:297–303.

42. Campell IG, Jones TA, Foulkes WD, et al. Folate-binding protein is a marker for ovarian cancer. *Cancer Res.* 1991;51:5329–5338.

43. Andersson H, Lindegren S, Bäck T, et al. Biokinetics of the monoclonal antibodies MOv18, OV185 and OV197 labelled with ^{125}I according to the m-MeATE method or the Iodogen method in nude mice with ovarian cancer xenografts. *Acta Oncol.* 1999;38:323–328.

44. Andersson H, Lindegren S, Bäck T, et al. Radioimmunotherapy of nude mice with intraperitoneally growing ovarian cancer xenograft utilizing [211]At-labelled monoclonal antibody MOv18. *Anticancer Res.* 2000;20:459–462.

45. Andersson H, Lindegren S, Bäck T, et al. The curative and palliative potential of the monoclonal antibody MOv18 labelled with [211]At in nude mice with intraperitoneally growing ovarian cancer xenografts—a long-term study. *Acta Oncol.* 2000;39:741–745.

46. Andersson H, Palm S, Lindegren S, et al. Comparison of the therapeutic efficacy of [211]At- and ^{131}I-labelled monoclonal antibody MOv18 in nude mice with intraperitoneal growth of human ovarian cancer. *Anticancer Res.* 2001;21:409–412.

47. Van Zanten-Przybysz I, Molthoff CF, Roos JC, et al. Radioimmunotherapy with intravenously administered ^{131}I-labeled chimeric monoclonal antibody MOvl8 in patients with ovarian cancer. *J Nucl Med.* 2000;41:1168–1176.

48. Van Zanten-Przybysz I, Moltoff CF, Roos JC, et al. Influence of the route of administration on targeting of ovarian cancer with the chimeric monoclonal antibody MOv18: i.v. VS. i.p. *Int J Cancer.* 2001;92:106–114.

49. Moltoff CF, Buist MR, Kenemans P, et al. Experimental and clinical analysis of the characteristics of a chimeric monoclonal antibody, MOv18, reactive with an ovarian cancer-associated antigen. *J Nucl Med.* 1992;33:2000–2005.

50. Moltoff CF, Prinssen HM, Kenemans P, et al. Escalating protein doses of chimeric monoclonal antibody MOv18 immunoglobulin G in ovarian carcinoma patients: a phase I study. *Cancer.* 1997;80:2712–2720.

51. Buist MR, Kenemans P, Hollander W, et al. Kinetics and tissue distribution of the radiolabeled chimeric monoclonal antibody MOv18 IgG and F(ab')2 fragments in ovarian cancer patients. *Cancer Res.* 1993;53:5413–5418.

52. Buijs WC, Tibben JG, Boerman OC, et al. Dosimetric analysis of chimeric monoclonal antibody cMOv18 IgG in ovarian carcinoma patients after intraperitoneal and intravenous administration. *Eur J Nucl Med.* 1998;25:1552–1561.

53. Welshinger M, Yin BWT, Lloyd KO. Initial immunochemical characterization of MX35 ovarian cancer antigen. *Gynecol Oncol.* 1997;67:188–192.

54. Rubin SC, Kostakoglu L, Divgi C, et al. Biodistribution and intraoperative evaluation of radiolabeled monoclonal antibody MX35 in patients with epithelial ovarian cancer. *Gynecol Oncol.* 1993;51:61–66.

55. Yin BW, Kiyamova R, Chua R, et al. Monoclonal antibody MX35 detects the membrane transporter NaPi2b (SLC34A2) in human carcinomas. *Cancer Immun.* 2008;8:3–11.

56. Elgqvist J, Andersson H, Bäck T, et al. Alpha-radioimmunotherapy of intraperitoneally growing OVCAR-3 tumors of variable dimensions: outcome related to measured tumor size and mean absorbed dose. *J Nucl Med.* 2006;47:1342–1350.

57. Elgqvist J, Andersson H, Bäck T, et al. Fractionated radioimmunotherapy of intraperitoneally growing ovarian cancer in nude mice with [211]At-MX35 F(ab')2: therapeutic efficacy and myelotoxicity. *Nucl Med Biol.* 2006;33:1065–1072.

58. Elgqvist J, Andersson H, Bernhardt P, et al. Administered activity and metastatic cure probability during radioimmunotherapy of ovarian cancer in nude mice with [211]At-MX35 F(ab')2. *Int J Radiat Oncol Biol Phys.* 2006;66:1228–1237.

59. Elgqvist J, Andersson H, Haglund E, et al. Intraperitoneal alpha-radioimmunotherapy in mice using different specific activities. *Cancer Biother Radiopharm.* 2009;24:509–513.

60. Elgqvist J, Andersson H, Jensen H, et al. Repeated intraperitoneal alpha-radioimmunotherapy of ovarian cancer in mice. *J Oncol.* 2010;2010:394913.

61. Bäck T, Andersson H, Divgi CR, et al. [211]At radioimmunotherapy of subcutaneous human ovarian cancer xenografts: evaluation of relative biologic effectiveness of an alpha-emitter in vivo. *J Nucl Med.* 2005;46:2061–2067.

62. Andersson H, Cederkrantz E, Bäck T, et al. Intraperitoneal α-particle radioimmunotherapy of ovarian cancer patients: pharmacokinetics and dosimetry of [211]At-MX35 F(ab')2—a phase I study. *J Nucl Med.* 2009;50:1153–1160.

63. Goldrosen MH, Biddle WC, Pancook J, et al. Biodistribution, pharmacokinetic, and imaging studies with [186]Re-labeled NR-LU-10 whole antibody in LS174T colonic tumor-bearing mice. *Cancer Res.* 1990;50:7973–7878.

64. Varki NM, Reisfeld RA, Walker LE. Antigens associated with a human lung adenocarcinoma defined by monoclonal antibodies. *Cancer Res.* 1984;44:681–687.

65. Breitz HB, Durham JS, Fisher DR, et al. Pharmacokinetics and normal organ dosimetry following intraperitoneal rhenium-186-labeled monoclonal antibody. *J Nucl Med.* 1995;36:754–761.

66. Jacobs AJ, Fer M, Su FM, et al. A phase I trial of a rhenium 186-labeled monoclonal antibody administered intraperitoneally in ovarian carcinoma: toxicity and clinical response. *Obstet Gynecol.* 1993;82:586–593.

67. Turner JH, Rose AH, Glancy RJ, et al. Orthotopic xenografts of human melanoma and colonic and ovarian carcinoma in sheep to evaluate radioimmunotherapy. *Br J Cancer.* 1998;78:486–494.

68. Edwards DP, Grzyb KT, Dressler LG, et al. Monoclonal antibody identification and characterization of a Mr 43,000 membrane glycoprotein associated with human breast cancer. *Cancer Res.* 1986;46:1306–1317.

69. Koprowski H, Steplewski Z, Mitchell H, et al. Colorectal carcinoma antigens detected by hybridoma antibodies. *Somat Cell Genet.* 1979;5:957–972.

70. Kievit E, Pinedo HM, Schlüper HM, et al. Comparison of the monoclonal antibodies 17-1A and 323/A3: the influence of the affinity on tumor uptake and efficacy of radioimmunotherapy in human ovarian cancer xenografts. *Br J Cancer.* 1996;73:457–464.

71. Baker TS, Bose SS, Caskey-Finney HM, et al. Humanisation of an anti mucin antibody for breast and ovarian cancer therapy. In: Ceriani RL, ed. *Antigen and Antibody Molecular Engineering in Breast Cancer Diagnosis and Treatment*. New York, NY: Plenum Press; 1994.

72. Zotter S, Hageman PC, Lossnitzer A, et al. Tissue and tumour distribution of human polymorphic epithelial mucin. *Cancer Rev*. 1988;11/12: 55–101.

73. Davis Q, Perkins AC, Roos JC, et al. An immunoscintigraphic evaluation of the engineered human monoclonal antibody (hCTMO1) for use in the treatment of ovarian carcinoma. *Br J Obst Gynaecol*. 1999; 106:31–37.

74. Poels LG, Peters D, van Megen Y, et al. Monoclonal antibody against human ovarian tumor-associated antigens. *J Nat Cancer Inst*. 1986; 76:781–787.

75. Buist MR, Kenemans P, Molthoff C, et al. Tumor uptake of intravenously administered radiolabeled antibodies in ovarian carcinoma patients in relation to antigen expression and other tumor characteristics. *Int J Cancer*. 1995;64:92–98.

76. Hilkens J. Biochemistry and function of mucins in malignant disease. *Cancer Rev*. 1988;11/12:25–54.

77. Molthoff C, Pinedo H, Schlüper H, et al. Influence of dose and schedule on the therapeutic efficacy of ^{131}I-labelled monoclonal antibody 139H2 in a human ovarian cancer xenograft model. *Int J Cancer*. 1992;50:474–480.

78. Knör S, Sato S, Huber T, et al. Development and evaluation of peptidic ligands targeting tumour-associated urokinase plasminogen activator receptor (uPAR) for use in alpha-emitter therapy for disseminated ovarian cancer. *Eur J Nucl Med Mol Imaging*. 2008;35: 53–64.

79. Song EY, Abbas Rizvi SM, Qu CF, et al. Pharmacokinetics and toxicity of [213]Bi-labeled PAI2 in preclinical targeted alpha therapy for cancer. *Cancer Biol Ther*. 2007;6:898–904.

80. Steffen AC, Orlova A, Wikman M, et al. Affibody-mediated tumour targeting of HER-2 expressing xenografts in mice. *Eur J Nucl Med Mol Imaging*. 2006;33:631–638.

81. Steffen AC, Almqvist Y, Chyan MK, et al. Biodistribution of [211]At labeled HER-2 binding affibody molecules in mice. *Oncol Rep*. 2006;17:1141–1147.

82. Tolmachev V, Orlova A, Pehrson R, et al. Radionuclide therapy of HER2-positive microzenografts using a ^{177}Lu-labeled HER2-specific affibody molecule. *Cancer Res*. 2007;67:2773–2782.

83. Elgqvist J, Bernhardt P, Hultborn R, et al. Myelotoxicity and RBE of [211]At-conjugated monoclonal antibodies compared with ^{99m}Tc-conjugated monoclonal antibodies and ^{60}Co irradiation in nude mice. *J Nucl Med*. 2005;46:464–471.

84. Elgqvist J, Andersson H, Bäck T, et al. Therapeutic efficacy and tumor dose estimations in radioimmunotherapy of intraperitoneally growing OVCAR-3 cells in nude mice with [211]At-labeled monoclonal antibody MX35. *J Nucl Med*. 2005;46:1907–1915.

85. Stewart JS, Hird V, Snook D, et al. Intraperitoneal yttrium-90-labeled monoclonal antibody in ovarian cancer. *J Clin Oncol*. 1990;8: 1941–1950.

86. Grana C, Bartolomei M, Handkiewicz D, et al. Radioimmunotherapy in advanced ovarian cancer: is there a role for pre-targeting with (90)Y-biotin? *Gynecol Oncol*. 2004;93:691–698.

87. Epenetos AA, Hird V, Lambert H, et al. Long term survival of patients with advanced ovarian cancer treated with intraperitoneal radioimmunotherapy. *Int J Gynecol Cancer*. 2000;10:44–46.

88. Hird V, Stewart JS, Snook D, et al. Intraperitoneally administered ^{90}Y-labelled monoclonal antibodies as a third line of treatment in ovarian cancer. A phase 1–2 trial: problems encountered and possible solutions. *Br J Cancer Suppl*. 1990;10:48–51.

89. Maraveyas A, Snook D, Hird V, et al. Pharmacokinetics and toxicity of an ^{90}Y-CITC-DTPA-HMFG1 radioimmunoconjugate for intraperitoneal radioimmunotherapy of ovarian cancer. *Cancer*. 1994;73:1067–1075.

90. Meredith RF, Alvarez RD, Partridge EE, et al. Intraperitoneal radioimmunotherapy of ovarian cancer: a phase I study. *Cancer Biother Radiopharm*. 2001;16:305–315.

91. Stewart JS, Hird V, Sullivan M, et al. Intraperitoneal radioimmunotherapy for ovarian cancer. *Br J Obstet Gynaecol*. 1989;96: 529–536.

92. Crippa F, Bolis G, Seregni E, et al. Single-dose intraperitoneal radioimmunotherapy with the murine monoclonal antibody ^{131}I MOv18: clinical results in patients with minimal residual disease of ovarian cancer. *Eur J Cancer*. 1995;31A:686–690.

93. Stewart JS, Hird V, Snook D, et al. Intraperitoneal radioimmunotherapy for ovarian cancer: pharmacokinetics, toxicity, and efficacy of ^{131}I labeled monoclonal antibodies. *Int J Radiat Oncol Biol Phys*. 1989;16: 405–413.

94. McDevitt MR, Finn RD, Sgouros G, et al. An [225]Ac/[213]Bi generator system for therapeutic clinical applications: construction and operation. *Appl Radiat Isot*. 1999;50:895–904.

95. Song EY, Qu CF, Rizvi SM, et al. Bismuth-213 radioimmunotherapy with C595 anti-MUC1 monoclonal antibody in an ovarian cancer ascites model. *Cancer Biol Ther*. 2008;7:76–80.

96. Zalutsky MR, Vaidyanathan G. Astatine-211-labeled radiotherapeutics: an emerging approach to targeted alpha-particle radiotherapy. *Curr Pharm Des*. 2000;6:1433–1455.

97. Zalutsky MR, Reardon DA, Akabani G, et al. Clinical experience with alpha-particle emitting [211]At: treatment of recurrent brain tumor patients with [211]At-labeled chimeric antitenascin monoclonal antibody 81C6. *J Nucl Med*. 2008;49:30–38.

98. Tolmachev V, Carlsson J, Lundqvist H. A limiting factor for the progress of radionuclide-based cancer diagnostics and therapy—availability of suitable radionuclides. *Acta Oncol*. 2004;43:264–275.

99. Pozzi OR, Zalutsky MR. Radiopharmaceutical chemistry of targeted radiotherapeutics. Part 1: Effects of solvent on the degradation of radiohalogenation precursors by [211]At alpha-particles. *J Nucl Med*. 2005;46:700–706.

100. Visser GWM, Diemer EL, Kaspersen FM. The nature of the astatine-protein bond. *Int J Appl Radiat Isot*. 1981;32:905–912.

101. Zalutsky MR, Garg PK, Friedman HS, et al. Labeling monoclonal antibodies and F(ab')2 fragments with the alpha-particle-emitting nuclide astatine-211: preservation of immunoreactivity and in vivo localizing capacity. *Proc Natl Acad Sci U S A*. 1989;86:7149–7153.

102. Pozzi OR, Zalutsky MR. Radiopharmaceutical chemistry of targeted radiotherapeutics. Part 3: Alpha-particle-induced radiolytic effects on the chemical behavior of [211]At. *J Nucl Med*. 2007;48:1190–1196.

103. Lindegren S, Frost S, Bäck T, et al. Direct procedure for the production of [211]At-labeled antibodies with an epsilon-lysyl-3-(trimethylstannyl)benzamide immunoconjugate. *J Nucl Med*. 2008;49:1537–1545.

104. Wilbur DS, Chyan MK, Hamlin DK, et al. Reagents for astatination of biomolecules. Conjugation of anionic boron cage pendant groups to a protein provides a method for direct labeling that is stable to in vivo deastatination. *Bioconjug Chem*. 2007;18:1226–1240.

105. Wilbur DS, Chyan MK, Hamlin DK, et al. Reagents for astatination of biomolecules: comparison of the in vivo distribution and stability of some radioiodinated/astatinated benzamidyl and nido-carboranyl compounds. *Bioconjug Chem*. 2004;15:203–223.

106. Palm S, Humm JL, Rundqvist R, et al. Microdosimetry of astatine-211 single-cell irradiation: role of daughter polonium-211 diffusion. *Med Phys*. 2004;31:218–225.

107. Ranson M, Tian Z, Andronicos NM, et al. In vitro cytotoxicity of [213]Bi-labeled-plasminogen activator inhibitor type 2 (alpha-PAI-2) on human breast cancer cells. *Breast Cancer Res Treat*. 2002;71:149–159.

108. Li Y, Rizvi SMA, Ranson M, et al. [213]Bi-PAI2 conjugate selectively induces apoptosis in PC3 metastatic prostate cancer cell line and shows anti-cancer activity in a xenograft animal model. *Br J Cancer*. 2002;86:1197–1203.

109. Song YJ, Qu CF, Rizvi SMA, et al. Cytotoxicity of PAI2, C595 and Herceptin vectors labeled with the alpha-emitting radioisotope Bismuth-213 for ovarian cancer cell monolayers and clusters. *Cancer Lett*. 2006;234:176–183.

110. Allen BJ, Tian Z, Rizvi SM, et al. Preclinical studies of targeted alpha therapy for breast cancer using [213]Bi-labelled-plasminogen activator inhibitor type 2. *Br J Cancer*. 2003;88:944–950.

111. Qu CF, Song EY, Li Y, et al. Preclinical study of [213]Bi labeled PAI2 for the control of micrometastatic pancreatic cancer. *Clin Exp Metastasis*. 2005;22:575–586.

112. Nicholson S, Gooden CS, Hird V, et al. Radioimmunotherapy after chemotherapy compared to chemotherapy alone in the treatment of advanced ovarian cancer: a matched analysis. *Oncol Rep*. 1998;5: 223–226.

113. Sgouros G, Roeske JC, McDevitt MR, et al. MIRD pamphlet no. 22 (abridged): radiobiology and dosimetry of alpha-particle emitters for targeted radionuclide therapy. *J Nucl Med*. 2010;51:311–328.

114. Sgouros G. Bone marrow dosimetry for radioimmunotherapy: theoretical considerations. *J Nucl Med*. 1993;34:689–694.

115. Paganelli G, Magnani P, Fazio F. Pretargeting of carcinomas with the avidin-biotin system. *Int J Biol Markers*. 1993;8:155–159.

116. Frost S, Jensen H, Lindegren S. In vitro evaluation of avidin antibody pretargeting using [211]At-labeled and biotinylated poly-L-lysine as effector molecule. *Cancer.* 2010;116:1101–1110.
117. Allen BJ. Clinical trials of targeted alpha therapy for cancer. *Rev Recent Clin Trials.* 2008;3:185–191.
118. Gaze MN. The current status of targeted radiotherapy in clinical practice. *Phys Med Biol.* 1996;41:1895–1903.
119. Kassis AI, Adelstein J, Mariani G. Radiolabeled nucleoside analogs in cancer diagnosis and therapy. *G J Nucl Med.* 1996;40:301–319.
120. Goldenberg DM. Targeted therapy of cancer with radiolabeled antibodies. *J Nucl Med.* 2002;43:693–713.
121. Kairemo K. Radioimmunotherapy of solid cancers. *Acta Oncol.* 1996;35:343–355.
122. Muto MG, Kassis AI. Monoclonal antibodies used in the detection and treatment of epithelial ovarian cancer. *Cancer.* 1995;15:2016–2027.
123. Oyen WJ, Bodei L, Giammarile F, et al. Targeted therapy in nuclear medicine—current status and future prospects. *Ann Oncol.* 2007;18:1782–1792.
124. Andersson H, Elgqvist J, Horvath G, et al. Astatine-211-labeled antibodies for treatment of disseminated ovarian cancer: an overview of results in an ovarian tumor model. *Clin Cancer Res.* 2003;9:3914–3921.
125. Meredith RF, Buchsbaum DJ, Alvarez RD, et al. Brief overview of preclinical and clinical studies in the development of intraperitoneal radioimmunotherapy for ovarian cancer. *Clin Cancer Res.* 2007;13:5643–5645.
126. Gadducci A, Cosio S, Conte PF, et al. Consolidation and maintenance treatments for patients with advanced epithelial ovarian cancer in complete response after first-line chemotherapy: a review of the literature. *Crit Rev Oncol Hematol.* 2005;55:153–166.
127. Zalutsky MR, Reardon DA, Pozzi OR, et al. Targeted alpha-particle radiotherapy with [211]At-labeled monoclonal antibodies. *Nucl Med Biol.* 2007;34:779–785.
128. Goldenberg DM, Sharkey RM. Advances in cancer therapy with radiolabeled monoclonal antibodies. *Q J Nucl Med Mol Imaging.* 2006;50:248–264.
129. Chérel M, Davodeau F, Kraeber-Bodéré F, et al. Current status and perspectives in alpha radioimmunotherapy. *Q J Nucl Med Mol Imaging.* 2006;50:322–329.
130. Sharkey RM, Goldenberg DM. Perspectives on cancer therapy with radiolabeled monoclonal antibodies. *J Nucl Med.* 2005;46:115–127.
131. Mulford DA, Sheinberg DA, Jurcic JG. The promise of targeted α-particle therapy. *J Nucl Med.* 2005;46:199–204.
132. Imam SK. Advancements in cancer therapy with alpha-emitters: a review. *Int J Radiat Oncol Biol Phys.* 2001;51:271–278.
133. Allen BJ, Raja C, Rizvi S, et al. Targeted alpha therapy for cancer. *Phys Med Biol.* 2004;4916:3703–3712.
134. Crippa F. Radioimmunotherapy of ovarian cancer. *Int J Biol Markers.* 1993;8:187–191.
135. Moltoff C, Calame J, Pinedo H, et al. Human ovarian cancer xenografts in nude mice: characterization and analysis of antigen expression. *Int J Cancer.* 1991;47:72–79.
136. Armstrong DK, Bundy B, Wenzel L, et al. Intraperitoneal cisplatin and paclitaxel in ovarian cancer. *N Engl J Med.* 2006;354:34–43.
137. Ward BG, Mather SJ, Hawkins LR, et al. Localization of radioiodine conjugated to the monoclonal antibody HMFG2 in human ovarian carcinoma: assessment of intravenous and intraperitoneal routes of administration. *Cancer Res.* 1987;47:4719–4723.
138. Horan Hand P, Shrivastav S, Colcher D, et al. Pharmacokinetics of radiolabeled antibodies following intraperitoneal and intravenous administration in rodents, monkeys and humans. *Antibody Immunoconj Radiopharm.* 1989;2:241–255.

Cancer of the Head and Neck

Marika Nestor

■ INTRODUCTION

Targeted therapy is gaining momentum for use in systemic therapy and also for treatment of head and neck cancer. In recent years, developments in fields such as antigen screening, protein engineering, and cancer biology have facilitated the rational design of targeted pharmaceuticals, with monoclonal antibodies (mAbs) forming the most rapidly expanding category. More than 25% of all pharmacologic agents currently under development are antibody based (1,2). Several engineered mAb fragments and nontraditional antibody-like scaffolds are under development. Several mAbs have received the US Food and Drug Administration (FDA) approval, some of which (cetuximab and bevacizumab) are also used in strategies for treatment of head and neck cancer. Clinical success with these therapeutic mAbs has boosted research and development on new mAbs enormously.

Challenges, however, still exist. Results to date have demonstrated weak activity with these agents as monotherapy, suggesting that combinations of targeted agents and other therapies will be necessary to achieve improved outcomes. Heterogeneous antigen expression, restricted penetration of the targeting agent into the tumor, limited tumor toxicity, or even resistance to the targeting agent might be some of the problems encountered in a monotherapy setting. Targeted radionuclide therapy (TRT) may be a promising way to improve targeted treatment of head and neck cancer (3). The potential of TRT may be particularly great in head and neck cancer, due to the intrinsic radiosensitivity of this tumor type. By using radionuclides as "warheads," the problem of multidrug resistance can be avoided. Because most radionuclides in use are cytotoxic at a distance of several cell diameters, the need to target every single tumor cell is reduced (4). TRT may also provide a good foundation upon which to build rational biologic combination therapies. In the next few years, the use of TRT might offer new opportunities for further improvement of the therapeutic ratio that potentially may obviate or reduce the need for conventional cytotoxic therapies. No doubt, there is a huge potential for TRT in the treatment of head and neck cancer.

■ HEAD AND NECK CANCER

Cancer can occur in any of the more than 30 different tissues or organs in the head and neck area. Subclasses are carcinoma, sarcoma, lymphoma, and melanoma, of which carcinoma is the most common type. About 85% of all head and neck tumors are carcinomas. Head and neck squamous cell carcinomas (HNSCCs) arise from the mucosa of the upper aerodigestive tract. Mainly, they include cancers of the oral cavities, the pharynx, and the larynx. Worldwide, HNSCCs represent the fifth most common malignancy, with more than 600,000 new cases diagnosed annually, and this incidence is rising (5,6).

The use of tobacco and alcohol has long been recognized as major risk factors for HNSCC, whereas chewing of betel quid, immunosuppression conditions, human papilloma viral infection, denture wear, or genetic factors are potential risk factors. Other risk factors for head and neck cancers, which have been explored but require more evidence, include passive smoking, marijuana use, and low body mass index (7–11).

Spread pattern and prognosis are dictated by the local anatomy. HNSCCs may have an origin in many different subsites. Each anatomic site will have a different clinical presentation, locoregional spread, and prognosis. Tumor recurrence, secondary tumors, and comorbidities contribute to therapy failure, in which local recurrence is the most common cause of treatment failure and death. Early-stage HNSCC is usually curable, with a 5-year survival rate of approximately 80%. However, about 50% of patients present with locally advanced disease (stages III to IV), with a 5-year survival rate of approximately 50%. Approximately 25% of these patients develop distant metastases (stage IVC), although autopsy studies have shown incidences as high as 57% (12,13). Only about 25% of these patients survive past 5 years. For the 50% of patients that develop recurrent disease, the overall median survival typically ranges from 6 to 9 months, and the 1-year survival is less than 33%. Patients with recurrent and/or metastatic disease who progress after treatment have the worst prognosis, with a median overall survival of 3 to 4 months and a 1-year survival of less than 5% (Table 30.1) (14–18).

The most important prognostic indicator of HNSCC is the presence or absence of lymph node metastases in the neck (19). The risk of distant metastases is more dependent on the status of the lymph nodes than on the primary tumor size. The sentinel node is the lymph node most likely to harbor metastatic disease and can act as a source for further dissemination into the surrounding lymphatics or the bloodstream. Distant metastases can also develop as a result of direct hematogenous spread from the primary tumor. The most common sites of distant metastases

Table **30.1**	Current treatment of head and neck cancer				
Setting	Patients (%) (16,18)	Treatment Objective	Standard-of-Care Treatment[a]	Survival (16–18)	Rate (%) Years
Initial diagnosis					
Early stage (I/II)	33	Cure	Single modality: RT or surgery	82	5
Locally advanced (III/IVA/IVB)	52	Cure	Combined modality: concurrent RT and CT.[b] Surgery if necessary	52	5
Metastatic (IVC)	10	Palliation	CT[b]	27	5
Recurrent/refractory	50	Palliation	CT[b]	33/>5	1/1

[a]RT, radiotherapy; CT, chemotherapy.

[b]Chemotherapy includes the option of cetuximab as an alternative (locally advanced and refractory head and neck squamous cell carcinoma [HNSCC] or adjuvant [recurrent and/or metastatic HNSCC] to conventional chemotherapeutics.
Adapted from Gold KA, Lee HY, Kim ES. Targeted therapies in squamous cell carcinoma of the head and neck. *Cancer.* 2009;115(5):922–935.

are the lungs and bones. Hepatic and brain metastases occur less frequently (20).

Evaluation of the neck is based on manual palpation. This method, however, is far from reliable for the detection of lymph node metastases. Although modern imaging techniques such as computed tomography, magnetic resonance imaging, ultrasound, and ultrasound-guided fine-needle aspiration cytology are more reliable than palpation, they also leave much room for improvement (21). Furthermore, sentinel lymph node biopsy is becoming an increasingly important alternative to elective neck dissection for staging clinically negative (N0) necks, showing high sensitivities in early-stage HNSCC (22).

Therapy for HNSCC presents many challenges since the head and neck region has many critical structures. Tumor or therapy can cause damage to tissues such as brain, brain stem, spinal cord, vertebral bodies, cranial nerves, carotid artery, pharynx, mandible, salivary glands, larynx, and pharynx, which can cause structural, cosmetic, and functional deficits that negatively impact quality of life. Therapy-related adverse events also have particular impact in HNSCC, in which several physical or mental conditions can complicate toxicity management, hinder treatment compliance, and have an adverse effect on survival rates (23,24). Generally, patients with stages I and II disease are treated with single local modalities such as surgery or radiation therapy (RT). Standard treatments for patients with advanced disease include surgical resection followed by adjuvant chemoradiotherapy for resectable, locally advanced HNSCC, or chemotherapy and/or radiation for unresectable disease (9). For patients with recurrent/metastatic disease, few effective treatment options other than palliative chemotherapy are available. For patients who have disease that progresses after platinum-based therapy, options are limited to modestly active agents or best supportive care (25).

Despite substantial laboratory and clinical efforts, survival rates of patients with advanced-stage head and neck

cancer appear to have plateaued, and local recurrences continue to occur at unacceptable rates. The use of more aggressive cytotoxic therapy may increase local control and survival but is associated with more significant acute and late toxicities. As fewer patients die from uncontrolled disease in the head and neck, more are exposed to the risk of disseminated disease below the clavicles (26). Among current therapy refinements, altered fractionation radiotherapy, integration of chemotherapy with radiotherapy, intensity-modulated radiotherapy, and the introduction of targeted biologic therapy can be found. Altered fractionation radiotherapy may improve overall survival and locoregional control compared with conventional (once-daily, standard fractionation) delivery. Intensity-modulated radiotherapy is another recent advancement that uses multiple-shaped radiation beams, which increases the dose delivered to tumor tissue while limiting exposure/scatter to normal structures. Advances such as the use of induction chemotherapy, concurrent chemotherapy and radiotherapy, and targeted therapy show promise to further improve outcomes. Recent incorporation of targeted therapies may also improve current therapy options and allow more tolerable treatment regimens. There is obviously a great demand for a systemic treatment effective in locating or treating metastases at distant sites and minimal residual disease at the local and regional level (27,28).

There are many potential diagnostic and therapeutic applications for radioimmunoconjugates. Depending which radiolabel is used, a targeting agent may be applied as an efficient and safe way to assess target expression, for accumulation in tumor lesions and normal tissues, to provide information about ideal dosing, to identify patients with the highest chance of treatment benefit, and finally to eradicate tumor cells. TRT of head and neck cancer is a realistic approach that contributes to a more effective treatment of advanced-stage disease (3). Small-volume disease might be the most suitable setting for TRT in solid cancers, as it has been demonstrated that mAb uptake and dose delivery are approximately four times higher in small-volume tumors (1 cm^3) than in large-volume tumors (50 cm^3) (29). Therefore, adjuvant treatment of patients who have been treated for their primary tumor, but who are at a high risk of developing locoregional recurrences and distant metastases, could be a very successful application for TRT. Furthermore, the combination of TRT with other molecular-targeted therapies, by additive or even synergistic effects, may further improve the benefits of therapy for patients with HNSCC without increasing toxicity.

ANTIGEN TARGETS

Targeted treatments are dependent on knowledge of suitable molecular targets and the relationships between their expression, pathogenesis, and clinical outcome. For TRT to be effective, the targeted antigen needs to be accessible to the antibody and should not be shed into circulation. The antigen must also have a high and preferably homogeneous expression in the tumor tissue, but a low or no expression in normal tissue, to obtain a high uptake ratio of tumor to healthy tissue (30).

Squamous-associated antigens are generally expressed in both HNSCC and normal squamous epithelia. Among these, the E48 (hLy-6D) and CD44v6 antigens have been most extensively studied. The E48 antigen is a 16- to 22-kDa glycosylphosphatidylinositol-anchored surface antigen thought to regulate interaction parameters between endothelial cells and HNSCC, but it has also been used as a target for colorectal cancer (31,32). This antigen is homogeneously expressed in approximately 70% of HNSCC tumors (33). However, since 30% of tumors have shown heterogeneous expression of this antigen, the applicability of this target may be limited (34). The CD44v6 antigen is an isoform of the membrane-associated glycoprotein CD44. It has been suggested to be involved in tumor formation, tumor cell invasion, metastasis formation, and cancer stem cell properties (35–38). Homogeneous expression of CD44v6 has been observed in a majority of primary and metastatic squamous cell carcinomas (SCCs) (in 96% of the HNSCC tumors, the mAb U36-defined CD44v6 antigen was expressed by more than 50% of the cells), whereas expression in nonmalignant tissues is essentially restricted to a subset of epithelia (39,40). Soluble v6-containing CD44 fragments have also been detected in the blood of cancer patients as well as of healthy individuals (41,42). The difference in expression between healthy and malignant cells makes the CD44v6 antigen an attractive target for antibody-based therapy. One drawback of these antigens, however, is the expression in normal squamous epithelia, which might cause uptake of radioactivity in normal oral mucosa. This can abrogate tumor detection in the head and neck areas when applied for imaging, while in TRT, mucositis might occur (43,44). In a phase 1 trial using the immunoconjugate bivatuzumab mertansine, consisting of a highly potent antimicrotubule agent coupled to an mAb against CD44v6, binding to

CD44v6 on skin keratinocytes mediated serious skin toxicity with a fatal outcome, leading to the termination of the development program of bivatuzumab mertansine (45). Instead, a fundamentally different approach, such as TRT, may be more promising toward this target, as the use of a radionuclide with a suitable half-life and energy can avoid skin toxicity.

The epidermal growth factor receptor (EGFR) has emerged as a promising antigen in HNSCC. EGFR is a member of the ErbB family, consisting of the EGFR (EGFR/erbB-1/HER1), HER2 (neu/erbB-2), HER3 (erbB-3), and HER4 (erbB-4). These are type 1 tyrosine kinase receptors and are important for mediating signals to control proliferation and differentiation (46). EGFR is a transmembrane cell-surface receptor found primarily on cells of epithelial origin. Overexpression occurs in up to 90% of HNSCC, and is also common in breast cancer, ovarian cancer, prostate cancer, bladder cancer, glioblastoma, and non-small-cell lung cancer. It has also been found to play a significant role in the progression of several human malignancies (47,48). EGFR has been shown to be essential for the upregulation of tumor cell proliferation, differentiation, and survival, and is associated with worse outcome in terms of locoregional tumor control, overall survival, and resistance to therapy (49–51). In addition, the level of EGFR expression has been shown to be inversely related to the effectiveness of RT to control cancer cell growth (52). Blocking of EGFR may interfere with signal transduction pathways and can result in disease stabilization and increased survival for patients with HNSCC. Studies have indicated that the expression of EGFR is higher in HNSCC tumor tissue versus normal tissue. One important exception is the expression of EGFRs in liver hepatocytes, which express about 10^5 to 10^6 EGFRs per cell (53,54). The expression in several normal tissues together with an occasional heterogenous reaction pattern with HNSCC may be a limitation for TRT.

Another appealing therapeutic approach is to target tumor vasculature. Angiogenesis is required for tumor progression and metastasis, and inhibiting this process has become an intensive focus of clinical investigation (55,56). This approach might be especially attractive since these markers are expressed by a diversity of tumor types and are well accessible for mAbs. Such targets are the vascular endothelial growth factor (VEGF) family, VEGF receptors, and the extra-domain B (EDB) of fibronectin. VEGF expression is upregulated in many tumors, favoring tumor vascularization and growth, and has been demonstrated to be highly correlated with worse prognosis in patients with HNSCC (57). Since VEGF is often bound to the extracellular matrix, both VEGF factors and its receptors may be possible TRT targets. The EDB-containing isoform of fibronectin is a marker of tumor angiogenesis, abundantly expressed around the neovasculature and in the stroma of the majority of malignant tumors of the head and neck. It is undetectable in normal tissues, with the exception of tissues undergoing physiologic remodeling and wound healing (58). In a study of 82 head and neck tissue biopsy specimens, a strong positive staining with the anti-EDB L19 antibody could be observed in 87% of the investigated malignant tumors, in only 38% of the benign tumors, and in 20% of the nontumoral lesions (59). Also for this category of antigens, heterogenous tumor expression as well as expression in normal tissues such as ovaries and endometrial tissues might form a limitation for TRT (60).

Other tumor cell and tumor stroma antigens, such as the A1 domain of tenascin-C, the tumor and cancer stem cell antigen EpCAM (epithelial cell adhesion molecule), the insulin growth factor type-1 receptor, and the hepatocyte growth factor receptor c-Met, have also shown promise as HNSCC targets, and their applicability for TRT warrants further evaluations (61–65).

■ TARGETING VECTORS

Targeting vectors are often antibodies or antibody derivatives. The progression in antibody engineering has enabled the production of murine, chimeric, humanized, or fully human antibodies for clinical use. The size of the targeting agent affects the residence time in the circulation. Small molecules are filtrated in glomerulus in the kidneys, whereas larger molecules will have a longer circulation time. Intact mAbs have a residence time in humans ranging from a few days to weeks, which results in optimal tumor-to-nontumor ratios at 2 to 4 days postinjection. Besides intact mAb molecules (molecular weight $\approx$150 kDa), several types of antibody fragments and engineered variants can be used as targeting vectors. Such constructs are F(ab')$_2$, Fab', single-chain Fv (scFv), and the covalent dimers (scFv)$_2$, diabodies, and minibodies (molecular weights ranging from 25 to 100 kDa). For a schematic picture of an immunoglobulin G (IgG) antibody and some of its derivatives, see Figure 30.1. Furthermore, several types of proteins based on nontraditional scaffolds, such as domain antibodies, affibodies, nanobodies, and anticalins, can be produced. Generally, intact mAbs are the choice for therapy, while other formats may be more suitable for diagnosis. A suitable mAb for adjuvant cancer therapy needs to accumulate selectively and to a high level in the tumor after administration to the patient, and should be able to target all tumor deposits, including tumor nodules, malignant cell clusters, and single tumor cells.

So far, more than 30 antibodies and antibody fragments directed against head and neck cancer have been described in the literature (21). However, most of these mAbs have demonstrated considerable limitations for application in tumor targeting, many showing considerable cross-reactivity with normal tissues. Also, despite promising preclinical results, it may appear at an early stage of clinical studies that the mAb is unsuitable for TRT. It is also possible that an antibody, although not selective enough for application in imaging or TRT, holds promise for other therapeutic approaches. To date, only a few mAbs have been administered in radioimmunoscintigraphy studies in HNSCC patients, and even less in TRT (66–88) studies (Table 30.2).

One extensively studied group of antibodies is predominantly reactive with SCC. Among these, the best-qualified antibodies for TRT are variants of U36 and BIWA. The murine mAbs U36 and BIWA-1 (formerly VFF18), binding to overlapping epitopes in the variable domain v6 of the cell-surface antigen CD44, were the first to be constructed. Eventually, chimeric derivatives of U36 (cMAb U36) and BIWA-1 (BIWA-2), as well as two humanized derivatives of BIWA-1 (BIWA-4 and BIWA-8), were produced. However, BIWA-1 showed complex formation with sCD44v6 present in the blood and heterogeneous uptake throughout the tumor, possibly related to the high affinity of this mAb (85). Another problem appeared to be the immunogenicity of these mAbs (40% human antichimeric antibody responses for cMAb U36 and 90% human antimouse antibody responses for BIWA-1). This led to the construction of the two humanized derivatives, and the intermediate-affinity hMAb BIWA-4 (bivatuzumab) was eventually selected as a candidate for further clinical development (39,89–91).

Blockade of EGFR pathways has been investigated as a rational anticancer strategy given the high numbers of EGFRs found in HNSCC. Several anti-EGFR agents have been developed in HNSCC, including mAbs, that target the extracellular domain of EGFR, such as cetuximab, panitumumab, and zalutumumab (92–97). Cetuximab (IMC-225, Erbitux) (92) is currently approved by the FDA as monotherapy or in combination with external radiotherapy for locally advanced head and neck cancer (93,98,99). This makes it the first and, currently, the only commercial targeted biologic available for use in head and neck cancer. Cetuximab binds to the extracellular domain of the receptor, competing with

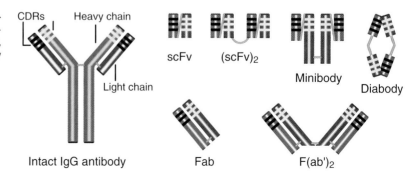

FIGURE 30.1 **A schematic representation of an immunoglobulin G antibody and some of its derivatives.** Fab and F(ab')$_2$ fragments are produced by enzymatic degradation, whereas ScFv, (ScFv)$_2$, diabodies, and minibodies are produced by antibody engineering.

Table **30.2** Agents used for radioimmunotargeting in HNSCC patients

Targeting Agent	Target	Radiolabel	Reference
Anti-CEA mAb IgG/F(ab')$_2$	Carcinoembryonic antigen	^{90}Y-biotin, ^{111}In-biotin, ^{131}I, ^{111}In	Paganelli et al. (66), Tranter et al. (67), Kairemo and Hopsu (68,69), Timon et al. (70), De Rossi et al. (71)
Anti-EGFR mAb	EGFR	^{111}In	Soo et al. (72)
mAb C225 (cetuximab)	EGFR	^{99m}Tc-EC	Schechte et al. (73)
mAb 174H.64	Cytokeratin-associated antigen	^{99m}Tc	Baum et al. (74), Heissler et al. (75), Adamietz et al. (76)
cMAb SF-25	Anti-SF-25	^{99m}Tc	de Bree et al. (34)
mMAb 323/A3 F(ab')$_2$	Epithelial cell adhesion molecule	^{99m}Tc	de Bree et al. (34)
mMAb K928	Anti-K928	^{99m}Tc	de Bree et al. (34)
mMAb E48 IgG/F(ab')$_2$	hLy-6D	^{99m}Tc	van Dongen et al. (77), de Bree et al. (78), de Bree et al. (79), de Bree et al. (80)
mMAb U36	CD44v6	^{99m}Tc	de Bree et al. (81), de Bree et al. (80)
cMAb U36	CD44v6	^{99m}Tc, ^{89}Zr, ^{186}Re	Colnot et al. (82), Borjesson et al. (83), Colnot et al. (82), Colnot et al. (84)
mMAb BIWA-1	CD44v6	^{99m}Tc	Stroomer et al. (85)
hMAb BIWA-4	CD44v6	^{99m}Tc, ^{186}Re	Colnot et al. (86), Borjesson et al. (87)
L19 (scFv)$_2$	Extra-domain B of fibronectin	^{123}I	Birchler et al. (88)

EGFR, epidermal growth factor receptor; HNSCC, head and neck squamous cell carcinoma.
Modified from Borjesson PK, Postema EJ, de Bree R, et al. Radioimmunodetection and radioimmunotherapy of head and neck cancer. *Oral Oncol.* 2004;40(8):761–772.

ligand binding and preventing receptor tyrosine kinase activation (100,101). This antibody has been shown to inhibit the growth of several EGFR-overexpressing cell lines of various histologies through cell cycle arrest, antiangiogenesis, apoptosis, and inhibition of tumor cell invasion and metastasis (102,103). Treatment with cetuximab has been shown to enhance the antitumor activity of several chemotherapeutic drugs in preclinical studies (95). In phase II and III studies, where cetuximab is used first or second line in combination with chemotherapy, a significant response has been shown in patients with SCC of the head and neck, non-small-cell lung cancer, and pancreatic cancer (28). Thus, cetuximab is also emerging as a promising new therapy to be used in combination with existing therapies for the treatment of several cancers. The combination of cetuximab and radiation is especially appealing. Recent data have shown that cetuximab may prevent the activation of deoxyribonucleic acid (DNA) repair mechanisms, and several preclinical studies have demonstrated that cetuximab augments the antitumor effects of both radiotherapy and conventional chemotherapeutics (101,104–107).

The targeted destruction of tumor vasculature is another appealing approach for TRT. Many ongoing trials are testing the potential role of angiogenesis inhibitors in HNSCC in combination with conventional approaches and with other targeted agents. One well-developed angiogenesis inhibitor

is the mAb bevacizumab, targeting the VEFG. It has FDA-approved indications in advanced colorectal, lung, and breast cancer and is in late-stage development in HNSCC (14). For TRT applications, different antibody formats targeting the EDB of fibronectin have recently emerged as interesting vectors. Several therapeutic derivatives of the human recombinant antibody fragment L19 scFv targeting EDB have been constructed, such as a complete human IgG1 and a bispecific L19 consisting of two L19 scFvs to form a divalent scFv small immunoprotein (L19-SIP) (108,109). At present, the therapeutic properties of ^{131}I-L19-SIP are being investigated in preclinical trials (61).

■ RADIONUCLIDES

Understanding that mAbs are currently the most reasonable choice for selective targeting of HNSCC and that the immune response to unconjugated antibodies is minimal in solid tumors, the next question is how to best "arm" these constructs. The choice of the radionuclide to be coupled to the mAb depends on the antibody used, antigen properties, and what targeting concept is to be considered. General factors such as decay half-life, type and energy spectrum of emitted radiation, and cost and availability of the nuclide must be considered. Additionally, the nuclide must match the properties of the targeting vehicle. When choosing a suitable nuclide for TRT, factors such as properties of the conjugate, radiation, and size of the tumor that is to be targeted must also be considered. The most commonly used radionuclides in TRT are beta-emitters, although Auger electron-emitting radionuclides and alpha-emitters can also be used. The path length of beta-particles is several millimeters, which will result in radiation from one targeted cell to hit surrounding cells, including poorly accessible cells or antigen-negative cells. In this fashion, there is no need to target every single tumor cell. On the other hand, the risk of irradiating adjacent healthy tissue will increase. Iodine-131 (^{131}I) and yttrium-90 (^{90}Y) are commonly used beta-emitters in TRT. Rhenium-186 (^{186}Re), rhenium-188 (^{188}Re), copper-67 (^{67}Cu), and lutetium-177 (^{177}Lu) are beta-emitters that have been considered for TRT more recently. The different path lengths make ^{177}Lu, ^{67}Cu, ^{131}I, and ^{186}Re particularly well suited for eradication of minimal residual disease, while ^{188}Re and ^{90}Y are the radionuclides of choice for treatment of bulky tumors (110,111).

If the objective is to eradicate single tumor cells, or very small cell clusters (up to a few hundred cells), an alpha-emitting nuclide might be preferred. Due to their short range, alpha-particles deposit all their energy within a few cell diameters from the location of the decay, thus sparing surrounding healthy tissues. Moreover, the high LET (linear energy transfer) of alpha-particles greatly increases the probability of double-strand breaks and cell death of the targeted cell and its closest neighbors (112). Among the alpha-emitting nuclides available, astatine-211 (^{211}At) has the most appropriate half-life (7.2 hours) for tumor targeting and has been successfully coupled to antibodies in a number of previous studies (112,113).

Radionuclides that emit Auger electrons might be an alternative for eradicating single tumor cells. However, Auger electrons have a very short range (nanometers), and need to be located in the nucleus or integrated into the DNA molecule itself in order to be cytotoxic.

Several radionuclide conjugates have been successfully created for therapeutic applications in HNSCC. For example, the cMAb U36 has been labeled with the alpha-emitter ^{211}At, as well as beta-emitters ^{131}I, ^{177}Lu, and ^{186}Re and the Auger emitters ^{125}I and ^{111}In in preclinical studies (89,114–117). A phase I therapy study was conducted to determine the safety, maximum tolerated dose (MTD), pharmacokinetics, dosimetry, immunogenicity, and therapeutic potential of ^{186}Re-cMAb U36. The study showed that ^{186}Re-cMAb U36 could be safely administered, with dose-limiting myelotoxicity at 41 mCi/m^2. The bone marrow doses ranged from 0.7 to 1.1 Gy. The MTD was established at 27 mCi/m^2 (82,118). In another study, further dose escalation in TRT was evaluated using a facile method of reinfusion of granulocyte colony-stimulating factor (G-CSF)-stimulated unprocessed whole blood. Results indicated that a doubling of the maximum tolerated activity and bone marrow dose of ^{186}Re-cMAb U36 could be achieved using this method (84).

mAbs BIWA-1, BIWA-2, BIWA-4, and BIWA-8 have been successfully labeled with ^{186}Re in preclinical studies (89). The safety and targeting potential of BIWA-1 was also assessed in 12 HNSCC patients by preoperative administration of ^{99m}Tc-labeled mAb BIWA-1 (85). Studies were continued with the humanized derivative BIWA-4. As a prelude to radioimmunotherapy (RIT), the safety, tumor-targeting potential, pharmacokinetics, and immunogenicity of ^{99m}Tc-labeled BIWA-4 in patients undergoing operations for primary HNSCC were evaluated, demonstrating the highest tumor uptake at the 50-mg dose (86). In a phase I TRT study, the safety, MTD, pharmacokinetics, immunogenicity, and therapeutic potential of ^{186}Re-labeled BIWA-4 on patients with inoperable recurrent or metastatic head and neck cancer were assessed. Dosimetric analysis of the data showed that the range of doses to normal organs seemed to be well within acceptable and safe limits. The only significant manifestations of toxicity were dose-limiting myelotoxicity consisting of thrombo- and leukocytopenia and, to a lesser extent, grade 2 oral mucositis. Grade 4 myelotoxicity was seen in two patients treated with 60 mCi/m^2. The MTD was established at 50 mCi/m^2, at which level dose-limiting myelotoxicity was seen in one of six patients (87,119).

The antibody variant L19-SIP has been radiolabeled with two candidate radionuclides for RIT, ^{177}Lu and ^{131}I, and evaluated in HNSCC tumor–bearing mice, in which ^{131}I-L19-SIP appeared most efficacious (120). As a base for future therapeutical applications in human beings, tumor targeting in HNSCC patients was evaluated using the ^{123}I-radiolabeled L19 (scFv)$_2$ antibody in a phase I/II clinical study. Five patients were injected with the conjugate and underwent scintigraphic detection with single-photon emission tomography with computerized tomography. Successful targeting of the primary tumor was achieved in four of five patients, comparable to positron emission tomography imaging. No side effects were observed (88).

PRECLINICAL AND CLINICAL EXPERIENCES

Preclinical studies

Several radiolabeled cMAb U36 conjugates have been created and assessed preclinically. For example, the potential of cMAb U36 labeled with the therapeutically interesting radiohalogens ^{211}At and ^{131}I was evaluated in cell toxicity assays. Studies demonstrated a dose-dependent and antigen-specific cellular toxicity for ^{211}At-cMAb U36, with about 10% cell survival at 50 decays per cell. As expected, the ^{131}I-labeled conjugate was less efficient in this monolayer setting, with a surviving cell fraction of about 50% at 55 decays per cell (116). These results indicate that ^{211}At-cMAb U36 might be a promising future candidate for eradicating HNSCC micrometastases in vivo. Possible disadvantages are the high cost and short physical half-life of this radionuclide.

A combination approach of TRT and anti-EGFR therapy has also been assessed preclinically, using ^{186}Re-labeled mAb U36 in combination with the anti-EGFR mAb 425. The combination treatment increased tumor growth delay as well as the maximum decrease in tumor volume in comparison to treatment with ^{186}Re-labeled mAb U36 or mAb 425 alone, without increase in toxicity (121). This study demonstrated both the efficacy of ^{186}Re-labeled mAb U36 and the potential for TRT anti-EGFR combination treatments.

The potential of TRT with the human mAb L19-SIP, directed against the EDB domain of fibronectin, has also been evaluated preclinically for treatment of HNSCC. L19-SIP was radiolabeled with two candidate radionuclides for RIT, ^{177}Lu and ^{131}I, and was evaluated in HNSCC-bearing nude mice. Radioiodinated L19-SIP performed better than ^{177}Lu-L19-SIP and was further exploited by assessing the efficacy of TRT with injected ^{131}I-L19-SIP, either alone or in combination with unlabeled cetuximab. TRT at the MTD level of 74 MBq caused significant tumor growth delay and improved survival. The best survival and cure rates were obtained, however, when TRT and cetuximab were combined, without increase in toxicity (Fig. 30.2) (120).

The mAb C215, targeting the transmembrane protein EpCAM, has been radiolabeled with ^{131}I and evaluated in HNSCC xenografts. For therapeutic approaches, 5, 15, or 25 MBq ^{131}I-labeled mAb was injected as a single bolus into tumor-bearing mice. Tumor growth was delayed in the groups receiving either 15 or 25 MBq ^{131}I-C215 relative to control groups and the 5 MBq group. However, animals in the high-dose groups suffered from treatment-related toxicity, which led to body weight loss of more than 20%, demonstrating the need to further increase efficacy and reduce toxicity of this therapeutic approach (122).

Clinical experiences

In the first clinical TRT trial using ^{186}Re-cMAb U36, 13 patients with recurrent or metastatic HNSCC were given a single dose of ^{186}Re-cMAb U36 (12 or 52 mg) in radiation dose-escalating steps of 0.4, 1.0, and 1.5 GBq/m^2. Administration was well tolerated, and excellent targeting of tumor lesions was seen in all patients (Fig. 30.3). A marked reduction in tumor size was observed in two patients with dose-limiting

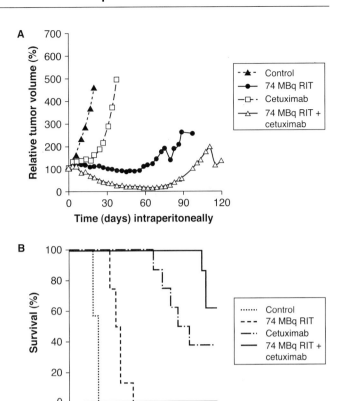

FIGURE 30.2 Mean tumor volume (A) and survival (B) of FaDu xenograft–bearing nude mice after intraperitoneal injection of ^{131}I-L19-SIP at day 0, cetuximab (1 mg given two times a week intraperitoneally for 4 weeks), or both. Standard deviations have been omitted for the sake of clarity. (Reprinted from Tijink BM, Neri D, Leemans CR, et al. Radioimmunotherapy of head and neck cancer xenografts using ^{131}I-labeled antibody L19-SIP for selective targeting of tumor vasculature. *J Nucl Med.* 2006;47(7):1127–1135.)

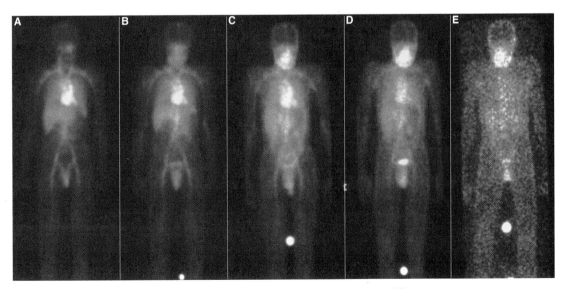

FIGURE 30.3 Whole-body scans of patient 4 acquired within 2 hours after administration of ^{186}Re-cMAb U36 and after 21, 72, and 144 hours and after 2 weeks. Immediately after injection, most prominent activity is in blood pool. This activity remains high up to 72 hours after injection. Relative uptake of radioimmunoconjugate in tumor in right oropharynx increases over time. Tumor becomes better delineated as background activity decreases. (Reprinted from Colnot DR, Quak JJ, Roos JC, et al. Phase I therapy study of ^{186}Re-labeled chimeric monoclonal antibody U36 in patients with squamous cell carcinoma of the head and neck. *J Nucl Med.* 2000;41(12):1999–2010.) (Please see Color Insert).

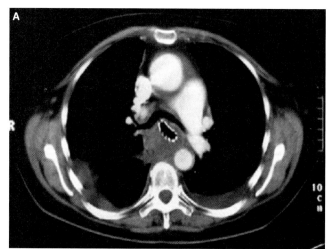

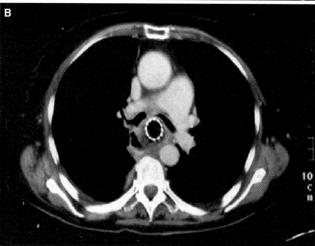

FIGURE 30.4 A: CT scan of patient 13 shows large tumor originating from esophagus compressing stent that was placed for palliation 12 months before RIT. B: CT scan of the same patient 3 weeks after administration of 2.15 GBq [186]Re-cMAb U36. Sixty percent decrease in tumor size was observed as well as relaxation of stent. (Reprinted from Colnot DR, Quak JJ, Roos JC, et al. Phase I therapy study of [186]Re-labeled chimeric monoclonal antibody U36 in patients with squamous cell carcinoma of the head and neck. *J Nucl Med.* 2000; 41(12):1999–2010.)

myelotoxicity (Fig. 30.4), and another patient showed stable disease for 6 months after treatment at the MTD (82,118), indicating that TRT with [186]Re-cMAb U36 in this form occasionally can cause antitumor effects. However, the radiation delivery to the lesions must be increased several times for complete tumor eradication.

To improve the potential of TRT with [186]Re-cMAb U36, a facile method of reinfusion of G-CSF-stimulated unprocessed whole blood was assessed in nine patients with recurrent or metastatic HNSCC. With this technique, the administered dose of [186]Re-cMAb U36 could be doubled, while no myelotoxicity greater than grade 3 was observed. Stable disease, ranging from 3 to 7 months, was observed in five of nine patients, including all three patients treated at the highest dose level (84).

Another way to increase the administered activity dose is by reduction of the circulation time of the radioactivity.

A possible way to do so was described by Paganelli et al. in 1998 (66), who successfully treated a case of locally advanced oropharyngeal carcinoma with a combination of various treatments including surgery, radiochemotherapy, and three-step TRT, with the avidin biotin pretargeting system. Nonradioactive biotinylated anti–carcinoembryonic antigen mAbs were infused, followed by administration of streptavidin. As the last step in this pretargeting approach, 70 mCi of ^{90}Y-DOTA-biotin was infused. The patient responded with a complete remission to TRT, and no hematologic toxicity was observed.

In a phase I study, the intermediate-affinity humanized mAb BIWA-4 (bivatuzumab) was labeled with [186]Re and studied in patients with recurrent HNSCC (87). Twenty patients received a single dose of [186]Re-labeled BIWA-4 in radiation dose-escalation steps of 20, 30, 40, 50, and 60 mCi/m^2. Administrations were well tolerated, and targeting of tumor lesions proved to be excellent (Fig. 30.5). A human antihuman antibody response was observed in only two patients, indicating that BIWA-4 can be used for repeated administrations. Stable disease, varying between 6 and 21 weeks, was observed in three of six patients treated at the MTD level. The fact that antitumor effects were seen in incurable patients with bulky disease is promising for further TRT studies with [186]Re-BIWA-4, especially in an adjuvant setting.

■ FUTURE DIRECTIONS

The appealing concept of systemically delivering targeted radiotherapy for the treatment of cancer has had a history of more than 50 years. Since then, a great number of molecular targets have been identified, and huge progress has been made in understanding the complexity and difficulties of this treatment modality. TRT is an effective addition to the arsenal against cancer for disseminated or metastatic disease. To date, TRT has emerged as an accepted treatment in lymphoma as well as neuroendocrine tumors. The therapeutic application of radiolabeled mAbs in solid tumors, however, has met considerable difficulties. In many clinical TRT studies, patients have suffered from advanced, mostly bulky disease, which is a highly unfavorable setting for the application of radiolabeled antibodies. Therefore, the modest therapeutic results of TRT in HNSCC patients with solid cancers may leave room for qualified optimism, and might suggest that TRT in patients with small-volume disease may be much more effective.

There is, however, much room for improvement. Appropriate patient selection is one important factor that may determine the eventual success of TRT. Here, pretherapy imaging may be used to predict patient response. This technique might be particularly suited to find routes to maximum synergism when mAb therapy is combined with other treatment modalities such as chemo- and radiotherapy (123). Several ways of increasing MTD without increasing toxicity are being explored. One option is to combine myeloablative doses of radiolabeled mAbs with stem cell

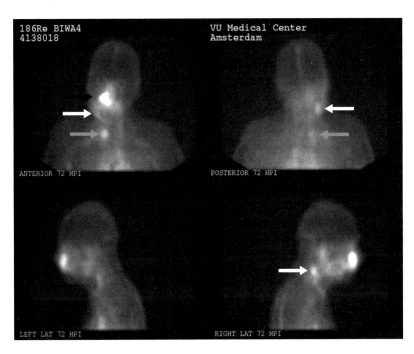

FIGURE 30.5 Frontal (*APPA*) and lateral (left and right) planar image of the head and neck region of patient after administration of [186]Re-BIWA-4. Accumulation of radiolabeled hMAb BIWA-4 is visible in tumor recurrence in the right nasal cavity and maxillary sinus (*black arrows*) and in two nodal metastases in the neck (*white arrows*, mid-neck; *grey arrows*, low neck). It should be noted that the right neck disease is not identified on the left lateral view due to patient attenuation. (Reprinted and modified from Borjesson PK, Postema EJ, Roos JC, et al. Phase I therapy study with [186]Re-labeled humanized monoclonal antibody BIWA-4 (bivatuzumab) in patients with head and neck squamous cell carcinoma. *Clin Cancer Res.* 2003; 9(10, pt 2):3961S–3972S.) (Please see Color Insert).

transplantation (124). Alternatively, stem cell–containing whole blood can be harvested, without separation of the stem cells from the blood (84). Another way to increase the administered activity dose is by reducing the circulation time of radioactivity, for example, by using a pretargeting approach (125). Other approaches to maximize the therapeutic index are fractionation, combined modality treatment, extracorporeal techniques and development of new approaches such as small molecules, and antibody alternatives (27). The use of alpha-emitting radionuclides is another interesting possibility for specific diseases, such as single disseminated tumor cells or small tumor clusters. Furthermore, the combination of TRT with other targeted therapies might be particularly attractive for application in head and neck cancer, by additive or even synergistic effects. Molecular-targeted therapies already belong to the treatment strategy for patients with HNSCC, and novel molecular targets and corresponding therapies continue to emerge. Agents such as the anti-EGFR mAb cetuximab and the proteasome inhibitor bortezomib have been shown to radiosensitize tumor cells, and the promise of combining TRT with such agents has been shown in several preclinical studies (126).

Although much remains to be elucidated, these efforts, combined with promising early-phase data in preclinical and clinical settings, promise advances of TRT in the near future that should further improve survival for patients with head and neck cancer.

■ REFERENCES

1. Carter P. Improving the efficacy of antibody-based cancer therapies. *Nat Rev Cancer.* 2001;1(2):118–129.
2. Reff ME, Hariharan K, Braslawsky G. Future of monoclonal antibodies in the treatment of hematologic malignancies. *Cancer Control.* 2002;9(2):152–166.
3. Potamianos S, Varvarigou AD, Archimandritis SC. Radioimmunoscintigraphy and radioimmunotherapy in cancer: principles and application. *Anticancer Res.* 2000;20(2A):925–948.
4. Carlsson J, Forssell Aronsson E, Hietala SO, et al. Tumour therapy with radionuclides: assessment of progress and problems. *Radiother Oncol.* 2003;66(2):107–117.
5. Parkin DM, Bray F, Ferlay J, et al. Global cancer statistics, 2002. *CA Cancer J Clin.* 2005;55(2):74–108.
6. Parkin DM, Bray F, Ferlay J, et al. Estimating the world cancer burden: Globocan 2000. *Int J Cancer.* 2001;94(2):153–156.
7. Browman GP, Wong G, Hodson I, et al. Influence of cigarette smoking on the efficacy of radiation therapy in head and neck cancer. *N Engl J Med.* 1993;328(3):159–163.
8. Weinberger PM, Yu Z, Haffty BG, et al. Molecular classification identifies a subset of human papillomavirus–associated oropharyngeal cancers with favorable prognosis. *J Clin Oncol.* 2006;24(5):736–747.
9. Chin D, Boyle GM, Porceddu S, et al. Head and neck cancer: past, present and future. *Expert Rev Anticancer Ther.* 2006;6(7):1111–1118.
10. Hashibe M, Straif K, Tashkin DP, et al. Epidemiologic review of marijuana use and cancer risk. *Alcohol.* 2005;35(3):265–275.
11. Lee YC, Boffetta P, Sturgis EM, et al. Involuntary smoking and head and neck cancer risk: pooled analysis in the International Head and Neck Cancer Epidemiology Consortium. *Cancer Epidemiol Biomarkers Prev.* 2008;17(8):1974–1981.
12. Dennington ML, Carter DR, Meyers AD. Distant metastases in head and neck epidermoid carcinoma. *Laryngoscope.* 1980;90(2):196–201.
13. Nishijima W, Takooda S, Tokita N, et al. Analyses of distant metastases in squamous cell carcinoma of the head and neck and lesions above the clavicle at autopsy. *Arch Otolaryngol Head Neck Surg.* 1993;119(1):65–68.
14. Gold KA, Lee HY, Kim ES. Targeted therapies in squamous cell carcinoma of the head and neck. *Cancer.* 2009;115(5):922–935.
15. SEER Cancer Statistics Review, 1975–2004. Based on November 2006 SEER data submission, posted to the SEER web site, 2007. Available at: http://seer.cancer.gov/csr/1975_2004/.
16. Argiris A, Li Y, Forastiere A. Prognostic factors and long-term survivorship in patients with recurrent or metastatic carcinoma of the head and neck. *Cancer.* 2004;101(10):2222–2229.
17. Jemal A, Siegel R, Ward E, et al. Cancer statistics, 2008. *CA Cancer J Clin.* 2008;58(2):71–96.
18. Leon X, Hitt R, Constenla M, et al. A retrospective analysis of the outcome of patients with recurrent and/or metastatic squamous cell carcinoma of the head and neck refractory to a platinum-based chemotherapy. *Clin Oncol (R Coll Radiol).* 2005;17(6):418–424.
19. Leemans CR, Tiwari R, Nauta JJ, et al. Regional lymph node involvement and its significance in the development of distant metastases in head and neck carcinoma. *Cancer.* 1993;71(2):452–456.

20. Laskar SG, Agarwal JP, Srinivas C, et al. Radiotherapeutic management of locally advanced head and neck cancer. *Expert Rev Anticancer Ther.* 2006;6(3):405–417.

21. Borjesson PK, Postema EJ, de Bree R, et al. Radioimmunodetection and radioimmunotherapy of head and neck cancer. *Oral Oncol.* 2004;40(8):761–772.

22. Cote V, Kost K, Payne RJ, et al. Sentinel lymph node biopsy in squamous cell carcinoma of the head and neck: where we stand now, and where we are going. *J Otolaryngol.* 2007;36(6):344–349.

23. Ko C, Citrin D. Radiotherapy for the management of locally advanced squamous cell carcinoma of the head and neck. *Oral Dis.* 2008;15: 121–132.

24. Lefebvre JL. Current clinical outcomes demand new treatment options for SCCHN. *Ann Oncol.* 2005;(16, suppl 6):vi7–vi12.

25. Vermorken JB, Mesia R, Rivera F, et al. Platinum-based chemotherapy plus cetuximab in head and neck cancer. *N Engl J Med.* 2008;359(11): 1116–1127.

26. Taneja C, Allen H, Koness RJ, et al. Changing patterns of failure of head and neck cancer. *Arch Otolaryngol Head Neck Surg.* 2002;128(3): 324–327.

27. Corvo R. Evidence-based radiation oncology in head and neck squamous cell carcinoma. *Radiother Oncol.* 2007;85(1):156–170.

28. Langer CJ. Targeted therapy in head and neck cancer: state of the art 2007 and review of clinical applications. *Cancer.* 2008;112(12): 2635–2645.

29. de Bree R, Kuik DJ, Quak JJ, et al. The impact of tumour volume and other characteristics on uptake of radiolabelled monoclonal antibodies in tumour tissue of head and neck cancer patients. *Eur J Nucl Med.* 1998;25(11):1562–1565.

30. Funaro A, Horenstein AL, Santoro P, et al. Monoclonal antibodies and therapy of human cancers. *Biotechnol Adv.* 2000;18(5):385–401.

31. Eshel R, Zanin A, Kapon D, et al. Human Ly-6 antigen E48 (Ly-6D) regulates important interaction parameters between endothelial cells and head-and-neck squamous carcinoma cells. *Int J Cancer.* 2002; 98(6):803–810.

32. Rubinfeld B, Upadhyay A, Clark SL, et al. Identification and immunotherapeutic targeting of antigens induced by chemotherapy. *Nat Biotechnol.* 2006;24(2):205–209.

33. Brakenhoff RH, Gerretsen M, Knippels EM, et al. The human E48 antigen, highly homologous to the murine Ly-6 antigen ThB, is a GPI-anchored molecule apparently involved in keratinocyte cell-cell adhesion. *J Cell Biol.* 1995;129(6):1677–1689.

34. de Bree R, Roos JC, Quak JJ, et al. Clinical screening of monoclonal antibodies 323/A3, cSF-25 and K928 for suitability of targeting tumours in the upper aerodigestive and respiratory tract. *Nucl Med Commun.* 1994;15(8):613–627.

35. Terpe HJ, Storkel S, Zimmer U, et al. Expression of CD44 isoforms in renal cell tumors. Positive correlation to tumor differentiation. *Am J Pathol.* 1996;148(2):453–463.

36. Gunthert U, Hofmann M, Rudy W, et al. A new variant of glycoprotein CD44 confers metastatic potential to rat carcinoma cells. *Cell.* 1991;65(1):13–24.

37. Prince ME, Sivanandan R, Kaczorowski A, et al. Identification of a subpopulation of cells with cancer stem cell properties in head and neck squamous cell carcinoma. *Proc Natl Acad Sci U S A.* 2007; 104(3):973–978.

38. Mack B, Gires O. CD44s and CD44v6 expression in head and neck epithelia. *PLoS ONE.* 2008;3(10):e3360.

39. Heider KH, Sproll M, Susani S, et al. Characterization of a high-affinity monoclonal antibody specific for CD44v6 as candidate for immunotherapy of squamous cell carcinomas. *Cancer Immunol Immunother.* 1996;43(4):245–253.

40. Heider KH, Kuthan H, Stehle G, et al. CD44v6: a target for antibody-based cancer therapy. *Cancer Immunol Immunother.* 2004;53:567–579.

41. Jung K, Lein M, Weiss S, et al. Soluble CD44 molecules in serum of patients with prostate cancer and benign prostatic hyperplasia. *Eur J Cancer.* 1996;32A(4):627–630.

42. Van Hal NL, Van Dongen GA, Ten Brink CB, et al. Evaluation of soluble CD44v6 as a potential serum marker for head and neck squamous cell carcinoma. *Clin Cancer Res.* 1999;5(11):3534–3541.

43. Heider KH, Mulder JW, Ostermann E, et al. Splice variants of the cell surface glycoprotein CD44 associated with metastatic tumour cells are expressed in normal tissues of humans and cynomolgus monkeys. *Eur J Cancer.* 1995;31A(13–14):2385–2391.

44. Schrijvers AH, Quak JJ, Uyterlinde AM, et al. MAb U36, a novel monoclonal antibody successful in immunotargeting of squamous

cell carcinoma of the head and neck. *Cancer Res.* 1993;53(18): 4383–4390.

45. Tijink BM, Buter J, de Bree R, et al. A phase I dose escalation study with anti-CD44v6 bivatuzumab mertansine in patients with incurable squamous cell carcinoma of the head and neck or esophagus. *Clin Cancer Res.* 2006;12(20, pt 1):6064–6072.

46. Walker RA. The erbB/HER type 1 tyrosine kinase receptor family. *J Pathol.* 1998;185(3):234–235.

47. Rikimaru K, Tadokoro K, Yamamoto T, et al. Gene amplification and overexpression of epidermal growth factor receptor in squamous cell carcinoma of the head and neck. *Head Neck.* 1992;14(1):8–13.

48. Santini J, Formento JL, Francoual M, et al. Characterization, quantification, and potential clinical value of the epidermal growth factor receptor in head and neck squamous cell carcinomas. *Head Neck.* 1991;13(2):132–139.

49. Ang KK, Berkey BA, Tu X, et al. Impact of epidermal growth factor receptor expression on survival and pattern of relapse in patients with advanced head and neck carcinoma. *Cancer Res.* 2002;62(24): 7350–7356.

50. Herbst RS. Review of epidermal growth factor receptor biology. *Int J Radiat Oncol Biol Phys.* 2004;59(2 suppl):21–26.

51. Mendelsohn J, Baselga J. Epidermal growth factor receptor targeting in cancer. *Semin Oncol.* 2006;33(4):369–385.

52. Akimoto T, Hunter NR, Buchmiller L, et al. Inverse relationship between epidermal growth factor receptor expression and radiocurability of murine carcinomas. *Clin Cancer Res.* 1999;5(10):2884–2890.

53. Dunn WA, Connolly TP, Hubbard AL. Receptor-mediated endocytosis of epidermal growth factor by rat hepatocytes: receptor pathway. *J Cell Biol.* 1986;102(1):24–36.

54. Gladhaug IP, Refsnes M, Christoffersen T. Regulation of surface expression of high-affinity receptors for epidermal growth factor (EGF) in hepatocytes by hormones, differentiating agents, and phorbol ester. *Dig Dis Sci.* 1992;37(2):233–239.

55. Neri D, Bicknell R. Tumour vascular targeting. *Nat Rev Cancer.* 2005;5(6):436–446.

56. Jain RK. Tumor angiogenesis and accessibility: role of vascular endothelial growth factor. *Semin Oncol.* 2002;29(6, suppl 16):3–9.

57. Lothaire P, de Azambuja E, Dequanter D, et al. Molecular markers of head and neck squamous cell carcinoma: promising signs in need of prospective evaluation. *Head Neck.* 2006;28(3):256–269.

58. Carnemolla B, Balza E, Siri A, et al. A tumor-associated fibronectin isoform generated by alternative splicing of messenger RNA precursors. *J Cell Biol.* 1989;108(3):1139–1148.

59. Birchler MT, Milisavljevic D, Pfaltz M, et al. Expression of the extra domain B of fibronectin, a marker of angiogenesis, in head and neck tumors. *Laryngoscope.* 2003;113(7):1231–1237.

60. Hasina R, Whipple ME, Martin LE, et al. Angiogenic heterogeneity in head and neck squamous cell carcinoma: biological and therapeutic implications. *Lab Invest.* 2008;88(4):342–353.

61. Brack SS, Silacci M, Birchler M, et al. Tumor-targeting properties of novel antibodies specific to the large isoform of tenascin-C. *Clin Cancer Res.* 2006;12(10):3200–3208.

62. Andratschke M, Hagedorn H, Luebbers CW, et al. Limited suitability of EpCAM for molecular staging of tumor borders in head and neck cancer. *Anticancer Res.* 2006;26(1A):153–158.

63. De Herdt MJ, Baatenburg de Jong RJ. HGF and c-MET as potential orchestrators of invasive growth in head and neck squamous cell carcinoma. *Front Biosci.* 2008;13:2516–2526.

64. Barnes CJ, Ohshiro K, Rayala SK, et al. Insulin-like growth factor receptor as a therapeutic target in head and neck cancer. *Clin Cancer Res.* 2007;13(14):4291–4299.

65. Hindermann W, Berndt A, Borsi L, et al. Synthesis and protein distribution of the unspliced large tenascin-C isoform in oral squamous cell carcinoma. *J Pathol.* 1999;189(4):475–480.

66. Paganelli G, Orecchia R, Jereczek-Fossa B, et al. Combined treatment of advanced oropharyngeal cancer with external radiotherapy and three-step radioimmunotherapy. *Eur J Nucl Med.* 1998;25(9):1336–1339.

67. Tranter RM, Fairweather DS, Bradwell AR, et al. The detection of squamous cell tumours of the head and neck using radio-labelled antibodies. *J Laryngol Otol.* 1984;98(1):71–74.

68. Kairemo KJ, Hopsu EV. Imaging of tumours in the parotid region with indium-111 labelled monoclonal antibody reacting with carcinoembryonic antigen. *Acta Oncol.* 1990;29(4):539–543.

69. Kairemo KJ, Hopsu EV. Imaging of pharyngeal and laryngeal carcinomas with indium-111-labeled monoclonal anti-CEA antibodies. *Laryngoscope.* 1990;100(10, pt 1):1077–1082.

70. Timon CI, McShane D, Hamilton D, et al. Head and neck cancer localization with indium labelled carcinoembryonic antigen: a pilot project. *J Otolaryngol.* 1991;20(4):283–287.

71. De Rossi G, Maurizi M, Almadori G, et al. The contribution of immunoscintigraphy to the diagnosis of head and neck tumours. *Nucl Med Commun.* 1997;18(1):10–16.

72. Soo KC, Ward M, Roberts KR, et al. Radioimmunoscintigraphy of squamous carcinomas of the head and neck. *Head Neck Surg.* 1987; 9(6):349–352.

73. Schechter NR, Wendt RE III, Yang DJ, et al. Radiation dosimetry of ⁹⁹ᵐTc-labeled C225 in patients with squamous cell carcinoma of the head and neck. *J Nucl Med.* 2004;45(10):1683–1687.

74. Baum RP, Adams S, Kiefer J, et al. A novel technetium-99m labeled monoclonal antibody (174H.64) for staging head and neck cancer by immuno-SPECT. *Acta Oncol.* 1993;32(7–8):747–751.

75. Heissler E, Grunert B, Barzen G, et al. Radioimmunoscintigraphy of squamous cell carcinoma in the head and neck region. *Int J Oral Maxillofac Surg.* 1994;23(3):149–152.

76. Adamietz IA, Baum RP, Schemann F, et al. Improvement of radiation treatment planning in squamous-cell head and neck cancer by immuno-SPECT. *J Nucl Med.* 1996;37(12):1942–1946.

77. van Dongen GA, Leverstein H, Roos JC, et al. Radioimmunoscintigraphy of head and neck cancer using ⁹⁹ᵐTc-labeled monoclonal antibody E48 F(ab')₂. *Cancer Res.* 1992;52(9):2569–2574.

78. de Bree R, Roos JC, Quak JJ, et al. Clinical imaging of head and neck cancer with technetium-99m-labeled monoclonal antibody E48 IgG or F(ab')₂. *J Nucl Med.* 1994;35(5):775–783.

79. de Bree R, Roos JC, Quak JJ, et al. Biodistribution of radiolabeled monoclonal antibody E48 IgG and F(ab')₂ in patients with head and neck cancer. *Clin Cancer Res.* 1995;1(3):277–286.

80. de Bree R, Roos JC, Verel I, et al. Radioimmunodiagnosis of lymph node metastases in head and neck cancer. *Oral Dis.* 2003;9(5):241–248.

81. de Bree R, Roos JC, Quak JJ, et al. Radioimmunoscintigraphy and biodistribution of technetium-99m-labeled monoclonal antibody U36 in patients with head and neck cancer. *Clin Cancer Res.* 1995; 1(6):591–598.

82. Colnot DR, Quak JJ, Roos JC, et al. Phase I therapy study of ¹⁸⁶Re-labeled chimeric monoclonal antibody U36 in patients with squamous cell carcinoma of the head and neck. *J Nucl Med.* 2000;41(12): 1999–2010.

83. Borjesson PK, Jauw YW, Boellaard R, et al. Performance of immunopositron emission tomography with zirconium-89-labeled chimeric monoclonal antibody U36 in the detection of lymph node metastases in head and neck cancer patients. *Clin Cancer Res.* 2006;12(7, pt 1): 2133–2140.

84. Colnot DR, Ossenkoppele GJ, Roos JC, et al. Reinfusion of unprocessed, granulocyte colony-stimulating factor-stimulated whole blood allows dose escalation of ¹⁸⁶Re-labeled chimeric monoclonal antibody U36 radioimmunotherapy in a phase I dose escalation study. *Clin Cancer Res.* 2002;8(11):3401–3406.

85. Stroomer JW, Roos JC, Sproll M, et al. Safety and biodistribution of ⁹⁹ᵐtechnetium-labeled anti-CD44v6 monoclonal antibody BIWA 1 in head and neck cancer patients. *Clin Cancer Res.* 2000;6(8): 3046–3055.

86. Colnot DR, Roos JC, de Bree R, et al. Safety, biodistribution, pharmacokinetics, and immunogenicity of ⁹⁹ᵐTc-labeled humanized monoclonal antibody BIWA 4 (bivatuzumab) in patients with squamous cell carcinoma of the head and neck. *Cancer Immunol Immunother.* 2003;52(9):576–582.

87. Borjesson PK, Postema EJ, Roos JC, et al. Phase I therapy study with (186)Re-labeled humanized monoclonal antibody BIWA 4 (bivatuzumab) in patients with head and neck squamous cell carcinoma. *Clin Cancer Res.* 2003;9(10, pt 2):3961S–3972S.

88. Birchler MT, Thuerl C, Schmid D, et al. Immunoscintigraphy of patients with head and neck carcinomas, with an anti-angiogenetic antibody fragment. *Otolaryngol Head Neck Surg.* 2007;136(4):543–548.

89. Verel I, Heider KH, Siegmund M, et al. Tumor targeting properties of monoclonal antibodies with different affinity for target antigen CD44V6 in nude mice bearing head-and-neck cancer xenografts. *Int J Cancer.* 2002;99(3):396–402.

90. Brakenhoff RH, van Gog FB, Looney JE, et al. Construction and characterization of the chimeric monoclonal antibody E48 for therapy of head and neck cancer. *Cancer Immunol Immunother.* 1995;40(3): 191–200.

91. Van Hal NL, Van Dongen GA, Rood-Knippels EM, et al. Monoclonal antibody U36, a suitable candidate for clinical immunotherapy of

92. squamous-cell carcinoma, recognizes a CD44 isoform. *Int J Cancer.* 1996;68(4):520–527.

92. Marshall J. Clinical implications of the mechanism of epidermal growth factor receptor inhibitors. *Cancer.* 2006;107(6):1207–1218.

93. Dutta PR, Maity A. Cellular responses to EGFR inhibitors and their relevance to cancer therapy. *Cancer Lett.* 2007;254(2):165–177.

94. Baselga J. Why the epidermal growth factor receptor? The rationale for cancer therapy. *Oncologist.* 2002;(7, suppl 4):2–8.

95. Mendelsohn J, Fan Z. Epidermal growth factor receptor family and chemosensitization. *J Natl Cancer Inst.* 1997;89(5):341–343.

96. Perez-Soler R, Donato NJ, Shin DM, et al. Tumor epidermal growth factor receptor studies in patients with non-small-cell lung cancer or head and neck cancer treated with monoclonal antibody RG 83852. *J Clin Oncol.* 1994;12(4):730–739.

97. Modjtahedi H, Dean C. Monoclonal antibodies to the EGF receptor act as betacellulin antagonists. *Biochem Biophys Res Commun.* 1996; 221(3):625–630.

98. Bonner JA, Harari PM, Giralt J, et al. Radiotherapy plus cetuximab for squamous-cell carcinoma of the head and neck. *N Engl J Med.* 2006;354(6):567–578.

99. Diaz Miqueli A, Blanco R, Garcia B, et al. Biological activity in vitro of anti-epidermal growth factor receptor monoclonal antibodies with different affinities. *Hybridoma (Larchmt).* 2007;26(6):423–431.

100. Cruz JJ, Ocana A, Del Barco E, et al. Targeting receptor tyrosine kinases and their signal transduction routes in head and neck cancer. *Ann Oncol.* 2007;18(3):421–430.

101. Fan Z, Baselga J, Masui H, et al. Antitumor effect of anti-epidermal growth factor receptor monoclonal antibodies plus cis-diamminedichloroplatinum on well established A431 cell xenografts. *Cancer Res.* 1993;53(19):4637–4642.

102. Fan Z, Lu Y, Wu X, et al. Antibody-induced epidermal growth factor receptor dimerization mediates inhibition of autocrine proliferation of A431 squamous carcinoma cells. *J Biol Chem.* 1994; 269(44):27595–27602.

103. Prewett M, Rockwell P, Rockwell RF, et al. The biologic effects of C225, a chimeric monoclonal antibody to the EGFR, on human prostate carcinoma. *J Immunother Emphasis Tumor Immunol.* 1996;19(6): 419–427.

104. Huang SM, Harari PM. Modulation of radiation response after epidermal growth factor receptor blockade in squamous cell carcinomas: inhibition of damage repair, cell cycle kinetics, and tumor angiogenesis. *Clin Cancer Res.* 2000;6(6):2166–2174.

105. Bianco C, Bianco R, Tortora G, et al. Antitumor activity of combined treatment of human cancer cells with ionizing radiation and anti-epidermal growth factor receptor monoclonal antibody C225 plus type I protein kinase A antisense oligonucleotide. *Clin Cancer Res.* 2000;6(11):4343–4350.

106. Milas L, Mason K, Hunter N, et al. In vivo enhancement of tumor radioresponse by C225 antiepidermal growth factor receptor antibody. *Clin Cancer Res.* 2000;6(2):701–708.

107. Huang SM, Bock JM, Harari PM. Epidermal growth factor receptor blockade with C225 modulates proliferation, apoptosis, and radiosensitivity in squamous cell carcinomas of the head and neck. *Cancer Res.* 1999;59(8):1935–1940.

108. Berndorff D, Borkowski S, Sieger S, et al. Radioimmunotherapy of solid tumors by targeting extra domain B fibronectin: identification of the best-suited radioimmunoconjugate. *Clin Cancer Res.* 2005;11(19, pt 2):7053s–7063s.

109. Borsi L, Balza E, Bestagno M, et al. Selective targeting of tumoral vasculature: comparison of different formats of an antibody (L19) to the ED-B domain of fibronectin. *Int J Cancer.* 2002; 102(1):75–85.

110. Sharkey RM, Blumenthal RD, Behr TM, et al. Selection of radioimmunoconjugates for the therapy of well-established or micrometastatic colon carcinoma. *Int J Cancer.* 1997;72(3):477–485.

111. Koppe MJ, Postema EJ, Aarts F, et al. Antibody-guided radiation therapy of cancer. *Cancer Metastasis Rev.* 2005;24(4):539–567.

112. Zalutsky MR, Vaidyanathan G. Astatine-211-labeled radiotherapeutics: an emerging approach to targeted alpha-particle radiotherapy. *Curr Pharm Des.* 2000;6(14):1433–1455.

113. Persson MI, Gedda L, Jensen HJ, et al. Astatinated trastuzumab, a putative agent for radionuclide immunotherapy of ErbB2-expressing tumours. *Oncol Rep.* 2006;15(3):673–680.

114. Nestor M, Andersson K, Lundqvist H. Characterization of (111)In and (177)Lu-labeled antibodies binding to CD44v6 using a novel automated radioimmunoassay. *J Mol Recognit.* 2008;21(3):179–183.

115. Nestor M, Persson M, Cheng J, et al. Biodistribution of the chimeric monoclonal antibody U36 radioiodinated with a closo-dodecaborate-containing linker. Comparison with other radioiodination methods. *Bioconjug Chem*. 2003;14(4):805–810.

116. Nestor M, Persson M, van Dongen GA, et al. In vitro evaluation of the astatinated chimeric monoclonal antibody U36, a potential candidate for treatment of head and neck squamous cell carcinoma. *Eur J Nucl Med Mol Imaging*. 2005;32(11):1296–1304.

117. Sandstrom K, Nestor M, Ekberg T, et al. Targeting CD44v6 expressed in head and neck squamous cell carcinoma: preclinical characterization of an ^{111}In-labeled monoclonal antibody. *Tumour Biol*. 2008;29(3):137–144.

118. Colnot DR, Quak JJ, Roos JC, et al. Radioimmunotherapy in patients with head and neck squamous cell carcinoma: initial experience. *Head Neck*. 2001;23(7):559–565.

119. Postema EJ, Borjesson PK, Buijs WC, et al. Dosimetric analysis of radioimmunotherapy with [186]Re-labeled bivatuzumab in patients with head and neck cancer. *J Nucl Med*. 2003;44(10):1690–1699.

120. Tijink BM, Neri D, Leemans CR, et al. Radioimmunotherapy of head and neck cancer xenografts using ^{131}I-labeled antibody L19-SIP for selective targeting of tumor vasculature. *J Nucl Med*. 2006;47(7):1127–1135.

121. van Gog FB, Brakenhoff RH, Stigter-van Walsum M, et al. Perspectives of combined radioimmunotherapy and anti-EGFR antibody therapy for the treatment of residual head and neck cancer. *Int J Cancer*. 1998;77(1):13–18.

122. Andratschke M, Gildehaus FJ, Johannson V, et al. Biodistribution and radioimmunotherapy of SCCHN in xenotransplanted SCID mice with a ^{131}I-labelled anti-EpCAM monoclonal antibody. *Anticancer Res*. 2007;27(1A):431–436.

123. van Dongen GA, Visser GW, Lub-de Hooge MN, et al. Immuno-PET: a navigator in monoclonal antibody development and applications. *Oncologist*. 2007;12(12):1379–1389.

124. Behr TM, Griesinger F, Riggert J, et al. High-dose myeloablative radioimmunotherapy of mantle cell non-Hodgkin lymphoma with the iodine-131-labeled chimeric anti-CD20 antibody C2B8 and autologous stem cell support. Results of a pilot study. *Cancer*. 2002;94(4 suppl):1363–1372.

125. Goldenberg DM, Sharkey RM. Novel radiolabeled antibody conjugates. *Oncogene*. 2007;26(25):3734–3744.

126. Shirai K, O'Brien PE. Molecular targets in squamous cell carcinoma of the head and neck. *Curr Treat Options Oncol*. 2007;8(3):239–251.

Targeted Radionuclide Therapy of Prostate Cancer: Targeting Prostate-Specific Membrane Antigen

Neil H. Bander, Shankar Vallabhajosula, Stanley J. Goldsmith, Scott T. Tagawa, and David M. Nanus

■ PROSTATE CANCER

▓ Clinical background

Prostate cancer (PC) is the most common cancer in men in the United States. It accounts for 25% of all cancers in men with an estimated 186,320 new cases and 28,660 deaths in 2008 (1). Since the advent of prostate-specific antigen (PSA) testing in the late 1980s to early 1990s, there has been a substantial and dramatic shift in the clinical stage of the disease at the time of diagnosis. Currently, in the United States, only 4% of newly diagnosed cases have demonstrable metastatic disease. The remainder has clinically localized disease. Indeed, the substantial majority has a palpably normal prostate and is diagnosed as a result of an abnormal PSA that leads to a biopsy. Localized PC is treated primarily with surgery or radiation therapy, the latter generally accompanied by hormonal therapy. In some cases, particularly where comorbidities are a factor, another option is active surveillance since some men will continue to be asymptomatic until death from another cause (2,3). Although surgery and/or radiotherapy is often successful at eradicating localized disease, approximately 30% of these patients will suffer recurrence. The vast majority of these local treatment failures result from occult micrometastatic disease present at the time of diagnosis (4).

For the past 60 years, first-line therapy for advanced PC has been androgen deprivation with a mean duration of efficacy of 12 to 18 months (5), although there is a wide variation in response in this heterogeneous disease. Following progression, taxane-based chemotherapy offers a quality of life as well as a survival benefit to those with metastatic castrate-resistant disease. Unfortunately, responses to chemotherapy are generally short lived, and there is no proven effective therapy beyond first-line chemotherapy (6–9).

▓ Biology of prostate cancer

The development of PC involves a multistep process, and specific genetic changes have been identified in PC. One such genetic change garnering considerable interest is the gene fusion that juxtaposes the androgen-regulated gene TMPRSS2 (21q22.3) and an erythroblast transformation specific transcription factor family member, either ERG (21q22.2), ETV1

(7p21.2), or ETV4 (17q21) (10). Among these, the TMPRSS2–ERG fusion is the most prevalent, occurring in up to 50% of clinically localized PCs, suggesting that the TMPRSS2–ERG fusion may be one of the most common somatic genomic alterations yet identified in any human malignancy.

Androgens are the primary regulators of PC cell growth and proliferation. Over the past few years, it has become clear that androgen and androgen receptor (AR) signaling pathways play a crucial role in both the development and progression of PC. Consequently, withdrawal of androgens remains a cornerstone of therapy for patients who develop advanced PC. Nevertheless, virtually all patients will progress to develop androgen-independent or castration-resistant disease, despite the lack of circulating androgens. It has recently become clear that AR signaling remains critical even in castrate-resistant PC progression (11–18). AR signaling under castrate conditions can occur through multiple pathways including (a) increased AR expression (amplification) and sensitivity, (b) AR mutations, (c) ligand-independent AR activation by polypeptide and neuropeptide growth factors (19), (d) overexpression of the HER-2/neu receptor tyrosine kinase (20–22), (e) alterations in AR coregulatory proteins, and (f) endogenous synthesis of androgen within the PC cell itself.

The molecular abnormalities may differ between primary, metastatic, and castrate-resistant PCs. As such, the targets relevant for the treatment of early-stage disease differ from those in late-stage cancers (23). For example, the frequency of expression of HER2 and BCL-2 is higher in castrate metastatic lesions than in untreated localized tumors (24,25). In contrast, the frequency of expression of prostate-specific membrane antigen (PSMA) is relatively constant across all clinical states, although the intensity of immunohistochemical staining is higher in castrate metastatic tumors (26).

▓ Prostate-specific membrane antigen

PSMA is the most well-established, PC-restricted, cell-surface antigen identified to date (27). In contrast to other well-known prostate-restricted molecules such as PSA and prostatic acid phosphatase that are secretory proteins, PSMA is a type II integral cell-surface membrane protein that is not secreted and not found in the blood. PSMA is expressed by virtually all PCs (28), and although first thought to be entirely prostate specific (29–33), subsequent studies have demonstrated that PSMA is also expressed by cells of the proximal renal tubules, small intestine, salivary glands, and a subset of astrocytes. However, the level of expression in these nonprostate tissues is 100- to 1000-fold less than in prostate tissue (33,34), and the site of PSMA expression in these normal cells (brush border/luminal location; behind the blood–brain barrier) is not typically exposed to circulating antibody. The PSMA gene has been cloned, sequenced, and mapped to chromosome 11p11, and recently, its three-dimensional crystal structure was determined (35,36). The 19 amino acid cytoplasmic domain of PSMA contains a novel MXXXL internalization motif (37,38) resulting in its internalization and endosomal recycling. PSMA is an ideal cell-surface antigen given its expression by virtually all PCs, its high degree of specificity, its high level of expression ($\pm 10^6$ sites per cell), its internalization, and the absence of a competing reservoir of antigen in the plasma (37).

PC represents a particularly favorable setting in which to test the relevance of radioimmunotherapy (RIT) in solid tumors. PC is a relatively radiosensitive malignancy with a propensity to form small foci in the bone marrow and lymph nodes. These small foci allow ready accessibility of circulating monoclonal antibody (mAb) to its target antigen, in contrast to other solid tumors that may be more radioresistant and where tumor masses are often bulky and poorly perfused. The availability of a sensitive blood test such as PSA provides a clinical indication for adjuvant mAb therapy at the first sign of relapse, years before clinical manifestations of disease, when tumor volume is small and ideally suited for antibody delivery. Furthermore, there exists a multitude of clinically validated measures to predict, even before PSA failure, those patients who are at high risk, allowing initiation of therapy in the face of an extremely small tumor burden. A surrogate marker such as PSA also allows rapid clinical evaluation of potential therapeutic efficacy in phase I and II trials.

PSMA has been validated as an in vivo target for immunoscintigraphy (39,40) using capromab (Prostascint) derived from the mAb 7E11. Molecular mapping revealed that mAb 7E11 targets an intracellular epitope of the PSMA molecule that is not exposed on the outer cell surface (41–43). As a result, 7E11/capromab does not bind to viable cells (41–44) with intact cell membranes. Recognition of this disadvantage led our group to propose that developing mAbs to the exposed, extracellular domain of PSMA had the potential to significantly improve in vivo targeting, likely leading to enhanced imaging and therapeutic benefit (43,45). This effort led to a series of antibodies (J591, J415, J533, and E99) to PSMA$_{ext}$ that demonstrate nanomolar-binding affinity to viable PSMA-expressing LNCaP cells in tissue culture followed by rapid internalization (38,43). Murine mAb J591 (muJ591) was chosen for clinical development and underwent extensive preclinical studies (46–49) outlined later in the text. The murine J591 antibody was deimmunized using a novel method involving specific deletion of human B- and T-cell-recognized epitopes (50).

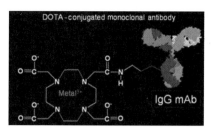

FIGURE 31.1 DOTA-conjugated Ig can be radiolabeled with a number of trivalent radiometals, such as ^{111}In, ^{90}Y, and ^{177}Lu. The metal will complex with DOTA with the four nitrogen atoms and the three carboxyl groups.

Given the optimal characteristics of the PSMA antigenic system plus the favorable clinical setting, PC offers an excellent model for the investigation and development of RIT as well as a litmus test of RIT in solid tumors. If RIT cannot succeed in PC, it will likely be very difficult to succeed in other solid tumors.

Preclinical studies

We reported the radiolabeling of three mAbs (J415, J533, and J591) with radionuclides useful for radioimmunodiagnosis and RIT: ^{131}I, ^{90}Y, and ^{177}Lu (46). To label mAbs with radiometals such as ^{111}In, ^{90}Y, and ^{177}Lu, the antibody was first conjugated with a macrocyclic chelating agent, DOTA (1,4,7,10-tetraazacyclododecane-N,N′,N″,N‴-tetraacetic acid). DOTA was conjugated to the mAbs via one of the carboxyl groups as shown in Figure 31.1. Based on LNCaP cell–binding assays, we demonstrated that J591 labeled with 10 to 20 mCi/mg of ^{90}Y or ^{177}Lu retained more than 80% immunoreactivity (51).

In vitro studies

In vitro saturation-binding studies with both PSMA-positive and PSMA-negative tumor cell lines demonstrated that radiolabeled mAbs J591, J415, and J533 recognize and bind with high affinity to PSMA$_{ext}$ (Fig. 31.2). Both J415 and J591 have similar nanomolar affinities to PSMA (46).

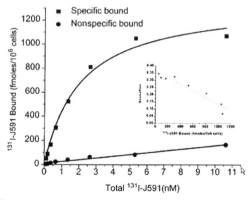

FIGURE 31.2 Specific binding of mAb J591 (^{131}I-labeled) to PSMA-expressing LNCaP cells. The same data are represented by a Scatchard plot, shown in the inset.

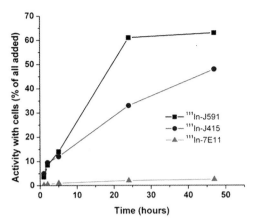

FIGURE 31.3 Binding and internalization of J591, J415, and 7E11 over time. 7E11 shows virtually no internalization by viable LNCaP cells.

In contrast to mAb 7E11/capromab, both J591 and J415 are far more readily bound and internalized by viable LNCaP cells (37,43,46) (Fig. 31.3). The in vitro studies clearly demonstrated that ^{111}In-labeled J591 and J415 retained more activity intracellularly than their radioiodinated counterparts; the latter lost most of the radiolabel due to dehalogenation. The $t_{1/2}$ of ^{111}In-DOTA-J591 from LNCaP cells was 520 hours compared to 38 hours for ^{131}I-J591 (46).

In vivo studies

We extended the study of radiolabeled mAbs to animal models. In nude mice bearing PSMA-positive xenografts (LNCaP), the tumor localization of ^{131}I- and ^{111}In-labeled anti-PSMA mAbs (J591, J415, and J533) was compared with that of radiolabeled 7E11. Autoradiographic studies demonstrated that 7E11 distinctly favors microlocalization to areas of necrosis, whereas J415 and J591 demonstrate a distinct preferential accumulation in areas of viable tumor (48).

Preclinical RIT efficacy studies were performed to assess in vivo antitumor and dose–response relationships of ^{131}I-, ^{90}Y-, and ^{177}Lu-labeled huJ591 preparations in nude mice bearing LNCaP xenografts (49). The RIT studies clearly demonstrated the antitumor effect of radiolabeled J591. Significant antitumor response and prolongation of median survival times were observed (Fig. 31.4). The antitumor effect of radiolabeled huJ591 was dose dependent. In addition, multiple dose treatments with either ^{90}Y- or ^{177}Lu-labeled J591 produced very high antitumor responses with a significant proportion of animals demonstrating apparent cure. All the theoretical and practical considerations strongly suggested that ^{90}Y- and ^{177}Lu-labeled J591 mAb would be more appropriate radiopharmaceuticals than ^{131}I-labeled J591 and supported our hypothesis that radiolabeled huJ591 was an appropriate agent for RIT studies in patients with PC.

▨ Human studies with radiolabeled J591

Initial phase I studies using huJ591-DOTA trace-labeled with ^{111}In showed that repetitive dosing was well tolerated with total doses of up to 500 mg/m^2 without the development of a human antihumanized (deimmunized) antibody (HAHA) response. No dose-limiting toxicity (DLT) occurred, and the maximum tolerated dose (MTD) of J591 was not reached (52,53). After the first dose, total body gamma

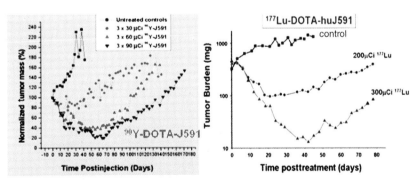

FIGURE 31.4 Decrease in tumor mass and increase in survival from single or multiple injections of ^{90}Y-J591 and ^{177}Lu-J591.

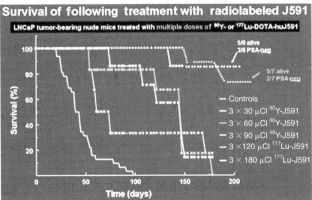

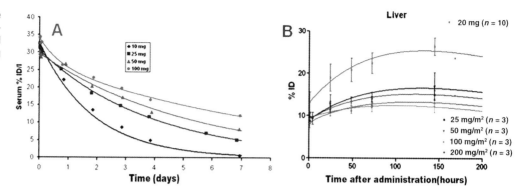

FIGURE 31.5 Increased dose (higher antibody mass) of ^{111}In-DOTA-J591 results in prolonged plasma clearance and decreasing liver uptake.

camera images were obtained within 1-hour postinfusion (day 0) and on three to four more occasions in the following week. Excellent tumor targeting could be detected at all dose levels of mAb. No mAb targeting to non-PC sites was observed although, as seen in other trials using radiometals, the liver is the primary site of excretion.

Pharmacokinetics and biodistribution

The effect of mass of J591 on the pharmacokinetics (PK) and biodistribution of J591 was studied over a range of 10 mg to 200 mg/m[2] using ^{111}In-DOTA-J591. Both the plasma clearance rate and the amount of liver uptake of ^{111}In activity were a function of antibody mass: the higher the mass, the slower the plasma clearance and lower the liver uptake (Fig. 31.5).

We subsequently compared the PK and biodistribution of [111]In- and ^{177}Lu-labeled DOTA-J591 (54) with a fixed 20 mg J591 mass. At this protein dose, both [111]In- and ^{177}Lu-J591 demonstrated a biexponential plasma clearance: less than 20% of activity had a fast component with a $t_{1/2}$ of less than 3 hours with the remaining 80% clearing from plasma slowly with an average $t_{1/2}$ of 44 ± 15 hours. The percentage of injected radioactivity excreted in the urine over a 3-day period was 7.3 ± 2.8%. The imaging studies showed similar biodistribution with both tracers (Fig. 31.6). Figure 31.7A and B shows that ^{111}In and ^{177}Lu appear equally effective in identifying metastatic lesions with a very high target-to-background contrast.

Biodistribution, PK, and tumor targeting remained consistent after sequential doses, confirming lack of an immune response to J591 (Fig. 31.8).

Radiation dosimetry

Using sequential studies, the biodistribution (percentage injected dose in several organs) of [111]In- and ^{177}Lu-labeled J591 was determined. Based on these data, ^{90}Y-J591 or ^{177}Lu-J591 radiation-absorbed dose (mGy/MBq) for a number of target organs was estimated based on the medical internal radiation dosimetry technique. The liver, the largest solid organ, receives the highest dose followed by spleen and kidney, as shown in Table 31.1.

Myelotoxicity: Dose–response relationship

The estimated radiation dose (mGy/MBq) to the bone marrow was three times higher with [90]Y (0.91 ± 0.43) than with [177]Lu (0.32 ± 0.10). The MTD was 647.5 MBq/m[2] with ^{90}Y-J591 and 2590 MBq/m[2] with ^{177}Lu-J591 (55). The proportion of patients with grades 3 to 4 myelotoxicity increased with increasing doses of [90]Y ($r = 0.91$) or [177]Lu ($r = 0.92$). There was a better correlation between the radioactive dose administered and the bone marrow radiation-absorbed dose (BM rad) with [177]Lu ($r = 0.91$) compared with [90]Y ($r = 0.75$) (Fig. 31.9). In addition, with ^{177}Lu, the

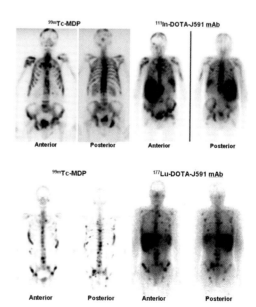

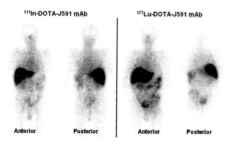

FIGURE 31.6 Similar biodistribution of ^{111}In-DOTA-J591 and ^{177}Lu-DOTA-J591 with a fixed antibody mass of 20 mg.

FIGURE 31.7 In comparison with a standard bone scan, ^{111}In and ^{177}Lu are equally effective in targeting metastatic sites.

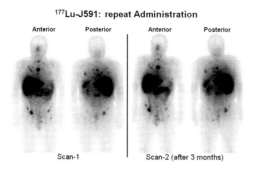

FIGURE 31.8 Consistent binding of metastatic sites after sequential dosing of ^{177}Lu-J591, indicating a lack of development of human antiglobulin (immune response) antibody to J591.

fractional decrease in platelets (FDP) correlates well with both the radioactive dose administered ($r = 0.88$) and the BM rad ($r = 0.86$). In contrast, with ^{90}Y, there was poor correlation between the FDP and the radioactive dose administered ($r = 0.20$) or the BM rad ($r = 0.26$). Similar results were also observed with leukocyte toxicity.

The radiation dose estimates described (Table 31.1) suggest that in patients with PC, myelotoxicity after treatment with ^{177}Lu-J591 can be predicted on the basis of the radioactive dose administered or the BM rad. The weaker correlation between myelotoxicity and ^{90}Y-J591 BM rad may be due to several factors. ^{90}Y-J591 may be less stable in vivo, and, as a result, higher amounts of free ^{90}Y may localize to the bone. In addition, the cross fire effect of high-energy β^- particles within the bone and the marrow may deliver a radiation dose nonuniformly within the marrow. Although a single large dose may deliver an optimal radiation dose to kill a larger fraction of tumor cells, fractionated therapy may offer the advantage of lower myelotoxicity and prolonged tumor response.

Clinical experience with radiolabeled J591

Two independent phase I clinical trials were performed using [90]Y- and ^{177}Lu-DOTA-huJ591 (56,57), each using a fixed huJ591 dose of 20 mg or 10 mg/m[2], respectively. Eligible patients had a prior histologic diagnosis of PC and evidence of progressing, recurrent, or metastatic disease, defined by at least three serially rising PSAs and/or radiographic studies. Briefly, the primary objectives of these trials were to define the MTDs as well as to further define dosimetry, PK, HAHA, and immunogenicity of the radiolabeled deimmunized mAb. Antitumor responses were assessed as a secondary end point.

The design and entry criteria of the two trials were identical. As prior studies had demonstrated that all PCs were PSMA positive (28), no determination of PSMA expression was done. Patients were required to have an absolute neutrophil count (ANC) of 2.0×10^9/L or more and a platelet count of 150×10^9/L or more. Prior radiation therapy of more than 25% of the skeleton or prior treatment with [89]strontium or [153]samarium was not permitted. Other standard laboratory exclusion criteria applied as well. DLT in the two trials was defined as hematologic toxicity consisting of grade 4 thrombocytopenia (platelet count of less than 10×10^9/L) and/or grade 4 neutropenia (ANC of less than 0.5×10^9) for greater than 5 days or nonhematologic toxicity of grade 3 or more attributable to radiolabeled J591.

[90]Y-J591 phase I trial (56): Patients received an initial dose of ^{111}In-J591 (20 mg, 5 mCi) for PK and biodistribution determinations, followed 1 week later with a dose of ^{90}Y-J591 (20 mg). The dose schedule was selected to allow multiple imaging sessions prior to ^{111}In decay as well as clearance of the initial dose of J591 prior to delivering the second dose. The ^{90}Y dose range was selected based on prior published experience with other antibodies.

A total of 29 subjects were entered at the following dose levels: 5, 10, 15, 17.5, and 20 mCi/m[2]. Based on two grade 3 non-life-threatening bleeding episodes with grade 3 thrombocytopenia at a ^{90}Y dose of 20 mCi/m[2], we chose to amend the predefined hematologic DLT criteria (grade 4 thrombocytopenia) and selected 17.5 mCi/m[2] as the MTD. This conservative approach may have underestimated the true

Table **31.1**	**Radiation dosimetry of radiolabeled J591 mAb**			
	Radiation Dosimetry with			
	^{90}Y-J591		**[177]Lu-J591**	
Organ	**mGy/MBq**	**Gy/MTD Dose[a]**	**mGy/MBq**	**Gy/MTD Dose[a]**
Liver	6.59 ± 2.27	8.534	2.10 ± 0.60	11.026
Spleen	4.92 ± 1.66	6.372	1.97 ± 0.92	10.342
Kidney	4.47 ± 1.08	5.788	1.41 ± 0.35	7.402
Lungs	2.87 ± 0.71	3.716	0.75 ± 0.22	3.938
Red marrow	0.91 ± 0.43	1.178	0.32 ± 0.10	1.68
Effective dose equivalent	1.78 ± 0.25	2.306	0.58 ± 0.09	3.046

[a]MTD: with [90]Y = 17.5 mCi or 647.5 MBq/m[2]; [177]Lu = 70 mCi or 2625 MBq/m[2]. Radiation dose at MTD dose was estimated for a subject with 2.0 m[2] body surface area; 1 mCi = 37 MBq; 1 Gray = 100 rads; 1 rad = 10 mGy or 10 mSv.

FIGURE 31.9 Fractional decrease in platelets corresponds better with ^{177}Lu in comparison with ^{90}Y.

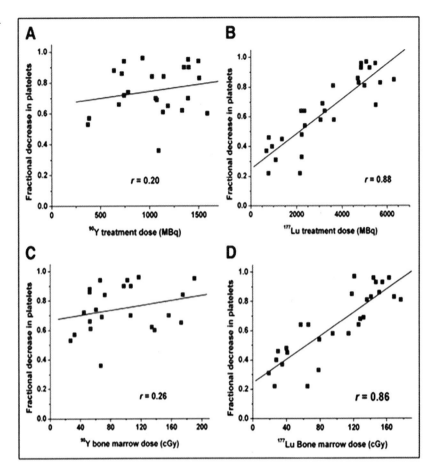

MTD, particularly in the context of two major responses seen at the 20 mCi/m^2 dose level. None of the patients in the trial experienced dose-limiting nonhematologic toxicity. As this was a phase I trial, our major concern was toxicity, and further trials may be necessary to clarify whether or not the 20 mCi/m^2 dose level can be administered safely.

Near the conclusion of the trial, after obtaining significant safety data, the protocol was amended to allow patients to receive up to three re-treatments if platelet and neutrophil recovery was satisfactory and if patients continued to meet the initial entry criteria. Ultimately, four patients in the trial were re-treated. None of the re-treated patients experienced DLT.

Among the 29 patients, 19 had bone lesions and 13 had soft tissue lesions. Seventeen of nineteen (89%) patients with bone lesions and 9 of 13 (69%) with soft tissue lesions were accurately targeted, resulting in an overall targeting sensitivity of 26 of 32 (81%).

Two patients treated at the 20 mCi/m^2 dose level exhibited 85% and 70% declines in PSA lasting 8 and 8.6 months, respectively, prior to returning to pretreatment values. In addition, these two patients had objective measurable disease responses with 90% and 40% decrease in the size of pelvic and retroperitoneal lymphadenopathy. Both patients were castrate resistant with lymph node–only disease; neither patient had received prior chemotherapy. The second

patient was re-treated with 20 mCi/m^2 ^{90}Y-J591 on day 119 and demonstrated evidence of a secondary response, although to a lesser magnitude than his initial response. Six additional patients experienced PSA stabilization during the initial 12-week posttreatment period.

PSA and objective measurable disease responses were seen in several patients. A high concordance was observed between PSA responses and measurable disease responses, implying that, with RIT, PSA may be used as a marker of response in patients without measurable disease in phase I and/or II trials.

DLT in RIT trials, in general, is limited to short-lived, reversible myelotoxicity. The consistency of findings across different tumor types, different antigenic systems, mAb derivation (mouse, chimeric, humanized), and site and bulk of tumor suggests that the myelotoxicity is a function of the physical characteristics of the isotope (half-life, energy, range) and presumably its plasma half-life. This can be explained by the fact that the overwhelming majority of the administered radiolabeled mAb circulates free in the plasma, unavoidably irradiating the marrow with nonspecific radiation, while only a very small proportion of the injected dose (≤0.01%/gm) localizes to tumor.

Also consistent with previous radiolabeled antibody experience, we found that within any given dose level, there was significant interpatient variability in the degree of hematologic toxicity. For example, at the MTD of 17.5 mCi/m^2, the mean platelet nadir was 41×10^9/L with a range of 15×10^9 to 77×10^9/L. Similarly, in a phase I/II trial with ^{90}Y-anti-CD20 (ibritumomab tiuxetan) in patients with non-Hodgkin lymphoma (NHL), at the MTD dose of 0.4 mCi/m^2, the median platelet nadir was 49.5×10^9/L with a range of 2×10^9 to 136×10^9/L (58). In a phase I study of ^{90}Y-anti-Lewis Y mAb B3, at the MTD, three of six patients had grade 1 platelet toxicity and the remaining three patients had grade 4 toxicity (59). In our study, we found no clear relationship between toxicity and prior chemotherapy or radiation treatment. In addition, there was no relationship to the extent of bone marrow involvement. The variability in the degree of myelotoxicity, despite the use of dosing adjusted to body weight or surface area, leads to the adoption of an (MTD) dose that, by definition, induces DLT-level toxicity in 17% or less patients and results in relative undertreatment of a significant proportion of patients who could tolerate higher, more effective doses. At our MTD of 17.5 mCi/m^2, three of the six patients treated experienced a mean platelet nadir of 62×10^9/L (range: 42×10^9 to 77×10^9/L) and could have tolerated a higher dose. ^{131}I tositumomab (Bexaar) attempts to overcome the interpatient variability in myelotoxicity by tailoring the administered dose based on a pretreatment dosimetry study in each patient. Despite this, myelotoxicity experienced with ^{131}I tositumomab remains quite variable and is consistent with our finding and of others that dosimetrically derived radiation dose to marrow was not highly predictive of the degree of myelotoxicity experienced (59).

In this study, as in RIT studies in general, nonhematologic toxicity was minimal and not dose limiting. Radiation dosimetry estimates of ^{90}Y-J591 indicate that administration of 20 mCi/m^2 of ^{90}Y dose would deliver less than 1000 cGy to the liver, spleen, and kidney, well below the acceptable radiation doses to these organs. No HAHA response was seen in any patient, including re-treated patients (56).

^{177}Lu-J591 phase I trial (57): Prior to our ^{177}Lu-J591 phase I trial, published experience with ^{177}Lu-labeled antibody was very limited. Only three previous trials had been reported, all of which used murine mAb CC49 (anti-TAG72) (60–62). Only one of these trials used intravenous administration (60), whereas the other two trials used an intraperitoneal approach (61,62).

We set out to study ^{177}Lu, with physical characteristics different from that of ^{90}Y, using the same preparation of J591-DOTA and a similar PC population. ^{177}Lu has the advantage over ^{90}Y of allowing direct imaging. In addition, the longer half-life, lower energy, and shorter range of the beta-emission of ^{177}Lu provide theoretical advantages in PC, where the metastases tend more often to be small-volume sites measured in microns to millimeters in bone marrow rather than bulky multicentimeter sites in lymph nodes or viscera. Thirty-five patients with castrate-resistant PC were entered. Patients received 10 mg/m^2 J591-DOTA with doses of ^{177}Lu ranging from 10 to 75 mCi/m^2. Of the three patients at the 75 mCi/m^2 dose level, one experienced dose-limiting (grade 4) thrombocytopenia, while the remaining two patients experienced grade 3 thrombocytopenia. All three of these patients experienced grade 4 neutropenia, one of which was dose-limiting neutropenia of 6 days' duration. As two of three patients at this dose level experienced DLT, no additional patients were entered at this dose. At the prior dose level of 70 mCi/m^2, six patients were entered. Two patients had transient grade 4 neutropenia not meeting the definition of DLT: one of these patients had grade 4 thrombocytopenia. As there was only one DLT in these six patients, the 70 mCi/m^2 dose level was determined to be the MTD. This MTD is significantly higher than the MTD of 17.5 mCi/m^2 we observed with ^{90}Y using the same J591-DOTA preparation in a similar patient population. This finding likely relates to the lower energy and range of ^{177}Lu resulting in less cross fire radiation to the bone marrow. Ultimately, of course, a higher MTD is irrelevant unless it results in an improved therapeutic ratio.

The nonhematologic toxicity in RIT trials, in general, and in this ^{177}Lu-J591 trial, was minimal and not dose limiting. Radiation dosimetry calculations indicate a radiation dose to the liver of 7.7 cGy/mCi or approximately 1088 cGy at the MTD of 70 mCi/m^2. This is well below the acceptable radiation limits to the liver. In this trial, 11 patients had transaminase elevations, 10 of which were grade 2 or less and 1 was grade 3, with 4 of these patients having pretreatment elevations. These elevations were transient and the patients experienced no related symptoms. The transaminase elevations in this trial were very similar to that seen with ^{90}Y-J591. In addition, in this ^{177}Lu-J591 trial, no significant hepatotoxicity was seen in patients who received multiple doses including eight patients who received cumulative doses between 90 and 120 mCi/m^2. Radiation doses to the kidney and spleen were also well within acceptable limits and no related organ toxicity was noted.

Sixteen of 35 patients in the trial received multiple doses. To our knowledge, this represented the largest experience with multiple dosing of RIT yet reported. Two doses of 45 or 60 mCi/m^2, totaling 90 to 120 mCi/m^2, proved to be quite toxic, with three of five patients experiencing prolonged and incomplete platelet recovery. Two or more doses of 30 mCi/m^2, however, were well tolerated and four patients received cumulative doses of 90 mCi/m^2, almost 30% higher than the single-dose MTD. Indeed, these four patients were eligible for a fourth dose of 30 mCi/m^2 but were not treated due to tumor progression. In this study, each dose was administered after allowing for hematologic recovery from the prior dose. It therefore took 3 to 4 months to administer the three doses, resulting in a higher cumulative dose but lower dose rate. Although there may be advantages to the higher cumulative dose, the time required to deliver this dose using this regimen may be offset by unrelenting tumor progression. Given the kinetics of platelet decline and recovery, a dose interval of 14 to 17 days may allow a two-dose regimen that might result in a higher cumulative dose (than a single-dose regimen) to be given over a shorter period of time than attempted in this trial. Such a schedule would result in the onset of platelet recovery from the first dose to coincide with platelet decline from the second dose, thereby resulting in a longer but shallower nadir than with a single MTD dose. We are currently exploring such a schedule (see "Dose Fractionation").

Among the 35 patients receiving ^{177}Lu-J591, 30 (86%) had metastatic disease detected on screening imaging studies. Specifically, 21 (60%) patients had bone-only metastases, 6 (17%) had soft tissue–only metastases, and 3 (9%) had both bone and soft tissue disease. In all of these 30 patients, all known sites of metastatic disease were successfully imaged by ^{177}Lu-J591 scintigraphy. In at least three cases, bone lesions were apparent on the J591 scan prior to becoming evident on conventional bone scan. Sequential imaging in patients who received multiple doses continued to consistently localize to tumor sites with no change in PK or biodistribution, consistent with laboratory assays that demonstrated a lack of J591 immunogenicity and human anti-J591 antibody development.

All 35 patients in this trial had abnormal, rising PSAs; seven patients had measurable disease. Although none of the seven patients with measurable disease had an objective tumor response or a 50% or more PSA decline, 20 of the 35 patients had evidence of biologic activity. Four patients had 50% or more PSA declines lasting 3+ to 8 months. The four PSA declines occurred in patients without measurable disease. This may be explained by responses to ^{177}Lu-J591, where the optimum tumor size is 1.2 to 3.0 mm (63), being more likely to occur in small-volume unmeasurable disease sites. Sixteen patients had PSA stabilization with a median duration of 60 days (range of 28 to more than 601 days). Fifteen patients demonstrated progressive disease (PSA increase of 25% or more) after treatment.

In this study, as in our ^{90}Y-J591 trial, we found (a) no clear relationship between a history of prior chemotherapy treatment and the degree of toxicity, (b) no correlation between prior radiotherapy and toxicity, and (c) no relationship between the extent of bone marrow involvement by cancer and toxicity. Although the lack of correlation between the extent of bone marrow involvement and toxicity differs from that seen in NHL, a similar observation in PC was made by Knox et al. (64) and O'Donnell et al. (65). In the latter trial of ^{90}Y-m170 in PC, the authors comment that "no obvious pretreatment parameter predicted hematological toxicity . . . ." This difference may be because NHL involves the marrow much more diffusely than PC where the disease tends to be more focal. As a result, radiolabeled-antibody localization in NHL may radiate the marrow more diffusely than in PC.

■ PHASE II RIT TRIAL IN METASTATIC CASTRATE-RESISTANT PC

Having explored both ^{90}Y- and ^{177}Lu-J591 in phase I trials and having documented that these agents were well tolerated, targeted tumor sites in virtually every patient despite the absence of any effort to select patients for PSMA expression were nonimmunogenic and displayed evidence of antitumor activity, we felt it was appropriate to proceed to a phase II trial. But for practical reasons, we felt we had to select only one of the isotopes to bring forward. Our decision to select ^{177}Lu was based on several factors. First, the myelosuppression resulting from ^{177}Lu-J591 seemed to have less interpatient variability than with ^{90}Y-J591. In addition, we were aware of the work of O'Donoghue et al. (63) that indicated ^{90}Y was better suited to larger lesions (with an optimal diameter of 2.8 to 4.2 cm), whereas ^{177}Lu was more ideally suited to lesions in the 1.2 to 3.0 mm diameter range. Indeed, their modeling fit well with our limited phase 1 data in that ^{90}Y resulted in both PSA and measurable responses in patients with 2 to 3 cm nodal disease, whereas the responses seen in the ^{177}Lu trial were PSA-only responses, and no larger, measurable lesions were identified for evaluation. We felt that the ideal clinical setting in PC, and where there was a great unmet medical need, was in the large segment of the PC population where patients have a progressively rising PSA but have not yet developed overt metastatic disease. These patients have small-volume lesions that are ideally suited for an antibody approach, have total tumor burdens that are small, have not yet been treated with mutagenic cytotoxic agents, and would be well suited for treatment with ^{177}Lu. Nevertheless, we felt that with the limited experience at that time, we should conduct an initial phase II study in late stage, metastatic patients, even though they were not optimal candidates for ^{177}Lu, to further assess the safety and activity before subjecting earlier stage, asymptomatic patients with a long anticipated survival, to this experimental therapy.

Based on phase I results (57) described earlier, a phase II trial of ^{177}Lu-J591 was conducted in subjects with progressive metastatic castration-resistant prostate cancer (CRPC), and preliminary results have recently been reported (66). Although the MTD of the phase I study (57) was 70 mCi/m^2 and because of limited experience at that time with ^{177}Lu-labeled antibodies, the US Food and Drug Administration required the initial cohort of 15 patients on this phase II trial be treated at 65 mCi/m^2 to confirm safety before escalating a second cohort of 17 patients to 70 mCi/m^2. The primary end point was PSA and/or measurable disease response; the secondary end point was toxicity. A ^{177}Lu-J591 imaging study was done to assess tumor targeting.

Median age of the 32 patients was 71 years (range 51 to 88), and median baseline PSA was 78 ng/mL (range 3.31 to 2184.6). Three patients achieved PSA declines of more than 50%. Based on retrospective analyses of patients on prospective docetaxel chemotherapy trials (67,68) demonstrating that any posttreatment decline in PSA correlated to a significantly longer survival than those patients without any PSA decline (20.7 vs. 11.7 months, respectively) (68) and that a 30% or more decline in PSA was the best survival surrogate (67,68), additional PSA response analyses were performed.

Overall, 10 of 32 patients (31%) experienced at least a 30% PSA decline. There also appeared to be a dose–response

Table **31.2** PSA response to ^{177}Lu-J591		
PSA Response	**Cohort 1:65 mCi/m^2 ($n = 15$)**	**Cohort 2:70 mCi/m^2 ($n = 17$)**
≥50% decline	1 (7%)	2 (12%)
≥30% decline	2 (13%)	8 (47%)
10%–29% decline	4 (26%)	2 (13%)
≥10% decline	6 (40%)	10 (63%)

relationship. Of the 15 subjects receiving 65 mCi/m^2, 6 (40%) had some PSA decline (Table 31.2).

A platelet nadir of less than 25×10^9/L occurred in 42% of patients, nine of whom required one to four platelet transfusions (median = 2). There were no hemorrhagic episodes. Twenty-nine patients recovered normal platelet counts; the remaining three patients had rapidly progressive disease with extensive bone marrow involvement. Neutropenia of 0.5×10^9/L or less occurred in 27% of patients, six of whom received brief treatment with growth factors. All 32 patients had normal neutrophil recovery and no patient experienced febrile neutropenia. No serious drug-related nonhematologic toxicity occurred.

All patients underwent planar ^{177}Lu-J591 scans after treatment. Excellent targeting of known sites of PC metastases was observed in 30 of 32 (94%) patients. In a preliminary analysis, the quality of imaging as determined by visual scale and semiquantitative tumor targeting index values (^{177}Lu tumor counts corrected for background/total body counts) correlated with PSA decline (69). This observation is being further studied prospectively in ongoing trials. No preselection of PSMA expression has been performed in any of the trials to date. If the intensity of radiolabeled J591 imaging predicts future response, studies examining the ability to preselect appropriate patients with an imaging study to enrich the target population may be appropriate.

Strategies to improve the success of anti-PSMA RIT

In radiotherapy, the antitumor response is primarily due to the induction of apoptosis (70–73). However, the degree of antitumor response following the administration of radiolabeled mAbs depends on several variables, especially total (cumulative) radiation dose to the tumor, dose rate, and tumor radiosensitivity. Single-agent RIT, although useful for slowing solid tumor growth, has not been effective in completely eliminating large, aggressive tumors, which often have p53 mutations and are less susceptible to apoptosis, the apparent mechanism of cell death from low dose-rate radiation (74). Therefore, strategies are being developed to optimize dosimetry to the bone marrow and tumor by dose fractionation and/or combining RIT with chemotherapy. In addition, studies to optimize patient selection are under way.

DOSE FRACTIONATION

The bone marrow is the dose-limiting organ in RIT in the absence of marrow reconstitution; dose fractionation is a practical strategy to decrease the dose to bone marrow while increasing the cumulative radiation dose to the tumor at an optimal dose rate (73,75,76). Dose fractionation may take advantage of the difference between early- and late-responding tissues. The radiation effect on early-responding tissue can be reduced by prolonging the treatment time and dose fractionation. The radiation effect on late-responding tissues will not be changed significantly if the total dose is not changed (73,76). Preclinical data have shown that dose fractionation or multiple low-dose treatments can decrease toxicity while increasing the efficacy (71,77,78). Similarly, there is some clinical evidence that bone marrow toxicity can be reduced with some modest increase in the cumulative MTD (79–81).

In a phase I dose escalation study supported by the Department of Defense Prostate Cancer Research Program, men with progressive metastatic castrate-resistant PC receive fractionated doses of ^{177}Lu-J591. Cohorts of three to six patients receive two doses of ^{177}Lu-J591 2 weeks apart: cohort 1 (20 mCi/m^2 × 2) with dose escalation 5 mCi/m^2 per dose per cohort. The primary end point is to determine DLT and the cumulative MTD of fractionated ^{177}Lu-J591 RIT with PK and dosimetry and a secondary end point of efficacy. DLT was defined as more than grade 3 hematologic toxicity or more than grade 2 nonhematologic toxicity.

Thirteen subjects have been treated to date, and preliminary results of the first 11 (cohorts 1 to 4) have been analyzed. Eighty-two percent had bone metastases, 45% lymph node metastases, and 36% extraosseous visceral metastases (lung). All patients had progressed after one to three hormonal therapies and 36% progressed on one to four lines of chemotherapy including docetaxel. No DLTs have occurred. Two patients experienced reversible grade 3 neutropenia and one grade 3 thrombocytopenia; no growth factors or transfusions were needed. There was no more than grade 1 nonhematologic toxicity. Overall, 5 of 11 patients have experienced a PSA decline. Excluding the lowest dose level (20 mCi/m^2 × 2), five of eight (63%) experienced a PSA decline (with median time to progression of 20 weeks), two with more than 30% decline, one with more than 50% decline. Excellent targeting of known sites of PC metastases has been seen in 85% of patients. This study continues to accrue.

COMBINATION RADIOIMMUNOTHERAPY WITH CHEMOTHERAPY

Although there is clear efficacy of anti-PSMA-based RIT in the treatment of metastatic CRPC, the results are limited, and all men treated to date with mature follow-up have developed disease progression. Following progression on primary hormonal therapy, chemotherapy offers a quality of life as well as survival benefit, although responses are transient and there is no proven therapy beyond first-line taxane chemotherapy (5–8). The combination of taxane chemotherapy with radiotherapy has been used in several diseases because of the radiosensitizing effects of taxanes (82–84). The combination of taxane chemotherapy with RIT has also been studied in preclinical and early clinical studies (85–87). In addition to favorable results from fractionated RIT, and the radiosensitizing effects of taxane-based chemotherapy, it is hypothesized that the additional debulking by chemotherapy will overcome some of the limits imposed by the physical characteristics of ^{177}Lu. Based on these data, a phase I trial of docetaxel and prednisone with escalating doses of fractionated ^{177}Lu-J591 is planned.

■ RADIOIMMUNOTHERAPY FOR BIOCHEMICALLY RELAPSED PROSTATE CANCER

In the current era, virtually all relapses after local therapy are initially "biochemical" only, that is, with a rising PSA in the absence of evidence of cancer on radiographic scans (88,89), affecting at least 50,000 men per year in the United States. It is estimated that the prevalence of this disease state in the United States is between 500,000 and 1,000,000 men. Although there is no proven overall survival benefit in a prospective randomized trial, radiotherapy as a salvage regimen can lead to long-term survival in selected individuals (89–93). However, most patients with biochemical relapse following surgery that receive local or regional radiotherapy with curative intent subsequently develop systemic progression because of subclinical micrometastatic disease outside of the radiation field. We have demonstrated J591-based therapy's ability to successfully target known sites of disease and have positive signals of ^{177}Lu-J591's efficacy in the advanced setting. Since forms of radiotherapy have been validated in the clinically localized as well as salvage settings, "targeted radiotherapy" in the form of RIT is an attractive option with the possibility being a higher yield therapy in the minimal disease (biochemical only) setting. The most studied form of RIT to date uses targeting of the CD20 antigen (^{131}I tositumomab and ^{90}Y ibritumomab tiuxetan) in NHL. Although approved in the relapsed setting, it appears that these therapies have their greatest impact in the minimal disease setting (94–99).

Based on acceptable toxicity and demonstrated antitumor activity, a multicenter, randomized phase II trial in castrate nonmetastatic biochemically progressive disease has been initiated in 2009. The primary objective of this trial is to prevent or delay radiographically evident metastatic disease. Secondary end points include PSA response and time to progression as well as correlative studies. Subjects with biochemically progressive PC after local therapy and initial hormonal therapy (testosterone level less than 50) at high risk for early development of metastatic disease (short PSA doubling time or elevated absolute PSA) (100) will be included. Subjects will be randomized to ketoconazole and hydrocortisone with ^{177}Lu-J591 or trace-labeled ^{111}In-J591 (i.e., placebo). One hundred forty subjects will be randomized in

a 2:1 fashion, stratified by investigational site and type of primary therapy (surgery vs. radiotherapy) to allow 80% power with a two-sided alpha of 5% to detect a 25% absolute difference (50% vs. 75% metastasis free) in radiographically apparent metastasis at 18 months. Radiolabeled J591 imaging will also be explored in these patients. This subset of patients has PSA progression, but no evidence of disease on traditional imaging modalities (bone scan and computed tomography/magnetic resonance imaging). We will explore the utility of radiolabeled J591 imaging to identify current and future clinical sites of disease. Patients with positive sites of imaging will be followed for the development of subsequent clinically detectable metastases in those locations to validate initial findings.

▨ Acknowledgments

The authors wish to acknowledge the Department of Defense for the following grants: CDMRP, PC000042, PC040566, PC970229, NCRR/NIH WCMC CTSC UL1RR024996. The authors also would like to acknowledge and thank the David H. Koch Foundation, the Cancer Research Institute, Prostate Cancer Foundation, and the Peter M. Sacerdote Foundation.

■ REFERENCES

1. Jemal A, Siegel R, Ward E, et al. Cancer statistics, 2008. *CA Cancer J Clin.* 2008;58(2):71–96.
2. Albertsen PC, Hanley JA, Gleason DF, et al. Competing risk analysis of men aged 55 to 74 years at diagnosis managed conservatively for clinically localized prostate cancer. *JAMA.* 1998;280(11):975–980.
3. Albertsen PC, Hanley JA, Fine J. 20-year outcomes following conservative management of clinically localized prostate cancer. *JAMA.* 2005;293(17):2095–2101.
4. Morgan TM, Lange PH, Porter MP, et al. Disseminated tumor cells in prostate cancer patients after radical prostatectomy and without evidence of disease predicts biochemical recurrence. *Clin Cancer Res.* 2009;15(2):677–683.
5. Scher HI, Leibel SA, Fuks Z, et al. Cancers of the prostate. In: DeVita VT Jr, Hellman S, Rosenberg SA, eds. *Cancer: Principles & Practice of Oncology.* 7th ed. Philadelphia, PA: Lippincott Williams & Wilkins; 2005.
6. Tannock IF, Osoba D, Stockler MR, et al. Chemotherapy with mitoxantrone plus prednisone or prednisone alone for symptomatic hormone-resistant prostate cancer: a Canadian randomized trial with palliative end points. *J Clin Oncol.* 1996;14(6):1756–1764.
7. Kantoff PW, Halabi S, Conaway M, et al. Hydrocortisone with or without mitoxantrone in men with hormone-refractory prostate cancer: results of the cancer and leukemia group B 9182 study. *J Clin Oncol.* 1999;17(8):2506–2513.
8. Petrylak DP, Tangen CM, Hussain MH, et al. Docetaxel and estramustine compared with mitoxantrone and prednisone for advanced refractory prostate cancer. *N Engl J Med.* 2004;351(15):1513–1520.
9. Tannock IF, de Wit R, Berry WR, et al. Docetaxel plus prednisone or mitoxantrone plus prednisone for advanced prostate cancer. *N Engl J Med.* 2004;351(15):1502–1512.
10. Tomlins SA, Rhodes DR, Perner S, et al. Recurrent fusion of TMPRSS2 and ETS transcription factor genes in prostate cancer. *Science.* 2005;310(5748):644–648.
11. Feldman BJ, Feldman D. The development of androgen-independent prostate cancer. *Nat Rev Cancer.* 2001;1(1):34–45.
12. Linja MJ, Visakorpi T. Alterations of androgen receptor in prostate cancer. *J Steroid Biochem Mol Biol.* 2004;92(4):255–264.
13. Edwards J, Bartlett JM. The androgen receptor and signal-transduction pathways in hormone-refractory prostate cancer. Part 2: Androgen-receptor cofactors and bypass pathways. *BJU Int.* 2005;95(9):1327–1335.

14. Edwards J, Bartlett JM. The androgen receptor and signal-transduction pathways in hormone-refractory prostate cancer. Part 1: Modifications to the androgen receptor. *BJU Int.* 2005;95(9):1320–1326.

15. Dehm SM, Tindall DJ. Regulation of androgen receptor signaling in prostate cancer. *Expert Rev Anticancer Ther.* 2005;5(1):63–74.

16. Schalken JA. Molecular aspects of hormone-independent prostate cancer. *BJU Int.* 2007;100(suppl 2):52–55.

17. Dehm SM, Tindall DJ. Androgen receptor structural and functional elements: role and regulation in prostate cancer. *Mol Endocrinol.* 2007;21:2855–2863.

18. Nieto M, Finn S, Loda M, et al. Prostate cancer: re-focusing on androgen receptor signaling. *Int J Biochem Cell Biol.* 2007;39(9):1562–1568.

19. Dai J, Shen R, Sumitomo M, et al. Synergistic activation of the androgen receptor by bombesin and low-dose androgen. *Clin Cancer Res.* 2002;8(7):2399–2405.

20. Craft N, Shostak Y, Carey M, et al. A mechanism for hormone-independent prostate cancer through modulation of androgen-receptor signaling by the HER-2/neu tyrosine kinase. *Nat Med.* 1999;5:280–285.

21. Yeh S, Lin HK, Kang HY, et al. From HER2/neu signal cascade to androgen receptor and its coactivators: a novel pathway by induction of androgen target genes through MAP kinase in prostate cancer cells. *Proc Natl Acad Sci U S A.* 1999;96(10):5458–5463.

22. Mellinghoff IK, Vivanco I, Kwon A, et al. HER2/neu kinase-dependent modulation of androgen receptor function through effects on DNA binding and stability. *Cancer Cell.* 2004;6(5):517–527.

23. Scher HI. Prostate carcinoma: defining therapeutic objectives and improving overall outcomes. *Cancer.* 2003;97(3 suppl):758–771.

24. McDonnell TJ, Troncoso P, Brisbay SM, et al. Expression of the proto-oncogene bcl-2 in the prostate and its association with emergence of androgen-independent prostate cancer. *Cancer Res.* 1992;52(24):6940–6944.

25. Morris MJ, Reuter VE, Kelly WK, et al. HER-2 profiling and targeting in prostate carcinoma. *Cancer.* 2002;94(4):980–986.

26. Ross JS, Gray KE, Webb IJ, et al. Antibody-based therapeutics: focus on prostate cancer. *Cancer Metastasis Rev.* 2005;24(4):521–537.

27. Bander NH, Nanus DM, Milowsky MI, et al. Targeted systemic therapy of prostate cancer with a monoclonal antibody to prostate specific membrane antigen (PSMA). *Semin Oncol.* 2003;30:667–677.

28. Bostwick DG, Pacelli A, Blute M, et al. Prostate specific membrane antigen expression in prostatic intraepithelial neoplasia and adenocarcinoma: a study of 184 cases. *Cancer.* 1998;82:2256–2261.

29. Israeli RS, Powell CT, Fair WR, et al. Expression of the prostate-specific membrane antigen. *Cancer Res.* 1994;54:1807–1811.

30. Wright GL Jr., Haley C, Beckett ML, et al. Expression of prostate-specific membrane antigen (PSMA) in normal, benign and malignant prostate tissues. *Urol Oncol.* 1995;1:18–28.

31. Wright GL Jr., Grob BM, Haley C, et al. Upregulation of prostate-specific membrane antigen after androgen-deprivation therapy. *Urology.* 1996;48:326–34.

32. Troyer JK, Beckett ML, Wright GL Jr. Detection and characterization of the prostate-specific membrane antigen (PSMA) in tissue extracts and body fluids. *Int J Cancer.* 1995;62:552–558.

33. Sokoloff RL, Norton KC, Gasior CL, et al. A dual-monoclonal sandwich assay for prostate-specific membrane antigen: levels in tissues, seminal fluid and urine. *Prostate.* 2000;43:150–157.

34. Sweat SD, Pacelli A, Murphy GP, et al. Prostate-specific membrane antigen expression is greatest in prostate adenocarcinoma and lymph node metastases. *Urology.* 1998;52:637–640.

35. Davis MI, Bennett MJ, Thomas LM, et al. Crystal structure of prostate-specific membrane antigen, a tumor marker and peptidase. *Proc Natl Acad Sci.* 2005;102:5981–5986.

36. Mesters JR, Barinka C, Li W, et al. Structure of glutamate carboxypeptidase II, a drug target in neuronal damage and prostate cancer. *EMBO J.* 2006;25:1375–1384.

37. Liu H, Rajasekaran AK, Moy P, et al. Constitutive and antibody-induced internalization of prostate-specific membrane antigen. *Cancer Res.* 1998;58:4055–4060.

38. Rajasekaran SA, Anilkuman G, Oshima E, et al. A novel cytoplasmic tail MXXXL motif mediates the internalization of prostate-specific membrane antigen. *Mol Biol Cell.* 2003;14:4835–4845.

39. Kahn D, Williams RD, Manyak MJ, et al. [111]Indium-capromab pendetide in the evaluation of patients with residual or recurrent prostate cancer after radical prostatectomy. The ProstaScint study group. *J Urol.* 1998;159:2041–2046.

40. Kahn D, Williams RD, Haseman MK, et al. Radioimmunoscintigraphy with in-111-labeled capromab pendetide predicts prostate cancer

response to salvage radiotherapy after failed radical prostatectomy. *J Clin Oncol.* 1998; 16:284–289.

41. Troyer JK, Feng Q, Beckett ML, et al. Biochemical characterization and mapping of the 7E11-C5.3 epitope of the prostate-specific membrane antigen. *Urol Oncol.* 1995;1(1):29–37.

42. Troyer JK, Beckett ML, Wright GL Jr. Location of prostate-specific membrane antigen in the LNCaP prostate carcinoma cell line. *Prostate.* 1997;30(4):232–242.

43. Liu H, Moy P, Kim S, et al. Monoclonal antibodies to the extracellular domain of prostate-specific membrane antigen also react with tumor vascular endothelium. *Cancer Res.* 1997;57(17):3629–3634.

44. Horoszewicz JS, Kawinski E, Murphy GP. Monoclonal antibodies to a new antigenic marker in epithelial prostatic cells and serum of prostate cancer patients. *Anticancer Res.* 1987;7:927–935.

45. Yao D, Trabulsi EJ, Kostakoglu L, et al. The utility of monoclonal antibodies in the imaging of prostate cancer. *Semin Urol Oncol.* 2002; 20(3):211–218.

46. Smith-Jones PM, Vallabhajosula S, Goldsmith SJ, et al. In vitro characterization of radiolabeled monoclonal antibodies specific for the extracellular domain of prostate-specific membrane antigen. *Cancer Res.* 2000;60(18):5237–5243.

47. McDevitt MR, Barendswaard E, Ma D, et al. An alpha-particle emitting antibody ([213Bi]J591) for radioimmunotherapy of prostate cancer. *Cancer Res.* 2000;60:6095–6100.

48. Smith-Jones PM, Vallabhajosula S, Navarro V, et al. Radiolabeled monoclonal antibodies specific to the extracellular domain of prostate-specific membrane antigen: preclinical studies in nude mice bearing LNCaP human prostate tumor. *J Nucl Med.* 2003;44(4):610–617.

49. Vallabhajosula S, Smith-Jones PM, Navarro V, et al. Radioimmunotherapy of prostate cancer in human xenografts using monoclonal antibodies specific to prostate specific membrane antigen (PSMA): studies in nude mice. *Prostate.* 2004;58:145–155.

50. Hamilton A, King S, Liu H, et al. A novel humanised antibody against prostate specific membrane antigen (PSMA) for in vivo targeting and therapy. *Proc Am Assoc Cancer Res.* 1998;39:440.

51. Konishi S, Hamacher K, Vallabhajosula S, et al. Determination of immunoreactive fraction of radiolabeled monoclonal antibodies: what is an appropriate method? *Cancer Biother Radiopharm.* 2004;19:706–715.

52. Bander NH, Nanus D, Bremer S, et al. Phase I clinical trial targeting a monoclonal antibody (mAb) to the extracellular domain of prostate specific membrane antigen (PSMAext) in patients with hormone-independent prostate cancer [abstract 1827]. 2000.

53. Bander NH, Nanus D, Goldstein S, et al. Phase I trial of humanized monoclonal antibody (mAb) to prostate specific membrane antigen/extracellular domain (PSMAext) [abstract 722]. 2001.

54. Vallabhajosula S, Kuji I, Hamacher KA, et al. Pharmacokinetics and biodistribution of ^{111}In and ^{177}Lu labeled J591 antibody specific to prostate specific membrane antigen: prediction of ^{90}Y-J591 radiation dosimetry based on ^{111}In and [177]Lu. *J Nucl Med.* 2005;46: 634–641.

55. Vallabhajosula S, Goldsmith SJ, Hamacher KA, et al. Prediction of myelotoxicity based on bone marrow radiation absorbed dose: radioimmunotherapy studies using ^{90}Y and ^{177}Lu labeled J591 antibodies specific to prostate specific membrane antigen (PSMA). *J Nucl Med.* 2005;46:850–858.

56. Milowsky MI, Nanus DM, Kostakoglu L, et al. Phase I trial of yttrium-90–labeled anti–prostate-specific membrane antigen monoclonal antibody J591 for androgen-independent prostate cancer. *J Clin Oncol.* 2003;22:2522–2531.

57. Bander NH, Milowsky MI, Nanus DM, et al. Phase I trial of [177]lutetium-labeled J591, a monoclonal antibody to prostate-specific membrane antigen, in patients with androgen-independent prostate cancer. *J Clin Oncol.* 2005;23:4591–4601.

58. Witzig TE, White CA, Gordon LI, et al. Safety of yttrium-90 ibritumomab tiuxetan radioimmunotherapy for relapsed low-grade, follicular, or transformed non-Hodgkin's lymphoma. *J Clin Oncol.* 2003;21: 1263–1270.

59. Pai-Scherf LH, Carrasquillo JA, Paik C, et al. Imaging and phase I study of [111]In- and ^{90}Y-labeled anti-LewisY monoclonal antibody B3. *Clin Cancer Res.* 2000;6:1720–1730.

60. Mulligan T, Carrasquillo JA, Chung Y, et al. Phase I study of intravenous Lu-labeled CC49 murine monoclonal antibody in patients with advanced adenocarcinoma. *Clin Can Res.* 1995;1:1447–1454.

61. Alvarez RD, Partridge EE, Khazaeli MB, et al. Intraperitoneal radioimmunotherapy of ovarian cancer with ^{177}Lu-CC49: a phase I/II study. *Gynecol Oncol.* 1997;65:94–101.

62. Meredith R, Alvarez RD, Partridge EE, et al. Intraperitoneal radioimmunochemotherapy of ovarian cancer: a phase I study. *Cancer Biotherapy Radiopharm.* 2001;16:305–315.

63. O'Donoghue JA, Bardies M, Wheldon TE. Relationships between tumor size and curability for uniformly targeted therapy with beta-emitting radionuclides. *J Nucl Med.* 1995;36:1902–1909.

64. Knox SJ, Goris ML, Trisler K, et al. Yttrium-90-labeled anti-CD20 monoclonal antibody therapy of recurrent B-cell lymphoma. *Clin Cancer Res.* 1996;2:457–470.

65. O'Donnell RT, DeNardo SJ, Yuan A, et al. Radioimmunotherapy with (111)In/(90)Y-2IT-BAD-m170 for metastatic prostate cancer. *Clin Cancer Res.* 2001;7:1561–1568.

66. Tagawa ST, Milowsky MI, Morris M, et al. Phase II trial of ^{177}lutetium radiolabeled anti-prostate-specific membrane antigen (PSMA) monoclonal antibody J591 (^{177}Lu-J591) in patients (pts) with metastatic castrate-resistant prostate cancer (metCRPC). In: *Proceedings of the American Society of Clinical Oncology.* American Society of Clinical Oncology; 2008:284s. [abstract 5140].

67. Petrylak DP, Ankerst DP, Jiang CS, et al. Evaluation of prostate-specific antigen declines for surrogacy in patients treated on SWOG 99-16. *J Natl Cancer Inst.* 2006;98(8):516–521.

68. Armstrong AJ, Garrett-Mayer E, Ou Yang YC, et al. Prostate-specific antigen and pain surrogacy analysis in metastatic hormone-refractory prostate cancer. *J Clin Oncol.* 2007;25(25):3965–3970.

69. Hynecek R, Goldsmith SJ, Vallabhajosula S, et al. ^{177}Lu-J591 monoclonal antibody (Lu-J591) therapy in metastatic castrate resistant prostate cancer (metCRPC): correlation of antibody-tumor targeting and treatment response. *J Nucl Med.* 2008;49(suppl 1):144P.

70. Meyn RE. Apoptosis and response to radiation: implications for radiation therapy. *Oncology (Williston Park)* 1997;11(3):349–356; discussion 356, 361, 365.

71. Kroger LA, DeNardo GL, Gumerlock PH, et al. Apoptosis-related gene and protein expression in human lymphoma xenografts (raji) after low dose rate radiation using 67Cu-2IT-BAT-lym-1 radioimmunotherapy. *Cancer Biother Radiopharm.* 2001;16(3):213–225.

72. Mirzaie-Joniani H, Eriksson D, Sheikholvaezin A, et al. Apoptosis induced by low-dose and low-dose-rate radiation. *Cancer.* 2002;94(4 suppl):1210–1214.

73. DeNardo GL, Schlom J, Buchsbaum DJ, et al. Rationales, evidence, and design considerations for fractionated radioimmunotherapy. *Cancer.* 2002;94(4 suppl):1332–1348.

74. Burke PA, DeNardo SJ, Miers LA, et al. Combined modality radioimmunotherapy. Promise and peril. *Cancer.* 2002;94(4 suppl):1320–1331.

75. O'Donoghue JA, Sgouros G, Divgi CR, et al. Single-dose versus fractionated radioimmunotherapy: model comparisons for uniform tumor dosimetry. *J Nucl Med.* 2000;41(3):538–547.

76. Shen S, Duan J, Meredith RF, et al. Model prediction of treatment planning for dose-fractionated radioimmunotherapy. *Cancer.* 2002;15;94(4 suppl):1264–1269.

77. Vriesendorp HM, Shao Y, Blum JE, et al. Fractionated intravenous administration of ^{90}Y-labeled B72.3 GYK-DTPA immunoconjugate in beagle dogs. *Nucl Med Biol.* 1993;20(5):571–578.

78. Buchsbaum D, Khazaeli MB, Liu T, et al. Fractionated radioimmunotherapy of human colon carcinoma xenografts with ^{131}I-labeled monoclonal antibody CC49. *Cancer Res.* 1995;55(23 suppl):5881s–5887s.

79. DeNardo GL, DeNardo SJ, Lamborn KR, et al. Low-dose, fractionated radioimmunotherapy for B-cell malignancies using ^{131}I-lym-1 antibody. *Cancer Biother Radiopharm.* 1998;13(4):239–254.

80. Steffens MG, Boerman OC, Oyen WJ, et al. Intratumoral distribution of two consecutive injections of chimeric antibody G250 in primary renal cell carcinoma: implications for fractionated dose radioimmunotherapy. *Cancer Res.* 1999;59(7):1615–1619.

81. Hindorf C, Linden O, Stenberg L, et al. Change in tumor-absorbed dose due to decrease in mass during fractionated radioimmunotherapy in lymphoma patients. *Clin Cancer Res.* 2003;9(10, pt 2):4003S–4006S.

82. Choy H, Rodriguez FF, Koester S, et al. Investigation of taxol as a potential radiation sensitizer. *Cancer.* 1993;71(11):3774–3778.

83. Tishler RB, Schiff PB, Geard CR, et al. Taxol: a novel radiation sensitizer. *Int J Radiat Oncol Biol Phys.* 1992;22(3):613–617.

84. Hennequin C, Giocanti N, Favaudon V. Interaction of ionizing radiation with paclitaxel (Taxol) and docetaxel (Taxotere) in HeLa and SQ20B cells. *Cancer Res.* 1996;56(8):1842–1850.

85. O'Donnell RT, DeNardo SJ, Miers LA, et al. Combined modality radioimmunotherapy for human prostate cancer xenografts with taxanes and ^{90}yttrium-DOTA-peptide-ChL6. *Prostate.* 2002;50(1):27–37.

86. Richman CM, Denardo SJ, O'Donnell RT, et al. High-dose radioimmunotherapy combined with fixed, low-dose paclitaxel in metastatic prostate and breast cancer by using a MUC-1 monoclonal antibody, m170, linked to indium-111/yttrium-90 via a cathepsin cleavable linker with cyclosporine to prevent human anti-mouse antibody. *Clin Cancer Res.* 2005;11(16):5920–5927.

87. Kelly MP, Lee FT, Smyth FE, et al. Enhanced efficacy of ^{90}Y-radiolabeled anti-Lewis Y humanized monoclonal antibody hu3S193 and paclitaxel combined-modality radioimmunotherapy in a breast cancer model. *J Nucl Med.* 2006;47(4):716–725.

88. Moul JW. Prostate specific antigen only progression of prostate cancer. *J Urol.* 2000;163(6):1632–1642.

89. Scher HI, Eisenberger M, D'Amico AV, et al. Eligibility and outcomes reporting guidelines for clinical trials for patients in the state of a rising prostate-specific antigen: recommendations from the prostate-specific antigen working group. *J Clin Oncol.* 2004;22(3):537–556.

90. Pazona JF, Han M, Hawkins SA, et al. Salvage radiation therapy for prostate specific antigen progression following radical prostatectomy: 10-year outcome estimates. *J Urol.* 2005;174(4, pt 1):1282–1286.

91. Buskirk SJ, Pisansky TM, Schild SE, et al. Salvage radiotherapy for isolated prostate specific antigen increase after radical prostatectomy: evaluation of prognostic factors and creation of a prognostic scoring system. *J Urol.* 2006;176(3):985–990.

92. Stephenson AJ, Shariat SF, Zelefsky MJ, et al. Salvage radiotherapy for recurrent prostate cancer after radical prostatectomy. *JAMA.* 2004;291(11):1325–1332.

93. Ward JF, Zincke H, Bergstralh EJ, et al. Prostate specific antigen doubling time subsequent to radical prostatectomy as a prognosticator of outcome following salvage radiotherapy. *J Urol.* 2004;172(6, pt 1):2244–2248.

94. Kaminski M, Estes J, Zasadny K, et al. Radioimmunotherapy with iodine ^{131}I tositumomab for relapsed or refractory B-cell non-Hodgkin lymphoma: updated results and long-term follow-up of the university of Michigan experience. *Blood.* 2000;96(4):1259–1266.

95. Kaminski MS, Zelenetz AD, Press OW, et al. Pivotal study of iodine I 131 tositumomab for chemotherapy-refractory low-grade or transformed low-grade B-cell non-Hodgkin's lymphomas. *J Clin Oncol.* 2001;19(19):3918–3928.

96. Press OW, Unger JM, Braziel RM, et al. A phase 2 trial of CHOP chemotherapy followed by tositumomab/iodine I 131 tositumomab for previously untreated follicular non-Hodgkin lymphoma: Southwest oncology group protocol S9911. *Blood.* 2003;102(5):1606–1612.

97. Kaminski MS, Tuck M, Estes J, et al. ^{131}I-tositumomab therapy as initial treatment for follicular lymphoma. *N Engl J Med.* 2005;352(5):441–449.

98. Leonard JP, Coleman M, Kostakoglu L, et al. Abbreviated chemotherapy with fludarabine followed by tositumomab and iodine I 131 tositumomab for untreated follicular lymphoma. *J Clin Oncol.* 2005;23(24):5696–5704.

99. Press OW, Unger JM, Braziel RM, et al. Phase II trial of CHOP chemotherapy followed by tositumomab/iodine I-131 tositumomab for previously untreated follicular non-Hodgkin's lymphoma: five-year follow-up of Southwest Oncology Group Protocol S9911. *J Clin Oncol.* 2006;24(25):4143–4149.

100. Smith MR, Kabbinavar F, Saad F, et al. Natural history of rising serum prostate-specific antigen in men with castrate nonmetastatic prostate cancer. *J Clin Oncol.* 2005;23(13):2918–2925.

Targeted Radionuclide Therapy in Renal Cell Carcinoma

Egbert Oosterwijk

■ RENAL CELL CARCINOMA: GENERAL ASPECTS

Renal cell carcinoma (RCC) is the most common renal malignant neoplasm in adults, accounting for approximately 85% of renal tumors and 2% of all adult malignancies (1). In 2008, it was estimated that more than 54,000 people will be diagnosed with and more than 13,000 people will die from cancer of the kidney and renal pelvis in the United States (1). RCC is the 3rd leading cause of death among genitourinary cancers and the 12th leading cause of cancer death overall in the United States (1). Kidney cancer is not a single disease; it is made up of a number of different types of cancer that occur in the kidney. They can be distinguished by different histology, have a different clinical course, and are associated with alterations of different genes. Based on morphologic and molecular considerations, four RCC subtypes are recognized: clear cell RCC (ccRCC), chromophobe RCC, papillary RCC, and renal oncocytoma (2). The molecular pathways involved in the development of these kidney cancers have been well established. ccRCC accounts for the vast majority of RCC (~75%), and genetic or epigenetic alterations in the Von Hippel Lindau (VHL) tumor suppressor gene can be found in greater than 90% of ccRCC, providing evidence that VHL alteration is an early event in ccRCC carcinogenesis. Of the remaining RCC, 15% are papillary where missense mutations in the proto-oncogene c-met lead to constitutive activation of the MET protein. Abberations in the folliculin gene have been linked with RCC belonging to the chromophobe and oncocytoma subtype (2). Preoperative identification of these different tumor types that occur within one organ might be beneficial and could have important implications for the choice of treatment for renal cancers.

When patients present with localized disease, radical or partial nephrectomy (dependent on the size and location of the lesion) is potentially curative. However, nearly one third of these patients develop recurrent disease, usually within 1 year. Approximately one third of newly diagnosed patients present with metastatic disease (mRCC). Thus, of all patients diagnosed, almost 50% need therapy for advanced (stage IV) RCC. For patients with mRCC, prognosis is poor with a median survival of approximately 10% and a 5-year survival less than 10%. This is a reflection of the lack of efficacy of standard therapies (chemotherapy and radiation therapy). Until recently, patients with advanced RCC were treated with various immunotherapeutic regimens that used recombinant human interleukin-2 (IL-2) and recombinant human interferon alpha-2b (IFN-alpha) either alone or in combination. The use of these cytokines is, however, limited by their toxicity and generally poor overall response rates. Based on the understanding of the molecular pathways that are involved in the biology of RCC, several novel therapeutic strategies have been developed. Indeed, the introduction of receptor tyrosine kinase inhibitors (TKI) has changed the clinical management of patients with mRCC substantially. Treatment with the antiangiogenic TKIs sorafenib and sunitinib significantly prolongs the progression-free survival (PFS) of mRCC patients. Additionally, treatment with bevacizumab, a humanized monoclonal antibody against vascular endothelial growth factor (VEGF) that binds and neutralizes all of the major isoforms of VEGF, significantly prolongs PFS (3). However, clinical responses mainly comprise stabilization of disease, and ultimately the majority of patients develop resistance to these drugs. There is currently no therapy that is effective in this situation. Therefore, there is still an urgent need to develop additional strategies that induce tumor regression rather than stabilization of disease.

■ MONOCLONAL ANTIBODIES IN RENAL CELL CANCER

Historically, RCC is considered an immunogenic tumor based on various lines of evidence: spontaneous regression of RCC has been observed, albeit very infrequent; several investigators have been able to isolate tumor-specific T cells; sera of RCC patients appear to contain RCC-specific IgG; and RCC-specific polyclonal antisera, not reactive with normal kidney tissue, have been described. Indeed, these considerations were the basis supporting the use of immunotherapy in advanced RCC. The fact that treatment of mRCC patients with expanded tumor-infiltrating lymphocytes led to antitumor responses highlighted the possibility that RCC-associated or RCC-specific molecules were expressed and might be used as therapeutic target.

Similar to other malignancies, monoclonal antibodies targeting renal cancer were developed without understanding the molecular events underlying the carcinogenic events leading to the malignancy, under the assumption that such molecules might be expressed based on the immunogenic profile of RCC. Several investigators described mAbs that recognized either kidney-associated molecules (4–7) or, in few cases, molecules expressed by RCC and not expressed by normal kidney tissue (5,8).

Several mechanisms to eradicate tumor cells by mAbs have been described. Destruction of tumor cells can be mediated via effector cells or complement, or conjugation of the mAb to toxins, drugs, or radionuclides. Since antigen expression within tumors is heterogeneous, antigen-negative tumor cells could evade tumor cell lysis by effector cell– or complement-mediated cytotoxicity. This could eventually lead to tumor recurrence in patients. The same applies to mAbs conjugated to toxins or drugs. Internalization of an mAb conjugated to a toxin or drug is required to mediate cell killing (9). Here I will focus on mAbs conjugated to radionuclides for the diagnosis and treatment of RCC.

Preclinical targeting studies have been restricted to mAbs A6H (10–12) and G250 (13–18). For A6H, relatively high tumor-to-blood ratios in mice with RCC xenografts were observed and radioimmunotherapy (RIT) with iodine 131-labeled A6H caused the tumor to regress or arrested the tumor growth in xenografts (10). In a clinical study the imaging and RIT abilities of this mAb were examined. Positive images were obtained in 5 of 15 patients only. This low number was attributed to circulating antigen and the expression of antigen in normal tissue, thereby diminishing adequate mAb accumulation into tumor tissue. An altered dose schedule resulted in an increase in the number of positive images, but the number of imaged lesions was still unsatisfactory (12). These findings halted the use of mAb A6H in the diagnosis and treatment of RCC.

MONOCLONAL ANTIBODY G250: PRECLINICAL EXPERIENCE

The preclinical experience with mAb G250 is quite extensive. This mAb was described as an mAb recognizing an RCC-associated antigen, absent in normal kidney and most other normal tissues and homogeneously expressed in most RCC (8), most notably ccRCC (19). Further extensive fine-specificity analyses have shown cross-reactivity to the (upper) gastrointestinal mucosa (stomach, ileum, and proximal and middle colon) and gastrointestinal-related structures (intra- and extrahepatic biliary system, and pancreas) in vitro.

Various animal and ex vivo experiments have shown the potential of G250 as a targeting modality of RCC (13–18,20,21): G250 demonstrated high homogeneous accumulation in RCC tissue, showed restricted uptake in non-RCC tissues in biodistribution experiments in animal models expression, and required a low protein dose for tumor antigen saturation in preclinical models. Thus, mAb G250 seemed a suitable candidate for further investigation in clinical studies. The first clinical studies with G250 were performed without any knowledge about the G250 target molecule. In 2000, the G250 antigen was molecular identified

and shown to be carbonic anhydrase 9 (CA9) (22). The molecular characterization allowed transcriptional regulation studies that revealed a strict dependence of G250 expression on HIF-1α (23). Thus, the mechanism responsible for CA9 expression in ccRCC is molecularly linked to the most prominent molecular defect in ccRCC, namely due to nonfunctional VHL protein leading to HIF-1α accumulation and gene expression. Indeed, this nicely explained the results of studies showing almost ubiquitous expression (greater than 90%) of G250-antigen in ccRCC and of gene expression studies demonstrating ubiquitous homogeneous G250 gene expression in all the ccRCC examined in contrast to G250 expression by oncocytomas, chromophobe, or papillary RCC, which was low or absent (19,24,25). These results have directed the scope of mAbG250 studies to ccRCC.

CLINICAL STUDIES WITH MURINE G250

In the first two clinical studies with radiolabeled G250, murine G250 was administered (26,27). In the first, biopsy-based protein-dose escalation study, G250 imaging and biodistribution were defined in 16 patients who received 10 mCi ^{131}I-mAbG250 1 week prior to nephrectomy (26). After 3 to 4 days, clear tumor images were seen in 12 patients, scanned with a gamma camera. Ten of these tumors turned out to be G250 positive, whereas the other two showed less than 5% G250 expression. The four tumors that were not visualized turned out to be of other histologic subtypes than clear cell. Importantly, at 2 mg protein doses, liver uptake was quite significant. This component turned out to be completely saturable, and at protein doses greater than 2 mg, G250-only tumors were visible by gamma camera. After nephrectomy, tumor samples showed high focal uptake of G250 accumulation in tumor tissue, up to 0.21% injected dose/gram (% ID/g). RCC is known as a tumor with high vessel density, and to exclude the possibility that the clear images were a reflection of high blood volume, patients received ^{99m}Tc-labeled human serum albumin before surgery. [99m]Tc images showed less tumor uptake than ^{131}I-mAbG250 that had been administered earlier and discordant images, indicative of true antibody targeting of the tumor by mAbG250. Second, in vitro analyses showed no uptake in G250-negative renal tumors, another indication that true antigen-specific antibody targeting was achieved.

As discussed, RCC is considered resistant to radiotherapy. Nevertheless, the observed G250 uptake levels were unprecedented in solid tumors, and dosimetric analysis suggested that tumor-sterilizing levels might be achieved. Therefore, a phase I/II dose-escalation RIT study was initiated (27). Patients were treated with increasing doses of ^{131}I-mAbG250. After reaching the maximum tolerated dose (MTD), 15 patients were enrolled and treated at the MTD to monitor any possible therapeutic effects. In this phase I dose-escalating study, hematologic toxicity prevented escalation beyond 90 mCi/m². Remarkably, transient hepatic toxicity occurred at dose levels of 45 mCi/m² and higher, most likely the result of ^{131}I-mAbG250 liver uptake, but was not dose limiting. No relation between the level of hepatic toxicity and 131-iodine dose could be seen. Of 33 patients treated (18 in the dose-escalating part of the study and another 15 at the MTD), 17 patients stabilized for 3 months, after which they received other treatments, making further follow-up impossible. Three patients showed regression of some of their lesions, but no partial or complete responses were noted (27). The effect of ^{131}I-mAbG250 on the disease was difficult to judge, particularly because it is well established that the growth velocity of RCC can fluctuate substantially.

■ CLINICAL STUDIES WITH CHIMERIC G250

Exposure of patients to the murine mAb G250 induced an immunologic response in all patients. Obviously, the formation of human antimouse antibodies (HAMA) in all patients prohibited retreatment as antibody immune complexes would be formed with rapid clearance of the radiolabeled mAb to liver and spleen (27). This, in combination with the high potential of G250 as a targeting agent in the treatment of metastasized RCC, led to the development of a chimeric form of G250 (cG250) (28). This mAb is composed of murine antigen-binding variable domains that recognize the tumor-associated antigen (TAA) and a human constant domain of heavy and light chains derived from the human IgG$_1$ isotype. The rationale behind this construction was the decrease in immunogenicity of the antibody, potentially allowing multiple administrations. Additionally, chimerization led to induction of tumor cell death through targeting of effector cells to the tumor cells via the Fc portion of the mAb through antibody-dependent cellular cytotoxicity (ADCC) (29,30). Several clinical studies with cold (unlabeled) cG250 have been performed (31,32), including a large phase III study in high-risk RCC patients (ARISER) in which more than 800 patients were included. In view of the emphasis on RIT, suffice it to say that treatment of patients suggested immunomodulation of the natural course of metastatic RCC. In the adjuvant setting, administration of cG250 led to a lower relapse rate than expected (http://www.wilex.de/News/2009/080409.htm), but this study still awaits the final analysis.

After the construction of the chimeric mAb G250 (cG250), the pharmacokinetics, biodistribution, imaging characteristics, and dosimetry were determined in a protein dose-escalating study similar to murine G250 (33). Presurgical RCC patients were entered in this phase I protein dose-escalation trial where five protein dose levels (2, 5, 10, 25, and 50 mg) were labeled with 6 mCi ^{131}I and administered i.v. 1 week before patients underwent nephrectomy. The highest relative tumor uptake was observed in patients receiving 5 mg ^{131}I-cG250, with tumor uptake as high as 0.52% ID/g. At higher protein doses, focal tumor uptake did not exceed 0.017% ID/g. This suggests that antigen saturation might have occurred at protein dose levels greater than 5 mg cG250. Similar to the murine G250 protein dose-escalation study, excellent, clear images were obtained in patients with G250-antigen-positive tumors, including

visualization of metastases. Dosimetric analysis revealed radiation-absorbed doses to primary tumors as well as to metastases up to 1.9 cGy/MBq. Human antichimeric antibody (HACA) responses were minimal: two patients demonstrated very low HACA levels, which were regarded clinically irrelevant, up to 20 weeks postinjection. Because the immunogenicity of the antibody was significantly diminished, multiple treatments became possible (33). Also, the results in this trial justified further investigation on the use of cG250 as a radioimmunotherapeutic agent.

The MTD of ^{131}I-cG250 in metastatic RCC was defined in a phase I trial in patients with progressive metastatic RCC at study entry (34). In contrast to the RIT study with murine G250, patients received a scout dose of 5 mg cG250 labeled with 5 mCi ^{131}I, followed by high-dose ^{131}I-cG250, only when accumulation of the scout dose was seen in target lesions. This prevented unnecessary toxicity in patients with CA9-negative tumors. The most remarkable difference between this dose-escalation trial and the murine G250 dose-escalation trial was the absence of hepatic toxicity. This most likely resulted from the saturation of the hepatic compartment by the diagnostic dose ^{131}I-cG250 (34). Besides mild nausea without vomiting and transient fatigue (both grade 1 common terminology criteria), no other side effects occurred. The MTD was established at 60 mCi/m^2, with hematologic toxicity as the dose-limiting factor. Of eight patients receiving high-dose ^{131}I-cG250 treatment, one showed stable disease and one had a partial response (34). One patient was excluded because of rapid disease progression; three did not receive the high-dose injection because of lack of tumor targeting, highlighting the necessity to prescreen patients for adequate cG250 targeting with the scout dose.

Subsequently two approaches were chosen in efforts to optimize RIT of metastatic ccRCC with ^{131}I-cG250: dose fractionation (35) and two sequential high-dose treatments (36). In the dose-fractionation study, patients received 30 mCi ^{131}I-cG250, and whole-body activity was measured after 2 to 3 days. Then, ^{131}I-cG250 was administered until the whole-body activity reached 30 mCi again. This schedule was continued until a whole-body absorbed dose of 0.50 Gy was reached. Patients without disease progression were retreated after recovery from hematologic toxicity. Cohorts consisted of three patients, and in subsequent cohorts the dose increased in 0.25-Gy increments. In this trial, 15 patients were included and HACA developed in two patients, leading to altered pharmacokinetics and excluding them from further treatment. Dose-limiting toxicity was hematopoietic, with the MTD at 0.75 Gy as whole-body absorbed dose. Of the 15 patients, 4 received multiple fractionated doses with disease stabilization occurring up to 7 and 13 months. Two other patients were alive 3 years after treatment (35). However, no partial or complete clinical responses were observed, and therefore the potential benefit of fractionation of RIT doses in treating ccRCC was not established.

In an independent study, the effects of two sequential high doses of ^{131}I-cG250 was investigated (36). Similar to the earlier RIT trial, patients needed to show a positive image after receiving a diagnostic dose with 5 mCi ^{131}I-cG250. Thereafter, patients received 60 mCi/m^2 ^{131}I-cG250. After 3 months, when hematopoietic blood count levels were restored, the same cycle was applied, including the scout dose to rule out rapid clearance of cG250 by HACA development. After establishing the MTD of the second RIT (45 mCi/m^2, i.e., 75% of the MTD of the first dose), 15 patients were treated at this dose level to evaluate tumor response. Higher doses were not possible in view of prolonged depression of leukocyte counts and platelet values. In total, 29 patients entered the study. Of these, 11 were excluded for evaluation of tumor response: 3 patients showed grade 4 hematologic toxicity after the first RIT, 2 patients received palliative treatment, 2 patients showed rapid progressive disease, and 4 patients developed HACA. Of the 18 patients evaluated (3 patients did not receive the second RIT at MTD), 5 patients showed stabilization of their disease, which lasted 3 to 12 months (36). Disappointingly, partial or complete responses were not observed.

■ RECENT DEVELOPMENTS

Indisputably, radionuclides other than ^{131}I such as ^{90}Y, ^{177}Lu, and ^{186}Re are potentially more effective: ^{131}I has been used to label antibodies for decades because it is an easy technique; it is inexpensive and widely available and emits γ-radiation, allowing imaging. However, this also results in high radiation burden to staff and relatives. Additionally, ^{131}I-labeled mAbs may degrade rapidly and the β-emission is of relatively low energy. Stable radiolabeling of mAbs with more potent radionuclides is cumbersome, but might result in more effective RIT.

Before initiating RIT with metallic radionuclides, a comparative ^{131}I/^{111}In-cG250 study was performed in four patients with metastatic RCC who were i.v. injected with 5 mCi ^{111}In-ITC-DTPA-cG250 on day 0 and 5 mCi ^{131}I-cG250 on day 4. Images were acquired on day 0 and day 4 after each injection and were compared (37). ^{111}In-ITC-DTPA-cG250 images revealed more lesions than ^{131}I-cG250 images (47 vs. 30), and quantitative analysis showed higher activities of ^{111}In-ITC-DTPA-cG250 in 20 of 25 lesions measured. Second, the therapeutic properties of four radionuclides (^{90}Y and ^{177}Lu [residualizing] and ^{131}I and ^{186}Re [nonresidualizing]) were explored in an animal model (13). Tumor growth and survival were monitored for each radionuclide. The most effective treatment was noted with ^{177}Lu-cG250, followed by ^{90}Y and ^{186}Re and least with ^{131}I (185, 125, 90, and 25 days, respectively). Additionally, ^{177}Lu-cG250 treatment showed the best median survival (300 days), with the control group having a median survival time of less than 150 days. Treatment with either residualizing radionuclide (^{177}Lu or ^{90}Y) led to higher radiation doses to the tumor. These radionuclides, therefore, were considered better candidates for RIT with cG250 than ^{131}I (13).

At present a phase I/II RIT study is ongoing and is very similar to the trial in which two sequential high doses of

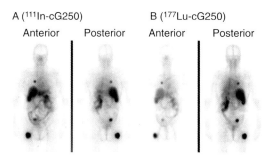

A (^{111}In-cG250) B (^{177}Lu-cG250)
Anterior Posterior Anterior Posterior

FIGURE 32.1 Immunoscintigram acquired 7 days after injection of 185 MBq ^{111}In-cG250 (A) and immunoscintigram of the same patient, acquired 7 days after injection of 3.256 MBq ^{177}Lu-cG250 (B). Left image, anterior view; right image, posterior view. Note the clear visualization of metastases in lung, remaining kidney, and lymph nodes. High tumor accumulation of the radiolabeled cG250 is evident and the ^{111}In and ^{177}Lu images are superimposable, demonstrating the predictive value of the injection of the scout dose.

^{131}I-cG250 were studied in metastatic RCC patients with progressive disease. Patients receive 5 mCi ^{111}In-cG250 to provide evidence that adequate target to lesions occurs, followed by high-dose ^{177}Lu-DOTA-cG250. When disease has not progressed after 3 months, this cycle is repeated, including the diagnostic ^{111}In-cG250. If tumor targeting is apparent, patients are retreated with 75% of the previous dose, for a maximum of three cycles. Thus far, ^{111}In-cG250/^{177}Lu-cG250 images have been highly similar (Fig. 32.1) and the ^{111}In-cG250 images could be used to estimate radiation doses to the tissues following injection of ^{177}Lu-cG250. MTD has now been reached, and currently patients are treated at MTD (60 mCi/m^2). Encouragingly, most patients (14/18) demonstrated stable disease 14 weeks after the first treatment cycle, and the average growth of all tumor lesions was reduced from 28.5% before treatment to 4.1% posttreatment ($p < .002$) (38). Despite this encouraging result, future strategies to improve clinical efficacy of cG250 need to be developed and might include pretargeting approaches, bone marrow support, transplantation, or use of high linear energy transfer (LET) particles emitting radionuclides.

Here, the focus has been on RIT with cG250. However, in view of the excellent imaging capacity of cG250, it may play a role in the diagnosis and monitoring of RCC. Preoperative identification of tumor type could have important implications for the choice of treatment for renal cancers. Divgi et al. demonstrated that positron emission tomography (PET) with ^{124}I-cG250 accurately identified ccRCC, with a negative scan highly predictive of a less aggressive (non-ccRCC) phenotype. The study suggests that stratification of patients with renal masses by ^{124}I-cG250 PET can identify aggressive tumors and help decide treatment (39).

In conclusion, mAb cG250 may have a role in diagnosing and/or treating metastatic RCC. Thus far no major responses have been noted, but the high homogeneous expression in RCC combined with the low cross-reactivity with normal tissue warrants further investigation on its use. Whether cG250 can play a role in the diagnosis and monitoring of ccRCC will become clear in the near future as a large randomized study addressing this issue is now being performed.

Acknowledgments

The author would like to thank the Departments of Urology and Nuclear Medicine of the Radboud University Medical Centre and the Ludwig Institute for Cancer Research, New York, for their very productive collaboration. The help of many technical research assistants working in various departments is gratefully acknowledged.

REFERENCES

1. Jemal A, Siegel R, Ward E, et al. Cancer statistics, 2008. *CA Cancer J Clin*. 2008;58:71–96.
2. Linehan WM, Grubb RL, Coleman JA, et al. The genetic basis of cancer of kidney cancer: implications for gene-specific clinical management. *BJU Int*. 2005;95(suppl 2):2–7.
3. Heng DY, Bukowski RM. Anti-angiogenic targets in the treatment of advanced renal cell carcinoma. *Curr Cancer Drug Targets*. 2008;8(8):676–682.
4. Bander NH, Finstad CL, Cordon-Cardo C, et al. Analysis of a mouse monoclonal antibody that reacts with a specific region of the human proximal tubule and subsets renal cell carcinomas. *Cancer Res*. 1989;49(23):6774–6780.
5. Finstad CL, Cordon-Cardo C, Bander NH, et al. Specificity analysis of mouse monoclonal antibodies defining cell surface antigens of human renal cancer. *Proc Natl Acad Sci USA*. 1985;82(9):2955–2959.
6. Oosterwijk E, Ruiter DJ, Wakka JC, et al. Immunohistochemical analysis of monoclonal antibodies to renal antigens. Application in the diagnosis of renal cell carcinoma. *Am J Pathol*. 1986;123(2):301–309.
7. Moon TD, Vessella RL, Palme DF, et al. A highly restricted antigen for renal cell carcinoma defined by a monoclonal antibody. *Hybridoma*. 1985;4(2):163–171.
8. Oosterwijk E, Ruiter DJ, Hoedemaeker PJ, et al. Monoclonal antibody G 250 recognizes a determinant present in renal-cell carcinoma and absent from normal kidney. *Int J Cancer*. 1986;38(4):489–494.
9. Oosterwijk E, Divgi CR, Brouwers A, et al. Monoclonal antibody-based therapy for renal cell carcinoma. *Urol Clin N Am*. 2003;30(3):623–631.
10. Chiou RK, Vessella RL, Limas C, et al. Monoclonal antibody-targeted radiotherapy of renal cell carcinoma using a nude mouse model. *Cancer*. 1988;61(9):1766–1775.
11. Vessella RL, Moon TD, Chiou RK, et al. Monoclonal antibodies to human renal cell carcinoma: recognition of shared and restricted tissue antigens. *Cancer Res*. 1985;45(12 pt 1):6131–6139.
12. Vessella RL, Chiou RK, Grund FM. Renal cell carcinoma (RCC) phase I-II trials with 131-I labeled monoclonal antibody A6H: imaging and pharmacokinetic studies. *Proc Am Assoc Cancer Res*. 1987;28:480.
13. Brouwers AH, van Eerd JE, Frielink C, et al. Optimization of radioimmunotherapy of renal cell carcinoma: labeling of monoclonal antibody cG250 with 131I, 90Y, 177Lu, or 186Re. *J Nucl Med*. 2004;45(2):327–337.
14. van Dijk J, Oosterwijk E, van Kroonenburgh MJ, et al. Perfusion of tumor-bearing kidneys as a model for scintigraphic screening of monoclonal antibodies. *J Nucl Med*. 1988;29(6):1078–1082.
15. van Dijk J, Zegveld ST, Fleuren GJ, et al. Localization of monoclonal antibody G250 and bispecific monoclonal antibody CD3/G250 in human renal-cell carcinoma xenografts: relative effects of size and affinity. *Int J Cancer*. 1991;48(5):738–743.
16. van Dijk J, Uemura H, Beniers AJ, et al. Therapeutic effects of monoclonal antibody G250, interferons and tumor necrosis factor, in mice with renal-cell carcinoma xenografts. *Int J Cancer*. 1994;56(2):262–268.
17. Kranenborg MH, Boerman OC, De Weijert MC, et al. The effect of antibody protein dose of anti-renal cell carcinoma monoclonal antibodies in nude mice with renal cell carcinoma xenografts. *Cancer*. 1997;80(12 suppl):2390–2397.
18. Steffens MG, Oosterwijk E, Kranenborg MH, et al. In vivo and in vitro characterizations of three 99mTc-labeled monoclonal antibody G250 preparations. *J Nucl Med*. 1999;40(5):829–836.
19. Uemura H, Nakagawa Y, Yoshida K, et al. MN/CA IX/G250 as a potential target for immunotherapy of renal cell carcinomas. *Br J Cancer*. 1999;81(4):741–746.
20. Steffens MG, Kranenborg MH, Boerman OC, et al. Tumor retention of 186Re-MAG3, 111In-DTPA and 125I labeled monoclonal antibody G250 in nude mice with renal cell carcinoma xenografts. *Cancer Biother Radiopharm*. 1998;13(2):133–139.
21. Steffens MG, Oosterwijk-Wakka JC, Zegwaart-Hagemeier NE, et al. Immunohistochemical analysis of tumor antigen saturation following injection of monoclonal antibody G250. *Anticancer Res*. 1999;19(2A):1197–1200.
22. Grabmaier K, Vissers JL, De Weijert MC, et al. Molecular cloning and immunogenicity of renal cell carcinoma-associated antigen G250. *Int J Cancer*. 2000;85(6):865–870.
23. Grabmaier K, A de Weijert MC, Verhaegh GW, et al. Strict regulation of CAIX(G250/MN) by HIF-1alpha in clear cell renal cell carcinoma. *Oncogene*. 2004;23(33):5624–5631.
24. Bismar TA, Bianco FJ, Zhang H, et al. Quantification of G250 mRNA expression in renal epithelial neoplasms by real-time reverse transcription-PCR of dissected tissue from paraffin sections. *Pathology*. 2003;35(6):513–517.
25. Chen YT, Tu JJ, Kao J, et al. Messenger RNA expression ratios among four genes predict subtypes of renal cell carcinoma and distinguish oncocytoma from carcinoma. *Clin Cancer Res*. 2005;11(18):6558–6566.
26. Oosterwijk E, Bander NH, Divgi CR, et al. Antibody localization in human renal cell carcinoma: a phase I study of monoclonal antibody G250. *J Clin Oncol*. 1993;11(4):738–750.
27. Divgi CR, Bander NH, Scott AM, et al. Phase I/II radioimmunotherapy trial with iodine-131-labeled monoclonal antibody G250 in metastatic renal cell carcinoma. *Clin Cancer Res*. 1998;4(11):2729–2739.
28. Oosterwijk E, Debruyne FM, Schalken JA. The use of monoclonal antibody G250 in the therapy of renal-cell carcinoma. *Semin Oncol*. 1995;22(1):34–41.
29. Surfus JE, Hank JA, Oosterwijk E, et al. Anti-renal-cell carcinoma chimeric antibody G250 facilitates antibody-dependent cellular cytotoxicity with in vitro and in vivo interleukin-2-activated effectors. *J Immunother Emphasis Tumor Immunol*. 1996;19(3):184–191.
30. Liu Z, Smyth FE, Renner C, et al. Anti-renal cell carcinoma chimeric antibody G250: cytokine enhancement of in vitro antibody-dependent cellular cytotoxicity. *Cancer Immunol Immunother*. 2002;51(3):171–177.
31. Bleumer I, Knuth A, Oosterwijk E, et al. A phase II trial of chimeric monoclonal antibody G250 for advanced renal cell carcinoma patients. *Br J Cancer*. 2004;90(5):985–990.
32. Bleumer I, Oosterwijk E, Oosterwijk-Wakka JC, et al. A clinical trial with chimeric monoclonal antibody WX-G250 and low dose interleukin-2 pulsing scheme for advanced renal cell carcinoma. *J Urol*. 2006;175(1):57–62.
33. Steffens MG, Boerman OC, Oosterwijk-Wakka JC, et al. Targeting of renal cell carcinoma with iodine-131-labeled chimeric monoclonal antibody G250. *J Clin Oncol*. 1997;15(4):1529–1537.
34. Steffens MG, Boerman OC, de Mulder PH, et al. Phase I radioimmunotherapy of metastatic renal cell carcinoma with 131I-labeled chimeric monoclonal antibody G250. *Clin Cancer Res*. 1999;5(10 suppl):3268s–3274s.
35. Divgi CR, O'Donoghue JA, Welt S, et al. Phase I clinical trial with fractionated radioimmunotherapy using 131I-labeled chimeric G250 in metastatic renal cancer. *J Nucl Med*. 2004;45(8):1412–1421.
36. Brouwers AH, Mulders PF, de Mulder PH, et al. Lack of efficacy of two consecutive treatments of radioimmunotherapy with 131I-cG250 in patients with metastatic clear cell renal cell carcinoma. *J Clin Oncol*. 2005;23(27):6540–6548.
37. Brouwers AH, Buijs WC, Oosterwijk E, et al. Targeting of metastatic renal cell carcinoma with the chimeric monoclonal antibody G250 labeled with (131)I or (111)In: an intrapatient comparison. *Clin Cancer Res*. 2003;9(10 pt 2):3953S–3960S.
38. Stillebroer A, Oosterwijk E, Boerman OC, et al. Interim analysis of a phase I radioimmunotherapy study in advanced renal cell carcinoma patients using Lutetium-177 labeled monoclonal antibody cG250. *24th Annual EAU Congress*, Stockholm, 2009.
39. Divgi CR, Pandit-Taskar N, Jungbluth AA, et al. Preoperative characterisation of clear-cell renal carcinoma using iodine-124-labelled antibody chimeric G250 (124I-cG250) and PET in patients with renal masses: a phase I trial. *Lancet Oncol*. 2007;8(4):304–310.

33

Radioimmunotherapy for Non-Hodgkin Lymphoma: A Clinical Update

Michael Burdick and Roger M. Macklis

◼ INTRODUCTION

An estimated 66,000 patients will be given a diagnosis of non-Hodgkin lymphoma (NHL) in the United States in 2008 (1). NHL is a heterogenous cluster of diseases with a myriad of clinical presentations, treatment options, and prognoses. Low-grade NHL typically is treatable but incurable once it progresses beyond stage I and usually has a protracted, indolent course. The majority of low-grade NHLs are follicular lymphomas (FLs). FL is a disease of the middle age and elderly with a median age of 60 at diagnosis and a slight female predominance (2). Median survival for FL is approximately 7 to 10 years. FL is initially sensitive to both chemotherapy and radiation. With each therapeutic failure, FL becomes progressively more aggressive and resistant to further therapeutic endeavors (3).

FL contains two main cell types: the centrocyte, or cleaved small cell, and the centroblast, the large noncleaved follicle center cell. The histologic pattern of FL resembles normal secondary lymphoid follicles, but differs in several ways: distortion of normal node architecture, absence of mantle zones, monomorphous population of centrocytes, and absence of tangible body macrophages (4). The Revised European American Lymphoma (REAL) system and World Health Organization (WHO) recommend histologic grading based on the number of centroblasts per high powered light microscopy field: 0 to 5 for grade 1, 6 to 15 for grade 2, and greater than 15 for grade 3 (5). Some institutions consider grade 3 FL a high-grade NHL and treat it similar to other aggressive NHL such as diffuse large B-cell lymphoma (DLBCL) (6). Immunohistochemistry usually reveals CD20+, CD10+, CD 43−, CD 5−, BCL-2+, and BCL-6+ (4). The classic cytogenetic translocation associated with FL is t(14:18), which involves juxtaposition of the BCL-2 gene next to the immunoglobulin heavy chain locus (7). This results in constitutive activation of the BCL-2 gene, an inner mitochondrial membrane–associated protein involved in preventing apoptosis (8). Occasionally, FLs transform into a higher grade NHL, such as DLBCL (9).

Staging for NHL is based on the Ann Arbor classification which was originally developed for Hodgkin lymphoma (10). Stage I has involvement of a single lymph node region (I) or single extralymphatic organ or site (IE) on one side of the diaphragm. Stage II has involvement of two or more lymph node regions (II) or localized involvement of an extralymphatic organ or site (IIE) on the same side of the diaphragm. Stage III has involvement of lymph node regions on both sides of the diaphragm (III) or localized involvement of an extralymphatic organ or site (IIIE) or spleen (IIIS) or both (IIIES). Stage IV disease involves diffuse or disseminated involvement of one or more extralymphatic organs with or without associated lymph node involvement. Stage IV includes bone marrow involvement. Associated "B" symptoms can be present in any stage and are designated with the addition of a B to the stage. B symptoms include persistent fevers greater than 38°C, drenching night sweats, and unexplained weight loss of greater than 10% over the preceding 6 months.

Early stage, localized FL is curable with conventional external beam radiation therapy (EBRT). Treatment options for advanced stage FL vary widely depending on patient age, patient medical comorbidities, disease burden, and institutional biases. In advanced stage disease, the National Comprehensive Cancer Network (NCCN) recommends observation, radiation therapy, immunotherapy, or chemotherapy depending on a variety of patient and tumor characteristics. Frontline chemotherapy regimens typically include the anti-CD20 chimeric antibody rituximab (R) as monotherapy or in combination with chemotherapy regimens such as CHOP-R (cyclophosphamide, Adriamycin, vincristine, and prednisone), CVP-R (cyclophosphamide, vincristine, and prednisone), FND-R (fludarabine, mitoxantrone, and dexamethasone), or fludarabine. NCCN recommends EBRT for symptomatic or bulky disease. Second-line therapy varies widely from additional chemotherapy, autologous or allogenic stem cell transplant (SCT), and radioimmunotherapy (RIT) (11). This chapter focuses on the use of RIT in low-grade B-cell NHL.

◼ BACKGROUND ON RADIOIMMUNOTHERAPY

The field of RIT has a surprisingly long history and is now finally becoming a realistic clinical option for the management of malignant lymphoma (12). Although some forms of chemically and biologically targeted radiopharmaceutical treatment actually extend back to the early decades of the 20th century, target-selective monoclonal antibody technology was developed and commercialized in the 1970s and the first cancer-selective RIT compounds finally received full Food and Drug Administration (FDA) clearance in 2002 (^{90}Y ibritumomab tiuxetan or Zevalin; Spectrum Pharmaceuticals, Inc., Irvine, CA) and in 2003 (^{131}I tositumomab or Bexxar; GlaxoSmithKline; Brentford, London, UK) (13–16). Both of these RIT compounds received their primary clinical indications for the treatment of relapsed or refractory CD20+ B-cell NHL. This apparent duplication of efforts relates both to the inherent cellular radiosensitivity of this disease group and to the burgeoning success of various biological treatments in the clinical management of sensitive hematopoietic diseases. Both ^{90}Y ibritumomab tiuxetan and ^{131}I tositumomab are based on monoclonal antibodies specific for the CD20 surface antigen found on normal B-cells and approximately 95% of B-cell malignancies. The chimeric anti-CD20 antibody rituximab is now enjoying increasing therapeutic prominence both as a single agent and as a component of multiagent treatment regimens for many different kinds of B-cell disorders (17). In an effort to improve the proportion of B-cell lymphoma patients achieving a remission and to extend the durability of these responses, investigators became interested in combining the powerful humoral immune system effects mediated by anti-CD20 antibodies with short-range molecular radiotherapy produced by high-energy beta emitters (notably ^{90}Y and ^{131}I) chemically attached to the antibody backbones (18,19). Although both of the currently approved antibody-targeted radiopharmaceuticals bind to the CD20 surface antigen, their specific pattern of clinical use is quite different due to major variances in the biologic effects and incorporated radionuclides. It is thus probable that both compounds will find a place in the therapeutic armamentarium for the management of malignant B-cell lymphomas and related diseases. These presumptive clinical niches, however, remain uncertain.

■ RADIOBIOLOGY

Dosimetry for clinical radioimmunotherapy

Clinical biodistribution and dosimetry studies in the RIT of lymphomas and other malignancies confirmed the ability of various radiolabeled antibodies to traffic through the vascular system and accumulate at major sites of disease without much normal tissue toxicity (20). However, the percentage of the injected dose localizing at the individual target sites was typically quite low, producing absorbed radiation dose rates on the order of 1 to 10 cGy/h (compared with ~100 to 600 cGy/min at isocenter for traditional external beam radiotherapy). Thus, the radiobiology of RIT can be understood as a special instance of the broader research area of low dose-rate radiation effects incorporating the physiology of ongoing cellular damage and nearly concurrent cellular damage repair (21). Moreover, the total absorbed radiation doses for many target disease sites in lymphoma patients treated with either ^{90}Y ibritumomab tiuxetan or ^{131}I tositumomab are typically on the order of 10 to 15 Gy. Thus, with respect to both radiation doses and radiation dose rates, it would appear that the

radiation dosimetry calculated using standard nuclear medicine unsealed source methodologies (such as the MIRD formalism) is probably at the lower end of the range of doses generally considered clinically effective (22). For malignant lymphomas, impressive antibody–based immunotherapy responses to compounds such as rituximab had already been broadly confirmed by earlier trials, and this clear evidence of immunoresponsiveness set the stage for further exploration of antibody-targeted radionuclides as a means of increasing therapeutic efficacy (23). Although the radiobiologic principles responsible for the clinical success of RIT in the management of B-cell malignant lymphoma are still not entirely clear, it appears that in many cases, a significant synergy develops between the continuous low dose-rate radioisotope–based radiation and the concurrent or sequential anti-CD20 antibody treatment (24,25). This sort of synergy is not readily demonstrable for experimental and clinical RIT of most common epithelial tumors despite the antibody-based delivery of comparable radiation doses (26). This radiobiologic difference in cellular physiologies may partially explain why the response rates for different malignancies vary so markedly. Major objective response rates for clinical single-agent RIT trials in reasonably radiosensitive adenocarcinomas rarely exceed 10% to 15%, whereas the same radiation doses and dose rates produce overall responses (ORs) in 60% to 80% of indolent B-cell lymphoma patients with complete response (CR) rates of 20% to 40% (25). This level of clinical responsiveness appears to be true for both ^{90}Y ibritumomab tiuxetan and ^{131}I tositumomab, thus lending support to the therapeutic potential of the entire RIT class of compounds in lymphoma management (27,28). Surprisingly, the dose intensity maps for antibody-targeted radiopharmaceuticals tracked on gamma camera images for both ^{131}I tositumomab and ^{90}Y ibritumomab tiuxetan may not correlate well with the likelihood of durable tumor response (29,30). It is thus not clear that the sites showing the most intense isotope accumulation activity will be the ones likely to show the most dramatic clinical effects (31). Thus, neither the unsealed source dosimetry nor the antibody-mediated radiobiology is currently felt to be predictive enough to derive reproducible clinical dose–response relationships. In all probability, the combinatorial physiology produced by the additional antibody effects on these target sites may have a greater impact on target tissue responsiveness than the calculated radiation absorbed doses (32). This is obviously an area in need of further clinical and preclinical investigation.

The CD20 surface antigen as a tumor target

CD20 is a nonglycosylated protein of unknown function encoded by the MS4A1 gene located on chromosome 11 (33,34). It appears to play an important role in cell cycle control, and some data suggest that it can function either singly or as a multimeric complex within a "lipid raft" organizational superstructure "floating" within the cell membrane. These lipid rafts are now thought to be platforms for biochemical signal transduction and are apparently involved in some of the major CD20 functions (35). Some evidence suggests a possible calcium channel function and this intracellular physiology may relate to data suggesting a role for CD20 in the induction of B-cell apoptosis (36). Under normal circumstances, CD20 is neither internalized nor shed and therefore makes an excellent target for immunotherapy and RIT. Although both tositumomab and rituximab can bind tightly to an extracellular domain of the CD20 molecule, these two antibodies appear to recognize different elements of the complex and appear to produce somewhat different cellular responses in vivo.

The CD20 molecule has been recognized as a tempting target antigen for B-cell immunotherapy since the 1990s when large-scale clinical trials with anti-CD20 monoclonal antibodies began at several academic sites. Rituximab, a genetically engineered chimeric monoclonal antibody, has been shown to produce B-cell lysis through several different in vivo mechanisms: complement-dependent cytotoxicity, antibody-dependent cell–mediated cytotoxicity, and direct induction of apoptosis (37). Although all of these mechanisms can be demonstrated in vitro, the relative importance of each in clinical cancer immunotherapy is unclear and may depend strongly on the integrity of the patient's immune system. Some investigators have produced evidence for a delayed cell-mediated cytotoxic effect for rituximab in animal studies and clinical trials. This delayed effect may represent cross presentation of lymphoma antigens with subsequent opsonization and tumor–directed cellular immune responses.

As a single agent, rituximab typically produces response rates of 50% or more in follicular NHL (38). When rituximab is used as a component of cytotoxic chemotherapy regimens such as CHOP-R, response rates for indolent B-cell NHL approach 100% (39). For very heavily pretreated patients, responses may be brief but retreatment is often possible. Nevertheless, it is clear that additional mechanisms must be developed both to increase the proportion of patients achieving a good clinical response and to increase the durability of the responses achieved.

Antibodies and isotopes

At present, only two RIT radiopharmaceuticals have received full FDA clearance for marketing (40,41). ^{90}Y ibritumomab tiuxetan (Zevalin) received FDA clearance in 2002 and ^{131}I tositumomab (Bexxar) received its clearance about one year later (Table 33.1). Both of these compounds received commercial clearance for the treatment of CD20+ indolent B-cell NHL and related conditions. Although both RIT compounds target the CD20 surface antigen, their pattern of use differs significantly, due in large part to differences in the radioisotopes incorporated into the compounds (Table 33.2).

For ^{90}Y ibritumomab tiuxetan, the incorporated isotope is yttrium-90, a pure beta-particle emitter with a half-life of approximately 2.7 days. The most energetic beta emission has energy of approximately 2.3 MeV, which corresponds to a maximum penetration in tissue of approximately 11.3 mm. It is noteworthy that 90% of the energy of the beta particle is actually delivered over 5.2 mm (R_{90}). Because there

Table **33.1**	Comparison of the two approved radioimmunotherapy compounds (19,20,42,43)	
	^{90}Y Ibritumomab Tiuxetan (Zevalin)	**^{131}I Tositumomab (Bexxar)**
Antibody used for RIT	Ibritumomab—murine IgG1-κ	Tositumomab—murine IgG2a-λ
Specificity	CD20	CD20
Linker molecule	Tiuxetan	None (directly halogenated)
"Cold" antibody	Chimeric rituximab 250 mg/m^2	Murine tositumomab 450 mg
Pretreatment imaging agent and dose	^{111}In ibritumomab tiuxetan—5 mCi	^{131}I tositumomab—5 mCi
Primary intent of imaging dose	Biodistribution safety assessment	Calculation of dose based on individual clearance patterns
Number of pretreatment scans	One^a	Three
Therapeutic isotope	Yttrium-90	Iodine-131
Major emission spectra	2.3 MeV β	0.6 MeV β and 0.36 MeV γ
Dosing parameters Platelets ≥150,000/μL Platelets 100,000–149,000/μL	0.4 mCi/kg 0.3 mCi/kg Maximum 32 mCi	75 cGy whole body dose 65 cGy whole body dose
Typical overall response rate (ORR)	60%–80%	60%–80%
Typical complete response rate (CR)	20%–40%	20%–40%

^{a}Additional scans are optional.

Table **33.2**	Physical properties of radioisotopes incorporated into ^{90}Y-ibritumomab tiuxetan (Zevalin) and ^{131}I-tositumomab (Bexxar)			
Radionuclide	Physical $t\frac{1}{2}$	Max Particle Energy (MeV)	Gamma Energy (MeV)	Max Range in Tissue (mm)
^{131}I	8.0 days	0.6	0.36	2.3
^{90}Y	64.1 hours	2.3	—	11.3

are no gamma emissions in the spectrum of this isotope, the radiopharmaceutical is very poorly visualized on routine gamma camera scans. For this reason, a replacement isotope (^{111}indium) with an appropriate gamma emission and similar radiometal chemistry is utilized as a surrogate to allow imaging and prediction of the biodistribution for the beta-emitting radiopharmaceutical. In the first year of FDA approval, review of the ^{90}Y ibritumomab tiuxetan imaging registry found only a 0.6% incidence of altered biodistribution (44). Radiopharmaceutical uptake on pretreatment ^{111}In ibritumomab tiuxetan scans was not shown to correlate with clinical response in a review of 20 patients with 105 cumulative disease sites at the Cleveland Clinic (31). Lack of predictive value for both toxicity and clinical outcomes has caused some to recommend that the pretreatment ^{111}In ibritumomab tiuxetan scans prior to administering therapeutic dose with ^{90}Y ibritumomab tiuxetan should be an optional safety step.

In contrast, ^{131}iodine tositumomab is a directly radiohalogenated mixed beta/gamma emitter with a gamma emission spike at 364 keV and a beta emission with energy of approximately 0.6 MeV. The maximum range in tissue for the beta particle is 2.3 mm (R_{90} = 0.7 mm). This radionuclide can thus be visualized directly on a properly collimated gamma camera, though the resolutions of the images obtained with the ^{131}I-iodinated compound are typically somewhat blurry. Although one can list a number of theoretical reasons why, based on the physical characteristics of the emission spectra for ^{131}I and ^{90}Y, one or the other isotope might be considered preferable as an incorporated component for RIT, there is really no convincing evidence that the use of either isotope provides a material benefit for the RIT of B-cell NHL. Both isotopes appear reasonably stable in their antibody linkages (45). ^{131}I tositumomab involves a covalent bond (Fig. 33.1), whereas ^{90}Y ibritumomab

tiuxetan makes use of an added chemical side-arm with a terminal chelation complex (tiuxetan) providing noncovalent linkage for the radiometal (Fig. 33.2). For both of the anti-CD20 radioimmunoconjugates, the treatment sequence begins with the preliminary infusion of an excess of a nonradioactive (cold) anti-CD20 antibody designed to saturate nonspecific uptake sites and thereby improve the more specific targeting. For ^{90}Y ibritumomab tiuxetan, the chimeric anti-CD20 antibody, rituximab, is utilized for this purpose. For ^{131}I tositumomab, the murine monoclonal antibody, tositumomab, is utilized for the same purpose. Although some in vitro studies show increased cytotoxic activity for tositumomab, the mouse–human chimeric antibody rituximab apparently survives longer in the bloodstream and also is able to activate other components of the immune system such as the complement system. Thus, in a patient with a reasonably intact immune system, it is unclear which of the cold antibodies would produce a higher degree of selective target cell cytotoxicity in vivo. For both of the radioimmunoconjugates, the treatment cycle is fairly similar (Figs. 33.3 and 33.4). Major pharmaceutical differences in the pattern of use for the two compounds include very different dosing paradigms, normal tissue protection strategies, and differing radiation safety provisions for the patient, the treatment team, and the public at large.

Investigational therapeutic antibodies

Given the clinical success of both ^{90}Y ibritumomab tiuxetan and ^{131}I tositumomab, several other agents now are under investigation for potential therapeutic use. Interestingly,

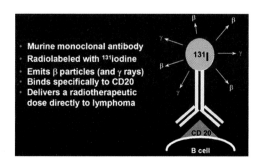

FIGURE 33.1 Summary of I^{131} tositumomab features.

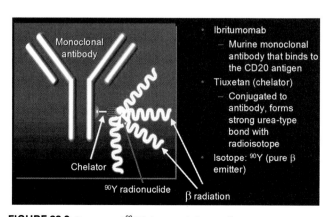

FIGURE 33.2 Summary of ^{90}Y ibritumomab tiuxetan features.

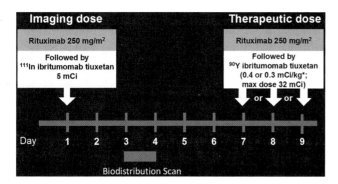

FIGURE 33.3 Schema for ^{90}Yibritumomab tiuxetan treatment protocol. *0.4 mCi/kg in patients with a platelet count ≥150,000/μl or 0.3 mCi/kg with a platelet count of 100,000-149,000/μl. Maximum dose is 32 mCi.

the original RIT study by Press et al. at the Fred Hutchinson Cancer Research Center was not with an anti-CD20 antibody, but rather with I^{131} radiolabeled MB-1 (anti-CD37) antibody (46). Lym-1 is an IgG$_{2a}$ mouse monoclonal antibody with high affinity for the HLA-DR membrane antigen found on B-cell malignancies (47). Radioisotopes used to label Lym-1 include ^{131}I and ^{67}Cu. Epratuzamab is a humanized antibody in which the antigen-binding portion of the antibody is derived from the murine parent, while the backbone has been replaced with human IgG$_1$ peptide sequences. Epratuzamab binds to CD22, another B-cell surface marker. RIT with epratuzamab involves conjugation of ^{90}Y through the chelating agent 1,4,7,10-tetra-azacyclodecane-N,N',N",N'''-tetraacetic acid (DOTA) (48). Targeting CD20 with radioisotopes other than B-emitters is also under investigation. Alpha emitters have the advantage of delivering high doses of ionizing radiation to very short distances. Concerns for safety with labeling, targeting, and radioactive decay products have limited clinical applications with alpha emitters in humans (49). Thorium-227, an alpha emitter, has been conjugated to rituximab through the bifunctional chelator pisothiocyanato-benzyl-DOTA and is under investigation. ^{90}Y ibritumomab tiuxetan and ^{131}I tositumomab thus are only the beginning in the field of clinical RIT for lymphoma management.

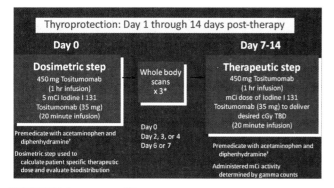

FIGURE 33.4 Schema for ^{131}I tositumomab treatment protocol. *Scans used for dosimetry and biodistribution evaluation. If biodistribution is altered, the therapeutic dose should not be administered. + Benefit of premedication in prevention infusion-related toxicity has not been evaluated.

Indications for treatment

Both ^{90}Y ibritumomab tiuxetan and ^{131}I tositumomab are FDA approved for the treatment of relapsed or refractory CD20+ B-cell NHL. ^{131}I tositumomab is also indicated for treatment of transformed CD20+ B-cell NHL. ^{90}Y ibritumomab has recently received FDA approval as first-line consolidation for advanced FL (see the section "Consolidation as Initial Treatment"). Other investigational uses will be highlighted later in this chapter. Contraindications to treatment include a platelet count of less than 100,000/mL, absolute neutrophil count of less than 1500/mL, KPS less than 60, pregnancy, inadequate renal or hepatic function, or lymphoma involvement of the bone marrow of a magnitude greater than 25%, as estimated from a bone marrow biopsy. The initial ^{90}Y ibritumomab tiuxetan registration trials also included a restriction on prior EBRT to greater than 25% of bone marrow. One group has reported treatment with dose attenuated ^{131}I tositumomab in patients with greater than 25% bone marrow involvement; this application remains investigational (50). Because ^{131}I tositumomab is a mouse–human chimeric antibody, roughly 10% patients will develop human anti-mouse antibodies (HAMAs) that can potentially alter the biodistribution of tositumomab and is considered a relative contraindication to treatment with ^{131}I tositumomab (51,52).

Radiopharmaceutical dosing strategy

For ^{131}I tositumomab, three serial gamma camera scans are obtained during the first week of the protocol after a preparatory infusion of a "tracer" activity of 5 mCi of the radiopharmaceutical (Fig. 33.4). These three scans are used to confirm the safety of the biodistribution pattern (no evidence of dangerous radioisotope pooling or large-scale dehalogenation) and to establish a predictive bioclearance curve for the subsequent high-activity therapeutic infusion. The clearance characteristics for ^{131}I tositumomab differ significantly from one patient to another, with some patients exhibiting very slow radiopharmaceutical clearance and other patients showing much faster clearance kinetics (Fig. 33.5). Because the ultimate absorbed radiation dose will depend on a "concentration multiplied by time" ($C \times T$) metric, this sort of variable pattern is utilized to choose the mCi activity infused for an individual patient, termed "individualized patient dosimetry" (42) (Fig. 33.6). These various mCi activities (doses) may differ by a factor of five or more. In contrast, for ^{90}Y ibritumomab tiuxetan, the chosen infused activity for the therapeutic dose is calculated based only on the patient's weight and hematopoietic status (typically indicated by pretreatment platelet count) (53). A single gamma camera scan is mandated (usually days 3 to 4; see Fig. 33.3) to confirm a safe biodistribution for the infusion (Fig. 33.7). As shown in this image, the 2-hour scan represents the typical vascular phase. The antibody is largely in the cardiac and body blood pool (large vessels easily identified). However, at 48 hours, the antibody begins to target disease in the

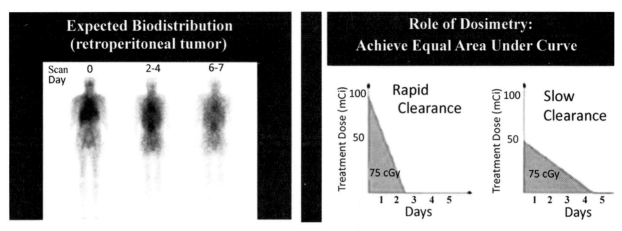

FIGURE 33.5 Comparable area under the curve data for fast vs. slow clearance of ^{131}I tositumomab.

left infraclavicular and axillary nodes, para-aortic and iliac regions. This represents the standard "slow" accretion of an intact, 150 kDa antibody (see Chapter 12), although tumor targeting may certainly begin earlier than 48 hours. Also, as illustrated in Figure 33.7, a large amount of antibody is

beginning to be consumed by the liver and spleen at 48 hours postinfusion. This process, however, appears to be significantly abrogated by "cold dosing" with unlabeled anti-CD20 antibody (see inset, Fig. 33.7). Interestingly, the typical range of ^{131}I tositumomab dose may vary between 50 and

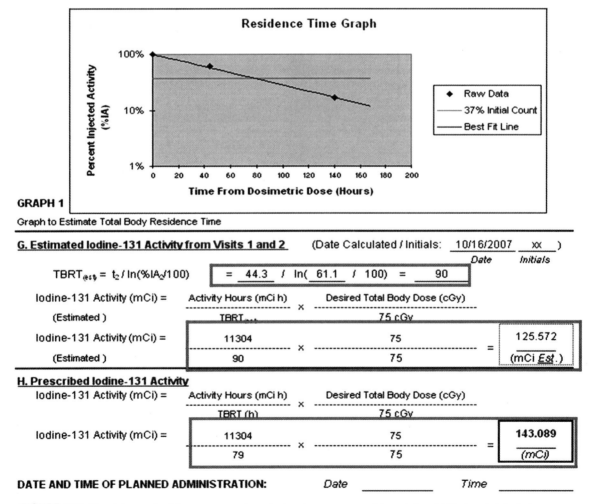

FIGURE 33.6 Pictorial example of the program used to calculate the necessary activity to deliver 65–75 cGy whole body dose (depending upon platelet count) for ^{131}I tositumomab treatment regimen.

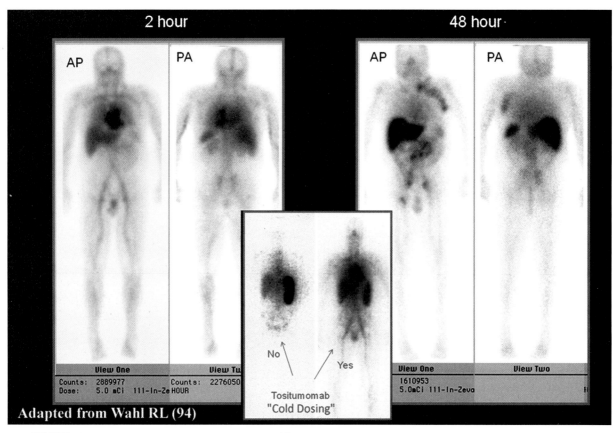

FIGURE 33.7 The normal 2 and 48 hour biodistributions of ^{111}In-ibritumomab (Zevalin). Cold antibody dosing (cold dosing), prior to imaging and therapy, will improve the biodistribution as shown in the inset (tositumomab prior to Bexxar; Rituxan prior to Zevalin).

200 mCi (Fig. 33.8) (54), whereas a ^{90}Y ibritumomab tiuxetan infusion would be 20 to 30 mCi of ^{90}Y radiopharmaceutical, up to a maximum of 32 mCi. For both ^{131}I tositumomab and ^{90}Y ibritumomab tiuxetan, there is a modest dose reduction if platelet counts are less than 150,000 (^{131}I tositumomab whole body dose calculation moves from 75 to 65 cGy; ^{90}Y ibritumomab activity calculation moves from 0.4 to 0.3 mCi/kg) and a standard safety contradiction for use if platelets are below 100,000 at the time of infusion. Note that for both of these radiopharmaceuticals, the infused activity does not depend on the quantitation of the activity taken up in the active target sites. In some cases, patients whose tumor

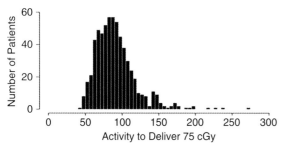

*Targeted total body radiation dose 75cGy for patients with platelets 150,000/mm³ or 65cGy for patients with platelet counts between 100,000 and 150,000/mm³.

FIGURE 33.8 Range of mCi required to deliver targeted total body radiation dose (*N* = 634). (Adapted from Wahl RL. Tositumomab and ^{131}I therapy in non-Hodgkin's lymphoma. *J Nucl Med.* 2005;46:128S–140S.)

sites image very poorly still show an excellent treatment response and thus at present calculated absorbed radiation doses for these unsealed sources are determined only as a protocol exercise and a safety check.

■ Radiation safety precautions

Because ^{90}Y ibritumomab tiuxetan is a pure beta emitter, shielding of the radiopharmaceutical compound can be accomplished using lightweight plastic or acrylic laboratory shields (typically about 1 cm in width). Radiation exposure for the patient's family and for the treatment team has been studied and is minimal. For the most part, the sorts of safety precautions necessary for ^{90}Y ibritumomab tiuxetan are essentially identical to those which would constitute "universal precautions" for the handling of any other bodily fluids obtained in the clinical environment. In contrast, the penetrating gamma emissions and longer half-life of ^{131}I tositumomab mandate more extensive shielding for the patient's family and for the health care team. Typically, lead bricks or custom shielding are utilized to surround the infusion syringe or infusion pump, and a special isolated or shielded location for the treatment may be mandated by the responsible radiation safety officers. Similarly, more stringent posttreatment safety instructions must be given to the patient and the patient's family for ^{131}I tositumomab compared with those suggested after ^{90}Y ibritumomab tiuxetan. In addition, because there is some degree of physiologic dehalogenation in vivo, the iodine-avid thyroid of the infused patient must first be chemically blocked to prevent treatment-induced hypothyroidism. Typically, a solution of super-saturated potassium iodide or equivalent is administered to the patient starting at least 24 hours prior to treatment with ^{131}I tositumomab. For both compounds, some anti-inflammatory premedication may be used to prevent or minimize the chance of a reaction against the murine antibody components (diphenhydramine and acetaminophen for instance). Under ordinary circumstances, virtually all RIT infusions involving either of the two commercially approved radiopharmaceuticals can be performed as outpatient procedures. In the rare instance that a patient infused with a high-dose radiopharmaceutical requires hospitalization, special training for the involved nurses and in some cases special shielding around the infused patient's bed may be mandated by the responsible radiation safety officer. Whether the patient is discharged the same day as the therapeutic infusion or retained in the hospital for an extra day (or more) prior to discharge, explicit going-home instructions should be given to the patient and the patient's family and it must be absolutely clear which member of the treatment team should be contacted in the event of either a medical problem or a public radiation safety question once a radioactive patient is discharged from the hospital or infusion center environment.

Treatment toxicities seen with anti-CD20 RIT

Compared with conventional cytotoxic chemotherapy, non-hematologic toxicities from either ^{90}Y ibritumomab tiuxetan or ^{131}I tositumomab are generally quite mild (55,56). Most of these side-effects relate to minor allergic responses to the protein components of the cold antibody. The likelihood of an infusion reaction is somewhat greater for patients treated with rituximab compared with tositumomab, and the cold antibody infusion process thus may take substantially longer and may require slower adjusted infusion rates for rituximab. Approximately 20% to 40% of patients report some level of asthenia and nausea after receiving either of the anti-CD20 radiopharmaceuticals. The rate of development of HAMA or human anti-chimeric antibody is approximately 10% for ^{131}I tositumomab and significantly lower (1% to 2%) for ^{90}Y ibritumomab tiuxetan. Posttreatment hypothyroidism occurs in approximately 10% to 20% of patients treated with ^{131}I tositumomab despite physiologic thyroid-blocking maneuvers.

Hematopoietic toxicity is the most common side effect seen with either antibody (57,58). Neutropenia and thrombocytopenia typically occur several weeks after infusion of the high-dose radiopharmaceutical and generally persist for 1 to 2 months after infusion. More than 50% of patients treated with either radiopharmaceutical will have a platelet nadir below 50,000/mL and approximately 20% will have a nadir below 25,000/mL and may require

platelet transfusions. Absolute neutrophil counts less than 500/mL are seen in approximately 25% to 30% of treated patients and the duration of this nadir is typically 1 month. Hospitalization for febrile neutropenia or similar treatment–related hematopoietic suppression occurs in less than 10% of patients.

Second malignancies after RIT

The most feared second malignancy risk that has been studied for lymphoma RIT involves treatment–related myelodysplastic syndrome (MDS) and acute myelogenous leukemia (AML) (59). This marrow syndrome is a well-recognized late problem in patients with a diagnosis of B-cell NHL no matter how they are treated. To date, most RIT-treated patient groups have not shown a statistically significant increase in the rate of these iatrogenic problems. An annualized incidence of approximately 1.6% per year with a crude overall incidence rate of approximately 2% to 3% per year is reported for patients treated with ^{131}I tositumomab for relapsed or refractory lymphoma (59). An analysis of 746 patients treated with ^{90}Y ibritumomab tiuxetan found that 2.5% of patients developed MDS or AML for an annualized rate of 0.7% per year after treatment. No increase in annualized incidence of MDS or AML was found when comparing patients receiving ^{90}Y ibritumomab tiuxetan with NHL patients receiving extensive chemotherapy regimens (60). Seventy-six patients treated with ^{131}I tositumomab as initial management found no cases of MDS or AML with a median follow-up of 5.1 years (61,62). Because most patients treated with RIT have received multiple chemotherapy regimens, separating the risk of leukemia attributable to RIT from the risk attributable to conventional chemotherapy is exceedingly difficult. Some experienced users would put the risk of these treatment-related diseases somewhere between the risk associated with conventional chemotherapy and the higher risk associated with stem cell transplantation. In any case, the risk of treatment-induced malignancies is certainly not out of line with that observed for other aggressive cancer treatment regimens.

RIT WITH ^{90}Y IBRITUMOMAB TIUXETAN OR ^{131}I TOSITUMOMAB: CLINICAL RESULTS

Table 33.3 summarizes the most significant prospective phase II/III clinical trials providing the evidence basis for the use of clinical lymphoma RIT (40,41). Together they comprise over 200 patients treated with each of the two biologically targeted radiopharmaceuticals (12). The data for these two radiopharmaceuticals are quite similar and mutually supportive. Both therapeutic agents suggest an OR of approximately 60% to 80% with a CR of 20% to 50% for indolent B-cell NHL. Unfortunately, even at very high administered doses, cures remain elusive.

Long-term efficacies with RIT for relapsed, refractory, or transformed low-grade NHL have been reported and are

Table **33.3**	Summary of major published trials of radioimmunotherapy (RIT) for relapsed or refractory low-grade non-Hodgkin lymphoma			
RIT	**Study Design**	**OR (%)**	**CR (%)**	**PFS (TTP) [MDR] (Months)**
^{90}Y-IT (19)	Treatment failure to an anthracycline or two prior regimens or intermediate grade or mantle cell NHL in relapse	67	26	(12.9 in responders) [11.7]
^{90}Y-IT (16)	No prior RTX. Phase III study comparing rituximab with ^{90}Y-IT	80	30	(11.2) [14.2]
^{90}Y-IT (63)	Prior treatment with RTX and either no response to RTX or time to progression after RTX of <6 months	74	15	(6.8) [6.4]
^{90}Y-IT (53)	RTX naive; platelet counts 100,000–150,000/mL	83	37	(9.4) [11.7]
^{90}Y-IT (64)	Prior RTX eligible	83	68	9.6
^{131}I-Tos (65)	Original report. Prior stem cell transplant allowed	71	34	12 for all responders
^{131}I-Tos (42)	No prior RTX	57	32	5.3 [9.9]
^{131}I-Tos (40)	At least two prior chemotherapy regimens with either no response or relapse within 6 months of completing their last regimen; no prior RTX	65	20	8.4 for all responders [6.5]
^{131}I-Tos (13)	No prior RTX	76	49	0.8 years [1.3 years]
^{131}I-Tos (66)	Trial comparing ^{131}I-Tos with unlabeled tositumomab	55	33	(6.3) [not reached]
^{131}I-Tos (56)	At least one prior course of RTX	65	38	10.4 [24.5]

OR, overall response; CR, complete response; PFS, progression-free survival; TTP, median time to progression for all patients in study; MDR, median duration of response in responders; ^{90}Y-IT, ^{90}Y ibritumomab tiuxetan; ^{131}I-Tos, ^{131}I tositumomab; LG, low grade; RTX, rituximab; NHL, non-Hodgkin lymphoma.

listed in Table 33.4. The data for ^{131}I tositumomab come from an analysis combining 250 patients from five registration trials (68), whereas the ^{90}Y ibritumomab tiuxetan data are obtained from an analysis combining 211 patients from four registration trials (67). Both analyses defined durable response as no evidence of progression for 1 year after RIT and found that disease bulk less than 5 cm predicted for long-term responders. For ^{90}Y ibritumomab tiuxetan, CR and stage I/II disease also predicted for long-term responders.

For ^{131}I tositumomab, normal pretreatment lactate dehydrogenase and response to last chemotherapy regimen predicted for long-term responders.

Due to differences in patient characteristics between the different registration trials, care should be taken when using this data to determine the relative efficacies of the two agents. However, one could comfortably conclude that both agents offer an excellent chance of success with the potential for intermediate- or long-term control for patients with

Table **33.4**	Meta-analyses of radioimmunotherapy (RIT) trials showing efficacy despite failure to previous conventional chemotherapy				
RIT Agent	**No. of Patients**	**LT Responders (%)**	**Median Duration of LT Response**	**LT Responders without Response to Previous Regimen (%)**	**LT Responders With Extensive Previous Chemotherapy Regimens**
^{90}Y ibritumomab tiuxetan (67)	211	37	28.1 months	37	33% (≥3 regimens)
^{131}I tositumomab (68)	250	32	45.8 months	36	43% (≥4 regimens)

Note: Long-term (LT) response in these trials was defined as lack of progression prior to 1 year after therapy.

relapsed or refractory low-grade B-cell NHL. Given the excellent responses in relapsed disease, the next logical question is whether initial treatment with RIT can improve clinical outcomes in this incurable disease.

Monotherapy as initial treatment

A phase II trial at the University of Michigan treated 76 patients with stage III or IV FL with ^{131}I tositumomab as initial management (61,62). OR was 95% with CR achieved in 75%. All patients with a partial response (PR) ultimately relapsed within 1.5 years with a median time to progression of 0.6 years. However, patients in CR had a median progression-free survival (PFS) of 9.2 years. Hematologic toxicity was moderate with no transfusions required, and no cases of MDS or AML developed. Interestingly, 63% of patients developed HAMA compared with the 10% seen in patients with relapsed disease. Perhaps, patients who have not received as much prior therapy have more active immune systems and are able to "cooperate" better with RIT to produce these impressive responses.

Consolidation as initial treatment

Given the impressive response of FL to ^{131}I tositumomab monotherapy, several investigators have attempted to optimize frontline therapy by combining induction chemotherapy with consolidation RIT. Phase II studies investigating the treatment of FL with conventional chemotherapy followed by consolidation with either ^{90}Y ibritumomab tiuxetan (69–71) or ^{131}I tositumomab (51,72,73) are summarized in Table 33.5. Several of these trials introduced qualitative

polymerase chain reaction (PCR) to detect the t(14:18) gene amplification as a method of measuring molecular response from samples in either the bone marrow (51,71,73,74) or peripheral blood (74). Debate remains on the question of whether rituximab should be included in the induction regimens, as it may decrease the efficacy of RIT through blocking tumor CD20 binding sites and debulking tumors, thus potentially preventing radiation delivery to some initial sites of disease. Clinically, this argument appears of marginal relevance given the excellent improvement in CR with consolidation RIT in the two studies that used induction rituximab.

In the initial management of low-grade lymphoma, early data show that RIT works reasonably well as monotherapy. In consolidation therapy, it may be unparalleled. Phase III randomized trials will determine whether RIT improves outcomes in comparison with chemotherapy and immunotherapy alone. Multiple multicenter trials are currently ongoing. Intergroup study S0016 is a joint effort by Southwest Oncology Group, Eastern Cooperation Oncology Group, and the Cancer and Leukemia Group B comparing six cycles of CHOP with six cycles of CHOP-R with six cycles of CHOP followed by ^{131}I tositumomab consolidation. Eligible patients have FL with bulky stage II to IV diseases. Concerning ^{90}Y ibritumomab tiuxetan, a proposed industry-sponsored trial has been designed to compare CVP-R with CVP-R and ^{90}Y ibritumomab tiuxetan.

Our European colleagues (75) have recently published a randomized phase III trial that investigated the safety and efficacy of ^{90}Y ibritumomab tiuxetan in 414 patients with stage III to IV FLs who had achieved a PR or CR/CR unconfirmed with chemotherapy (The "Frontline Indolent Trial or FIT"). Initial chemotherapy was not designated on protocol

Table **33.5**	Phase II studies investigating the use of induction chemotherapy followed by consolidation radioimmunotherapy (RIT) with either ^{90}Y ibritumomab tiuxetan or ^{131}I tositumomab in the initial management of low-grade NHL						
Group	RIT	Patients	Chemotherapy	CR after Induction Chemotherapy (%)	CR after Consolidation RIT (%)	PFS (%) (Time Point)
Minnie Pearl Cancer Research Network (69)	^{90}Y ibritumomab tiuxetan	42 stage II–IV	CHOP-R × 3	28	67	77 (2 years)
Pittsburgh (71)	^{90}Y ibritumomab tiuxetan	60 bulky stage II–IV	CHOP-R × 3	46	89	
Italian (70)	^{90}Y ibritumomab tiuxetan	61 stage III–IV	Fludarabine & mitoxantrone × 6	75	96	76 (3 years)
Iowa, Michigan, Cornell (72)	^{131}I tositumomab	30 bulky stage II–IV	CVP × 6	50	80	
Cornell (51)	^{131}I tositumomab	35 stage III–IV	Fludarabine × 3	9	86	60 (5 years)
SWOG S9911 (73)	^{131}I tositumomab	90 bulky stage II–IV	CHOP × 6	39	69	67 (5 years)

NHL, non-Hodgkin lymphoma; RIT, radioimmunotherapy; CR, complete response; PFS, progression-free survival; CHOP-R, cyclophosphamide, hydroxydaunomycin (doxorubicin or Adriamycin), oncovin (vincristine), prednisone, and rituximab; CVP, cyclophosphamide, vincristine, prednisone.

Table 33.6 Data regarding repeat treatment with either ^{90}Y ibritumomab tiuxetan or ^{131}I tositumomab for relapsed NHL

RIT Agent	No. of Patients	Initial OR (%)	Initial CR (%)	Initial Median DR (months)	Median Time between RIT Courses (Months)	Retreatment OR (%)	Retreatment CR (%)	Retreatment Median DR (Months)
^{90}Y ibritumomab tiuxetan (76)	18	89	56	11.3	16.6	77	33	8.4
^{131}I tositumomab (52)	32	94	56	13.6	21	56	25	15.2
^{131}I rituximab (77)	16	100	69	14	19	88	56	10.5

NHL, non-Hodgkin lymphoma; RIT, radioimmunotherapy; OR, overall response; CR, complete response; DR, duration of response.

and instead was a practitioner's choice of first-line therapies including CVP, CHOP, chlorambucil, fludarabine combinations, and rituximab combinations. ^{90}Y ibritumomab tiuxetan consolidation led to improved CR and PFS. Patients in PR status converted to CR in 77% of cases with ^{90}Y ibritumomab tiuxetan consolidation compared with 17% in the control arm ($p < 0.001$). Among 186 patients assessed for the BCL-2 gene rearrangement with PCR, 127 were positive at the time of random assignment. In the ^{90}Y ibritumomab tiuxetan consolidation arm, 90% (61/68) of patients converted to PCR-negative status, whereas only 36% (21/59) of patients in the control arm converted to PCR-negative status. Median PFS was improved by approximately 2 years with ^{90}Y ibritumomab tiuxetan consolidation (36.5 months vs. 13.3 months, $p < 0.0001$). Median follow-up in this trial was only 3.5 years; longer follow-up should confirm whether there is a survival advantage to ^{90}Y ibritumomab tiuxetan consolidation. As a result of these data, ^{90}Y ibritumomab tiuxetan has received FDA approval and a category 1 recommendation from the NCCN clinical practice guidelines for first-line consolidation therapy in advanced FL. One criticism of this trial is that only 14% of patients received rituximab during the chemotherapy portion of the trial. However, ^{90}Y ibritumomab tiuxetan has been proved superior to rituximab in a phase III study for relapsed FL (16). Furthermore, two phase II studies have shown improved CR rates with ^{90}Y ibritumomab tiuxetan consolidation after CHOP-R × 3 (Table 33.5) (69,71). Given these additional data regarding the additional benefit of ^{90}Y ibritumomab tiuxetan to rituximab, one might argue that there would still be improved response with ^{90}Y ibritumomab tiuxetan consolidation if the protocol had mandated rituximab–based induction regimens. Current and future clinical trials have been proposed to investigate the degree to which rituximab maintenance could substitute for ^{90}Y ibritumomab tiuxetan. Data are not yet available on this important question.

■ RETREATMENT WITH RIT

Because of the excellent response with RIT in NHL and the tendency for NHL to ultimately relapse, several investigators have examined whether repeat treatment with RIT is feasible

(52,76,77). Results from selected studies are shown in Table 33.6. Patients included in these studies had been heavily treated prior to their second RIT dose, some even having had high-dose chemotherapy with autologous stem cell rescue. Dosing in these studies followed the same rules of dosing for the initial treatment with dose reductions for thrombocytopenia. Hematologic toxicity in these studies was similar between the initial RIT treatment and retreatment. Five patients retreated with ^{131}I tositumomab developed MDS or AML; it is unclear what role RIT may have played in the pathogenesis of their leukemia given their prior chemotherapy history. Interestingly, there is a subset of patients who will respond more favorably on second RIT treatment than the first. These reports show that RIT can be a successful salvage therapy for patients who initially responded to RIT.

■ CONSOLIDATION THERAPY FOR NONFOLLICULAR NON-HODGKIN LYMPHOMA

With such impressive results for RIT consolidation in the initial management of FL, several investigators are exploring the use of RIT with other CD20+ B-cell malignancies. Phase II studies involving nonfollicular low-grade NHL and DLBCL have already been published.

The Italian Leukemia, Lymphoma, and Multiple Myeloma Association has performed a phase II study for nonfollicular NHL with six cycles of fludarabine and mitoxantrone followed by consolidation with ^{90}Y ibritumomab tiuxetan (70). Eligible histology included marginal zone lymphoma, lymphoblastic lymphoma, and small lymphocytic lymphoma. OR was 80.5% with 50% achieving CR. Toxicity was primarily hematologic as seen in prior studies. Three-year PFS was 89.5% with 3-year overall survival (OS) of 100%.

RIT has also been investigated in aggressive NHL. The Italian Leukemia, Lymphoma, and Multiple Myeloma Association has treated 20 elderly patients with DLBCL with six cycles of CHOP-R chemotherapy followed by consolidation with ^{90}Y ibritumomab tiuxetan (78). Initial OR with CHOP-R was 100%, with 75% of patients achieving CR. After ^{90}Y ibritumomab tiuxetan consolidation, four of the five initial PR converted to CR for an OR of 95%. ^{90}Y ibritumomab tiuxetan consolidation was safe and had a similar toxicity profile to earlier studies with no treatment-related deaths on study. With a median follow-up of 15 months, three patients progressed: the patient who never achieved CR, one patient who achieved CR after CHOP-R, and one patient who converted to CR after ^{90}Y ibritumomab tiuxetan. Two-year PFS was 75% and 2-year OS was 95%. SWOG protocol S0433 is a phase II study for DLBCL NHL. Patients with stage II bulky, III, or IV will receive CHOP-R followed by ^{131}I tositumomab. Longer follow-up and randomized trials should determine the role of consolidation RIT in DLBCL.

RIT AFTER AUTOLOGOUS STEM CELL TRANSPLANT

Disseminated FL is currently considered a treatable but incurable entity. With each subsequent relapse, further treatment becomes less effective. Once disease progresses after a regimen that includes SCT, patients have few options. The initial RIT trials that led to FDA approval largely excluded patients with prior SCT (79). However, results of RIT treatment for patients who have received previous SCT have been reported.

In a single center phase I/II study for treatment of relapsed FL with ^{131}I tositumomab, 14 patients had received a prior SCT. The maximally tolerated dose in these patients was 45 cGy total body radiation equivalent dose. Response rate was 50% with a median PFS of 4.7 years (65).

The University of Pittsburgh reported a series of eight patients treated with ^{90}Y ibritumomab tiuxetan who had received prior SCT. Dosing was standard 0.4 mCi/kg with dose reduction for platelets less than 150,000/mL. Hematologic toxicity was similar to previous reports. Response, however, was poor. Two patients had a CR and an additional patient had a PR. One of the reports of retreatment with ^{90}Y ibritumomab tiuxetan included five patients who had also had prior SCT (76).

A phase I dose escalation study found that the optimal dose of ^{90}Y ibritumomab tiuxetan for patients previously treated with SCT was 0.2 mCi/kg with a maximum dose of 32 mCi (80). Most of these patients (89%) had failed rituximab, and 58% had DLBCL. Grades 3 to 4 thrombocytopenia occurred in 10 of 13 patients at the 0.2 mCi/kg dose level. Outcomes for the 0.2 mCi/kg dose level included a 1-year event-free survival of 38% and 1-year OS of 52%.

A series of eight patients with FL treated with nine courses of ^{90}Y ibritumomab tiuxetan after SCT showed a 77% response rate and 1-year OS of 83%. Four patients had previously received total body irradiation (TBI). The investigators used standard dosing. Despite demonstrating higher hematologic toxicity than the phase I study conducted by Vose et al. (80), it was argued that standard dosing was safe and effective (81).

Differences in response rates between these studies could be related to heterogeneity of disease, including histology, previous therapy, and response to previous therapy. Given the dismal circumstances involved with treatment

failure after SCT, it is encouraging that RIT can provide benefit to some patients. Whether dose reduction will be necessary due to limited bone marrow capacity in these heavily pretreated patients remains a topic of further investigation.

RIT WITH SCT SUPPORT

Patients with malignant lymphoma refractory to multiple regimens have limited treatment options. RIT as previously discussed is one management option. High-dose chemotherapy followed by autologous SCT is another alternative available to patients with relapsed or refractory disease. Autologous SCT typically begins with the mobilization of peripheral stem cells after a low dose of priming chemotherapy. This is followed by a myeloablative dose of cytoxic therapy aimed at eliminating all tumor cells in the body. The cytotoxic therapy utilized in previous protocols includes high-dose chemotherapy, TBI, or a combination of chemotherapy and TBI. RIT is a promising weapon in the armament of autologous SCT, as it allows for the use of targeted radiation to sites of disease. Press et al. estimated a 10-fold increase in dose to tumor compared with TBI with escalated dose ^{131}I tositumomab and bone marrow support (82). The prospect of replacing external beam TBI with radiopharmaceutical TBI to achieve greater tumoricidal effect with lower collateral damage has led several investigators to attempt incorporation of RIT into the preparative regimen for autologous SCT protocols.

Several studies have previously been published regarding the use of ^{90}Y ibritumomab tiuxetan or ^{131}I tositumomab in combination with autologous SCT. Lymphomas eligible for these protocols include patients with relapsed, refractory, or transformed FL, DLBCL, and mantle cell lymphoma. These protocols have involved the use of high-dose chemotherapy combined with standard dose RIT or the use of escalated dose RIT. Some regimens have included etoposide/cyclophosphamide followed by high-dose ^{90}Y ibritumomab tiuxetan (83) or high-dose ^{131}I tositumomab (84), BEAM (carmustine, etoposide, cytarabine, melphalan) chemotherapy followed by standard dose ^{131}I tositumomab (85) or ^{90}Y ibritumomab tiuxetan (86,87), high-dose ^{131}I tositumomab (88,89), and high-dose ^{90}Y ibritumomab tiuxetan (90). Escalated dose RIT dosimetry has been based on dosing to critical organs, with critical organ target doses of 10 Gy with ^{90}Y ibritumomab tiuxetan (83) and 25 Gy with ^{131}I tositumomab (88,89). Doses of ^{90}Y ibritumomab tiuxetan in these trials reached 100 mCi (90) compared with the standard maximum dose of 32 mCi. A recent dose escalation trial of high-dose BEAM, ^{90}Y ibritumomab tiuxetan, and autologous SCT found that 15 Gy to critical organs was the maximum tolerated dose of ^{90}Y ibritumomab tiuxetan (91). In these protocols, ^{90}Y ibritumomab tiuxetan was administered on day 13 or 14 prior to infusion of stem cells, whereas ^{131}I tositumomab was administered between 2 and 19 days prior to SCT. Despite concerns of stem cell ablation by the radiopharmaceutical, RIT conditioning has fortunately not prevented engraftment in these clinical trials. Toxicity has been comparable with chemotherapy regimens (85,86), with treatment-related mortality ranging from 0% to 9% (83,87,88). OR rates have been on the order of 60% to 80%, with 2-year PFS of 50% to 70%, and 2-year OS ranging from 60% to 90%. High-dose ^{131}I tositumomab has produced long-term remissions in 14 of 29 patients at 27+ and 87+ months after RIT (92). Patients treated on a protocol of cyclophosphamide, etoposide, and high-dose ^{131}I tositumomab had improved OS when compared with a cohort of patients treated at the same institution and time period on a protocol of cyclophosphamide, etoposide, and TBI (84). Like standard dose RIT in relapsed disease, three or more previous chemotherapy regimens predict for poor response when RIT is used with SCT (87,90). Longer follow-up along with phase III randomized trials should help define the role of RIT with autologous SCT.

Equally interesting is the use of RIT in preparation for allogeneic SCT where the infused stem cells come from an HLA-matched donor. Lymphoma patients who are candidates for allogeneic SCT typically have a poorer prognosis than those who receive autologous SCT. Shimoni et al. have published a report of 12 patients treated with fludarabine and either busulfan or melphalan chemotherapy and standard dose ^{90}Y ibritumomab tiuxetan (93). OR rate was 83% with a 2-year PFS of 33%. Nonrelapse mortality with this protocol was 42%, primarily related to graft-versus-host disease. RIT used as a form of preparative therapy for allogeneic SCT protocols appears promising and warrants further investigation.

CONCLUSIONS

RIT initiatives with anti-CD20 radioimmunoconjugates have produced excellent clinical results for patients with low-grade B-cell NHL, both as single-agent treatment and in combination with chemotherapy. In addition to the two FDA-approved anti-CD20 radiopharmaceuticals, Zevalin and Bexxar, new anti-CD20 constructs and treatment strategies have emerged in clinical trials. In some cases, these biologically targeted radiopharmaceuticals make use of new antibodies or isotopes, while others rely on different cytotoxic combinations or sequencing strategies. Despite improved clinical results observed to date in phase I, II, and III clinical trials, RIT has had remarkably poor market penetration. Some have ascribed this underperformance to the difficulty in putting together the necessary multidisciplinary teams, including members from hematology–oncology, radiation oncology, and nuclear medicine, necessary for safe and effective RIT use. Others have expressed concern over potential hematopoietic toxicity or difficulty administering subsequent systemic treatment regimes (94). Still others have proposed that some of the newer members of the anti-CD20 targeted therapy biopharmaceuticals might be capable of reproducing the excellent clinical results seen with RIT without the clinical and logistic radiation concerns of a high-energy radiolabeled product. Some cynics have voiced the

contention that the real driver relates more to the economic and political turf incentives and disincentives affecting referral patterns for some gatekeeper doctors. Whatever the case, the class of targeted anti-CD20 radiopharmaceutical constructs has apparently produced exceptional clinical results with surprisingly low short-term and long-term toxicity. Current phase III clinical trials suggest that the ideal role for these agents may be in consolidation phase after initial chemotherapy. In this case, RIT is used as a facilitator rather than as a competitive replacement for more conventional nonradioactive systemic agents. When used in combination with chemotherapy, some of the newer types of biological agents, and limited field conformal EBRT, radiolabeled anti-CD20 agents may finally produce the long sought–after tail on the survival curve, thus implying that at least some types of disseminated low-grade B-cell NHL may reasonably be treated with curative intent using combination therapies. This would allow low-grade NHL to be removed from the list of highly responsive but categorically incurable lesions, a result that we have sought for over a century.

REFERENCES

1. Jemal A, Siegel R, Ward E, et al. Cancer statistics, 2008. *CA Cancer J Clin*. 2008;58(2):71–96.
2. Armitage JO, Weisenburger DD. New approach to classifying non-Hodgkin's lymphomas: clinical features of the major histologic subtypes. Non-Hodgkin's Lymphoma Classification Project. *J Clin Oncol*. 1998;16(8):2780–2795.
3. Fisher RI. Overview of non-Hodgkin's lymphoma: biology, staging, and treatment. *Semin Oncol*. 2003;30(2, suppl 4):3–9.
4. Mauch PM. *Non-Hodgkin's Lymphomas*. Philadelphia, PA: Lippincott Williams & Wilkins; 2004.
5. Mann RB, Berard CW. Criteria for the cytologic subclassification of follicular lymphomas: a proposed alternative method. *Hematol Oncol*. 1983;1(2):187–192.
6. Wendum D, Sebban C, Gaulard P, et al. Follicular large-cell lymphoma treated with intensive chemotherapy: an analysis of 89 cases included in the LNH87 trial and comparison with the outcome of diffuse large B-cell lymphoma. Groupe d'Etude des Lymphomes de l'Adulte. *J Clin Oncol*. 1997;15(4):1654–1663.
7. Tsujimoto Y, Finger LR, Yunis J, et al. Cloning of the chromosome breakpoint of neoplastic B cells with the t(14;18) chromosome translocation. *Science*. 1984;226(4678):1097–1099.
8. Hockenbery D, Nunez G, Milliman C, et al. Bcl-2 is an inner mitochondrial membrane protein that blocks programmed cell death. *Nature*. 1990;348(6299):334–336.
9. Traweek ST, Liu J, Johnson RM, et al. High-grade transformation of chronic lymphocytic leukemia and low-grade non-Hodgkin's lymphoma. Genotypic confirmation of clonal identity. *Am J Clin Pathol*. 1993;100(5):519–526.
10. Carbone PP, Kaplan HS, Musshoff K, et al. Report of the Committee on Hodgkin's Disease Staging Classification. *Cancer Res*. 1971;31(11):1860–1861.
11. Zelenetz AD, Advani RH, Byrd JC, et al. Non-Hodgkin's lymphomas. *J Natl Compr Canc Netw*. 2008;6(4):356–421.
12. Pohlman B, Sweetenham J, Macklis RM. Review of clinical radioimmunotherapy. *Expert Rev Anticancer Ther*. 2006;6(3):445–461.
13. Davies AJ, Rohatiner AZ, Howell S, et al. Tositumomab and iodine I 131 tositumomab for recurrent indolent and transformed B-cell non-Hodgkin's lymphoma. *J Clin Oncol*. 2004;22(8):1469–1479.
14. Macklis RM. Radithor and the era of mild radium therapy. *JAMA*. 1990;264(5):614–618.
15. Press OW. Radioimmunotherapy for non-Hodgkin's lymphomas: a historical perspective. *Semin Oncol*. 2003;30(2, suppl 4):10–21.
16. Witzig TE, Gordon LI, Cabanillas F, et al. Randomized controlled trial of yttrium-90-labeled ibritumomab tiuxetan radioimmunotherapy

versus rituximab immunotherapy for patients with relapsed or refractory low-grade, follicular, or transformed B-cell non-Hodgkin's lymphoma. *J Clin Oncol.* 2002;20(10):2453–2463.

17. McLaughlin P, Grillo-Lopez AJ, Link BK, et al. Rituximab chimeric anti-CD20 monoclonal antibody therapy for relapsed indolent lymphoma: half of patients respond to a four-dose treatment program. *J Clin Oncol.* 1998;16(8):2825–2833.

18. Kaminski MS, Zasadny KR, Francis IR, et al. Radioimmunotherapy of B-cell lymphoma with [131I]anti-B1 (anti-CD20) antibody. *N Engl J Med.* 1993;329(7):459–465.

19. Witzig TE, White CA, Wiseman GA, et al. Phase I/II trial of IDEC-Y2B8 radioimmunotherapy for treatment of relapsed or refractory CD20(+) B-cell non-Hodgkin's lymphoma. *J Clin Oncol.* 1999;17(12):3793–3803.

20. Leichner PK, Yang NC, Frenkel TL, et al. Dosimetry and treatment planning for ^{90}Y-labeled antiferritin in hepatoma. *Int J Radiat Oncol Biol Phys.* 1988;14(5):1033–1042.

21. Dillehay LE. A model of cell killing by low-dose-rate radiation including repair of sublethal damage, G2 block, and cell division. *Radiat Res.* 1990;124(2):201–207.

22. Yorke ED, Wessels BW, Bradley EW. Absorbed dose averages and dose heterogeneities in radioimmunotherapy. *Antibody Immunoconjugates Radiopharm.* 1991;4:623–626.

23. Witzig TE, Vukov AM, Habermann TM, et al. Rituximab therapy for patients with newly diagnosed, advanced-stage, follicular grade I non-Hodgkin's lymphoma: a phase II trial in the North Central Cancer Treatment Group. *J Clin Oncol.* 2005;23(6):1103–1108.

24. Hernandez MC, Knox SJ. Radiobiology of radioimmunotherapy: targeting CD20 B-cell antigen in non-Hodgkin's lymphoma. *Int J Radiat Oncol Biol Phys.* 2004;59(5):1274–1287.

25. Macklis RM. How and why does radioimmunotherapy work? *Int J Radiat Oncol Biol Phys.* 2004;59(5):1269–1271.

26. DeNardo SJ. Radioimmunodetection and therapy of breast cancer. *Semin Nucl Med.* 2005;35(2):143–151.

27. Kaminski MS, Zasadny KR, Francis IR, et al. Iodine-131-anti-B1 radioimmunotherapy for B-cell lymphoma. *J Clin Oncol.* 1996;14(7):1974–1981.

28. Knox SJ, Goris ML, Trisler K, et al. Yttrium-90-labeled anti-CD20 monoclonal antibody therapy of recurrent B-cell lymphoma. *Clin Cancer Res.* 1996;2(3):457–470.

29. Koral KF, Kaminski MS, Wahl RL. Correlation of tumor radiation-absorbed dose with response is easier to find in previously untreated patients. *J Nucl Med.* 2003;44(9):1541–1543.

30. Wiseman GA, Kornmehl E, Leigh B, et al. Radiation dosimetry results and safety correlations from ^{90}Y-ibritumomab tiuxetan radioimmunotherapy for relapsed or refractory non-Hodgkin's lymphoma: combined data from 4 clinical trials. *J Nucl Med.* 2003;44(3):465–474.

31. Gokhale AS, Mayadev J, Pohlman B, et al. Gamma camera scans and pretreatment tumor volumes as predictors of response and progression after Y-90 anti-CD20 radioimmunotherapy. *Int J Radiat Oncol Biol Phys.* 2005;63(1):194–201.

32. Du Y, Honeychurch J, Cragg MS, et al. Antibody-induced intracellular signaling works in combination with radiation to eradicate lymphoma in radioimmunotherapy. *Blood.* 2004;103(4):1485–1494.

33. O'Keefe TL, Williams GT, Davies SL, et al. Mice carrying a CD20 gene disruption. *Immunogenetics.* 1998;48(2):125–132.

34. Shan D, Ledbetter JA, Press OW. Signaling events involved in anti-CD20-induced apoptosis of malignant human B cells. *Cancer Immunol Immunother.* 2000;48(12):673–683.

35. Hofmeister JK, Cooney D, Coggeshall KM. Clustered CD20 induced apoptosis: src-family kinase, the proximal regulator of tyrosine phosphorylation, calcium influx, and caspase 3-dependent apoptosis. *Blood Cells Mol Dis.* 2000;26(2):133–143.

36. Li H, Ayer LM, Lytton J, et al. Store-operated cation entry mediated by CD20 in membrane rafts. *J Biol Chem.* 2003;278(43):42427–42434.

37. Bellosillo B, Villamor N, Lopez-Guillermo A, et al. Complement-mediated cell death induced by rituximab in B-cell lymphoproliferative disorders is mediated in vitro by a caspase-independent mechanism involving the generation of reactive oxygen species. *Blood.* 2001;98(9):2771–2777.

38. Hainsworth JD, Litchy S, Burris HA III, et al. Rituximab as first-line and maintenance therapy for patients with indolent non-Hodgkin's lymphoma. *J Clin Oncol.* 2002;20(20):4261–4267.

39. Czuczman MS, Weaver R, Alkuzweny B, et al. Prolonged clinical and molecular remission in patients with low-grade or follicular non-Hodgkin's lymphoma treated with rituximab plus CHOP chemotherapy: 9-year follow-up. *J Clin Oncol.* 2004;22(23):4711–4716.

40. Kaminski MS, Zelenetz AD, Press OW, et al. Pivotal study of iodine I 131 tositumomab for chemotherapy-refractory low-grade or transformed low-grade B-cell non-Hodgkin's lymphomas. *J Clin Oncol.* 2001;19(19):3918–3928.

41. Gordon LI, Molina A, Witzig T, et al. Durable responses after ibritumomab tiuxetan radioimmunotherapy for CD20+ B-cell lymphoma: long-term follow-up of a phase 1/2 study. *Blood.* 2004;103(12):4429–4431.

42. Vose JM, Wahl RL, Saleh M, et al. Multicenter phase II study of iodine-131 tositumomab for chemotherapy-relapsed/refractory low-grade and transformed low-grade B-cell non-Hodgkin's lymphomas. *J Clin Oncol.* 2000;18(6):1316–1323.

43. Mach JP, Buchegger F, Pelegrin A. *Progress in Radiolabeled Monoclonal Antibodies for Cancer Diagnosis and Potential for Therapy.* Philadelphia, PA: Lippincott Williams & Wilkins; 1989.

44. Conti PS, White C, Pieslor P, et al. The role of imaging with (111) In-ibritumomab tiuxetan in the ibritumomab tiuxetan (zevalin) regimen: results from a Zevalin Imaging Registry. *J Nucl Med.* 2005;46(11):1812–1818.

45. Kassis AI, Adelstein SJ. Radiobiologic principles in radionuclide therapy. *J Nucl Med.* 2005;46(suppl 1):4S–12S.

46. Press OW, Eary JF, Badger CC, et al. Treatment of refractory non-Hodgkin's lymphoma with radiolabeled MB-1 (anti-CD37) antibody. *J Clin Oncol.* 1989;7(8):1027–1038.

47. Melhus KB, Larsen RH, Stokke T, et al. Evaluation of the binding of radiolabeled rituximab to CD20-positive lymphoma cells: an in vitro feasibility study concerning low-dose-rate radioimmunotherapy with the alpha-emitter ^{227}Th. *Cancer Biother Radiopharm.* 2007;22(4):469–479.

48. Linden O, Hindorf C, Cavallin-Stahl E, et al. Dose-fractionated radioimmunotherapy in non-Hodgkin's lymphoma using DOTA-conjugated, 90Y-radiolabeled, humanized anti-CD22 monoclonal antibody, epratuzumab. *Clin Cancer Res.* 2005;11(14):5215–5222.

49. Shen S, DeNardo GL, Yuan A, et al. Splenic volume change and nodal tumor response in non-Hodgkin's lymphoma patients after radioimmunotherapy using radiolabeled Lym-1 antibody. *Cancer Biother Radiopharm.* 2005;20(6):662–670.

50. Mones JV, Coleman M, Kostakoglu L, et al. Dose-attenuated radioimmunotherapy with tositumomab and iodine 131 tositumomab in patients with recurrent non-Hodgkin's lymphoma (NHL) and extensive bone marrow involvement. *Leuk Lymphoma.* 2007;48(2):342–348.

51. Leonard JP, Coleman M, Kostakoglu L, et al. Abbreviated chemotherapy with fludarabine followed by tositumomab and iodine I 131 tositumomab for untreated follicular lymphoma. *J Clin Oncol.* 2005;23(24):5696–5704.

52. Kaminski MS, Radford JA, Gregory SA, et al. Re-treatment with I-131 tositumomab in patients with non-Hodgkin's lymphoma who had previously responded to I-131 tositumomab. *J Clin Oncol.* 2005;23(31):7985–7993.

53. Wiseman GA, Gordon LI, Multani PS, et al. Ibritumomab tiuxetan radioimmunotherapy for patients with relapsed or refractory non-Hodgkin lymphoma and mild thrombocytopenia: a phase II multicenter trial. *Blood.* 2002;99(12):4336–4342.

54. Wahl RL. Tositumomab and ^{131}I therapy in non-Hodgkin's lymphoma. *J Nucl Med.* 2005;46:128S–140S.

55. Witzig TE, White CA, Gordon LI, et al. Safety of yttrium-90 ibritumomab tiuxetan radioimmunotherapy for relapsed low-grade, follicular, or transformed non-Hodgkin's lymphoma. *J Clin Oncol.* 2003;21(7):1263–1270.

56. Horning SJ, Younes A, Jain V, et al. Efficacy and safety of tositumomab and iodine-131 tositumomab (Bexxar) in B-cell lymphoma, progressive after rituximab. *J Clin Oncol.* 2005;23(4):712–719.

57. Gregory SA, Leonard JP, Knox SL, et al. The iodine I-131 tositumomab therapeutic regimen: summary of safety in 995 patients with relapsed/refractory low grade (LG) and transformed LG non-Hodgkin's lymphoma (NHL) [ASCO Annual Meeting Proceedings (Post-Meeting Edition)]. *J Clin Oncol.* 2004;22(suppl):14S.

58. Sweetenham JW, Dicke K, Arcaroli J, et al. Efficacy and safety of yttrium 90 (^{90}Y) ibritumomab tiuxetan (Zevalin(R)) therapy with rituximab in patients with untreated low-grade follicular lymphoma. *Blood.* 2004;104(11):2633.

59. Bennett JM, Kaminski MS, Leonard JP, et al. Assessment of treatment-related myelodysplastic syndromes and acute myeloid leukemia in patients with non-Hodgkin lymphoma treated with tositumomab and iodine I^{131} tositumomab. *Blood.* 2005;105(12):4576–4582.

60. Czuczman MS, Emmanouilides C, Darif M, et al. Treatment-related myelodysplastic syndrome and acute myelogenous leukemia in patients treated with ibritumomab tiuxetan radioimmunotherapy. *J Clin Oncol.* 2007;25(27):4285–4292.

61. Kaminski MS, Tuck M, Estes J, et al. ^{131}I-tositumomab therapy as initial treatment for follicular lymphoma. *N Engl J Med.* 2005;352(5):441–449.

62. Kaminski MS, Estes J, Tuck M, et al. I131-tositumomab monotherapy as frontline treatment for follicular lymphoma: updated results after a median follow-up of 8 years. *J Clin Oncol.* 2007 ASCO Annual Meeting Proceedings (Post-Meeting Edition). 2007;25(18 suppl):8033.

63. Witzig TE, Flinn IW, Gordon LI, et al. Treatment with ibritumomab tiuxetan radioimmunotherapy in patients with rituximab-refractory follicular non-Hodgkin's lymphoma. *J Clin Oncol.* 2002;20(15):3262–3269.

64. Tobinai K, Watanabe T, Ogura M, et al. Japanese phase II study of 90Y-ibritumomab tiuxetan in patients with relapsed or refractory indolent B-cell lymphoma. *Cancer Sci.* 2009;100(1):158–164.

65. Kaminski MS, Estes J, Zasadny KR, et al. Radioimmunotherapy with iodine (131)I tositumomab for relapsed or refractory B-cell non-Hodgkin lymphoma: updated results and long-term follow-up of the University of Michigan experience. *Blood.* 2000;96(4):1259–1266.

66. Davis TA, Kaminski MS, Leonard JP, et al. The radioisotope contributes significantly to the activity of radioimmunotherapy. *Clin Cancer Res.* 2004;10(23):7792–7798.

67. Witzig TE, Molina A, Gordon LI, et al. Long-term responses in patients with recurring or refractory B-cell non-Hodgkin lymphoma treated with yttrium 90 ibritumomab tiuxetan. *Cancer.* 2007;109(9):1804–1810.

68. Fisher RI, Kaminski MS, Wahl RL, et al. Tositumomab and iodine-131 tositumomab produces durable complete remissions in a subset of heavily pretreated patients with low-grade and transformed non-Hodgkin's lymphomas. *J Clin Oncol.* 2005;23(30):7565–7573.

69. Shipley DL, Greco FA, Spigel DR, et al. Rituximab with short duration chemotherapy followed by 90Y ibritumomab tiuxetan as first-line treatment for patients with follicular lymphoma: update of a Minnie Pearl Cancer Research Network phase II trial. *J Clin Oncol.* 2005 ASCO Annual Meeting Proceedings. 2005;23(16 suppl):6577.

70. Zinzani PL, Tani M, Fanti S, et al. A phase 2 trial of fludarabine and mitoxantrone chemotherapy followed by yttrium-90 ibritumomab tiuxetan for patients with previously untreated, indolent, nonfollicular, non-Hodgkin lymphoma. *Cancer.* 2008;112(4):856–862.

71. Jacobs SA, Swerdlow SH, Kant J, et al. Phase II trial of short-course CHOP-R followed by 90Y-ibritumomab tiuxetan and extended rituximab in previously untreated follicular lymphoma. *Clin Cancer Res.* 2008;14(21):7088–7094.

72. Link B, Kaminski MS, Coleman M, et al. Phase II study of CVP followed by tositumomab and iodine I 131 tositumomab (Bexxar therapeutic regimen) in patients with untreated follicular non-Hodgkin's lymphoma (NHL). *J Clin Oncol.* 2004 ASCO Annual Meeting Proceedings. 2004;22(14 suppl):6520.

73. Press OW, Unger JM, Braziel RM, et al. Phase II trial of CHOP chemotherapy followed by tositumomab/iodine I-131 tositumomab for previously untreated follicular non-Hodgkin's lymphoma: five-year follow-up of Southwest Oncology Group Protocol S9911. *J Clin Oncol.* 2006;24(25):4143–4149.

74. Zinzani PL, Tani M, Pulsoni A, et al. Fludarabine and mitoxantrone followed by yttrium-90 ibritumomab tiuxetan in previously untreated patients with follicular non-Hodgkin lymphoma trial: a phase II non-randomised trial (FLUMIZ). *Lancet Oncol.* 2008;9(4):352–358.

75. Morschhauser F, Redford J, Van Hoof A, et al. Phase III trial of consolidation therapy with yttrium-90-ibritumomab tiuxetan compared with no additional therapy after first remission in advanced follicular lymphoma. *J Clin Oncol.* 2008;26:5156–5164.

76. Shah J, Wang W, Harrough VD, et al. Retreatment with yttrium-90 ibritumomab tiuxetan in patients with B-cell non-Hodgkin's lymphoma. *Leuk Lymphoma.* 2007;48(9):1736–1744.

77. Bishton MJ, Leahy MF, Hicks RJ, et al. Repeat treatment with iodine-131-rituximab is safe and effective in patients with relapsed indolent B-cell non-Hodgkin's lymphoma who had previously responded to iodine-131-rituximab. *Ann Oncol.* 2008;19(9):1629–1633.

78. Zinzani PL, Tani M, Fanti S, et al. A phase II trial of CHOP chemotherapy followed by yttrium 90 ibritumomab tiuxetan (Zevalin) for previously untreated elderly diffuse large B-cell lymphoma patients. *Ann Oncol.* 2008;19(4):769–773.

79. Jacobs SA, Vidnovic N, Joyce J, et al. Full-dose 90Y ibritumomab tiuxetan therapy is safe in patients with prior myeloablative chemotherapy. *Clin Cancer Res.* 2005;11(19, pt 2):7146s–7150s.

80. Vose JM, Bierman PJ, Loberiza FR Jr, et al. Phase I trial of (90)Y-ibritumomab tiuxetan in patients with relapsed B-cell non-Hodgkin's lymphoma following high-dose chemotherapy and autologous stem cell transplantation. *Leuk Lymphoma.* 2007;48(4):683–690.

81. Peyrade F, Triby C, Slama B, et al. Radioimmunotherapy in relapsed follicular lymphoma previously treated by autologous bone marrow transplant: a report of eight new cases and literature review. *Leuk Lymphoma.* 2008;49(9):1762–1768.

82. Press OW, Eary JF, Appelbaum FR, et al. Radiolabeled-antibody therapy of B-cell lymphoma with autologous bone marrow support. *N Engl J Med.* 1993;329(17):1219–1224.

83. Nademanee A, Forman S, Molina A, et al. A phase 1/2 trial of high-dose yttrium-90-ibritumomab tiuxetan in combination with high-dose etoposide and cyclophosphamide followed by autologous stem cell transplantation in patients with poor-risk or relapsed non-Hodgkin lymphoma. *Blood.* 2005;106(8):2896–2902.

84. Press OW, Eary JF, Gooley T, et al. A phase I/II trial of iodine-131-tositumomab (anti-CD20), etoposide, cyclophosphamide, and autologous stem cell transplantation for relapsed B-cell lymphomas. *Blood.* 2000;96(9):2934–2942.

85. Vose JM, Bierman PJ, Enke C, et al. Phase I trial of iodine-131 tositumomab with high-dose chemotherapy and autologous stem-cell transplantation for relapsed non-Hodgkin's lymphoma. *J Clin Oncol.* 2005;23(3):461–467.

86. Krishnan A, Nademanee A, Fung HC, et al. Phase II trial of a transplantation regimen of yttrium-90 ibritumomab tiuxetan and high-dose chemotherapy in patients with non-Hodgkin's lymphoma. *J Clin Oncol.* 2008;26(1):90–95.

87. Shimoni A, Zwas ST, Oksman Y, et al. Yttrium-90-ibritumomab tiuxetan (Zevalin) combined with high-dose BEAM chemotherapy and autologous stem cell transplantation for chemo-refractory aggressive non-Hodgkin's lymphoma. *Exp Hematol.* 2007;35(4):534–540.

88. Gopal AK, Rajendran JG, Gooley TA, et al. High-dose [131I]tositumomab (anti-CD20) radioimmunotherapy and autologous hematopoietic stem-cell transplantation for adults > or = 60 years old with relapsed or refractory B-cell lymphoma. *J Clin Oncol.* 2007;25(11):1396–1402.

89. Press OW, Eary JF, Appelbaum FR, et al. Phase II trial of 131I-B1 (anti-CD20) antibody therapy with autologous stem cell transplantation for relapsed B cell lymphomas. *Lancet.* 1995;346(8971):336–340.

90. Ferrucci PF, Vanazzi A, Grana CM, et al. High activity 90Y-ibritumomab tiuxetan (Zevalin) with peripheral blood progenitor cells support in patients with refractory/resistant B-cell non-Hodgkin lymphomas. *Br J Haematol.* 2007;139(4):590–599.

91. Winter JN, Inwards DJ, Spies S, et al. Yttrium-90 ibritumomab tiuxetan doses calculated to deliver up to 15 Gy to critical organs may be safely combined with high-dose BEAM and autologous transplantation in relapsed or refractory B-cell non-Hodgkin's lymphoma. *J Clin Oncol.* 2009;27(10):1653–1659.

92. Liu SY, Eary JF, Petersdorf SH, et al. Follow-up of relapsed B-cell lymphoma patients treated with iodine-131-labeled anti-CD20 antibody and autologous stem-cell rescue. *J Clin Oncol.* 1998;16(10):3270–3278.

93. Shimoni A, Zwas ST, Oksman Y, et al. Ibritumomab tiuxetan (Zevalin) combined with reduced-intensity conditioning and allogeneic stem-cell transplantation (SCT) in patients with chemorefractory non-Hodgkin's lymphoma. *Bone Marrow Transplant.* 2008;41(4):355–361.

94. Maloney DG. Factors leading to rituximab resistance and how to overcome them. *Clin Adv Hematol Oncol.* 2009;7(2):3–7.

Targeted Radionuclide Therapy for Leukemia

Roland B. Walter and John M. Pagel

■ INTRODUCTION

The term *leukemia* was introduced in 1847 by the German pathologist, Rudolf Virchow, to describe a rapidly fatal disease entity presenting with fever, exhaustion, abdominal swelling, edema, and bleeding that was characterized microscopically by a predominance of white cells ("weisses Blut") in the peripheral blood (1). Soon thereafter, the distinction between acute and chronic forms was appreciated based on the observed duration of patient survival; and, subsequently, a splenic form of the disease (later called myeloid after bone marrow changes were seen in one patient with this type of leukemia) was distinguished from a lymphatic form based on morphologic similarities of the leukemic cells to cells normally residing in the spleen (1). This empirically derived classification system has survived over time, and the leukemias are still broadly categorized into acute and chronic myeloid and lymphoid leukemias. However, morphologic, cytohistochemical, cytogenetic, and, more recently, molecular and immunologic information has led to the recognition that the leukemias are a very heterogeneous group of diseases that, although uniformly characterized by infiltration of the blood, bone marrow, and other tissues by neoplastic cells of the hematopoietic system, vary significantly with regard to etiology, pathogenesis, natural course, treatment strategies, and therapy outcome. This recognition is at least partly reflected by the increasingly complex classification systems currently proposed for myeloid and lymphoid neoplasms, for example, by the World Health Organization (WHO; Table 34.1) (2,3). For example, the WHO classification considers chronic lymphocytic leukemia to be identical, that is, one disease at different stages, to the mature (peripheral) B-cell neoplasm small lymphocytic lymphoma (CLL/SLL) (2), thus overlapping with the group of low-grade non-Hodgkin lymphomas discussed elsewhere in this book.

Leukemia is currently the most common fatal cancer in males under age 40 and females under age 20 in the United States (4). Overall, it is estimated that 44,270 individuals (25,180 men, 19,090 women) in this country developed leukemia, while 21,710 individuals (12,460 men, 9,250 women) died from the disease in 2008 (4). These figures should not distract from the fact that our understanding of the pathophysiologic basis of many leukemias has advanced

considerably, and significant improvements in treatment success have been achieved over the last several decades. The introduction of effective chemotherapeutics, cytokines, differentiating agents, hematopoietic stem cell transplantation, antibody-based immunotherapeutics, and small molecule inhibitors has resulted in durable responses or even cure in many patients. For example, the use of tyrosine kinase inhibitors such as imatinib mesylate in Philadelphia-chromosome positive chronic myeloid leukemia (CML), all-trans retinoic acid (ATRA) and arsenic trioxide in acute promyelocytic leukemia (APL), and chlorodeoxyadenosine in hairy cell leukemia has resulted in 5- to 10-year survival rates in affected patients that exceed 80% (5). Nevertheless, treatment of many forms of leukemia remains challenging, and many patients ultimately die of their disease or have significant complications of their antileukemia treatment. Thus, alternative treatment strategies are needed for this group of diseases. To this end, radiation-based approaches have been attempted for more than 100 years; since the advent of hybridoma technology, these efforts have focused on radioimmunotherapy for the last two decades; in fact, leukemias are particularly attractive targets for radioimmunotherapy because of their exquisite radiosensitivity, their well-defined surface antigenic structures, the multitude of available monoclonal antibodies, the ready accessibility of the marrow space, and the relative infrequency of human antiglobulin responses as compared with solid tumors.

■ HISTORICAL PERSPECTIVE OF RADIATION-BASED THERAPY FOR LEUKEMIA

Less than 10 years after Roentgen's discovery of x-rays in 1895, the first cases of successful treatment of leukemia with radiation were reported (1), documenting the sensitivity of these diseases to radiation. For several decades, radiation remained the mainstay of therapy for enlarged spleens and lymph nodes in chronic leukemias; remissions were often complete, and the patient's quality of life improved, even though relapses inevitably occurred and survival was not prolonged (1,6). By comparison, radiation was only marginally effective for acute leukemias (1,7). Concerns about nuclear warfare and nuclear accidents after World War II ushered into the era of hematopoietic cell transplantation (HCT) (8). It soon became evident that HCT might be of use

Table **34.1** **WHO classification of myeloid and lymphoid leukemias**

Myeloid Leukemias	Lymphoid Leukemias
Myeloproliferative diseases	B-cell neoplasms
Chronic myelogenous leukemia, Philadelphia chromosome positive with t(9;22)(qq34;q11), BCR/ABL	Precursor B-cell neoplasm
Chronic neutrophilic leukemia	Precursor B-lymphoblastic leukemia/lymphoma (precursor B-cell acute lymphoblastic leukemia)
Chronic eosinophilic leukemia/hypereosinophilic syndrome	t(9;22)(a34;q11); BCR/ABL
Myelodysplastic/myeloproliferative diseases	t(v;11q23); MLL rearranged
Chronic myelomonocytic leukemia	t(1;19)(q23;p13) E2A/PBX1
Atypical chronic myelogenous leukemia	t(12;21)(p12;q22) ETV/CBF-alpha
Juvenile myelomonocytic leukemia	Mature (peripheral) B-cell neoplasms
Acute myeloid leukemias	B-cell chronic lymphocytic leukemia/small lymphocytic lymphoma
AMLs with recurrent cytogenetic translocations	B-cell prolymphocytic leukemia
AML with t(8;21)(q22;q22), AML1(CBF-alpha)/ETO	Hairy cell leukemia
Acute promyelocytic leukemia (AML with t(15;17)(q22;q11-12) and variants, PML/RAR-alpha)	Burkitt lymphoma/Burkitt cell leukemia
AML with abnormal bone marrow eosinophils (inv(16)(p13q22) or t(16;16)(p13;q11), CBFb/MYH11X)	T-cell and NK-cell neoplasms
AML with 11q23 (MLL) abnormalities	Precursor T-cell neoplasm
AML with multilineage dysplasia	Precursor T-lymphoblastic lymphoma/leukemia (precursor T-cell acute lymphoblastic leukemia)
With prior myelodysplastic syndrome	Mature (peripheral) T-cell neoplasms
Without prior myelodysplastic syndrome	T-cell prolymphocytic leukemia
AML and myelodysplastic syndromes, therapy related	Small cell variant
Alkylating agent related	Cerebriform cell variant
Epipodophyllotoxin related (some may be lymphoid)	T-cell granular lymphocytic leukemia
Other types	Aggressive NK-cell leukemia
AML not otherwise categorized	Adult T-cell lymphoma/leukemia (HTLV-1+)
AML minimally differentiated	Acute
AML without maturation	Lymphomatous
AML with maturation	Chronic
Acute myelomonocytic leukemia	Smoldering
Acute monocytic leukemia	Hodgkin-like
Acute erythroid leukemia	
Acute megakaryocytic leukemia	
Acute basophilic leukemia	
Acute panmyelosis with myelofibrosis	
Acute biphenotypic leukemias	

Modified from Harris NL, Jaffe ES, Diebold J, et al. World Health Organization classification of neoplastic diseases of the hematopoietic and lymphoid tissues: report of the Clinical Advisory Committee meeting, Airlie House, Virginia, November 1997. *J Clin Oncol.* 1999;17:3835–3849.

not only in radiation protection but also in the therapeutic application to leukemias (8). Early experience of HCT in humans demonstrated the effectiveness of total body irradiation (TBI) as an antileukemic agent when used in the setting of HCT (9). Several studies since then documented the importance of the TBI dose for therapeutic response. For example, two separate randomized trials, one in acute and one in

CML, showed that it is possible to decrease the incidence of relapse by increasing the dose of TBI from 12 to 15.75 Gy, indicating a steep dose–response of leukemia cells to radiation (10–12). However, this benefit was offset by an increased incidence of severe or fatal toxicities, principally involving lung, liver, and mucous membranes, leading to increased early transplant-related mortality (10–12). Nevertheless, these studies suggested the possibility of improved treatment outcomes if additional radiation therapy could be directed to hematopoietic and lymphoid tissue while sparing normal organs, particularly liver and lung, and formed the rational basis for radioimmunotherapy in leukemias.

ANTIGENS AND RADIONUCLIDES FOR TARGETED THERAPY OF LEUKEMIA

While leukemias oftentimes express aberrant types or abundances of cell surface antigens relative to their normal cell counterparts, no truly leukemia-specific antigens have been identified so far that currently serve as targets for radioimmunotherapy. However, the expression pattern of cell surface antigens is well characterized on both normal and malignant hematopoietic cells, including cells of different forms of leukemia, and serves as important diagnostic tool (13). An increasing number of these antigens have been exploited for use as targets for radioimmunotherapy of leukemias, most notably CD33, CD45, and the CD66 antigens (Table 34.2).

CD33 is a sialic acid-dependent cell adhesion molecule and member of the immunoglobulin superfamily subset of sialic acid binding immunoglobulin-related lectins (Siglecs; CD33 is also referred to as Siglec-3) (14,15). CD33 is normally expressed on early multilineage hematopoietic progenitors and myelomonocytic precursors but not on multipotent hematopoietic stem cells. CD33 is downregulated to low levels on peripheral granulocytes and resident macrophages but retained on circulating monocytes as well as dendritic cells (16–18); some studies suggested that CD33 can also be found on subsets of B lymphocytes and mitogen- or alloantigen-activated human T and natural killer (NK) cells (19–26). In addition to its physiologic expression, 85% to 90% of adult and pediatric acute myeloid leukemia (AML) cases are considered CD33-positive, as defined by the presence of CD33 on greater than 20% to 25% of the leukemic blasts (17,27). CD33 is also found in CML and may

be aberrantly expressed on B-cell neoplasms, including acute lymphoblastic leukemia (ALL) (13). The usefulness of CD33 for radioimmunotherapy is limited by its relative low abundance: quantitative studies estimated a mean of about 10^4 CD33 molecules per AML cells, and expression in CML appeared even lower (28), resulting in rapid saturation of antigenic targets. Furthermore, CD33 is rapidly internalized and modulated, and anti-CD33 antibodies are quickly degraded (29).

CD45, also known as leukocyte common antigen, is a cell surface glycoprotein (size 180 to 220 kDa) with tyrosine phosphatase activity (30,31). Absent on non-hematopoietic cells, almost all hematopoetic cell lineages express CD45, except mature thrombocytes, mature erythrocytes, and some of their progenitors (31). Most hematologic malignancies, including 85% to 90% of acute lymphoid and myeloid leukemias express CD45 (31–34). This antigen is expressed in a relatively high copy number (200,000 binding sites per cell) and is not appreciably internalized or shed after ligand binding (29,35). CD45 exists in several isoforms; however, while isoform-specific antibodies have been developed and investigated for immunotherapy, the CD45-targeting antibodies used so far for radioimmunotherapy are pan specific (31).

Similar to CD45, CD66 antigens are neither internalized nor shed (36). They are expressed on members of the carcinoembryonic-antigen-related cell-adhesion molecule (CEACAM) family of proteins that play a role in various intercellular-adhesion and intracellular signalling-mediated effects involved in cellular growth and differentiation (37). Some of these glycoproteins, namely CD66a (CEACAM1, biliary glycoprotein), CD66b (CEACAM8, CGM6), CD66c (CEACAM6, nonspecific crossreacting antigen), and CD66d (CEACAM3, CGM1), are expressed on hematopoietic cells but can also be found on epithelial or endothelial cells. CD66 antigens are found in myeloid cells from the late myeloblast or early promyelocyte stage and reach highest levels in myelocytes and metamyelocytes, while early

Table **34.2** Radionuclides for radioimmunotherapy of leukemias (110)				
Radionuclide	**Half-Life**	**Path Length (mm)**[a]	**Particle Energy (MeV)**	**Antigenic Target Used in Clinical Studies**
β-Emitters				
Iodine-131	8.1 days	0.8	0.6	CD20, CD22, CD33, CD37, CD45, HLA-DR
Yttrium-90	2.5 days	5.3	2.2	CD5, CD20, CD22, CD25, CD45, CD66
Rhenium-188	17 hours	4.4	2.1	CD66
Copper-67	61.5 days	0.4–0.6	0.6	HLA-DR
α-Emitters				
Bismuth-213	46 minutes	0.04–0.08	8.0	CD33, CD45
Actinum-225	10 days	0.05–0.08	8.0	CD33

[a] The path length whereby 90% of the energy is deposited.

myeloid progenitors or multipotent progenitors do not express CD66 antigens (38–40). CD66 antigens are only occasionally found on AML cells; however, many B-cell acute lymphoblastic leukemias and some cases of lymphoid blast crisis CML express these antigens (39,41). Studies with a CD66c-specific antibody suggested restriction primarily to CD10-positive early B-cell ALL (42). However, many anti-CD66 antibodies recognize several CD66 antigens; for example, BW 250/183, the most widely used antibody for CD66-targeted radioimmunotherapy, recognizes CD66a, b, and c (43). Thus, although the exact expression patterns may differ between the individual CD66 antigens (37,42), this is currently of limited significance for radioimmunotherapeutic approaches.

Since CD33 and CD45 are expressed by both normal and malignant cells, antibodies targeting these antigens can deliver radiation to marrow, spleen, and lymph nodes in patients with measureable disease as well as in patients in remission. Malignant cells that do not express these antigens may be killed if they are in close proximity to other radiolabeled malignant cells. The eradication of cells that are not directly targeted by the antibody is termed the cross-fire effect. This cross-fire effect is particularly important for radioimmunotherapy of myeloid leukemias using CD66, as these antigens are oftentimes not expressed by the malignant clone.

Besides, CD33, CD45, and CD66, a number of other antigens have been used in clinical studies of radioimmunotherapy of leukemias. These include HLA-DR, CD5, CD20, CD22, CD25, and CD37. For example, CD5 is a surface antigen present on T-cells, a subset of B-cells, as well as on subsets of CLL (44). CD25 (interleukin-2 receptor, alpha subunit) is felt to be an attractive target for radioimmunotherapy as it is only weakly expressed in some normal tissues, including epithelial tissues and lymphocyte subsets, but is found on malignant cells in several diseases, including adult T-cell leukemia, cutaneous T-cell lymphoma, anaplastic large-cell lymphoma, hairy cell B-cell leukemia, and the Reed Sternberg and associated polyclonal T-cells in Hodgkin disease as well as some AML (45).

A variety of radionuclides have been used for radioimmunotherapy of leukemias (Table 34.2). The types of emissions employed have primarily focused on the use of β-particles (^{131}I, ^{90}Y, ^{188}Re) (46). The use of β-emitters that deposit energy over a relatively long distance allows irradiation of many cells adjacent to the decay position, provided that sufficient radiation is deposited. This offers the advantage of targeting cells that express limited amounts of the target antigen, or lack it completely. However, as not only targeted but also surrounding hematopoietic cells, including normal pluripotent stem cells, are affected, stem cell rescue is required (47). Some of these β-emitters also have γ emission, which can be used to provide in vivo antibody biodistribution images; however, γ emission, if in high abundance, can significantly contribute to irradiation of normal tissues. More recent studies have used α-emitters (^{213}Bi, ^{225}Ac, ^{211}At). The deposition of energy over a much

shorter range than β-emitters is of interest as targeted cells might be destroyed while neighboring cells are spared; this would offer an advantage if avoidance of marrow toxicity is a goal (46). The short half-lives, particularly of bismuth radionuclides, limit the clinical use to diseases in which cancer cells are readily accessible by antibodies. Thus, leukemias are thus among the best candidates for radioimmunotherapy using α-emitters.

■ CLINICAL STUDIES OF TARGETED RADIONUCLIDE THERAPY

Clinical studies on radioimmunoconjugate therapy of leukemias have mainly focused on CD33, CD45, and CD66. Two main strategies have emerged, both attempting to intensify the dose of irradiation to hematopoietic sites in order to increase the response rates and reduce the likelihood of relapse without increasing treatment-related toxicities. The first approach includes radioimmunotherapy as an addition to fully myeloablative conditioning regimens. The second approach uses radioimmunotherapy as an addition to reduced-intensity conditioning regimens.

▓ Radioimmunotherapy targeting CD33

Despite promising results from animal models, results from clinical trials using unconjugated anti-CD33 antibodies have been disappointing (47,48). Although such antibodies reduced blast counts in patients with AML, only few complete remissions (CRs) were observed and were restricted to patients with low initial tumor burden, and there is some evidence that unconjugated anti-CD33 antibodies have activity against minimal residual disease in APL (47,48). Nevertheless, these studies demonstrated the feasibility and safety of anti-CD33 antibody administration in patients with leukemia, and spurred interest in labeling antileukemia antibodies with radionuclides. Initial studies of radioimmunotherapy in leukemia came from the Fred Hutchinson Cancer Research Center (FHCRC) and Memorial Sloan-Kettering Cancer Center (MSKCC) and have focused on the use of anti-CD33 antibodies (p67 and M195) labeled with ^{131}I. ^{131}I was chosen in these early studies because of its ready availability, low cost, and simple radiochemistry. Appelbaum and colleagues at the FHCRC employed ^{131}I-p67 followed by a standard preparative regimen of cyclophosphamide (Cy) plus 12 Gy TBI for patients with recurrent or refractory AML (49). Only four of nine patients had favorable biodistribution studies, that is, more radiation would be delivered to marrow and spleen than any other nonhematopoietic organ. These four patients eventually underwent transplantation and tolerated the procedure well; ^{131}I-p67 delivered between 1.79 and 5.56 Gy of radiation to the marrow, as compared to 1.75 Gy that was delivered to the normal organ with the highest radiation (liver or lung). Three of the four patients remained initially in CR (195 to 477 days posttransplant), and one patient remained long-term disease free (46,49). Simultaneously, the MSKCC group studied ^{131}I-M195, a radioimmunoconjugate with a biodistribution similar to ^{131}I-p67 (50). In an initial dose-escalation study on 24 patients, ^{131}I-M195 was given in two to four divided doses at least 48 hours apart to allow for reexpression of the CD33 antigen between infusions. A marked decrease in peripheral and marrow blasts was observed in 23/24 and 17/19 patients, respectively. Profound cytopenia of at least 12 days duration occurred at doses greater than 135 mCi/m^2; 8 patients achieved sufficient cytoreduction to proceed with HCT (51). ^{131}I-M195 has later been used by the MSKCC group as addition to myeloablative conditioning with busulfan and cyclophosphamide. Out of 19 patients with advanced AML or CML treated, 18 achieved a CR; 3 patients remained in CR 18 to 29 months posttransplant, whereas 6 patients relapsed (3 to 21 months posttransplant) and another 10 patients died in CR of graft-versus-host disease (GVHD) or infection (52). ^{131}I-M195 was further used in seven patients with relapsed APL in second CR after ATRA induction for minimal residual disease (52). The maximum tolerated dose, resulting in neutropenic periods less than 14 days, was approximated at 50 mCi/m^2. The median disease-free survival (DFS) was 8 months (range 3 to 14.5 months), an outcome that appeared favorable relative to patients treated with alternative approaches, although no direct comparisons were done (Table 34.3) (52).

A humanized version of M195, HuM195, was later developed to avoid immune responses, which limited repeated dosing. Compared to M195, HuM195 displayed an increased binding avidity and mediated antibody-dependent cellular cytotoxicity against leukemic target cells as an unconjugated antibody (53,54). In a trace-labeling phase 1b study, ^{131}I-HuM195 could be repeatedly administrated (up to 12 doses over 4 months) without development of human antiglobulin responses and with only minor acute side effects, predominantly fever and rigor (54). The serum half-life was found to be shorter for ^{131}I-HuM195 compared to ^{131}I-M195, possibly due to more rapid targeting of CD33 binding sites because of the higher avidity of the humanized antibody (54). However, similar to M195, rapid internalization of HuM195 within 1 hour was observed, and significant degradation of the radioimmunoconjugate was evidenced by free ^{131}I in blood and urine (54). In 2003, the MSKCC group reported their extended experience in using either ^{131}I-M195 or ^{131}I-HuM195 to intensify busulfan/cyclophosphamide-containing pretransplant conditioning; this study contained updated information on those 19 patients reported in the earlier study but also contained information on 13 patients that received ^{131}I-HuM195 in two to four individual doses 48 to 72 hours apart (55). Thirty-one of these 32 patients proceeded to transplantation and received between 2.72 and 14.7 Gy of radiation to the marrow. The median survival of all 31 patients who underwent transplant was 4.9 months (range 0.3 to 90+ months). Of the 25 patients that survived longer than 42 days posttransplant, 24 had no evidence of leukemia on at least one follow-up marrow examination. Six patients relapsed at a median of

161 days (range 90 to 479 days) posttransplant. Among the 17 patients with AML or MDS, three (18%) remain in remission at 59+, 87+, and 90+ months posttransplant, while none of the 14 patients with advanced CML achieved long-term remission. A total of 20 (65%) patients died of treatment-related causes, including infections, GVHD, interstitial pneumonia, hemorrhage, veno-occlusive disease (VOD) of the liver, and multiple organ failure. Intensified conditioning resulted in few toxicities beyond those expected with busulfan/cyclophosphamide alone. However, the most common extramedullary toxicity was hyperbilirubinemia (at least grade 2 in 69% of patients); since the liver received between 2.63 and 6.51 Gy of radiation, additional liver toxicity could not be ruled out (55).

Together, these studies with ^{131}I-labeled anti-CD33 antibodies demonstrated the feasibility of using radioimmunotherapy as part of a HCT preparative regimen, and that the marrow and spleen could be preferentially targeted to absorb greater amounts of radioactivity than the liver (usually the normal organ receiving the highest radiation dose), lungs, or kidneys. CRs were achieved in the majority of patients transplanted in these trials without engraftment complications and with little toxicity related to the radioisotope. Similar to later studies, however, the lack of appropriate control groups makes it difficult to estimate whether inclusion of radioimmunotherapy indeed conferred a benefit compared to standard preparative regimens. These early studies further identified important limitations of ^{131}I-labeled anti-CD33 antibodies, in particular the short marrow residence time (9 to 41 hours with ^{131}I-p67) (49,50). This phenomenon is most likely explained by modulation of the CD33-radioimmunoconjugate internalization with subsequent intracellular deiodination and release of ^{131}I from the marrow space, as suggested by preclinical studies (29). Furthermore, the limited abundance of CD33 binding sites resulted in saturation at doses of 3 to 5 mg/m^2, rendering dose escalations by use of higher individual doses impossible (50,54). However, studies by the MSKCC group indicated that surface CD33 levels returned to pretreatment levels within 72 hours, which would allow repeated dosing in 72-hour intervals as the most appropriate dosing schedule (54).

Acknowledging the limitations of short residence time of ^{131}I-labeled anti-CD33 antibodies, the MSKCC group explored the use of radionuclides that are retained intracellular once internalized, such as ^{90}Y, which provided superior retention of radioactivity relative to ^{125}I when conjugated to anti-CD33 antibodies in preclinical studies (56). In a phase I study, 19 patients with relapsed or refractory AML were treated with a single-dose ^{90}Y-HuM195 (0.1 to 0.3 mCi/kg) without marrow support (57). Thirteen patients had reductions in bone marrow blasts, and 5 of the 10 patients treated at the highest dose levels had hypocellular bone marrow biopsies without evidence of AML 2 or 4 weeks after treatment. A CR was observed in one of the seven patients treated at the maximum tolerated dose of 0.275 mCi/kg (57). These data suggested a

Table 34.3 Radioimmunotherapy targeting CD33

Study	N	Age (Median)	Disease	Isotope	Target	Other Therapy	Results
Scheinberg (50)	10	20–74 (38.5)	AML (9), CMML (1)	131-I	CD33 (M195)	None	Phase I trace-labeling study; rapid internalization of radioimmunoconjugate; no tumor regressions
Appelbaum (49)	9	16–53	AML	131-I	CD33 (P67)	Cy/TBI	Short marrow residence time; favorable biodistribution in 4/9; 3/4 alive and in remission 195–477 days posttransplant
Schwartz (51)	24	2–76 (40)	Advanced AML (18), MDS (5), blast-crisis CML (1)	131-I	CD33 (M195)	None	Dose-escalation study: profound cytopenia for 131-I doses >135 mCi/m^2; 8 patients with sufficient cytoreduction to proceed with HCT
Caron (54)	10	20–80 (47)	AML (12), blast crisis CML (1)	131-I	CD33 (HuM195)		Phase Ib trace-labeling study; repeated antibody administration without human antiglobulin responses; rapid internalization of radioimmuno-conjugate; binding site saturation at 3 mg/m^2; blast reduction in 1 patient, stable disease in 1 patient
Jurcic (52)	19	(38)	AML (10), CML (9)	131-I	CD33 (M195)	Bu/Cy	18/19 achieved CR; 3 patients remain in CR 18–29 months posttransplant; 6 patients relapsed (3–21 months posttransplant); 10 patients died in complete remission of GVHD or infection
Jurcic (52)	7	(53)	Relapsed APL in second remission after ATRA	131-I	CD33 (M195)	None	Median DFS 8 (range 3–14.5) months
Jurcic (61)	18	17–74 (56)	Advanced AML (17), CMML (1)	213-Bi	CD33 (HuM195)	None	Phase I dose-escalation study; maximum tolerated dose not reached; myelosuppression in all 17 evaluable patients; peripheral blood blast count reduction in 14/15 patients; bone marrow blast reduction in 14/18 patients
Burke (55)	32	4–60 (38)	AML (17), CML (14), MDS (1)	131-I	CD33 (M195, 19; HuM195, 13)		31/32 transplanted; median survival 4.9 months; 24/25 patient surviving >42 days posttransplant achieved CR; 3/16 patients with AML remain in CR 59, 87, and 90 months after transplant; all patients with CML relapsed; 20/31 died of treatment-related causes
Mulford (62)	25	49–80 (67)	AML	213-Bi	CD33 (HuM195)	Cytarabine	2 CR; 3 CRp; 2 PR
Rosenblat (65)	7	46–77 (61)	Relapsed AML (3), refractory AML (4)	225-Ac	CD33 (HuM195)	None	Phase I dose escalation trial; elimination of peripheral blood blasts in 3 of 6 evaluable patients; dose-related reductions of >33% of bone marrow blasts in 4 patients at 4 weeks; one patient had 3% bone marrow blasts after therapy

AML, acute myeloid leukemia; APL, acute promyelocytic leukemia; Bu, busulfan; CML, chronic myeloid leukemia; CMML, chronic myelomonocytic leukemia; CR, complete remission; CRp, CR with incomplete platelet recovery; Cy, cyclophosphamide; GVHD, graft-versus-host disease; MDS, myelodysplastic syndrome; PR, partial remission; TBI, total body irradiation.

potential role of ^{90}Y-HuM195 as part of a pretransplant preparative regimen.

To reduce the amount of cross-fire toxicity and allow selective leukemia cell kill, particularly in the setting of minimal residual disease, the MKSCC group also explored the potential use of α-emitting anti-CD33 antibodies (58,59). Preclinical studies with ^{212}Bi-HuM195 and ^{213}Bi-HuM195 demonstrated that both constructs were rapidly internalized, similar to ^{131}I-HuM195; however, the bismuth radioimmunoconjugates were retained about two- to threefold longer than the iodine-radiolabeled HuM195, likely because of binding to transferrin and other metal-binding intracellular proteins (58). Dose- and specific activity-dependent killing was observed in cytotoxicity assays, in which ^{212}Bi-HuM195 proved slightly more toxic than ^{213}Bi-HuM195 because of its longer physical half-life. Calculations indicated that both bismuth radionuclides showed approximately 50% killing of the CD33-positive human HL-60 AML cell line when two bismuth atoms were bound to the target cell surface, demonstrating the potent cytotoxic activity of α-emitting anti-CD33 antibodies (58). Early clinical studies in patients with relapsed AML showed that ^{213}Bi-HuM195, given in three to six fractions over 48 hours, allowed imaging of patients and enabled determination of pharmacokinetic parameters and dosimetry (60). Subsequently, a phase I dose-escalation trial was conducted in 18 patients with relapsed/refractory AML or chronic myelomonocytic leukemia (CMML) that were treated with 10.36 to 37.0 MBq/kg ^{213}Bi-HuM195, given in three to seven injections over 2 to 4 days (61). No significant extramedullary toxicity was seen, and the maximum tolerated dose was not reached because escalation beyond the highest dose was restricted by availability and cost of the ^{225}Ac/^{213}Bi generator. Nearly all the ^{213}Bi-HuM195 rapidly localized and was retained in areas of leukemic involvement; absorbed dose ratios between these sites and the whole body were 1000-fold greater than those seen with β-emitting anti-CD33 antibodies (61). All 17 evaluable patients developed myelosuppression with a median time to recovery of 22 days. ^{213}Bi-HuM195 had clear antileukemic activity: 14 of 15 evaluable patients had reductions in circulating blasts, and 14 of 18 patients had reductions in the percentage of bone marrow blasts (61). However, no CR was achieved. It was calculated that approximately 1 in 2700 molecules of HuM195 carried the radiolabel at the specific activities injected, which rendered it difficult to deliver the 1 to 2 ^{213}Bi atoms necessary for cell kill to every leukemia cell (61). A second phase I/II study then evaluated the effects of ^{213}Bi-HuM195 after partial cytoreduction with cytarabine (200 mg/m^2/day for 5 days) in 25 patients with AML (62). Patients received between 0.5 and 1.25 mCi/kg; the maximum tolerated dose was 1 mCi/kg. Seven of the 19 patients who received either 1 or 1.25 mCi/kg responded (two CRs lasting 9 and 12 months; three CRs with incomplete platelet recovery [CRps] lasting 1, 2, and 6 months; two partial remissions lasting 3 and 8 months). The median time from initiation of chemotherapy to recovery of leukocyte counts was 34 days (range,

21 to 59 days), with delayed count recovery attributable to persistent leukemia. Side effects were relatively mild and transient (62), suggesting that this approach may deserve further testing in more controlled studies.

Recognizing that ^{213}Bi is short lived and may thus result in a short marrow residence time, a HuM195 conjugated with ^{225}Ac has been developed (63,64). Preclinical studies showed that ^{225}Ac-containing immunoconjugates could kill in vitro at radioactivity doses 1000 times lower than ^{213}Bi analogs and prolong survival of animals in several xenograft models (63). Subsequent studies in cynomolgus monkeys indicated that high doses of ^{225}Ac nanogenerators can cause renal toxicity, in particular renal tubular damage associated with interstitial fibrosis, as well as anemia, and suggested the hematologic and renal function would need to be monitored closely during clinical use (64). A phase I dose-escalation feasibility trial was conducted in seven patients with relapsed/refractory AML treated with a single dose of ^{225}Ac-HuM195 (0.5 to 2 μCi/kg) (65). Myelosuppression, including grade 4 thrombocytopenia and neutropenia, was observed. Antileukemic effects included elimination of peripheral blood blasts in three of six evaluable patients and dose-related reductions of greater than 33% of bone marrow blasts in four patients at 4 weeks following treatment. One patient had 3% bone marrow blasts after therapy (65). This approach holds considerable promise for advancing the field of α-particle radioimmunotherapy because of the longer half-life and the generation of short-lived daughter therapeutic α-particles (^{221}Fr, ^{217}At, ^{213}Bi) from ^{225}Ac inside a targeted leukemia cell, which largely accounts for the increased potency of ^{225}Ac-atomic nanogenerators over ^{213}Bi constructs (66).

Radioimmunotherapy targeting CD45

As discussed above, two major problems with using CD33 as the target antigen for radioimmunotherapy are the limited expression of CD33 on leukemia cells and its internalization upon antibody binding. In an alternative approach to concentrate radiation to sites of hematopoiesis, the FHCRC group has focused its efforts on CD45, which is expressed at a much higher copy number than CD33 (at least 10- to 20-fold higher) on both leukemic and normal cells and is not significantly internalized upon antibody binding (29,35). Theoretically, this expression pattern should provide an opportunity to deliver radiation to the marrow space in a patient with either low or high tumor burden, and the antigen stability should prolong the exposure of targeted cells and surrounding hematopoietic tissues to radiation. Indeed, early preclinical studies demonstrated that ^{131}I-anti-CD45 antibodies target AML cells with longer cell surface retention and provided superior tumor targeting of AML xenografts in athymic mice compared to ^{131}I-anti-CD33 antibodies (29). Parallel studies in normal mice and healthy primates (*Macaca nemestrina*) established that radiolabeled anti-CD45 antibody can deliver radiation with relative specificity to the hematopoietic and lymphoid tissues (two- to threefold more to marrow, up to 12-fold more to spleen, and two- to eight-fold more to lymph nodes than to critical normal organs) (67,68). Since targeting this antigen leads to significant myelosuppression, clinical studies with anti-CD45 antibody-mediated radioimmunotherapy, to date, have relied on HCT to reconstitute hematopoiesis. An initial phase I dose-escalation study was conducted with BC8, a murine anti-pan-CD45 IgG1 monoclonal antibody, in 23 patients with advanced acute leukemia or MDS (69). Biodistribution studies showed that the antibody was rapidly cleared from plasma, presumably due to rapid antigen binding; patients with relapsed disease achieved higher marrow doses than patients in remission due to higher uptake and longer retention of the radionuclide in the marrow (69). Tolerable side effects (chills, nausea, vomiting, diarrhea, headache, hypotension) occurred in 78% of the patients. Twenty of these 23 patients had favorable biodistribution, and received treatment doses of ^{131}I-BC8 in combination with cyclophosphamide (120 mg/kg) and 12.0 Gy of TBI (69). Estimated radiation doses provided by the radioimmunoconjugate ranged from 3.5 to 7 Gy to the liver, 4 to 30 Gy to bone marrow, and 7 to 60 Gy to spleen. Toxicities were not felt to be appreciably greater than what would have been expected with this preparative regimen alone and the maximum tolerated dose was not reached. However, one patient, who received 30.7 Gy to the marrow, died on day +29 from infection without evidence of engraftment despite the use of myeloid growth factors. Four patients died before day +100 (day 20, 29, 36, 40). Of 10 patients with AML or MDS that survived beyond day 100, 9 are surviving disease-free 8 to 41 (median, 17) months posttransplant; 2 of 6 patients with ALL remained relapse free 9 and 22 months posttransplant (69). A study update was later provided that included 44 patients, of which 84% had favorable biodistribution (70). The radiation dose to the liver from the tracer study was used to limit dose escalation. Therefore, the maximum tolerated dose was 10.5 Gy with the occurrence of grade 3/4 mucositis as the dose-limiting toxicity. This approach to the MTD resulted in 24 Gy more radiation delivered to the marrow and approximately 50 Gy to the spleen, without excessive toxicity in a setting of conventional cyclophosphamide/TBI. Of 25 treated patients with AML/MDS, 7 survived disease-free 15 to 89 (median, 65) months posttransplant; of 9 treated patients with ALL, 3 survived disease-free 19, 54, and 66 months posttransplant. Together, these studies demonstrated that ^{131}I-labeled anti-CD45 antibody could deliver an estimated 2.3- to 4.8-fold higher radiation dose to the bone marrow and spleen, as compared to the liver. The liver is the normal organ receiving the highest dose (in all but one patient) and can be safely evaluated in a myeloablative transplant regimen containing cyclophosphamide and TBI (70). The same preparative regimen was used in a later study for patients with AML beyond first remission, relapsed/primary refractory AML, or advanced MDS (71). Results suggested that a greater radiation absorbed dose delivered to marrow may lead to lower posttransplant relapse rates for patients with high-risk AML/MDS. Half of the patients treated received a dose to marrow less than 7 cGy/mCi while the remaining half of patients received greater than 7 cGy/mCi to marrow. Although the number of patients was limited, only one of nine patients relapsed in the high marrow-absorbed dose group while six of nine patients relapsed in the lower dose cohort. The hazard of relapse in the group that received less than 7 cGy/mCi to marrow was more than six times higher than that seen in the group that received the higher marrow dose (Table 34.4) (71).

Table **34.4**	**Radioimmunotherapy targeting CD45**						
Study	**N**	**Age (Median)**	**Disease**	**Isotope**	**Target**	**Other Therapy**	**Results**
Matthews (69)	23	16–52 (40)	AML (15), ALL (7), MDS (1)	131-I	CD45 (BC8)	Cy/TBI	9/13 patients with AML/MDS and 2/7 patients with ALL alive disease free at 8–41 (median 17) months
Matthews (70)	44	16–55 (38)	AML (31), ALL (10), MDS (3)	131-I	CD45 (BC8)	Cy/TBI	34 patients received therapeutic dose: 7/25 treatment-related deaths; 17/34 relapse; 10/34 disease-free survival 15–89 months posttransplant
Pagel (73)	33	50–71 (61)	Advanced AML (24), high-risk MDS (9)	131-I	CD45 (BC8)	Cy/TBI	Day 100 NRM 12%; 18 patients disease-free 2–16 months posttransplant; 9 patients with relapse 3–38 months posttransplant
Pagel (72)	52	16–55 (41)	AML in first CR	131-I	CD45 (BC8)	Bu/Cy	Estimated 3-year NRM 21%, estimated 3-year DFS 61%
Glatting (74)	8	44–61 (54)	AML (7), ALL (1)	111-In, 90-Y	CD45 (YAML568))	Bu/Cy; Cy/TBI	Favorable biodistribution with 111-In if preloaded with unlabeled Ab (0.5mg/kg); 4/8 received 90-Y and achieved CR

ALL, acute lymphoblastic leukemia; AML, acute myeloid leukemia; Bu, busulfan; CR, complete remission; Cy, cyclophosphamide; DFS, disease-free survival; MDS, myelodysplastic syndrome; NRM, nonrelapse mortality; TBI, total body irradiation.

A phase I/II trial was performed that incorporated this therapeutic approach for patients with AML in first remission (72). Of 59 patients evaluated, 52 (88%) had favorable biodistribution and 46 received therapeutic doses of ^{131}I-BC8. The radiolabeled antibody delivered 5.3 to 19.0 (mean 11.3) Gy radiation to the marrow, 17 to 72 (mean 29.7) Gy to the spleen, and 3.5 to 5.25 Gy to the liver. The estimated 3-year nonrelapse mortality and disease-free survival were 21% and 61%, respectively (72). Similar to previous studies, this trial did not contain any direct control groups. The results from this radioimmunoconjugate study were compared with those from 509 similar patients from the International Bone Marrow Transplant Registry and it was estimated that the hazard of mortality was 0.65 (95% confidence interval: 0.39 to 1.08, $p = 0.09$) that of the Registry patients (72). Despite these comparative studies, carefully controlled randomized trials will be necessary to definitively assess the contribution of the ^{131}I-anti-CD45 antibody to standard transplant regimens.

These encouraging results suggested that this approach might be applied to older patients. Given the reduced toxicity of a low-intensity conditioning regimen in high-risk older patients, the antileukemic effect of a nonablative approach might also be improved by the addition of targeted hematopoietic irradiation delivered by a radiolabeled antibody. Therefore, a phase I dose-escalation trial using ^{131}I-BC8 combined with fludarabine (30 mg/m^2/day for 3 days) and 200 cGy TBI followed by reduced-intensity HCT (matched related in 10, matched unrelated in 23) was conducted for a particularly poor risk population of 33 patients with advanced AML and high-risk MDS that were older than 50 years of age (73). This study demonstrated that ^{131}I-BC8 could deliver 5.2 to 45.9 (mean 27.5) Gy to bone marrow, 17.3 to 155 (mean 81.2) Gy to spleen, and 12 to 24 Gy to the liver (dose-limiting organ), in addition to a standard reduced intensity transplant regimen, without a marked increase in day 100 mortality (73). A remission was achieved in all patients, and all had 100% donor CD3$^+$ and CD33$^+$ cell engraftment by day 28 posttransplant. Median time to neutrophil and platelet engraftment was 14 (10 to 19) and 17 (15 to 43) days, respectively. The day 100 nonrelapse mortality was 12%. Eighteen patients are disease-free 2 to 16 months (median 9.5 months) posttransplant, whereas the disease recurred in nine patients 3 to 38 months posttransplant (73). Whether use of a radiolabeled antibody combined with a nonmyeloablative transplant will reduce posttransplant relapse rates for these older patients with high-risk AML/MDS, however, remains to be determined.

So far, all clinical experience in targeting CD45 with radioimmunoconjugates has been accumulated with ^{131}I. However, limited data obtained with YAML568, a rat IgG2a monoclonal antibody that recognizes all CD45 isoforms, suggest that anti-CD45 antibodies can selectively deliver radiation to hematopoietic tissues when labeled with ^{90}Y, provided that patients are preloaded with unlabeled antibody (74).

Radioimmunotherapy targeting CD66

While lymphoid leukemias often express CD66, myeloid leukemias only occasionally stain positive for these antigens. Therefore, radioimmunotherapy primarily depends on crossfire effects. A group from the University of Ulm has pioneered the use of ^{188}Re-labeled BW 250/183, an anti-CD66 (a, b, c, e) antibody as part of a conditioning regimen prior to HCT (43). ^{188}Re was chosen as the therapeutic radionuclide because it is an almost pure β-emitter, has a high energy of β-emissions, and has a shorter half-life compared to ^{131}I (43). In an initial phase I–II study, 36 patients with high-risk AML or MDS received ^{188}Re-BW 250/183 in combination with either intravenous busulfan (128 mg/kg)/cyclophosphamide (120 mg/kg) or TBI (12 Gy)/cyclophosphamide (for matched family or unrelated donor allogeneic HCT or autologous HCT) or TBI (12 Gy)/cyclophosphamide with thiotepa (10 mg/kg; for haploidentical family donor HCT). Thirty of the 32 allogeneic stem cell grafts were T-cell depleted. A favorable dosimetry was observed in all patients. Radioimmunotherapy delivered a mean of 15.3 ± 4.9 Gy of additional radiation to the marrow, 19.5 ± 17.5 Gy to the spleen, 6.0 ± 2.3 Gy to the liver, and 7.4 ± 2.3 Gy to the kidney. Infusion-related toxicities were minimal, and no increase in treatment-related mortality due to the radioimmunoconjugate was observed. Median time to neutrophil and platelet engraftment was 11 and 12 days, respectively. Day 30 and day 100 mortalities were 3% and 6%, respectively, and after a median follow-up of 18 months treatment-related mortality was 22%; at that time, disease-free survival was 45%. The relapse rate was 20% for patients transplanted in first or second remission, and 30% if the patients were in relapse at the time of transplant. In contrast to radiolabeled anti-CD45 antibodies, the normal organ that received the highest radiation was the kidney, and late renal toxicity was observed in 17% of the patients (43). In fact, as demonstrated later, the application of ^{188}Re-BW 250/183 at the doses used leads to excess renal toxicity despite a concomitant 50% reduction of the external-beam contribution to the kidney dose (75). A study update was later reported that comprised data on 50 patients with acute leukemia, CML, or MDS (76). In these 50 patients, transplant-related mortality was 26%; 9 out of 50 patients relapsed; however, with a follow-up of 3.8 to 23.4 (mean 11.0) months, 28 of 50 patients were still in ongoing clinical remission with a disease-free survival of 10.4 ± 7.2 months (76). A second update of this study cohort from Ulm focused on patients with acute leukemia (77). In this study update, that comprised 57 patients, 53 of which had AML, the transplant-related mortality was 30% after a median follow-up of 26 months and 14% late renal toxicity; 25% of these patients developed grade 2 to 4 acute GVHD, and 29% developed chronic GVHD. This study demonstrated a significant difference between the 64% disease-free survival for 44 patients that were in either CR or had less than 15% blasts in the marrow at the time of transplant as compared to 8% for 13 patients that had greater than 15% blasts at the time of transplant (77). These findings suggested that ^{188}Re-BW

250/183 containing preparative regimens may be particularly effective if the tumor burden is low (77); however, better controlled studies will be necessary, as patients with low tumor burden at the time of transplantation have intrinsically a better outcome (Table 34.5).

These encouraging results can be contrasted to a study on 19 similar patients that were treated with similar doses of [188]Re-BW 250/183 in combination with various preparative regimens (TBI/cyclophosphamide, melphalan alone, or combination of chemotherapeutics) followed by HCT (78). Unlike the patients treated by the Ulm group, 13 patients received unmanipulated grafts in combination with immunosuppressive therapy, while the remaining 6 patients received allografts with CD34+ selected cells but received T-cells back every 4 to 6 weeks starting at day +28 post-transplant. Fifteen out of 19 patients developed acute

GVHD, with 8 having grade 3 or 4 disease. Eleven of the 19 patients had intestinal GVHD, which was fatal in at least four cases. Overall, treatment-related mortality was high (9 or 19 patients) (78). Given the apparent differences in outcome between this study and earlier studies using T-cell depleted grafts, it was initially thought that the presence of T-cell in donor grafts might account for the high treatment-related mortality and incidence of severe acute GVHD (78). However, more recent data obtained by the group from Hannover Medical School appear to contradict this hypothesis (79). Specifically, 21 patients with AML or MDS were treated with [188]Re-BW 250/183 followed by myeloablative HCT with busulfan/cyclosphosphamide (in 11 patients) or reduced-intensity HCT with fludarabine/busulfan or fludarabine/melphalan. On average, the radioimmunoconjugate delivered 10.9 (4.95 to 21.3) Gy to the bone marrow,

Table **34.5**		**Radioimmunotherapy targeting CD66**					
Study	N	Age (Median)	Disease	Isotope	Target	Other Therapy	Results
Bunjes (43)	36	17–63 (48)	High-risk AML (32), MDS (4)	188-Re	CD66 (BW 250/183)	Bu/Cy, Cy/TBI, Cy/TBI/TT	30/32 allogeneic grafts T-cell depleted; 8/36 (22%) TRM; day 100 mortality 6%; DFS 45% at median of 18 months; 17% late renal toxicity
Bunjes (77)	57	17–63 (45)	High-risk AML (53), MDS (4)	188-Re	CD66 (BW 250/183)	Bu/Cy, Cy/TBI, Cy/TBI/TT	T-cell depletion; at median of 26 months: TRM 30%; relapse 35%; DFS 47%; 64% DFS if <15% blasts at time of transplant; 8% DFS if >15% blasts at time of transplant; 25% acute GVHD, 29% chronic GVHD
Klein (78)	19	25–60 (42)	ALL (12), AML (5), CML (1), MDS (1)	188-Re	CD66 (BW 250/183)	Cy/TBI, melphalan, other chemotherapy	No T-cell depletion; 15/19 developed acute GVHD (8/19 grade 3/4); intestinal GVHD in 11/19; TRM 9/19
Buchmann (76)	50	17–59 (40.5)	AML (26), ALL (11), CML (9), MDS (4)	188-Re	CD66 (BW 250/183)	Cy/TBI, Cy/TBI/TT, Bu/Mel/Flu, Bu/Flu	T-cell depletion; 28/50 patients in clinical remission with follow-up of 3.8–23.4 months; mean DFS 10.4 months; 9/50 patients relapsed; TRM 26%
Ringhoffer (80)	20	56–67 (63)	AML (15), MDS (3), ALL (2)	188-Re (8); 90-Y (12)	CD66 (BW 250/183)	Flu/ATG (MRD); Flu/ATG/ Mel (MUD)	Cumulative incidence of relapse 55% at 30 months; NRM 25% at 2 years; probability of survival 70% at 1 year, 52% at 2 years; 1/20 acute GVHD; 3/20 chronic GVHD
Koenecke (79)	21	21–62 (48)	High-risk AML (14), secondary AML (6), advanced MDS (1)	188-Re	CD66 (BW 250/183)	Bu/Cy (Conv, 11), Flu/Bu (RIC, 7), Flu/Mel (RIC, 3)	DFS 43% with median follow-up of 42 months (23–60); TRM 28.6%; 6/21 relapsed (41–367 days posttransplant); 8/21 acute GVHD, 9/16 chronic GVHD

ALL, acute lymphoblastic leukemia; AML, acute myeloid leukemia; ATG, antithymocyte globulin; Bu, busulfan; CML, chronic myeloid leukemia; Conv, conventional-intensity conditioning; Cy, cyclophosphamide; DFS, disease-free survival; Flu, fludarabine; GVHD, graft-versus-host disease; Mel, melphalan; MDS, myelodysplastic syndrome; MRD, matched related donor; MUD, matched unrelated donor; RIC, reduced-intensity conditioning; TBI, total body irradiation; TRM, treatment-related mortality; TT, thiotepa.

17.09 (7.27 to 40.92) Gy to the spleen, 3.61 (1.07 to 11.45) Gy to the liver, and 7.81 (3.94 to 12.21) Gy to the kidney. All patients received an unmanipulated allogeneic graft. Median time to neutrophil engraftment was 20 (12 to 28) days. Interestingly, three patients developed VOD of the liver. Six patients died from treatment-related causes. Acute and chronic GVHD developed in 8/21 and 9/16 patients, respectively. Six patients relapsed 41 to 367 days posttransplant. At a median follow-up of 42 months, the disease-free survival was 43% (79).

For older high-risk AML or MDS patients, radioimmunotherapy with BW 250/183 labeled with either ^{188}Re or ^{90}Y was also combined with a reduced intensity conditioning regimen followed by transplant using T-cell-depleted allografts (80). A phase I–II study comprised 20 patients, in which fludarabine or fludarabine/melphalan-based conditioning was used for matched-related and matched-unrelated donor grafts. All grafts were T-cell depleted with alemtuzumab-based strategies (80). The radioimmunoconjugates provided a mean of 21.9 ± 8.4 Gy radiation to the marrow space. Despite the low level of toxicities seen in older patients using this approach (day 100 mortality 15%), the cumulative incidence of relapse remained high (55% at 30 months posttransplant). The risk of relapse was almost 20% higher for patients not in remission compared to those in either first or second remission (60% vs. 42%) (80). These studies may highlight the difficulty of targeting multiple low-energy beta emissions to neighboring leukemic blasts by relying on cross fire from normal targeted CD66-positive myeloid cells.

Together, the accumulated clinical experience demonstrates the feasibility of integrating radioimmunoconjugates targeting CD33, CD45, or CD66 antigens into treatment regimens for leukemias. Given the proof-of-principle character of most clinical studies performed with radioimmunoconjugates so far, important questions remain. Most importantly, it remains to be unequivocally documented that such radioimmunotherapy approaches indeed lead to better patient outcomes. Indeed, while the data suggest a potential benefit, very few attempts have been undertaken to document such a benefit, and controlled clinical trials addressing this important question are lacking altogether. Furthermore, assuming a beneficial role of radioimmunoconjugates, it remains unclear which antigen should be targeted and which radionuclide should be used. So far, no comparative trials testing radioimmunoconjugate targeting of different antigens have been reported. There is some evidence using technetium-99m labeling that anti-CD66 antibody-based radioimmunoconjugates may provide a higher selectivity of delivering radiation to the marrow space as compared to extramedullary organs such as liver or kidneys than anti-CD45 antibody-based radioimmunoconjugates in patients with low leukemia tumor load (81). However, it remains to be determined whether this holds true for other radionuclides, and whether this increased selectivity indeed translates into a clinical benefit. Furthermore, the benefits of individual radionuclides need to be evaluated in a more

controlled fashion. A first step in this direction was undertaken by Ringhoffer et al. who used both ^{188}Re and ^{90}Y-labeled anti-CD66 antibody in a series of 20 patients undergoing reduced-intensity conditioning for acute leukemias or MDS (80). The results of the dosimetry differed between the two radionuclides in that ^{90}Y delivered a significantly higher radiation dose to bone marrow (26.0 ± 8.0 Gy vs. 15.9 ± 4.3 Gy, $p < 0.01$) and liver (12.8 ± 4.6 Gy vs. 5.1 ± 1.2 Gy, $p < 0.001$), whereas the kidney dose was not significantly lower (4.8 ± 2.9 Gy vs. 7.0±2.9 Gy). This difference was thought to be due to a higher in vivo stability of the ^{90}Y conjugate, which would reduce exposure of the renal cortex to dissociated radionuclides and indirectly increase the bone marrow dose (80). A later study confirmed that the absorbed renal dose was lower in patients receiving BW 250/183 labeled with ^{90}Y relative to those receiving ^{188}Re-labeled antibody (82). This may have clinical significance as only patients receiving ^{188}Re-BW 250/183 developed posttransplant nephropathy (incidence about 20%), particularly when the radioimmunoconjugate was used in combination with TBI (82).

Radioimmunotherapy targeting other antigens

A few additional antigens have been explored for used in targeting leukemias with radionuclides. Most importantly, the overlap between CLL/SLL and low-grade non-Hodgkin lymphomas has resulted in the inclusion of patients with CLL in lymphoma studies. An early study on 10 lymphoma patients, including three patients with SLL, explored the usefulness of ^{131}I-labeled anti-CD37 antibody (MB-1) (83). Biodistribution studies in the five patients with splenomegaly and large tumor burdens indicated that not all tumor sites would receive more radiation, and these patients were therefore not treated with high-dose radioimmunotherapy. Four of the other five patients, including one patient with SLL, received therapeutic ^{131}I-MB-1 and achieved CRs (83). Later small studies suggested the usefulness of CD37-targeted radioimmunotherapy in selected cases (84,85). However, further studies were not pursued because of the perceived superiority of radioimmunotherapy using anti-CD20 antibodies due to more favorable biodistribution with smaller doses and slower internalization and degradation of the radioimmunoconjugates by tumor cells leading to longer serum half-times (85). Notwithstanding, CD37 remains an appealing target in CLL (86), and recent preclinical studies may spur renewed interest in CD37-directed therapy (87).

Single-agent activity of the unconjugated anti-CD20 antibody, rituximab, in relapsed or refractory CLL/SLL has been disappointing, possibly due to relatively low expression levels of CD20 on these malignant cells (88). Nevertheless, many patients with CLL/SLL have been treated on studies investigating CD20-targeted radioimmunoconjugates. Extensive clinical evaluations have been performed with ^{131}I-labeled and ^{90}Y-labeled anti-CD20 antibodies (tositumomab and ibritumomab tiuxetan, respectively).

These studies are discussed in the chapter on lymphomas in detail. However, the use of radioimmunotherapy in CLL/SLL is limited by the oftentimes very extensive bone marrow involvement, and the use of both radiolabeled anti-CD20 antibodies is typically restricted to patients with less than 25% bone marrow involvement due to safety concerns (88).

HLA-DR has been used as carrier for radionuclides because its expression on normal B-lymphocytes is about 100-fold lower than on malignant B-lymphocytes (89,90). A ^{131}I-labeled anti-HLA-DR antibody (Lym-1) has been used in a small number of patients with CLL/SLL. A high proportion of the patients responded, and responses appeared to be associated with improved survival; the dose-limiting toxicity was thrombocytopenia (91–93). In a study on 51 patients with B-cell malignancies, including six patients with CLL, treated with ^{131}I-HLA-DR (Lym-1), human anti-mouse antibody (HAMA) developed in 18 (35%). Interestingly, development of elevated HAMA titers was associated with a survival benefit, even in multivariate analyses; HAMA titers correlated negatively with the number of previous treatments, and seroconversion was directly related to pretreatment absolute lymphocyte counts (94). Potential HAMA-related mechanisms underlying this beneficial effect remain unclear, although detailed study in one of these patients suggests that activation of the idiotype cascade with generation of an anti-idiotype antibody with ability to exert antibody-dependent cellular toxicity could be involved (95). An alternative radionuclide, ^{67}Cu, has also been used with promising results as radiolabel for Lym-1 in a limited number of patients with lymphoid neoplasms (96,97), and additional studies suggest that this radionuclide might be of use in combination with anti-CD25 antibodies (98–100).

The experience with CD25 as target for radioimmunotherapy is quite limited. A phase I/II study has investigated a ^{90}Y-labeled anti-CD25 antibody (Tac) in 18 patients with adult T-cell leukemia, an aggressive form of leukemia with a median survival time of 9 months (101). These patients received a total of 55 doses of ^{90}Y-Tac. Nine out of 16 evaluable patients showed a clinical response to this radioimmunoconjugate (seven partial responses, two complete responses), which was felt to be an improvement in outcome when compared with previous results with unmodified anti-Tac antibody (101). Even more limited than with HLA-DR is the clinical experience with CD5, a rapidly internalizing antigen: only one phase I study has investigated the potential usefulness of targeting CD5 with a ^{90}Y-labeled antibody (T101) in 10 patients, including two patients with CLL (102). Partial responses were observed in 5 of the 10 patients, including both CLL patients, with a median duration of response of 23 weeks (102).

An antigen of high interest is CD22, another member of the Siglec family of proteins (Siglec-2) (15). Similar to CD33, CD22 is internalized upon antibody binding. Anti-CD22-based immunotoxins have shown high efficacy in the treatment of patients with fludarabine-refractory hairy

cell leukemia, and has activity against B-cell ALL in preclinical models (103–105). In a phase I trial using ^{131}I-labeled LL2, a murine IgG2a anti-CD22 monoclonal antibody, patients with various forms of lymphoid malignancies, including some CLL patients, were studied. Among 18 assessable patients, six showed responses, including one patient who only received diagnostic doses of the radioimmunoconjugate (106). A similar group of 20 patients was later treated with humanized LL2 (hLL2; epratuzumab) labeled with ^{131}I or ^{90}Y. Objective tumor responses were seen in 2 of 13 and 2 of 7 patients given ^{131}I-hLL2 or ^{90}Y-hLL2, respectively. ^{90}Y-hLL2 resulted in a more favorable tumor dosimetry compared with ^{131}I-hLL2 (107). A response in 5 out of 15 patients with relapsed or refractory CD22-positive non-Hodgkin lymphoma, including CLL, was observed when epratuzumab was labeled with ^{186}Re (108). Finally, a more recent study used fractionated doses of ^{90}Y-epratuzumab in 16 patients (1 CLL) found an overall response rate of 62% (95% confidence interval, 39% to 86%) and a complete response rate of 25% (109).

■ RECENT PRECLINICAL STUDIES OF TARGETED RADIONUCLIDE THERAPY

Preclinical studies in experimental animals, both rodents and primates, were instrumental in demonstrating the feasibility and potential efficacy of radioimmunotherapy as treatment modality (110). Undoubtedly, preclinical studies remain critical for the development of radioimmunotherapeutic approaches of leukemia. This research will focus its efforts in several different directions, including the identification of alternative target antigens that demonstrate enhanced efficacy for radioimmunotherapy as well as the exploration of alternative radionuclides that offer improved specificity of tumor targeting and lower nonspecific toxicities. Other attempts will focus on improving the specificity of radiation delivery and enhancing the tumor penetration with targeted radionuclides.

The number of antigens targeted with radioimmunotherapy may expand significantly over the next years. Many are under active investigation, including CD25, CD30, and CD52. Even though CD25 has so far not gained major importance for radioimmunotherapy of leukemias (101), it remains an attractive target due to its relatively selected expression on a high proportion of malignant cells in certain forms of lymphoid neoplasms, including adult T-cell leukemia. Given this expression pattern, α-particle therapy may be particularly appealing in an attempt to spare normal hematopoietic tissue. To this end, a ^{211}At-labeled murine anti-CD25 IgG2a monoclonal antibody (7G7/B6) has been developed and tested with promising results in immunodeficient mice bearing CD25-positive leukemia and lymphoma cells (111). Using a similar model, the same group also achieved promising results using a ^{211}At-labeled murine anti-CD30 IgG1 monoclonal antibody (HeFi-1) in prolonging survival of immunodeficient mice bearing tumors that express CD30, an antigen that is found on some lymphocyte subsets but is also expressed on some lymphoid neoplasms (112). Together, these findings may set the foundation for progression to clinical studies using [211]At-labeled antibodies for the treatment of patients with either CD25 or CD30 expressing leukemias. CD52 is normally expressed on B and T lymphocytes, monocytes, macrophages, eosinophils, NK cells, dendritic cells, as well as on cells of the male reproductive tract (113). However, CD52 is also expressed by a variety of lymphoid neoplasms and has thus been exploited as target for antibody-based therapies, in particular for CLL. Alemtuzumab (Campath-1H), a humanized rat IgG1 monoclonal antibody directed against CD52, has shown promising activity alone and in combination with other therapeutics for untreated and previously treated patients with CLL (113–115). In 2001, it has been approved in the United States and Europe for use in fludarabine-refractory CLL patients. More recently, this antibody has been explored for radioimmunotherapy using [188]Re (116). Preclinical studies found [188]Re-alemtuzumab to have good in vitro stability, and showed high uptake in blood with biexponential clearance, with some increased uptake observed in kidneys and heart (116). Among the targets explored for treatment of CLL/SLL is also CD23. An unconjugated anti-CD23 antibody, lumiliximab (IDEC-152), has shown promising activity in clinical studies (88,115,117), and it is conceivable that this, or other antibodies under development for CLL, will be used to deliver radiation to tumor sites.

Parallel efforts are ongoing to identify novel radionuclides and radionuclide–antibody conjugates, and define their antileukemic properties. For example, a [213]Bi-labeled anti-CD45 antibody (YAML568) is under preclinical development that shows interesting properties regarding induction of apoptosis and breakage of chemoresistance and radioresistance by overcoming DNA repair mechanisms in leukemia cells (118). The high linear energy transfer of [213]Bi-radiotherapy may also provide synergistic cytotoxic activity when combined with antileukemic chemotherapeutics, for example, for the treatment of CLL/SLL (119). Other examples of radioimmunoconjugates that potentially are exploited in the clinical setting include ^{90}Y-B4, ^{90}Y-BU12, and ^{90}Y-HD37 (mouse IgG1 anti-CD19 antibodies), ^{90}Y-RFB4 (mouse IgG1 anti-CD22 antibody), [211]At-hTac (humanized anti-CD25 antibody), [213]Bi-rituximab (humanized anti-CD20 antibody), and ^{177}Lu-labeled anti-CD20, anti-CD22, and anti-HLA-DR antibodies (120–126).

While clinical evidence demonstrates that radioimmunotherapy can deliver a prolonged, exponentially decreasing low dose rate of radiation that may result in the accumulation of DNA damage in leukemia cells and cytotoxic effects, a general limitation of radioimmunotherapy is the suboptimal therapeutic index (risk-to-benefit ratio) currently achievable with conventional methodologies (127). An important strategy that is actively pursued to overcome some of these shortcomings in the treatment of leukemias is pretargeting, that is, the sequential use of "cold" antibody prior to delivery or a therapeutic radionuclide attached to a small molecule that allows for rapid tumor uptake and rapid excretion of nontumor bound radioactivity (127). This strategy is discussed elsewhere in this book in detail. Promising data from experimental animal models using either a recombinant single-chain or conventional anti-CD45 antibody–streptavidin conjugate followed by a dendrimeric N-acetylgalactosamine-containing clearing agents and radiobiotin (^{90}Y-DOTA-biotin) have been shown (128,129). Similarly promising preclinical data are available for pretargeting strategies for other antigens, such as CD20 and CD25 (130–132). Potential advantages using pretargeting strategies, which allow flexibility with respect to radionuclide and antigen target, include the achievement of more favorable biodistribution and enhanced blood clearance, leading to a higher target-to-nontarget organ ratio. Hurdles remain that will need to be addressed in future research, such as challenges in manufacturing, decreased tumor residence time if monovalent fragment constructs are used, cross-linking phenomena if multivalent constructs are used, and immunogenicity and hapten release from processed antibody (127).

An exciting new avenue to improve the efficacy of radioimmunoconjugates and potentially reduce nonspecific toxicities entails antibody modifications that could allow clinical use of the Auger electron-emitting radionuclide ^{111}In in combination with anti-CD33 antibodies. Specifically, M195 and HuM195 were modified with a 13-mer peptide (CGYG-PKKKRKVGG) harboring the nuclear localization sequence (NLS) of SV-40 large T-antigen (133). This resulted in efficient internalization and improved routing of the radioimmunoconjugate to the nucleus of leukemia cells compared to antibody constructs lacking the NLS. This effect was associated with enhanced killing of drug-sensitive and drug-resistant AML cell lines and primary AML cells by the radioimmunoconjugates containing NLSs (133,134). An equally exciting avenue to explore is the development of small synthetic multidentate ligands that mimic properties of antibodies and bind to cell surface antigens with high affinity and specificity, as shown for example for the HLA-DR antigen, and due to the smaller size may provide better tumor penetration (135,136). Such small, engineered molecules may therefore provide an alternative way of targeted delivery of radiation to sites of leukemic involvement. Finally, an alternative approach to increase accessibility of leukemias to radioimmunoconjugates lies in the manipulation of tumor blood flow, and early studies with interleukin-2 suggest that increasing vascular permeability to achieve this goal might be a valid strategy worth exploring in the future (137).

■ FUTURE DIRECTIONS

An increasing number of proof-of-principle clinical studies demonstrate that radioimmunotherapy for leukemia is safe, feasible, and has acceptable toxicities, even in older adults. Research over the last two decades established important principles of directing radiolabeled antibodies to leukemias, and has provided encouraging results. Nevertheless, radioimmunotherapy is a complex, multidisciplinary effort that still faces many challenges on the road to success: significant obstacles remain that must be overcome to achieve optimal targeting and elimination of leukemia cells by radioimmunoconjugates. For example, the optimal therapeutic radionuclide–antibody–antigen combination for leukemia radioimmunotherapy remains unclear, and better-controlled clinical trials will ultimately be required to address this question and to determine whether addition of radioimmunoconjugates truly improves patient outcomes over standard treatment. Undoubtedly, future studies will explore alternative antigenic targets and novel radionuclides to improve imaging, dosimetry, and therapy. Furthermore, innovative strategies such as pretargeting and extracorporeal immunoabsorption may optimize the administration of radionuclide therapy and allow more widespread use of very short half-life materials such as the α-emitters for radioimmunotherapy of leukemia. With continued research, radioimmunotherapy holds the potential to establish itself as first-line treatment in leukemias for small volume disease or as a radiation boost in combination with other treatments, such as stem cell rescue or as adjuvant therapy. Thereby, radioimmunotherapy-based approaches may become an important cornerstone to improve the outcome of patients with leukemias, and will remain an exciting avenue due to constant methodologic refinements.

■ REFERENCES

1. Henderson ES. History of leukemia. In: Henderson ES, Lister TA, Greaves MF, eds. *Leukemia.* 6th ed. Philadelphia, PA: W.B. Saunders Company; 1996:1–7.
2. Harris NL, Jaffe ES, Diebold J, et al. World Health Organization classification of neoplastic diseases of the hematopoietic and lymphoid tissues: report of the Clinical Advisory Committee meeting, Airlie House, Virginia, November 1997. *J Clin Oncol.* 1999;17:3835–3849.
3. Vardiman JW, Harris NL, Brunning RD. The World Health Organization (WHO) classification of the myeloid neoplasms. *Blood.* 2002;100: 2292–2302.
4. Jemal A, Siegel R, Ward E, et al. Cancer statistics, 2008. *CA Cancer J Clin.* 2008;58:71–96.
5. Kantarjian H, O'Brien S, Cortes J, et al. Therapeutic advances in leukemia and myelodysplastic syndrome over the past 40 years. *Cancer.* 2008;113:1933–1952.
6. Goldman JM, Gordon MY. A history of the chronic leukemias. In: Wiernik PH, Goldman JM, Dutcher JP, et al., eds. *Neoplastic Diseases of the Blood.* Vol. 1, 1st ed. Cambridge: Cambridge University Press; 2003:3–8.
7. Gunz FW. Leukemia in the past. In: Henderson ES, Lister TA, eds. *William Dameshek and Frederick Gunz's Leukemia.* Vol. 1. Philadelphia, PA: W.B. Saunders Company; 1990:3–11.
8. Thomas ED. A history of bone marrow transplantation. In: Blume KG, Forman SJ, Appelbaum FR, eds. *Thomas' Hematopoietic Cell Transplantation.* Vol. 1, 3rd ed. Malden, MA: Blackwell Publishing; 2004:3–8.
9. Thomas ED, Storb R, Clift RA, et al. Bone-marrow transplantation (first of two parts). *N Engl J Med.* 1975;292:832–843.
10. Clift RA, Buckner CD, Appelbaum FR, et al. Allogeneic marrow transplantation in patients with acute myeloid leukemia in first remission: a randomized trial of two irradiation regimens. *Blood.* 1990;76:1867–1871.
11. Clift RA, Buckner CD, Appelbaum FR, et al. Allogeneic marrow transplantation in patients with chronic myeloid leukemia in the chronic phase: a randomized trial of two irradiation regimens. *Blood.* 1991;77: 1660–1665.
12. Clift RA, Buckner CD, Appelbaum FR, et al. Long-term follow-up of a randomized trial of two irradiation regimens for patients receiving allogeneic marrow transplants during first remission of acute myeloid leukemia. *Blood.* 1998;92:1455–1456.
13. Craig FE, Foon KA. Flow cytometric immunophenotyping for hematologic neoplasms. *Blood.* 2008;111:3941–3967.
14. Freeman SD, Kelm S, Barber EK, et al. Characterization of CD33 as a new member of the sialoadhesin family of cellular interaction molecules. *Blood.* 1995;85:2005–2012.
15. Crocker PR, Paulson JC, Varki A. Siglecs and their roles in the immune system. *Nat Rev Immunol.* 2007;7:255–266.
16. Andrews RG, Torok-Storb B, Bernstein ID. Myeloid-associated differentiation antigens on stem cells and their progeny identified by monoclonal antibodies. *Blood.* 1983;62:124–132.
17. Griffin JD, Linch D, Sabbath K, et al. A monoclonal antibody reactive with normal and leukemic human myeloid progenitor cells. *Leukemia Res.* 1984;8:521–534.
18. Andrews RG, Takahashi M, Segal GM, et al. The L4F3 antigen is expressed by unipotent and multipotent colony-forming cells but not by their precursors. *Blood.* 1986;68:1030–1035.
19. Handgretinger R, Schafer HJ, Baur F, et al. Expression of an early myelopoietic antigen (CD33) on a subset of human umbilical cord blood-derived natural killer cells. *Immunol Lett.* 1993;37:223–228.
20. Nakamura Y, Noma M, Kidokoro M, et al. Expression of CD33 antigen on normal human activated T lymphocytes. *Blood.* 1994;83: 1442–1443.
21. Schmidt-Wolf IG, Grimm B, Lefterova P, et al. Propagation of large numbers of cells of a human mixed-lineage T-lymphoid/myeloid. *Br J Haematol.* 1995;90:512–517.
22. Márquez C, Trigueros C, Franco JM, et al. Identification of a common developmental pathway for thymic natural killer cells and dendritic cells. *Blood.* 1998;91:2760–2771.
23. Dworzak MN, Fritsch G, Froschl G, et al. Four-color flow cytometric investigation of terminal deoxynucleotidyl transferase-positive lymphoid precursors in pediatric bone marrow: CD79a expression precedes CD19 in early B-cell ontogeny. *Blood.* 1998;92:3203–3209.
24. Eksioglu-Demiralp E, Kibaroglu A, Direskeneli H, et al. Phenotypic characteristics of B cells in Behcet's disease: increased activity in B cell subsets. *J Rheumatol.* 1999;26:826–832.
25. Tricarico M, Macchi S, D'Atri S, et al. In vitro infection of CD4+ T lymphocytes with HTLV-I generates immortalized cell lines coexpressing lymphoid and myeloid cell markers. *Leukemia.* 1999;13: 222–229.
26. Hernández-Caselles T, Martínez-Esparza M, Pérez-Oliva AB, et al. A study of CD33 (SIGLEC-3) antigen expression and function on activated human T and NK cells: two isoforms of CD33 are generated by alternative splicing. *J Leukoc Biol.* 2006;79:46–58.
27. Dinndorf PA, Andrews RG, Benjamin D, et al. Expression of normal myeloid-associated antigens by acute leukemia cells. *Blood.* 1986;67: 1048–1053.
28. Jilani I, Estey E, Huh Y, et al. Differences in CD33 intensity between various myeloid neoplasms. *Am J Clin Pathol.* 2002;118:560–566.
29. van der Jagt RHC, Badger CC, Appelbaum FR, et al. Localization of radiolabeled antimyeloid antibodies in a human acute leukemia xenograft tumor model. *Cancer Res.* 1992;52:89–94.
30. Omary MB, Trowbridge IS, Battifora HA. Human homologue of murine T200 glycoprotein. *J Exp Med.* 1980;152:842–852.
31. Dahlke MH, Larsen SR, Rasko JE, et al. The biology of CD45 and its use as a therapeutic target. *Leukemia Lymphoma.* 2004;45:229–236.
32. Andres TL, Kadin ME. Immunologic markers in the differential diagnosis of small round cell tumors from lymphocytic lymphoma and leukemia. *Am J Clin Pathol.* 1983;79:546–552.
33. Nakano A, Harada T, Morikawa S, et al. Expression of leukocyte common antigen (CD45) on various human leukemia/lymphoma cell lines. *Acta Pathol Jpn.* 1990;40:107–115.
34. Taetle R, Ostergaard H, Smedsrud M, et al. Regulation of CD45 expression in human leukemia cells. *Leukemia.* 1991;5:309–314.
35. Press OW, Howell-Clark J, Anderson S, et al. Retention of B-cell-specific monoclonal antibodies by human lymphoma cells. *Blood.* 1994;83:1390–1397.
36. Becker W, Goldenberg DM, Wolf F. The use of monoclonal antibodies and antibody fragments in the imaging of infectious lesions. *Semin Nucl Med.* 1994;24:142–153.
37. Gray-Owen SD, Blumberg RS. CEACAM1: contact-dependent control of immunity. *Nat Rev Immunol.* 2006;6:433–446.
38. Wahren B, Gahrton G, Hammarstrom S. Nonspecific cross-reacting antigen in normal and leukemic myeloid cells and serum of leukemic patients. *Cancer Res.* 1980;40:2039–2044.
39. Noworolska A, Harlozinska A, Richter R, et al. Non-specific cross-reacting antigen (NCA) in individual maturation stages of myelocytic cell series. *Br J Cancer.* 1985;51:371–377.

40. Watt SM, Sala-Newby G, Hoang T, et al. CD66 identifies a neutrophil-specific epitope within the hematopoietic system that is expressed by members of the carcinoembryonic antigen family of adhesion molecules. *Blood*. 1991;78:63–74.

41. Carrasco M, Munoz L, Bellido M, et al. CD66 expression in acute leukaemia. *Ann Hematol*. 2000;79:299–303.

42. Boccuni P, Di Noto R, Lo Pardo C, et al. CD66c antigen expression is myeloid restricted in normal bone marrow but is a common feature of CD10+ early-B-cell malignancies. *Tissue Antigens*. 1998;52:1–8.

43. Bunjes D, Buchmann I, Duncker C, et al. Rhenium 188-labeled anti-CD66 (a, b, c, e) monoclonal antibody to intensify the conditioning regimen prior to stem cell transplantation for patients with high-risk acute myeloid leukemia or myelodysplastic syndrome: results of a phase I-II study. *Blood*. 2001;98:565–572.

44. Royston I, Majda JA, Baird SM, et al. Human T cell antigens defined by monoclonal antibodies: the 65,000-dalton antigen of T cells (T65) is also found on chronic lymphocytic leukemia cells bearing surface immunoglobulin. *J Immunol*. 1980;125:725–731.

45. Waldmann TA. Daclizumab (anti-Tac, Zenapax) in the treatment of leukemia/lymphoma. *Oncogene*. 2007;26:3699–3703.

46. Matthews DC, Appelbaum FR. Radioimmunotherapy and hematopoietic cell transplantation. In: Blume KG, Forman SJ, Appelbaum FR, eds. *Thomas' Hematopoietic Cell Transplantion*. Vol. 1, 3rd ed. Malden, MA: Blackwell Publishing; 2004:198–208.

47. Appelbaum FR. Antibody-targeted therapy for myeloid leukemia. *Semin Hematol*. 1999;36:2–8.

48. Abutalib SA, Tallman MS. Monoclonal antibodies for the treatment of acute myeloid leukemia. *Curr Pharm Biotechnol*. 2006;7:343–369.

49. Appelbaum FR, Matthews DC, Eary JF, et al. The use of radiolabeled anti-CD33 antibody to augment marrow irradiation prior to marrow transplantation for acute myelogenous leukemia. *Transplantation*. 1992;54:829–833.

50. Scheinberg DA, Lovett D, Divgi CR, et al. A phase I trial of monoclonal antibody M195 in acute myelogenous leukemia: specific bone marrow targeting and internalization of radionuclide. *J Clin Oncol*. 1991;9:478–490.

51. Schwartz MA, Lovett DR, Redner A, et al. Dose-escalation trial of M195 labeled with iodine 131 for cytoreduction and marrow ablation in relapsed or refractory myeloid leukemias. *J Clin Oncol*. 1993;11:294–303.

52. Jurcic JG, Caron PC, Nikula TK, et al. Radiolabeled anti-CD33 monoclonal antibody M195 for myeloid leukemias. *Cancer Res*. 1995;55:5908s–5910s.

53. Caron PC, Co MS, Bull MK, et al. Biological and immunological features of humanized M195 (anti-CD33) monoclonal antibodies. *Cancer Res*. 1992;52:6761–6767.

54. Caron PC, Jurcic JG, Scott AM, et al. A phase 1B trial of humanized monoclonal antibody M195 (anti-CD33) in myeloid leukemia: specific targeting without immunogenicity. *Blood*. 1994;83:1760–1768.

55. Burke JM, Caron PC, Papadopoulos EB, et al. Cytoreduction with iodine-131-anti-CD33 antibodies before bone marrow transplantation for advanced myeloid leukemias. *Bone Marrow Transplant*. 2003;32:549–556.

56. Press OW, Shan D, Howell-Clark J, et al. Comparative metabolism and retention of iodine-125, yttrium-90, and indium-111 radioimmunoconjugates by cancer cells. *Cancer Res*. 1996;56:2123–2129.

57. Jurcic JG. Antibody therapy for residual disease in acute myelogenous leukemia. *Crit Rev Oncol Hematol*. 2001;38:37–45.

58. Nikula TK, McDevitt MR, Finn RD, et al. Alpha-emitting bismuth cyclohexylbenzyl DTPA constructs of recombinant humanized anti-CD33 antibodies: pharmacokinetics, bioactivity, toxicity and chemistry. *J Nucl Med*. 1999;40:166–176.

59. McDevitt MR, Finn RD, Ma D, et al. Preparation of alpha-emitting 213Bi-labeled antibody constructs for clinical use. *J Nucl Med*. 1999;40:1722–1727.

60. Sgouros G, Ballangrud AM, Jurcic JG, et al. Pharmacokinetics and dosimetry of an alpha-particle emitter labeled antibody: 213Bi-HuM195 (anti-CD33) in patients with leukemia. *J Nucl Med*. 1999;40:1935–1946.

61. Jurcic JG, Larson SM, Sgouros G, et al. Targeted alpha particle immunotherapy for myeloid leukemia. *Blood*. 2002;100:1233–1239.

62. Mulford DA, Pandit-Taskar N, McDevitt MR, et al. Sequential therapy with cytarabine and bismuth-213 (213Bi)-labeled-HuM195 (anti-CD33) for acute myeloid leukemia (AML). *Blood*. 2004;104:Abstract #1790.

63. McDevitt MR, Ma D, Lai LT, et al. Tumor therapy with targeted atomic nanogenerators. *Science*. 2001;294:1537–1540.

64. Miederer M, McDevitt MR, Sgouros G, et al. Pharmacokinetics, dosimetry, and toxicity of the targetable atomic generator, 225Ac-HuM195, in nonhuman primates. *J Nucl Med*. 2004;45:129–137.

65. Rosenblat TL, McDevitt MR, Pandit-Taskar N, et al. Phase I trial of the targeted alpha-particle nano-generator actinium-225 (225Ac)-HuM195 (anti-CD33) in acute myeloid leukemia (AML). *Blood*. 2007;110:Abstract #910.

66. Mulford DA, Scheinberg DA, Jurcic JG. The promise of targeted {alpha}-particle therapy. *J Nucl Med*. 2005;46(suppl 1):199S–204S.

67. Matthews DC, Appelbaum FR, Eary JF, et al. Radiolabeled anti-CD45 monoclonal antibodies target lymphohematopoietic tissue in the macaque. *Blood*. 1991;78:1864–1874.

68. Matthews DC, Badger CC, Fisher DR, et al. Selective radiation of hematolymphoid tissue delivered by anti-CD45 antibody. *Cancer Res*. 1992;52:1228–1234.

69. Matthews DC, Appelbaum FR, Eary JF, et al. Development of a marrow transplant regimen for acute leukemia using targeted hematopoietic irradiation delivered by 131I-labeled anti-CD45 antibody, combined with cyclophosphamide and total body irradiation. *Blood*. 1995;85:1122–1131.

70. Matthews DC, Appelbaum FR, Eary JF, et al. Phase I study of (131)I-anti-CD45 antibody plus cyclophosphamide and total body irradiation for advanced acute leukemia and myelodysplastic syndrome. *Blood*. 1999;94:1237–1247.

71. Pagel J, Gooley T, Rajendran J, et al. Targeted radiotherapy using 131I-anti-CD45 antibody followed by allogeneic hematopoietic cell transplantation (HCT): the relationships among dosimetry, bone marrow uptake, and relapse [abstract]. *Eur J Nucl Med Mol Imaging*. 2006;33:S193.

72. Pagel JM, Appelbaum FR, Eary JF, et al. 131I-anti-CD45 antibody plus busulfan and cyclophosphamide before allogeneic hematopoietic cell transplantation for treatment of acute myeloid leukemia in first remission. *Blood*. 2006;107:2184–2191.

73. Pagel JM, Appelbaum FR, Sandmaier BM, et al. 131I-anti-CD45 antibody plus fludarabine, low-dose total body irradiation and peripheral blood stem cell infusion for elderly patients with advanced acute myeloid leukemia (AML) or high-risk myelodysplastic syndrome (MDS). *Blood*. 2005;106:Abstract #397.

74. Glatting G, Muller M, Koop B, et al. Anti-CD45 monoclonal antibody YAML568: a promising radioimmunoconjugate for targeted therapy of acute leukemia. *J Nucl Med*. 2006;47:1335–1341.

75. Rottinger EM, Bartkowiak D, Bunjes D, et al. Enhanced renal toxicity of total body irradiation combined with radioimmunotherapy. *Strahlenther Onkol*. 2003;179:702–707.

76. Buchmann I, Bunjes D, Kotzerke J, et al. Myeloablative radioimmunotherapy with Re-188-anti-CD66-antibody for conditioning of high-risk leukemia patients prior to stem cell transplantation: biodistribution, biokinetics and immediate toxicities. *Cancer Biother Radiopharm*. 2002;17:151–163.

77. Bunjes D. 188Re-labeled anti-CD66 monoclonal antibody in stem cell transplantation for patients with high-risk acute myeloid leukemia. *Leukemia Lymphoma*. 2002;43:2125–2131.

78. Klein SA, Hermann S, Dietrich JW, et al. Transplantation-related toxicity and acute intestinal graft-versus-host disease after conditioning regimens intensified with Rhenium 188-labeled anti-CD66 monoclonal antibodies. *Blood*. 2002;99:2270–2271.

79. Koenecke C, Hofmann M, Bolte O, et al. Radioimmunotherapy with [(188)Re]-labelled anti-CD66 antibody in the conditioning for allogeneic stem cell transplantation for high-risk acute myeloid leukemia. *Int J Hematol*. 2008;87(4):414–421.

80. Ringhoffer M, Blumstein N, Neumaier B, et al. 188Re or 90Y-labelled anti-CD66 antibody as part of a dose-reduced conditioning regimen for patients with acute leukaemia or myelodysplastic syndrome over the age of 55: results of a phase I-II study. *Br J Haematol*. 2005;130:604–613.

81. Buchmann I, Kull T, Glatting G, et al. A comparison of the biodistribution and biokinetics of (99m)Tc-anti-CD66 mAb BW 250/183 and (99m)Tc-anti-CD45 mAb YTH 24.5 with regard to suitability for myeloablative radioimmunotherapy. *Eur J Nucl Med Mol Imaging*. 2003;30:667–673.

82. Zenz T, Schlenk RF, Glatting G, et al. Bone marrow transplantation nephropathy after an intensified conditioning regimen with radioimmunotherapy and allogeneic stem cell transplantation. *J Nucl Med*. 2006;47:278–286.

83. Press OW, Eary JF, Badger CC, et al. Treatment of refractory non-Hodgkin's lymphoma with radiolabeled MB-1 (anti-CD37) antibody. *J Clin Oncol*. 1989;7:1027–1038.

84. Kaminski MS, Fig LM, Zasadny KR, et al. Imaging, dosimetry, and radioimmunotherapy with iodine 131-labeled anti-CD37 antibody in B-cell lymphoma. *J Clin Oncol.* 1992;10:1696–1711.

85. Press OW, Eary JF, Appelbaum FR, et al. Radiolabeled-antibody therapy of B-cell lymphoma with autologous bone marrow support. *N Engl J Med.* 1993;329:1219–1224.

86. Belov L, de la Vega O, dos Remedios CG, et al. Immunophenotyping of leukemias using a cluster of differentiation antibody microarray. *Cancer Res.* 2001;61:4483–4489.

87. Zhao X, Lapalombella R, Joshi T, et al. Targeting CD37-positive lymphoid malignancies with a novel engineered small modular immunopharmaceutical. *Blood.* 2007;110:2569–2577.

88. Mavromatis B, Cheson BD. Monoclonal antibody therapy of chronic lymphocytic leukemia. *J Clin Oncol.* 2003;21:1874–1881.

89. Rose LM, Gunasekera AH, DeNardo SJ, et al. Lymphoma-selective antibody Lym-1 recognizes a discontinuous epitope on the light chain of HLA-DR10. *Cancer Immunol Immunother.* 1996;43:26–30.

90. Rose LM, Deng CT, Scott SL, et al. Critical Lym-1 binding residues on polymorphic HLA-DR molecules. *Mol Immunol.* 1999;36:789–797.

91. DeNardo GL, Lewis JP, DeNardo SJ, et al. Effect of Lym-1 radioimmunoconjugate on refractory chronic lymphocytic leukemia. *Cancer.* 1994;73:1425–1432.

92. DeNardo GL, Lamborn KR, Goldstein DS, et al. Increased survival associated with radiolabeled Lym-1 therapy for non-Hodgkin's lymphoma and chronic lymphocytic leukemia. *Cancer.* 1997;80:2706–2711.

93. DeNardo GL, DeNardo SJ, Lamborn KR, et al. Low-dose, fractionated radioimmunotherapy for B-cell malignancies using 131I-Lym-1 antibody. *Cancer Biother Radiopharm.* 1998;13:239–254.

94. Azinovic I, DeNardo GL, Lamborn KR, et al. Survival benefit associated with human anti-mouse antibody (HAMA) in patients with B-cell malignancies. *Cancer Immunol Immunother.* 2006;55:1451–1458.

95. Bradt BM, DeNardo SJ, Mirick GR, et al. Documentation of idiotypic cascade after Lym-1 radioimmunotherapy in a patient with non-Hodgkin's lymphoma: basis for extended survival? *Clin Cancer Res.* 2003;9:4007S–4012S.

96. O'Donnell RT, DeNardo GL, Kukis DL, et al. 67Copper-2-iminothiolane-6-[p-(bromoacetamido)benzyl-TETA-Lym-1 for radioimmunotherapy of non-Hodgkin's lymphoma. *Clin Cancer Res.* 1999;5:3330s–3336s.

97. Dowell JA, Korth-Bradley J, Liu H, et al. Pharmacokinetics of gemtuzumab ozogamicin, an antibody-targeted chemotherapy agent for the treatment of patients with acute myeloid leukemia in first relapse. *J Clin Pharmacol.* 2001;41:1206–1214.

98. Kroger LA, DeNardo GL, Gumerlock PH, et al. Apoptosis-related gene and protein expression in human lymphoma xenografts (Raji) after low dose rate radiation using 67Cu-2IT-BAT-Lym-1 radioimmunotherapy. *Cancer Biother Radiopharm.* 2001;16:213–225.

99. DeNardo GL, DeNardo SJ, O'Donnell RT, et al. Are radiometal-labeled antibodies better than iodine-131-labeled antibodies: comparative pharmacokinetics and dosimetry of copper-67-, iodine-131-, and yttrium-90-labeled Lym-1 antibody in patients with non-Hodgkin's lymphoma. *Clin Lymphoma.* 2000;1:118–126.

100. DeNardo GL, Kukis DL, Shen S, et al. 67Cu-versus 131I-labeled Lym-1 antibody: comparative pharmacokinetics and dosimetry in patients with non-Hodgkin's lymphoma. *Clin Cancer Res.* 1999;5:533–541.

101. Waldmann TA, White JD, Carrasquillo JA, et al. Radioimmunotherapy of interleukin-2R alpha-expressing adult T-cell leukemia with Yttrium-90-labeled anti-Tac. *Blood.* 1995;86:4063–4075.

102. Foss FM, Raubitschek A, Mulshine JL, et al. Phase I study of the pharmacokinetics of a radioimmunoconjugate, 90Y-T101, in patients with CD5-expressing leukemia and lymphoma. *Clin Cancer Res.* 1998;4:2691–2700.

103. Herrera L, Farah RA, Pellegrini VA, et al. Immunotoxins against CD19 and CD22 are effective in killing precursor-B acute lymphoblastic leukemia cells in vitro. *Leukemia.* 2000;14:853–858.

104. Herrera L, Yarbrough S, Ghetie V, et al. Treatment of SCID/human B cell precursor ALL with anti-CD19 and anti-CD22 immunotoxins. *Leukemia.* 2003;17:334–338.

105. Kreitman RJ, Wilson WH, Bergeron K, et al. Efficacy of the anti-CD22 recombinant immunotoxin BL22 in chemotherapy-resistant hairy-cell leukemia. *N Engl J Med.* 2001;345:241–247.

106. Juweid M, Sharkey RM, Markowitz A, et al. Treatment of non-Hodgkin's lymphoma with radiolabeled murine, chimeric, or humanized LL2, an anti-CD22 monoclonal antibody. *Cancer Res.* 1995;55:5899s–5907s.

107. Juweid ME, Stadtmauer E, Hajjar G, et al. Pharmacokinetics, dosimetry, and initial therapeutic results with 131I- and (111)In-/90Y-labeled humanized LL2 anti-CD22 monoclonal antibody in patients with relapsed, refractory non-Hodgkin's lymphoma. *Clin Cancer Res.* 1999;5:3292s–3303s.

108. Postema EJ, Raemaekers JM, Oyen WJ, et al. Final results of a phase I radioimmunotherapy trial using (186)Re-epratuzumab for the treatment of patients with non-Hodgkin's lymphoma. *Clin Cancer Res.* 2003;9:3995S–4002S.

109. Linden O, Hindorf C, Cavallin-Stahl E, et al. Dose-fractionated radioimmunotherapy in non-Hodgkin's lymphoma using DOTA-conjugated, 90Y-radiolabeled, humanized anti-CD22 monoclonal antibody, epratuzumab. *Clin Cancer Res.* 2005;11:5215–5222.

110. Grossbard ML, Press OW, Appelbaum FR, et al. Monoclonal antibody-based therapies of leukemia and lymphoma. *Blood.* 1992;80:863–878.

111. Zhang M, Yao Z, Zhang Z, et al. The anti-CD25 monoclonal antibody 7G7/B6, armed with the alpha-emitter 211At, provides effective radioimmunotherapy for a murine model of leukemia. *Cancer Res.* 2006;66:8227–8232.

112. Zhang M, Yao Z, Patel H, et al. Effective therapy of murine models of human leukemia and lymphoma with radiolabeled anti-CD30 antibody, HeFi-1. *Proc Natl Acad Sci U S A.* 2007;104:8444–8448.

113. Alinari L, Lapalombella R, Andritsos L, et al. Alemtuzumab (Campath-1H) in the treatment of chronic lymphocytic leukemia. *Oncogene.* 2007;26:3644–3653.

114. Tam CS, Keating MJ. Chemoimmunotherapy of chronic lymphocytic leukemia. *Best Pract Res Clin Haematol.* 2007;20:479–498.

115. Robak T. Recent progress in the management of chronic lymphocytic leukemia. *Cancer Treat Rev.* 2007;33:710–728.

116. De Decker M, Bacher K, Thierens H, et al. In vitro and in vivo evaluation of direct rhenium-188-labeled anti-CD52 monoclonal antibody alemtuzumab for radioimmunotherapy of B-cell chronic lymphocytic leukemia. *Nucl Med Biol.* 2008;35:599–604.

117. Cheson BD. Monoclonal antibody therapy of chronic lymphocytic leukemia. *Cancer Immunol Immunother.* 2006;55:188–196.

118. Friesen C, Glatting G, Koop B, et al. Breaking chemoresistance and radioresistance with [213Bi]anti-CD45 antibodies in leukemia cells. *Cancer Res.* 2007;67:1950–1958.

119. Vandenbulcke K, Thierens H, De Vos F, et al. In vitro screening for synergism of high-linear energy transfer 213Bi-radiotherapy with other therapeutic agents for the treatment of B-cell chronic lymphocytic leukemia. *Cancer Biother Radiopharm.* 2006;21:364–372.

120. Ma D, McDevitt MR, Barendswaard E, et al. Radioimmunotherapy for model B cell malignancies using 90Y-labeled anti-CD19 and anti-CD20 monoclonal antibodies. *Leukemia.* 2002;16:60–66.

121. Vallera DA, Elson M, Brechbiel MW, et al. Radiotherapy of CD19 expressing Daudi tumors in nude mice with Yttrium-90-labeled anti-CD19 antibody. *Cancer Biother Radiopharm.* 2004;19:11–23.

122. Vallera DA, Brechbiel MW, Burns LJ, et al. Radioimmunotherapy of CD22-expressing Daudi tumors in nude mice with a 90Y-labeled anti-CD22 monoclonal antibody. *Clin Cancer Res.* 2005;11:7920–7928.

123. Wesley JN, McGee EC, Garmestani K, et al. Systemic radioimmunotherapy using a monoclonal antibody, anti-Tac directed toward the alpha subunit of the IL-2 receptor armed with the alpha-emitting radionuclides (212)Bi or (211)At. *Nucl Med Biol.* 2004;31:357–364.

124. Vandenbulcke K, De Vos F, Offner F, et al. In vitro evaluation of 213Bi-rituximab versus external gamma irradiation for the treatment of B-CLL patients: relative biological efficacy with respect to apoptosis induction and chromosomal damage. *Eur J Nucl Med Mol Imaging.* 2003;30:1357–1364.

125. Michel RB, Andrews PM, Rosario AV, et al. 177Lu-antibody conjugates for single-cell kill of B-lymphoma cells in vitro and for therapy of micrometastases in vivo. *Nucl Med Biol.* 2005;32:269–278.

126. Postema EJ, Frielink C, Oyen WJ, et al. Biodistribution of 131I-, 186Re-, 177Lu-, and 88Y-labeled hLL2 (Epratuzumab) in nude mice with CD22-positive lymphoma. *Cancer Biother Radiopharm.* 2003;18:525–533.

127. Pagel JM. Radioimmunotherapeutic approaches for leukemia: the past, present and future. *Cytotherapy.* 2008;10:13–20.

128. Lin Y, Pagel JM, Axworthy D, et al. A genetically engineered anti-CD45 single-chain antibody-streptavidin fusion protein for pretargeted radioimmunotherapy of hematologic malignancies. *Cancer Res.* 2006;66:3884–3892.

129. Pagel JM, Hedin N, Drouet L, et al. Eradication of disseminated leukemia in a syngeneic murine leukemia model using pretargeted anti-CD45 radioimmunotherapy. *Blood.* 2008;111:2261–2268.

130. Sharkey RM, Karacay H, Chang CH, et al. Improved therapy of non-Hodgkin's lymphoma xenografts using radionuclides pretargeted with a new anti-CD20 bispecific antibody. *Leukemia*. 2005;19:1064–1069.

131. Zhang M, Zhang Z, Garmestani K, et al. Pretarget radiotherapy with an anti-CD25 antibody-streptavidin fusion protein was effective in therapy of leukemia/lymphoma xenografts. *Proc Natl Acad Sci U S A*. 2003;100:1891–1895.

132. Zhang M, Yao Z, Garmestani K, et al. Pretargeting radioimmunotherapy of a murine model of adult T-cell leukemia with the alpha-emitting radionuclide, bismuth 213. *Blood*. 2002;100:208–216.

133. Chen P, Wang J, Hope K, et al. Nuclear localizing sequences promote nuclear translocation and enhance the radiotoxicity of the anti-CD33 monoclonal antibody HuM195 labeled with 111In in human myeloid leukemia cells. *J Nucl Med*. 2006;47:827–836.

134. Kersemans V, Cornelissen B, Minden MD, et al. Drug-resistant AML cells and primary AML specimens are killed by 111In-anti-CD33 monoclonal antibodies modified with nuclear localizing peptide sequences. *J Nucl Med*. 2008;49:1546–1554.

135. DeNardo GL, Hok S, Van Natarajan A, et al. Characteristics of dimeric (bis) bidentate selective high affinity ligands as HLA-DR10 beta antibody mimics targeting non-Hodgkin's lymphoma. *Int J Oncol*. 2007; 31:729–740.

136. Balhorn R, Hok S, Burke PA, et al. Selective high-affinity ligand antibody mimics for cancer diagnosis and therapy: initial application to lymphoma/leukemia. *Clin Cancer Res*. 2007;13:5621s–5628s.

137. DeNardo GL, Kukis DL, DeNardo SJ, et al. Enhancement of 67Cu-2IT-BAT-LYM-1 therapy in mice with human Burkitt's lymphoma (Raji) using interleukin-2. *Cancer*. 1997;80:2576–2582.

35

Hodgkin Lymphoma

John Okosun and Christopher McNamara

■ INTRODUCTION

Hodgkin lymphoma (HL) affects approximately 8500 new patients in the United States annually (1). The incidence of HL varies considerably but has a bimodal pattern, with the highest incidence seen in young adults and elderly patients (2). HL is a unique malignancy considering its histology. Tumor cells (Hodgkin Reed Sternberg, H-RS) constitute only a minority of the cellular population. The H-RS cells occur among a pleiomorphic background of mixed reactive and inflammatory cells (3).

Selection of the appropriate therapy is based on accurate assessment of disease stage. The treatment of HL has evolved over several decades with advances in combination chemotherapy, radiation techniques, and disease assessment tools rendering the disease as being highly curable (4). Currently, more than 80% of all patients with newly diagnosed HL are likely to be cured of their disease. However, patients with relapsed or refractory disease have a poorer prognosis and pose a significant therapeutic challenge (5). The persistence of residual tumor cells after first-line therapy has been suggested as a reason for this poor outcome (6,7). The introduction of targeted therapeutic approaches offers more options to eradicate residual tumor cells. One such approach is the use of radioimmunotherapy (RIT). HL is an ideal tumor for an RIT approach, given the inherent radiosensitivity of the disease and the differential expression of cell surface antigens on H-RS and background tumor cells, which allow for efficient tumor targeting.

■ PRINCIPLES OF RADIOIMMUNOTHERAPY

RIT dates back more than 20 years and offers a novel strategy of delivering systemic radiation therapy concurrently with immunotherapy to tumor cells by using monoclonal antibodies (MAbs) as tumor-specific targeting constructs. MAbs selected to target tumor-specific antigens are conjugated with a radioactive moiety and are delivered to the target tumor cells. RIT offers several advantages over its individual therapies, that is, MAbs (immunotherapy) and external beam radiotherapy. Since RIT is administered intravenously, multiple tumor sites can be targeted simultaneously with reduced toxicity to normal tissue (i.e., liver, lung, and heart) compared with conventional external beam radiotherapy. A unique feature of radioimmunoconjugates (RIC) not seen with "naked" or "cold" MAbs is the cross-fire

effect, from the particulate radiation, that contributes to increased antitumor cytotoxicity. Through the cross-fire effect, not only are antibody bound cells affected but neighboring cells such as antigen-negative or low-antigen-expressing tumor cells, as well as those that fail to be targeted because of inadequate monoclonal antibody penetration, are killed by the cytocidal energy released by nearby radionuclide decay. The clinical impact of RIT is determined by various factors including the selection of the targeted antigen, type of antibody, and radioisotope used (8,9).

The selection of RIC and their clinical impact is determined by various factors, including the expression of the antigen density in the tumor, availability of specific antibodies, the path length and half-life of the isotope as well as the type of energy the isotope emits. The optimal target antigen for RIT has to fulfill several criteria: (a) it has to be preferentially expressed on the surface of the tumor cells (or in the abnormal tumor stoma or vasculature) in order to allow for targeting of diseased tissue and relative sparing of normal cells, (b) the density or concentration of antigen expression should be such that a threshold amount of radionuclide can be delivered to the tumor, and (c) it should not be secreted into the circulation or undergo modulation on the cell surface. Note that with the use of RIC, internalization of the target after binding to the antibody is not required to be effective, in contrast to targeted delivery of immunotoxins to HL disease sites.

H-RS express high amounts of specific surface antigens such as CD15, CD25, and CD30 and hence provides numerous targets for RIT (10,11).

The effect of the radioisotope is dependent on the following features: (a) nature of the particle energy emitted—isotopes with a long path length of emission are more likely to be effective in large "bulky" tumors, (b) isotope half-life—a short half-life is likely to reduce radiation hazard (exposure and toxicity), and (c) affinity for normal tissue—a lack of binding or reduced accumulation in specific tissues is likely to be safer for clinical use.

The radioisotopes most commonly used in the clinical setting are iodine-131 (^{131}I) or yttrium-90 (^{90}Y). They exhibit relatively simple conjugation chemistry and the energetic particulate radiation, such as β-emission, focuses the radiation dose to defined areas and takes advantage of the cross-fire effect.

The targeting antibody is usually an IgG of murine origin. Chimeric and humanized antibodies for RIT are currently being investigated.

■ EARLY STUDIES AND ANTIFERRITIN

As early as the 1960s, Bonadonna et al. experimented with the use of radiolabeled (^{131}I) lipiodol fluide as endolymphatic radiotherapy by infusing the radionuclide in patients with Hodgkin disease to treat lymphadenopathy (12). Building upon this approach in the 1970s, ferritin was identified as a tumor-associated antigen in many human tumors including HL. Ferritin was synthesized and secreted by tumor infiltrates present in the interstitium but not on the cell surface as a membrane antigen (13). The ferritin molecule consists of a protein shell (apoferritin) composed of heavy (H) and light (L) subunits, which surrounds a crystalline core containing iron oxide and phosphate. Radiolabeled antiferritin (AF) will target the tumor interstitium and "shrink" tumors by the radiation effect, not by an immunologic process (14).

The first clinical trial documenting activity of antibodies against this tumor-associated antigen came from a phase II study using low-dose ^{131}I-labeled polyclonal AF antibody in 38 patients with relapsed or refractory HL (15). In this study, the patients received a total of 50 mCi (30 mCi initially on day 0 and an additional 20 mCi on day 5). Tumor regression was seen in 40% with 1 patient obtaining a complete remission (CR) and 14 patients obtaining a partial remission (PR). Of the 23 patients who underwent a second cycle of therapy, only 2 had improvement in response. The main toxicities

associated with this therapy were hematologic (5% and 10% grade 4 leucopenia and thrombocytopenia, respectively). There were no toxic deaths in this trial (Table 35.1).

A subsequent study used ^{90}Y RIC. The selection of this isotope has theoretical advantages with a higher and more uniform dose distribution and a greater path length, offering the potential for use in patients with disease bulk. Vriesendorp and colleagues performed a phase I/II study with ^{90}Y-labeled polyclonal AF immunoglobulins (20 to 50 mCi) with ($n = 19$) or without ($n = 16$) autologous bone marrow transplantation for patients with refractory HL (16). Seventeen patients (two patients did not target with ^{111}In monoclonal murine antihuman ferritin and were not treated) received doses ranging from 20 to 50 mCi followed by autologous bone marrow support on day 18 with an overall response rate (ORR) of 65% (7 out of 17 achieved a CR and 4 out of 17 achieved a PR). Thirteen patients were treated without bone marrow support (3 patients did not target and were not treated) and received a lower dose (20 mCi) and achieved an ORR of 53% (2 out of 13 achieved a CR and 5 out of 13 achieved a PR). Responses were better in patients with a smaller tumor burden (less than 30 cm^3) compared to large tumors (greater than 500 cm^3). Comparably, the use of lower dose (2 mCi) was just as effective as the higher dose (4 mCi) with reduced bone marrow suppression. All patients experienced hematologic toxicities with three

Table **35.1**	Summary of clinical RIT trials in advanced, relapsed, refractory and heavily pre-treated Hodgkin lymphoma patients					
Reference	**Construct**	**No. of Patients**	**Application**	**Response Rates**	**Toxicity**	**Antigen**
Lenhard et al. (15)	^{131}I-AF	38	Bolus IV 30 mCi D0 Bolus IV 20 mCi D5	40% (1 CR, 14 PR)	Myelosuppression Grade 4 leucopenia 5%	Ferritin
Vriesendorp et al. (16)	^{90}Y-AF	35	Bolus IV 20–50 mCi D1 ± ABMT	62% (9 CR, 9 PR)	Myelosuppression	
Bierman et al. (19)	^{90}Y-AF	12	Bolus IV 20–50 mCi D1 + CBV + ABMT	33% (1 CR, 3 PR, 4 deaths)	Myelosuppression	
Herpst et al. (18)	^{90}Y-AF	39	Bolus IV 10–50 mCi D1	51% (10 CR, 10 PR)	Myelosuppression, mild fever, and fatigue	
Vriesendorp et al. (20)	^{90}Y-AF	90	IV 0.3–0.5 mCi/kg D1 or 2 × 0.25 mCi/kg D1 + 8	42% fr/20% to 86% unfr (15 CR, 29 PR)	Myelosuppression, mild fever, and fatigue	
Decaudin et al. (21)	^{90}Y-AF	10^a	IV 0.2–0.4 mCi/kg D1	70% (1 CR, 6 PR)	Myelosuppression	
Schnell et al. (26)	^{131}I-Ki-4	22	Bolus IV 20–100 mCi D1	41% (1 CR, 5 PR, 3 MR)	Myelosuppression, mild fever, and fatigue	CD30
Dancey et al. (30)	^{131}I-CHT25	11	MTD 1200 MBq/m^2	54% (3 CR, 3 PR)	Myelosuppression, mild fever, and fatigue	CD25
O'Mahony et al. (31–33)	^{90}Y-daclizumab	30	MTD 15 mCi	63% (12 CR, 7 PR)	Myelosuppression, mild fever, and fatigue	

AF, antiferritin; D, day; CR, complete remission; PR, partial remission; MR, minor response (decrease of 25% to 50% of tumor mass); ABMT, autologous bone marrow transplantation; fr, fractionated; unfr, unfractionated; MTD, maximum tolerated dose.
^{a}One patient expired prior to treatment.

patients dying after prolonged bone marrow aplasia. The use of autologous bone marrow infusion did not shorten the duration of the cytopenias. In a follow up of this trial in the same group, after additional accrual with 39 patients evaluable, an ORR of 51% (20/39) was achieved (17,18).

Another trial evaluated the feasibility of combining RIT with high dose chemotherapy followed by autologous bone marrow transplantation. This trial of 12 patients however showed marked toxicity with a 30% (4/12) mortality associated with transplantation (19). Based on these early data, another clinical trial explored the role of fractionating the dose of ^{90}Y-labelled AF. Ninety patients with HL received either fractionated (2 × 0.25 mCi/kg) or unfractionated (0.3 to 0.5 mCi/kg) ^{90}Y-labelled AF. The outcome of the study demonstrated no decrease in hematologic toxicity despite fractionation. The tumor response rate was dose-related with response rates ranging from 22% to 86% and fractionation did not demonstrate considerable benefit in response rates (20).

More recently, Decaudin et al. revisited the safety and efficacy of radiolabeled polyclonal AF antibody in relapsed or refractory HL. Ten patients were entered onto the study with intent to treat, but one patient expired prior to initiating the therapy. The ORR was 78% (1 CR, 6 PR out of 9 treated patients) with a median duration of response of 8 months (21). The experience obtained in the above studies indicates that a low amount of radiolabeled protein can induce a tumor response. It supports the argument of a radiation effect of this particular RIC as opposed to an immunologic process. In addition, a limitation of ^{90}Y-labeled AF therapy highlighted by some of the above studies was its failure to eradicate small-volume disease (less than 1 cm in diameter). These areas of small-volume disease seemed to be the site of recurrence in at least one third of the patients in these studies. The explanations postulated for the lack of targeting of small-volume disease were that such small tumors contained insufficient ferritin or did not possess the tumor neovascularization required for targeting. Of course, it must also be considered that there may be a diminished build up of electronic equilibrium in preangiogenic metastases when using high energy particulate emitters with a maximum range in tissue measured in millimeters. Although ^{90}Y-labeled AF could play a role in the development of less toxic HL therapy, its future is unclear with the advent of specific MAbs directed against cell surface proteins.

ANTI-CD30

The CD30 antigen is an integral membrane glycoprotein (120 kDa) belonging to the tumor necrosis factor (TNF)-receptor superfamily (22). In normal tissues, CD30 is restricted to activated T and B lymphocytes and NK cells. The biological function of CD30/CD30L is not fully understood; it may be involved in stimulation of cell growth and induction of apoptosis (23). In HL, the CD30 ligand CD153 induces signaling via TNF receptor-associated factors 2 and 6 (TRAF-2 and -6) with subsequent NF-κB activation (24,25).

In the only study using an anti-CD30 radioimmunoconstruct, 22 patients with refractory HL and prior CD30 positive biopsies were treated with ^{131}I-Ki-4 (a radioimmunoconstruct consisting of the murine anti-CD30 monoclonal antibody, labeled with iodine-131) targeting the cell surface marker CD30. The ORR was only 41% (9 of 22 patients). A total of 57% of patients experienced progressive disease. Hematologic toxicity was significant and prolonged with 33% (7 of 22 patients) experiencing a grade IV hematologic event. Eighteen percent of the patients developed human antimurine antibodies (HAMA) (26).

ANTI-CD25

Certain hematologic malignancies express abnormally high levels of interleukin (IL)-2Rα (CD25, Tac) including HL. The CD25 molecule is a 55-kDa low affinity IL-2 receptor alpha with expression seen only on activated lymphocytes within normal tissues (27–29). Since CD25 is expressed on H-RS cells as well as bystander T-cells infiltrating the tumor, it provides another target antigen for RIT.

A phase I study was performed to evaluate safety and clinical activity utilizing CHT25 (a chimeric antibody to the alpha chain of the IL2 receptor, CD25) conjugated to iodine-131 (^{131}I) in patients with relapsed or refractory CD25-positive lymphomas. The data were presented at the 2007 meeting of the American Society of Hematology (ASH) by Dancey et al. (30). Eleven patients with HL and three patients with other lymphomas were treated. A maximum tolerated dose (MTD) of 1200 MBq/m^2 was established, defined by an accelerated titration design. Of nine patients treated with a dose of 1200 MBq/m^2 or higher, six responded to therapy (3 CR, 3 PR). The principal toxicity was hematologic, as with previous RIC (Table 35.1). Figures 35.1 and 35.2 represent a PET/CT of a patient with HL before and after treatment with ^{131}I-CHT25, respectively.

Preliminary results of a phase II study were presented at the 2008 meeting of the ASH. In this study, ^{90}Y-radiolabeled humanized monoclonal antibody to CD25 (daclizumab) was used in refractory and relapsed HL. An MTD of 15 mCi ^{90}Y-daclizumab was established and administered every 6 weeks until disease progression. Ca-DTPA was used to reduce bone marrow exposure to free ^{90}Y. Thirty patients with relapsed/refractory HL achieved an ORR of 63% (12 CR, 7 PR). It was noted that many of those that responded were in patients with CD25 negative malignant cells but with surrounding CD25 positive T-cells within the tumor microenvironment. Five patients developed nonsymptomatic human antihuman antibody (HAHA). Thrombocytopenia developed in several patients with seven patients failing to recover their count to above 75 and therapy was halted. Three patients developed MDS (31–33).

FUTURE DIRECTIONS

One of the major issues in the design of future clinical trials is deciding which phase of the therapeutic algorithm RIT should be applied, other than at a time of advanced and progressive chemorefractoriness. Earlier, upfront treatment in patients with poor risk disease may result in a prolonged

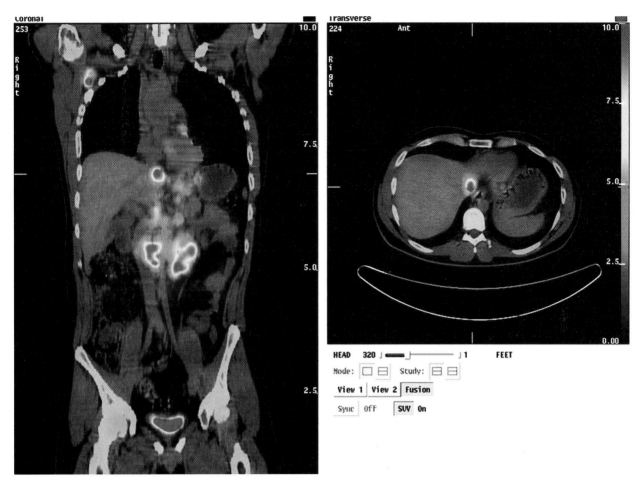

FIGURE 35.1 Fused PET imaging pre-CHT25 treatment in a Hodgkin lymphoma patient showing FDG-avid uptake above and below the diaphragm. (Please see Color Insert).

reduction in bone marrow reserve and may limit or preclude subsequent systemic therapies in the short term. It should be noted, however, that a retrospective review of patients diagnosed with non-Hodgkin lymphoma (NHL), and previously treated with ^{90}Y ibritumomab tiuxetan, revealed that these patients can reasonably undergo other forms of therapy, including autologous stem cell transplantation (34). RIT in HL may also be included alongside already established chemotherapy regimes, as part of first-line treatment but there is a risk of additional toxicity if the side-effect profiles of the two strategies overlap. Finally, RIT in other lymphoproliferative disorders has been approved to consolidate first response in chemosensitive patients, in effect deepening the response to conventional therapies by treating minimal residual disease. So far, trials in HL have limited the use of RIT to the relapsed/refractory disease setting when patients have failed several lines of therapy.

Future developments will require improved efficacy and a decrease of associated toxicities. Although the currently available antibodies are "targeted," there remains an element of nonspecific radiation injury to normal tissue as the RIT constructs circulate to find their target, contributing to toxicity. Although higher doses of RIT tend to be associated with better disease control, the hematologic toxicity becomes

severe and limits use without stem cell rescue strategies. Avenues for development are multiple—new antibody targets, new radionuclides, new molecular constructs, improved dosimetry, fractionation, pretargeting, and newer strategies to prevent or overcome host toxicities. An example is the use of new α-emitters; astatine 211 has a path length that will traverse several cell diameters making it efficient against small cell clusters and its high linear energy transfer increases the probability for cytotoxicity even when targeting low-density antigens.

A very interesting approach is the application of pretargeted RIT to increase the therapeutic window of RIT. The administration of the nonradioactive antitumor antibody is separated in time from the injection of small, radioactive molecules that can bind to the antibody. Thus, the tumor is targeted by the monoclonal antibody, which is allowed to clear from circulation and normal organs. The small radioactive molecules that have affinity to bind to the pretargeted antibody have the advantage that they clear very fast from organs, tissues, and the circulation where no antibody is present, thereby reducing radiation-induced toxicity of normal organs, especially the bone marrow. Thus, these strategies provide increased tumor-to-background ratios and the delivery of a higher therapeutic dose. The use of pretargeted RIT holds promise by reducing toxicity without

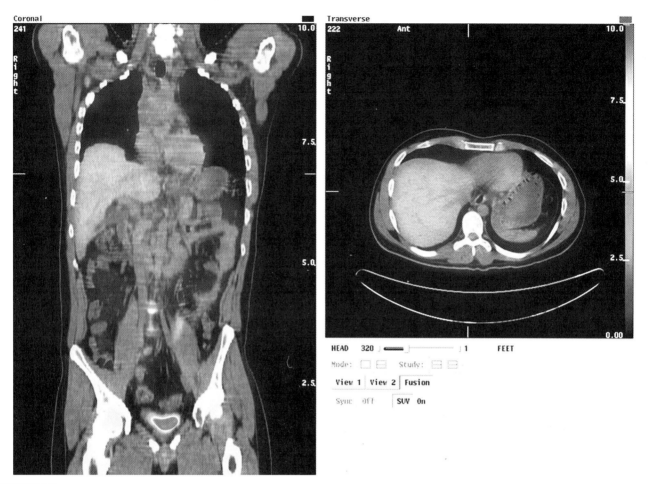

FIGURE 35.2 Same patient post-CHT25 treatment with resolution of FDG uptake in previously diseased areas. Small residual uptake remained in the right axilla. (Please see Color Insert).

sacrificing efficacy. Other methods being considered for reducing toxicities include fractionating the dose of RIT.

It is not established what the long-term side effects of RIT are and it may take several years before its full safety profile is known. One safety issue includes the induction of secondary cancers, such as acute myeloid leukemia (AML) and myelodysplastic syndrome (MDS). The difficulty of defining the rate of MDS or AML associated with RIT is complicated by the fact that nearly all patients have had numerous prior therapies. It is noteworthy that others have not identified an increase in AML or MDS after radionuclide therapy for well-differentiated thyroid cancer (^{131}I) and NHL (^{90}Y ibritumomab or ^{131}I tositumomab), below standard administered activities (35–37). We eagerly await further clinical trials to evaluate these and other questions regarding long-term outcomes of HL patients treated with RIT.

CONCLUSIONS

RIT in Hodgkin disease is still a relatively undefined treatment modality. Despite numerous trials investigating varying RICs, none have advanced into phase III trials. In general, a comparison of RIT techniques of HL and NHL reveals that the HL trials treated patients late in the evolution of disease, used lower antibody mass, and used polyclonal immunoglobulins. As a result, tumor response durations have been measured in months for HL versus years for NHL (38). However, there is growing evidence that RIT can have a significant impact on the treatment of Hodgkin disease. It certainly adds to the therapeutic armory against HL with a targeted approach. With the advent of newer antigen targets and improvement of radioimmunoconstructs, it seems likely that a precise role for RIT will be further refined and our current treatment algorithms may favorably change in the years to come.

REFERENCES

1. Horner MJ, Ries LAG, Krapcho M, et al., eds. *SEER Cancer Statistics Review, 1975–2006*. Bethesda, MD: National Cancer Institute; 2006.
2. Glaser SL, Jarrett RF. The epidemiology of Hodgkin's disease. *Baillieres Clin Haematol*. 1996;9:401–416.
3. Jaffe ES, Harris NL, Stein H, et al., eds. *Pathology and Genetics of Tumours of Haematopoietic and Lymphoid Tissues*. Lyon: IARC Press; 2001.
4. Devita VT Jr, Serpick AA, Carbone PP. Combination chemotherapy in the treatment of advanced Hodgkin's disease. *Ann Intern Med*. 1970;73:881–895.
5. Josting A, Reiser M, Rueffer U, et al. Treatment of primary progressive Hodgkin's and aggressive non-Hodgkin's lymphoma: is there a chance for cure? *J Clin Oncol*. 2000;18:332–339.

6. Gribben JG, Neuberg D, Freedman AS, et al. Detection by polymerase chain reaction of residual cells with the bcl-2 translocation is associated with increased risk of relapse after autologous bone marrow transplantation for B-cell lymphoma. *Blood.* 1993;15:3449–3457.
7. Vockerodt M, Soares M, Kanzler H, et al. Detection of clonal Hodgkin and Reed-Sternberg cells with identical somatically mutated and rearranged VH genes in different biopsies in relapsed Hodgkin's disease. *Blood.* 1998;92:2899–2907.
8. Wilder RB, DeNardo GL, DeNardo SJ. Radioimmunotherapy: recent results and future directions. *J Clin Oncol.* 1996;14:1383–1400.
9. DeNardo SJ, Williams LE, Leigh BR, et al. Choosing an optimal radioimmunotherapy dose for clinical response. *Cancer.* 2002;94(suppl 4):1275–1286.
10. Agnarsson BA, Kadin ME. The immunophenotype of Reed-Sternberg cells: a study of 50 cases of Hodgkin's disease using fixed frozen tissues. *Cancer.* 1989;63:2083–2087.
11. Stein H, Mason DY, Gerdes J, et al. The expression of the Hodgkin's disease associated antigen Ki-1 in reactive and neoplastic lymphoid tissue: evidence that Reed-Sternbery cells and histiocytic malignancies are derived from activated lymphoid cells. *Blood.* 1985;66:848–858.
12. Bonadonna G, Chiappa S, Musumeci R, et al. Endolymphatic radiotherapy in malignant lymphomas. A clinical evaluation of 285 patients. *Cancer.* 1968;22:885–898.
13. Order SE, Porter M, Hellman S. Hodgkin's disease: evidence for a tumor-associated antigen. *N Engl J Med.* 1971;285:471–474.
14. Eshbar Z, Order SE, Katz DH. Ferritin, a Hodgkin's disease associated antigen. *Proc Natl Acad Sci U S A.* 1974;71:3956–3960.
15. Lenhard RE Jr, Order SE, Spunberg JJ, et al. Isotopic immunoglobulin: a new systemic therapy for advanced Hodgkin's disease. *J Clin Oncol.* 1985;3:1296–1300.
16. Vriesendorp HM, Herpst JM, Germack MA, et al. Phase I–II studies of ytrrium-labeled antiferritin treatment for end-stage Hodgkin's disease, including Radiation Therapy Oncology Group 87-01. *J Clin Oncol.* 1991;9:918–928.
17. Vriesendorp HM, Quadri SM, Andersson BS, et al. Recurrence of Hodgkin's disease after indium-111 and ytrrium-90 labeled antiferritin administration. *Cancer.* 1997;80:2721s–2727s.
18. Herpst JM, Klein JL, Leichner PK, et al. Survival of patients with resistant Hodgkin's disease after polyclonal yttrium 90-abeled antiferritin treatment. *J Clin Oncol.* 1995;13:2394–2400.
19. Bierman PJ, Vose JM, Leichner PK, et al. Ytrrium 90-labeled antiferritin followed by high-dose chemotherapy and autologous bone marrow transplantation for poor-prognosis Hodgkin's disease. *J Clin Oncol.* 1993;11:698–703.
20. Vriesendorp HM, Quadri SM, Wyllie CT, et al. Fractionated radiolabelled antiferritin therapy for patients with recurrent Hodgkin's disease. *Clin Cancer Res.* 1999;5:3324s–3329s.
21. Decaudin D, Levy R, Lokiec F, et al. Radioimmunotherapy of refractory or relapsed Hodgkin's lymphoma with 90Y-labelled antiferritin antibody. *Anticancer Drugs.* 2007;18:725–731.
22. Chiarle R, Podda A, Prolla G, et al. CD30 overexpression enhances negative selection in the thymus and mediates programmed cell death via a Bcl-2-sensitive pathway. *J Immunol.* 1999;163:194–205.
23. Chiarle R, Podda A, Prolla G, et al. CD30 in normal and neoplastic cells. *Clin Immunol.* 1999;90:157–164.
24. Wiley SR, Goodwin RG, Smith CA. Reverse signaling via CD30 ligand. *J Immunol.* 1996;157:3635–3639.
25. Horie R, Watanabe T. CD30: expression and function in health and disease. *Semin Immunol.* 1998;10:457–470.
26. Schnell R, Dietlein M, Staak JO, et al. Treatment of refractory Hodgkin's lymphoma patients with an iodine-131-labelede murine anti-CD30 monoclonal antibody. *J Clin Oncol.* 2005;23:4669–4678.
27. Robb RJ, Munck A, Smith KA. T-cell growth factor receptors. *J Exp Med.* 1982;154:1455–1474.
28. Waldmann TA. The structure, function, and expression of interleukin-2 receptors on normal and malignant T-cells. *Science.* 1986;232:727–732.
29. Robb RJ, Kutny RM. Structure-function relationships for the IL-2 receptor system. *J Immunol.* 1987;139:855–862.
30. Dancey G, Violet J, Othman S, et al. Phase I Trial of the ^{131}I-labelled anti-CD25 antibody basiliximab in the treatment of patients with relapsed or refractory lymphoma. *Blood.* 2007(ASH Annual Meeting Abstracts) 110: Abstract 648.
31. O'Mahony D, Morris J, Carrasquillo J, et al. Phase I/II study of yttrium-90 labeled humanized anti-Tac (HAT) monoclonal antibody and calcium DTPA in CD25-expressing malignancies. *J Nucl Med.* 2006;47(suppl 1):98P.
32. O'Mahony D, Janik J, Carrasquillo J, et al. Phase I/II study of yttrium-90 labeled humanized anti-Tac (HAT) monoclonal antibody and calcium DTPA in adult T-cell leukaemia/lymphoma (ATL). *J Nucl Med.* 2006;47(suppl 1):483P.
33. O'Mahony D, Janik JE, Carrasquillo JA, et al. Yttrium-90 radiolabeled humanized monoclonal antibody to CD25 in refractory and relapsed Hodgkin's lymphoma. 2008; ASH Annual Meeting Abstracts: Abstract 231.
34. Ansell SM, Schilder RJ, Pieslor PC, et al. Antilymphoma treatments given subsequent to yttrium 90 ibritumomab tiuxetan are feasible in patients with progressive non-Hodgkin's lymphoma: a review of the literature. *Clin Lymphoma.* 2004;5:202–204.
35. Verkooijen RB, Smit JW, Romijn JA, et al. The incidence of second primary tumors in thyroid cancer patients is increased, but not related to treatment of thyroid cancer. *Eur J Endocrinol.* 2006;155:801–806.
36. Czuczman MS, Emmanouilides C, Darif M, et al. Treatment-related myelodysplastic syndrome and acute myelogenous leukemia in patients treated with ibritumomab tiuxetan radioimmunotherapy. *J Clin Oncol.* 2007;25:4285–4292.
37. Kaminski MS, Tuck M, Estes J, et al. ^{131}I-Tositumomab therapy as initial treatment for follicular lymphoma. *N Engl J Med.* 2005;352:441–449.
38. Vriesendorp HM, Quadri SM. Radiolabeled immunoglobulin therapy in patients with Hodgkin's disease. *Cancer Biother Radiopharm.* 2000;15:431–445.

Targeted Radiotherapy for the Treatment of Multiple Myeloma

Kim Orchard

INTRODUCTION

Multiple myeloma (MM) is a malignant condition characterized by the clonal proliferation of plasma cells. In the last decade, several small molecule agents have been introduced that are highly effective in tumor reduction; consequently, the treatment options for patients have increased with improved remission rates and duration of response, but despite these developments the condition remains incurable. A characteristic of the disease is the acquisition of drug resistance leading to treatment failure and eventually untreatable disease. External beam radiotherapy has been used to control localized disease activity and is highly effective even in late-stage disease as malignant plasma cells retain sensitivity to radiation after acquiring resistance to chemotherapy. High-dose therapy with stem cell transplantation has been shown to improve response rates and leads to longer lasting remissions. The addition of radiation to high-dose chemotherapy prior to stem cell transplantation would seem to be a logical treatment strategy; however, conventional external beam total body irradiation (TBI) causes excessive toxicity with no overall benefit. Targeted radiotherapy would seem to be an appropriate approach retaining the benefits of radiation but potentially avoiding the toxicity of TBI. Phase I trials using targeted radiotherapy have had some encouraging results, but the future of this form of radiation delivery in treatment pathways for patients with myeloma will depend upon carefully constructed randomized clinical trials.

INCIDENCE AND SURVIVAL

MM is the second commonest hematologic malignancy after non–Hodgkin lymphoma causing approximately 1% of all cancers and 15% of hematologic malignancies. In the United Kingdom, the nonadjusted annual incidence per 100,000 population was 6.6, and there were nearly 4000 new cases reported in 2006 (data from CRUK *weblink* (1)). In the USA, the overall incidence is similar at 6.0 per 100,000 with nearly 20,000 new cases reported in 2008. In both countries there is a distinct sex difference with a lower incidence in females than in males (5.9 vs. 7.3), while USA data show a higher incidence in African-Americans than in Caucasians

(13 vs. 7.1). The reasons for these gender and ethical influences on the incidence are unknown. There is also a clear age relationship; the incidence increases steadily from age of 50 years rising to a peak incidence in the population over 80 years at 60 cases per annum per 100,000 population. It is relatively uncommon for the first three decades of life. In the USA, in 2005, it was estimated that 56,000 individuals were living with myeloma (data from MMRF *weblink* (2)). Survival figures for myeloma appear to be disappointing reflecting the fact that with current treatment options, despite major advances in the last decade, the condition remains incurable. At 1 year following diagnosis 65% of patients are alive, by 5 years this has fallen to 25%, and at 10 years only 15% of patients survive. Although many of these patients are older than 70 years of age, most of the deaths are due to myeloma or from complications arising from the disease.

DISEASE CHARACTERISTICS AND DIAGNOSTIC CRITERIA

MM is characterized by the clonal proliferation of plasma cells. In the majority of cases, the disease arises in the plasma cell population residing within red marrow and dissemination throughout all red marrow sites is usual, but extramedullary disease is not uncommon. The distribution of the disease in the marrow is often patchy and variable; at one extreme the plasma cell population may appear to be much localized forming a solitary collection of tumor cells termed a plasmacytoma, but in most patients at diagnosis there is a distinct plasma cell infiltration throughout the marrow. The variation of tumor burden, disease distribution at the time of presentation together with biologic diversity of the disease has led to the need for a set of diagnostic criteria formalized by the International Myeloma Working Group (3,4). These diagnostic criteria help to discriminate between clonal plasma cell disorders that do not require treatment, such as monoclonal gammopathy of uncertain significance (MGUS) and smoldering myeloma, from active MM that requires therapy. At presentation, MM is classified using disease-specific parameters that relate to the tumor burden and that also have some significance for prognosis. The Durie–Salmon Staging System (5) was extensively used, but more recently the International Staging System was introduced, which has a more direct link to prognosis (6,7). MM is diagnosed from a combination of factors that include the presence of a monoclonal band in serum (paraprotein) or urine (either kappa or lambda light chains termed "Bence-Jones protein") detected by electrophoresis, elevated serum free light chains (either kappa or lambda), suppression of normal antibody production (immuneparesis), an increase in plasma cells in the bone marrow (BM), and lytic bone lesions detected by skeletal imaging (plain x-ray, computed tomography, or magnetic resonance imaging [MRI]) (8). Patients frequently present with or develop complications such as anemia, infection, renal impairment, and electrolyte disturbances such as hypercalcemia, hyperviscosity, and pathologic fractures (often vertebral bodies) with associated severe pain. Localized lesions can cause direct organ damage; cord compression is not uncommon and requires urgent treatment, usually involving external beam radiotherapy.

BIOLOGY

Although MM is a malignant condition of mature plasma cells, there is considerable evidence that the malignant cell population is intimately dependent on nonmalignant cells and structural proteins within the BM microenvironment. These nonmalignant elements include BM stromal cells, endothelial cells, and the extracellular matrix all of which interact with the malignant plasma cells through direct contact and secreted cytokines (9). Key to the malignant process is the acquisition of certain cytogenetic changes that may precede the full malignant phenotype. Patients with MGUS and symptomatic MM have demonstrated similar chromosomal changes (10). A wide range of analytical methods have been used to untangle the complexities of MM genetics, including G-band karyotyping, fluorescent in situ hybridization, expression array profiling, and comparative genomic hybridization. These techniques and others have transformed the understanding of the underlying genetic changes that cause myeloma and have led to the creation of a molecular classification system (10). One model of the disease is of a progression from MGUS to smoldering myeloma, symptomatic myeloma, and in the later stages of the disease loss of dependence for the BM microenvironment with the appearance of extramedullary disease and plasma cell leukemia (11,12). These genetic analytical technologies have not only given insights into disease pathogenesis but also generated prognostic information that may form the basis for individualized treatment decisions in the future. Expression profiling could, in theory, be used to discover not only new disease-specific targets for small molecule development but also targets for radioimmunotherapy.

The tumor cell characteristically has the morphologic appearance of a mature plasma cell (Fig. 36.1), but abnormal forms can be found with multiple nuclei and prominent intracellular vacuoles. A feature of poor-prognosis MM is the presence of less mature plasmablastic cells. In parallel

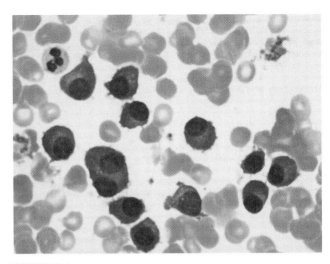

FIGURE 36.1 Malignant plasma cells from a patient with de novo myeloma. (Please see Color Insert).

with the mature phenotype, malignant plasma cells express surface antigens that are present on normal plasma cells. These could potentially be used as targets for radioimmunotherapy. Some of these plasma cell surface antigens are detailed in Table 36.1.

TREATMENT AND OUTCOMES

For many years the standard treatment of MM was with melphalan and prednisolone, inducing responses but with a median duration of response of only 24 months and median survival of approximately 3 years (13,14). More intensive combinational drug therapy schedules were introduced using agents that were considered to have activity against plasma cells—vincristine, adriamycin, prednisolone (VAD) and cyclophosphamide (C-VAD) or adriamycin, carmustine, cyclophosphamide, and melphalan (ABCM). Although able to induce remissions, these were of relatively short duration and had little impact on the duration of survival (13,15,16). A number of trials completed in the 1990s showed that the use of high-dose chemotherapy followed by autologous BM or peripheral blood stem cell rescue increased the response rate, disease- free survival, and overall survival, but the majority of patients relapse within 5 years (17–19) (reviewed in (20,21)). The origin of cells causing relapse in these patients is not known but must arise either from the reinfusion of tumor cells contaminating autologous material or from inadequate elimination of disease by the conditioning regimen or a combination of the two. Increased tumor reduction in vivo could, in theory, be possible by further increasing the conditioning therapy. This has been tested in a number of studies using additional chemotherapeutic agents or with the addition of external beam radiotherapy as TBI (22). However, intensification of conditioning therapy has been associated with significant increase in toxicity (22,23).

Table **36.1**	Surface antigens expressed by plasma cells (PC)				
CD Number	Alternative Name	Size	Expression	Function	Expression Level on PC
CD38	T10	45 kD	Plasma cells T and B lymphocytes Variable level on other hematopoietic cells Malignant plasma cells	ecto-ADP-ribosyl cyclase, cell activation	High
CD56	NCAM	175–185 kD	NK, T-cell subset, neuron Large granular lymphocyte leukemia Myeloid leukemias	Cell adhesion	Moderate
CD66a	CEACAM-6	160–180 kD	Plasma cells Myeloid cells Epithelial cells	Cell adhesion	Moderate
CD126	IL-6R	80 kD	Plasma cells Activated B cells Most leukocytes[a] Fibroblasts	IL-6 receptor alpha chain	Moderate
CD138	Syndecan-1	80–150 kD	Plasma cells Pre-B lymphocytes Basolateral surface of epithelial cells Neurons	Receptor for ECM	High
SIg	Surface immunoglobulin	150 kD	Plasma cells B lymphocytes	Antigen recognition	High
BLyS receptor			Plasma cells B lymphocytes	Receptor for BlyS Cell signaling/activation	Moderate

[a]Also low level or variable expression of the following: CD9, CD19, CD20, CD10, CD28.

Since the late 1990s, research into new agents active against malignant plasma cells has rapidly expanded, introducing small molecule agents such as thalidomide, bortezomib (Velcade), and lenalidomide (Revlimid). These drugs have greater activity against malignant plasma cells and after initially being used for relapsed disease are now being tested in de novo disease. Early results indicate improved disease responses and duration of response compared with established induction schedules (24,25); however, it is very unlikely that they will be curative and high-dose therapy with stem cell transplantation remains an important treatment modality.

The toxicity associated with increasing the components of high-dose therapy has led to the development of tandem autologous transplants, which allows the delivery of treatment intensification with less toxicity than the equivalent treatment in a single transplant event (21,26,27). Some trials have shown a clear benefit of such approaches, while in other clinical trials the results are less obvious (28). This may, in part, be due to the heterogeneity of MM and the fact that due to excessive toxicity in some trials few patients received the second transplant.

A feature of disease progression in myeloma is the appearance of chemotherapy resistance, due to the expression of the multidrug resistance mediated by P-glycoprotein, multidrug resistance–related protein, or the major vault protein (29–32). Resistance to the more recently developed drugs does occur and although the overall survival period appears to be extended by these agents, the disease invariably recurs. In the later stages of the disease, secondary mutational events appear in MYC, RAS family, TP53, RB1 loss of function of cyclin-dependent kinase inhibitors, and other genes (8). These changes may be the cause for an increasingly aggressive phenotype characteristic of late-stage myeloma with reduced responses to chemotherapy, shorter response periods, and preterminal complications arising from the disease.

■ THE ROLE OF RADIOTHERAPY IN MYELOMA

Radiotherapy has an important role in the management of patients with myeloma and is frequently used to treat localized disease–causing pain or serious disease-related complications such as lytic bone lesions, pathologic fracture, or spinal cord compression. The external beam total body radiotherapy has been used as a component of high-dose therapy prior to hematopoietic stem cell transplantation (HSCT), in both autologous and allogeneic transplantation. In autologous HSCT, the role of TBI has been formally tested in a randomized trial by the Intergroupe Francophone du Myélome (22). Patients were randomized after induction therapy with three cycles of VAD to undergo an autologous HSCT with either TBI 8 Gy plus melphalan 140 mg/m^2 or melphalan 200 mg/m^2 for conditioning. The median duration of event-free survival was similar in both arms (21 vs. 20.5 months), but there was a significant difference in the incidence of gastrointestinal (GI) toxicity grades 3 or 4 in the TBI-containing arm. In addition, there were five toxicity-related deaths in the TBI group but none in the melphalan alone group, although this did not reach statistical significance. The results suggested that TBI in this patient group (median age was 60 years in arm A and 61 years in arm B) has excessive toxicity with no overall benefit with remission rates similar in each arm (CR for arm A 29%, arm B 35% $p = 0.41$).

In the allogeneic transplant setting, a combination of TBI and melphalan conditioning can produce high CR rates and long-term disease-free survival. Russell et al. published the results of a small series of younger patients (median age 49 years) with myeloma who had received a combination of melphalan 110 mg/m^2 and a TBI dose of 12 Gy given as six fractions (33). There were no deaths due to organ toxicity but six deaths due to viral pneumonitis. A high remission rate was achieved with 18 of 19 surviving patients achieving CR. This is in contrast to the results of allogeneic stem cell transplantation using conditioning schedules that lack TBI where the relapse rate is high (34). These results suggest that TBI may have an important role in the preparative conditioning prior to allogeneic HSCT for younger patients and those with an available donor. However, the majority of patients with MM are elderly and although autologous HSCT may be possible, they are unlikely to tolerate the full toxicities associated with an allogeneic transplant using TBI. The implication from these data is that radiation, if it can be delivered effectively to all sites of disease, can result in major responses that are sustained.

Therapeutic strategies that exploit the inherent radiosensitivity of malignant plasma cells while reducing the nonspecific toxicity caused by total body external beam irradiation have been tested clinically. These fall into three broad types:

1. Total marrow irradiation using helical tomography in combination with chemotherapy in either autologous or allogeneic transplantation conditioning protocols (35–37).
2. Targeted radiotherapy using radiolabeled bone-seeking agents.
3. Targeted radiotherapy targeting the cellular component of BM.

Total marrow irradiation

Total marrow (and lymphatic) irradiation (TMI) using helical tomography is essentially a form of TBI with modified organ shielding. A detailed description of this technique lies

outside of this chapter, however the procedure has been previously well described (38,39). TMI is technically difficult, but it has the potential to reduce radiation dose exposure of nonhematopoietic organs while maintaining the proper dose to the marrow and lymphatic system. A number of small studies have reported a reduction in the median radiation dose received by nonhematopoietic organs of between 35% and 70% while delivering an estimated 12 Gy to the BM (38,40). One of the first reports of TMI in the context of HSCT for myeloma was from Tübingen in 2003. Einsele et al. reported the use of TMI combined with busulphan (12 mg/kg) and cyclophosphamide (120 mg/kg) as conditioning prior to autologous HSCT. TMI radiation dose was 9 Gy in six fractions with 90% of lung and liver were shielded and separate electron beam treatment given to rib areas protected from the TMI (35). Overall response rates were good with 39 out of 89 (44%) patients achieving CR and 50 out of 89 (56%) a PR. In patients with de novo myeloma, the CR rate was similar at 48%. However, toxicity to nonhematopoietic tissues was high with 68 out of 89 (76%) patients experiencing GI toxicity grade 3 to 4. Durations of stay in hospital were also longer than for high-dose melphalan due to the long (12 days) pretreatment before stem cell infusion.

Wong et al. described the use of image-guided TMI in 13 patients undergoing autologous HSCT. They used a tandem transplant approach with the first transplant using high-dose melphalan (200 mg/m^2) followed after an interval of 6 weeks by a TMI-alone conditioned transplant. This was a phase I radiation dose escalation study with dose levels of 10, 12, 14, and 16 Gy to the target volume. They report a reduction of critical organ doses between 15% and 65% of the gross target volume dose. All patients engrafted and toxicities were acceptable with no grade 4 toxicity to nonhematopoietic organs (37). TMI would appear to be an acceptable form of therapy prior to HSCT but requires considerable planning of dose delivery in each patient. The radiation dose delivered to the BM is similar to that achieved by TBI but without the same degree of toxicity to nonhematopoietic organs.

Targeted radiotherapy

Targeted radiotherapy, selectively delivering therapeutic doses of radiation by intravenous infusion, is a logical development for the treatment of MM. The site of disease is largely within the BM, which is highly vascular and readily accessible to agents delivered via the bloodstream. In addition, the continuous, low dose rate delivered by the natural decay of a targeted radionuclide may have a greater destructive effect on tumor cells than single-dose or fractionated external beam radiation (41,42). Malignant plasma cells may be targeted by either indirect or direct routes. The indirect method may involve the delivery of a radionuclide to close proximity of malignant plasma cells either by targeting the mineral component of trabecular bone or by targeting the cellular elements of the marrow, which is composed predominantly of hematopoietic tissue. Direct targeting would require the targeting of plasma cell–specific antigens as described in Table 36.1. The indirect routes have some inherent weaknesses; for example, malignant plasma cells can form large aggregates within the marrow space and may also expand outside of the bone into soft tissues. In addition, true extramedullary disease can occur, which develops in nonosseous sites. In these situations, the indirect targeting routes will result in reduced irradiation of these nonbone and nonhematopoietic deposits.

Indirect targeting via bone-seeking agents

Radiation may be directed to sites of disease by the use of bone-seeking agents such as bisphosphonates. The concept behind this form of targeted radiotherapy is that malignant plasma cells are often associated with areas of bone destruction and are present in the marrow adjacent to trabecular bone. These agents have a high affinity for areas of active bone turnover and by binding to the mineral component of bone localize the chelated radioisotope at this anatomical site. The cross-fire effect of the delivered radiation will irradiate not only the peritrabecular cells but also deeper into the cellular marrow space. These agents can be readily radiolabeled with a number of radiometals as they also function as chelating agents. Two such agents have been used clinically in patients with MM: 1,4,7,10-tetraazcyclododecane-1,4,7,10-tetramethylenephosphonate (DOTMP) labeled with the radionuclide holmium-166 (^{166}Ho-DOTMP) (43) and ethylenediaminetetramethylenephosphonate (EDTMP) labeled with Samarium-153 (^{153}Sm-EDTMP, Quadramet) (44). ^{166}Ho emits a high-energy beta particle and has a relatively short half-life of 26.8 hours. It has been used as complexed to EDTMP or DOTMP in a canine model and caused marrow aplasia that could be reversed by BM transplantation (45,46). ^{153}Sm has a slightly longer half-life of 46.3 hours and emits a beta particle of medium energy and a gamma photon allowing dosimetry.

^{166}Ho complexed to DOTMP has been used clinically as part of the conditioning in addition to high-dose melphalan prior to autologous stem cell transplantation for patients with myeloma (47). In a phase I radiation dose escalation study, patients received increasing doses of ^{166}Ho-DOTMP; the infused dose of ^{166}Ho was determined from initial dosimetry and calculated to deliver an absorbed radiation dose of 20, 30, or 40 Gy to the marrow. Patients were randomized to receive in addition 140- or 200-mg/m^2 melphalan or 140-mg/m^2 melphalan plus 800-cGy TBI. Fifty-four patients received treatment, 43% achieving a complete remission. There were no differences in response rates between the various treatment arms. The most significant problems were renal toxicity and hemorrhagic cystitis. These toxicities may have been a consequence of using an isotope with a relatively short half-life, the high energy of the beta emission, and the high renal excretion rate for the complex. Of particular concern in a subsequent phase I/II trial was renal toxicity with grades 2 to 4 in 30% of patients and late renal toxicity in 18% of patients, largely associated with a dose of ^{166}Ho greater than 1200 mCi/m^2 (40 Gy to

BM) (47). In addition, 7 of 83 patients experienced complications considered due to thrombotic microangiography, but this complication was apparent only in patients who had received a dose of ^{166}Ho-DOTMP calculated to deliver 30 Gy to the BM. Significant dose inhomogeneity was also seen, probably due to the unequal uptake of the bisphosphonate by the skeleton (43,48). In a later retrospective analysis, 41 patients who had received ^{166}Ho-DOTMP as part of the conditioning prior to autologous HSCT were compared with 63 patients who had received high-dose melphalan alone in the same institution over a similar period of time (49). Although this form of analysis can be criticized on several levels, there were some interesting trends demonstrated. An arbitrary cutoff was made between patients receiving less than 2400 mCi (group A) and more than 2400 mCi (group B) total infused dose of ^{166}Ho-DOTMP. The nonrelapse mortality in group A was 5% and was similar to that seen with high-dose melphalan alone (3.2%) but was an unusually high 20% in group B. In addition, there was a trend toward improved PR to CR conversion rates in the ^{166}Ho-DOTMP-treated groups of patients. This was neither a randomized study nor a case-match retrospective analysis; however, some tentative conclusions could be drawn. The addition of ^{166}Ho-DOTMP may result in improved responses and too much radiation may be detrimental due to increased nonrelapsed mortality as well as probable increased morbidity.

Other groups have used the same concept but utilized ^{153}Sm complexed to EDTMP, available as an agent used for the control of bone pain due to metastatic malignancies (Quadramet). The lower energy of the beta radiation and the longer half-life of the isotope may contribute to the apparently lower toxicity of this agent when used in high doses in the setting of HSCT. Initial preclinical evaluation was performed in a murine myeloma model using the 5T33 cell line and autologous HSCT. Tumor-bearing mice undergoing HSCT received conditioning with melphalan alone or combined with ^{153}Sm-EDTMP. Those receiving the combined conditioning had median survivals 40% longer than those receiving melphalan only and 75% longer than control animals (50). In a phase I radiation dose escalation study, 10 patients were treated with 19 to 45 GBq of ^{153}Sm-EDTMP 12 to 14 days before the standard transplant regimen. Seven of these patients were undergoing HSCT for myeloma. After transplantation, four of seven patients achieved CR (by EBMT criteria), two a PR, and one had stable disease. These initial results were promising with high CR rate and low toxicity (44). An estimated 62% of the infused radiation dose was retained in the skeleton at 24 hours. However, higher infused radiation doses resulted in reduced percentage retention, suggesting that the available binding sites in the skeleton were saturated. Because of this, the maximum radiation dose of ^{153}Sm-EDTMP that could be efficiently infused was 35 GBq (946 mCi). Dosimetry indicated a mean BM absorbed dose of 0.78 and 0.22 Gy/GBq to the bladder and 0.2 Gy/GBq to the liver. A mean absorbed radiation dose of 12 Gy was delivered to the BM for 35-GBq infused radiation

(48). Radiation dose delivered to the limb skeleton was low and external beam limb irradiation was added.

In a separate phase I dose escalation study, 12 patients received doses of ^{153}Sm-EDTMP from 6 to 30 mCi/kg (222 to 1110 MBq/kg) body weight together with high-dose melphalan as the conditioning prior to autologous HSCT. Again toxicities were low and no dose-limiting toxicity was reported, but red marrow absorbed radiation dose varied widely between patients at each dose level with up to fivefold difference. An additional six patients received a dose of ^{153}Sm-EDTMP calculated to deliver 40 Gy to the marrow based on dosimetry determined 1 week prior to therapy. In this dose escalation scenario, the median absorbed radiation dose to the red marrow rose from 6.68 Gy at the first dose level up to 65.25 Gy at the highest dose level. Responses were excellent with 94% of patients achieving either a CR (5 of 18) or very good PR (7 of 18). There were no graft failures and no evidence of late BM fibrosis, suggesting that the BM microenvironment was preserved (51). In contrast to the results of trials with the higher energy/shorter half-life ^{166}Ho-DOTMP, estimated absorbed renal doses were low at all infused dose levels. A phase II trial has been initiated and the results are awaited.

A further refinement of the use of ^{153}Sm-EDTMP to improve on tumor cell reduction was tested in the murine 5TGM1 model of myeloma combining the proteasome inhibitor PS-341 (bortezomib or Velcade) as a radiosensitizing agent (52). A small nontransplant phase I clinical study has been performed combining bortezomib with ^{153}Sm-EDTMP using relatively low doses of infused radiation. A total of 24 patients with relapsed or treatment refractory myeloma were entered into the study, receiving either 1.0 or 1.3 mg/m^2 of bortezomib following a standard treatment schedule (days 1, 4, 8, and 11) with an infusion of ^{153}Sm-EDTMP on day 3 of a 56-days cycle. There were three radiation dose levels, 0.25, 0.5, and 1.0 mCi/kg (9.25, 18.5, and 37 MBq/kg) body weight. Toxicities were mainly hematologic with grade 4 neutropenia (neutrophils less than 0.5×10^9/L) in 12.5% of patients and grade 4 thrombocytopenia (platelets less than 25×10^9/L) in 8.3%. Response rates in this poor-risk group of patients were good with three patients achieving a CR (53). These results indicate that for patients who are unsuitable for high-dose therapy and autologous HSCT an alternative effective salvage using a bone-seeking radionuclide can be safely given with good effect. It would be interesting to see whether further increases in the infused radiation dose combined with bortezomib would result in improved CR rates in a transplant setting.

Targeted radiotherapy directed at bone marrow and/or tumor cells

Targeted radiotherapy, using a monoclonal antibody as vector targeting hematopoietic tissues, could allow treatment intensification without toxicity to nonhematologic tissues and may improve dose distribution to red marrow. Several groups have used targeted radiotherapy directed

against antigens associated with hematopoietic cells, in the setting of stem cell transplantation for acute leukemia and lymphoma but not specifically for patients with myeloma (reviewed in (54–56)). The published trials have exploited antigens such as CD45, CD33, and CD66 for myeloid malignancies or CD20 for lymphoma. Potential antigenic targets on plasma cells are listed in Table 36.1 with some of their characteristics. However, excellent potential target antigens present on plasma cells such as CD38 and CD138 do not seem to have as yet been exploited. In patients with myeloma, the post–induction therapy tumor cell burden may be low and theoretically targeting myeloid antigens such as CD45 or CD33 would indirectly irradiate plasma cells interspersed with normal marrow elements. However, this does not seem to have been attempted in published trials. Our own group has tested the potential of an anti-CD138 (anti-syndecan-1) monoclonal antibody as a vector for targeted radiotherapy specifically in patients with myeloma. Three patients with variable levels of plasma cell percentage in the marrow were imaged using ^{111}In-labeled murine anti-CD138 (provided by Dr John Wijdenes, Besançon). Figure 36.2 shows a gamma image of one patient who had approximately 30% plasma cells in the marrow. The image shows good BM localization of the labeled antibody and binding in the spleen, but the uptake by the liver was also high, possibly due to expression of the antigen on hepatocytes or liver endothelial cells. This would result in unacceptable radiation doses to the liver if a therapeutic dose of a radioisotope such as ^{90}Y was used. There was a correlation

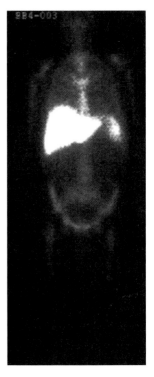

FIGURE 36.2 Gamma camera image of patient with de novo myeloma 24 hours following infusion of 2-mg anti-Syndecan-1 antibody radiolabeled with ^{111}In. Although there is uptake in the red marrow, the uptake by the liver is high.

between the plasma cell percentage in the BM and estimated radiation dose.

THE POTENTIAL OF CD66 AS A TARGET IN MYELOMA THERAPY

CD66 is a member of the carcinoembryonic antigen (CEA) family of membrane proteins which is itself a member of the immunoglobulin superfamily of receptors. CD66 actually consists of several structurally related glycoproteins, CD66a to f, four of which (CD66a to d) are expressed by neutrophils (57). CD66 cluster members also have other designations—CD66a is also termed biliary glycoprotein or cell adhesion molecule-1 (CEACAM-1); CD66b as CGM6, nonspecific crossreacting antigen 95 (NCA95) or CEACAM-8; CD66c as NCA50/90 or CEACAM-6; and CD66d as CGM1 or CEACAM-3. CD66 family members are thought to function as cell adhesion molecules interacting with E-selectin, galectins, and type 1 fimbriae of *Escherichia coli* (58). The CD66 antigens a to d are expressed on normal myeloid cells from the promyelocyte stage through to mature neutrophils. They are also upregulated by neutrophil activation signals. Expression of CD66 isoforms on hematopoietic tissue was thought to be restricted to the myeloid lineage.

Since 2002, a targeted radiotherapy program in Southampton has tested the use of a radiolabeled anti-CD66 murine monoclonal antibody as part of the conditioning therapy prior to stem cell transplantation. In a similar fashion to other groups, the approach adopted was to use ^{111}In-labeled anti-CD66 for imaging and dosimetry and ^{90}Y-labeled anti-CD66 for therapy. In a phase I radiation dose escalation study, 20 patients received the radiolabeled anti-CD66 as part of the conditioning prior to either an autologous HSCT ($n = 16$) for MM, or an allogeneic HSCT for MM ($n = 2$) or acute myeloid leukemia ($n = 2$). Figure 36.3 shows a typical gamma camera image from one of the patients after infusion of the ^{111}In-labeled anti-CD66. Excellent BM localization is shown, with minimal uptake by nonhematopoietic organs such as the liver and kidneys. At the highest radiation dose in the phase I study, 37.5 MBq/kg body weight of ^{90}Y-labeled anti-CD66 was infused delivering an estimated dose of radiation to the BM of 25 Gy, 6 Gy to the liver, and 2 Gy to the kidneys. We noted an unusual localization of ^{111}In-labeled antibody in one patient (Fig. 36.4). This patient had active myeloma at the time of imaging with a detectable paraprotein. In addition, they had pain in the right knee, the site of particularly intensive antibody localization. Following treatment with ^{90}Y-labeled anti-CD66, the pain resolved. A subsequent MRI scan revealed a small lytic lesion in the distal right femur. This suggested the possibility that CD66 was present on malignant plasma cells and in vivo directly targeting foci of plasma cells. Flow cytometry confirmed the presence of CD66 on myeloma cell lines and plasma cells from patients with myeloma, more specifically only CD66a (CEACAM-1) was detected on plasma cells (59). The favorable pharmacokinetics of the anti-CD66 and the presence of the target

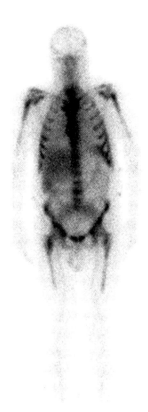

FIGURE 36.3 Gamma camera images of a patient with myeloma prior to autologous HSCT. Images generated following infusion of 1.5 mg of ^{111}In-labeled anti-CD66 monoclonal antibody (185 MBq). The ^{111}In-labeled antibody localizes in red marrow with little uptake in nonhaematopoietic organs.

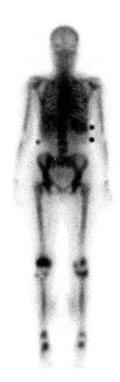

FIGURE 36.4 Gamma camera image of a patient with active myeloma: the image was generated following the infusion of 185 MBq of ^{111}In-labeled anti-CD66 monoclonal antibody. Note the unusual distribution of uptake and focal localization in the right distal femur, the site of a lytic lesion revealed by MRI scan.

antigen on malignant plasma cells make this a particularly interesting target for antibody-delivered radionuclide therapy. A randomized phase II clinical trial is now open, testing the efficacy of the ^{90}Y-labeled anti-CD66 when used with high-dose melphalan in the conditioning prior to autologous HSCT compared to high-dose melphalan alone in the control arm.

CONCLUDING REMARKS

Although the treatment of myeloma has radically changed in the last decade with the development of several new small molecule agents, stem cell transplantation remains an important therapy for consolidation of responses induced by chemotherapy. Retrospective analysis of outcomes following autologous stem cell transplantation indicates that the achievement of complete remission appears to result in longer disease-free survival. Targeted radiotherapy using bone-seeking agents or targeting the cellular components of marrow has been shown to be well tolerated and, for some agents, with little or no additional toxicity. These early-phase clinical trials have demonstrated that targeted radiotherapy can be safely used in conjunction with standard conditioning prior to transplantation. The hope is that this additive approach can further increase the response rates after high-dose therapy leading to greater improvements in response duration. These early clinical trials have established some of the treatment parameters, whether the addition of the best performing agents to HSCT protocols can result in better response rates and longer duration of remission needs to be tested in randomized clinical trials.

REFERENCES

1. CRUK. Multiple myeloma statistics—UK [web page]. 2009; Available at: http://info.cancerresearchuk.org/cancerstats/types/multiple-myeloma/index.htm?script=true. Accessed January 8, 2010.
2. MMRF. Causes and incidence of multiple myeloma [web page]. 2009; Available at: http://www.themmrf.org/living-with-multiple-myeloma/newly-diagnosed-patients/what-is-multiple-myeloma/causes-and-incidence.html. Accessed January 8, 2010.
3. Group IMW. Criteria for the classification of monoclonal gammopathies, multiple myeloma and related disorders: a report of the International Myeloma Working Group. *Br J Haematol.* 2003;121(5):749–757.
4. Kyle RA, Rajkumar SV. Criteria for diagnosis, staging, risk stratification and response assessment of multiple myeloma. *Leukemia.* 2009;23(1):3–9.
5. Durie BG, Salmon SE. A clinical staging system for multiple myeloma. Correlation of measured myeloma cell mass with presenting clinical features, response to treatment, and survival. *Cancer.* 1975;36(3):842–854.
6. Greipp PR, San Miguel J, Durie BG, et al. International staging system for multiple myeloma. *J Clin Oncol.* 2005;23(15):3412–3420.
7. Hari PN, Zhang MJ, Roy V, et al. Is the International Staging System superior to the Durie-Salmon staging system? A comparison in multiple myeloma patients undergoing autologous transplant. *Leukemia.* 2009;23(8):1528–1534.
8. Raab MS, Podar K, Breitkreutz I, et al. Multiple myeloma. *Lancet.* 2009;374(9686):324–339.
9. Burger JA, Ghia P, Rosenwald A, et al. The microenvironment in mature B-cell malignancies: a target for new treatment strategies. *Blood.* 2009;114(16):3367–3375.
10. Fonseca R, Bergsagel PL, Drach J, et al. International Myeloma Working Group molecular classification of multiple myeloma: spotlight review. *Leukemia.* 2009;23(12):2210–2221.
11. Kuehl WM, Bergsagel PL. Multiple myeloma: evolving genetic events and host interactions. *Nat Rev Cancer.* 2002;2(3):175–187.
12. Kyle RA, Therneau TM, Rajkumar SV, et al. A long-term study of prognosis in monoclonal gammopathy of undetermined significance. *N Engl J Med.* 2002;346(8):564–569.
13. Alexanian R, Dimopoulos M. Drug therapy: the treatment of multiple myeloma. *N Engl J Med.* 1994;330(7):484–489.
14. Barlogie B, Jagannath S, Epstein J, et al. Biology and therapy of multiple myeloma in 1996. *Semin Hematol.* 1997;34(1 suppl 1):67–72.
15. Myeloma Trialists' Collaborative Group. Combination chemotherapy versus melphalan plus prednisone as treatment for multiple myeloma: an overview of 6,633 patients from 27 randomized trials. *J Clin Oncol.* 1998;16(12):3832–3842.
16. Diagnosis and management of multiple myeloma. *Br J Haematol.* 2001;115(3):522–540.
17. Attal M, Harousseau JL, Stoppa AM, et al. A prospective, randomized trial of autologous bone marrow transplantation and chemotherapy in multiple myeloma. Intergroupe Francais du Myelome. *N Engl J Med.* 1996;335(2):91–97.
18. Child JA, Morgan GJ, Davies FE, et al. High-dose chemotherapy with hematopoietic stem-cell rescue for multiple myeloma. *N Engl J Med.* 2003;348(19):1875–1883.
19. Lenhoff S, Hjorth M, Holmberg E, et al. Impact on survival of high-dose therapy with autologous stem cell support in patients younger than 60 years with newly diagnosed multiple myeloma: a population-based study. Nordic Myeloma Study Group. *Blood.* 2000;95(1):7–11.
20. Barlogie B, Shaughnessy J, Tricot G, et al. Treatment of multiple myeloma. *Blood.* 2004;103(1):20–32.
21. Samson D. High-dose therapy in multiple myeloma. *Curr Opin Hematol.* 1996;3(6):446–452.
22. Moreau P, Facon T, Attal M, et al. Comparison of 200 mg/m(2) melphalan and 8 Gy total body irradiation plus 140 mg/m(2) melphalan as conditioning regimens for peripheral blood stem cell transplantation in patients with newly diagnosed multiple myeloma: final analysis of the Intergroupe Francophone du Myelome 9502 randomized trial. *Blood.* 2002;99(3):731–735.
23. Abraham R, Chen C, Tsang R, et al. Intensification of the stem cell transplant induction regimen results in increased treatment-related mortality without improved outcome in multiple myeloma. *Bone Marrow Transplant.* 1999;24(12):1291–1297.
24. Kyle RA, Rajkumar SV. Treatment of multiple myeloma: a comprehensive review. *Clin Lymphoma Myeloma.* 2009;9(4):278–288.
25. Laubach JP, Mahindra A, Mitsiades CS, et al. The use of novel agents in the treatment of relapsed and refractory multiple myeloma. *Leukemia.* 2009;23(12):2222–2232.
26. Barlogie B, Jagannath S, Desikan KR, et al. Total therapy with tandem transplants for newly diagnosed multiple myeloma. *Blood.* 1999;93(1):55–65.
27. Barlogie B, Jagannath S, Vesole DH, et al. Superiority of tandem autologous transplantation over standard therapy for previously untreated multiple myeloma. *Blood.* 1997;89(3):789–793.
28. Kumar A, Kharfan-Dabaja MA, Glasmacher A, et al. Tandem versus single autologous hematopoietic cell transplantation for the treatment of multiple myeloma: a systematic review and meta-analysis. *J Natl Cancer Inst.* 2009;101(2):100–106.
29. Grogan TM, Spier CM, Salmon SE, et al. P-glycoprotein expression in human plasma cell myeloma: correlation with prior chemotherapy. *Blood.* 1993;81(2):490–495.
30. Rimsza LM, Campbell K, Dalton WS, et al. The major vault protein (MVP), a new multidrug resistance associated protein, is frequently expressed in multiple myeloma. *Leuk Lymphoma.* 1999;34(3–4):315–324.
31. Schwarzenbach H. Expression of MDR1/P-glycoprotein, the multidrug resistance protein MRP, and the lung-resistance protein LRP in multiple myeloma. *Med Oncol.* 2002;19(2):87–104.
32. Sonneveld P. Multidrug resistance in haematological malignancies. *J Intern Med.* 2000;247(5):521–534.
33. Russell N, Bessell E, Stainer C, et al. Allogeneic haematopoietic stem cell transplantation for multiple myeloma or plasma cell leukaemia using fractionated total body radiation and high-dose melphalan conditioning. *Acta Oncol.* 2000;39(7):837–841.
34. Crawley C, Iacobelli S, Bjorkstrand B, et al. Reduced-intensity conditioning for myeloma: lower nonrelapse mortality but higher relapse rates compared with myeloablative conditioning. *Blood.* 2007;109(8):3588–3594.

35. Einsele H, Bamberg M, Budach W, et al. A new conditioning regimen involving total marrow irradiation, busulfan and cyclophosphamide followed by autologous PBSCT in patients with advanced multiple myeloma. *Bone Marrow Transplant.* 2003;32(6):593–599.

36. Shueng PW, Lin SC, Chong NS, et al. Total marrow irradiation with helical tomotherapy for bone marrow transplantation of multiple myeloma: first experience in Asia. *Technol Cancer Res Treat.* 2009;8(1):29–38.

37. Wong JY, Rosenthal J, Liu A, et al. Image-guided total-marrow irradiation using helical tomotherapy in patients with multiple myeloma and acute leukemia undergoing hematopoietic cell transplantation. *Int J Radiat Oncol Biol Phys.* 2009;73(1):273–279.

38. Hui SK, Kapatoes J, Fowler J, et al. Feasibility study of helical tomotherapy for total body or total marrow irradiation. *Med Phys.* 2005;32(10):3214–3224.

39. Wong JY, Liu A, Schultheiss T, et al. Targeted total marrow irradiation using three-dimensional image-guided tomographic intensity-modulated radiation therapy: an alternative to standard total body irradiation. *Biol Blood Marrow Transplant.* 2006;12(3):306–315.

40. Schultheiss TE, Wong J, Liu A, et al. Image-guided total marrow and total lymphatic irradiation using helical tomotherapy. *Int J Radiat Oncol Biol Phys.* 2007;67(4):1259–1267.

41. Knox SJ. Overview of studies on experimental radioimmunotherapy. *Cancer Res.* 1995;55(23 suppl):5832s–5836s.

42. Wessels BW, Vessella RL, Palme DF II, et al. Radiobiological comparison of external beam irradiation and radioimmunotherapy in renal cell carcinoma xenografts. *Int J Radiat Oncol Biol Phys.* 1989;17(6):1257–1263.

43. Breitz H, Wendt R, Stabin M, et al. Dosimetry of high dose skeletal targeted radiotherapy (STR) with 166Ho-DOTMP. *Cancer Biother Radiopharm.* 2003;18(2):225–230.

44. Macfarlane DJ, Durrant S, Bartlett ML, et al. 153Sm EDTMP for bone marrow ablation prior to stem cell transplantation for haematological malignancies. *Nucl Med Commun.* 2002;23(11):1099–1106.

45. Appelbaum FR, Brown PA, Sandmaier BM, et al. Specific marrow ablation before marrow transplantation using an aminophosphonic acid conjugate 166Ho-EDTMP. *Blood.* 1992;80(6):1608–1613.

46. Parks NJ, Kawakami TG, Avila MJ, et al. Bone marrow transplantation in dogs after radio-ablation with a new Ho-166 amino phosphonic acid bone-seeking agent (DOTMP). *Blood.* 1993;82(1):318–325.

47. Giralt S, Bensinger W, Goodman M, et al. 166Ho-DOTMP plus melphalan followed by peripheral blood stem cell transplantation in patients with multiple myeloma: results of two phase 1/2 trials. *Blood.* 2003;102(7):2684–2691.

48. Bartlett ML, Webb M, Durrant S, et al. Dosimetry and toxicity of Quadramet for bone marrow ablation in multiple myeloma and other haematological malignancies. *Eur J Nucl Med Mol Imaging.* 2002;29(11):1470–1477.

49. Christoforidou AV, Saliba RM, Williams P, et al. Results of a retrospective single institution analysis of targeted skeletal radiotherapy with (166)Holmium-DOTMP as conditioning regimen for autologous stem cell transplant for patients with multiple myeloma. Impact on transplant outcomes. *Biol Blood Marrow Transplant.* 2007;13(5):543–549.

50. Turner JH, Claringbold PG, Manning LS, et al. Radiopharmaceutical therapy of 5T33 murine myeloma by sequential treatment with samarium-153 ethylenediaminetetramethylene phosphonate, melphalan, and bone marrow transplantation. *J Natl Cancer Inst.* 1993;85(18):1508–1513.

51. Dispenzieri A, Wiseman GA, Lacy MQ, et al. A phase I study of 153Sm-EDTMP with fixed high-dose melphalan as a peripheral blood stem cell conditioning regimen in patients with multiple myeloma. *Leukemia.* 2005;19(1):118–125.

52. Goel A, Dispenzieri A, Geyer SM, et al. Synergistic activity of the proteasome inhibitor PS-341 with non-myeloablative 153-Sm-EDTMP skeletally targeted radiotherapy in an orthotopic model of multiple myeloma. *Blood.* 2006;107(10):4063–4070.

53. Berenson JR, Yellin O, Patel R, et al. A phase I study of samarium lexidronam/bortezomib combination therapy for the treatment of relapsed or refractory multiple myeloma. *Clin Cancer Res.* 2009;15(3):1069–1075.

54. Buchmann I, Meyer RG, Mier W, et al. Myeloablative radioimmunotherapy in conditioning prior to haematological stem cell transplantation: closing the gap between benefit and toxicity? *Eur J Nucl Med Mol Imaging.* 2009;36(3):484–498.

55. Orchard K, Cooper M. Targeting the bone marrow: applications in stem cell transplantation. *Q J Nucl Med Mol Imaging.* 2004;48(4):267–278.

56. Pagel JM, Matthews DC, Appelbaum FR, et al. The use of radioimmunoconjugates in stem cell transplantation. *Bone Marrow Transplant.* 2002;29(10):807–816.

57. Klein ML, McGhee SA, Baranian J, et al. Role of nonspecific cross-reacting antigen, a CD66 cluster antigen, in activation of human granulocytes. *Infect Immun.* 1996;64(11):4574–4579.

58. Skubitz KM, Campbell KD, Skubitz AP. Synthetic peptides of CD66a stimulate neutrophil adhesion to endothelial cells. *J Immunol.* 2000;164(8):4257–4264.

59. Lee C, Guinn BA, Brooks SE, et al. CD66a (CEACAM1) is the only CD66 variant expressed on the surface of plasma cells in multiple myeloma: a refined target for radiotherapy trials? *Br J Haematol.* 2010;149(5):795–796.

Osteosarcoma: An Opportunity for Targeted Radiotherapy

Peter Anderson

Osteosarcoma is a unique tumor in that pathologic diagnosis requires not only recognition of the cancer cell in the tumor but also recognition of a product, osteoid (bone formed by the tumor), to achieve the diagnosis. This characteristic of osteosarcoma, formation of bone by malignant cells, provides the opportunity for radioisotopes to image and treat these tumors. Table 37.1 describes clinical characteristics of osteosarcoma biology and therapy that are important in understanding the role of different modalities of imaging and treatment in the multidisciplinary care of these young patients. Osteosarcoma is treated with surgery and amputations tend to be less common today (1–4). Chemotherapy is extremely important for eradication of micrometastases (5–7) and the addition of the macrophage activator L-MTP-PE (MEPACT) has recently shown a benefit with an increased overall survival in newly diagnosed patients (8–10). Despite the known effectiveness of radiation against osteosarcoma (11,12), this tumor is not particularly radiation sensitive and until recently the trend seemed to be less utilization of radiation and a greater reliance on surgery (1). Nevertheless, recent clinical results indicate that radiation can provide benefit in a variety of situations including limb salvage (13), treatment of unresectable tumors (14–19), and control of metastases (19–21). Surgery, if possible, is very important in the goal to eradicate metastases (22,23). The combination of chemotherapy and radiotherapy is probably more effective than either modality alone (12,15,19,21). Bone–seeking radioisotope therapy is currently used for the palliation of pain and as part of multidisciplinary approaches for treatment of unresectable osteosarcoma tumors (19–21,24–28). Alkaline phosphatase is a serum marker for osteosarcoma in humans that reflects tumor burden and potentially the effectiveness of treatment (29–34).

^{99m}Tc-MDP (i.e., standard "bone scan") (35–37) and ^{18}FDG (i.e., PET-CT) are very useful for the staging of osteosarcoma, including evaluation of the primary tumor and metastases (38,39). Response as determined by PET-CT has been shown to have prognostic significance in osteosarcoma (40,41). Because the diphosphonate moiety of ^{99m}Tc-MDP is taken up selectively by osteosarcoma cells that are forming osteoid in the tumor mass, both bone and soft-tissue components of osteosarcoma are avid and images indicate how well the neoplastic cells function as bone-forming cells. Although most osteosarcoma primary tumors image fairly well with ^{99m}Tc-MDP, uptake in lung metastases can be minimal or absent (42). The author has observed that some cases of osteosarcoma with metastases are discordant in terms of ^{18}FDG uptake (PET-CT scan) and bone scan. Thus, a bone scan may be considered as a good screening test of whether bone–seeking radioisotope therapy could be of benefit. PET-CT is more useful for following response than bone scintigraphy. Increased uptake of ^{99m}Tc-MDP by unresectable or metastatic osteosarcoma indicates a potential opportunity for a targeted therapy with a bone–seeking therapeutic isotope that is specifically taken up by the neoplastic cells. All of the clinically useful beta emitters, except for ^{89}SrCl, emit gamma radiation, which is useful for imaging and providing a quantitative estimate of radiation dose to the tumor, if serial scans are performed (Table 37.2).

The physical half-life and the bone and red marrow biodistribution are important characteristics in the choice of a bone–seeking radiopharmaceutical for the treatment of osteosarcoma; characteristics of available radiopharmaceuticals are summarized in Table 37.3. Considering high-dose radiopharmaceutical therapy, the instillation of stem cells should occur when the decay of the radionuclide has reached a level that is not cytotoxic to circulating stem cells. The author used a body burden of 3.6 mCi as an acceptable amount of residual radioactivity of ^{153}Sm-EDTMP for safe stem cell infusion (43). Because alpha emitters are high linear energy transfer (LET) and exhibit less "cross-fire effect" (Table 37.4), ^{223}Ra may become a more useful agent for osteosarcoma therapy.

Of all the clinically available radiopharmaceuticals, ^{153}Sm-EDTMP has had the most clinical success in the treatment of osteosarcoma. This isotope was initially developed by William Goeckeler (44). Treatment of dogs with osteosarcoma resulted in a significant clinical usefulness in this disease, with smaller tumors having more durable responses (45,46). Other investigators have used ^{153}Sm-EDTMP to provide a benefit in dogs with osteosarcoma (46–48). Isolated limb perfusion studies of ^{153}Sm-EDTMP at Colorado State (Nicole Ehrhart, DVM, personal communication) showed nonhomogenous distribution of ^{153}Sm-EDTMP deposition. Thus, ^{153}Sm-EDTMP plus external beam RT may be the most effective combination to provide radiation to all

Table **37.1**	Clinical observations of osteosarcoma biology and current therapy approaches

Characteristic	Observation
Age	Peak incidence in 2nd and 3rd decade (i.e., during rapid growth of long bones)
Bone formation	High formation in osteoblastic primary osteosarcoma tumors and bone metastases
	Often low formation in osteosarcoma lung metastases
Initial therapy	Neoadjuvant chemotherapy, surgery, then adjuvant chemotherapy (established paradigm for nonmetastatic tumors)
Recurrence	Surgery
Metastases	Very poor prognosis for bone metastases
	Pain palliation and quality of life are major goals
	Often "chemotherapy resistant"
	Bone–seeking radionuclide therapy may reduce pain and serum alkaline phosphatase
Radiotherapy (RT)	External beam: usually daily fractionated treatments in 1–5 weeks; retreatment is difficult
	Bone–seeking isotopes: low dose rate; repeated treatments may be possible
Unresectable tumors	External beam RT + bone–seeking radioisotope may help control

portions of osteosarcoma tumors. Because of the "bone-only" distribution and short half-life of ^{153}Sm-EDTMP, autologous peripheral blood stem cells or marrow infusion have also been investigated as a means to increase dose of ^{153}Sm-EDTMP (26–28,43,49). A recent dose-finding study showed 1.2 mCi/kg was the maximum tolerated dose in osteosarcoma patients with prior treatment (50). The use of stem cell infusions allowed 30 mCi/kg to be safely infused compared to the standard 1 mCi/kg (43,49). Gemcitabine is a powerful radiosensitizer and is capable of increasing radiation damage to cells (51,52). Thus, when using a bone–seeking radioisotope with a radiosensitizer, the protocol should consist of administering the radiosensitizer only after unbound radiopharmaceutical has been eliminated from the

Table **37.2**	Gamma scintigraphy using bone–seeking radiopharmaceuticals (photon emissions for "bone scans" showing targeted radioisotopes)

	Decay		
Drug	Energy (keV)	Abundance (%)	Imaging
^{99m}Tc-MDP	141	89	Yes
^{153}Sm-EDTMP	103	29	Yes
^{186}Re-HEDP	137	10	Yes
^{223}RaCl	81	15	Yes
	84	26	Yes
	269	14	Yes
^{89}SrCl$_2$	None	0	No

circulation; this should reduce the toxicity to organs such as the kidney and bladder. Thus, when a radiosensitizer is given 1 day after ^{153}Sm-EDTMP (i.e., after ^{153}Sm-EDTMP is bound to bone and unbound has passed out of the kidney and bladder), an increased radiation effect is seen (49). The clinical use of ^{153}Sm-EDTMP in osteosarcoma with and without external beam radiotherapy has been reviewed previously (21,24,25). An example of a patient with osteoblastic osteosarcoma metastases treated with ^{153}Sm-EDTMP is shown in Figure 37.1.

^{223}Ra is a powerful, but very selective bone–seeking alpha emitter (53). It has an improved bone surface: red marrow biodistribution ratio compared to ^{89}SrCl and ^{153}Sm-EDTMP (Table 37.2). The ^{223}Ra decay pathway is depicted in Figure 37.2. Selective targeting of osseous sites by ^{223}Ra was initially described by Henriksen et al. (54). Mechanism of selective sequestration in bone appears to be via a more general pathway involving osteoblastic cell metabolism having a large quantity of a ferritin isoform involved in long-term storage of heavy metals (55). Relative marrow sparing in preclinical studies was shown by dose-related depletion of osteoblasts; ablation of marrow and blood production was not seen (56). Canine biodistribution studies of ^{223}Ra also showed affinity and stability within calcified tissue (53). Unbound ^{223}Ra is eliminated via the gastrointestinal system. Because of the short range of the emitted alpha particle, the intestinal wall dose is low and comparable to other soft tissue (53). Since very high ^{223}Ra accumulations are seen in osteoblastic bone (53), ^{223}Ra may be an ideal candidate for osteosarcoma therapy (Fig. 37.3).

Because of rarity of osteosarcoma compared to other skeletal metastases, clinical development of ^{223}Ra has been

Table **37.3** Decay and marrow/bone ratios of clinically useful bone–seeking isotopes				
			MeV Particle	
RadioPharmaceutical	Half-Life (Days)	Ratio of Surface Bone: Red Marrow	Particle	Emission Energy Range (mm)
153Sm-EDTMP	2	4.4	Beta	0.66 max
				0.6
				0.22 average
89SrCl2	50.5	1.6	Beta	0.58
				2.4
223RaCl	11.4	10.3	Alpha	27.4
				<0.1
			+Beta	

*a*Bone surface to red bone marrow radioactivity dose ratio.

Table **37.4** Comparison of alpha and beta emissions of bone–seeking radioisotopes		
Characteristic	Alpha	Beta
Range (μm)	40–90	50–6000
Linear energy transfer (LET; keV/μm)	60–230	0.015–0.4
Relative mass	7000*a*	1*a*
DNA hits to kill a cell	1–5	100–1000
Cytotoxic against G0 cells	Yes	No
Effective against "radio-resistant" cells	Yes	No

*a*Alpha particles are dense particles (helium nucleus); beta particles are electrons.

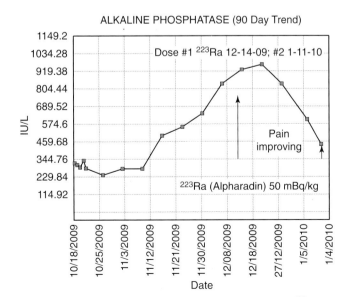

FIGURE 37.1 Osteoblastic osteosarcoma after treatment with 223Ra. The graph depicts a decrease in alkaline phosphatase after treatment in a 22-year old with osteosarcoma metastatic to the right mandible, left maxilla, right femur, sacrum, and spine. Pain was also improved after therapy with the alpha emitter.

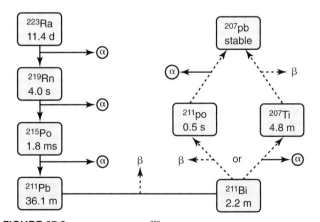

FIGURE 37.2 Decay cascade of 223Ra. The initial ejection of the high LET alpha particle takes a relatively long time ($t_{1/2}$ 11.4 days). Subsequent quick decay of radon daughters (minutes, seconds, milliseconds) yields an additional 3 alpha particles + 2 beta particles before the stable 207Pb isotope is formed. Alpha emissions account for about 94% of the emitted energy of 223Ra. In 2 months (~5 half-lives), only about 1/32 of initial 223Ra radioactivity remains. The 223Ra isotope is more safe than 224Ra because the radon daughter of 223Ra (219Rn) has a half-life of only 4 seconds compared to 56 seconds for the 220Rn daughter of 224Ra; thus there is less chance for diffusion away from the osteosarcoma tumor or bone.

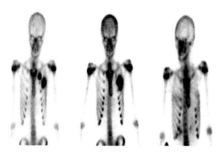

FIGURE 37.3 Osteosarcoma of the chest wall, presenting with a malignant pleural effusion, became localized to rib/chest wall after chemotherapy. **Left:** After 1 mCi/kg[153]Sm-EDTMP. Gamma imaging shows uptake in two sites; the patient also received 48 Gy external beam radiation. **Middle:** 14 months later 1 mCi/kg [153]Sm-EDTMP scan of solitary lesion recurrence and retreatment. **Right:** ^{99m}Tc-MDP bone scan 3 and 4 years after samarium scans (**left, middle**) and subsequent resection of chest wall mass. This patient also received L-MTP-PE (8–10) and has had no local recurrence in the lungs or chest wall.

with more common clinical problems, prostate and breast cancer bone metastases. Excellent pain relief was reported in these cancer patients with skeletal metastases in the initial phase I trial of [223]Ra (57). Production of the isotope for clinical use, dose estimates in humans, and development of [223]Ra as a bone–seeking radiopharmaceutical was described by Bruland et al. (53). A randomized phase II study in prostate cancer bone metastases using 50 kBq/kg showed clinical benefit without significant myelotoxicity and significantly reduced bone alkaline phosphatase (p less than 0.001) (58). Because of these promising results, [223]Ra is currently in phase III clinical trials. In 2009, the first patient was treated with [223]Ra on a compassionate basis (Oyvind Bruland, personal communication). The second patient was treated at MD Anderson; in both patients a decreased alkaline phosphatase and pain improvement were seen (Fig. 37.3). Thus, the era of using [223]Ra for osteoblastic osteosarcoma, which should selectively accumulate [223]Ra at disease sites, has just begun.

■ REFERENCES

1. Aksnes LH, Hall KS, Folleraas G, et al. Management of high-grade bone sarcomas over two decades: the Norwegian Radium Hospital experience. *Acta Oncol.* 2006;45(1):38–46.
2. Lewis VO. What's new in musculoskeletal oncology. *J Bone Joint Surg Am.* 2007;89(6):1399–1407.
3. Lewis VO. Limb salvage in the skeletally immature patient. *Curr Oncol Rep.* 2005;7(4):285–292.
4. Bielack S, Carrle D, Jost L. Osteosarcoma: ESMO clinical recommendations for diagnosis, treatment and follow-up. *Ann Oncol.* 2008; 19(suppl 2):ii94–ii96.
5. Ferguson WS, Goorin AM. Current treatment of osteosarcoma. *Cancer Invest.* 2001;19(3):292–315.
6. Marina N, Gebhardt M, Teot L, et al. Biology and therapeutic advances for pediatric osteosarcoma. *Oncologist.* 2004;9(4):422–441.
7. Gorlick R, Anderson P, Andrulis I, et al. Biology of childhood osteogenic sarcoma and potential targets for therapeutic development: meeting summary. *Clin Cancer Res.* 2003;9(15):5442–5453.
8. Meyers PA, Schwartz CL, Krailo MD, et al. Osteosarcoma: the addition of muramyl tripeptide to chemotherapy improves overall survival—a report from the Children's Oncology Group. *J Clin Oncol.* 2008;26(4):633–638.
9. Chou AJ, Kleinerman ES, Krailo MD, et al. Addition of muramyl tripeptide to chemotherapy for patients with newly diagnosed metastatic osteosarcoma: a report from the Children's Oncology Group. *Cancer.* 2009;115(22):5339–5348.
10. Meyers PA. Muramyl tripeptide (mifamurtide) for the treatment of osteosarcoma. *Expert Rev Anticancer Ther.* 2009;9(8):1035–1049.
11. Anderson P. Osteosarcoma relapse: expect the worst, but hope for the best. *Pediatr Blood Cancer.* 2006;47(3):231.
12. Anderson P, Salazar-Abshire M. Improving outcomes in difficult bone cancers using multimodality therapy, including radiation: physician and nursing perspectives. *Curr Oncol Rep.* 2006;8(6):415–422.
13. Dincbas FO, Koca S, Mandel NM, et al. The role of preoperative radiotherapy in nonmetastatic high-grade osteosarcoma of the extremities for limb-sparing surgery. *Int J Radiat Oncol Biol Phys.* 2005;62(3):820–828.
14. Machak GN, Tkachev SI, Solovyev YN, et al. Neoadjuvant chemotherapy and local radiotherapy for high-grade osteosarcoma of the extremities. *Mayo Clin Proc.* 2003;78(2):147–155.
15. Anderson PM. Effectiveness of radiotherapy for osteosarcoma that responds to chemotherapy. *Mayo Clin Proc.* 2003;78(2):145–146.
16. DeLaney TF, Park L, Goldberg SI, et al. Radiation therapy for local control of osteosarcoma. *Int J Radiat Oncol Biol Phys.* 2003;57(2 suppl):S449.
17. DeLaney TF, Park L, Goldberg SI, et al. Radiotherapy for local control of osteosarcoma. *Int J Radiat Oncol Biol Phys.* 2005;61(2):492–498.
18. Kamada T, Tsujii H, Tsuji H, et al. Efficacy and safety of carbon ion radiotherapy in bone and soft tissue sarcomas. *J Clin Oncol.* 2002;20(22):4466–4471.
19. Anderson P, Kornguth D, Ahrar K, et al. Recurrent, refractory, metastatic, and/or unresectable pediatric sarcomas: treatment options for young people that are off the roadmap. *Pediatr Health.* 2008;2:605–615.
20. Mahajan A, Woo SY, Kornguth DG, et al. Multimodality treatment of osteosarcoma: radiation in a high-risk cohort. *Pediatr Blood Cancer.* 2008;50(5):976–982.
21. Anderson P, Aguilera D, Pearson M, et al. Outpatient chemotherapy plus radiotherapy in sarcomas: improving cancer control with radiosensitizing agents. *Cancer Control.* 2008;15(1):38–46.
22. Bielack SS, Kempf-Bielack B, Branscheid D, et al. Second and subsequent recurrences of osteosarcoma: presentation, treatment, and outcomes of 249 consecutive cooperative osteosarcoma study group patients. *J Clin Oncol.* 2009;27(4):557–565.
23. Kempf-Bielack B, Bielack SS, Jurgens H, et al. Osteosarcoma relapse after combined modality therapy: an analysis of unselected patients in the Cooperative Osteosarcoma Study Group (COSS). *J Clin Oncol.* 2005;23(3):559–568.
24. Anderson P. Samarium for osteoblastic bone metastases and osteosarcoma. *Expert Opin Pharmacother.* 2006;7(11):1475–1486.
25. Anderson P, Nunez R. Samarium lexidronam ([153]Sm-EDTMP): skeletal radiation for osteoblastic bone metastases and osteosarcoma. *Expert Rev Anticancer Ther.* 2007;7(11):1517–1527.
26. Franzius C, Bielack S, Flege S, et al. High-activity samarium-153-EDTMP therapy followed by autologous peripheral blood stem cell support in unresectable osteosarcoma. *Nuklearmedizin.* 2001;40(6):215–220.
27. Franzius C, Bielack S, Sciuk J, et al. High-activity samarium-153-EDTMP therapy in unresectable osteosarcoma. *Nuklearmedizin.* 1999; 38(8):337–340.
28. Franzius C, Schuck A, Bielack SS. High-dose samarium-153 ethylene diamine tetramethylene phosphonate: low toxicity of skeletal irradiation in patients with osteosarcoma and bone metastases. *J Clin Oncol.* 2002;20(7):1953–1954.
29. Ehrhart N, Dernell WS, Hoffmann WE, et al. Prognostic importance of alkaline phosphatase activity in serum from dogs with appendicular osteosarcoma: 75 cases (1990–1996). *J Am Vet Med Assoc.* 1998; 213(7):1002–1006.
30. Ferrari S, Bertoni F, Mercuri M, et al. Predictive factors of disease-free survival for non-metastatic osteosarcoma of the extremity: an analysis of 300 patients treated at the Rizzoli Institute. *Ann Oncol.* 2001; 12(8):1145–1150.
31. Wang J, Pei F, Tu C, et al. Serum bone turnover markers in patients with primary bone tumors. *Oncology.* 2007;72(5–6):338–342.
32. Anh DJ, Dimai HP, Hall SL, et al. Skeletal alkaline phosphatase activity is primarily released from human osteoblasts in an insoluble form, and the net release is inhibited by calcium and skeletal growth factors. *Calcif Tissue Int.* 1998;62(4):332–340.
33. Bacci G, Ferrari S, Longhi A, et al. High-grade osteosarcoma of the extremity: differences between localized and metastatic tumors at presentation. *J Pediatr Hematol Oncol.* 2002;24(1):27–30.

34. Bacci G, Longhi A, Ferrari S, et al. Prognostic significance of serum alkaline phosphatase in osteosarcoma of the extremity treated with neoadjuvant chemotherapy: recent experience at Rizzoli Institute. *Oncol Rep.* 2002;9(1):171–175.

35. Malmud LS, Charkes ND. Bone scanning: principles, technique and interpretation. *Clin Orthop Relat Res.* 1975;107:112–122.

36. Toegel S, Hoffmann O, Wadsak W, et al. Uptake of bone-seekers is solely associated with mineralisation! A study with ^{99m}Tc-MDP, ^{153}Sm-EDTMP and 18F-fluoride on osteoblasts. *Eur J Nucl Med Mol Imaging.* 2006;33(4):491–494.

37. Soderlund V. Radiological diagnosis of skeletal metastases. *Eur Radiol.* 1996;6(5):587–595.

38. Brenner W, Bohuslavizki KH, Eary JF. PET imaging of osteosarcoma. *J Nucl Med.* 2003;44(6):930–942.

39. Peterson JJ, Kransdorf MJ, O'Connor MI. Diagnosis of occult bone metastases: positron emission tomography. *Clin Orthop Relat Res.* 2003(415 suppl):S120–S128.

40. Costelloe CM, Macapinlac HA, Madewell JE, et al. 18F-FDG PET/CT as an indicator of progression-free and overall survival in osteosarcoma. *J Nucl Med.* 2009;50(3):340–347.

41. Franzius C, Bielack S, Flege S, et al. Prognostic significance of (18)F-FDG and (99m)Tc-methylene diphosphonate uptake in primary osteosarcoma. *J Nucl Med.* 2002;43(8):1012–1017.

42. Rees CR, Siddiqui AR, duCret R. The role of bone scintigraphy in osteogenic sarcoma. *Skeletal Radiol.* 1986;15(5):365–367.

43. Anderson PM, Wiseman GA, Dispenzieri A, et al. High-dose samarium-153 ethylene diamine tetramethylene phosphonate: low toxicity of skeletal irradiation in patients with osteosarcoma and bone metastases. *J Clin Oncol.* 2002;20(1):189–196.

44. Goeckeler WF, Troutner DE, Volkert WA, et al. ^{153}Sm radiotherapeutic bone agents. *Int J Rad Appl Instrum B.* 1986;13(4):479–482.

45. Lattimer JC, Corwin LA Jr., Stapleton J, et al. Clinical and clinicopathologic response of canine bone tumor patients to treatment with samarium-153-EDTMP. *J Nucl Med.* 1990;31(8):1316–1325.

46. Barnard SM, Zuber RM, Moore AS. Samarium Sm 153 lexidronam for the palliative treatment of dogs with primary bone tumors: 35 cases (1999–2005). *J Am Vet Med Assoc.* 2007;230(12):1877–1881.

47. Milner RJ, Dormehl I, Louw WK, et al. Targeted radiotherapy with Sm-153-EDTMP in nine cases of canine primary bone tumours. *J S Afr Vet Assoc.* 1998;69(1):12–17.

48. Moe L, Boysen M, Aas M, et al. Maxillectomy and targeted radionuclide therapy with ^{153}Sm-EDTMP in a recurrent canine osteosarcoma. *J Small Anim Pract.* 1996;37(5):241–246.

49. Anderson PM, Wiseman GA, Erlandson L, et al. Gemcitabine radiosensitization after high-dose samarium for osteoblastic osteosarcoma. *Clin Cancer Res.* 2005;11(19 pt 1):6895–6900.

50. Loeb DM, Garrett-Mayer E, Hobbs RF, et al. Dose-finding study of ^{153}Sm-EDTMP in patients with poor-prognosis osteosarcoma. *Cancer.* 2009;115(11):2514–2522.

51. McGinn CJ, Shewach DS, Lawrence TS. Radiosensitizing nucleosides. *J Natl Cancer Inst.* 1996;88(17):1193–1203.

52. Lawrence TS, Eisbruch A, McGinn CJ, et al. Radiosensitization by gemcitabine. *Oncology (Huntingt).* 1999;13(10 suppl 5):55–60.

53. Bruland OS, Nilsson S, Fisher DR, et al. High-linear energy transfer irradiation targeted to skeletal metastases by the alpha-emitter ^{223}Ra: adjuvant or alternative to conventional modalities? *Clin Cancer Res.* 2006;12(20 pt 2):6250s–6257s.

54. Henriksen G, Fisher DR, Roeske JC, et al. Targeting of osseous sites with alpha-emitting 223Ra: comparison with the beta-emitter 89Sr in mice. *J Nucl Med.* 2003;44(2):252–259.

55. Atkinson MJ, Spanner MT, Rosemann M, et al. Intracellular sequestration of 223Ra by the iron-storage protein ferritin. *Radiat Res.* 2005;164(2):230–233.

56. Larsen RH, Saxtorph H, Skydsgaard M, et al. Radiotoxicity of the alpha-emitting bone-seeker ^{223}Ra injected intravenously into mice: histology, clinical chemistry and hematology. *In Vivo.* 2006;20(3):325–331.

57. Nilsson S, Larsen RH, Fossa SD, et al. First clinical experience with alpha-emitting radium-223 in the treatment of skeletal metastases. *Clin Cancer Res.* 2005;11(12):4451–4459.

58. Nilsson S, Franzen L, Parker C, et al. Bone-targeted radium-223 in symptomatic, hormone-refractory prostate cancer: a randomised, multicentre, placebo-controlled phase II study. *Lancet Oncol.* 2007;8(7):587–594.

38

I-131-MIBG Therapy for Neuroendocrine Tumors

H. Bulstrode and John R. Buscombe

■ INTRODUCTION

Neuroendocrine tumors (NETs) are typically derived from gastrointestinal origin and are often metastatic at presentation. For the classic carcinoid syndrome to occur, serotonin (5-HT) must be secreted into the systemic circulation. This syndrome is usually associated with systemic disease, particularly liver metastases where the serotonin is not subject to hepatic first-pass metabolism. Greater than 90% of patients with carcinoid syndrome will exhibit metastatic disease. The tumors tend to be slow growing, especially if they originate from the midgut. This presentation can result in a polysymptomatic patient with an unresectable tumor, in whom chemotherapy is often of limited benefit (1). Embolization can help palliate symptoms if the tumor is limited to the liver (2). The management of patients with NETs is based on the attempt to palliate symptoms and provide the best quality of life.

NETs were originally described as APUDomas (amine precursor uptake decarboxylase) due to their preferential uptake of amines. One such amine which exhibits preferential uptake into NETs but minimal clearance is metaiodobenzylguanidine (MIBG). MIBG is a guanethidine derivative and accumulates in place of noradrenalin within neural crest-derived tissues, including a range of NETs, pheochromocytomas, and paragangliomas (3).

MIBG may be radiolabeled with I-123 or I-131, the latter emitting beta particles at a maximum energy of 0.81 MeV, yielding a maximum depth of 2.0 mm tissue penetration. Although originally used for imaging, I-131-MIBG is now employed as a therapeutic agent in patients with metastatic NETs unsuitable for curative resection (4). The tumor types that have been treated with systemic radiotherapy include gastroenteropancreatic tumors, various NETs, paragangliomas, pheochromocytomas, medullary carcinoma of the thyroid, and neuroblastoma.

The general principle of treating unresectable NETs with I-131-MIBG has been that if "the tumor can be imaged, then it is treatable." Imaging can be performed with I-131, but dosimetry is not reliable and I-131 emits therapeutic beta particles. Therefore, the administered activity needs to be kept to a minimum, often no more than 35 MBq (~1 mCi). I-123 is a pure gamma-emitting version of iodine and thus can be used to label MIBG for imaging. The count rate is

often sufficient to allow for single photon emission computed tomography (SPECT) (Fig. 38.1).

The decision of whether or not to treat a patient will depend on standard oncologic parameters. It is important that both the treating physician and the patient understand the goals of treatment, potential side effects and complications, and the probability of success. If the aim of treatment is to palliate symptoms, then a reasonable assessment of those symptoms must be undertaken. It must also be determined what type of prior treatments the patient has received and if they were successful or not. For example, in patients with carcinoid type NETs, the main reasons for treatment with I-131-MIBG will be symptoms related to carcinoid syndrome (uncontrollable with injected somatostatin) or the presence of disease progression documented with radiographic imaging.

Considering pheochromocytomas and paragangliomas, which have a more aggressive natural history, it may be decided that these tumors will eventually progress and that treatment should be initiated earlier and should be more aggressive. There is often a fine line between wanting to treat a patient while the tumor is small and the probability of success is improved, compared to treating too early and then the patient is exposed to the risks of therapy without being able to obviously benefit. These approaches, however, are not evidence based and rely upon historical patterns of practice. In most large centers that treat patients with NETs, such as in Europe and Australia, radiolabeled somatostatins are available; therefore I-131-MIBG may be reserved for the small number of patients who have negative somatostatin imaging but a positive I-123-MIBG scan.

■ EVIDENCE OF TREATMENT BENEFIT

As one is discussing the treatment option of I-131-MIBG with a patient, it is vital that the patient be involved in the treatment decision. Not only do they have to give informed consent but they need to comply with the requirements and complexities of treatment. Therefore, it is important to impart information to the patient which represents a realistic view of outcomes. Symptomatic benefit is well expected from I-131-MIBG therapy, with 40% to 70% of patients reporting improvement in clinical symptoms such

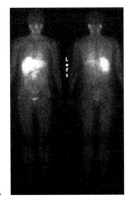

A

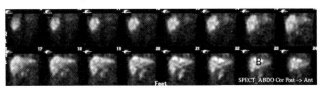

FIGURE 38.1 A: Whole body SPECT I-123-MIBG in a patient with carcinoid syndrome. The scan identifies para-aortic nodes, but the disease within the liver is not clearly seen. B: Coronal SPECT I-123-MIBG images showing further detail within the liver. There are multiple small areas of focal uptake identified. C: Contrast enhanced CT scan confirms multiple liver metastases. D: Posttherapy I-131-MIBG scan. This study shows good uptake in the liver metastases and para-aortic nodes but does not have the resolution to show individual tumor sites.

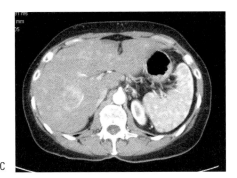

C

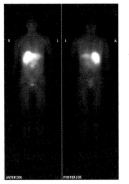

D

as flushing and diarrhea (carcinoid syndrome) or pain relief (5,6). This response is maintained for at least 6 months in the majority of patients (7). What is interesting is that the relief from symptoms appears to be unrelated to any effect on tumor size identified on CT imaging. This contradicts conventional wisdom in oncology where reduction in tumor size is taken as the determinant of treatment success. Some emerging data (8,9) have revealed that symptom relief, not tumor response as shown on imaging studies, is related to improved survival. However, what is clear is that tumor progression during treatment is a poor prognostic sign. Therefore, our standard therapeutic regime consists of three treatments, 3 months apart and a CT scan performed 6 weeks after the second treatment. This scan is compared to the baseline CT scan obtained prior to the first treatment and if progression is identified the third treatment is not given and alternative therapies are sought.

Unfortunately neither randomized controlled trials have been performed using I-131 MIBG for treating NETs, nor is this an ethical possibility in view of the apparent benefits of I-131-MIBG and the fact that symptomatic patients are often successfully palliated. The closest approximation has been a case control study by Sywak et al. (8), who compared outcomes from two different centers that treated patients with metastatic carcinoid arising from midgut tumors. All patients were treated with multimodality therapy (surgery, biotherapy, and chemotherapy) with (center A; $n = 58$) or without (center B; $n = 58$) I-131-MIBG. The 5-year survivals were 63% and 47% for center A and B, respectively. It should be noted that the 5-year survival of

47% for center B is comparable to the 5-year survival of 44% quoted in a study of over 13,000 midgut carcinoid cases (9). However, the different survival rates between centers A and B did not attain statistical significance. It was again noted that early symptomatic relief was related to long-term survival. Also, it was determined that treatment with I-131-MIBG caused few side effects or toxicity. Of course, comparisons between different institutions should be cautiously viewed as patient selection may differ. The results of recent studies are summarized in Table 38.1 (7,8,10–12). From these studies, what appears to be emerging, in order to have a reasonable chance of symptom relief and improved survival, is that a minimum of 15 GBq (405.4 mCi) of I-131-MIBG must be given in two to three treatments over a maximum of 6 months.

■ TREATMENT PROCEDURE

Treatment procedures may vary in different centers but the principles are the same. Delivery of the product must be safe for the operator, other staff, and the patient's immediate caregiver. With most patients this will mean that they will need to be self-caring because they will be admitted to the hospital for at least 5 days and will need their own toilet and shower facilities. The room that they occupy may need additional shielding depending on its location and proximity to nursing staff and other patient rooms. If a patient requires nursing assistance it is best that this be provided by a comforter who knows the patient. This will reduce the radiation dose to the staff. Any such comforter must be

Table **38.1** Comparative results of the use of I-131-MIBG in neuroendocrine tumors					
Study	n	Symptomatic Response (%)	Median Survival from Initial Treatment for Symptomatic Responders (Months)	Median Survival from Initial Treatment for Nonresponders (Months)	Bone Marrow Suppression (%)
Nwosu et al. (10)	48	56.3	59.0 ± 13.9	22.0 ± 5.3	25
Safford et al. (11)	98	48.6	69.1	25.1	13
Sywak et al. (8)	58	N/A	99.6	49.2	30
Navalkissoor et al. (12)	38	42.8	62 (mean)	29 (mean)	5
Buscombe et al. (7)	25	N/A	18		0

briefed to ensure they reduce exposure to themselves, especially from urine or feces. This may be particularly relevant when children are being treated for neuroblastoma.

As some drugs interfere with the uptake of MIBG these should be discontinued before therapy. These types of drugs typically are of the following classes: drugs with an alpha blocking action, monoamine oxidase inhibitors, methyldopa, and guanethidine (antihypertensive medication that should no longer be used). The only drug in which withdrawal may cause a problem is phenoxybenzamine, an alpha-adrenergic blocking agent, used in the treatment of secreting pheochromocytomas. Withdrawal of this drug could result in a hypertensive crisis, stroke, and death. The best approach is to reduce the dose gradually, titrating the dose reduction against the patient's blood pressure, keeping the systolic below 180 mm Hg and the diastolic below 90 mm Hg. This may reduce the efficacy of the I-131-MIBG therapy but it is a compromise that has to be accepted. Prior to therapy, patients are treated with either potassium perchlorate or potassium iodide/iodate for 3 hours and this is continued for at least 5 days, and potentially up to 10 days if activities over 7 GBq are administered. Also, as the treatment can cause nausea, ondansetron (8 mg) can be given about 30 minutes before the start of treatment.

When I-131-MIBG treatment was first initiated in the 1980s, patients had continuous monitoring of vital signs with an electrocardiogram and blood pressure assessment. This is because MIBG in high doses can cause hypotension, tachycardia, and tachyarrhythmias. Modern preparations contain less unlabelled MIBG and as such, the actual dose of the MIBG has been reduced. Therefore, except in children and some patients with pheochromocytomas with unstable blood pressure, cardiac and vital sign monitoring is not required. If monitoring is necessary, then automatic monitoring systems should be used.

Excluding children with neuroblastoma, most centers use a standard activity of I-131-MIBG between 5.5 GBq (148.6 mCi) and 11 GBq (297.3 mCi) administered in a dispensing system designed to reduce the radiation exposure and dose to staff (Fig. 38.2). The dispensing rate depends on the administered activity and the type of dispensing method. Regardless, usual treatment times are between 45 minutes and 4 hours. Approximately 10% of the initial activity remains in the system due to dead space losses.

The patient should be asked to remain well hydrated and if they cannot accomplish this, intravenous fluids can be provided. They may feel nauseous for 2 to 3 days and need treatment. The patient is discharged to home when national legal limits for radiation exposure have been achieved, normally at 5 days for 5.5 GBq (148.6 mCi) I-131-MIBG and 8 days for 11 GBq (297.3 mCi) I-131-MIBG. Subsequent follow-up will track both efficacy and possible toxicity to the thyroid or bone marrow. A full course of treatment would include two to four cycles of I-131-MIBG. Imaging can occur at any point after administration of I-131-MIBG and can be used to assess response (Fig. 38.3). Occasionally, it can be used for dosimetry. The procedure requires isolation facilities, and treatment is undertaken by appropriately trained medical and nursing staff. Medical physics support, as well

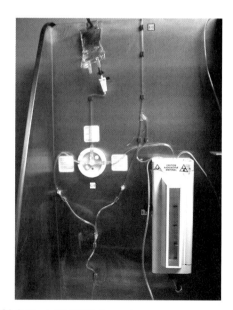

FIGURE 38.2 The I-131-MIBG dispensing system provided by Amersham Bucher (mid-1990s). The system relies on the ability to flush activity into a pediatric burette (seen encased in lead and lead glass). The activity is then infused into the patient followed by a "saline flush" of the burette in order to improve delivery efficiency.

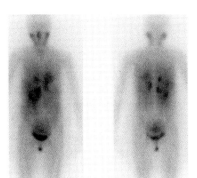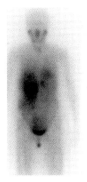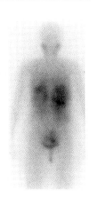

A   B

FIGURE 38.3 A: Posttherapy scan showing uptake of activity of I-131-MIBG in the liver of a patient with a malignant gastrinoma after the first cycle of treatment. B: Posttherapy scan of the same patient after the third cycle of treatment showing a good functional response. This was reflected in the patient's serum level of gastrin returning to normal and being able to reduce her medication.

as appropriate equipment and procedures for administration and disposal of waste are necessary. The European Association of Nuclear Medicine (EANM) guidelines for treatment are reviewed in a recent publication (13), and utilization of these guidelines is legally bound by the European Energy Council Directive 97/43/EURATOM.

Role of dosimetry

One major controversy in I-131-MIBG therapy is the role of dosimetry. There are two approaches used to calculate the necessary activity of I-131-MIBG: a weight–based administration method and a calculated administration based upon whole-body retention data (14). The first approach delivers an activity based upon the patient's weight. The second approach calculates a whole-body dose (equating to bone marrow dose) to try and reduce toxicity. This can be performed by using standardized dosimetric techniques such as the MIRD system. To date, almost all of the efforts of the dosimetric approach have been accomplished in children with neuroblastoma where it is possible to limit whole-body doses to 3 to 4 Gy. This can subsequently result in tumor doses up to 103 Gy (14). However, although this approach results in a more uniform whole-body dose calculation and a consistent effect in reducing toxicity, it cannot predict efficacy. In addition, there is no evidence that such a dosimetric approach will offer an advantage in improving treatment outcomes in adults with NETs. There is clearly a great need for further research in this area.

New advances in I-131-MIBG therapy

Two recent developments have begun to reshape the "thinking" about I-131-MIBG. The main reason that large administered activities of I-131-MIBG cannot be given is not related to radiation toxicity but to the fact that for every molecule of radioactive MIBG there may be 1000 nonradioactive molecules. Using a patented gel separation column it has been possible to concentrate the radioactive I-131-MIBG so that approximately 1 in 5 to 10 molecules is radioactive. This so-called "carrier free" MIBG has undergone early clinical trials. In a phase I trial it was shown that carrier free I-131-MIBG (ultratrace) had excellent and rapid tumor uptake with manageable bone marrow and kidney toxicity (15). A phase II

study is now under way in which activities as high as 26 GBq (702.7 mCi) I-131-MIBG are to be given as a single therapeutic dose in NETs. This project should report its results in 2012/2013.

The second development is to combine two therapies using the radiation sensitization advantages of some types of chemotherapy in conjunction with I-131-MIBG. This concept has been successful in combined modality approaches of external beam radiotherapy delivered concurrently with chemotherapy. Some preclinical data has suggested that the combined use of simultaneous therapy with I-131-MIBG and topotecan results in a higher rate of nonrepairable DNA damage than either of the treatments alone (16). Although there has been some early work in the use of combined therapies in neuroblastoma there are no randomized clinical trials showing the benefit of chemotherapy and I-131-MIBG over conventional monotherapy. In addition, the timing and dose of the two treatments can be crucial as topotecan given before or after I-131-MIBG was less effective in tumor kill than the simultaneous therapy. This could lead to practical issues as patients receiving chemotherapy may need intensive nursing, the very scenario that we try to avoid with I-131-MIBG therapies.

■ CONCLUSIONS

The available evidence suggests symptomatic benefit from I-131-MIBG therapy in the majority of patients diagnosed with metastatic NETs, an effect sustained over at least 6 months. Survival is difficult to assess in the absence of randomized control studies, but a relative improvement in 5-year survival of the order of 30% appears likely. This benefit appears to be predicted by symptomatic response to initial therapy.

■ REFERENCES

1. Oberg K. The use of chemotherapy in neuroendocrine tumours. *Endocrinol Metab Clin North Am.* 1993;22:941–952.
2. Kim YH, Ajani JA, Carrasco CH, et al. Selective hepatic arterial chemoembolization for liver metastases in patients with carcinoid tumor or islet cell carcinoma. *Cancer Invest.* 1999;17:474–478.
3. Wafelman AR, Hoefnagel CA, Maes RA, et al. Radioiodinated meta-iodobenzylguanidine: a review of its biodistribution and pharmacokinetics, drug interactions, cytotoxicity and dosimetry. *Eur J Nucl Med.* 1994;21:545–559.

4. Castellani MR, Di Bartolomeo M, Maffioli L, et al. ^{131}I-metaiodobenzylguanidine therapy in carcinoid tumors. *J Nucl Biol Med.* 1991;35: 349–351.

5. Prvulovich EM, Stein RC, Bomanji JB, et al. Iodine-131-MIBG therapy of a patient with carcinoid liver metastases. *J Nucl Med.* 1998;39:1743–1745.

6. Mukherjee JJ, Kaltsas GA, Islam N, et al. Treatment of metastatic carcinoid tumours, phaeochromocytoma, paraganglioma and medullary carcinoma of the thyroid with (131)I-meta-iodobenzylguanidine. *Clin Endocrinol (Oxf).* 2001;55:47–60.

7. Buscombe JR, Cwikla JB, Caplin ME, et al. Long-term efficacy of low activity meta-[131]Iiodobenzylguanidine therapy in patients with disseminated neuroendocrine tumours depends on initial response. *Nucl Med Commun.* 2001;26:969–976.

8. Sywak MS, Pasieka JL, McEwan A, et al. ^{131}I-meta-iodobenzylguanidine in the management of metastatic midgut carcinoid tumors. *World J Surg.* 2004;28:1157–1162.

9. Modlin IM, Lye KD, Kidd M. A 5-decade analysis of 13,715 carcinoid tumors. *Cancer.* 2005;97(4):934–959.

10. Nwosu AC, Jones L, Vora J, et al. Assessment of the efficacy and toxicity of ^{131}I-metaiodobenzylguanidine therapy for metastatic neuroendocrine tumors. *Br J Cancer.* 2008;98:1053–1058.

11. Safford SD, Coleman RE, Gockerman JO, et al. Iodine-131 metaiodobenzylguanidine treatment for metastatic carcinoid. *Cancer.* 2004;101: 1987–1993.

12. Navalkissoor S, Alhashimi DM, Quigley AM, et al. Efficacy of using a standard activity of (131)I-MIBG therapy in patients with disseminated neuroendocrine tumours. *Eur J Nucl Med Mol Imaging.* 2010;37: 904–912.

13. Giammarile F, Chiti A, Lassmann M, et al. EANM procedure guidelines for ^{131}I-meta-iodobenzylguanidine (^{131}I-mIBG) therapy. *Eur J Nucl Med Mol Imaging.* 2008;35(5):1039–1047.

14. Buckley SE, Saran FH, Gaze MN, et al. Dosimetry for fractionated (131)I-mIBG therapies in patients with primary resistant high-risk neuroblastoma: preliminary results. *Cancer Biother Radiopharm.* 2007; 22:105–112.

15. Coleman RE, Stubbs JB, Barrett JA, et al. Radiation dosimetry, pharmacokinetics, and safety of ultratrace Iobenguane I-131 in patients with malignant pheochromocytoma/paraganglioma or metastatic carcinoid. *Cancer Biother Radiopharm.* 2009;24:469–475.

16. McCluskey AG, Boyd M, Ross SC, et al. [131]I]meta-iodobenzylguanidine and topotecan combination treatment of tumors expressing the noradrenaline transporter. *Clin Cancer Res.* 2005;11:7929–7937.

Malignancies Treated with Peptides

Denise Zwanziger and Annette G. Beck-Sickinger

The diagnosis of human cancers at an early stage is an important prerequisite to increase the survival rate of patients. The selective targeting of primary tumors and metastases may result in more evaluable images, outcomes largely achieved with radiopharmaceuticals that exhibit high tumor to background ratios. Recently, peptide hormones have become increasingly important for targeting tumor cells for diagnostic as well as therapeutic applications (1,2). The basis for peptide-based radiopharmaceuticals in oncology is the strong overexpression of peptide receptors in different human cancers accompanied with a promising selectivity strategy (2,3). In addition, normal cells are often characterized by the absence or only a low peptide receptor expression (4,5). Accordingly, by using peptide hormones a more selective delivery for tumor diagnosis and therapy is given compared to conventional strategies, for example, chemotherapy. Furthermore, conventional strategies are often limited by drug resistance of tumor cells and toxicity of normal cells (6–8). However, relevant features for peptide receptor imaging (PRI) include high peptide receptor expression in the corresponding tumor cell, preferentially high affinity of the peptide hormone for a distinct receptor, high accumulation in the tumor compared to low accumulation in nontarget tissues, and a rapid clearance from nontarget tissues and the blood to preclude toxicity of the peptide-based radiopharmaceutical. Furthermore, peptide receptor radiation therapy (PRRT) also requires a long-lasting tumor washout for successful therapy (9).

The use of peptide-based radiopharmaceuticals is common and peptides are advantaged by numerous features compared to antibodies (10,11). Peptide synthesis is easily accomplished by using the well-established solid phase peptide synthesis technique, resulting in large quantities of peptides with high levels of purity. Furthermore, peptides survive strong chemical reaction conditions often needed for radionuclide introduction. Because of their small size, peptides are characterized by a good permeability into tumors and fast clearance from the body. Another prerequisite, the high tumor to background ratio, is realized by the selectivity and high binding affinity to the corresponding peptide receptor and results in decreased side effects. The low antigenicity as well as the fact that peptides are unable to penetrate the blood–brain barrier are also preferable characteristics. Despite these advantages, the successful use of peptides as imaging tools and therapeutic agents is influenced by different chemical and pharmacokinetic properties of the peptide-based radiopharmaceutical and, by all

means, is not trivial (2,10,12). The low metabolic stability in vivo as a result of fast proteolytic degradation has as much hampered their application in tumor diagnosis and therapy as the often-described influence of the modifications needed to create the peptide-based radiopharmaceutical. Furthermore, side effects of endogenous receptors have been observed and peptides often show a limited bioavailability. For clinics, a nonoral application is preferred. It is crucial to develop enzymatically stable peptides, with modifications of the naturally existing ligand, in order to overcome the most important disadvantage of peptide hormones, their metabolic instability. Commonly used strategies are the introduction of unnatural amino acids (D-amino acids, N-methyl amino acids), an amidated C-terminus, the partial or complete cyclization of the peptide, the introduction of phosphorylated amino acids, the association to a stabilizing protein, the insertion of an amino alcohol, or the introduction of unusual side chains (1,2). Despite the preferably higher metabolic stability it is also an important prerequisite to preserve the nearly original binding affinity of the peptide to the receptor.

A typical peptide-based radiopharmaceutical can be subdivided into several different parts (2). The main component is the peptide itself that binds with high affinity and selectivity to the peptide receptor expressed on tumor cells. Positioned between the peptide and the conjugated bifunctional chelator (BFC), a spacer is frequently attached to increase the steric distance. In the process, the spacer minimizes possible side effects by improving the pharmacologic profile of the peptide–radionuclide moiety and by allowing for maximum function of the BFC. Moreover, it has been found that the spacer positively exerts an influence on the body clearance, especially in the renal–urinary or hepatobilary system. Of course, the ultimate result is a radionuclide that is complexed to a peptide by the BFC that potentially enables tumor diagnosis as well as tumor therapy. Figure 39.1 shows the schematic illustration of the principal strategy for peptide-based radionuclide therapy.

■ BIFUNCTIONAL CHELATORS AND RADIONUCLIDES

A wide range of BFCs (see Chapter 7) have been developed for the conjugation of targeting constructs with several radionuclides (13,14). A useful BFC is characterized not only by easy and fast labeling procedures, but also by its ability to obtain large, expedient, and stable yields in radiolabeling.

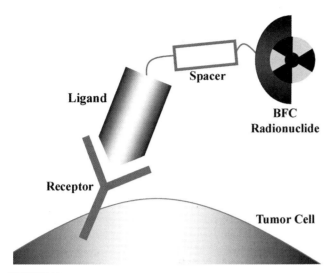

FIGURE 39.1 Illustration of the principal strategy for peptide-based radionuclide therapy.

Because of the short physical half-life of some radionuclides, lengthy reaction conditions and additional purification steps are unfavorable. To create peptide-based radiopharmaceuticals the post- and the prelabeling approaches can be distinguished (see Chapter 3). The most widely used approach comprises the covalent attachment of the BFC to the peptide followed by the complexation of the radionuclide via the ligation group of the BFC, named the postlabeling approach. The less frequently applied prelabeling approach can be described by a BFC radionuclide formation and an additional covalent bond formation of this complex to the peptide. Several macrocyclic agents have been developed for stable radionuclide complexation, frequently based on 1,4,7,10-tetraazacyclododecane-1,4,7,10-tetraacetic acid (DOTA) or DOTA monoamide (DOTAMA) (Fig. 39.2). The high numbers of variations of functional groups include amines, aldehydes and ketones, alkynes, carboxyls, isothiocyanates, maleimides, and vinyl sulfone and have led to suitable BFCs for peptide radiolabeling (15–18). Radionuclides can be separated into diagnostic and therapeutic radionuclides, in which therapeutic efficacy of the internal radiation induces damage to tumor cells in the target tissue by using high- or medium-energy β-emitters. Different physical and biologic characteristics, for example, half-life, availability, particle emission, or the maximum tissue penetration, have led to numerous suitable radionuclides. Moreover, therapeutic applications require the injection of higher activities and, at times, some form of pretherapeutic dosimetry studies or evaluation, when compared to the use of diagnostic radionuclides. Positron emission tomography (PET) can therefore be used with the suitable β^+/β^--emitting radionuclides $^{124}I/^{131}I$, $^{86}Y/^{90}Y$, or $^{64}Cu/^{67}Cu$. In contrast, α-emitting radionuclides, for example, ^{212}Bi or ^{211}At, may be preferable due to their short emission range, high linear energy transfer, and ultimately a larger relative biologic effectiveness (Chapters 6 and 27), but limited due to their

low availability (19), cost, and difficult chemistry. More promising radionuclides, created by using commercially available radionuclide generators, include, for example, ^{68}Ga or ^{99m}Tc. Furthermore, radionuclides either without or with a low gamma emission (^{90}Y, ^{177}Lu, or ^{67}Cu) are also of great interest as therapeutic radionuclides.

PEPTIDE HORMONES

The discovery of specific peptide receptors on human cancers has opened the new field of peptide hormones in tumor diagnosis and therapy. Historically, the first peptide hormone used in clinical studies was ^{123}I-[Tyr^3]-octreotide (^{123}I-TOC), a somatostatin analogue (Fig. 39.3) (20). Accordingly, somatostatin receptor scintigraphy started in the late 1980s by using the more preferable [^{111}In-DTPA]-octreotide (OctreoScan) (21). By now, many other peptide hormones have been identified as potential peptide-based radiopharmaceuticals (2,22). Among others, they act as hormones, neurotransmitters, neuromodulators, cytokines, as well as growth hormone inhibitors. Furthermore, high affinity binding is imparted to various peptide receptors that frequently belong to the class of G protein–coupled receptors (GPCRs) (23). GPCRs belong to the superfamily of heptahelix transmembrane proteins consisting of a single protein chain with seven transmembrane helices. Apart from the first and most widely used peptide hormone, somatostatin, more peptides are currently being investigated as peptide-based radiopharmaceuticals in tumor diagnosis and therapy because of the distinct occurrence of their peptide receptors. Preclinical and clinical investigations are currently performed with bombesin (BBS)/gastrin-releasing peptide (GRP), vasoactive intestinal peptide (VIP), neurotensin, α-melanotropin-stimulating hormone (α-MSH), cholecystokinin (CCK), and neuropeptide Y (NPY) (24). Table 39.1 gives an overview of the peptide hormones and the tumor localization sites of their corresponding receptors. Amino acid sequences of the peptide hormones are given in Figure 39.4.

Moreover, multireceptor targeting has become more and more important due to simultaneous receptor overexpression in numerous human cancers (20,25). This method often leads to an increased accumulation of radioactivity in the tumor. Furthermore, the unsuccessful tumor uptake based on low homogeneously expressed receptors, tumor dedifferentiation, and subsequent loss of receptors can be minimized by multireceptor targeting, especially for PRRT.

Somatostatin

The cyclic peptide hormone somatostatin consists of 14 amino acids and was first isolated in the 1970s from the hypothalamus of sheep (26). As a ubiquitously diffused peptide in the body, somatostatin was found in the peripheral nervous system, gut, multiple endocrine glands, gastrointestinal tract, as well as the immune system. The biologic functions that are characterized by inhibitory

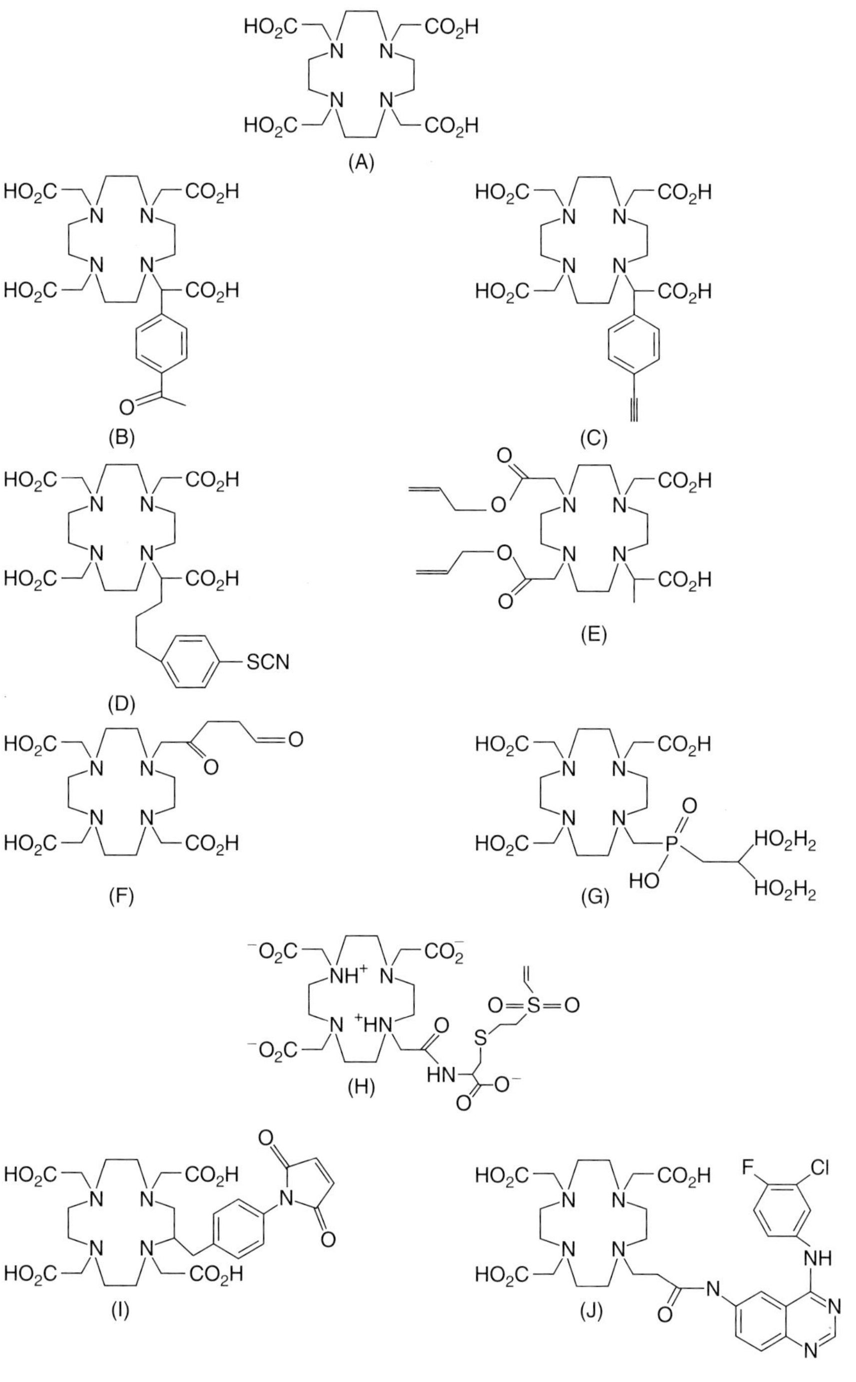

FIGURE 39.2 Chemical structures of the bifunctional chelator 1,4,7,10-tetraazacyclododecane-1,4,7,10-tetraacetic acid (DOTA) and DOTA functionalized derivatives. **A:** DOTA; **B:** 4-acetylphenyl-DOTA derivative; **C:** ethynylphenyl-DOTA derivative; **D:** isothiocyanate-DOTA derivative; **E:** tris-allyl-DOTA derivative; **F:** aldehyde-DOTA derivatives; **G:** bis(phosphonicacid)-DOTA derivative; **H:** vinyl sulfone-cysteinamide-DOTA derivative; **I:** maleinamide-DOTA derivative; **J:** quinazoline-based DOTA derivative.

effects and physiologic functions in the hormone system are transmitted by five different somatostatin receptor subtypes (sst$_1$ to sst$_5$) (27). They all belong to the class A of the family of GPCRs (28). Somatostatin activates all these somatostatin receptor subtypes with a nanomolar affinity followed by internalization. The tumor diagnostic as well as therapeutic potential of somatostatin started when the overexpression of different receptor subtypes was found in human cancers (29). The strong overexpression has been determined in neuroendocrine tumors (NETs), neuroblastomas, renal cell carcinomas, breast cancer, prostate cancer, small cell lung cancer (SCLC), brain tumors, and malignant lymphoma (1). Moreover, the sst$_2$ receptor is predominantly expressed in

gastroenteropancreatic neuroendocrine tumors (GEP-NETs) that have led to the development of sst$_2$ receptor–specific somatostatin analogues (1). Unfortunately, the native ligand somatostatin is rapidly inactivated by a fast enzymatic degradation within few minutes (30). Within recent years, research has concentrated on the development of metabolically more stable somatostatin analogues (Table 39.2) (31). By the introduction of D-amino acids and the shortening of the original peptide sequence an improved set of somatostatin analogues showing variable receptor-binding affinities and selectivities has been designed and characterized, in vitro and in vivo. Somatostatin analogues are metabolically more stable than the native ligand due to the numerous

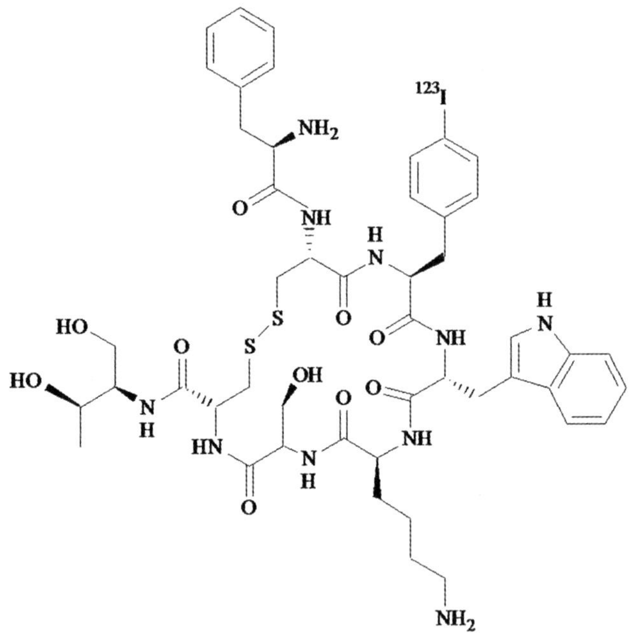

FIGURE 39.3 Chemical structure of the somatostatin analogue, ^{123}I-[Tyr^3]-octreotide.

modifications, whereas the truncation of the original peptide sequence leads to an enhanced clearance from the blood. It has been shown that the truncated somatostatin (7–14) is the shortest sequence needed for activity (32). The somatostatin analogues lanreotide and vapreotide (RC-160) contain only eight amino acids of the native sequence and have been found to be more stable than somatostatin because of the lack of the key enzyme cleavage sites (33). Krenning et al. described the ^{123}I-labeled octapeptide

octreotide that was the first somatostatin analogue used for tumor diagnosis. In 1994, the commercially available peptide [^{111}In-DTPA]-octreotide (^{111}In-OctreoScan) replaced the ^{123}I-labeled octreotide in tumor imaging due to the observed unfavorable radioiodination procedures as well as the significant hepatobiliary excretion (34). Now, ^{111}In-OctreoScan is a routinely used tool for the detection of NETs. However, the therapeutic benefit of ^{111}In-OctreoScan is limited by the small particle range of ^{111}In that results in poor energy absorption in tumors. The replacement of Phe^3 by Tyr^3 to obtain TOC revealed a higher sst$_2$ receptor affinity, whereas sst$_3$ receptor affinity decreased significantly (35). By using the BFC DOTA conjugated to TOC, several clinical studies have shown the potential application of this somatostatin analogue for tumor diagnosis (^{111}In, ^{68}Ga) and therapy (^{90}Y). [^{90}Y-DOTA^0,Tyr^3]-octreotide or more simply, ^{90}Y-DOTA-TOC, has been found to be therapeutically more potent compared to ^{111}In-OctreoScan in which a complete and partial tumor remission in 7% to 29% has been observed for ^{90}Y-DOTA-TOC compared to 0% to 8% for ^{111}In-OctreoScan (24). ^{90}Y-DOTA-TOC has also been used for the treatment of other tumors, for example, meningiomas (36). In this case, PRRT has been performed in 29 patients with a strong sst$_2$ receptor overexpression in tumors. After 3 months complete disease stabilization was found in 66% of the patients. Another somatostatin analogue has been achieved by the substitution of the C-terminal Thr(ol) with Thr that resulted not only in a higher binding affinity and faster internalization, but also in a higher tumor uptake (37,38). Treatment of the somatostatin analogue [^{177}Lu-DOTA^0,Tyr^3]-octreotate (^{177}Lu-DOTA-[Tyr^3]-TATE) in patients with GEP-NETs resulted in a tumor remission in 47% of 125 patients (39). Due to the lower energy and shorter particle ranges of ^{177}Lu

Table **39.1**	Peptide hormones, receptors, and tumor localization sites		
Class	**Peptide Hormone**	**Receptor**	**Tumor**
A	Somatostatin	sst$_1$-sst$_5$	Neuroendocrine tumors (NETs), neuroblastoma, small cell lung cancer (SCLC), prostate, breast, astrocytoma, renal cell carcinoma, lymphoma
B	Bombesin/gastrin-releasing peptide	BB$_1$, BB$_2$, and BB$_3$	SCLC, breast, gastric, prostate, colon, glioblastoma, melanoma
C	Vasoactive intestinal peptide	VPAC$_1$ and VPAC$_2$	Breast, prostate, colon, lung, rectum, pancreatic ducts, liver, and urinary neoplasms
D	Neurotensin	NTR$_1$	Breast, colon, thyroid cancer, SCLC, astrocytoma, medulloblastoma, meningioma, Ewing sarcoma
E	α-Melanotropin-stimulating hormone	MC$_1$	Melanoma
F	Cholecystokinin	CCK$_1$ and CCK$_2$	SCLC, astrocytoma, ovarian stromal tumors, colorectal, pancreatic cancer, medullary thyroid carcinomas
G	Neuropeptide Y	NPY Y$_1$ and Y$_2$	Neuroblastoma, breast, gastrointestinal stromal tumor, renal cell carcinoma, paraganglioma, pheochromocytoma, ovarian sex cord-stromal tumor, ovarian adenocarcinoma

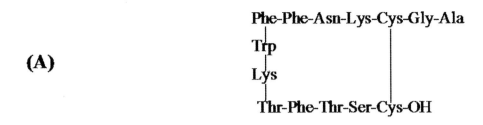

(A)

Phe-Phe-Asn-Lys-Cys-Gly-Ala
Trp
Lys
Thr-Phe-Thr-Ser-Cys-OH

(B) pyro-Glu-Gln-Arg-Leu-Gly-Asn-Gln-Trp-Ala-Val-Gly-His-Leu-Met-NH₂

(C) His-Ser-Asp-Ala-Val-Phe-Thr-Asp-Asn-Tyr-Thr-Arg-Leu-Arg-Lys
-Gln-Met-Ala-Val-Lys-Lys-Tyr-Leu-Asn-Ser-Ile-Leu-Asn-NH₂

(D) pyro-Glu-Leu-Tyr-Gln-Asn-Lys-Pro-Arg-Arg-Pro-Tyr-Ile-Leu

(E) Ac-Ser-Tyr-Ser-Met-Gln-His-Phe-Arg-Trp-Gly-Lys-Pro-Val-NH₂

(F) Asp-Tyr(SO₃H)-Met-Gly-Trp-Met-Asp-Phe-NH₂

(G) Tyr-Pro-Ser-Lys-Pro-Asp-Asn-Pro-Gly-Glu-Asp-Ala-Pro-Ala-Glu-Asp-Leu-Ala-Arg
-Tyr-Tyr-Ser-Ala-Leu-Arg-His-Tyr-Ile-Asn-Leu-Ile-Thr-Arg-Gln-Arg-Tyr-NH₂

FIGURE 39.4 Amino acid sequences of the peptide hormones. **A:** Somatostatin; **B:** bombesin; **C:** vasoactive intestinal peptide; **D:** neurotensin; **E:** α-melanotropin-stimulating hormone; **F:** cholecystokinin; **G:** neuropeptide Y (porcine).

compared to ⁹⁰Y, this somatostatin analogue has a better energy absorption in smaller tumors (9). Interestingly, quality of life was significantly improved after treatment with ⁹⁰Y-DOTA-NOC and ¹⁷⁷Lu-DOTA-TATE, respectively, whereas side effects were few and mild (37,38). These somatostatin analogues seem to be promising tools, especially for patients with inoperable or metastatic NETs. For numerous somatostatin analogues, a significant growth reduction of NETs expressing sst₂ receptors has been demonstrated. Promising targeting and therapeutic results of NET-positive patients

Peptide	Amino Acid Sequence
Somatostatin	Ala-Gly-cyclo(Cys-Lys-Asn-Phe-Phe-Trp-Lys-Thr-Phe-Thr-Ser-Cys)
Lanreotide	D-β-Nal-cyclo(Cys-Tyr-DTrp-Lys-Val-Cys)-Thr-NH₂
Vapreotide (RC-160)	DPhe-cyclo(Cys-Tyr-DTrp-Lys-Val-Cys)-Trp-NH₂
Octreotide	DPhe-cyclo(Cys-Phe-DTrp-Lys-Thr-Cys)-Thr-ol
[Tyr³]-octreotide (TOC)	DPhe-cyclo(Cys-Tyr-DTrp-Lys-Thr-Cys)-Thr-ol
[Tyr³]-octreotate	DPhe-cyclo(Cys-Tyr-DTrp-Lys-Thr-Cys)-Thr
[1-Nal³]-octreotide (NOC)	DPhe-cyclo(Cys-1-Nal-DTrp-Lys-Thr-Cys)-Thr-ol
[1-Nal³,Thr⁸]-octreotide (NOC-ATE)	DPhe-cyclo(Cys-1-Nal-DTrp-Lys-Thr-Cys)-Thr
[BzThi³,Thr⁸]-octreotide (BOC-ATE)	DPhe-cyclo(Cys-BzThi-DTrp-Lys-Thr-Cys)-Thr
ANT	Phe(4-NO₂)-cyclo(DCys-Tyr-DTrp-Lys-Thr-Cys)-DTyr-NH₂
RC-121	DPhe-cyclo(Cys-Thr-DTrp-Lys-Val-Cys)-Thr-NH₂

Table **39.2** Amino acid sequences of somatostatin and analogues

Nal, naphthylalanine; BzThi, (3-benzothienyl)-alanine.

could be achieved, but further developments for more appropriate treatments with fewer side effects are preferable. Therefore, van Essen et al. investigated the combination of ^{177}Lu-DOTA-TATE and capecitabine (Chapter 16), an oral prodrug of 5-fluorouracil (5-FU), in seven GEP-NET tumor patients (40). As an oral drug, capecitabine is more convenient when compared to intravenous 5-FU. This combination is safe and feasible with regard to short-term side effects. However, the expression of other somatostatin receptor subtypes, for example, sst$_3$ or the combination of sst receptor subtype expression in various tumors, has been identified. For a broader somatostatin receptor subtype targeting profile [DOTA]-[1-Nal^3,Thr^8]-octreotide (DOTA-NOC-ATE) and [DOTA]-[BzThi^3,Thr^8]-octreotide (DOTA-BOC-ATE) have been developed and successfully investigated (41). In addition, the small cyclic hexapeptide depreotide can also be used for a broader range of tumors because of its sst$_2$, sst$_3$, and sst$_5$ receptor affinity (42). It can be subdivided into a somatostatin receptor binding sequence and into a linear tetrapeptide and then conjugated to a radionuclide.

In 2006, Ginj et al. found sst$_2$ receptor affinity for the somatostatin antagonist sst$_2$-ANT, as well as tumor uptake and slow clearance of [^{111}In-DOTA]-sst$_2$-ANT in nude mice that bear human embryonic kidney cells (43). The comparison of this antagonist with an agonist revealed a lower receptor affinity of the antagonist but significantly higher tumor retention. It is hypothesized that the antagonist binds to a larger variety of receptor conformations that might increase tumor retention. With a physical half-life of 12.7 hours and its availability by a cyclotron, ^{64}Cu is a promising PET nuclide. Ultrastable ^{64}Cu complexes can be achieved by the use of the cross-bridged BFC CB-TE2A, whereas the ^{64}Cu-DOTA complex only shows moderate stability (44). Therefore, ^{64}Cu-CB-TE2A-sst$_2$-ANT has been used as PET radiopharmaceutical for sst$_2$ receptor–positive tumor diagnosis (45). The application of the somatostatin antagonist resulted in lower uptake in sst receptor–positive tissues and tumors compared to the agonist ^{64}Cu-CB-TE2A-Y3-TATE. In contrast to these findings, higher tumor to blood and tumor to muscle ratios have been observed for the antagonist resulting because of the increased chemical stability and increased hydrophobicity of sst$_2$-ANT. Furthermore, small animal imaging of AR42J tumors led to good tumor to background images and high standardized uptake tumor values for the target tissue.

In 2007, Gabriel et al. compared ^{68}Ga-DOTA-Tyr^3-octreotide PET with the conventional scintigraphy and computed tomography (CT) in 84 patients with NETs (46). For PET imaging they found a sensitivity of 97%, a specificity of 92%, and an accuracy of 96%. This demonstrates a significantly higher efficacy compared to the conventional scintigraphy or CT. However, the authors suggest that best results will be achieved by the combination of PET and CT. Moreover, in recent studies of the same group, they compared ^{68}Ga-DOTA-TOC PET with CT and magnetic resonance imaging in solid tumors (47). In 5 of the 46 patients with NETs the development

of new metastases during therapy was detected earlier by PET than by other methods and therefore PET is a promising tool as an early predictor.

Recently, ^{68}Ga-DOTA-TATE, as an sst$_2$ receptor–selective somatostatin analogue, has been compared with ^{18}F-FDG in NETs by using PET/CT (48). Clinical studies in 18 patients showing different types of carcinoids revealed a high and selective uptake of the somatostatin analogue in low-grade bronchial carcinoid tumors, whereas ^{18}F-FDG showed negative or minimal uptake. In contrast, atypical and higher grade tumors revealed a better accumulation for ^{18}F-FDG.

Non-small-cell lung cancer (NSCLC) is an aggressive tumor type that was investigated for therapy by Treszl et al. (49). Therefore, the effect of the cytotoxic somatostatin analogue AN-162 has been investigated in different human NSCLC cell lines in vitro as well as in nude mice xenografted with H460 or H1299 NSCLC cells in vivo. AN-162 contains the somatostatin analogue RC-121 for receptor-selective targeting and a conjugated doxorubicin for cytotoxicity. In vitro decreased cell proliferation has been found. A significant in vivo tumor growth inhibition has been observed after treatment with AN-162, in a xenograph, nude mouse model (H640 and H1229 cells). Furthermore, real-time PCR in cell lines and tumors revealed an induction of several apoptosis-related genes by using AN-162.

The often-observed high renal uptake and high retention of radiolabeled peptides is known to be a limiting factor for successful PRI and PRRT (50). Different mechanisms have been suggested for the nontarget accumulation (51,52). In 2007, a relationship between the number of charged amino acid residues of the radiolabeled peptide and the renal retention has been identified (53). Several studies explored the coinfusion of different agents (e.g., the positively charged amino acids L-lysine or L-arginine) that appeared to significantly reduce renal toxicity from radiation (54). Furthermore, by using the plasma expander succinylated gelatin (Gelofusine) a reduction of the renal reabsorption has been shown for ^{111}In-octreotide in humans (55). However, none of these agents showed complete inhibition of the reabsorption. Vegt et al. investigated the correlation of the most abundant plasma protein albumin in reducing the renal uptake of ^{111}In-labeled octreotide and other radiolabeled peptides (56). In a detailed study, they selected a set of albumin-derived peptides to identify fragments that show strong inhibition of renal reabsorption (57). In addition, one of these albumin-derived peptides showed promising characteristics for kidney protection, especially in PRRT, whereas a combination of inhibitors seems to be useful for complete inhibition.

Bombesin

BBS is a 14-amino acid peptide hormone that was first isolated from frog's skin in 1971, whereas the mammalian counterpart, the 27-amino acid GRP, was isolated from porcine stomach in 1979 (58,59). The peptides are characterized by their identical C-terminal. BBS is physiologically involved in various functions, such as the regulation of the smooth muscle concentration, the thermoregulation in the central nervous system, the pancreatic and gastric acid secretion, as well as the release of gut hormones (60,61). The corresponding receptor subtypes include the neuromedin B receptor subtype (BB1), the orphan receptor subtype (BB3), and the BBS receptor subtype (BB4). BBS binds with high affinity to these receptor subtypes that belong to the class A of GPCRs (62). The native ligand and BBS-derived analogues can be used as peptide-based radiopharmaceuticals because of the overexpression of BBS receptor subtypes in various human tumors including SCLC, breast cancer, colon cancer, prostate cancer, and gastric cancer (63).

Due to the fast proteolytic degradation of the native ligand BBS with a half-life in the plasma of only a few minutes, metabolically more stable BBS analogues have been developed (2,22). The C-terminal amino acids 7 to 14 have been shown to play an important role in high and specific binding affinity of BBS to the receptor subtypes (64). Recently, numerous BBS analogues have been developed and investigated, in vitro and in vivo (65). Despite the tumor uptake, peptides are often limited by their high accumulation in nontarget tissues leading to unfavorable tumor to background ratios (56,66). Accordingly, strategies to improve the target to nontarget ratios have been performed in which spacers have been introduced between the peptide and the BFC–radionuclide moiety. Aliphatic amino acid spacers have been shown to enhance efficacy significantly (67,68). Moreover, by the introduction of two β-alanine residues as a spacer, improved tumor uptake, as well as a lower accumulation in the liver, will result. Furthermore, to avoid the fast proteolytic degradation of the BBS analogue BBS(7–14)

Leu13 was replaced by cyclohexylalanine (Cha) and Met14 by norleucine (Nle), respectively (65). These modifications resulted in enhanced metabolic stability of the peptide. Schweinsberg et al. investigated the influence of hydrophilic carbohydrate spacer moieties, especially to reduce the nontarget accumulation (69). In vivo biodistribution studies in nude mice bearing PC-3 tumor xenografts showed an improved tumor to liver ratio and, moreover, a higher tumor uptake and retention over 5 hours of [^{99m}Tc(CO)$_3$]-(N$^\alpha$His-ac)-(Ala(^{N}TG))-(βAla)$_2$-[Cha^{13},Nle^{14}]BBS(7–14) compared to [^{99m}Tc(CO)$_3$]-(N$^\alpha$His-ac)-(βAla)$_2$-[Cha^{13},Nle^{14}]BBS(7–14). These results are in agreement with previous studies with a series of BBS analogues containing the ^{99m}Tc(I)-tricarbonyl core and a polar serylserylserine spacer that also showed a longer tumor retention compared to BBS analogues containing β-Ala or glycylglycylglycine spacer moieties (70). Another study investigated several ^{99m}Tc(CO)$_3$-DTMA-(X)-BBS(7–14) analogues, where X represents GGG, SSS, or β-Ala spacer moieties (Fig. 39.5A). The tridentate BFC DTMA stably coordinates fac-[^{99m}Tc(CO)$_3$]$^+$. The highest tumor uptake has been observed for the β-Ala containing BBS analogue in PC-3 tumor-bearing mice. Unfortunately, the biodistribution results in normal mice were not nearly as favorable as were observed in the in vitro studies. Only low values of tumor uptake comparable to other reported tridentate ^{99m}Tc-conjugated BBS analogues could be achieved (65,70).

The design of potent BBS-based radiopharmaceuticals has focused not only on peptide modifications, ideal spacers, and radionuclides, but also on suitable BFCs. A comparative study between ^{99m}Tc-HYNIC-BBS and ^{99m}TcN(PNP6)-Cys-BBS has been reported recently (71). In the synthesis procedure,

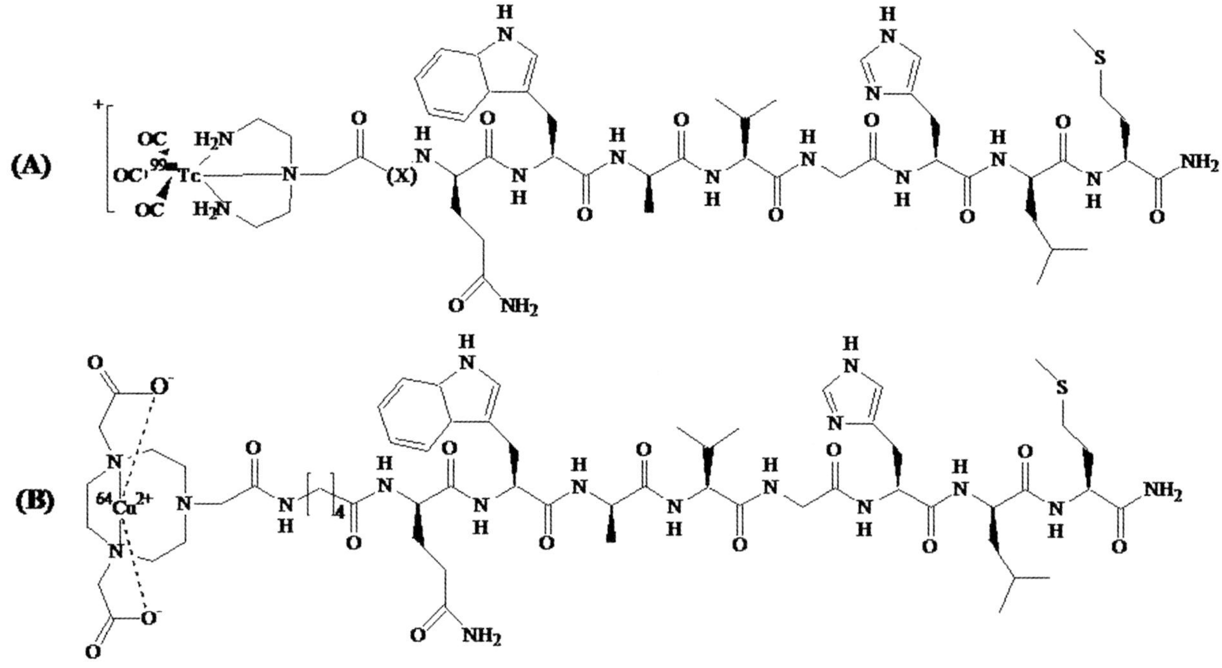

FIGURE 39.5 Chemical structures of two BBS-based radiopharmaceuticals. **A:** ^{99m}Tc(CO)$_3$-DTMA-(X)-BBS(7–14) (X = GGG, SSS, or βAla); **B:** ^{64}Cu-NO2A-Aoc-BBS(7–14).

HYNIC was more advantageous than PNP6 because of the long preparation time, lower radiochemical yield, and additional purification steps. Furthermore, biodistribution studies in PC-3 tumor-bearing mice resulted in a higher tumor uptake of ^{99m}Tc-HYNIC-BBS.

Due to the relatively low tumor accumulation as well as an unfavorable hepatobiliary excretion of BBS analogues, multireceptor tumor targeting can be a preferable strategy for optimization. In 2008, a BBS-RGD (RGD; arginyl-glycyl-aspartic acid) heterodimer was designed and investigated in biodistribution studies (72). Integrin is involved in angiogenesis and, moreover, most solid tumors are angiogenesis dependent. Accordingly, RGD-containing peptides are useful for tumor targeting due to their ability to bind integrin (73). PC-3 tumor-bearing mice biodistribution studies showed a significantly higher tumor uptake of the heterodimer with more than an additive effect compared to the monomeric agents BBS or RGD. In addition, the pharmacokinetic profile was enhanced, especially for the liver and the kidney uptake. Further investigations by using a ^{18}F-labeled RGD-BBS heterodimer have been performed recently (74). In this case PEG$_3$ was used as a spacer that has been described to increase the hydrophilicity, to facilitate the sterical hindrance, and to enhance the body clearance. Studies led to improved yields in radiolabeling after the introduction of PEG$_3$. Moreover, a higher body clearance in PC-3 tumor-bearing mice could be detected. More recently, Liu et al. evaluated ^{64}Cu-labeled RGD-BBS heterodimers for PET (75). They compared the suitability of the two BFCs, DOTA and NOTA, for stable ^{64}Cu complexation. In vivo characteristics in a PC-3 tumor model led to a significantly higher tumor uptake of ^{64}Cu-NOTA-RGD-BBS compared to ^{64}Cu-NOTA-RGD, ^{64}Cu-NOTA-BBS, the mixture of both, as well as ^{64}Cu-DOTA-RGD-BBS. The chemical structure of the RGD-BBS heterodimer is shown in Figure 39.6.

In some cases human breast cancer overexpresses BBS receptors (4). Accordingly, ^{64}Cu-labeled BBS analogues have been investigated for their targeting efficacy (76). In T-47D tumor-bearing SCID mice, ^{64}Cu-NO2A-Aoc-BBS(7–14)

(Fig. 39.5B) showed a higher relative accumulation in the tumor for nearly all tissues compared to ^{64}Cu-DOTA-Aoc-BBS(7–14). The liver uptake is of important relevance as it is the major site of copper metabolism (77). Furthermore, it has been suggested that different results in the tumor to liver ratios are derived from the more hydrophobic nature of the ^{64}Cu-NO2A complex compared to the ^{64}Cu-DOTA complex. A more unstable ^{64}Cu-DOTA formation could lead to the loss of ^{64}Cu that is preferentially metabolized in the liver.

The promising findings of a somatostatin antagonist as a peptide-based radiopharmaceutical resulted in the comparison of the BBS agonist [^{99m}Tc]-Demobesin 4 and the BBS antagonist [^{99m}Tc]-Demobesin 1 (Fig. 39.7) (78). The biodistribution studies in PC-3 tumor-bearing mice showed advantages for the antagonist because of its reduced physiologic activity and a much longer washout from the tumor compared to the agonist. It was suggested that this might be due to the more efficient receptor labeling of the antagonist compared to the agonist or the often-described higher metabolic stability of antagonists as well as the slower dissociation rate from the tumor (43,79). These results have been confirmed by a recent comparison of the [^{111}In/^{68}Ga]-labeled BBS antagonist RM-1 and the BBS agonist [^{111}In]-AMBA (80). The pharmacokinetic profiles were investigated in the same tumor model by using single photon emission computed tomography (SPECT)/CT and PET/CT. The antagonist showed not only a high tumor uptake, but also high tumor to normal tissue ratios. Its use also resulted in an improved tumor to kidney ratio compared to the agonist. With respect to the two different radionuclides, the ^{68}Ga-labeled RM-1 resulted in a lower kidney uptake as well as lower kidney retention than the ^{111}In-labeled RM-1.

^{90}Y and ^{177}Lu are widely used radionuclides showing suitable physical characteristics and have been successfully evaluated by using different BBS analogues (81,82). More recently, the DOTA-BBS analogue BBS(2–14) has been radiolabeled with both ^{90}Y and ^{177}Lu (83). For ^{90}Y and ^{177}Lu high radiochemical yields were obtained. In contrast, the

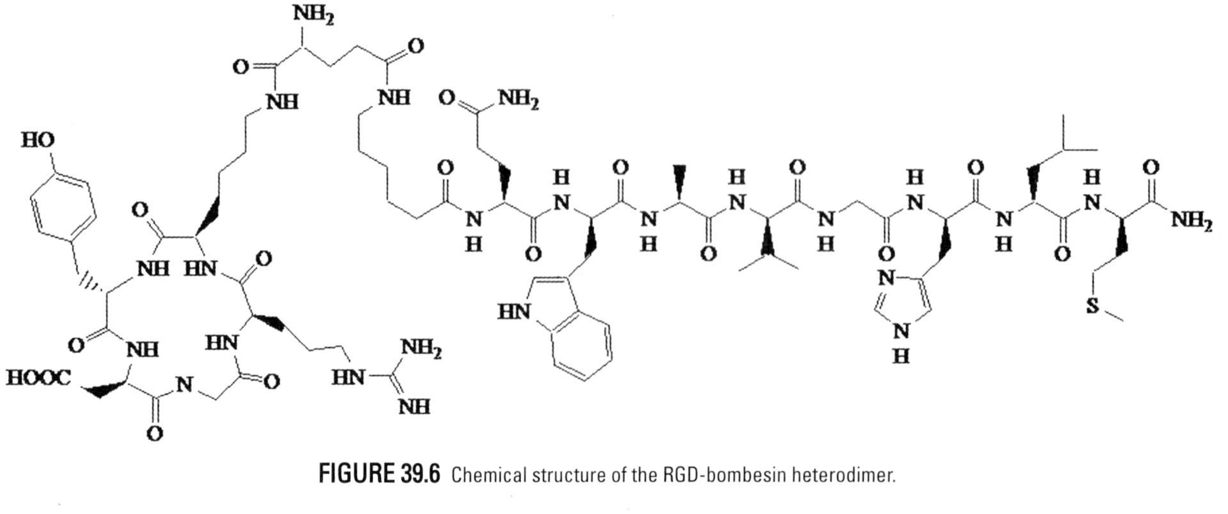

FIGURE 39.6 Chemical structure of the RGD-bombesin heterodimer.

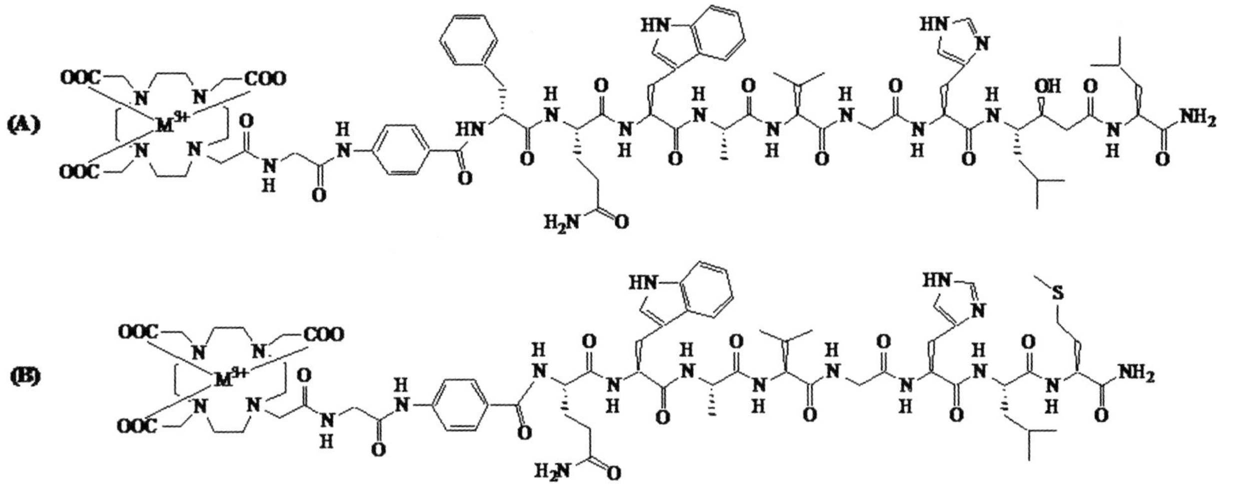

FIGURE 39.7 Chemical structures of the BBS antagonist and the BBS agonist from the comparison study. **A:** [M^{3+}]DOTA-RM-1 antagonist (M^{3+} = ^{68}Ga and ^{111}In); **B:** [M^{3+}]DOTA-AMBA agonist (M^{3+} = ^{111}In).

biologic behavior revealed a metal-mediated influence with a significant preference for the ^{177}Lu-labeled BBS analogue.

The circumvention of radiolytic damage of the peptide-based radiopharmaceutical including oxidation, hydroxylation, aggregation, or bond scission is also of great interest. The BBS analogue ^{177}Lu-AMBA is a very promising agent with high therapeutic efficacy in PC-3 tumor-bearing nude mice and currently is in clinical trials (84). However, this peptide showed high radiosensitivity and the oxidation of methionine residues resulted in complete inactivation. Recently, several radiostabilizers have been evaluated to decrease radiolytic damage of ^{177}Lu-AMBA (85). With a radiochemical purity of greater than 90% for at least 2 days at room temperature, a mixture of selenomethionine and ascorbic acid showed predominance over other investigated radiostabilizers. In this combination, selenomethionine has stabilizer functions, whereas the ascorbic acid solution is used to dilute and further stabilize the radioreaction solution. Because of the low toxicity, free radical scavenger properties, as well as antioxidant characteristics of selenium compounds, selenomethionine is a promising radiostabilizer. In 2009, a study evaluated the therapeutic potential of ^{177}Lu-AMBA in low GRP receptor–expressing prostate cancer models (86). Maddalena et al. compared the biodistribution in LNCaP, DU145, and PC-3 tumor-bearing mice. A 10-fold reduced tumor uptake was observed for the LNCaP and DU145 cell lines compared to the high GRP receptor–expressing PC-3 cell line. Interestingly, both low GRP receptor–expressing cell lines showed a significant reduction in proliferation after treatment with ^{177}Lu-AMBA.

Other peptide hormones

The 26-amino acid VIP, which belongs to the class of secretin-like peptides, was first isolated from small bowel in 1970 (87). VIP triggers numerous physiologic functions, for example, inflammation, mucosal immune functions,

secretion of different hormones, electrolyte secretion in the gut, or gastrointestinal blood flow (88). Furthermore, VIP binds to the VIP receptor subtypes VPAC$_1$ and VPAC$_2$ with high affinity, which belong to the family B of GPCRs (89). Because of high VIP receptor expression in human tumors (breast, prostate, colon, lung, liver, rectal, pancreatic ducts, as well as urinary neoplasm), this peptide hormone shows promising characteristics as a peptide-based radiopharmaceutical (90). For the first time, the ^{123}I-labeled VIP was investigated in vivo in 1994 (91). Unfortunately, a fast proteolytic degradation has been observed, which limited further applications. Accordingly, several metabolically more stable VIP analogues have been developed (92,93). Despite successful clinical studies within the last years, the often-detected lung uptake is a critical disadvantage because of the high VIP receptor expression in normal lung tissues (94). However, VIP has also been implicated in tumor cell proliferation by increasing the expression of angiogenic factors (95,96). Furthermore, it may also function as a cytokine, especially in the early metastatic stage of human prostate cancer induction, mediated by the NF-κB/MMPs-RECK/E-cadherin (NF-κB, nuclear factor-κB; MMPs, matrix metalloproteases; RECK, reversion inducing cystein rich protein with kazal motifs) system (97). Recently, cross talk has been investigated between VPAC receptors and the transactivation of the epidermal growth factor receptor (EGFR) and the human epidermal growth factor receptor 2 (HER2) in estrogen-dependent (T47D) and estrogen-independent (MDA-MB-468) human breast cancer cells (98). Interestingly, it has been found that EGFR/HER2 are transactivated by VPAC receptors that might lead to a potential application of VIP antagonists as inhibitors for human breast cancer itself.

Neurotensin

The tridecapeptide, neurotensin, was first isolated from calf hypothalamus in 1973 (99). As a neurotransmitter and a neuromodulator, several physiologic functions, including analgesic effects, paracrine and endocrine modulation, and growth stimulation in normal cells, have been determined (100). Neurotensin binds with high affinity to the three neurotensin receptor subtypes NTR_1, NTR_2, and NTR_3. NTR_1 and NTR_2 belong to the family of GPCRs, whereas NTR_3 is a single transmembrane domain type I receptor (101). The overexpression of the most important receptor subtype NTR_1 has been found in numerous human tumors including breast cancer, colon cancer, SCLC, thyroid cancer, astrocytoma, medulloblastoma, meningioma, and Ewing sarcoma (102). Due to the fast proteolytic degradation of neurotensin, analogues with improved metabolic stability have been developed in which NT(8–13) is the minimal sequence with high efficacy (103). Furthermore, neurotensin contains three enzymatic cleavage sites (104). By the stabilization of these positions, the resulting ^{99m}Tc-NT-XIX analogue shows a high tumor uptake, low nontarget accumulations (especially in the kidney), and a fast body clearance in nude mice with HT-29 xenografts (105). Furthermore, the ^{188}Re-NT-XIX analogue shows significant inhibition of the HT-29 tumor xenografts in nude mice. Recently, a set of neurotensin analogues labeled with ^{111}In-DTPA has been designed and characterized (106). In this study, the labeling position changed from the α-amino group of NT(8–13) analogues to the ε-amino group of NT(6–13) analogues in which the α-amino group was acetylated. The three enzymatic cleavage sites of neurotensin were modified by several substitutions. The most promising neurotensin analogue was a doubly stabilized [Lys^6(DTPA)] NT(6–13) analogue containing an acetylation at the α-amino group and stabilization of the Arg^8-Arg^9 bond. This analogue showed a high affinity and stability as well as a specific tumor uptake and high tumor to nontarget tissue ratios in nude mice with HT-29 xenografts.

α-Melanotropin-stimulating hormone

The first isolation of the linear tridecapeptide α-MSH was achieved from the porcine pituitary in 1956 (107). It binds to the melanocortin receptor subtypes MC_1, MC_2, MC_3, MC_4, and MC_5 that belong to the class A of GPCRs (108). The primary physiologic function of α-MSH is the regulation of skin pigmentation (109). The proven expression of MC_1 receptors in melanoma led to the potential application of α-MSH as peptide-based radiopharmaceutical (110). Unfortunately, only a low receptor density between 900 and 7000 receptors per cell has been observed (111). However, because melanoma is the most aggressive type of skin cancer and due to the lack of other applicable conventional diagnostic and therapeutic strategies, α-MSH analogues were investigated (111,112). Moreover, α-MSH analogues have been studied in preclinical and early clinical investigations (113,114). It was found that lactam bridged-cyclized α-MSH analogues were more affine and more stable compared to noncyclized peptides (115). Furthermore, after radiolabeling with ^{99m}Tc or ^{111}In small-animal SPECT/CT

in sacrificed melanoma-engrafted mice revealed successful noninvasive imaging of the tumor (113). Recently, the ^{111}In-labeled DOTA-GlyGlu-CycMSH peptide has been synthesized and investigated in vivo (116). Biodistribution studies in B16/F1 pulmonary metastatic melanoma-bearing C57 mice exhibited the successful detection of tumors. The renal uptake was 44% reduced due to the introduction of the negatively charged spacer GlyGlu. DOTA-conjugated peptides generally require higher temperatures and longer incubation times for effective radiolabeling that is in conflict with the stability of most peptides. Therefore, Wei et al. used the mono-N-hydroxysuccinimidyl penta-*tert*-butyl derivative of N-(2-aminoethyl)-*trans*-1,2-diamino-cyclohexane-N,N',N''-pentaacetic acid (CHX-A'') as BFC for ^{111}In-, ^{86}Y-, and ^{68}Ga-radiolabeling of the cyclic version of (Arg11) CCMSH (117). They obtained the radiolabeled CHX-A''-Re(Arg11)CCMSH peptides with more than 95% radiolabeling efficiency. The biodistribution in B16/F1 melanoma-bearing mice showed a fast but only moderate tumor uptake due to the low specific activity. High specific activity is much more important for α-MSH analogues because of the low receptor expression in melanoma cells. Another limitation is the high kidney uptake that was significantly reduced by the preinjection of D-lysine (114). To increase the specific activity of short half-life radiolabeled peptides microwave techniques for rapid synthesis can be applied. Cantorias et al. synthesized the ^{68}Ga-labeled CHX-A''-Re(Arg11)CCMSH peptide by using this approach, which also allowed an additional purification step to obtain high specific activity (118). The peptide was then investigated in biodistribution studies in B16/F1 murine melanoma-bearing C57 mice. Interestingly, an increased tumor uptake as well as enhanced pharmacokinetics could be observed. Moreover, the tumor retention was also significantly increased. By the separation of the radiolabeled peptide from the nonradiolabeled counterpart the unfavorable kidney uptake was 50% reduced. Due to the higher binding affinity and in vivo metabolic stability, Guo et al. investigated a cyclized α-MSH analogue labeled with ^{111}In-DOTA at the α-amino group of Lys in which the N-terminus was acetylated, Ac-GluGlu-CycMSH(DOTA), and compared it with ^{111}In-DOTA-GlyGlu-CysMSH (119). Similar MC_1 receptor binding affinities were determined. Biodistribution studies in B16/F1 melanoma-bearing C57 mice showed an increased uptake and a prolonged tumor retention for the MSH analogue labeled with DOTA at the lactam bridge-cyclic ring and can therefore be used as a suitable radiopharmaceutical for melanoma targeting.

Cholecystokinin

The peptide hormone CCK exists in three different lengths (CCK58, CCK33, and CCK8), whereas CCK33 was first isolated from porcine small intestine in 1967 (120). Physiologically, CCK8 is the predominantly active form including its activity in stimulation of the digestion of fat and proteins or its hunger suppressor functions (121). As a gastrointestinal peptide hormone CCK shows high similarity to gastrin and binds with high affinity to the CCK receptor subtypes CCK_1 and CCK_2. In addition, CCK receptor overexpression has been found in SCLC, astrocytomas, some stromal ovarian cancer, colorectal cancer, medullary thyroid carcinomas (MTC), and pancreatic cancer, whereas receptor subtype expression levels change from cancer type to cancer type (122,123). A high CCK_2 receptor density has been identified in MTC and has led to the development of CCK_2 receptor–selective peptides for tumor diagnosis and therapy (124). Despite the suitable tumor uptake and therapeutic efficacy, limitations were found due to the high toxicity of the compound, especially in the kidney and the bone barrow (125). Recently, a novel promising compound, DOTA-MG11 radiolabeled with ^{111}In, showed enhanced tumor to kidney ratios (126). Breeman et al. compared the pharmacokinetic efficacy of three different CCK_2 receptor peptides, the ^{111}In-labeled DOTA-MG11, the ^{111}In-labeled DOTA-CCK, as well as the ^{99m}Tc-labeled demogastrin 2 (127). Clinical studies in six MTC patients showed a rapid clearance by the kidney as well as a low metabolic stability of only a few minutes. The best results were obtained with the ^{99m}Tc-labeled demogastrin 2 that had the longest half-life and the highest resolution imaging of the CCK_2 receptor–positive targets. With respect to the findings of the promising application of the somatostatin antagonists, very recently, in an in vitro study two 1,4-benzodiazepine derivatives were investigated as antagonistic CCK_1 and CCK_2 receptor–selective compounds labeled with ^{125}I and compared to the ^{125}I-labeled agonist CCK (128). Moreover, these compounds only differed by their distinct R/S-isomerism. The R-isomer exhibited good specificities, affinities, and selectivities for the CCK_2 receptor. Interestingly, the S-isomer led to comparable results for the CCK_1 receptor in receptor-bearing membrane preparations as well as in Chinese hamster ovary kidney cells. In addition, the S-isomer showed a significant identification of a higher number of CCK_1 receptors compared to the agonist and might be a suitable tool for CCK_1 receptor–expressing tumors.

Neuropeptide Y

The 36-amino acid amide NPY was isolated for the first time from the brain of pig in 1982 (129). Together with the peptide YY (PYY) and the pancreatic polypeptide (PP) it forms the NPY family. As one of the most abundant peptides in the brain (the peripheral and central nervous system), NPY transmits numerous physiologic functions including regulation of food intake, control of anxiolytic and antiepileptic reactions, vasoconstriction, and the increase in memory retention (130,131). The activities are transmitted by different Y receptor subtypes, named Y_1, Y_2, Y_4, and Y_5, which belong to the family A of GPCRs (131,132). Due to the overexpression of Y_1 and/or Y_2 receptor in neuroblastoma, breast cancer, gastrointestinal stromal tumor, renal cell carcinoma, nephroblastoma, paraganglioma, pheochromocytoma, ovarian sex cord-stromal tumor, and ovarian

adenocarcinoma, NPY has been suggested to be a useful peptide-based radiopharmaceutical (133,134). It also has been shown that NPY acts as growth hormone factor in Y_1 receptor–expressing human neuroblastoma (SK-N-MC) cells. However, an important limitation is the fast proteolytic degradation of NPY and as a result metabolically more stable NPY analogues are required. Within recent years, numerous peptide and nonpeptide Y_1 and Y_2 receptor–selective derivatives have been developed (135,136). In vitro and in vivo studies have been performed for the investigation of the enzymatic cleavage sites (137,138). Moreover, breast cancer diagnosis as well as therapy is the most promising strategy by using NPY analogues due to the strong Y_1 receptor overexpression found in these tissues, whereas normal breast tissues only express Y_2 receptors (139). Therefore, current research concentrates on the development of highly potent Y_1 receptor–selective derivatives. In 2008, the Y_1 receptor–selective $[Phe^7, Pro^{34}]$NPY analogue was labeled with ^{111}In-DOTA at the N^ε side chain of Lys^4 and investigated in vitro and in vivo (Fig. 39.8A) (140). In vitro, a nanomolar-selective Y_1 receptor binding as well as a metabolic stability of several hours was identified. In addition, in vivo biodistribution studies in human breast adenocarcinoma (MCF-7) tumor-bearing mice showed a clear uptake of the ^{111}In-labeled peptide in the tumor. Unfortunately, a high accumulation in the kidney has been observed as well. Recently, $[Phe^7, Pro^{34}]$NPY and NPY were modified with N^α-histidinyl-acetyl (N^αHis-ac) at two distinct positions for Re and ^{99m}Tc labeling (Fig. 39.8B) (141). The Re-labeled peptides were investigated with respect to their binding affinities, signal transduction, and internalization that led to

(A)

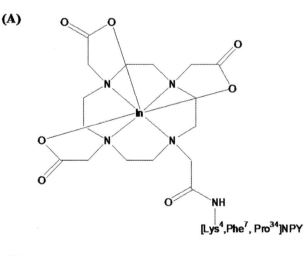

$[Lys^4,Phe^7, Pro^{34}]$NPY

(B)

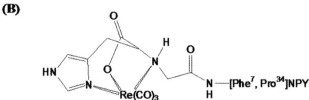

FIGURE 39.8 Chemical structures of the modified Y_1 receptor–selective $[Phe^7, Pro^{34}]$NPY analogue. **A:** $[Lys^4(In-DOTA),Phe^7,Pro^{34}]$NPY; **B:** $Re(CO)_3$-N^αHis-ac-$[Phe^7,Pro^{34}]$NPY.

Y_1 receptor–selective Re-labeled [Phe^7, Pro^{34}] NPY agonists. Moreover, in vitro studies in human blood plasma resulted in metabolically stable peptides, and the incubation of the ^{99m}Tc-labeled Y_1 receptor–selective NPY analogues showed a distinct radiostability. Optimal tumor to background ratios and a fast clearance from organs have been observed in in vivo biodistribution studies in normal rabbits. The most promising NPY analogue, the N-terminally modified [Phe^7, Pro^{34}]NPY, has been used in the first clinical studies in human breast cancer patients. For the first time, clear tumor uptake and a detection of metastases, derived from the tumor, were observed. These results highlight the potential for Y_1 receptor–selective peptides in breast cancer diagnosis and imaging. Due to the higher labeling efficiencies and lower costs, the synthesis of smaller Y_1 receptor–selective peptides is needed. In 2009, the first truncated agonistic Y_1 receptor–selective agent has been designed and characterized (142). The ligand is based on the C-terminal fragment of NPY(28–36) containing four substitutions (Pro^{30}, Nle^{31}, Bpa^{32}, and Leu^{34}) compared to the original peptide sequence. It exhibited nanomolar and selective Y_1 receptor binding. Microscopy studies revealed an agonistic behavior. A half-life of several hours was observed in vitro, in human blood plasma.

FUTURE DIRECTIONS

Due to the fact that peptide hormones are involved in tumor cell growth, the use of antagonists can inhibit cell proliferation and, moreover, can lead to tumor reduction. Multireceptor targeting strategies can significantly improve the therapeutic efficacy compared to single receptor targeting. Jaggi et al. investigated the anticancer activity in several human tumor cells of four peptide hormone analogues by coadministration (143). The peptide hormone combination, named DRF7295, contains a somatostatin, BBS, VIP, and substance P analogue. After injection of DRF7295 the gastrointestinal (colon, duodenum, and pancreas) tumor cell death exceeded 80%. Furthermore, in animal studies no toxic effects have been observed.

Tumor diagnosis and therapy appear to be very promising due to the efficacy of distinct receptor selectivity. However, despite the promising results obtained in recent years, only few peptide-based radiopharmaceuticals are commercially available and routinely used in the clinic. Future directions thus need to focus on further optimizations for the successful clinical application of PRI and PRRT. Tumor visualization and the biodistribution of the peptide-based radiopharmaceutical must be improved. Furthermore, an acceptable nontarget accumulation is required, especially for PRRT, due to the need to inject high radiation activities. Currently, only patients with small tumors or minimal residual disease have shown promising results. Because of the low and heterogeneous uptake of peptides in larger tumors, the therapeutic potential can be significantly decreased for peptide-based radiopharmaceuticals in this particular setting (144). Otherwise, the detection and therapy of not only primary tumors, but also subclinical tumors and metastases by PRRT, which are too small for conventional strategies, is a promising advantage of peptide hormones. Moreover, to increase the PRI and PRRT efficacy, combinatorial approaches are suitable tools, including the conjugation of radionuclides and chemotherapy to peptides (20,143), multiple radionuclides (145), and peptide-based radiopharmaceuticals containing an additional cytotoxic (antineoplastic) agent (40).

REFERENCES

1. Reubi JC. Peptide receptors as molecular targets for cancer diagnosis and therapy. *Endocr Rev.* 2003;24:389–427.
2. Zwanziger D, Beck-Sickinger AG. Radiometal targeted tumor diagnosis and therapy with peptide hormones. *Curr Pharm Des.* 2008;14:2385–2400.
3. Blok D, Feitsma RI, Vermeij P, et al. Peptide radiopharmaceuticals in nuclear medicine. *Eur J Nucl Med.* 1999;26:1511–1519.
4. Giacchetti S, Gauville C, de Cremoux P, et al. Characterization, in some human breast cancer cell lines, of gastrin-releasing peptide-like receptors which are absent in normal breast epithelial cells. *Int J Cancer.* 1990;46:293–298.
5. Papotti M, Croce S, Bello M, et al. Expression of somatostatin receptor types 2, 3 and 5 in biopsies and surgical specimens of human lung tumours. Correlation with preoperative octreotide scintigraphy. *Virchows Arch.* 2001;439:787–797.
6. Stinchcombe TE, Lee CB, Socinski MA. Current approaches to advanced-stage nonsmall-cell lung cancer: first-line therapy in patients with a good functional status. *Clin Lung Cancer.* 2006;7(suppl 4):S111–S117.
7. Kaida H, Ishibashi M, Fujii T, et al. Improved detection of breast cancer on FDG–PET cancer screening using breast positioning device. *Ann Nucl Med.* 2008;22:95–101.
8. Schally AV, Nagy A. Chemotherapy targeted to cancers through tumoral hormone receptors. *Trends Endocrinol Metab.* 2004;15:300–310.
9. Kaltsas GA, Papadogias D, Makras P, et al. Treatment of advanced neuroendocrine tumours with radiolabelled somatostatin analogues. *Endocr Relat Cancer.* 2005;12:683–699.
10. Okarvi SM. Peptide-based radiopharmaceuticals: future tools for diagnostic imaging of cancers and other diseases. *Med Res Rev.* 2004;24:357–397.
11. Heppeler A, Froidevaux S, Eberle AN, et al. Receptor targeting for tumor localisation and therapy with radiopeptides. *Curr Med Chem.* 2000;7:971–994.
12. Benedetti E, Morelli G, Accardo A, et al. Criteria for the design and biological characterization of radiolabeled peptide-based pharmaceuticals. *BioDrugs.* 2004;18:279–295.
13. Liu S, Edwards DS. Bifunctional chelators for therapeutic lanthanide radiopharmaceuticals. *Bioconjug Chem.* 2001;12:7–34.
14. Fichna J, Janecka A. Synthesis of target-specific radiolabeled peptides for diagnostic imaging. *Bioconjug Chem.* 2003;14:3–17.
15. Barge A, Tei L, Upadhyaya D, et al. Bifunctional ligands based on the DOTA-monoamide cage. *Org Biomol Chem.* 2008;6:1176–1184.
16. Knor S, Modlinger A, Poethko T, et al. Synthesis of novel 1,4,7,10-tetraazacyclodecane-1,4,7,10-tetraacetic acid (DOTA) derivatives for chemoselective attachment to unprotected polyfunctionalized compounds. *Chemistry.* 2007;13:6082–6090.
17. Li L, Tsai SW, Anderson AL, et al. Vinyl sulfone bifunctional derivatives of DOTA allow sulfhydryl- or amino-directed coupling to antibodies. Conjugates retain immunoreactivity and have similar biodistributions. *Bioconjug Chem.* 2002;13:110–115.
18. Lewis MR, Shively JE. Maleimidocysteineamido-DOTA derivatives: new reagents for radiometal chelate conjugation to antibody sulfhydryl groups undergo pH-dependent cleavage reactions. *Bioconjug Chem.* 1998;9:72–86.
19. Couturier O, Supiot S, Degraef-Mougin M, et al. Cancer radioimmunotherapy with alpha-emitting nuclides. *Eur J Nucl Med Mol Imaging.* 2005;32:601–614.
20. Reubi JC, Waser B. Concomitant expression of several peptide receptors in neuroendocrine tumours: molecular basis for in vivo multireceptor tumour targeting. *Eur J Nucl Med Mol Imaging.* 2003;30:781–793.

21. Krenning EP, Kwekkeboom DJ, Bakker WH, et al. Somatostatin receptor scintigraphy with [^{111}In-DTPA-D-Phe^1]- and [^{123}I-Tyr^3]-octreotide: the Rotterdam experience with more than 1000 patients. *Eur J Nucl Med.* 1993;20:716–731.

22. Weiner RE, Thakur ML. Radiolabeled peptides in diagnosis and therapy. *Semin Nucl Med.* 2001;31:296–311.

23. McAfee JG, Neumann RD. Radiolabeled peptides and other ligands for receptors overexpressed in tumor cells for imaging neoplasms. *Nucl Med Biol.* 1996;23:673–676.

24. Ansquer C, Kraeber-Bodere F, Chatal JF. Current status and perspectives in peptide receptor radiation therapy. *Curr Pharm Des.* 2009;15:2453–2462.

25. Reubi C, Gugger M, Waser B. Co-expressed peptide receptors in breast cancer as a molecular basis for in vivo multireceptor tumour targeting. *Eur J Nucl Med Mol Imaging.* 2002;29:855–862.

26. Brazeau P, Vale W, Burgus R, et al. Hypothalamic polypeptide that inhibits the secretion of immunoreactive pituitary growth hormone. *Science.* 1973;179:77–79.

27. Hoyer D, Bell GI, Berelowitz M, et al. Classification and nomenclature of somatostatin receptors. *Trends Pharmacol Sci.* 1995;16:86–88.

28. Patel YC. Somatostatin and its receptor family. *Front Neuroendocrinol.* 1999;20:157–198.

29. Dorr U, Wurm K, Horing E, et al. Diagnostic reliability of somatostatin receptor scintigraphy during continuous treatment with different somatostatin analogs. *Horm Metab Res Suppl.* 1993;27:36–43.

30. Sheppard M, Shapiro B, Pimstone B, et al. Metabolic clearance and plasma half-disappearance time of exogenous somatostatin in man. *J Clin Endocrinol Metab.* 1979;48:50–53.

31. Reubi JC, Schar JC, Waser B, et al. Affinity profiles for human somatostatin receptor subtypes SST$_1$-SST$_5$ of somatostatin radiotracers selected for scintigraphic and radiotherapeutic use. *Eur J Nucl Med.* 2000;27:273–282.

32. Reubi JC. Somatostatin and other peptide receptors as tools for tumor diagnosis and treatment. *Neuroendocrinology.* 2004;80(suppl 1):51–56.

33. Virgolini I, Traub T, Novotny C, et al. New trends in peptide receptor radioligands. *Q J Nucl Med.* 2001;45:153–159.

34. Reubi JC, Lamberts SJ, Krenning EP. Receptor imaging of human diseases using radiolabeled peptides. *J Recept Signal Transduct Res.* 1995;15:379–392.

35. de Jong M, Bakker WH, Krenning EP, et al. Yttrium-90 and indium-111 labelling, receptor binding and biodistribution of [DOTA^0, D-Phe^1,Tyr^3]octreotide, a promising somatostatin analogue for radionuclide therapy. *Eur J Nucl Med.* 1997;24:368–371.

36. Bartolomei M, Bodei L, De Cicco C, et al. Peptide receptor radionuclide therapy with $^{(90)}$Y-DOTATOC in recurrent meningioma. *Eur J Nucl Med Mol Imaging.* 2009;36:1407–1416.

37. de Jong M, Breeman WA, Bakker WH, et al. Comparison of $^{(111)}$In-labeled somatostatin analogues for tumor scintigraphy and radionuclide therapy. *Cancer Res.* 1998;58:437–441.

38. Forrer F, Uusijarvi H, Waldherr C, et al. A comparison of $^{(111)}$In-DOTATOC and $^{(111)}$In-DOTATATE: biodistribution and dosimetry in the same patients with metastatic neuroendocrine tumours. *Eur J Nucl Med Mol Imaging.* 2004;31:1257–1262.

39. Kwekkeboom DJ, Teunissen JJ, Bakker WH, et al. Radiolabeled somatostatin analog [^{177}Lu-DOTA^0,Tyr^3]octreotate in patients with endocrine gastroenteropancreatic tumors. *J Clin Oncol.* 2005;23:2754–2762.

40. van Essen M, Krenning EP, Kam BL, et al. Report on short-term side effects of treatments with ^{177}Lu-octreotate in combination with capecitabine in seven patients with gastroenteropancreatic neuroendocrine tumours. *Eur J Nucl Med Mol Imaging.* 2008;35:743–748.

41. Ginj M, Chen J, Walter MA, et al. Preclinical evaluation of new and highly potent analogues of octreotide for predictive imaging and targeted radiotherapy. *Clin Cancer Res.* 2005;11:1136–1145.

42. Virgolini I, Leimer M, Handmaker H, et al. Somatostatin receptor subtype specificity and in vivo binding of a novel tumor tracer, ^{99m}Tc-P829. *Cancer Res.* 1998;58:1850–1859.

43. Ginj M, Zhang H, Waser B, et al. Radiolabeled somatostatin receptor antagonists are preferable to agonists for in vivo peptide receptor targeting of tumors. *Proc Natl Acad Sci USA.* 2006;103:16436–16441.

44. Boswell CA, Sun X, Niu W, et al. Comparative in vivo stability of copper-64-labeled cross-bridged and conventional tetraazamacrocyclic complexes. *J Med Chem.* 2004;47:1465–1474.

45. Wadas TJ, Eiblmaier M, Zheleznyak A, et al. Preparation and biological evaluation of ^{64}Cu-CB-TE2A-sst$_2$-ANT, a somatostatin antagonist for PET imaging of somatostatin receptor-positive tumors. *J Nucl Med.* 2008;49:1819–1827.

46. Gabriel M, Decristoforo C, Kendler D, et al. ^{68}Ga-DOTA-Tyr^3-octreotide PET in neuroendocrine tumors: comparison with somatostatin receptor scintigraphy and CT. *J Nucl Med.* 2007;48:508–518.

47. Gabriel M, Oberauer A, Dobrozemsky G, et al. ^{68}Ga-DOTA-Tyr^3-octreotide PET for assessing response to somatostatin-receptor-mediated radionuclide therapy. *J Nucl Med.* 2009;50:1427–1434.

48. Kayani I, Conry BG, Groves AM, et al. A comparison of ^{68}Ga-DOTA-TATE and ^{18}F-FDG PET/CT in pulmonary neuroendocrine tumors. *J Nucl Med.* 2009;50:1927–1932.

49. Treszl A, Schally AV, Seitz S, et al. Inhibition of human non-small cell lung cancers with a targeted cytotoxic somatostatin analog, AN-162. *Peptides.* 2009;30:1643–1650.

50. Bodei L, Cremonesi M, Ferrari M, et al. Long-term evaluation of renal toxicity after peptide receptor radionuclide therapy with ^{90}Y-DOTA-TOC and ^{177}Lu-DOTATATE: the role of associated risk factors. *Eur J Nucl Med Mol Imaging.* 2008;35:1847–1856.

51. de Jong M, Barone R, Krenning E, et al. Megalin is essential for renal proximal tubule reabsorption of $^{(111)}$In-DTPA-octreotide. *J Nucl Med.* 2005;46:1696–1700.

52. Baines RJ, Brunskill NJ. The molecular interactions between filtered proteins and proximal tubular cells in proteinuria. *Nephron Exp Nephrol.* 2008;110:e67–e71.

53. Gotthardt M, van Eerd-Vismale J, Oyen WJ, et al. Indication for different mechanisms of kidney uptake of radiolabeled peptides. *J Nucl Med.* 2007;48:596–601.

54. Behr TM, Goldenberg D, Becker W. Reducing the renal uptake of radiolabeled antibody fragments and peptides for diagnosis and therapy: present status, future prospects and limitations. *Eur J Nucl Med.* 1998;25:201–212.

55. Rolleman EJ, Bernard BF, Breeman WA, et al. Molecular imaging of reduced renal uptake of radiolabelled [DOTA^0,Tyr^3]octreotate by the combination of lysine and Gelofusine in rats. *Nuklearmedizin.* 2008;47:110–115.

56. Vegt E, van Eerd JE, Eek A, et al. Reducing renal uptake of radiolabeled peptides using albumin fragments. *J Nucl Med.* 2008;49:1506–1511.

57. Vegt E, Eek A, Oyen WJ, et al. Albumin-derived peptides efficiently reduce renal uptake of radiolabelled peptides. *Eur J Nucl Med Mol Imaging.* 2009;37:226–234.

58. Anastasi A, Erspamer V, Bucci M. Isolation and structure of bombesin and alytesin, 2 analogous active peptides from the skin of the European amphibians *Bombina* and *Alytes. Experientia.* 1971;27:166–167.

59. McDonald TJ, Jornvall H, Nilsson G, et al. Characterization of a gastrin releasing peptide from porcine non-antral gastric tissue. *Biochem Biophys Res Commun.* 1979;90:227–233.

60. Cuttitta F, Carney DN, Mulshine J, et al. Bombesin-like peptides can function as autocrine growth factors in human small-cell lung cancer. *Nature.* 1985;316:823–826.

61. Aprikian AG, Tremblay L, Han K, et al. Bombesin stimulates the motility of human prostate-carcinoma cells through tyrosine phosphorylation of focal adhesion kinase and of integrin-associated proteins. *Int J Cancer.* 1997;72:498–504.

62. Ohki-Hamazaki H, Iwabuchi M, Maekawa F. Development and function of bombesin-like peptides and their receptors. *Int J Dev Biol.* 2005;49:293–300.

63. Gugger M, Reubi JC. Gastrin-releasing peptide receptors in non-neoplastic and neoplastic human breast. *Am J Pathol.* 1999;155:2067–2076.

64. Hoffman TJ, Quinn TP, Volkert WA. Radiometallated receptor-avid peptide conjugates for specific in vivo targeting of cancer cells. *Nucl Med Biol.* 2001;28:527–539.

65. Garcia Garayoa E, Ruegg D, Blauenstein P, et al. Chemical and biological characterization of new Re(CO)$_3$/[^{99m}Tc](CO)$_3$ bombesin analogues. *Nucl Med Biol.* 2007;34:17–28.

66. Kunstler JU, Veerendra B, Figueroa SD, et al. Organometallic ^{99m}Tc(III) '4 + 1' bombesin(7–14) conjugates: synthesis, radiolabeling, and in vitro/in vivo studies. *Bioconjug Chem.* 2007;18:1651–1661.

67. Parry JJ, Kelly TS, Andrews R, et al. In vitro and in vivo evaluation of ^{64}Cu-labeled DOTA-linker-bombesin(7–14) analogues containing different amino acid linker moieties. *Bioconjug Chem.* 2007;18:1110–1117.

68. Smith CJ, Gali H, Sieckman GL, et al. Radiochemical investigations of $^{(99m)}$Tc-N(3)S-X-BBN[7–14]NH$_{(2)}$: an in vitro/in vivo structure–activity relationship study where X = 0-, 3-, 5-, 8-, and 11-carbon tethering moieties. *Bioconjug Chem.* 2003;14:93–102.

69. Schweinsberg C, Maes V, Brans L, et al. Novel glycated [^{99m}Tc(CO)$_3$]-labeled bombesin analogues for improved targeting of gastrin-releasing peptide receptor-positive tumors. *Bioconjug Chem.* 2008;19:2432–2439.

70. Alves S, Correia JD, Santos I, et al. Pyrazolyl conjugates of bombesin: a new tridentate ligand framework for the stabilization of fac-$[M(CO)_3]^+$ moiety. *Nucl Med Biol.* 2006;33:625–634.

71. Faintuch BL, Teodoro R, Duatti A, et al. Radiolabeled bombesin analogs for prostate cancer diagnosis: preclinical studies. *Nucl Med Biol.* 2008;35:401–411.

72. Li ZB, Wu Z, Chen K, et al. ^{18}F-labeled BBN–RGD heterodimer for prostate cancer imaging. *J Nucl Med.* 2008;49:453–461.

73. Haubner R, Weber WA, Beer AJ, et al. Noninvasive visualization of the activated alphavbeta3 integrin in cancer patients by positron emission tomography and [^{18}F]galacto-RGD. *PLoS Med.* 2005;2:e70.

74. Liu Z, Yan Y, Chin FT, et al. Dual integrin and gastrin-releasing peptide receptor targeted tumor imaging using ^{18}F-labeled PEGylated RGD–bombesin heterodimer ^{18}F-FB-PEG$_3$-Glu-RGD-BBN. *J Med Chem.* 2009;52:425–432.

75. Liu Z, Li ZB, Cao Q, et al. Small-animal PET of tumors with $^{(64)}$Cu-labeled RGD–bombesin heterodimer. *J Nucl Med.* 2009;50:1168–1177.

76. Prasanphanich AF, Retzloff L, Lane SR, et al. In vitro and in vivo analysis of [$^{(64)}$Cu-NO2A-8-Aoc-BBN(7–14)NH$_{(2)}$]: a site-directed radiopharmaceutical for positron-emission tomography imaging of T-47D human breast cancer tumors. *Nucl Med Biol.* 2009;36:171–181.

77. Wadas TJ, Wong EH, Weisman GR, et al. Copper chelation chemistry and its role in copper radiopharmaceuticals. *Curr Pharm Des.* 2007;13: 3–16.

78. Cescato R, Maina T, Nock B, et al. Bombesin receptor antagonists may be preferable to agonists for tumor targeting. *J Nucl Med.* 2008;49: 318–326.

79. Vauquelin G, Van Liefde I. Slow antagonist dissociation and long-lasting in vivo receptor protection. *Trends Pharmacol Sci.* 2006;27: 356–359.

80. Mansi R, Wang X, Forrer F, et al. Evaluation of a 1,4,7,10-tetraazacyclododecane-1,4,7,10-tetraacetic acid-conjugated bombesin-based radioantagonist for the labeling with single-photon emission computed tomography, positron emission tomography, and therapeutic radionuclides. *Clin Cancer Res.* 2009;15:5240–5249.

81. Gourni E, Paravatou M, Bouziotis P, et al. Evaluation of a series of new ^{99m}Tc-labeled bombesin-like peptides for early cancer detection. *Anticancer Res.* 2006;26:435–438.

82. Panigone S, Nunn AD. Lutetium-177-labeled gastrin releasing peptide receptor binding analogs: a novel approach to radionuclide therapy. *Q J Nucl Med Mol Imaging.* 2006;50:310–321.

83. Koumarianou E, Mikolajczak R, Pawlak D, et al. Comparative study on DOTA-derivatized bombesin analog labeled with ^{90}Y and ^{177}Lu: in vitro and in vivo evaluation. *Nucl Med Biol.* 2009;36:591–603.

84. Lantry LE, Cappelletti E, Maddalena ME, et al. ^{177}Lu-AMBA: synthesis and characterization of a selective ^{177}Lu-labeled GRP-R agonist for systemic radiotherapy of prostate cancer. *J Nucl Med.* 2006;47: 1144–1152.

85. Chen J, Linder KE, Cagnolini A, et al. Synthesis, stabilization and formulation of [^{177}Lu]Lu-AMBA, a systemic radiotherapeutic agent for gastrin releasing peptide receptor positive tumors. *Appl Radiat Isot.* 2008;66:497–505.

86. Maddalena ME, Fox J, Cheng J et al. ^{177}Lu-AMBA biodistribution, radiotherapeutic efficacy, imaging, and autoradiography in prostate cancer models with low GRP-R expression. *J Nucl Med.* 2009;50: 2017–2024.

87. Said SI, Mutt V. Polypeptide with broad biological activity: isolation from small intestine. *Science.* 1970;169:1217–1218.

88. Schwartz CJ, Kimberg DV, Sheerin HE, et al. Vasoactive intestinal peptide stimulation of adenylate cyclase and active electrolyte secretion in intestinal mucosa. *J Clin Invest.* 1974;54:536–544.

89. Vaudry D, Gonzalez BJ, Basille M, et al. Pituitary adenylate cyclase-activating polypeptide and its receptors: from structure to functions. *Pharmacol Rev.* 2000;52:269–324.

90. Hoshino M, Yanaihara C, Ogino K, et al. Production of VIP- and PHM (human PHI)-related peptides in human neuroblastoma cells. *Peptides.* 1984;5:155–160.

91. Virgolini I, Raderer M, Kurtaran A, et al. Vasoactive intestinal peptide-receptor imaging for the localization of intestinal adenocarcinomas and endocrine tumors. *N Engl J Med.* 1994;331:1116–1121.

92. Pallela VR, Thakur ML, Chakder S, et al. ^{99m}Tc-labeled vasoactive intestinal peptide receptor agonist: functional studies. *J Nucl Med.* 1999;40:352–360.

93. Rao PS, Thakur ML, Pallela V, et al. ^{99m}Tc labeled VIP analog: evaluation for imaging colorectal cancer. *Nucl Med Biol.* 2001;28:445–450.

94. Thakur ML, Marcus CS, Saeed S, et al. ^{99m}Tc-labeled vasoactive intestinal peptide analog for rapid localization of tumors in humans. *J Nucl Med.* 2000;41:107–110.

95. Moody TW, Jensen RT. Breast cancer VPAC$_1$ receptors. *Ann N Y Acad Sci.* 2006;1070:436–439.

96. Valdehita A, Carmena MJ, Collado B, et al. Vasoactive intestinal peptide (VIP) increases vascular endothelial growth factor (VEGF) expression and secretion in human breast cancer cells. *Regul Pept.* 2007;144:101–108.

97. Fernandez-Martinez AB, Bajo AM, Sanchez-Chapado M, et al. Vasoactive intestinal peptide behaves as a pro-metastatic factor in human prostate cancer cells. *Prostate.* 2009;69:774–786.

98. Valdehita A, Bajo AM, Schally AV, et al. Vasoactive intestinal peptide (VIP) induces transactivation of EGFR and HER2 in human breast cancer cells. *Mol Cell Endocrinol.* 2009;302:41–48.

99. Carraway R, Leeman SE. The isolation of a new hypotensive peptide, neurotensin, from bovine hypothalami. *J Biol Chem.* 1973;248:6854–6861.

100. Vincent JP, Mazella J, Kitabgi P. Neurotensin and neurotensin receptors. *Trends Pharmacol Sci.* 1999;20:302–309.

101. Pelaprat D. Interactions between neurotensin receptors and G proteins. *Peptides.* 2006;27:2476–2487.

102. Reubi JC, Waser B, Schaer JC, et al. Neurotensin receptors in human neoplasms: high incidence in Ewing's sarcomas. *Int J Cancer.* 1999;82: 213–218.

103. Bergmann R, Scheunemann M, Heichert C, et al. Biodistribution and catabolism of $^{(18)}$F-labeled neurotensin(8–13) analogs. *Nucl Med Biol.* 2002;29:61–72.

104. Garcia-Garayoa E, Blauenstein P, Bruehlmeier M, et al. Preclinical evaluation of a new, stabilized neurotensin(8–13) pseudopeptide radiolabeled with $^{(99m)}$Tc. *J Nucl Med.* 2002;43:374–383.

105. Garcia-Garayoa E, Blauenstein P, Blanc A, et al. A stable neurotensin-based radiopharmaceutical for targeted imaging and therapy of neurotensin receptor-positive tumours. *Eur J Nucl Med Mol Imaging.* 2009;36:37–47.

106. Alshoukr F, Rosant C, Maes V, et al. Novel neurotensin analogues for radioisotope targeting to neurotensin receptor-positive tumors. *Bioconjug Chem.* 2009;20:1602–1610.

107. Harris JI, Roos P. Amino-acid sequence of a melanophore-stimulating peptide. *Nature.* 1956;178:90.

108. Schioth HB, Haitina T, Ling MK, et al. Evolutionary conservation of the structural, pharmacological, and genomic characteristics of the melanocortin receptor subtypes. *Peptides.* 2005;26:1886–1900.

109. Sawyer TK, Staples DJ, Castrucci AM, et al. Alpha-melanocyte stimulating hormone message and inhibitory sequences: comparative structure–activity studies on melanocytes. *Peptides.* 1990;11:351–357.

110. Siegrist W, Solca F, Stutz S, et al. Characterization of receptors for alpha-melanocyte-stimulating hormone on human melanoma cells. *Cancer Res.* 1989;49:6352–6358.

111. Rampen FH, Casparie-van Velsen JI, van Huystee BE, et al. False-negative findings in skin cancer and melanoma screening. *J Am Acad Dermatol.* 1995;33:59–63.

112. Dadachova E, Casadevall A. Renaissance of targeting molecules for melanoma. *Cancer Biother Radiopharm.* 2006;21:545–552.

113. Miao Y, Benwell K, Quinn TP. ^{99m}Tc- and ^{111}In-labeled alpha-melanocyte-stimulating hormone peptides as imaging probes for primary and pulmonary metastatic melanoma detection. *J Nucl Med.* 2007;48: 73–80.

114. Wei L, Miao Y, Gallazzi F, et al. Gallium-68-labeled DOTA–rhenium-cyclized alpha-melanocyte-stimulating hormone analog for imaging of malignant melanoma. *Nucl Med Biol.* 2007;34:945–953.

115. Fung S, Hruby VJ. Design of cyclic and other templates for potent and selective peptide alpha-MSH analogues. *Curr Opin Chem Biol.* 2005;9:352–358.

116. Guo H, Shenoy N, Gershman BM, et al. Metastatic melanoma imaging with an $^{(111)}$In-labeled lactam bridge-cyclized alpha-melanocyte-stimulating hormone peptide. *Nucl Med Biol.* 2009;36:267–276.

117. Wei L, Zhang X, Gallazzi F, et al. Melanoma imaging using $^{(111)}$In-, $^{(86)}$Y- and $^{(68)}$Ga-labeled CHX-A″-Re(Arg^{11})CCMSH. *Nucl Med Biol.* 2009;36:345–354.

118. Cantorias MV, Figueroa SD, Quinn TP, et al. Development of high-specific-activity $^{(68)}$Ga-labeled DOTA–rhenium-cyclized alpha-MSH peptide analog to target MC$_1$ receptors overexpressed by melanoma tumors. *Nucl Med Biol.* 2009;36:505–513.

119. Guo H, Yang J, Gallazzi F, et al. Effect of DOTA position on melanoma targeting and pharmacokinetic effect of ^{111}In-labeled lactam bridge-

cyclized α-melanocyte stimulating hormone peptide. *Bioconjug Chem.* 2009;20:2162–2168.

120. Mutt V, Jorpes JE. Contemporary developments in the biochemistry of the gastrointestinal hormones. *Recent Prog Horm Res.* 1967;23: 483–503.

121. Hakanson R, Sundler F. Trophic effects of gastrin. *Scand J Gastroenterol Suppl.* 1991;180:130–136.

122. Jensen RT. Involvement of cholecystokinin/gastrin-related peptides and their receptors in clinical gastrointestinal disorders. *Pharmacol Toxicol.* 2002;91:333–350.

123. Weinberg DS, Ruggeri B, Barber MT, et al. Cholecystokinin A and B receptors are differentially expressed in normal pancreas and pancreatic adenocarcinoma. *J Clin Invest.* 1997;100:597–603.

124. Reubi JC, Waser B. Unexpected high incidence of cholecystokinin-B/gastrin receptors in human medullary thyroid carcinomas. *Int J Cancer.* 1996;67:644–647.

125. Behe M, Behr TM. Cholecystokinin-B (CCK-B)/gastrin receptor targeting peptides for staging and therapy of medullary thyroid cancer and other CCK-B receptor expressing malignancies. *Biopolymers.* 2002;66:399–418.

126. Good S, Walter MA, Waser B, et al. Macrocyclic chelator-coupled gastrin-based radiopharmaceuticals for targeting of gastrin receptor-expressing tumours. *Eur J Nucl Med Mol Imaging.* 2008;35:1868–1877.

127. Breeman WA, Froberg AC, de Blois E, et al. Optimised labeling, preclinical and initial clinical aspects of CCK-2 receptor-targeting with 3 radiolabeled peptides. *Nucl Med Biol.* 2008;35:839–849.

128. Akgun E, Korner M, Gao F, et al. Synthesis and in vitro characterization of radioiodinatable benzodiazepines selective for type 1 and type 2 cholecystokinin receptors. *J Med Chem.* 2009;52:2138–2147.

129. Tatemoto K, Carlquist M, Mutt V. Neuropeptide Y—a novel brain peptide with structural similarities to peptide YY and pancreatic polypeptide. *Nature.* 1982;296:659–660.

130. Pedrazzini T, Pralong F, Grouzmann E. Neuropeptide Y: the universal soldier. *Cell Mol Life Sci.* 2003;60:350–377.

131. Magni P. Hormonal control of the neuropeptide Y system. *Curr Protein Pept Sci.* 2003;4:45–57.

132. Michel MC, Beck-Sickinger A, Cox H, et al. XVI. International Union of Pharmacology recommendations for the nomenclature of neuro-peptide Y, peptide YY, and pancreatic polypeptide receptors. *Pharmacol Rev.* 1998;50:143–150.

133. Korner M, Waser B, Reubi JC. Neuropeptide Y receptor expression in human primary ovarian neoplasms. *Lab Invest.* 2004;84:71–80.

134. Korner M, Waser B, Reubi JC. Neuropeptide Y receptors in renal cell carcinomas and nephroblastomas. *Int J Cancer.* 2005;115:734–741.

135. Leban JJ, Heyer D, Landavazo A, et al. Novel modified carboxy terminal fragments of neuropeptide Y with high affinity for Y_2-type receptors and potent functional antagonism at a Y_1-type receptor. *J Med Chem.* 1995;38:1150–1157.

136. Koglin N, Zorn C, Beumer R, et al. Analogues of neuropeptide Y containing beta-aminocyclopropane carboxylic acids are the shortest linear peptides that are selective for the Y_1 receptor. *Angew Chem Int Ed Engl.* 2003;42:202–205.

137. Khan IU, Reppich R, Beck-Sickinger AG. Identification of neuropeptide Y cleavage products in human blood to improve metabolic stability. *Biopolymers.* 2007;88:182–189.

138. Abid K, Rochat B, Lassahn PG, et al. Kinetic study of neuropeptide Y (NPY) proteolysis in blood and identification of NPY3-35: a new peptide generated by plasma kallikrein. *J Biol Chem.* 2009;284:24715–24724.

139. Reubi JC, Gugger M, Waser B, et al. Y(1)-mediated effect of neuropeptide Y in cancer: breast carcinomas as targets. *Cancer Res.* 2001;61:4636–4641.

140. Zwanziger D, Khan IU, Neundorf I, et al. Novel chemically modified analogues of neuropeptide Y for tumor targeting. *Bioconjug Chem.* 2008;19:1430–1438.

141. Khan IU, Zwanziger DZ, Böhme I, et al. Breast-cancer diagnosis by neuropeptide Y analogs: from synthesis to clinical application. *Angew Chem Int Ed Engl.* 2010;49(6):1155–1158.

142. Zwanziger D, Böhme I, Lindner D, et al. First selective agonist of the neuropeptide Y_1 receptor with reduced size. *J Pept Sci.* 2009;15:856–866.

143. Jaggi M, Prasad S, Singh AT, et al. Anticancer activity of a peptide combination in gastrointestinal cancers targeting multiple neuropeptide receptors. *Invest New Drugs.* 2008;26:489–504.

144. Chatal JF, Le Bodic MF, Kraeber-Bodere F, et al. Nuclear medicine applications for neuroendocrine tumors. *World J Surg.* 2000;24:1285–1289.

145. de Jong M, Breeman WA, Valkema R, et al. Combination radionuclide therapy using ^{177}Lu- and ^{90}Y-labeled somatostatin analogs. *J Nucl Med.* 2005;46(suppl 1):13S–17S.

Radioimmunotherapy of Melanoma

Ekaterina Dadachova and Arturo Casadevall

■ INTRODUCTION

Melanoma is a malignancy with increasing incidence that affects ~60,000 new patients each year in the United States and an estimated 132,000 worldwide (1). Melanoma is particularly notable as an important cause of cancer among individuals 30 to 50 years of age, and the impact on this relatively young age group imposes economic losses to society that further compound the human loss and suffering caused by this disease. While primary tumors that are localized to the skin can be successfully treated by surgical removal, there is no satisfactory treatment for metastatic melanoma, a condition that currently has an estimated 5-year survival of only 6% (2).

The pioneers of targeted radionuclide therapy recognized the potential of radioimmunotherapy (RIT) in the treatment of metastatic melanoma from its earliest days. Already in 1981, only 5 years after Köhler and Milstein described the hybridoma technology for production of larger quantities of monoclonal antibodies (mAbs), DeNardo and colleagues published encouraging results on curative radiation therapy delivered to melanoma in mice by ^{131}I-labeled mAbs against P-51 murine melanoma (3). RIT of melanoma quickly moved into the clinic when in 1985 Larsen observed a 50% reduction in tumor size in a patient with metastatic melanoma treated with ^{131}I-labeled Fab' fragments of a mAb against high molecular weight melanoma–associated antigen (HMW MAA) (4). Despite early successes during the 1980s, RIT of melanoma did not develop into a clinical modality for a variety of reasons that included the complexity of therapy, and disappointing results in clinical trials of different solid tumors.

Within the last decade RIT has made an impressive comeback as evidenced by the approval in 2003 to 2004 of Zevalin and Bexxar (anti-CD20 mAbs labeled with ^{90}Y and ^{131}I, respectively) for the treatment of relapsed or refractory B-cell non-Hodgkin lymphoma (5). The encouraging reports on the use of RIT as an initial treatment for follicular lymphoma which followed these developments (6) have contributed to the 2009 FDA approval making Zevalin a part of first-line therapy of NHL. Simultaneously, there has been little change over the past 25 years in the dismal prognosis for patients with metastatic melanoma. Here we review the early encouraging results in the treatment of melanoma with radiolabeled mAbs, provide an analysis of the reasons for the downturn in melanoma RIT during the 1990s and of the subsequent developments, which have lead to renewed

interest in developing RIT of melanoma. Also, recent encouraging clinical and preclinical results in melanoma treatment with radiolabeled mAbs and peptides will be described.

■ OVERVIEW OF THE EARLY ENCOURAGING RESULTS IN RIT OF MELANOMA

The first panel of mAbs to melanoma with the aim of using them for RIT was generated against P51 murine melanoma in 1981 by SJ and GL DeNardo and colleagues (3,5). The antigens to which the mAbs were binding were located on melanoma tumor cell membranes in high concentration (~3×10^5 binding sites per cell). The tissue distribution of ^{131}I-mAb in P51 melanoma-bearing C57 black mice demonstrated a ratio of tumor to muscle uptake of 20 to 1 and tumor-injected dose per gram (ID/g) of 15% at 72 hours. When therapeutic doses of ^{131}I-mAb were administered to mice the tumors regressed from 0.4 cm to nonpalpable in 5 days and the animals survived 6 months without evidence of recurrence. In 1982 to 1983, the DeNardos formulated the general approach to successful RIT of cancer when "judicious choice of tumor antigens for targets must be made and well characterized; avid antibody fragment carriers must be produced; radionuclides appropriate to the biokinetics must be selected; and radiochemical attachment of the nuclide and antibody carrier performed in a manner that will assure a stable, safe and dependable radiopharmaceutical"(7,8). This group also recognized the great potential of computer modeling in RIT and used three-compartmental model system to investigate the interplay between renal clearance, tumor uptake, and radioactive decay of a radiolabeled mAb (7).

The identification of target antigens on melanoma cells and the development of mAbs against these antigens for radioimmunodetection of malignant melanoma received considerable attention in the early 1980s. Several important antigens were identified such as the 94 kDa membrane-bound glycoprotein; HMW MAA (9) (which consists of two noncovalently associated glycopolypeptides, the apparent MW of which is 280 and over 440 kDa, respectively); an 85 kDa membrane-bound glycoprotein; a four-chain cytoplasmic antigen; Ia antigens (which are the human counterparts of the murine I-E subregion antigens) (10); and the 97 kDa p97 sialoglycoprotein located on the outer surface of the plasma membrane (11). The 94 kDa glycoprotein (HMW MAA) and the 85 kDa antigen and cytoplasmic antigen are similar in their distribution on cells of the melanocyte lineage so they are not detectable on resting melanocytes but are expressed by nevi and melanoma cells.

In the prewhole body positron emission tomography (PET) era mAbs labeled with ^{99m}Tc, ^{111}In, as well as with ^{131}I were used extensively for radioimmunoimaging of metastatic melanoma, as it is possible to survey the entire body for metastases in a single study and to detect a substantial number of otherwise occult lesions. HMW MAA became by far the most widely used antigen for radioimmunoimaging. A review by Kang and Yong (12) summarizes 58 patient trials (excluding case studies) involving a total of 3638 patients with the majority of these studies (greater than 80%) utilizing mAbs to HMW MAA. MAb to HMW MAA became the choice for clinical RIT of melanoma when ^{131}I-labeled Fab' of a mAb to HMW MAA was used to treat a patient with bulky metastatic disease. Administration of a total dose of 374 mCi ^{131}I-labeled Fab' fragment resulted in a greater than 50% reduction in the size of pelvic and pericaval nodes (4). These early studies provide remarkably strong evidence that radiolabeled mAbs can be effective in treatment of melanoma in animal models and in patients.

■ DECLINE OF MELANOMA RIT IN THE 1990S

There are four major reasons for the decline of melanoma RIT during the 1990s, with two of them related to the state of nuclear medicine field in general and the other two being melanoma specific. First, in the 1990s PET started to be introduced into clinical practice for whole body imaging, proving to be superior to the radiolabeled antibodies. Disillusionment with the mAbs as imaging agents also resulted in abandoning many of these agents for further therapeutic development. Second, the RIT field in general was plagued by disappointing results in clinical trials of different solid tumors. Third, RIT of melanoma might have been discouraged by the perception that melanoma is a radiation-resistant tumor (13), given the inefficacy of radiation therapy of melanoma with external beam sources. In fact, inadequate external radiation therapy can promote metastatic spread in human melanoma (14). And fourth, dosimetry calculation performed by using the biodistribution data in patients showed that if therapeutic doses of radiolabeled mAb are administered, the dose to the tumor will be relatively low while the dose to the whole body and liver will be unacceptably high.

Taylor et al. (15) imaged patients with metastatic melanoma with ^{111}In-labeled ZME-018 mAb to HMW MAA and performed calculations based on obtained biodistributions. The results indicate that an average tumor uptake of 0.01% ID/g was obtained from a delivered activity of 100 mCi ^{90}Y-labeled ZME-018. The calculated doses were 1830, 220, and 790 cGy to the tumor, whole body, and liver, respectively. Of note, the high whole body and liver doses could be decreased by fractionation. At that time, it was assumed that the tumoricidal doses should be in the 10,000 to 20,000 cGy range (following external radiation beam therapy requirements) thus it appeared that RIT was nonviable. However,

the authors also noted that in some patients the uptake into the tumor was as high as 0.67% ID/g, which meant that five times lower activity of 20 mCi ^{90}Y-labeled ZME-018 would deliver approximately 20,000 cGy to the tumor. This last observation highlights the need for patient-specific dosimetry, which was not widely practiced in the late 1980s and 1990s but which since then has become state of the art in clinical RIT.

■ RENAISSANCE OF RIT OF MELANOMA IN THE LAST DECADE

In the last decade we have witnessed the renewed effort in developing RIT for melanoma treatment. This is a consequence of the fact that RIT is currently experiencing a renaissance as a treatment modality. RIT is now equipped with much better "tools" in regard to better mAbs (16), radioisotopes with a variety of emission types and half-lives, novel antigenic targets, bifunctional chelators and linkers to attach those radioisotopes to mAbs (17), as well as with much more advanced administration protocols such as pretargeting (18). During the early days of RIT it was suggested that more efficient "delivery vehicles" such as mAb fragments and radioisotopes with superior to emission characteristics and with a shorter half-life (compared to ^{131}I) would be more efficacious in treatment of tumors while less toxic to normal organs (8). Enormous advances have been made in understanding the mechanisms of RIT. Finally it has been realized that the radiobiological mechanisms of cancer RIT are different from those involved in killing the cancer cells during external beam radiation therapy (EBRT). For example, high-dose rate radiation, which is typical for EBRT, delivers 6 krad/h (60 Gy/h). In contrast, clinical RIT has a peak dose rate of only 10 cGy/h (0.1 Gy/h) and sometimes even lower (19). Thus, from the viewpoint of radiation therapy, RIT delivers suboptimal doses to tumors but is still effective by promoting apoptosis and cell death in irradiated tumor cells. Additionally, there are a number of phenomenon that increase the efficacy of low dose, low-dose rate radiotherapy such as the radiation–induced biological bystander effect (death of adjacent, nonirradiated cells), the cross-fire effect, low dose/dose rate apoptosis, low-dose hyperradiosensitivity-increased radioresistance (LDH-IRR), G_2 synchronization (inverse dose–rate effect), and cell cycle arrest (20–22). This realization is especially important for melanoma RIT because it removes the necessity to deliver doses of 10,000 cGy to the tumors—the "perceived" requirement which was particularly discouraging for those attempting RIT of melanoma. Here are some examples of the recent work on the reintroduction of melanoma RIT into the clinic.

▓ Targeting "traditional" surface antigens in melanoma

Scott et al. (23) conducted a phase I trial of KM871 chimeric mAb against a novel cell surface ganglioside antigen GD3, which is highly expressed on melanoma cells. This mAb is also known to have some innate cytotoxic effect on the cells which it binds. The patients were given five dose levels of mAb (from 1 to 40 mg/m^2) which were traced with ^{111}In-labeled KM871 to assess biodistribution in vivo. The authors concluded that targeting of an anti-GD3 mAb to metastatic melanoma in patients was specific and that the lack of immunogenicity of KM871 makes this mAb an attractive potential therapy for patients with metastatic melanoma.

Urbano and colleagues (24) investigated the feasibility of using a pretargeting strategy for developing melanoma RIT. They utilized novel biotin–DOTA conjugates (r-BHD: reduced biotinamidohexylamine-DOTA) labeled with ^{90}Y or ^{177}Lu as an agent to deliver radiation to the pretargeted mAb. The preliminary evaluation of the conjugate was performed in an animal model while a pilot study was conducted in a patient with metastatic melanoma. There was a total body clearance of the antibody of approximately 85% in 24 hours and a kidney to tumor (10 mm diameter) absorbed dose of 1.5 and 12 mGy/MBq, respectively. The conclusion was that the new biotin–DOTA conjugate may be a suitable candidate for pretargeted therapy of metastatic melanoma.

The last decade in RIT has also been characterized by the introduction of mAb–targeted alpha-emitting radionuclides such as ^{213}Bi, ^{211}At, and ^{225}Ac into the clinical practice. A number of clinical trials have demonstrated safety, feasibility, and therapeutic activity of targeted alpha therapy, despite having to traverse complex obstacles (25). Allen et al. (26) reported the development of intralesional-targeted alpha therapy for melanoma. For labeling of mAb 9.2.27 the group used ^{213}Bi, a powerful alpha-particle emitter which has become available to the RIT community. Their objective was to investigate the safety and efficacy of intralesional injections of ^{213}Bi-9.2.27 in patients with melanoma metastatic to the skin. Sixteen patients received intralesional doses of 50 to 450 mCi, which resulted in cell death as observed by the presence of tumor debris, decline in serum marker melanoma-inhibitory-activity protein at 2 weeks posttherapy, apoptosis, and ki67 proliferation marker tests. Such therapy can be promising for the control of inoperable secondary melanoma or primary ocular melanoma.

Not every mAb that targets broad classes of surface antigens is useful for melanoma RIT. Milenic et al. evaluated the potential of radiolabeled cetuximab, an FDA-approved mAb that binds to the epidermal growth-factor receptor, as a potential radiotherapeutic agent in mice bearing xenografts of LS-174T (colorectal), SHAW (pancreatic), SKOV3 (ovarian), DU145 (prostate), HT-29 (colorectal), and A375 (melanoma) cell lines. Excellent tumor targeting was observed in each of these cell lines except for melanoma (27). This highlights the need of careful preclinical evaluation of every potential target antigen for melanoma RIT.

Targeting melanin antigen in melanoma

Melanoma RIT has been traditionally performed with mAbs that bind cell surface antigens. Melanin, the pigment from which melanoma derives its name, has not been considered a target for RIT because it is generally regarded to be an intracellular pigment beyond the reach of specific mAbs. However, since melanomas are rapidly growing tumors we hypothesized that cell turnover would release melanin pigment into the extracellular space that could be available as a target for mAbs delivering cytotoxic radiation (28). In this approach the cytotoxic radiation emanating from labeled mAb bound to melanin is presumably delivered by "crossfire" effect to the adjacent viable tumor cells. Furthermore, this strategy is attractive because melanin in normal tissues should not be accessible to the mAb by virtue of its intracellular location. To test this hypothesis we employed a murine mAb known as 6D2 that had been generated from mice immunized with melanin produced by the fungus *Cryptococcus neoformans* (29). This mAb also binds human melanin since both fungal and human melanins have structural similarities (30), and are negatively charged. Scatchard plot analysis of 6D2 binding to melanin released from MNT1-pigmented human melanoma cells found its association constant (K_a) to be 1.8×10^8 M^{-1}, which is close to association constants reported for anti-HMW MAA mAbs (31). Nude mice bearing MNT1 tumors were treated with mAb 6D2 labeled with 1.5 mCi of the beta-emitter ^{188}Re and subsequently manifested inhibition of tumor growth and prolonged survival. MAb 6D2 bound tumor melanin but did not bind to normal melanized tissues in black mice. The mechanism of mAb 6D2 targeting to melanoma involved mAb binding to extracellular melanin released during tumor cell turnover by penetrating dying cells with damaged or permeable membranes. These results established the feasibility of targeting melanin released from dead melanoma cells in tumors with radiolabeled mAbs to achieve a therapeutic effect (28).

In preparation for a clinical trial of RIT for melanoma with ^{188}Re-labeled mAb 6D2 it became necessary to model the factors, which may determine the efficacy of mAb therapy in a patient: the effect of the wide range of melanin concentrations in the tumors on mAb–antigen complex formation, determination of rate-limiting factors in the formation of mAb–antigen complex within the tumor as a function of time, and estimation of the absorbed dose to the tumor. Using finite-element analysis (FEA), we created a pharmacokinetic model that describes melanin-targeting RIT of melanoma. The model describes the uptake of intravenously delivered ^{188}Re-6D2 mAb within a melanoma micrometastasis (1.3 mm radius) surrounded by normal tissue (2.6 mm radius) for four different melanin concentrations of 76, 7.6, 0.76, and 0.076 μM. A 76 μM melanin concentration was experimentally determined for the highly melanized human MNT1 melanoma. The lower values of 0.076 to 7.6 μM were used to investigate the dose–response effect of lower melanin concentration. The modeling predicted that the penetration of the radiolabeled mAb into the tumor was inversely proportional to the melanin concentration of the tumor, while the formation of mAb–melanin complex per total tumor volume was remarkably similar within a 1000-fold range of melanin concentration. This resulted in almost similar doses of approximately 3000 rad (cGy) delivered to the tumors with melanin concentrations of 0.076 to 76 μM. This study provided crucial data showing that RIT of melanoma can be effective over a wide range of melanin concentrations in tumors (32).

Following several years of preclinical development (33), a phase I clinical trial of ^{188}Re-labeled melanin–binding 6D2 mAb was conducted in patients with stage IV metastatic melanoma who failed prior therapy. Patients had lesions in the bones, soft tissues (lungs, skin, lymph nodes, stomach), liver, and pancreas as per ^{18}FDG PET/CT. They received a 10 mCi dose of ^{188}Re-6D2 mAb and a cold mAb preload escalated in each of four cohorts of three patients (0, 10, 20, 50 mg). Whole body planar scintigraphy followed by SPECT/CT of the area of interest was performed immediately, 3 to 5, 7 to 9, and 18 to 24 hours after injection. Although γ emission represents only 15% of the injected 10 mCi ^{188}Re-6D2, the normal biodistribution (liver, spleen, kidneys, and bladder) was visible up to 24 hours postinjection on planar scintigraphy. SPECT/CT visualized uptake of ^{188}Re-6D2 in most soft tissue metastases and no dose-limiting toxicities were observed (34). Based on the promising results of phase I trial, a dose-escalation phase I/II trial in patients with metastatic melanoma has been initiated and is currently ongoing.

Finally, in an effort to improve the outcomes of melanoma RIT with melanin-binding mAbs, the efficacy of RIT with ^{188}Re-6D2 was compared to chemotherapy with dacarbazine and to combined chemotherapy and RIT in human metastatic melanoma-bearing nude mice (35). This study was based on the hypothesis that as melanin targeting involves the mAb binding to extracellular melanin released from necrotic melanoma cells, the administration of a chemotherapeutic agent followed by RIT would facilitate the delivery of radiation to the tumors due to the increased presence of free melanin in dead cells. Comparison of chemotherapy with dacarbazine and RIT with ^{188}Re-6D2 mAb in A2058 human metastatic melanoma tumor–bearing nude mice revealed that RIT was more effective in slowing tumor growth in mice. Administration of dacarbazine followed by RIT was more effective than either modality alone. These observations might be useful for selection of patients for clinical trials, as those patients who have recently undergone a course of chemotherapy might respond more favorably to antimelanin RIT.

■ THERAPY OF MELANOMA WITH RADIOLABELED PEPTIDES

Closely related to RIT is the domain of tumor therapy with radiolabeled peptides, which are capable of specifically delivering their radioactive "cargo" to the tumors. During the last decade radiolabeled peptides that bind to different receptors on tumors have been investigated as potential therapeutic agents both in preclinical and clinical settings (36). Advantages of radiolabeled peptides over mAbs include relatively straightforward chemical synthesis, versatility, easier radiolabeling, rapid clearance from the circulation, faster

penetration into tumors, more uniform distribution in normal tissues, and less immunogenicity (37). On the other hand, peptides have very short serum half-lives and lack the effector functions conferred by an Fc region of a mAb.

Melanocyte-stimulating hormone (MSH) receptor, a melanogenesis regulating protein, is under investigation as a target for radionuclide therapy of melanoma. This effort has been directed primarily at the synthesis of metal-cyclized alpha-MSH peptide analogues such as Re-(Arg^{11})CCMSH and Re-CCMSH, which are suitable for the incorporation of Re isotopes such as ^{188}Re or ^{186}Re (38), radioiodination (39), or attachments of various radiometals such as ^{177}Lu via bifunctional chelating agents such as DOTA (1,4,7, 10-tetraazacyclododecane-N,N',N'',N'''-tetraacetic acid) (40,41) (Fig. 40.1A). Both ^{177}Lu-DOTA-Re(Arg^{11})CCMSH and ^{188}Re-(Arg^{11})-CCMSH treatment yielded quantitative therapeutic effects in B16/F1 murine melanoma-bearing C57 mice (41,42). The best therapeutic results were achieved when metal-cyclized alpha-MSH peptide analogue was radiolabeled with alpha-emitter ^{212}Pb. ^{212}Pb-DOTA-Re(Arg^{11}) CCMSH peptide exhibited superior therapeutic efficacy when compared to ^{188}Re or ^{177}Lu-labeled peptides, with 45% of B16/F1 melanoma-bearing C57 mice surviving a 120-day study disease-free after the treatment with 7.4 MBq of ^{212}Pb-DOTA-Re(Arg^{11})CCMSH (40).

Melanin can also be targeted by peptide-directed radiotherapy of melanoma. Melanoma tumors in mice were treated with ^{188}Re-labeled melanin–binding decapeptide 4B4 (TyrGlyArgLysPheTrpHisGluArgHis) and a comprehensive safety evaluation of this treatment was subsequently performed. Similar to 6D2 melanin-binding mAb described above, the 4B4 decapeptide was originally developed against fungal melanin (43). The decapeptide was radiolabeled with ^{188}Re via chelating agent HYNIC (hydrazinonicotinamide) (Fig. 40.1B). Administration of 1 mCi (37 MBq) ^{188}Re-HYNIC-4B4 to human MNT1 melanoma-bearing mice significantly slowed tumor growth (44). Importantly, there was no difference in uptake of ^{188}Re-HYNIC-4B4 in melanized tissues of black C57BL6 mice in comparison with white BALB/C mice and no histologically apparent damage to these tissues. Treatment of C57BL6 mice with ^{188}Re-HYNIC-4B4 did not change mice behavior, as established by SHIRPA protocol (45), and did not cause damage to neurons and glial cells. These results indicate that radiolabeled melanin–binding peptides are efficient and safe in treatment of melanoma and could be potentially useful against this tumor.

Though the results indicated that radiolabeled melanin-binding decapeptide had activity against melanoma, that peptide also manifested high kidney uptake and this might become a concern during clinical trials. We hypothesized that by identifying peptides with different amino acid composition against tumor melanin we might be able to decrease their kidney uptake. Using the Heptapeptide Ph.D.-7 Phage Display Library we identified three heptapeptides that bind to human tumor melanin. These peptides were radiolabeled with ^{188}Re via HYNIC ligand and their comprehensive biodistribution in A2058 human metastatic melanoma

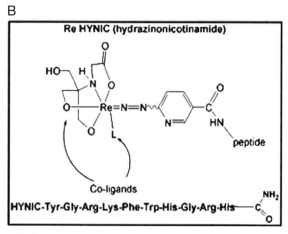

FIGURE 40.1 Structures of radiolabeled peptides used for radiotherapy of melanoma. **A:** Metal-cyclized alpha-MSH peptide analogue ^{177}Lu-DOTA-Re(Arg[11])CCMSH; **B:** melanin–binding decapeptide [188]Re-HYNIC-4B4.

tumor-bearing nude mice was compared to that of [188]Re-4B4 decapeptide (46). While tumor uptake of heptapeptides was quite similar to that of [188]Re-4B4 decapeptide, there was dramatically less uptake in the kidneys at both 3 hours (6% ID/g vs. 38%) and 24 hours (2% ID/g vs. 15%) postinjection. Administration of one of the generated heptapeptides, [188]Re-HYNIC-AsnProAsnTrpGlyProArg, to A2058 human metastatic melanoma–bearing nude mice resulted in significant retardation of the tumor growth. Immunofluorescence showed that in spite of their relatively small size, heptapeptides were not able to penetrate through the membranes of viable melanoma cells and bound only to extracellular melanin, which provides assurance that they will be safe to healthy melanin-containing tissues during radionuclide therapy. Thus, these heptapeptides appear to have potentially significant advantages for targeted therapy of melanoma relative to existing melanin-binding peptides.

■ CONCLUSIONS

RIT for melanoma remains an underdeveloped area despite the promise of several approaches reviewed in the chapter above and lack of therapeutic options for metastatic forms of this malignancy. There are several potentially promising avenues for development of such therapies—mAbs to melanoma surface antigens, mAbs and peptides to melanin, variety of radiolabeled compounds belonging to the groups of melanin binders, melanin precursors and binders to melanogenesis-related proteins (47). We are hopeful that when RIT finally "comes of age," RIT of metastatic melanoma will become a clinical reality.

■ REFERENCES

1. Linos E, Swetter SM, Cockburn MG, et al. Increasing burden of melanoma in the United States. *J Invest Dermatol.* 2009;129:1666–1674.
2. Sun W, Schuchter LM. Metastatic melanoma. *Curr Treat Options Oncol.* 2001;1:193–202.
3. DeNardo SJ, Erickson KL, Benjamin E, et al. Radioimmunotherapy for melanoma. *Clin Res.* 1981;29:434–440.
4. Larson SM, Carrasquillo JA, McGuffin RW, et al. Use of I-131 labeled, murine Fab against a high molecular weight antigen of human melanoma: preliminary experience. *Radiology.* 1985;155:487–492.
5. DeNardo GL. Treatment of non-Hodgkin's lymphoma (NHL) with radiolabeled antibodies (mAbs). *Semin Nucl Med.* 2005;35:202–211.
6. Kaminski MS, Tuck M, Estes J, et al. 131I-tositumomab therapy as initial treatment for follicular lymphoma. *N Engl J Med.* 2005;352:441–449.
7. DeNardo SJ, Hines HH, Erickson KL, et al. The evaluation of radiolabeled monoclonal antibody parameters necessary for cancer immunotherapy. In: Chabner BA, ed. *Rational Basis for Chemotherapy.* New York: Alan R. Liss; 1983.
8. DeNardo SJ, DeNardo GL, Peng J-S, et al. Monoclonal antibody radiopharmaceuticals for cancer radioimmunotherapy. In: Burchiel S, Rhodes B, eds. *Radioimmunoimaging and Radioimmunotherapy.* New York: Elsevier Publishing; 1983.
9. Buraggi GL. Radioimmunodetection of malignant melanoma with the 225.28S monoclonal antibody to HMW-MAA. *Nuklearmedizin.* 1986; 25:220–224.
10. Imai K, Wilson BS, Bigotti A, et al. A 94,000-Dalton glycoprotein expressed on human melanoma and carcinoma cells. *J Nation Cancer Inst.* 1982;68:761–769.
11. Brown JP, Nishiyama K, Hellstrom I, et al. Structural characterization of human melanoma-associated antigen p97 with monoclonal antibodies. *J Immunol.* 1981;127:539–546.
12. Kang NV, Yong A. New techniques for imaging metastatic melanoma. *Surgery (St. Louis).* 1998;16:5–7.
13. Rofstad EK. Radiation biology of malignant melanoma. *Acta Radiol Oncol.* 1986;25:1–10.
14. Rofstad EK, Mathiesen B, Galappathi K. Increased metastatic dissemination in human melanoma xenografts after subcurative radiation treatment: radiation-induced increase in fraction of hypoxic cells and hypoxia-induced up-regulation of urokinase-type plasminogen activator receptor. *Cancer Res.* 2004;64:13–18.
15. Taylor A Jr, Milton W, Eyre HP, et al. Radioimmunodetection of human melanoma with indium-111-labeled monoclonal antibody. *J Nucl Med.* 1988;29:329–337.
16. Milenic DE. Radioimmunotherapy: designer molecules to potentiate effective therapy. *Semin Radiat Oncol.* 2000;10:139–155.
17. Milenic DE, Brady ED, Brechbiel MW. Antibody-targeted radiation cancer therapy. *Nat Rev Drug Discov.* 2004;3:488–498.
18. Sharkey RM, Goldenberg DM. Perspectives on cancer therapy with radiolabeled monoclonal antibodies. *J Nucl Med.* 2005;46(suppl 1): 115–127S.
19. Murtha AD. Review of low-dose-rate radiobiology for clinicians. *Semin Radiat Oncol.* 2000;10:133–138.
20. Knox SJ, Goris ML, Wessels BW. Overview of animal studies comparing radioimmunotherapy with dose equivalent external beam radiation. *Radiother Oncol.* 1992;23:111–117.

21. Xue LY, Butler NJ, Makrigiorgos GM, et al. Bystander effect produced by radiolabeled tumor cells *in vivo*. *Proc Natl Acad Sci U S A*. 2002;99:13765–13770.
22. Macklis RM. How and why does radioimmunotherapy work? *Int J Radiat Oncol Biol Phys*. 2004;59:1269–1271.
23. Scott AM, Lee FT, Hopkins W, et al. Specific targeting, biodistribution, and lack of immunogenicity of chimeric anti-GD3 monoclonal antibody KM871 in patients with metastatic melanoma: results of a phase I trial. *J Clin Oncol*. 2001;19:3976–3987.
24. Urbano N, Papi S, Ginanneschi M, et al. Evaluation of a new biotin-DOTA conjugate for pretargeted antibody-guided radioimmunotherapy (PAGRIT). *Eur J Nucl Med Mol Imaging*. 2007;34:68–77.
25. Brechbiel MW. Targeted alpha-therapy: past, present, future? *Dalton Trans*. 2007;21(43):4918–4928.
26. Allen BJ, Raja C, Rizvi S, et al. Intralesional targeted alpha therapy for metastatic melanoma. *Cancer Biol Ther*. 2005;4:1318–1324.
27. Milenic DE, Wong KJ, Baidoo KE, et al. Cetuximab: preclinical evaluation of a monoclonal antibody targeting EGFR for radioimmunodiagnostic and radioimmunotherapeutic applications. *Cancer Biother Radiopharm*. 2008;23:619–631.
28. Dadachova E, Nosanchuk JD, Shi L, et al. Dead cells in melanoma tumors provide abundant antigen for targeted delivery of ionizing radiation by a monoclonal antibody to melanin. *Proc Natl Acad Sci U S A*. 2004;101:14865–14870.
29. Rosas AL, Nosanchuk JD, Feldmesser M, et al. Synthesis of polymerized melanin by *Cryptococcus neoformans* in infected rodents. *Infect Immun*. 2000;68:2845–2853.
30. Wakamatsu K, Ito S. Advanced chemical methods in melanin determination. *Pigment Cell Res*. 2002;15:174–183.
31. Matzku S, Kirchgessner H, Schmid U, et al. Melanoma targeting with a cocktail of monoclonal antibodies to distinct determinants of the human HMW-MAA. *J Nucl Med*. 1989;30:390–397.
32. Schweitzer AD, Rakesh V, Revskaya E, et al. Computational model predicts effective delivery of 188-Re-labeled melanin-binding antibody to the metastatic melanoma tumors with wide range of melanin concentrations. *Melanoma Res*. 2007;17:291–303.
33. Dadachova E, Revskaya E, Sesay MA, et al. Pre-clinical evaluation and efficacy studies of a melanin-binding IgM antibody labeled with (188)Re against experimental human metastatic melanoma in nude mice. *Cancer Biol Ther*. 2008;7:1116–1127.
34. Klein M, Shibli N, Friedmann N, et al. Imaging of metastatic melanoma (MM) with a 188Rhenium(188Re)-labeled melanin binding antibody. *J Nucl Med*. 2008;49(suppl 1):52P. Abstract.
35. Revskaya E, Jongco AM, Sellers RS, et al. Radioimmunotherapy of experimental human metastatic melanoma with melanin-binding antibodies and in combination with dacarbazine. *Clin Cancer Res*. 2009;15:2373–2379.
36. Krenning EP, Kwekkeboom DJ, Valkema R, et al. Peptide receptor radionuclide therapy. *Ann N Y Acad Sci*. 2004;1014:234–240.
37. Blok D, Feitsma RI, Vermeij P, et al. Peptide radiopharmaceuticals in nuclear medicine. *Eur J Nucl Med*. 1999;26:1511–1521.
38. Miao Y, Whitener D, Feng W, et al. Evaluation of the human melanoma targeting properties of radiolabeled alpha-melanocyte stimulating hormone peptide analogues. *Bioconjug Chem*. 2003;4:1177–1184.
39. Cheng Z, Chen J, Quinn TP, et al. Radioiodination of rhenium cyclized alpha-melanocyte-stimulating hormone resulting in enhanced radioactivity localization and retention in melanoma. *Cancer Res*. 2004;64:1411–1418.
40. Miao Y, Hylarides M, Fisher DR, et al. Melanoma therapy via peptide-targeted alpha-radiation. *Clin Cancer Res*. 2005;11:5616–5621.
41. Miao Y, Shelton T, Quinn TP. Therapeutic efficacy of a 177Lu-labeled DOTA conjugated alpha-melanocyte-stimulating hormone peptide in a murine melanoma-bearing mouse model. *Cancer Biother Radiopharm*. 2007;22:333–341.
42. Miao Y, Owen NK, Fisher DR, et al. Therapeutic efficacy of a 188Re-labeled alpha-melanocyte-stimulating hormone peptide analog in murine and human melanoma-bearing mouse models. *J Nucl Med*. 2005;46:121–129.
43. Nosanchuk JD, Valadon P, Feldmesser M, et al. Melanization of *Cryptococcus neoformans* in murine infection. *Mol Cell Biol*. 1999;19:745–752.
44. Dadachova E, Moadel T, Schweitzer AD, et al. Radiolabeled melanin-binding peptides are safe and effective in treatment of human pigmented melanoma in a mouse model of disease. *Cancer Biother Radiopharm*. 2006;21:117–129.
45. Rogers DC, Fisher EM, Brown SD, et al. Behavioral and functional analysis of mouse phenotype: SHIRPA, a proposed protocol for comprehensive phenotype assessment. *Mamm Genome*. 1997;8:711–718.
46. Howell RC, Revskaya E, Pazo V, et al. Phage display library derived peptides that bind to human tumor melanin as potential vehicles for targeted radionuclide therapy of metastatic melanoma. *Bioconjug Chem*. 2007;18:1739–1748.
47. Dadachova E, Casadevall A. Melanin as a potential target for radionuclide therapy of metastatic melanoma. *Future Oncol*. 2005;1:541–549.

41

Radioimmunotherapy of Pediatric Malignancies

Nidale Tarek and Shakeel Modak

■ INTRODUCTION

The radiation sensitivity of most pediatric malignancies makes them attractive candidates for radioimmunotherapy (RIT). Toxicities associated with external beam radiotherapy are often more severe and profound in children than in adults: growth failure and musculoskeletal asymmetry, learning difficulties and other neurological and neuroendocrine sequelae, and the increased risk of secondary malignancies are of particular importance in younger patients. RIT has the potential to diminish some of these toxicities by sparing normal tissue damage associated with external beam radiation. Treatment failure in most children is due to the inability of sophisticated combination therapies to eradicate minimal residual disease, which is typically distant and occult. Therefore, RIT may be an effective adjunct to the established modalities of chemotherapy, external beam radiotherapy, and surgery, particularly against minimal residual disease. Moreover, since most children with cancer are treated with immunosuppressive, high-dose chemotherapy, passive immunotherapy with monoclonal antibodies (mAbs), is feasible without rapid induction of human antimouse antibody or human antichimeric antibody responses, potentially permitting repeated administration of RIT. Despite these potential advantages, few mAbs are currently available for RIT specifically for children with cancer, and most pediatric patients are treated suboptimally on RIT protocols targeted to adult tumors. Reasons for this include different antigen repertoire of childhood neoplasms, particularly solid tumors, when compared with common adult tumors, and the "orphan" status of pediatric cancers for which approaches and objectives of RIT may differ significantly from those for adult tumors. We discuss the current state of clinical trials of RIT for pediatric malignancies in the following sections (Tables 41.1 and 41.2).

■ RADIOIMMUNOTHERAPY OF HEMATOLOGIC MALIGNANCIES

Leukemia

Leukemia is the most common cancer diagnosed in children and adolescents, accounting for approximately 3250 new cases a year. Acute lymphoblastic leukemia (ALL), being the most prevalent type of leukemia, has a peak incidence at 13 years of age (1). Treatment of ALL is based on risk stratification. Long-term survival rates for patients with low-risk ALL are more than 80%, though treatment extends over 2 to 3 years and has serious long-term side effects (2). However, prognosis is significantly worse in patients with poor biological markers and those who relapse despite intensification of multiagent chemotherapy, additional radiotherapy, and/or hematopoietic stem cell transplant (3). The central nervous system (CNS) is a known sanctuary site for ALL cells and the advent of intrathecal chemotherapy resulted in a significant improvement in survival. However, a small minority of patients with chemoresistant CNS leukemia

Table **41.1**	Antigens targeted for radioimmuno-detection	
Radiolabeled Antibody	**Antigen Targeted**	**Tumor Binding**
[111]In R11D10 F(ab)	Myosin	Rhabdomyosarcoma Leiomyosarcoma Rhabdoid tumor
[131]I-14G2A	GD2	Neuroblastoma Osteosarcoma
^{131}I-TP1 ^{131}I-TP3	TP1/TP3	Osteosarcoma Malignant histiocytoma Synovial sarcoma
^{99m}Tc-IMMU-30	Alpha-fetoprotein	Germ cell tumor Hepatoblastoma
[99m]Tc-ch14.18	GD2	Neuroblastoma
[131]I-chCE7	L1-CAM	Neuroblastoma Renal cell carcinoma
[131]8H9	Gp58	Osteosarcoma Rhabdomyosarcoma DSRCT Ewing family Wilms tumor Hepatoblastoma Leiomyosarcoma Malignant histiocytoma Rhabdoid tumor
[131]I-3F8	GD2	Osteosarcoma DSRCT

Table **41.2** Antigens targeted for radioimmunotherapy

Radiolabeled Antibody	Targeted Antigen	Tumor Binding
Hematologic malignancies		
^{131}I-WCMH15.14	CD10	Acute lymphoblastic lymphoma
^{131}I-HD37	CD19	Acute lymphoblastic lymphoma
[131]I-P67	CD33	Acute myeloid leukemia
^{131}I-OKB7	CD21	Non-Hodgkin lymphoma
^{131}I-BC8	CD45	Acute myeloid leukemia, acute lymphoblastic lymphoma, myelodysplastic syndrome
[90]Y-T101	CD5	T-cell acute lymphoblastic leukemia
[90]Y-ibritumomab tiuxetan	CD20	Non-Hodgkin lymphoma, Hodgkin disease
[131]I-tositumomab	CD20	Non-Hodgkin lymphoma, Hodgkin disease
[90]Y-HuM195 ^{131}I-HuM195 [213]Bi HuM195	CD33	Acute myeloid leukemia
[188]Re BW250/183	CD66	Acute myeloid leukemia, acute lymphoblastic lymphoma
[90]Y-epratuzumab ^{131}I-epratuzumab [186]Re epratuzumab	CD22	Non-Hodgkin lymphoma
[67]Cu Lym-1 ^{131}I-Lym-1 ^{90}Y-Lym-1	HLA-DR	Non-Hodgkin lymphoma
[90]Y-B9E9FP fusion protein	CD20	Non-Hodgkin lymphoma, Hodgkin disease
Primary brain tumors, leptomeningeal neoplasm		
^{90}Y-ERIC-1	NCAM	Malignant glioma
[131]I-81C6 [211]At 81C6 [90]Y-81C6	Tenascin	High-grade glioma, astrocytoma, ependymoma, medulloblastoma
^{131}I-UJ181.4	L1	Primitive neuroectodermal tumor, pinealoblastoma
[131]I-M340	L1	Primitive neuroectodermal tumor, pinealoblastoma
^{131}I-UJ13A	NCAM	Primitive neuroectodermal tumor
[131]I-3F8	GD2	Medulloblastoma, ependymoma, primitive neuroectodermal tumor, meningioma, rhabdoid tumor, retinoblastoma, neuroblastoma
[131]I-8H9	Gp58	Glioma, ependymoma, astrocytoma, primitive neuroectodermal tumor, Schwannoma, meningioma, neurofibroma, pinealoblastoma
[125]I-425	EGF-R	High-grade glioma, astrocytoma
[90]Y-biotinylated BC4	Tenascin	High-grade glioma
Solid tumors		
[131]I-3F8	GD2	Neuroblastoma

NCAM, neural cell adhesion molecule.

require craniospinal radiotherapy (CRT) which is associated with major toxicities including growth and learning disorders in young children (4). The CNS compartment is uniquely amenable to targeted radiotherapy and can be exploited for RIT. CD10, CD19, and CD20 are surface antigens expressed on pediatric ALL. RIT with ^{131}I-labeled anti-CD10 (WCMH15.14) and anti-CD19 (HD37) mAbs

administered intrathecally was associated with transient clearing of the cerebrospinal fluid (CSF) lymphoblasts in five out of six patients. Toxicities included headaches, nausea, vomiting, fever, and myelosuppression (5). Radiation dose to the CSF was 12.2 to 25.3 Gy: more than 6 times higher than dose to the brain surface and 40 to 140 times higher than dose to the whole brain (5,6).

Acute myeloid leukemia (AML) has a much worse prognosis than ALL despite intensive chemotherapy and/or hematopoietic stem cell transplant (7). Treatment of patients with high-risk factors and those who relapse remains suboptimal and complicated by transplant-related toxicities. Novel targeted approaches added to frontline or salvage regimens may have a role in decreasing toxicity and improving overall survival. Pediatric and adult AML share surface antigens that may be targeted by mAbs: CD33, CD45, and CD66 which are expressed at different stages of hematopoietic differentiation. CD33 is expressed on myeloid progenitor cells and myeloid leukemic blasts but not on primitive hematopoietic stem cells. CD45 is highly expressed in nearly all cells of hematopoietic origin, myeloblasts, and lymphoblasts, and CD66 is expressed on maturing myeloid cells beyond promyelocyte stage, but not on myeloid blasts (8). Radiolabeled anti-CD33, anti-CD45, and anti-CD66 mAbs were used in different trials as part of conditioning regimens for adults with relapsed or refractory myeloid leukemia with favorable results (9). However, the pediatric experience is very limited: two children with multiple relapsed AML were treated with the anti-CD33 mAb M195. Therapy was well tolerated with targeting to bone marrow (BM) (10). Phase I/II trials using ^{213}Bi-labeled human mAb to CD33 (11) (^{213}Bi-HuM195) (Clinicaltrials.gov NCT00014495) and ^{131}I-labeled BC8 targeted to CD45 (12) (NCT00002554) open for children and adults with advanced myeloid leukemias were recently completed, but it is not clear if pediatric patients received RIT.

Lymphoma

Lymphomas are the third most common pediatric malignancies; they constitute 10% to 12% of childhood cancers and are classified into Hodgkin lymphomas (HLs) and non-Hodgkin lymphomas (NHLs). Both are chemosensitive and radiosensitive tumors (13) and current treatment includes combined chemotherapy with or without low-dose involved-field radiation therapy. Five-year progression survival for both lymphomas is more than 80% (14,15), but salvage rates for NHL are poor (16,17). The Children's Cancer Group (CCG) study CCG-5961 observed that cell surface CD20 was present in 100% of Burkitt and high-grade B-cell lymphomas and 98% of diffuse large B-cell lymphoma (18), making CD20 an ideal target for immunotherapy in children with high-risk B-cell NHL. However, rituximab-mediated anti-CD20 immunotherapy is of limited efficacy for these aggressive, rapidly growing tumors. A phase I study of ^{90}Y-ibritumomab-tiuxetan was conducted by the Children's Oncology Group (COG) (NCT00036855) in children and adolescents with relapsed/refractory CD20-positive NHL. Five patients with recurrent/refractory verified CD20-positive lymphoma were enrolled; intervention consisted of rituximab (250 mg/m² i.v.) on days 0 and 7, ^{111}In-ibritumomab-tiuxetan (5 mCi i.v.) on day 0, and ^{90}Y-ibritumomab-

tiuxetan on day 7. Three patients with good BM reserve received 0.4 mCi/kg and two patients with poor marrow reserve received 0.1 mCi/Kg of ^{90}Y-ibritumomab-tiuxetan. Treatment was well tolerated and side effects included BM suppression but none of the patients required growth factor support. Evaluation of the primary tumor showed stable disease; however, no patient achieved complete or partial response. Solid organ and red BM exposure was below the maximal accepted dose (19). A phase II study using ^{90}Y-ibritumomab-tiuxetan is planned in order to determine further safety and efficacy in children with B-NHL. Other radiolabeled mAb conjugates with rituximab (anti-CD20), epratuzumab (anti-CD22), and Lym-1 (anti HLA-DR) have been tested in adults but not yet in the pediatric population. An anecdotal report of pretargeted antibody-guided RIT using biotinylated antitenascin murine IgG2b mAb tenatumomab and ^{90}Y-biotin-DOTA in a 6-year-old girl with chemoresistant anaplastic large cell lymphoma described complete remission durable for 10 months posttreatment (20). Although tenascin is expressed on a subpopulation of NHL in adults (21), little is known about its expression on pediatric lymphomas.

■ RADIOIMMUNOTHERAPY OF SOLID TUMORS

RIT in adult patients with solid tumors has failed to show responses similar to those in patients with hematologic malignancies, in part related to the reduced radiosensitivity of these tumors. The radiosensitivity of most pediatric tumors renders them a good target for RIT; however, its use is still very limited. Neuroblastoma (NB) is the only pediatric solid tumor that has been treated with RIT thus far.

■ Neuroblastoma

Neuroblastoma (NB) is the most common extracranial solid tumor of childhood and 60% to 70% of patients have metastatic disease at diagnosis; most have a very poor prognosis with long-term survival of 10% to 40% despite the use of aggressive multiagent chemotherapy, surgery, and radiation therapy (22,23). Antibody-mediated immunotherapy targeting disialoganglioside (GD2) antigen on NB cells has shown promising results (24–26). GD2 is ubiquitous and homogeneously expressed on NB cells (27) with normal human tissue expression limited to the peripheral and central neural tissues; neurons are protected from intravenous GD2-targeted antibodies by the blood–brain barrier (28). Additional important characteristics make GD2 an ideal target for RIT: it is not modulated from the cell surface after antibody binding; circulating levels of GD2 are minimal and do not interfere with tumor antibody binding (27,29). Anti-GD2 mAbs, 3F8, and ch14.18 are now considered to be standard of care, as consolidation therapy after surgery and chemotherapy have achieved remission. Their safety profile has been well established: acute toxicities include severe but transient pain and allergic reactions. Long-term toxicities have not been encountered (24–26). However, as "naked" antibodies or in combination with cytokines, they have limited utility for relapsed or refractory disease. 3F8 is a murine IgG3 mAb selective for GD2 and was the first mAb to be studied in patients with NB (30). It has the slowest dissociation rate among anti-GD2 antibodies (31) and mediates dose-dependent destruction of NB by human complement and by human lymphocytes (32), cultured monocytes (33), and granulocytes (34). It utilizes both FcγRII and FcγRIII Fc receptors for neutrophil antibody-dependent cell-mediated cytotoxicity and the CR3 receptor for iC3b mediated cytotoxicity (35,36). 3F8 has shown clinical utility for two groups of NB patients in particular. (a) In patients with chemorefractory osteomedullary NB with a low disease burden disease, the combination of 3F8 and granulocyte macrophage colony-stimulating factor (GM-CSF) (37) demonstrated a CR rate of more than 80% by histology in the marrow (38). (b) This combination was associated with a significant improvement of long-term extended free survival (EFS) compared with historical controls when used to treat ultra–high-risk stage 4 NB patients in first remission (24). However, it has limited clinical utility for patients with recurrent NB and for those with refractory soft tissue or significant osteomedullary NB.

The known radiosensitivity of NB cells and their limited repair mechanisms after radiation-induced damage led to the investigation of RIT for NB. Furthermore, in this disease of young children, the potential of RIT to target radiation to metastatic sites while avoiding the toxicities of external beam radiation is an attractive property. In initial radioimmunodetection (RID) studies, ^{131}I-3F8 showed excellent tumor targeting in patients with NB localizing to NB at primary and metastatic sites in lymph nodes, BM, and bone in 42 patients. When compared with ^{131}I-MIBG or with magnetic resonance imaging (MRI) scans, anti-G$_{D2}$ (^{131}I-3F8) was more sensitive and more specific in detecting sites of metastatic disease (39). ^{131}I-3F8 had a relatively high tumor uptake in patients of 0.08% to 0.1% injected dose per gram (40). Similarly, two other anti-G$_{D2}$ antibodies, ^{131}I-14G2a (41) and ^{99m}Tc-ch14.18, and the anti-L1 Ab ^{131}I-chCE7 have been used for RID in patients with NB. ^{99m}Tc-ch14.18 and ^{131}I-chCE7 have been reported to have higher sensitivity and specificity than ^{131}I-MIBG in the detection of NB (42). In comparison with ^{131}I-MIBG, recurrent metastases were detected earlier with ^{99m}Tc-ch14.18 and tumor uptake persisted for a shorter duration after initiation of anti-NB chemotherapy, indicating possible disease response (43).

^{131}I-3F8 is the only Ab that has been used for RIT of pediatric solid tumors thus far. Toxicities were evaluated at MSKCC in a phase I dose-escalating study (doses 6 to 28 mCi/kg) conducted on 24 patients with NB (23 patients with refractory stage IV and 1 patient with unresectable stage III with ascites). Acute toxicities included expected grade 4 myelosuppression requiring autologous BM rescue or GM-CSF therapy, fever, mild diarrhea, and pain during infusion; the only late toxicity observed was hypothyroidism in spite of thyroid suppression. The maximum tol-

erated dose (MTD) was not reached. The calculated tumor average dose was 150 cGy/mCi/kg, the average cumulative blood radiation dose was 740 to 888 MBq/kg, and the total body dose was estimated at 500 to 700 cGy. Six patients survived for more than 20 months after antibody treatment and 1 patient died of progressive disease before BM infusion; 10 patients were evaluated for response, 2 patients demonstrated complete response of the BM disease, and 2 patients demonstrated partial response of soft tissue disease (27,44). Based on the phase I study results, ^{131}I-3F8 was added to a multimodality program for high-risk NB patients (n = 35): the MSKCC N7 protocol. Reported toxicities were identical to the phase I trial including myelosuppression, fever, and hypothyroidism; one patient died of infection and the overall survival of newly diagnosed patients older than 18 months was approximately 40% with a follow-up of 6 to 10 years from diagnosis. The average radiation dose based on tracer dosimetry was estimated at 0.37 cGy/MBq to the tumor, 0.05 cGy/MBq to the lung, 0.06 cGy/MBq to the liver and BM, and 0.07 cGy/MBq to the spleen (29,45,46).

Preclinical studies indicate that the combination of targeted radiotherapy and antiangiogenesis effectively suppressed NB xenografts even at relatively low doses of ^{131}I-3F8 (47). A clinical trial based on these observations has recently been completed at MSKCC in 24 patients with resistant NB (NCT01114555). ^{131}I-3F8 was dose escalated from 4 to 8 mCi/kg/dose, while the dose of the antiangiogenic agent bevacizumab was maintained at 15 mg/kg/dose. MTD for ^{131}I-3F8 was not reached. All patients developed grade 4 myelosuppression and nine patients required autologous stem cell rescue, all of whom engrafted at a median of 11 (range 4 to 15) days. Preliminary assessment of data indicate that bevacizumab did not appear to impair ^{131}I-3F8 targeting to sites of NB nor impair BM recovery after autologous stem cells rescue (48).

Desmoplastic small round cell tumor

Desmoplastic small round cell tumor (DSRCT) is a rare sarcoma of adolescents and young adults that arises from serosal surfaces typically as disseminated, bulky intra-abdominal tumors arising from the peritoneum. It is characterized by the t(11;22)(p13:q12) chromosomal translocation (49) that leads to fusion of the amino terminus of the Ewing sarcoma gene (EWS) to the carboxy terminus of the tumor suppressor Wilms tumor gene WT1 (50). The resultant chimeric protein acts as an aberrant transcription factor and is probably tumorigenic (51). Despite demonstrated chemosensitivity, optimal therapy for this rare disease remains to be determined, and prognosis is currently extremely poor (52–56) with a long-term survival rate of less than 20% despite aggressive chemoradiotherapy and surgery. The most common cause of treatment failure in DSRCT is local or peritoneal relapse. Since DSRCT is a radiosensitive tumor (57,58), RIT has the potential to target and deliver effective therapy to DSRCT cells. The murine monoclonal IgG1 antibody 8H9, first developed at MSKCC, binds to a novel, as-yet-incompletely characterized glycoprotein antigen, 4Ig-B7H3, which is expressed on a wide range of pediatric solid tumors with restricted expression on normal tissues (59,60). 4Ig-B7H3 is thought to regulate tumor cell migration and invasion (61), known to inhibit NK cells and T cells (62,63). 4Ig-B7H3 transcript is ubiquitously expressed in tumors and normal tissues by qRT-PCR, but B7H3 protein was found only on tumors and not on most normal tissues both by Western blot and by immunohistochemistry (5,64,65). Binding kinetics studied by Biacore testing revealed that mAb 8H9 has a slow dissociation rate (k_{off}) which is crucial for sustained in vivo drug efficacy (60,66). Radioiodinated 8H9 targets and suppresses rhabdomyosarcoma xenografts in mouse models (67). 8H9 was demonstrated to react with 96% DSRCT (68). Radioiodinated 8H9 is currently being studied as intra-Ommaya (IO) therapy for patients with leptomeningeal malignancies (Clinicaltrials.gov NCT00089245) as described in section on "Leptomeningeal metastases". Intraperitoneal RIT can potentially direct radiation to sites of occult or obvious peritoneal disease that are inaccessible to intravenous (i.v.) chemotherapy, enhancing local control by targeted delivery of radiation to micrometastases while potentially achieving high tumor to nontumor ratios and sparing normal tissues. Based on this rationale, a phase I study investigating ^{131}I-8H9 administered intraperitoneally for patients with DSRCT and other B7-H3 expressing intraperitoneal tumors has been initiated at MSKCC and is currently accruing patients (NCT01099644).

Thyroid carcinoma

Thyroid neoplasms, although very rare, are the most common endocrine malignancies in children and adolescents. Papillary and follicular carcinomas account for more than 90% of thyroid malignancies in children. They tend to be well differentiated, respond well to conventional therapy, including surgery and radioactive iodine, and are associated with a long-term survival of 83% to 100%. Medullary thyroid cancer (MTC) accounts for only 5% of thyroid neoplasms and presents in children with multiple endocrine neoplasia types IIA and IIB. MTC is more resistant to chemoradiotherapy and the 10 years survival rate of affected children is 68% (69). Patients with MTC are known to have a high tissue and serum expression of carcinoembryonic antigen (CEA) (70). There are anecdotal reports of children being treated on phase I trials of the anti-CEA antibodies ^{131}I NP-4 and ^{131}I MN-14 without unexpected toxicities and with variable antitumor effect (71).

Other solid tumors

Radioconjugated antibodies have been used for the RID of other pediatric solid tumors. However, there are no published reports of their therapeutic use. These include ^{111}In-labeled antimyosin Fab fragments (^{111}In-R11D10) for rhabdomyosarcoma, leiomyosarcoma, and other types of soft tissue sarcomas. Although myosin is an intracellular protein, in sarcomas due to alteration in membrane permeability, F(ab) fragments can access their target. Conversely, there is no binding to normal muscle tissues which have intact cell membranes. Three different studies using ^{111}In-R11D10 for RID in patients with soft tissue sarcomas including rhabdomyosarcoma, leiomyosarcoma, and alveolar soft tissue sarcoma have reported favorable targeting when compared with standard imaging modalities with variable specificities and sensitivities (72–74).

^{131}I-labeled F(ab) antibody targeting TP-1, an osteosarcoma cell surface antigen associated with the bone alkaline phosphatase, was used for RID in five patients with bone sarcomas. Antibody uptake was higher in sarcoma cells compared with healthy cells with a tumor to blood ratio ranging from 1.2 to 4.2 compared with 0.1 to 0.8 in normal tissues. Tumor detection was positive in one patient with primary osteogenic sarcoma of the femur and two-fourth patients with lung metastases (75).

Finally, ^{99m}Tc anti-AFP (^{99m}Tc-IMMU-30) was used to determine the sensitivity and specificity of AFP scans in patients with germ cell tumors including some pediatric patients. Forty-five patients with testicular or mediastinal tumors were evaluated, comparing serum levels of AFP, conventional imaging, and radioimmunoscintigraphy for detection capabilities. Radioimmunoscintigraphy showed higher sensitivity at 86% but lower specificity at 58% (76). ^{99m}Tc-IMMU-30 has also detected hepatic lesions correlating with MRI scan findings in a child with hepatoblastoma, with possible extrahepatic lesions, who was being considered for a liver transplant (77).

■ RADIOIMMUNOTHERAPY OF BRAIN TUMORS

Primary central nervous system tumors

Primary CNS tumors are the most common solid tumors in childhood. With current combination therapies including surgery, radiation therapy, and chemotherapy, about 50% of children diagnosed with primary brain tumors survive for more than 5 years from diagnosis; however, survival rates vary widely with tumor type and stage at diagnosis and prognosis remains very poor for cases of relapse. For most malignant brain tumors, a dose–response relationship exists between survival and the total external beam radiation dose administered, but the dose is limited by the debilitating long-term effects on growth and neurodevelopment, especially in younger children. Since most CNS tumors recur at or near the primary site, local therapy may have a role in controlling primary tumors and preventing relapse. Radiolabeled mAbs recognizing brain tumor antigens have been used mostly in adult patients with poor-prognosis brain tumors; a few children were treated on the same protocols, since many of the tumors also occur in the pediatric age group. However, exact data on toxicity and/or efficacy of these agents specifically in children are usually unavailable.

[131]I-labeled antitenascin murine mAb 81C6 was used intrathecally or directly within the tumor resection cavity in two different dose-escalation phase 1 trials. In the first study, 10 pediatric patients (18 years or younger) with ependymoma, medulloblastoma, astrocytoma, anaplastic astrocytoma, and glioblastoma multiforme were treated. A dose of 40 mCi was achieved without MTD being reached in the pediatric population, whereas in adults, grade 4 neutropenia and thrombocytopenia were dose-limiting toxicities (DLTs). Overall, younger patients tended to have a better outcome, and a total of five patients (all children) did not show any evidence of disease progression at a median follow-up of 409 days posttreatment. In a second study, 34 patients, aged 6 to 64 years, with recurrent glioblastoma multiforme, anaplastic astrocytomas, and anaplastic oligodendrogliomas, were injected ^{131}I-labeled 81C6 within the tumor resection cavity. MTD was 100 mCi and the DLT was severe neurologic complications such as seizures, aphasia, and hemiparesis. The number of children treated on this study is unclear (78). Subjects of subsequent phase II studies of [131]I-81C6 (79) and of [211]At-81C6 (80) have not included children. Anecdotal descriptions of pediatric patients treated on predominantly adult studies report on the applications of the anti–neural cell adhesion molecule (NCAM) mAb ^{90}Y-ERIC1 (1/15 patients) administered by intratumoral injection (81); the antiepidermal growth factor receptor mAb [12]vI-425 (2/180 patients) administered i.v. or intra-arterially (82). Although toxicity and dosimetry data are available for the entire group, details for pediatric patients have not been separately described.

[131]I-chTNT-1/B specific for histone H1, an intracellular antigen that gets exposed in malignant solid tumors, was used via convection-enhanced delivery for the treatment of patients with high-grade gliomas. Fifty-one patients were treated as the initial cohort on a phase I dose-escalation study, followed by an expanded cohort, with the dose being calculated to a clinical target volume of tumor. Nine patients had ages between 15 and 40 years but exact number of pediatric patients is not reported. The antibody was infused by a microinfusion pump over 1 to 2 days through a catheter with the tip ending at the center of the tumor. In the entire cohort, an average of 8% to 10% of patients developed grade 3 to 4 CNS toxicity described as headaches, hemiparesis, seizures, and brain edema. The overall median survival was 37.9 weeks; of the 11 patients evaluated for response, 1 patient had a partial response, 6 had stable disease, and 4 had disease progression (83).

Leptomeningeal metastases

Leptomeningeal metastases are often terminal events in adults with high-risk systemic malignancies and are being increasingly described in children with high-risk malignancies including acute leukemia, NHL, Ewing sarcoma, NB, Wilms tumor, rhabdomyosarcoma, osteosarcoma, melanoma, hepatoblastoma, retinoblastoma, and germ cell

tumors (84). The overall incidence of brain metastasis in children with pediatric malignancies is estimated to range between 1% and 10% (84); this incidence is increasing with improvement of systemic therapy with the CNS emerging as a sanctuary site for cancer relapse. As in adults, leptomeningeal metastasis is associated with significant mortality. Many pediatric tumors that metastasize to the CNS are radiosensitive, but external beam radiation is often ineffective because of the DLT to normal tissues. Radiolabeled mAbs reactive with tumor-associated antigens constitute a promising strategy, providing targeted radiation specifically to malignant cells and limiting toxicity to the normal cells.

Initial studies targeted cell adhesion molecules: NCAM (mAb ^{131}I-UJ13A) and L1 (^{131}I-UJ181.4 and ^{131}I-M340). These cell adhesion molecules are expressed on tissues of neuroectodermal origin, fetal brain, muscle, and kidney and also on embryonic tumors such as NB, Ewing tumor, Wilms tumor, medulloblastoma, retinoblastoma, and rhabdomyosarcomas but not on hematopoietic cell lines and pediatric or adult brain (85). Thirteen pediatric patients with relapsed refractory medulloblastoma, pineoblastoma, and primitive neuroectodermal tumors were treated with ^{131}I-UJ13A (n = 1), ^{131}I-UJ181.4 (n = 2), or ^{131}I-M340 (n = 10 patients) administered into the CSF. The ^{131}I activity range was between 20 and 71 mCi and 50% of treated patients showed either stabilization or improvement of disease, but response to therapy was transient and patient survival was between 1 and 39 months. Treatment-related toxicities were aseptic meningitis presenting as headaches, fever and cervical rigidity, grade 1 to 4 reversible myelosuppression, and seizures. No chronic complications were observed and no radiation damage to the spinal cord, brain, or meninges was described (86).

The anti-GD2 antibody 3F8 binds to several other pediatric tumors besides NB: medulloblastoma, retinoblastoma, melanoma, high-grade astrocytoma, osteosarcoma, and DSRCT. Fifteen patients with refractory GD2-positive leptomeningeal malignancies (13 patients younger than 18 years) were treated on a phase I clinical trial with IO [131]I-3F8 after demonstration of adequate CSF flow (87) (NCT00003022). Diagnoses included ependymoma, NB, rhabdoid, retinoblastoma, primitive neuroectodermal tumor, and medulloblastoma. Patients initially received a 1 to 2 mCi tracer dose of [131]I-3F8 followed by a therapeutic dose of 10 to 20 mCi. Pharmacokinetic studies were based on CSF and blood sampling and dosimetry on gamma camera scans. MTD (activity) was determined to be 10 mCi. The DLT at 20 mCi was transient chemical meningitis and increased intracranial pressure experienced by two different patients; no long-term toxicities were observed in two patients who remained in remission 3.5 years posttreatment. Tracer studies reliably predicted therapeutic dose to the CSF, and the total absorbed CSF dose was calculated as 1.12 to 13.00 Gy by sampling and 1.00 to 13.70 Gy by region of interest. CSF half-life was 3 to 12.9 hours. Objective responses were noted in 3 of the 13 evaluable patients: 2 had CSF clearing of malignant cells and a further patient had radiological improvement of leptomeningeal disease. A mathematical model has been developed to predict dosimetry and kinetics for IO ^{131}I-3F8 (88).

Based on the completed phase I study, IO ^{131}I-3F8 is part of two currently open phase II studies: (a) a phase II study of multiple doses of ^{131}I-3F8 each administered at 10 mCi in patients with GD2-positive CNS or metastatic leptomeningeal malignancies (NCT00445965), and (b) a pilot phase II study of postoperative IO ^{131}I-3F8 in conjunction with reduced intensity CRT plus chemotherapy for patients with standard-risk medulloblastoma (NCT00058370). The objective of the latter study is to investigate if the dose of external beam CRT can be decreased in patients receiving RIT without adversely effecting outcome in patients with standard-risk medulloblastoma, the most common CNS tumor in children.

The anti-B7H3 mAb 8H9 targets a range of pediatric embryonic tumors and has limited reactivity with normal tissues, in particular, and it does not react with any neural tissues. ^{124}I-8H9 (2 mCi tracer dose) and ^{131}I-8H9 are currently being investigated in a phase I dose-escalation study (NCT00089245) in patients with leptomeningeal CNS disease. DLT has not yet been encountered. Toxicities include transient hepatic transaminitis, biochemical hypothyroidism, and self-limited myelosuppression observed at doses 40 mCi or more. ^{124}I-8H9-mediated positron emission tomography (PET) scans facilitated detailed imaging of leptomeningeal targeting and CSF biodistribution of 8H9 (89) (Fig. 41.1), and enhanced pharmacokinetic calculations. Relatively close agreement was observed between PET dosimetry estimates and the mean dose calculated by serial CSF sampling for the (subsequent) ^{131}I-8H9 IO injections. ^{131}I-8H9 (as utilized in the earlier trial) and ^{131}I-3F8 are integral components of the current salvage regimen for NB relapsing in the CNS at MSKCC. This includes (a) resection of CNS parenchymal disease when possible, with concurrent placement of an intraventricular Ommaya catheter to deliver intrathecal therapy, (b) craniospinal irradiation with a boost to parenchymal masses, (c) adjuvant chemotherapy with irinotecan and temozolomide, (d) IO RIT with ^{131}I-8H9

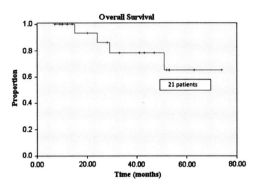

FIGURE 41.2 Kaplan–Meier curve for overall survival from CNS disease detection for 21 patients with neuroblastoma treated with radioimmunotherapy-based treatment planning, utilizing intra-Ommaya ^{131}I-8H9 or^{131}I-3F8.

or ^{131}I-3F8, (e) systemic immunotherapy with 3F8 plus GM-CSF and oral 13-*cis*-retinoic acid, and (f) oral temozolomide. Out of 21 patients treated with the above regimen, 2 received ^{131}I-3F8, 18 received ^{131}I-8H9, and 1 received both ^{131}I-8H9 and ^{131}I-3F8. Currently, 17 patients remain alive, 7 to 74 months (median 33) from the time of CNS NB diagnosis (Fig. 41.2), all without evidence of CNS disease. Three deaths occurred from non-CNS events related to systemic recurrences or prior therapies. Only one patient (no. 9) progressed in the CNS, 14 months after the initial CNS recurrence. He died of both progressive CNS and systemic disease 35 months after the CNS event. These data (EFS of more than 60% at 5 years) are in stark contrast to prior therapeutic approaches not including IO RIT which were associated with a median survival of 2 to 6.7 months after CNS recurrence (90,91) (5-year OS = 0%) indicating an important role for RIT in treatment of NB recurrent to CNS (92,93).

■ FUTURE OF RADIOIMMUNOTHERAPY FOR PEDIATRIC TUMORS

Pediatric malignancies present unique opportunities and challenges as targets for RIT. Successful radiotargeting to radiation-sensitive pediatric tumors may alleviate the considerable toxicities of external beam radiotherapy in young patients. However, safety and efficacy profiles of available radioimmunoconjugates in children remain to be defined and require careful evaluation in phase I/II studies. The rapid development of other radiolabeled mAbs for hematological malignancies in adults also has exciting implications for future therapy of pediatric leukemia and lymphoma which share target antigens with their adult counterparts. It is encouraging to see that the COG has initiated multicenter phase I/II studies to evaluate anti-CD20 RIT for pediatric lymphomas. In contrast to hematological malignancies, the antigen repertoire of pediatric solid tumors differs substantially from malignancies in adults, probably because of their differing lineage: pediatric solid tumors are typically of embryonal origin, whereas adult tumors are usually carcinomas of endothelial origin. Hence, RIT agents specific to pediatric solid tumors will need to be developed and investigated. New routes of

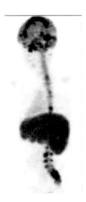

FIGURE 41.1 ^{124}I-8H9 positron emission tomography scan obtained 48 hours post–intra-Ommaya injection demonstrating distribution throughout the thecal space and activity within leptomeningeal neuroblastoma deposits.

administration may permit improved targeting of malignancies in "sanctuary" sites. Novel methodologies such as multistep targeting and use of alpha emitters with their favorable microdosimetry, especially for minimal residual disease, are being explored for pediatric tumors. However, unless there are substantial policy changes in drug development for orphan indications, the relatively small number of patients with pediatric malignancies will likely not have these therapeutic agents available in the very near future.

REFERENCES

1. Altekruse SF, Kosary CL, Krapcho M, et al., eds. *SEER Cancer Statistics Review, 1975-2007.* Bethesda, MD: National Cancer Institute. Available at: http://seer.cancer.gov/csr/1975_2007/.
2. Moricke A, Reiter A, Zimmermann M, et al. Risk-adjusted therapy of acute lymphoblastic leukemia can decrease treatment burden and improve survival: treatment results of 2169 unselected pediatric and adolescent patients enrolled in the trial ALL-BFM 95. *Blood.* 2008;111:4477–4489.
3. Tallen G, Ratei R, Mann G, et al. Long-term outcome in children with relapsed acute lymphoblastic leukemia after time-point and site-of-relapse stratification and intensified short-course multidrug chemotherapy: results of trial ALL-REZ BFM 90. *J Clin Oncol.* 2010;28:2339–2347.
4. Pui CH, Thiel E. Central nervous system disease in hematologic malignancies: historical perspective and practical applications. *Semin Oncol.* 2009;36:S2–S16.
5. Pizer B, Papanastassiou V, Hancock J, et al. A pilot study of monoclonal antibody targeted radiotherapy in the treatment of central nervous system leukaemia in children. *Br J Haematol.* 1991;77:466–472.
6. Pizer BL, Kemshead JT. The potential of targeted radiotherapy in the treatment of central nervous system leukaemia. *Leuk Lymphoma.* 1994;15:281–289.
7. Lange BJ, Smith FO, Feusner J, et al. Outcomes in CCG-2961, a children's oncology group phase 3 trial for untreated pediatric acute myeloid leukemia: a report from the children's oncology group. *Blood.* 2008;111:1044–1053.
8. Nemecek ER, Matthews DC. Antibody-based therapy of human leukemia. *Curr Opin Hematol.* 2002;9:316–321.
9. Pagel JM. Radioimmunotherapeutic approaches for leukemia: the past, present and future. *Cytotherapy.* 2008;10:13–20.
10. Schwartz MA, Lovett DR, Redner A, et al. Dose-escalation trial of M195 labeled with iodine 131 for cytoreduction and marrow ablation in relapsed or refractory myeloid leukemias. *J Clin Oncol.* 1993;11:294–303.
11. Jurcic JG, Larson SM, Sgouros G, et al. Targeted alpha particle immunotherapy for myeloid leukemia. *Blood.* 2002;100:1233–1239.
12. Pagel JM, Gooley TA, Rajendran J, et al. Allogeneic hematopoietic cell transplantation after conditioning with 131I-anti-CD45 antibody plus fludarabine and low-dose total body irradiation for elderly patients with advanced acute myeloid leukemia or high-risk myelodysplastic syndrome. *Blood.* 2009;114:5444–5453.
13. Magrath IT. Malignant non-Hodgkin's lymphomas in children. *Hematol Oncol Clin North Am.* 1987;1:577–602.
14. Thomson AB, Wallace WH. Treatment of paediatric Hodgkin's disease: a balance of risks. *Eur J Cancer.* 2002;38:468–477.
15. Burkhardt B, Zimmermann M, Oschlies I, et al. The impact of age and gender on biology, clinical features and treatment outcome of non-Hodgkin lymphoma in childhood and adolescence. *Br J Haematol.* 2005;131:39–49.
16. Attarbaschi A, Dworzak M, Steiner M, et al. Outcome of children with primary resistant or relapsed non-Hodgkin lymphoma and mature B-cell leukemia after intensive first-line treatment: a population-based analysis of the Austrian Cooperative Study Group. *Pediatr Blood Cancer.* 2005;44:70–76.
17. Cairo MS, Sposto R, Hoover-Regan M, et al. Childhood and adolescent large-cell lymphoma (LCL): a review of the Children's Cancer Group experience. *Am J Hematol.* 2003;72:53–63.
18. Perkins SL, Lones MA, Davenport V, et al. B-cell non-Hodgkin's lymphoma in children and adolescents: surface antigen expression and clinical implications for future targeted bioimmune therapy: a children's cancer group report. *Clin Adv Hematol Oncol.* 2003;1:314–317.
19. Cooney-Qualter E, Krailo M, Angiolillo A, et al. A phase I study of 90yttrium-ibritumomab-tiuxetan in children and adolescents with relapsed/refractory CD20-positive non-Hodgkin's lymphoma: a Children's Oncology Group study. *Clin Cancer Res.* 2007;13:5652s–5660s.
20. Palumbo G, Grana CM, Cocca F, et al. Pretargeted antibody-guided radioimmunotherapy in a child affected by resistant anaplastic large cell lymphoma. *Eur J Haematol.* 2007;79:258–262.
21. Vacca A, Ribatti D, Fanelli M, et al. Expression of tenascin is related to histologic malignancy and angiogenesis in b-cell non-Hodgkin's lymphomas. *Leuk Lymphoma.* 1996;22:473–481.
22. Haupt R, Garaventa A, Gambini C, et al. Improved survival of children with neuroblastoma between 1979 and 2005: a report of the Italian Neuroblastoma Registry. *J Clin Oncol.* 2010;28:2331–2338.
23. Modak S, Cheung NK. Neuroblastoma: therapeutic strategies for a clinical enigma. *Cancer Treat Rev.* 2010;36:307–317.
24. Cheung NK, Kushner BH, Cheung IY, et al. Anti-G(D2) antibody treatment of minimal residual stage 4 neuroblastoma diagnosed at more than 1 year of age. *J Clin Oncol.* 1998;16:3053–3060.
25. Gilman AL, Ozkaynak MF, Matthay KK, et al. Phase I study of ch14.18 with granulocyte-macrophage colony-stimulating factor and interleukin-2 in children with neuroblastoma after autologous bone marrow transplantation or stem-cell rescue: a report from the Children's Oncology Group. *J Clin Oncol.* 2009;27:85–91.
26. Yu A, Gilman A, Ozkaynak MF, et al. A phase III randomized trial of the chimeric anti-GD2 antibody ch14.18 with GMCSF and IL2 as immunotherapy following dose intensive chemotherapy for high-risk neuroblastoma. *Proc ASCO.* 2009;27:10067z.
27. Modak S, Cheung NK. Disialoganglioside directed immunotherapy of neuroblastoma. *Cancer Invest.* 2007;25:67–77.
28. Hakomori S. Tumor-associated carbohydrate antigens defining tumor malignancy: basis for development of anti-cancer vaccines. *Adv Exp Med Biol.* 2001;491:369–402.
29. Modak S, Cheung NK. Antibody-based targeted radiation to pediatric tumors. *J Nucl Med.* 2005;46(suppl 1):157S–163S.
30. Cheung NK, Saarinen UM, Neely JE, et al. Monoclonal antibodies to a glycolipid antigen on human neuroblastoma cells. *Cancer Res.* 1985;45:2642–2649.
31. Xu H, Hu J, Cheung NK. Induction of tumor cell death by anti-GD2 monoclonal antibodies: requirement of antibody Fc and a long residence time (slow k off). *J Clin Oncol.* (ASCO Annual Meeting Proceedings) 2007;25:13507.
32. Munn DH, Cheung NK. Interleukin-2 enhancement of monoclonal antibody-mediated cellular cytotoxicity (ADCC) against human melanoma. *Cancer Res.* 1987;47:6600–6605.
33. Munn DH, Cheung NK. Antibody-dependent antitumor cytotoxicity by human monocytes cultured with recombinant macrophage colony-stimulating factor. Induction of efficient antibody-mediated antitumor cytotoxicity not detected by isotope release assays. *J Exp Med.* 1989;170:511–526.
34. Kushner BH, Cheung NK. GM-CSF enhances 3F8 monoclonal antibody-dependent cellular cytotoxicity against human melanoma and neuroblastoma. *Blood.* 1989;73:1936–1941.
35. Kushner BH, Cheung NK. Absolute requirement of CD11/CD18 adhesion molecules, FcRII and the phosphatidylinositol-linked FcRIII for monoclonal antibody-mediated neutrophil antihuman tumor cytotoxicity. *Blood.* 1992;79:1484–1490.
36. Hong F, Yan J, Baran JT, et al. Mechanism by which orally administered beta-1,3-glucans enhance the tumoricidal activity of antitumor monoclonal antibodies in murine tumor models. *J Immunol.* 2004;173:797–806.
37. Kushner BH, Cheung NK. GM-CSF enhances 3F8 monoclonal antibody-dependent cellular cytotoxicity against human melanoma and neuroblastoma. *Blood.* 1989;73:1936–1941.
38. Kushner B, Kramer K, Modak S, et al. Anti-GD2 monoclonal antibody 3F8 plus granulocyte macrophage colony stimulating factor for primary refractory neuroblastoma in bone marrow. *Proc ASCO.* 2007;25:9502.
39. Yeh SD, Larson SM, Burch L, et al. Radioimmunodetection of neuroblastoma with iodine-131-3F8: correlation with biopsy, iodine-131-metaiodobenzylguanidine (MIBG) and standard diagnostic modalities. *J Nucl Med.* 1991;32:769–776.

40. Larson SM, Pentlow KS, Volkow ND, et al. PET scanning of iodine-124-3F8 as an approach to tumor dosimetry during treatment planning for radioimmunotherapy in a child with neuroblastoma. *J Nucl Med.* 1992;33:2020–2023.

41. Murray JL, Cunningham JE, Brewer H, et al. Phase I trial of murine monoclonal antibody 14G2a administered by prolonged intravenous infusion in patients with neuroectodermal tumors. *J Clin Oncol.* 1994;12:184–193.

42. Hoefnagel CA, Rutgers M, Buitenhuis CK, et al. A comparison of targeting of neuroblastoma with mIBG and anti L1-CAM antibody mAb chCE7: therapeutic efficacy in a neuroblastoma xenograft model and imaging of neuroblastoma patients. *Eur J Nucl Med.* 2001;28:359–368.

43. Reuland P, Geiger L, Thelen MH, et al. Follow-up in neuroblastoma: comparison of metaiodobenzylguanidine and a chimeric anti-GD2 antibody for detection of tumor relapse and therapy response. *J Pediatr Hematol Oncol.* 2001;23:437–442.

44. Cheung NK, Kushner BH, LaQuaglia M, et al. N7: a novel multimodality therapy of high risk neuroblastoma (NB) in children diagnosed over 1 year of age. *Med Pediatr Oncol.* 2001;36:227–230.

45. Larson SM, Divgi C, Sgouros G, et al. Monoclonal antibodies: basic principles—radioisotope conjugates. In: DeVita VT, Hellman S, Rosenberg SA, eds. *Biologic Therapy of Cancer—Principles and Practice.* Philadelphia, PA: J.B. Lippincott Co.; 2000:396–412.

46. Cheung NK, Pentlow K, Graham MC, et al. Radioimmunotherapy of human neuroblastoma using monoclonal antibody 3F8. In: *Fifth International Radiopharmaceutical Dosimetry Symposium.* Oak Ridge, TN: Oak Ridge Associated Universities; 1992:95–112.

47. Modak S, Chung J, Cheung NK. Targeting of vascular endothelial growth factor (VEGF) synergizes with ^{131}I-3F8 in radioimmunotherapy of human neuroblastoma. Abstract accepted for presentation at AACR 2006; 2006.

48. Modak S, Cheung NK, Abramson SJ, et al. Lack of early bevacizumab-related skeletal radiographic changes in children with neuroblastoma. *Pediatr Blood Cancer.* 2008;52(2):304–305.

49. Sawyer JR, Tryka AF, Lewis JM. A novel reciprocal chromosome translocation t(11;22)(p13;q12) in an intraabdominal desmoplastic small round-cell tumor. *Am J Surg Pathol.* 1992;16:411–416.

50. Ladanyi M, Gerald W. Fusion of the EWS and WT1 genes in the desmoplastic small round cell tumor. *Cancer Res.* 1994;54:2837–2840.

51. Gerald WL, Haber DA. The EWS-WT1 gene fusion in desmoplastic small round cell tumor. *Semin Cancer Biol.* 2005;15:197–205.

52. Modak S. Myeloablative chemotherapy with autologous stem cell rescue for desmoplastic small round cell tumor. *Pediatr Blood Cancer.* 2005;45S:500.

53. Saab R, Khoury JD, Krasin M, et al. Desmoplastic small round cell tumor in childhood: the St. Jude Children's Research Hospital experience. *Pediatr Blood Cancer.* 2007;49:274–279.

54. Lal DR, Su WT, Wolden SL, et al. Results of multimodal treatment for desmoplastic small round cell tumors. *J Pediatr Surg.* 2005;40:251–255.

55. Livaditi E, Mavridis G, Soutis M, et al. Diffuse intraabdominal desmoplastic small round cell tumor: a ten-year experience. *Eur J Pediatr Surg.* 2006;16:423–427.

56. Stuart-Buttle CE, Smart CJ, Pritchard S, et al. Desmoplastic small round cell tumour: a review of literature and treatment options. *Surg Oncol.* 2008;17:107–112.

57. Jahraus CD, Glisson SD, St Clair WH. Treatment of desmoplastic small round cell tumor with image-guided intensity modulated radiation therapy as a component of multimodality treatment. *Tumori.* 2005;91:253–255.

58. Goodman KA, Wolden SL, La Quaglia MP, et al. Whole abdominopelvic radiotherapy for desmoplastic small round-cell tumor. *Int J Radiat Oncol Biol Phys.* 2002;54:170–176.

59. Modak S, Kramer K, Gultekin SH, et al. Monoclonal antibody 8H9 targets a novel cell surface antigen expressed by a wide spectrum of human solid tumors. *Cancer Res.* 2001;61:4048–4054.

60. Xu H, Cheung I, Cheung NK. 4Ig-B7H3: a target for monoclonal antibody therapy of human neuroblastoma. In: *Advances in Neuroblastoma Research: Eleventh Conference*; 2008:158.

61. Chen YW, Tekle C, Fodstad O. The immunoregulatory protein human B7H3 is a tumor-associated antigen that regulates tumor cell migration and invasion. *Curr Cancer Drug Targets.* 2008;8:404–413.

62. Sun X, Vale M, Leung E, et al. Mouse B7-H3 induces antitumor immunity. *Gene Ther.* 2003;10:1728–1734.

63. Flies DB, Chen L. The new B7s: playing a pivotal role in tumor immunity. *J Immunother.* 2007;30:251–260.

64. Sun M, Richards S, Prasad DV, et al. Characterization of mouse and human B7-H3 genes. *J Immunol.* 2002;168:6294–6297.

65. Chapoval AI, Ni J, Lau JS, et al. B7-H3: a costimulatory molecule for T cell activation and IFN-gamma production. *Nat Immunol.* 2001;2:269–274.

66. Xu H, Cheung I, Cheung NK. 4Ig-B7H3: a target for monoclonal antibody of human solid tumors. *Proc AACR.* 2008:2139.

67. Modak S, Guo HF, Humm JL, et al. Radioimmunotargeting of human rhabdomyosarcoma using monoclonal antibody 8H9. *Cancer Biother Radiopharm.* 2005;20:534–546.

68. Modak S, Gerald W, Cheung NK. Disialoganglioside GD2 and a novel tumor antigen: potential targets for immunotherapy of desmoplastic small round cell tumor. *Med Pediatr Oncol.* 2002;39:547–551.

69. Chadha NK, Forte V. Pediatric head and neck malignancies. *Curr Opin Otolaryngol Head Neck Surg.* 2009;17:471–476.

70. Ishikawa N, Hamada S. Association of medullary carcinoma of the thyroid with carcinoembryonic antigen. *Br J Cancer.* 1976;34:111–115.

71. Juweid M, Sharkey RM, Behr T, et al. Radioimmunotherapy of medullary thyroid cancer with iodine-131-labeled anti-CEA antibodies. *J Nucl Med.* 1996;37:905–911.

72. Hoefnagel CA, Kapucu O, de Kraker J, et al. Radioimmunoscintigraphy using [^{111}In]antimyosin Fab fragments for the diagnosis and follow-up of rhabdomyosarcoma. *Eur J Cancer.* 1993;29A:2096–2100.

73. Koscielniak E, Reuland P, Schilling F, et al. Radio-immunodetection of myosarcoma using 111-indium anti-myosin. *Klin Paediatr.* 1990;202:230–234.

74. Planting A, Verweij J, Cox P, et al. Radioimmunodetection in rhabdo- and leiomyosarcoma with ^{111}In-anti-myosin monoclonal antibody complex. *Cancer Res.* 1990;50:955s–957s.

75. Bruland OS, Fodstad O, Aas M, et al. Immunoscintigraphy of bone sarcomas—results in 5 patients. *Eur J Cancer.* 1994;30A:1484–1489.

76. Amato R, Kim EE, Prow D, et al. Radioimmunodetection of residual, recurrent or metastatic germ cell tumors using technetium-99 anti-(alpha-fetoprotein) Fab´ fragment. *J Cancer Res Clin Oncol.* 2000; 126:161–167.

77. Kairemo KJ, Lindahl H, Merenmies J, et al. Anti-alpha-fetoprotein imaging is useful for staging hepatoblastoma. *Transplantation.* 2002;73:1151–1154.

78. Bigner DD, Brown MT, Friedman AH, et al. Iodine-131-labeled antitenascin monoclonal antibody 81C6 treatment of patients with recurrent malignant gliomas: phase I trial results. *J Clin Oncol.* 1998; 16:2202–2212.

79. Reardon DA, Akabani G, Coleman RE, et al. Phase II trial of murine (131)I-labeled antitenascin monoclonal antibody 81C6 administered into surgically created resection cavities of patients with newly diagnosed malignant gliomas. *J Clin Oncol.* 2002;20:1389–1397.

80. Zalutsky MR, Reardon DA, Akabani G, et al. Clinical experience with alpha-particle emitting ^{211}At: treatment of recurrent brain tumor patients with ^{211}At-labeled chimeric antitenascin monoclonal antibody 81C6. *J Nucl Med.* 2008;49:30–38.

81. Hopkins K, Chandler C, Bullimore J, et al. A pilot study of the treatment of patients with recurrent malignant gliomas with intratumoral yttrium-90 radioimmunoconjugates. *Radiother Oncol.* 1995;34:121–131.

82. Emrich JG, Brady LW, Quang TS, et al. Radioiodinated (I-125) monoclonal antibody 425 in the treatment of high grade glioma patients: ten-year synopsis of a novel treatment. *Am J Clin Oncol.* 2002;25:541–546.

83. Patel SJ, Shapiro WR, Laske DW, et al. Safety and feasibility of convection-enhanced delivery of Cotara for the treatment of malignant glioma: initial experience in 51 patients. *Neurosurgery.* 2005;56:1243–1252; discussion 1252–1253.

84. Goldman S, Echevarria ME, Fangusaro J. Pediatric brain metastasis from extraneural malignancies: a review. *Cancer Treat Res.* 2007;136:143–168.

85. Patel K, Rossell RJ, Bourne S, et al. Monoclonal antibody UJ13A recognizes the neural cell adhesion molecule (NCAM). *Int J Cancer.* 1989;44:1062–1068.

86. Coakham HB, Kemshead JT. Treatment of neoplastic meningitis by targeted radiation using (131)I-radiolabelled monoclonal antibodies. Results of responses and long term follow-up in 40 patients. *J Neurooncol.* 1998;38:225–232.

87. Kramer K, Humm JL, Souweidane MM, et al. Phase I study of targeted radioimmunotherapy for leptomeningeal cancers using intra-Ommaya 131-I-3F8. *J Clin Oncol.* 2007;25:5465–5470.

88. Lv Y, Cheung NK, Fu BM. A pharmacokinetic model for radioimmunotherapy delivered through cerebrospinal fluid for the treatment of leptomeningeal metastases. *J Nucl Med.* 2009;50:1324–1331.

89. Kramer K, Smith-Jones PM, Humm J, et al. Intra-Ommaya 124I-8H9 positron emission tomography for detection and dosimetry of neuroblastoma metastases in the CNS. In: *Advances in Neuroblastoma Research: Eleventh Conference*; 2008:172.

90. Matthay KK, Brisse H, Couanet D, et al. Central nervous system metastases in neuroblastoma: radiologic, clinical, and biologic features in 23 patients. *Cancer.* 2003;98:155–165.

91. Kramer K, Kushner B, Heller G, et al. Neuroblastoma metastatic to the central nervous system. The Memorial Sloan-Kettering Cancer Center Experience and A Literature Review. *Cancer.* 2001;91: 1510–1519.

92. Croog VJ, Kramer K, Cheung NK, et al. Whole neuraxis irradiation to address central nervous system relapse in high-risk neuroblastoma. *Int J Radiat Oncol Biol Phys.* 2010. DOI: 10.1016/j.ijrobp.2009.09.005.

93. Kramer K, Kushner BH, Modak S, et al. Compartmental intrathecal radioimmunotherapy: results for treatment for metastatic CNS neuroblastoma. *J Neurooncol.* 2010;97:409–418.

Palliative Use of Radioimmunotherapy

Frits Aarts, Robert P. Bleichrodt, Thijs Hendriks, Wim J.G. Oyen, and Otto C. Boerman

■ INTRODUCTION

In clinical oncology, the majority of the patients are treated with a palliative intent. The goal of treating these patients is to maintain or improve their quality of life, in the face of progressive, advanced disease, with pain being the dominant symptom (1). Recently, the use of biologics, such as monoclonal antibodies (MAb), in the treatment of cancer has increased. In radioimmunotherapy (RIT), MAbs are labeled with radionuclides to selectively irradiate tumor cells. In addition to the intravenous administration, the radiolabeled MAb in RIT may also be administered regionally (intraperitoneally, intrathecally) in order to reduce systemic side effects and enhance tumor targeting. The vast majority of both clinical and preclinical studies on the use of RIT have focused on the improvement of survival. When therapeutic options are no longer available, however, RIT may offer patients a chance of minimally invasive palliation, mainly as a result of the inherent targeted nature as compared to contemporary chemotherapy regiments and the low degree of treatment-related toxicity, mainly hematologic. The following sections will focus on the regional administration of RIT for palliation in patients suffering from end-stage malignancy.

■ INTRATHORACIC RADIOIMMUNOTHERAPY

The thoracic cavity is lined with a pleural surface that consists of mesothelial cells. These mesothelial cells, like the peritoneal mesothelium, play a role in the lubrication of the parietal and visceral surfaces. For RIT of intrapleural lesions, the administration of radiolabeled antibodies into the pleural space is advantageous as compared to their systemic infusion, because higher concentrations of the antibody can be delivered to the tumor.

▓ Malignant pleural mesothelioma

The prognosis of patients with malignant pleural mesothelioma (MPM) is poor. In general, median survival is 6 to 16 months. The malignant form can be classified into two categories: diffuse and localized, and both are essentially insensitive to most treatments (2). Although different agents for intracavitary chemotherapy to treat mesothelioma have been applied, response rates were poor (15% to 37%) and

without effect on survival. Clinical data on studies investigating intrathoracic chemotherapy adjuvant to surgical debulking were disappointing (3,4). Therefore, the intrathoracic application of chemotherapeutic agents is mainly used to treat malignant pleural effusion (MPE) (5,6). Postoperative external beam radiotherapy, following an extrapleural pneumonectomy, results in reduced ipsilateral thoracic failures and appears to alter the pattern of relapse. Thus, it does appear that radiotherapy may indeed be an effective adjunctive therapy.

The obstacle, however, for the application of RIT for the treatment of mesothelioma is low tumor antigen (mesothelin, tenascin-c) expression in this type of malignancy. Efforts to enhance antigen expression with proinflammatory cytokines did not improve survival after immunotherapy (7,8). Normal mesothelial cells express mesothelin, a 40-kDa cell surface glycosylated phosphatidylinositol-anchored glycoprotein with a function in cell–cell adhesion. Mesothelin is highly overexpressed in cancers such as malignant mesothelioma, pancreatic or ovarian carcinoma, sarcomas, and in some gastrointestinal and pulmonary carcinomas (9).

Preclinically, the use of antimesothelin antibodies and antibody fragments linked to exotoxins was investigated to treat mesothelin-expressing tumors in nude mice, resulting in inhibition of the development of experimental metastases and even complete regression of the tumor (10,11). This antigen may therefore be an attractive target for the intrathoracic application of RIT. Currently, a clinical trial is being conducted, using a chimeric monoclonal antibody (MORAb-009) directed against a cell surface glycoprotein, GP-9, that is overexpressed in cancers as mesothelioma, ovarian, and pancreatic cancer (http://www.clinicaltrials.gov). GP-9 may therefore be a potentially suitable target for radiolabeled MORAb-009 for RIT of MPM.

▓ Malignant pleural effusion

MPE is thought to arise from tumor emboli detaching from visceral tumor nodules and subsequent attachment to the parietal pleura. Also direct tumor invasion (in lung cancers, chest wall neoplasms, and breast carcinoma), hematogenous spread to the parietal pleura, and lymphatic involvement may be a mechanism for development of MPE. The effusion is composed of extracellular matrix proteins, cytokines, and growth factors, thereby promoting cell proliferation and invasion (12). In women, the most common causes of these effusions are breast and ovarian cancer, whereas in men, these are lung cancer and MPM. Treatment of this specific entity can be done by either therapeutic pleural aspiration (in patients with a short life expectancy), pleurodesis, or catheters. MPM with MPE is also an indication for intrapleural therapy, as is the case with MPE arising from ovarian cancer.

Using the ^{90}Y-labeled anti-carcinoembryonic antigen (CEA) antibody cT84.66 in a phase I study in seven women with metastatic, CEA-expressing breast cancer, resolution of MPE was observed in one patient (13). Schmidt et al. described the successful intrapleural application of rituximab, an anti-CD20 monoclonal antibody, in a patient with non-Hodgkin lymphoma who was free of symptoms for 8 months after this treatment (14). In a case report, the authors described treatment failure of repeated percutaneous drainage and bilateral continuous chest tube drainage. This result may be promising, in particular when considering the possibilities of the effects of the application of radiolabeled antibodies. This is the case with ^{90}Y-labeled ibritumomab tiuxetan for the treatment of non-Hodgkin lymphoma (NHL), where the radioimmunoconjugate produces better responses than the unlabeled MAb alone (15).

■ RADIOIMMUNOTHERAPY FOR PALLIATION OF BONE METASTASES

Bone metastases, regardless of the primary malignancy, cause severe morbidity and mortality, including severe pain and bone fractures. The mechanisms that mediate skeletal pain are thought to be multifactorial: tumor-induced osteolysis and tumor-induced nerve injury. Traditionally, pain arising from bone metastases is treated with bisphosphonates, bone-seeking radiometals, chemotherapy, or external beam radiotherapy.

Research on the different processes and steps of the development of metastases has revealed several new targets that can potentially be used for targeted therapy: integrins, the process of angiogenesis, and transforming growth factor-β. In addition, tumor cells themselves can be targeted.

Prostate cancer is complicated by the presence of bone metastases in 68% of the patients and could therefore be an excellent clinical model for targeted therapy.

In 26 patients with hormone refractory metastatic prostate cancer, 25 patients had all known sites of metastases visualized. A total of 50% of the patients experienced palliation of bone pain after treatment with a ^{90}Y-labeled anti-MUC1 antibody (16). In another study, using the ^{177}lutetium-labeled anti-PSMA (prostate-specific membrane antigen) antibody hJ591 was used to treat 35 patients with hormone refractory prostate cancer. All known metastatic sites were visualized in all patients. Four patients had ≥50% PSA declines lasting 3 to 8 months and 16 patients showed PSA stabilization of ≥28 days (17).

Since bone metastases are the most common location of metastases in women with breast cancer, the palliative use

of RIT may be of value to these patients as well. After performing imaging studies that confirmed tumor targeting in patients with CEA-expressing breast cancer, six patients received a single dose of the ^{90}Y-labeled anti-CEA antibody cT84.66 (15 to 22.5 mCi/m^2) in combination with stem cell support. This resulted in disease stabilization of up to 4 months in one patient, and stable disease and reduction of bone pain for 3 months in one patient; the remaining patients showed improvement in bone scans, a 50% reduction of metastasis, the reduction of a pleural effusion, and bone pain palliation for 3 to 14 months (13).

A chimeric version of the L6 Ab (ChL6), radiolabeled with ^{131}I in a dose of 20 to 70 mCi/m^2 per cycle, was administered in four monthly cycles in 10 patients with metastatic breast cancer who failed standard therapy. The Ab L6 is directed against a 24-kDa cell surface antigen that is expressed in high levels in lung, breast, colon, and ovarian carcinomas. This resulted in a clinically measurable response in 6/10 patients, lasting for 1.5 to 5 months and in one patient, in a marked reduction of bone pain lasting for a period of 9 months (18).

In recent years, trastuzumab, a monoclonal antibody that specifically binds to HER-2 (human epidermal growth factor receptor-2), exerting an inhibitory effect on the growth of HER-2-positive breast cancer, has become part of standard treatment of women with HER-2-positive breast cancer. More recently, trastuzumab was radiolabeled in order to investigate the therapeutic potential of anti-HER-2 based RIT. Until now, these agents have only been used preclinically and the results of clinical data on their use are not yet available.

■ LEPTOMENINGEAL METASTASES

Leptomeningeal metastases (LMM) involve the meninges of the central nervous system, most commonly arise from primary solid tumors such as breast, lung, melanoma, gastrointestinal tract, and primary central nervous system malignancies, and represent a terminal phase of these malignancies. When clinically apparent, survival is limited with a median survival of 4 to 14 months. Generally, LMM are treated with steroids, external beam radiotherapy, and intrathecal or intravenous administration of chemotherapy. Occasionally, decompressive neurosurgical intervention or a combination of the aforementioned therapies is utilized. The application of RIT in patients with primary central nervous system (CNS) malignancy has been discussed elsewhere (Chapter 27) and is beyond the scope of this chapter.

In a phase I dose-searching trial, a single intrathecal administration of an ^{131}I-labeled antitenascin monoclonal antibody (81C6) was delivered in 31 patients with either leptomeningeal neoplasms or primary brain tumor resection cavities with subarachnoid communication (19). Administered activities ranged from 40 to 100 mCi. Hematologic toxicity was the dose-limiting side effect. Eighteen patients had glioblastoma (58%). A partial response was observed in 1 patient and 13 (42%) exhibited stabilization of disease.

Targeted treatment with 30 to 60 mCi of intrathecally administered ^{131}I-labeled HMFG1 (an anti-MUC1 antibody) in seven patients with neoplastic meningitis (ovarian, bladder, lung, and breast cancer) resulted in a partial response in two patients (one breast and one ovarian cancer patient). In addition, two patients with meningitis arising from melanoma were treated with 45 or 60 mCi ^{131}I-Mel-14 (an antimelanoma antibody), resulting in a complete response in both patients with a disease-free survival of 12 and 46 months (20).

Neuroblastoma commonly results in LMM and expresses ganglioside D (GD2). 3F8 is an antibody against GD2, expressed on neuroblastoma and primary central nervous system tumors. Kramer et al. performed a phase I study in 15 patients with LMM from neuroblastoma using 10 to 20 mCi ^{131}I-labeled 3F8, administered through an Ommaya reservoir (21). This resulted in decreased headaches in two patients, clearance of malignant cells from CNS fluid for the duration of 1 month, and two complete remissions for the duration of 45 months.

Currently, a study is recruiting patients with refractory, recurrent, or advanced CNS or leptomeningeal disease (NCT00089245). Unlike trials using antibodies against the tenascin antigen (extracellular matrix), this study employs the ^{131}I-labeled 8H9 monoclonal antibody. This antibody reacts to a tumor-restricted surface antigen that is overexpressed on tumors that arise from neuroectodermal, epithelial, and mesenchymal tissues. This murine G1 MAb (8H9) demonstrates immunoreactivity to a majority of glioblastoma and anaplastic astrocytoma cell lines and shows no cross-reactivity to human CNS tissue (22,23).

Based on this information, the use of RIT as minimally invasive treatment for patients with LMM may be promising.

■ CONCLUSIONS

Despite the fact that both clinical studies and preclinical research on the use of RIT are mainly focused on curative intent in patients with malignant disease, the limited data on the results of phase I studies as discussed in this chapter indicate that the use of RIT in patients with metastatic disease of various malignancies can be a good adjunct to standard therapy in the setting of palliative treatment. The future of RIT may therefore also reside in the setting of palliative treatment as a supplement or even substitution for present-day treatment of metastatic cancer.

■ REFERENCES

1. Goudas LC, Bloch R, Gialeli-Goudas M, et al. The epidemiology of cancer pain. *Cancer Invest.* 2005;23:182–190.
2. Sterman DH, Kaiser LR, Albelda SM. Advances in the treatment of malignant pleural mesothelioma. *Chest.* 1999;116:504–520.
3. van Ruth S, Baas P, Haas RL, et al. Cytoreductive surgery combined with intraoperative hyperthermic intrathoracic chemotherapy for stage I malignant pleural mesothelioma. *Ann Surg Oncol.* 2003;10:176–182.
4. van Ruth S, van TO, Korse CM, et al. Pharmacokinetics of doxorubicin and cisplatin used in intraoperative hyperthermic intrathoracic chemotherapy after cytoreductive surgery for malignant pleural mesothelioma and pleural thymoma. *Anticancer Drugs.* 2003;14:57–65.
5. Kasahara K, Shibata K, Shintani H, et al. Randomized phase II trial of OK-432 in patients with malignant pleural effusion due to non-small cell lung cancer. *Anticancer Res.* 2006;26:1495–1499.
6. Eitan R, Levine DA, Abu-Rustum N, et al. The clinical significance of malignant pleural effusions in patients with optimally debulked ovarian carcinoma. *Cancer.* 2005;103:1397–1401.
7. Fitzpatrick DR, Peroni DJ, Bielefeldt-Ohmann H. The role of growth factors and cytokines in the tumorigenesis and immunobiology of malignant mesothelioma. *Am J Respir Cell Mol Biol.* 1995;12:455–460.
8. Robinson BW, Lake RA. Advances in malignant mesothelioma. *N Engl J Med.* 2005;353:1591–1603.
9. Scherpereel A, Grigoriu B, Conti M, et al. Soluble mesothelin-related peptides in the diagnosis of malignant pleural mesothelioma. *Am J Respir Crit Care Med.* 2006;173:1155–1160.
10. Hassan R, Viner JL, Wang QC, et al. Anti-tumor activity of K1-LysPE38QQR, an immunotoxin targeting mesothelin, a cell-surface antigen overexpressed in ovarian cancer and malignant mesothelioma. *J Immunother.* 2000;23:473–479.
11. Fan D, Yano S, Shinohara H, et al. Targeted therapy against human lung cancer in nude mice by high-affinity recombinant antimesothelin single-chain Fv immunotoxin. *Mol Cancer Ther.* 2002;1:595–600.
12. Lynch CC, Matrisian LM. Matrix metalloproteinases in tumor–host cell communication. *Differentiation.* 2002;70:561–573.
13. Wong JY, Somlo G, Odom-Maryon T, et al. Initial clinical experience evaluating yttrium-90-chimeric T84.66 anticarcinoembryonic antigen antibody and autologous hematopoietic stem cell support in patients with carcinoembryonic antigen-producing metastatic breast cancer. *Clin Cancer Res.* 1999;5:3224s–3231s.
14. Schmidt HH, Renner H, Linkesch W. Intrapleural instillation of rituximab for the treatment of malignant pleural effusions in NHL. *Haematologica.* 2004;89:ECR39.
15. Witzig TE, Gordon LI, Cabanillas F, et al. Randomized controlled trial of yttrium-90-labeled ibritumomab tiuxetan radioimmunotherapy versus rituximab immunotherapy for patients with relapsed or refractory low-grade, follicular, or transformed B-cell non-Hodgkin's lymphoma. *J Clin Oncol.* 2002;20:2453–2463.
16. Denardo SJ, Richman CM, Albrecht H, et al. Enhancement of the therapeutic index: from nonmyeloablative and myeloablative toward pretargeted radioimmunotherapy for metastatic prostate cancer. *Clin Cancer Res.* 2005;11:7187s–7194s.
17. Bander NH, Milowsky MI, Nanus DM, et al. Phase I trial of [177]lutetium-labeled J591, a monoclonal antibody to prostate-specific membrane antigen, in patients with androgen-independent prostate cancer. *J Clin Oncol.* 2005;23:4591–4601.
18. Denardo SJ, O'Grady LF, Richman CM, et al. Radioimmunotherapy for advanced breast cancer using I-131-ChL6 antibody. *Anticancer Res.* 1997;17:1745–1751.
19. Brown MT, Coleman RE, Friedman AH, et al. Intrathecal ^{131}I-labeled antitenascin monoclonal antibody 81C6 treatment of patients with leptomeningeal neoplasms or primary brain tumor resection cavities with subarachnoid communication: phase I trial results. *Clin Cancer Res.* 1996;2:963–972.
20. Coakham HB, Kemshead JT. Treatment of neoplastic meningitis by targeted radiation using (131)I-radiolabelled monoclonal antibodies. Results of responses and long term follow-up in 40 patients. *J Neurooncol.* 1998;38:225–232.
21. Kramer K, Humm JL, Souweidane MM, et al. Phase I study of targeted radioimmunotherapy for leptomeningeal cancers using intra-Ommaya 131-I-3F8. *J Clin Oncol.* 2007;25:5465–5470.
22. Luther N, Cheung NKV, Dunkel IJ, et al. Intraparenchymal and intratumoral interstitial infusion of anti-glioma monoclonal antibody 8H9. *Neurosurgery.* 2008;63:1166–1174.
23. Modak S, Kramer K, Gultekin SH, et al. Monoclonal antibody 8H9 targets a novel cell surface antigen expressed by a wide spectrum of human solid tumors. *Cancer Res.* 2001;61:4048–4054.

Note: Page numbers in *italics* denote figures; those followed by a t denote tables.

CNT. *See* Carbon nanotubes (CNT)
Cobalt gray-equivalent (CGE), 110
Code of Federal Register (CFR), 307
COG. *See* Children's Oncology Group (COG)
Cold antibody, 179
Collagen, 186–187
Colominic acid (polysialylation), 26
Colon-specific antigen-p (CSAp), 199
  trials, 333
Colorectal cancer
  clinical trials in, results of, 327–334, 328t–329t, 330t
    A33 trials, 332–333
    CEA trials, 331–332
    colon-specific antigen-p trials, 333
    DNA histone trials, 333–334
    Ep-CAM trials, 333
    TAG-72 trials, 332
  radioembolization, 310–311
  radioimmunotherapy in, 321–343
    antibody factors, 321–324
    antigen factors, 324–325
    host factors, 327
    radionuclides, 325–327, 326t
    strategies to optimize, 334–343
    tumor factors, 327
Combined modality therapy (CMT)
  biology of targeted radionuclide, 221–222
  extrinsic tumor targets of, 228–230
  intrinsic tumor targets of, 222–228
  overview, 220
  rationale for, 220–221
  selective tumor cell death, with targeted radionuclide therapy, 230–232
  synthetic lethal approaches, 227–228
Combretastatin A-4- phosphate (CA4P), 337
Common Toxicity Criteria of Adverse Events (CTCae), 307
Complement 5a (C5a), 185
Complementarity-determining regions (CDRs), 22, 191
Complementary MORF (cMORF), 203
Complement-dependent cytotoxicity (CDC), 9, 27
Complete remission (CR), 381, 444
Complete response (CR) rates, 427
Compton effect, 74
Computational combinatorial ligand design (CCLD), 35
Computed tomography (CT), 117, 362
  in head and neck cancer, 398, *404*
  medullary thyroid cancer and, 377
Computed tomography (CT) scanner for small animal, 215
//φ—ψ conformational map, 32–33, *33*
Constructs, 337–338
  route of delivery for, 367
  targeting, 366t, 381–382

Continuous slowing down approximation (CSDA), 132
Coordination chemistry
  history of, 88
  of radiopharmaceuticals, 36
Coster–Kronig electrons, 138, 139, 250
CPE. *See* Charged particle equilibrium (CPE)
CPP. *See* Cell-penetrating peptides (CPP)
Cp tricarbonyl complexes, 100
CR. *See* Complete remission (CR)
Craniospinal radiotherapy (CRT), 505
Crossfire effect, 366, 468, 500
Crosspresentation of TA, 7
CRPC. *See* Castration-resistant prostate cancer (CRPC)
CR rates. *See* Complete response (CR) rates
CRT. *See* Craniospinal radiotherapy (CRT)
Cryptococcus neoformans, 500
CSAp. *See* Colon-specific antigen-p (CSAp)
CSDA. *See* Continuous slowing down approximation (CSDA)
CSF. *See* Cerebrospinal fluid (CSF)
CT. *See* Computed tomography (CT)
Ct. *See* Calcitonin (Ct)
CTCae. *See* Common Toxicity Criteria of Adverse Events (CTCae)
CTL. *See* CD8+ T cells (CTL)
CTLA-4 mAb. *See* Anticytotoxic T lymphocyte-associated antigen 4 (CTLA-4) mAb
CTLA-4–specific ipilimumab (MDX-010), 17
CTLs. *See* Cytotoxic T lymphocytes (CTLs)
^{64}Cu-CB-TE2A-sst2-ANT, 488
Curie, Marie, 357
Curie, Pierre, 357
Curies (Ci), 281
Cyclam. *See* 1,4,8, 11-tetraazacyclotetradecane (cyclam)
trans-Cyclohexyldiethylenetriamine pentaacetic acid (CyDPTA), 95
CyDPTA. *See trans*-cyclohexyldiethylenetriamine pentaacetic acid (CyDPTA)
Cytokines, 11
Cytotoxic radiosensitizing agents
  antimetabolites, 222–223
  clinical studies, 224–225
  gemcitabine, 223
  preclinical studies, 223–224
  tubule-targeting drugs, 223
Cytotoxic therapy, delivery of
  dose density of, 259–260
  Norton–Simon hypothesis, 259–260
  validation of, 259–260
Cytotoxic T lymphocytes (CTLs), 3

D-amino acid peptide (D-KRYRR), 188
"Danger" model, 5
DCs. *See* Dendritic cells (DCs)
Deferoxamine. *See* "Desferal"
"Degree of freedom," 120
Dehalogenation, 326
Delta particles, 74
DeNardo, GL, 498
DeNardo, SJ, 498
Dendritic cells (DCs), 7–9
  activation of, 9
  elimination, tumor microenvironment, 13
  immunotherapy employing for, 164
  interaction with dying tumor cells, 8, *8*
Densely ionizing radiations, 109, 251, 265, 357
Deoxyribonucleic acid (DNA), 59, 137, 249
Department of Defense Prostate Cancer Research Program, 417
"Desferal," 98
Desmoplastic small round cell tumor (DSRCT)
  radioimmunotherapy of, 507–508
DFS. *See* Disease-free survival (DFS)
Diabodies, 323
Dianhydride (*N*,*N*-bis[2-(2,6-dioxo-4-morpholinyl)ethyl] glycine) (DTPA), 37–38, *38*, *94*, 94–95
  history of, 94
Diazenido, 99–100, *100*
Dichlorovinyl arsine (Lewisite), 88
Diethylenetriamine pentaacetic acid (DPTA), 94–95
  structure of, *94*
Differentiation antigens, 161, 163
Diffuse large B-cell lymphoma (DLBCL), 426
2,3-dimercaptopropanol, 88
Direct priming, 7
Discrete-ordinates method (DOM), 83
Disease-free survival (DFS), 445
Disialoganglioside (GD2) antigen, 506
Display technologies
  human antibody generation using
    eukaryotic cell display, 24–25
    phage display, 23–24, *24*
    ribosome display, 24
Distant metastases, in neck, 397–398
D-KRYRR. *See* D-amino acid peptide (D-KRYRR)
DLBCL. *See* Diffuse large B-cell lymphoma (DLBCL)
DLT. *See* Dose-limiting toxicity (DLT)
DNA. *See* Deoxyribonucleic acid (DNA)
DNA histone trials, 333–334
DNA lesions, 227
DNAPK. *See* DNA-protein kinase (DNAPK)
DNAPK-deficient SCID mice, 228